S0-BXK-570

Silicon VLSI Technology

Fundamentals, Practice and Modeling

James D. Plummer
Michael D. Deal
Peter B. Griffin
Department of Electrical Engineering
Stanford University

Prentice Hall

Prentice Hall
Upper Saddle River, NJ 07458

Library of Congress Cataloging-in-Publication Data
Silicon VLSI technology
p. cm.
ISBN 0–13–085037–3
1. Integrated circuits—Very large scale integration—Design and construction. 2. Silicon. 3. Silicon oxide films. 4. Metal oxide semiconductors. 5. Silicon technology.
TK7874.75.S54 2000
621.39'5—dc21 99-42745
CIP

Publisher: Tom Robbins
Associate Editor: Alice Dworkin
Editorial/Production Supervision: Rose Kernan
Vice President and Editorial Director, ECS: Marcia Horton
Vice President of Production and Manufacturing: David W. Riccardi
Executive Managing Editor: Vince O'Brien
Marketing Manager: Danny Hoyt
Managing Editor: David A. George
Manufacturing Buyer: Pat Brown
Manufacturing Manager: Trudy Pisciotti
Art Director: Jayne Conte
Cover Design: Bruce Kenselaar
Editorial Assistant: Jesse Power
Copy Editor: Martha Williams
Composition: D&G Limited, LLC

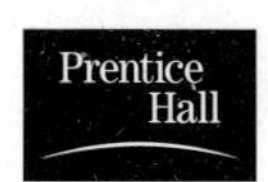

Printed in the United States of America

10 9 8 7 6 5 4 3

ISBN 0-13-085037-3

Prentice Hall International (UK) Limited, *London*
Prentice Hall of Australia Pty. Limited, *Sydney*
Prentice Hall Canada Inc., *Toronto*
Prentice Hall Hispanoamericana, S.A., *Mexico*
Prentice Hall of India Private Limited, *New Delhi*
Prentice Hall of Japan, Inc., *Tokyo*
Pearson Education Pte., Ltd. , *Singapore*
Editora Prentice† Hall do Brasil, Ltda., *Rio de Janeiro*

Contents

Preface

The silicon integrated circuit is surely one of the wonders of our age. The ability to fabricate tens of millions of individual components on a silicon chip with an area of a few cm^2 has enabled the information age.

Basic discoveries and inventions between 1945 and 1970 laid the foundations for these chips. In the past 30 years, chip complexity has increased at an exponential rate, primarily because of the constant shrinking of device geometries, improved manufacturing practice, and clever inventions enabling specific functions to be implemented in new ways. Shrinking geometries permit more devices to be placed in a given area of silicon; improved manufacturing permits larger chips to be economically fabricated; and clever inventions permit functions to be realized in smaller areas. It is widely expected that these historical trends will continue for at least another 10–20 years, resulting in chips that contain billions of components. Such chips will have extraordinary capabilities. We will likely find ourselves in 10–20 years thinking of today's chips as primitive precursors to the chips that will be in manufacturing at that time.

The technology that is used to build silicon integrated circuits today has evolved largely through empirical methods. It often seems that the chip industry moves so rapidly and new products are introduced so often that there is little time to worry about the scientific basis of the technologies used to build these chips. Yet in parallel with the rapid pace of this industry, a strong effort has been proceeding, often behind the scenes, to develop a solid, physically based understanding of the many technologies used in chip manufacturing. Because of the feature sizes of structures in modern chips, this understanding often needs to be on a molecular or atomic level. It is not sufficient any longer to think of silicon oxidation as simply a chemical reaction between silicon and oxygen that grows SiO_2. Today we must understand the detailed bonding between silicon and oxygen atoms and the kinetics that drive this reaction on an atomic basis.

Silicon integrated circuit technology makes use of many diverse fields of science and engineering. The optical steppers which print microscopic patterns on wafers, represent one of the most advanced applications of the principles of Fourier optics. Plasma etching involves some of the most complex chemistries used in manufacturing today. Ion implantation draws upon understanding from research in high energy physics. Thin films on the silicon wafer surface exhibit complex mechanical behavior which stretches our understanding of basic materials properties. And of course, silicon devices themselves are approaching physical sizes at which molecular and atomic scale phenomena involving ideas from quantum mechanics are important. One of the great challenges in integrated circuit manufacturing is the need to draw on scientific principles and engineering developments from such an extraordinarily wide range of disciplines. Integrating the knowledge from these diverse disciplines has been and will continue to be a great challenge. Scientists and engineers who work in this field need broad understanding and the ability to seek out, integrate and use ideas from many fields.

Over the past 20 years much has been learned about silicon and the other materials that are used in modern chips. Often new knowledge is incorporated in a "model" which may be a mathematical equation describing a process or an atomistic picture of how a particular process works. Models codify knowledge and are an elegant way of expressing what is known. They also provide a way of exchanging ideas between researchers in a particular field, and can be tested experimentally to assess their predictive capability.

Within the last decade, a serious attempt has been made to develop computer simulation tools which can simulate the various technologies used in fabricating chips. These simulation tools are built around models of the physical processes involved. Some simulation tools today use well-established scientific principles to predict experimental results. Optical lithography simulators, which are based on mathematical descriptions of Fourier optics, are a good example. Such tools today can accurately predict the image that will be printed in resist on a silicon wafer, given a particular mask design and a specific exposure system. Other simulation tools rest on less solid ground. Models of dopant diffusion in silicon, for example, use models which are still debated in the scientific community and which are clearly incomplete in terms of describing all the physical phenomena involved. Nevertheless, even these models are very useful today.

This book attempts to describe not only the manufacturing practice associated with the technologies used in silicon chip fabrication, but also the underlying scientific basis for those technologies. Those scientific principles are described in terms of models of the process in many cases. In most chapters, models are discussed in the context of computer simulation programs which have incorporated the models and which use them to simulate technology steps. We make extensive use of simulation examples to illustrate how technologies work and to help in visualizing features of the technologies that are not easily seen any other way. We have found these tools to be powerful teaching aids.

Simulation tools are widely used in the semiconductor industry today to supplement traditional experimental methods. While it is unlikely that simulation will completely eliminate the need for experiments, especially in a fast moving industry like the IC industry, simulators can result in very substantial cost savings in developing new generations of technology and in solving manufacturing problems. It is widely believed that simulation tools will be essential in the future if the rapid progress that has characterized the semiconductor industry is to continue.

This book is organized somewhat differently than other texts on this general topic, in two principal ways. The first is the extensive use of simulation examples throughout the text. These serve several purposes. The first is simply to help explain the scientific principles involved in each chapter. Simulations help to illustrate things like the time evolution of a growing oxide layer, a diffusing dopant profile or a depositing thin film. They are also very useful in illustrating the effects of specific physical phenomena in a process step because it is straightforward in simulators to add or eliminate specific physical models. Simulators provide the only real way in which complex interactions between process steps can be illustrated and understood. Finally, students who spend their careers in this industry will certainly use these tools and understanding their capabilities and limitations will be important in their future work.

The second way in which this book is organized differently is the discussion of a complete process flow early in the book (Chapter 2). While readers new to this field may not appreciate many of the complexities of a CMOS process before studying the later chapters, we have found that an early broad exposure to a complete chip manufacturing process is very helpful in establishing the context for the specific technologies discussed in later chapters. In teaching the material in this book, we usually cover the CMOS process in the first or second lecture somewhat superficially, and then return to the same topic in the last lecture, at which point the details can be more fully discussed.

We have also attempted in each chapter to include some discussion of future trends. Predicting the future is obviously difficult and there is some risk that including this material will simply serve to date this book. Nevertheless, we have found that students are often interested in this topic and at least in general terms, we believe it is possible to predict where silicon technology is heading. The semiconductor industry *National Technology Roadmap for Semiconductors* (the NTRS) provides some guidance in looking to the future.

The material in this book can be covered in a one quarter senior/graduate level course, although not all of the material in each chapter can be covered in one quarter. A semester long course would provide more time to cover the full range of material in the book. If the book is used in connection with a one quarter long course, one option is to minimize the amount of time spent on the Manufacturing Methods and Measurement Techniques sections in each chapter. A set of lecture notes based on figures from the text is available to instructors by contacting the publisher or the authors by email. We have used these notes several times in a one quarter course at Stanford.

Follow-on courses to a basic IC fabrication course can make more extensive use of the simulation tools discussed in this text. We have not used the simulation tools described in this book for homework assignments or for lab assignments in connection with a first course in IC fabrication. We believe that the simulation examples are better used simply as teaching tools in such courses, to illustrate ideas and to clarify physical principles. But in a follow-on course, hands-on experience with these simulation tools is easily possible. Most of the computer tools we use in the book are commercially available and the vendors of these tools are generally anxious to work with university instructors to make the tools available for teaching purposes.

Finally, we acknowledge the many students at Stanford who have helped refine the material in this book by using various draft versions of the text in classes we have taught. Their inputs and suggestions have hopefully made this a better book. For many years we have worked with an energetic group of Ph.D. students and faculty colleagues at Stanford who have helped to develop some of the models and software tools described in this book. We particularly acknowledge Professor Bob Dutton and former Ph.D. students Professor Mark Law (now at the U. Florida) and Dr. Conor Rafferty (now at Lucent Technologies). We are also very grateful to a number of individuals who reviewed draft versions of this book and who provided technical inputs to various chapters. Paul Rissman of Hewlett Packard, Jim McVittie of Stanford, and Mark Law all provided substantial inputs and comments. Our own work in this field has been supported over many years by DARPA (the Defense Advanced Research Projects Agency) and by the Semiconductor Research Corporation (SRC) . We owe them a considerable debt of gratitude for making our work possible. We welcome comments or suggestions on this text by email at plummer@ee.stanford.edu, deal@ee.stanford.edu, or griffin@stanford.edu.

Introduction and Historical Perspective

1

1.1 Introduction

Since its invention about 40 years ago, the Integrated Circuit (IC) has literally changed our world. From a modest beginning, which permitted the integration of a few semiconductor devices and passive components on a common substrate, has come a technology which can integrate tens of millions of components in a square cm of silicon. From a beginning in which integrated circuits were applied only to a very small set of specialized applications has come a technology which is pervasive in today's world. Many have referred to these events as a true revolution, the beginning of the information age. Most industrialized nations today believe that integrated circuits will be one of the basic building blocks for their future economies. Global competition for a share of these market opportunities is intense today and will remain so for the foreseeable future.

What are the factors that have contributed to this remarkable growth in integrated circuit capability? Fundamentally, integrated circuits (chips) consist of a large number of individual components (transistors, resistors, capacitors, etc.), fabricated side by side in a common substrate and wired together to perform a particular circuit function. Over time, more complex circuits are built simply by making the individual components smaller which allows more of them to be integrated in a given area, and by making the overall size of chips larger. The higher levels of integration permitted by these smaller devices and bigger chips have made it possible to build progressively more complex, higher-performance, and more economical integrated systems as time has passed.

Figure 1–1 illustrates the increasing complexity of integrated circuits over the past 35 years. Technology improvements over that period have resulted in a doubling of the number of transistors on a chip roughly every two years, a "law" that has become known as "Moore's law" [1.1]. Decreasing component size is often characterized in IC technology by the minimum line width. This is usually defined as the smallest lateral feature size that is printed on the wafer surface during the fabrication process. This dimension is plotted in Figure 1–2 over the past 35 years and extrapolated into the future. On average, this dimension has decreased by 13% each year. In recent years, this reduction has been closer to 10% per year. The other principal contributor to increasing chip complexity, overall chip size, has risen by about 16% each year over the past 35 years. In recent years this number has also slightly decreased, ranging from about 6.3% per year for microprocessors, to 12% per year for dynamic memory or DRAMs.

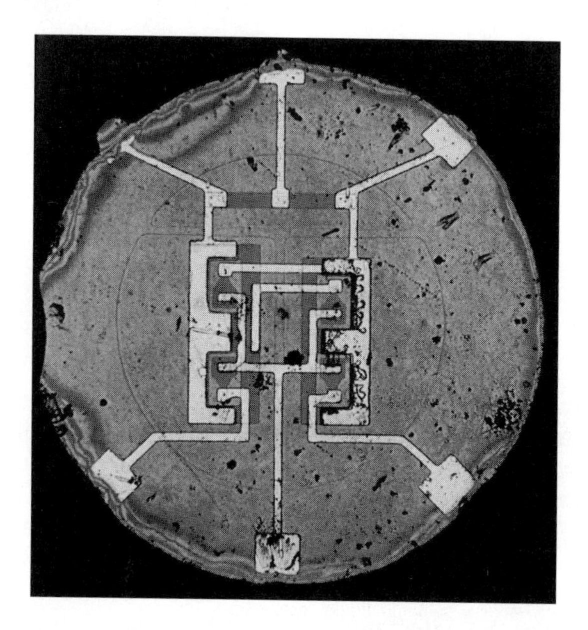

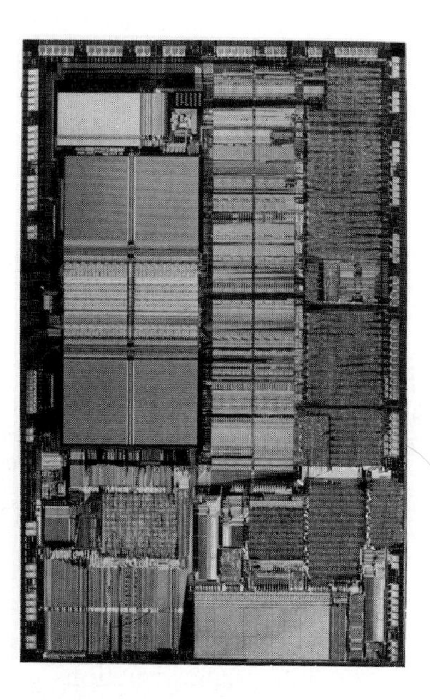

Figure 1–1 Photomicrographs of state-of-the-art ICs manufactured in the early 1960s (left) and in the early 1990s (right). The 1960s IC contains four bipolar transistors and several resistors. The 1990s chip contains over a million MOS transistors.

In 1994 the Semiconductor Industry Association (SIA) organized a workshop in Boulder, Colorado which was chartered to produce a roadmap for the semiconductor industry. The result was the National Technology Roadmap for Semiconductors or NTRS [1.2]. This roadmap was updated in 1997 through a series of industrywide meetings [1.3] and is being updated again in 1999. The NTRS is currently the most widely cited "strategic plan" for the semiconductor industry. The fundamental premise of the NTRS is that industry history as described by Moore's law should be maintained through 2012. In other words, a new generation of technology should appear on average every three years, starting with 0.25-μm technology today and extending to 0.05-μm technology in 2012. The NTRS is a needs-driven document which assumes that silicon CMOS technology will dominate the semiconductor industry for this entire period. The starting point is a standard set of industry products—DRAMs, static memory or SRAMs, microprocessors, and Application-Specific Integrated Circuits or ASICs—which result in the technology requirements in Table 1–1, abstracted from the 1997 roadmap.

Several trends can be observed from this table. First, of course, are the steady progressions to smaller feature sizes and larger chips. Together these make possible the increases in transistors per chip. Note that a factor greater than 100X is expected in the complexity of microprocessor chips over the next 15 years. The number of wiring levels is projected to steadily increase over this time period as well. This is because of the great difficulty in connecting all the components in these very complex chips. This is the same trend that has occurred in the number of wiring levels in printed circuit boards over the

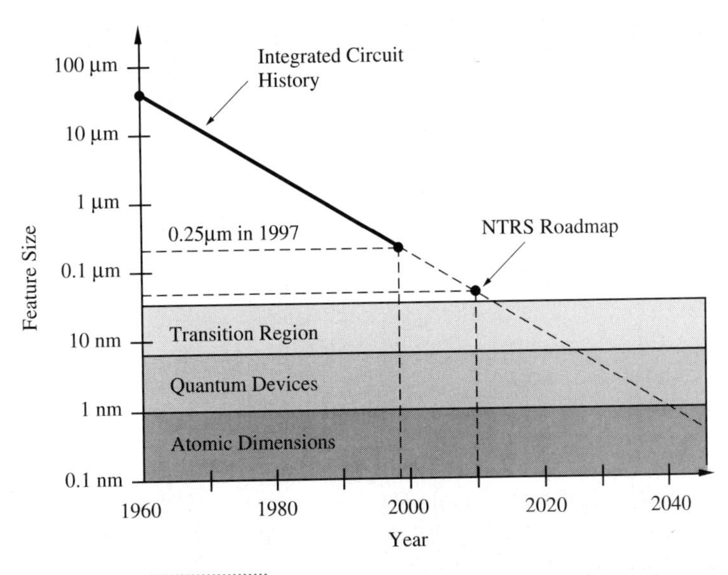

Figure 1–2 Historical trends and future projections for the minimum feature size used in integrated circuits in manufacturing.

years, for the same reasons. The mask count is a measure of the number of lithography or printing operations required to manufacture the chips. It is really a measure of the complexity of the manufacturing process. Here the trend is obviously upward as well, primarily to accommodate the increased wiring levels needed in the chips. Finally, the operating voltage of future chips is expected to decrease significantly. This is driven by the fact that as transistors get smaller, the electric fields in these devices will increase to unacceptable levels unless operating voltages are reduced. Just as important, the power dissipation of chips is proportional to the square of the operating voltage and this is also becoming a major issue as more and more complexity is packed onto a single chip.

Table 1–1 Future projections for silicon technology taken from the SIA NTRS [1.3]

Year of first DRAM shipment	1997	1999	2003	2006	2009	2012
Minimum Feature Size	250 nm	180 nm	130 nm	100 nm	70 nm	50 nm
DRAM Bits/Chip	256M	1G	4G	16G	64G	256G
DRAM Chip Size (mm^2)	280	400	560	790	1120	1580
Microprocessor Transistors/chip	11M	21M	76M	200M	520M	1.40G
Maximum Wiring Levels	6	6–7	7	7–8	8–9	9
Minimum Mask Count	22	22–24	24	24–26	26–28	28
Minimum Supply Voltage (volts)	1.8–2.5	1.5–1.8	1.2–1.5	0.9–1.2	0.6–0.9	0.5–0.6

One final point about the NTRS is worth making. This is the assumption that in the future, silicon will remain the basic material used in the fabrication of ICs. There are many other material possibilities that have been investigated over the years, ranging from elemental semiconductors like Ge to compound materials like GaAs. None of these, however, has the combination of properties that together provide a viable alternative to silicon. We will see why this is so throughout this text as we discuss the various processing technologies used to make silicon ICs today. Simply stated, silicon will be the dominant material used for chips for as far into the future as we can reliably see.

The primary devices used in today's integrated circuits are Metal Oxide Semiconductor (MOS) transistors and Bipolar Junction Transistors (BJTs). The basic physical principles underlying these devices were understood before the invention of the integrated circuit. The field effect mechanism on which the MOS device is based was first investigated in the 1930s. The operating principles of the BJT device were first described in the late 1940s. While the first ICs were built with BJT devices, the MOS transistor has become the dominant device in the past two decades. MOS devices offer higher density, lower power operation, and considerably greater design flexibility than do BJT devices. BJT devices are still used today in analog and a few other applications, but their market share will likely continue to shrink. As a result, most efforts to develop new IC technologies today focus on MOS technologies and that is the emphasis we will take in this book.

Many studies have probed the question of how small MOS devices can be made before their basic operating principles change. Stated another way, how long can the historical trends of shrinking transistors and increasing chip complexity continue? While there is still disagreement about the exact answers to these questions, it is clear that quantum mechanical effects will become important when device dimensions reach 10 or 20 nanometers. It is also clear that toward the end of the NTRS or perhaps just beyond it, today's MOS device structures will begin to encounter significant problems. Lateral devices dimensions between 0.05 μm (50 nm) and about 0.01 μm (10 nm) fall into this category, labeled the "transition region" in Figure 1–2. An example of an issue that is important at these dimensions is that gate oxides in MOS devices likely cannot be shrunk below about 1–1.5 nm because electrons can easily tunnel through such thin insulators. (A 1-nm oxide thickness would be required in MOS devices with lateral dimensions on the order of 0.05 μm or 50 nm according to the NTRS.) Also at these dimensions, it is very difficult to keep the depletion regions associated with PN junctions from interacting with each other. In any case, device innovations will be required in order to continue shrinking dimensions in integrated circuits much beyond the NTRS. If history is any guide, these innovations will occur, resulting in the ability to continue shrinking device dimensions and increasing chip capability well into the next century. In fact the 1999 version of the NTRS has added another technology generation at 35 nm.

Many researchers today believe that the ultimate limits of silicon CMOS technology lie well beyond the above roadmap. Theoretical studies have indicated that fairly standard silicon transistor structures can work properly down to dimensions of 20–30 nm. If such devices can be manufactured economically, they will become the basis of chips with 10^{10} to 10^{12} devices around 2020. Such extraordinary "systems on a chip" will allow products that we cannot even envision clearly today.

It is interesting to note that even though there are device problems related to continued scaling, there are no known fundamental fabrication limitations until far into the

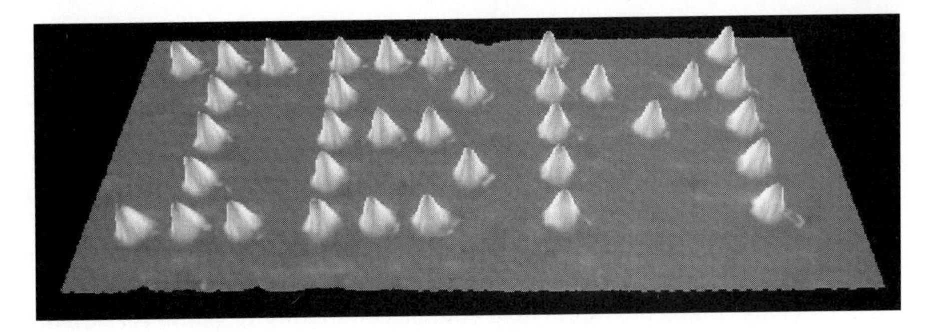

Figure 1–3 Xenon atoms individually placed on a nickel single crystal surface to spell IBM. The spacing between xenon atoms is about 1nm. Reprinted with permission of IBM.

future. Integrated circuits today are built using optical techniques to produce the fine line patterns required for device structures. These techniques will likely have to be replaced at dimensions below 0.1 μm (although continued innovation may reduce this limit). There are a number of possibilities that have been shown to work at smaller dimensions, such as electron-beam and X-ray lithography. Other possibilities also exist, including some very recent and quite remarkable work (Figure 1–3) in which a scanning tunneling microscope was used to control the placement of individual atoms on a single-crystal Ni surface [1.4]. It is clear that technology options will allow smaller structures and continued device innovation far into the future.

In addition to shrinking individual device sizes, overall chip sizes have increased dramatically over the past three decades. Larger chips permit more complex functions to be integrated, improving system reliability and generally also producing higher system performance. This is because it is often the case that driving signals over the relatively large distances between chips is the limiting factor in overall system speed. Eliminating these long signal paths by combining functions on a single chip can therefore improve performance. It is also the case that the smaller devices characteristic of improved technologies are also intrinsically faster than their larger counterparts and hence also contribute to higher-performance systems.

At any point in time, there is an upper bound on the size of a chip which is economically manufacturable. Defects during the manufacturing process can arise from a number of sources including airborne particulates, machine introduced particles, or the printing or lithographic process. Such defects tend to be randomly distributed over a wafer and are often characterized with an average defect density per square centimeter. Since in most ICs redundancy is not used, a single defect larger than some critical size usually means that the chip will not function correctly. Manufacturing ICs with high yield therefore requires low defect densities. This has been the driving force for the ultra clean facilities in which ICs are manufactured today. When new chips are introduced to the marketplace, their manufacturing yield may be less than 20%. However, as experience is gained with manufacturing the part and as improvements are made in manufacturing processes, yields often approach 80% or more in mature products. There are no fundamental reasons why chips much larger than those built today cannot be manufactured. We should expect the historical trends in this regard to continue for the foreseeable future.

There is, however, one byproduct of this drive for larger chips and higher manufacturing yields that should be mentioned. The cost of the factories in which such chips are built has also risen astronomically in the past three decades. In 1970, a state-of-the-art fabrication facility could be built for a few million dollars. The costs today are over $1 billion. Concerns have been expressed that these very high costs will necessarily drive many companies out of high volume commodity IC markets (memory chips, for example) in the future. This has not happened as yet. Innovations in manufacturing such as designing and building plants so that capacity can be added in phases as the market grows, or sharing the costs of large plants across a broader product spectrum have helped to mitigate the high plant costs. The recent surge in foundries, which manufacture chips for a wide spectrum of customers, is an interesting development in this regard. In the foundry scenario, an independent company builds an expensive chip fabrication plant and then fabricates products using standard processes for many other companies which often do not have their own chip manufacturing plants. Also, of course, because of the economic importance of semiconductors, governments around the world have chosen to invest substantial resources in establishing chip manufacturing in their countries.

As the complexity of integrated circuits has increased, so have the costs associated with designing them. Gordon Moore pointed out in 1979 [1.5] that the cost required to design an IC was increasing at about the same rate as the complexity of the technology. Transistor count was doubling in ICs every two years; design costs were not far behind. Had this continued, there would be very few ICs being designed today at the capability of the technology (tens of millions of transistors), simply because it would be difficult to define products that could return the huge investment needed to design such chips. Beginning in the late 1970s however, a revolution took place, which dramatically reduced design costs. That revolution was the introduction of very powerful Computer-Aided Design (CAD) tools, which take care of many of the design details. CAD tools continue to be refined today and they have opened up the opportunity to design ICs to a wide range of people who do not necessarily have to know about the details of transistor physics or IC technology. This CAD revolution has included the introduction of ideas like gate arrays, programmable logic arrays, standard cells, and powerful tools to design fully custom ICs. The net result has been that IC design costs have remained low enough that thousands of new chips are introduced each year. In fact the number of new chip designs introduced each year continues to increase.

In the remainder of this chapter we will discuss some of the important inventions, particularly in the 1940s and 50s, that made integrated circuits possible. We will also review basic ideas about semiconductors, materials, devices and circuit families. This review is not intended to be comprehensive since there are many complete references, which cover these topics in detail. However, since we will make use of many of these concepts in later chapters, the background provided here will be important to those discussions.

1.2 Integrated Circuits and the Planar Process—Key Inventions That Made It All Possible

The devices which are used in today's integrated circuits, primarily MOS and bipolar transistors, were invented long before the technologies were available to manufacture them in high volume. Many of the basic properties of semiconductors such as rectification and photoconductivity were discovered before 1900 although they were not understood at that time. Simple devices based on these properties were available in the form of selenium rectifiers and photodetectors by the mid 1930s. It was also during this time period when the physical principles underlying the behavior of metal/semiconductor contacts began to be understood, particularly through the work of Schottky and Mott.

The behavior of semiconductor surfaces plays a key role in all modern devices. Liandrat first proposed in 1935 that the conductivity of a surface region in a semiconductor could be modulated by the application of a perpendicular electric field. This "field effect" concept led to many studies of semiconductor surfaces over the next three decades.

The Second World War interrupted much of the basic work on semiconductors that was ongoing at the time, particularly at Bell Telephone Laboratories where an effort was underway to find a solid-state device for switching telephone signals. Shortly after the end of the war, this effort resumed, and it was not long until a major breakthrough was made with the demonstration of the point contact transistor in December 1947 (Figure 1–4). This and subsequent work, which resulted in the invention of the bipolar transistor, resulted in the Nobel Prize in physics for John Bardeen, Walter Brattain, and William Shockley in 1956. An interesting historical account of many of these events can be found in [1.6].

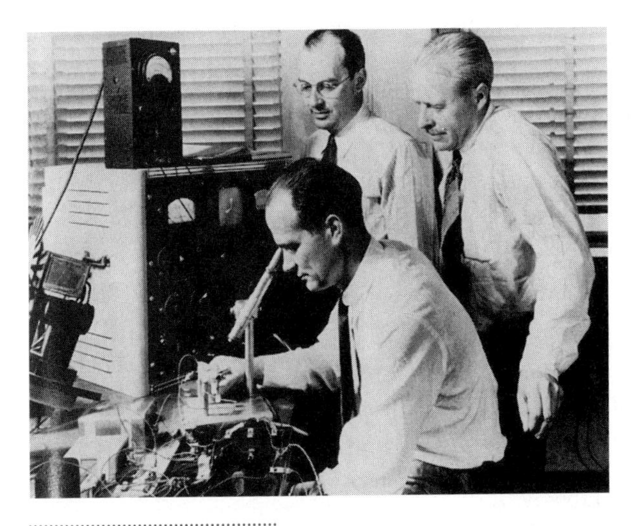

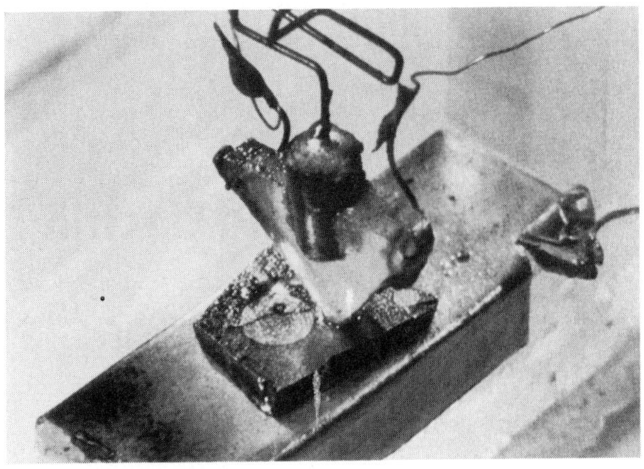

Figure 1–4 The point contact transistor invented at Bell Telephone Laboratories in 1947 by Bardeen, Brattain, and Shockley. Reprinted with permission of Lucent Technologies, Bell Labs Innovations.

In the 1950s, interest in semiconductor surfaces was renewed when it became apparent that reliability problems associated with the new transistor structures were related to surface effects. In a classic experiment in 1953, Brattain and Bardeen found that the surface properties of semiconductors could be controlled by exposing them to oxygen, water, or ozone ambients. Many experiments over the next few years led to the first high-quality SiO_2 layers grown on Si substrates around 1960. At about this same time, the stable properties of SiO_2 layers on Si began to be understood theoretically.

Although the first point contact transistors in 1947 were built in polycrystalline germanium, within a year or two after that the device was also demonstrated in silicon and in single-crystal material. These two changes would also have a major impact on future integrated circuits. Single crystals provide uniform and reproducible device characteristics and thus provide the ability to integrate millions of identical components side by side on a chip. Silicon provides a controllable, stable, and reproducible surface passivation layer (SiO_2) which has made possible modern IC technology. Much of the credit for developing single crystal source material (Si and Ge) belongs to Gordon Teal of Bell Labs. Chapter 3 describes these developments in more detail.

By the mid 1950s, both grown junction and alloy junction bipolar transistors were commercially available. Ge was still the dominant material used at this time. Figures 1–5 and 1–6 illustrate the methods used to fabricate these devices. In the grown junction process, a single crystal of silicon or germanium was grown which contained a thin region (P type in Figure 1–5) of opposite doping to the main part of the crystal. Sawing removed most of the upper and lower N-type material, leaving a thin wafer with an NPN structure. Further sawing of this wafer resulted in a number of individual transistor structures to which leads were attached to provide external connections. In silicon-based devices, it was common to use Al wires to connect to the middle base (P) region since Al forms an ohmic (conducting) contact to P-type material and a rectifying

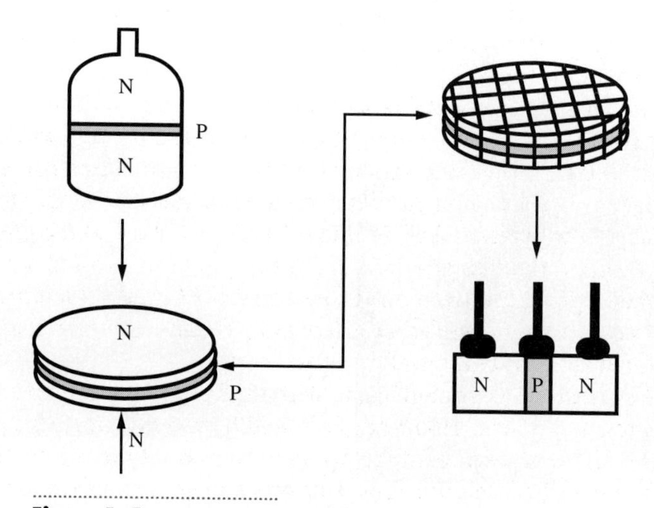

Figure 1–5 Grown junction transistor technology of the 1950s.

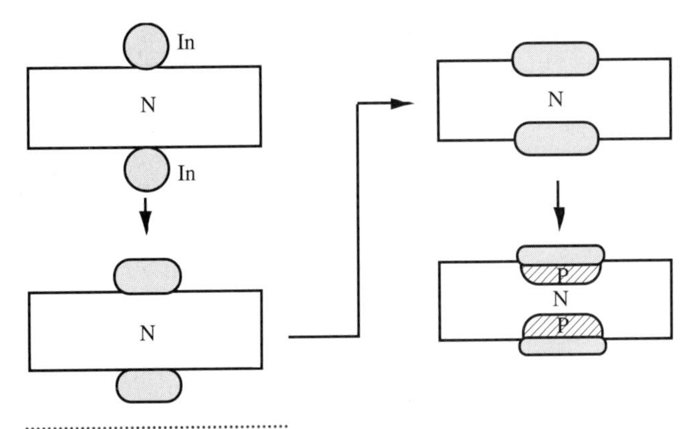

Figure 1–6 Alloy junction technology of the 1950s.

(Schottky) contact to lightly doped N regions. As a result it was not critical that the middle connection be placed exactly on the P region. In Ge based structures of this type, PNP type devices were usually made, with Au contacts to the middle N region.

The alloy junction technology illustrated in Figure 1–6 was even simpler. A metal such as indium was placed on the semiconductor (usually Ge). The structure was then heated, melting the In and allowing it to dissolve into the Ge. Indium is a P-type dopant so P regions were formed creating a PNP structure along with contacts to the P regions.

While such devices were very useful components, the technologies used to build them were not extendible to multitransistor integrated circuits. Exposed junctions were present on the semiconductor surface and no means to interconnect multiple devices was provided. New inventions were needed to overcome these problems.

Part of the solution was provided by the invention of gas phase diffusion processes, again at Bell Laboratories. That led to the commercial availability of diffused mesa bipolar transistors by 1957. Figure 1–7 illustrates this device structure. Beginning with an N-type crystal, the wafer was exposed in a high temperature furnace to a gaseous source of a P-type dopant such as boron. The boron diffused into the crystal by solid-state diffusion, resulting in the P-type layer. The process was then repeated with an N-type source, producing the final NPN structure. After contacts were alloyed to the surface N and P regions, a Si etch created the mesa structure to localize the N and P regions on the surface. This double diffused process had the great advantage that multiple devices could be produced from a single substrate and multiple substrates (wafers) could be produced from one grown crystal. However, all of the processes described to this point still had the great disadvantage that exposed junctions were present on the wafer surface or at the wafer edges.

The next breakthrough came with the invention of the planar process, illustrated in Figure 1–8, by Jean Hoerni of Fairchild Semiconductor. This process relied on the gas phase diffusion of dopants to produce N- and P-type regions, but also on the ability of SiO_2 to mask these diffusions. This was a major advance and it was largely responsible for the switch from Ge to Si. Silicon is unique among semiconductor materials in its

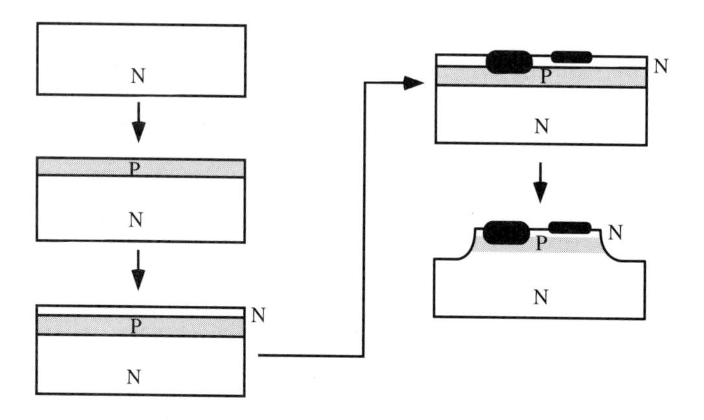

Figure 1–7 Double diffused mesa transistor technology of the late 1950s.

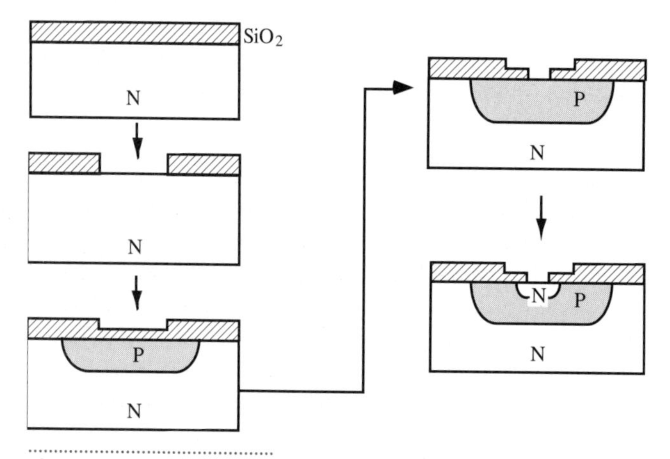

Figure 1–8 The planar process invented by Jean Hoerni of Fairchild in the late 1950s.

ability to be oxidized to produce a stable insulating coating. SiO_2 has many properties that make it almost an ideal surface layer for semiconductor devices. We will discuss oxidation and SiO_2 in much more detail in Chapter 6, but one of those properties is the ability to mask most of the common dopants that are used in semiconductor fabrication. In other words, most dopants like As, B, and P have much smaller rates of diffusion in SiO_2 than they do in silicon. The planar process makes use of this property by using SiO_2 to selectively block the dopants from diffusing into the silicon substrate. This produces junctions that terminate under an SiO_2 surface and which as a result are passivated. (We will define passivation more carefully in Chapter 6, but we basically mean by this term that the junction electrical properties are not significantly degraded at the surface, compared to their bulk properties.)

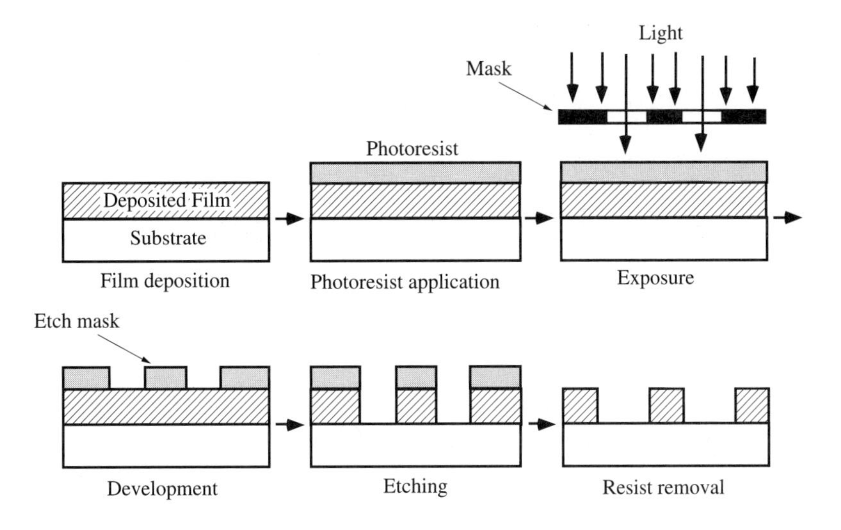

Figure 1–9 Basic photolithography process. The IC pattern is transferred from a mask to the silicon by printing it on the wafer using a light sensitive resist material.

A second essential part of the planar process, illustrated in Figure 1–9, is the ability to pattern the SiO_2. This is normally accomplished by a process called photolithography that we will discuss in detail in Chapter 5. The essence of this process involves the use of a light sensitive resist (or "film"), which is deposited onto the SiO_2 surface. The resist is then exposed through a mask and developed to produce a pattern in the resist. During the developing, the resist washes away in the regions where diffusions are desired. The resist is then used as a mask to selectively etch the SiO_2 layer.

One final key invention was needed to make modern IC technology possible. That was the ability to integrate multiple components on the same chip and to interconnect them to form a circuit. The invention of the integrated circuit occurred in 1959 and was due to Jack Kilby of Texas Instruments and Robert Noyce of Fairchild Semiconductor. An interesting historical account of these events is given in [1.7]. The key ideas were the extensions of the ideas in Figures 1–8 and 1–9 to using masking and lithography to provide multiple devices and interconnects on the same chip. Figure 1–10 illustrates these extensions for a simple circuit example. Kilby and Noyce have been widely recognized for their work leading to the integrated circuit. By combining P- and N-type diffusions and SiO_2 passivation layers, many types of devices including transistors, resistors, and capacitors are possible in modern IC structures.

Although it is perhaps obvious from Figure 1–10, it should be noted that when multiple diffusions and thin film layers are used to construct an integrated circuit, the masks associated with each of the layers must be precisely aligned with respect to each other. That is, the N-type diffusion in the center NPN transistor must be placed inside the P-type region and the contact holes which allow the Al metal to contact the device regions must be placed inside those regions. In general the placement accuracy during

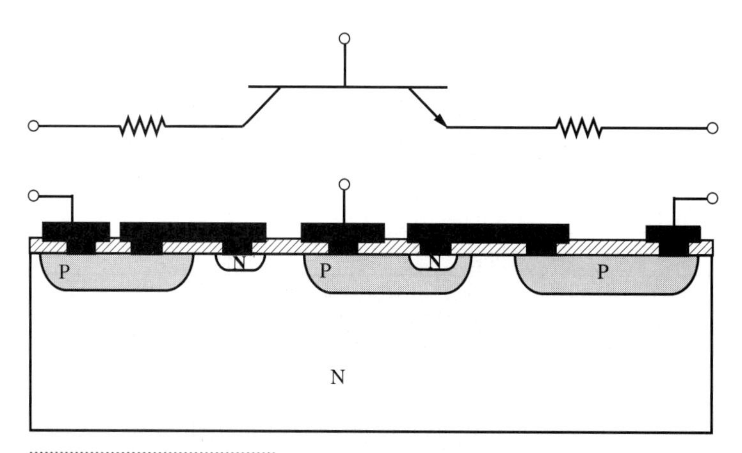

Figure 1–10 Integrated circuits use photolithography and masking to fabricate multiple components in a common substrate.

photolithography must be on the order of 1/4 to 1/3 of the linewidth being printed. In today's modern factories, this alignment process is carried out automatically in machines called steppers which we will discuss in more detail in Chapter 5.

Since 1960, the basic technologies used to manufacture integrated circuits have not changed. They have, of course, been significantly improved and many new ways of depositing, etching, diffusing, and patterning have been developed. These improvements have been more evolutionary than revolutionary however. In spite of this fact, the cumulative impact of rapid evolutionary developments over the past 35 years in IC technology has been enormous and we should expect many more years of the same kinds of developments.

Figure 1–11 shows a schematic cross section of a modern silicon integrated circuit. The silicon wafer is typically > 500 μm thick; the layers on the top surface are typically 1 μm or thinner. Thus the full wafer thickness is not normally shown in these drawings. The N and P regions have been selectively doped to change their conductivity and they form the electrically active parts of the devices. The layers above the surface may be insulators like SiO_2 or Si_3N_4, conductors like Al, or semiconductors like polycrystalline silicon. All of these layers are either selectively deposited only in certain areas or are patterned after a blanket deposition using photolithography and etching so that they remain only in local areas. The lateral scale of the various features is determined by the patterning capability of the technology. In high-volume manufacturing today, such features might have a minimum size of perhaps 0.25 μm. The particular technology illustrated in Figure 1–11 is called CMOS (Complementary MOS) since it integrates both N- and P-type MOS devices side by side on the same chip. This is the technology that forms the basis of the NTRS discussed earlier and outlined in Table 1–1. Figure 1–12 shows an actual cross section of a modern CMOS IC. Note that the interconnect layers dominate the overall chip cross section. The devices themselves are all located in a thin layer near the bottom of the photomicrograph. Most of the silicon wafer itself is not shown and is off the bottom of the photograph.

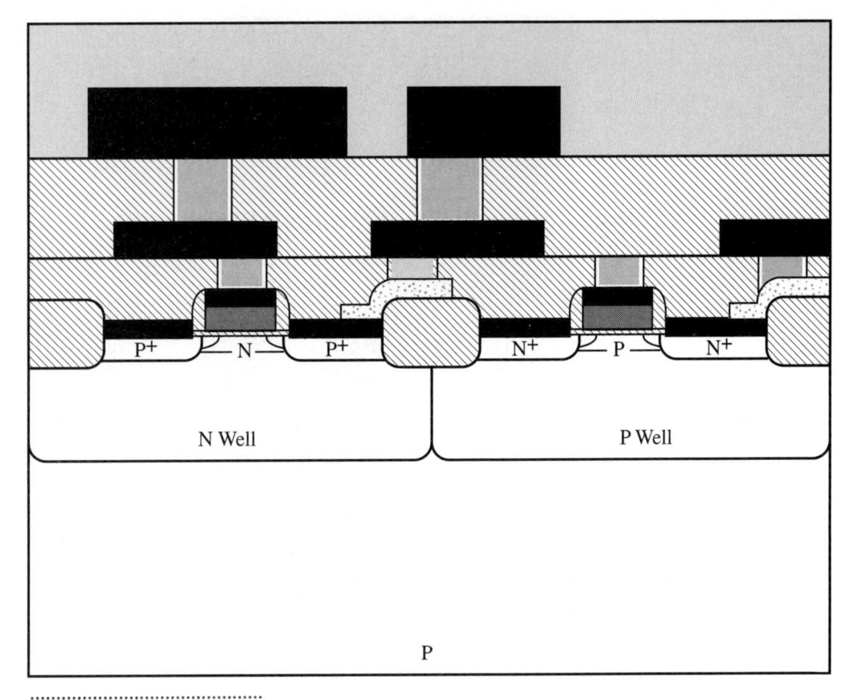

Figure 1–11 Schematic cross section of a modern silicon integrated circuit. The particular technology shown is CMOS with an NMOS device on the right and a PMOS device on the left. There are two levels of wiring shown. We will discuss this technology in detail in Chapter 2.

1.3 Semiconductors

This section provides a brief review of the basic properties of semiconductor materials. Many of the ideas discussed here will be used throughout this book. For readers already familiar with this material, this section can be skimmed or skipped.

Semiconductors are a class of materials which have the unique property that their electrical conductivity can be controlled over a very wide range by the introduction of dopants. While this property can easily be observed in crystalline, polycrystalline, or amorphous semiconductor materials, crystalline materials provide the most reproducible properties and the highest performance devices and are almost always used in integrated circuits. Dopants are atoms that generally contain either one more or one fewer electrons in their outermost shell than the host semiconductor. They provide one extra electron or one missing electron (a "hole") compared to the host atoms. These excess electrons and holes are the carriers, which carry current in semiconductor devices. The key to building semiconductor devices and integrated circuits lies in the ability to control the local doping and hence the local electronic properties of a semiconductor crystal.

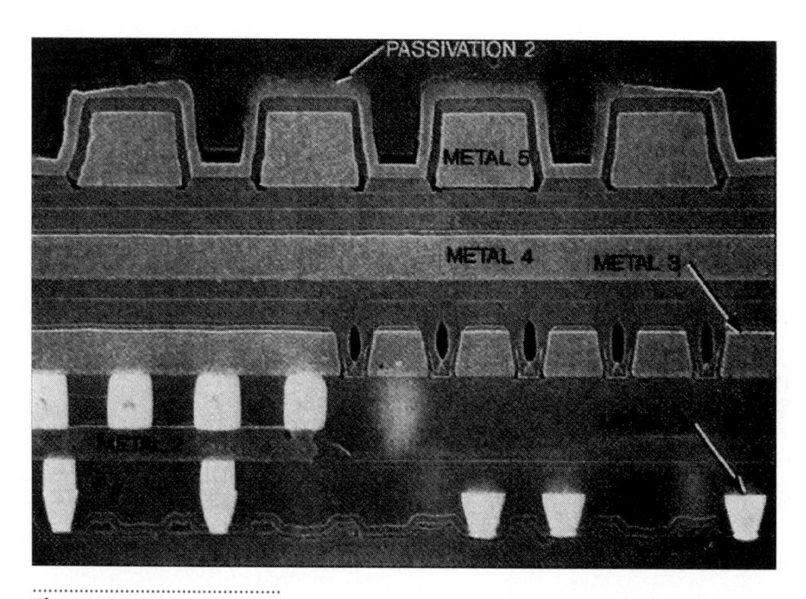

Figure 1–12 Actual cross section of a modern IC (IBM's PowerPC chip). Note the multiple layers of metal for wiring above the silicon surface. The active parts of the transistors are barely visible at the bottom of the photograph. Reprinted with permission of Integrated Circuit Engineering Corporation.

Consider silicon as a representative semiconductor. As illustrated in Figure 1–13, silicon has four electrons in its outermost shell. These are known as the valence electrons since they are the participants in chemical reactions and chemical bonding. When silicon atoms combine to form a solid crystal, a particularly stable electronic arrangement can be formed if the silicon atoms form covalent or shared electron bonds with their four nearest neighbors as illustrated in Figure 1–13. This arrangement is favored because each silicon atom can then "fill up" its outermost shell to a total of eight shared electrons. (In the periodic table, elements with full outer electron shells are the inert gases like Ar and Ne which are chemically rather inert and very stable.) The covalent bonding or sharing arrangement in essence populates the entire outer shell for each Si atom, resulting in a stable structure in which all electrons are bound to atoms, at least at very low temperatures.

Elemental semiconductors, all of which have this same bonding arrangement, lie in Column IV of the periodic table as shown in Figure 1–14. This same type of bonding arrangement can be produced using mixtures of elements from other columns of the periodic table. For example GaAs consists of alternating Ga (column III) and As (column V) atoms which have an average of four electrons per atom and so the same covalent bonding arrangement works. More complex examples like $Hg_xCd_{1-x}Te$ are also possible. Thus nature provides many possible materials which can act as semiconductors.

At temperatures above absolute zero, thermal energy can break some of the Si-Si bonds as illustrated in Figure 1–15. This creates both a free or mobile electron and a mobile hole (or missing electron). The concentrations of electrons and holes are exactly equal in pure semiconductors and are referred to as the intrinsic carrier concentration

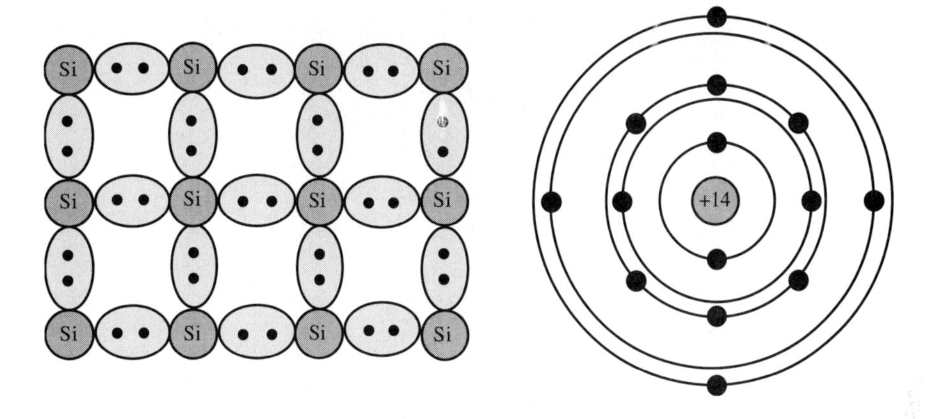

Figure 1–13 Simple representation of silicon atoms bonded in a crystal (left). The dotted areas are covalent or shared electron bonds. The electronic structure of a single Si atom is shown conceptually on the right. The four outermost electrons are the valence electrons that participate in the covalent bonds.

II B	III A	IV A	V A	VI A
	5 B 10.81	6 C 12.01	7 N 14.01	8 O 16.00
	13 Al 26.98	14 Si 28.09	15 P 30.97	16 S 32.06
30 Zn 65.39	31 Ga 69.72	32 Ge 72.59	33 As 74.92	34 Se 78.96
48 Cd 112.4	49 In 114.8	50 Sn 118.7	51 Sb 121.8	52 Te 127.6
80 Hg 200.6	81 Tl 204.4	82 Pb 207.2	83 Bi 209.0	84 Po 209

Figure 1–14 Portion of the periodic table relevant to semiconductor materials and doping. Elemental semiconductors are in column IV. Compound semiconductors are combinations of elements from columns III and V (or II and VI).

n_i. Figure 1–16 plots this concentration as a function of temperature. At room temperature, n_i has a value of about 1.4 x 10^{10} cm^{-3} in silicon. Since there are about 5 x 10^{22} cm^{-3} atoms in silicon, fewer than 1 in 10^{12} bonds are broken at room temperature. As a result, pure silicon is a very poor conductor. The mobile carriers carry electrical currents in devices. With so few of these present in pure silicon, the currents would be far too small to be useful in devices.

Fortunately, semiconductors have the property that they can be doped. This process is illustrated in Figure 1–17. Doping could be accomplished by the gas phase diffusion process we discussed in connection with Figures 1–7 and 1–8. However, today it is generally accomplished by a process called ion implantation that we will discuss in detail in

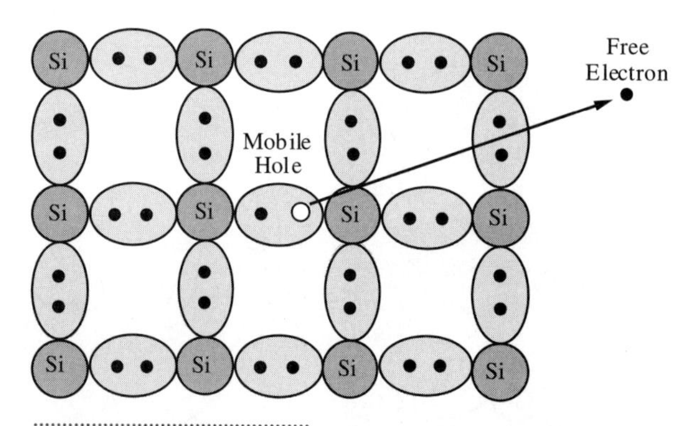

Figure 1–15 Electron (-) and hole (+) pair generation represented by a broken bond in the crystal. Both carriers are mobile and can carry currents in devices.

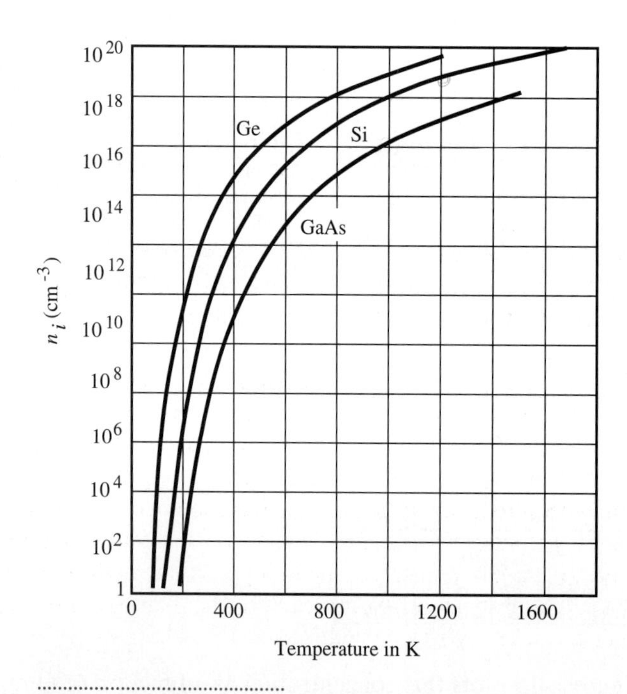

Figure 1–16 Intrinsic carrier concentration versus temperature in common semiconductors. After [1.9].

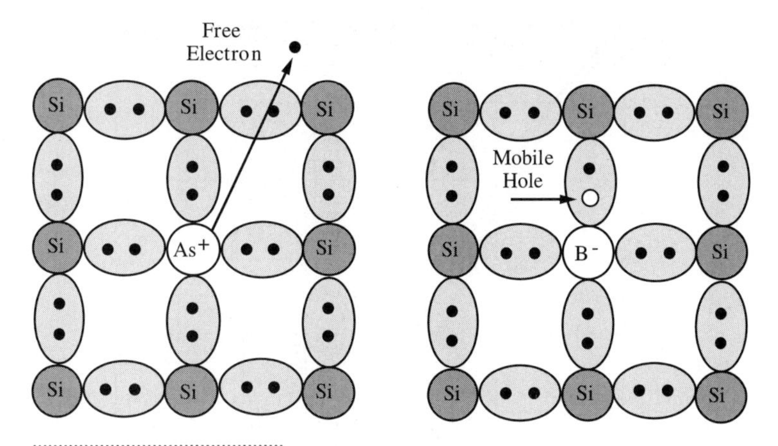

Figure 1–17 Doping of group IV semiconductors using elements from column V (arsenic) or III (boron) of the periodic table.

Chapter 8. Doping results in a column V (As, for example) or a column III (B, for example) atom replacing a silicon atom in the crystal structure. Such dopants either contribute an extra electron (column V) to the crystal and become N-type dopants, or they contribute a hole (column III) and become P-type dopants. The electrons or holes are introduced on a one for one basis by the dopants. As a result, to the extent that we can control the doping concentration accurately, we can precisely control the free electron and hole concentrations and therefore the conductivity of the silicon. N_D and N_A are used to refer to the N-type (donor) and P-type (acceptor) concentrations, respectively. In semiconductor devices, this doping is done locally as illustrated in Figure 1–11 using photolithography and masking.

Modern integrated circuit technology generally uses ion implantation to dope the semiconductor. This permits the controlled introduction of parts per million to parts per hundred of dopant atoms. As a result, the conductivity of silicon can be controlled over a very wide range, permitting many types of semiconductor devices to be fabricated. Figure 1–18 illustrates the range of conductivity it is possible to achieve in silicon by doping. The terms N^+, N^-, P^{++}, and so on are often used in semiconductor devices to describe relative levels of doping in a particular region. While there are no formal definitions of the ranges of doping each of these terms represents, the following approximate definitions are often used:

$$N^{--} \text{ or } P^{--}: \quad N_D \text{ or } N_A < 10^{14}\text{ cm}^{-3}$$

$$N^{-} \text{ or } P^{-}: 10^{14}\text{ cm}^{-3} < N_D \text{ or } N_A < 10^{16}\text{ cm}^{-3}$$

$$N \text{ or } P: 10^{16}\text{ cm}^{-3} < N_D \text{ or } N_A < 10^{18}\text{ cm}^{-3}$$

$$N^{+} \text{ or } P^{+}: 10^{18}\text{ cm}^{-3} < N_D \text{ or } N_A < 10^{20}\text{ cm}^{-3}$$

$$N^{++} \text{ or } P^{++}: \quad N_D \text{ or } N_A > 10^{20}\text{ cm}^{-3}$$

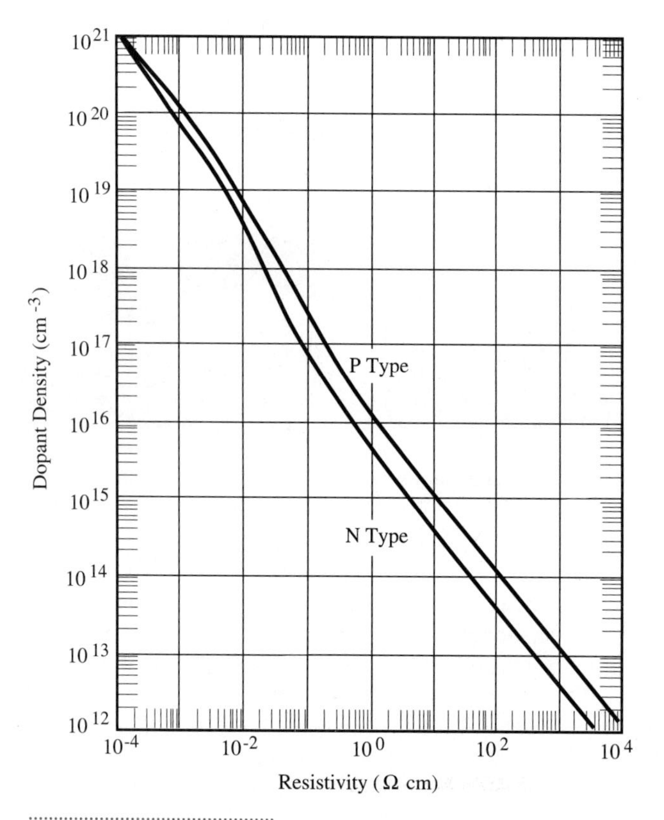

Figure 1–18 Resistivity versus doping for N- and P-type silicon. After [1.10].

Since the lattice density in silicon is 5 x 10^{22} cm^{-3}, even the heaviest doped regions, N^{++} and P^{++}, normally use doping concentrations less than 1%.

The resistivity plotted in Figure 1–18 is inversely proportional to the carrier concentrations and is defined as

$$\rho = \frac{1}{q\mu_n n + q\mu_p p} \tag{1.1}$$

where n and p are the electron and hole concentrations and μ_n and μ_p are the electron and hole mobilities, respectively. μ_n and μ_p vary with temperature, doping, and electric field in semiconductors. In silicon at room temperature, with low doping concentration and small fields, maximum values of $\mu_n \approx 1500$ cm^2 $volt^{-1}$ sec^{-1} and $\mu_p \approx 500$ cm^2 $volt^{-1}$ sec^{-1} are observed. n and p are determined by the dopant concentrations N_D and N_A through relationships we will describe shortly. In general only one of the two terms in Eq. (1.1) is significant since $n >> p$ in N-doped material and $p >> n$ in P-doped material.

The electrical properties of semiconductors are often described through the use of two types of models. The first of these is the "bond" model that we used beginning with Figure 1–13. The second model is the "band" model. Both of these approaches model the

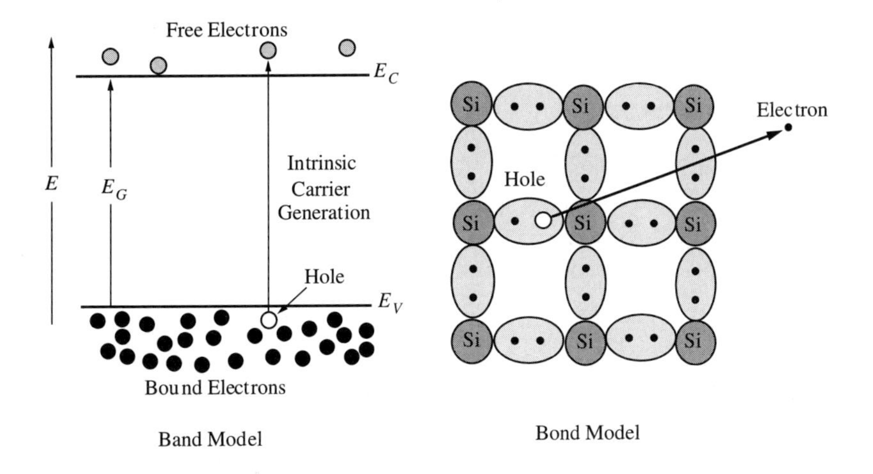

Figure 1–19 Simple band and bond diagram representations of pure silicon. Bonded electrons lie at energy levels below E_V; free electrons are above E_C. The process of intrinsic carrier generation is illustrated in each model.

same physical phenomena. They are simply different ways of explaining the same underlying mechanisms. We will make use of both approaches in this book because some concepts are easier to understand with the bond model, others with the band model.

Figure 1–19 illustrates both models for the case of pure silicon. In the band model representation, the vertical direction is the potential energy of electrons in the crystal. From the bond model, we can see that in a perfect crystal, electrons are either bound to host silicon atoms or they are free. A finite amount of energy is required to free the electron (that is, to break a Si-Si bond). In the band diagram, we represent this with the bound electron energy levels below the valence band (E_V) and the free electron energy levels above the conduction band (E_C). The energy gap between E_V and E_C represents the energy needed to free the electron. In a perfect crystal, there are no allowed energy levels between E_V and E_C (an electron is either free or it is bound). Thus the breaking of a Si-Si bond, which creates one free electron and one free hole, is illustrated in the band model by elevating an electron up to the conduction band.

In Figure 1–20, the introduction of dopants is represented in the bond model and in the band diagram by the E_D and E_A energy levels. Consider the E_D level first, which represents a donor atom (As for example). When an As atom is introduced into the crystal, it brings with it an extra electron in its outermost shell, beyond the four needed for covalent bonding in the silicon lattice. This electron will be bound weakly to the As atom because the As atom also brings along with it a positive charge in its nucleus (proton) to balance each electron. The binding energy of this fifth valence electron is usually rather small since it is not needed for the four covalent bonds the As atom forms in the silicon lattice. As a result, the fifth electron can be quite easily freed. We represent this in the band diagram with an energy level E_D that is close to E_C. The small difference in energy between E_C and E_D represents the energy, which must be supplied to free the fifth electron. When $E_C - E_D$ is small, we refer to the dopant as a "shallow" donor. For

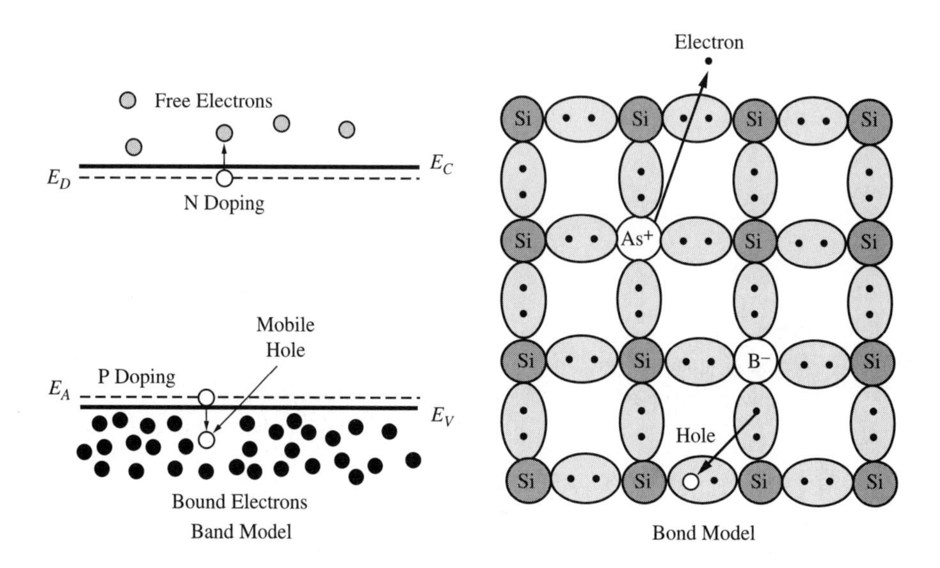

Figure 1–20 Simple band and bond diagram representations of doped silicon. E_A and E_D represent acceptor and donor energy levels respectively. P- and N-type doping are illustrated in each model, using As as the donor and B as the acceptor.

such donors, except at very low temperatures, this energy is always available due to the thermal energy of the crystal and so each donor provides one free electron in the crystal. Note that once the As atom has donated its extra electron to the crystal, the As will have a net positive charge As^+.

$$As \rightarrow As^+ + e^- \qquad \text{or} \qquad As \rightarrow As^+ + n \tag{1.2}$$

P-type dopants are represented in an analogous manner as also shown in Figure 1–20 for both the bond and band models. E_A represents the energy level introduced into the crystal by the P-type dopant (B, for example). Such dopants have one fewer valence electrons per atom than the host crystal. The hole or missing electron is weakly bound to the B atom. An electron from a neighboring Si atom can exchange positions with the hole, effectively allowing the hole to move through the crystal as a positively charged carrier. The energy difference between E_V and E_A represents this binding energy of the hole to the B atom and is small in the case of a "shallow" acceptor. As is the case with N-type dopants, thermal energy supplies enough energy to free the hole at all but the very lowest temperatures.

An analogy to bubbles in a liquid is often used to describe hole behavior in the band model. Bubbles tend to rise to the surface. Thus energy needs to be provided to these bubbles or holes to push them down from the E_A level into the valence band where they become mobile positively charged carriers.

Once the boron gives up its hole to the crystal, it has a net negative charge B^-.

$$\mathrm{B} \rightarrow \mathrm{B}^{-} + \mathrm{h}^{+} \qquad \text{or} \qquad \mathrm{B} \rightarrow \mathrm{B}^{-} + \mathrm{p} \tag{1.3}$$

We can quantify these ideas a little more carefully. The intrinsic carrier concentration in silicon is given by [1.8]

$$n_i = 3.1 \times 10^{16} T^{3/2} \exp\left(-\frac{0.603\mathrm{eV}}{kT} \right) \mathrm{cm}^{-3} \tag{1.4}$$

This equation is an empirical fit to experimental data. It describes the process by which an electron can be excited from the valence band (bound states) to the conduction band (free states). As we saw in Figure 1–16, the number of such carriers in materials like silicon is relatively small at room temperature. Since the process responsible for generating n_i is bond breaking, we would expect that semiconductors that have weaker bonds also have higher n_i values. This is indeed the case. Weaker bonds are represented in the band model by smaller bandgaps. Table 1–2 summarizes these key numbers for three typical semiconductors. n_i depends exponentially on the bandgap with wider bandgap materials having smaller values of n_i.

Table 1–2 Bandgap and intrinsic carrier concentration of three common semiconductors.

Material	E_G at Room Temp	n_i at Room Temp
Germanium	0.66 eV	2.5×10^{13} cm^{-3}
Silicon	1.12 eV	1.45×10^{10} cm^{-3}
GaAs	1.42 eV	2×10^{6} cm^{-3}

In an undoped material, it is also the case that $n = p$, so it must be true that

$$np = n_i^2 \tag{1.5}$$

Although we have not proven it, Eq. (1.5) holds in doped as well as in undoped semiconductors. This is often called the law of mass action and is an important relationship in describing carrier concentrations in semiconductors. An important implication of this equation is that if we increase the electron population in the crystal by introducing N-type dopants, n will increase and p will decrease. Physically, the reason for this is that the processes of generation of hole-electron pairs by Si-Si bond breaking and the reverse recombination process are constantly occurring in a crystal to produce an equilibrium number of carriers. If we introduce more electrons by doping, we will increase the probability of electrons and holes encountering each other in the crystal and hence the probability of recombination. An increase in n will therefore drive the hole population down as described by Eq. (1.5).

At very high doping concentrations, the n_i value used in Eq. (1.5) must be changed to account for what are called "heavy doping effects." Fundamentally such effects occur because the simple picture of a Si crystal with widely separated doping atoms is not a correct picture at high doping concentrations. At n or p values greater than about 10^{19} cm^{-3}, the doping atoms are on average close enough to each other that they begin to interact and to affect the Si crystal structure. (See problem 1.2.) Generally this results in a reduction in the Si bandgap and an increase in n_i.

While shallow donors or acceptors are always ionized at room temperature (that is they contribute free electrons or holes to the crystal), this is not always the case at low temperatures. Also, for atoms that introduce energy levels deeper in the bandgap, full ionization often does not occur even at room temperature because thermal energy is not large enough to excite the extra electron or hole up to E_C (or down to E_V).

Figure 1–21 illustrates the general behavior of the free carrier concentration versus temperature, for a specific case of a shallow donor in silicon. At temperatures below about 100K, freezeout of the As donor is observed and the free electron concentration drops. At temperatures above about 600K, n_i begins to dominate the doping and n increases. We refer to this n_i dominated regime as the intrinsic region. For lower temperatures, the material is extrinsic or dopant dominated. Devices are almost always operated in the temperature regime in which the material is extrinsic, that is, the doping controls the behavior. In the processing world, however, much higher temperatures are involved and the material is often intrinsic. This difference will have significant impact throughout this book. Note also that the value of n_i that is appropriate for device operation is the room temperature value of 1.45×10^{10} cm^{-3} in silicon, whereas much higher values ($10^{16} - 10^{18}$ cm^{-3}) are appropriate in the processing world.

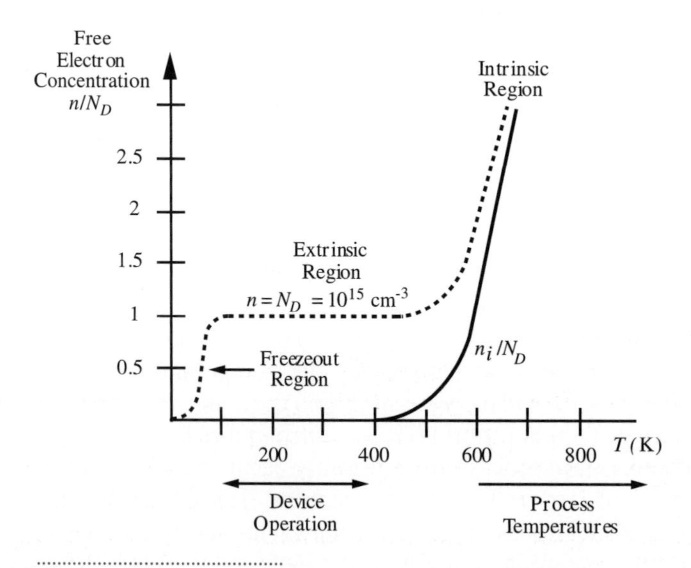

Figure 1–21 Behavior of free carrier concentration versus temperature. Arsenic in silicon is qualitatively illustrated as a specific example ($N_D = 10^{15}$ cm^{-3}). Note that at high temperatures n_i becomes larger than the 10^{15} doping and $n \approx n_i$. Devices are normally operated where $n = N_D^+$. Fabrication occurs at much higher temperatures where n is often $\approx n_i$.

The probability of an electron occupying any particular energy level E in a system of discrete energy levels, when the electrons are subject to the Pauli exclusion principle is given by the Fermi-Dirac probability function:

$$F(E) = \frac{1}{1 + \exp\left(\frac{E - E_F}{kT}\right)} \tag{1.6}$$

This is the appropriate expression for electrons and holes in a semiconductor crystal. The quantity E_F in this equation is called the Fermi level and is defined by this equation to be simply the energy level at which the probability of finding an electron is exactly 0.5. $1 - F(E)$ is the probability of not finding an electron at energy E, or in other words, the probability of finding a hole there.

Figure 1–22 illustrates the concept of the Fermi level. The left-hand case represents an undoped semiconductor. In that case, $n = p$ and typically there will be a very small number of electrons in the conduction band and holes in the valence band. Thus the probability of a valence band energy level being occupied by an electron is essentially 1; the probability of finding an electron in the conduction band is essentially 0. Therefore, E_F must be located somewhere in the forbidden band between E_V and E_C. In fact, it is almost exactly in the middle of the bandgap. E_F is usually called the intrinsic Fermi level E_{Fi} or E_i in this case. If we add N-type doping (middle case in Figure 1–22), we know that the number of electrons in the conduction band increases, so the probability of finding an electron above E_C also increases. The Fermi level will move up in the bandgap to reflect this. In fact, a little experience with these sorts of band diagrams will allow the reader to quickly estimate the electron or hole populations in a given situation from a picture, which shows E_F. The higher E_F is in the bandgap, the higher n is.

Note also in Figure 1–22 that we are now showing (schematically) only the holes in the valence band rather than all the bound electrons as we have in earlier figures. The holes are the mobile charge carriers in the valence band and they are what we care about when we describe device operation or process physics issues. From this point forward we will show only the mobile carriers in these diagrams—holes in the valence band and electrons in the conduction band.

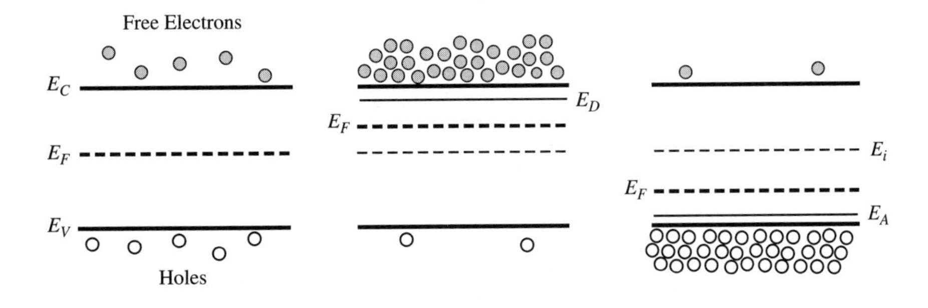

Figure 1–22 Fermi level position in an undoped (left), N-type (center), and P-type (right) semiconductor. The dots represent free electrons; the open circles represent mobile holes.

P-type doping is analogous (right side of Figure 1–22). Introducing P-type dopants increases the hole population in the valence band and decreases the free electron population in the conduction band. E_F moves down in the bandgap to reflect the lower free electron population. The closer E_F is to E_V, the higher the hole population is. Thus, while E_F is a well-defined mathematical quantity, perhaps its greatest use in semiconductors is in visualizing the electronic properties (carrier concentrations and type) through the band diagram concept.

To actually calculate n and p in a given situation, we need to know not only the probability of finding them at an energy level E [Eq. (1.6)], but also the number and position of allowed energy levels. Quantum mechanics tells us how the electrons fill the energy levels in an atom or in a system of atoms like a crystal. In such a system the energy levels are not continuous (no two electrons can have exactly the same set of quantum numbers). From these concepts comes an approximate expression for the allowed electron energy levels at an energy E:

$$N(E) = \frac{4\pi}{h^3}(m_e^*)^{\frac{3}{2}}(E - E_C)^{\frac{1}{2}} \text{ for } E > E_c \tag{1.7}$$

$$N(E) = \frac{4\pi}{h^3}(m_h^*)^{\frac{3}{2}}(E_V - E)^{\frac{1}{2}} \text{ for } E < E_V \tag{1.8}$$

where the first equation describes the allowed energy levels for electrons in the conduction band and the second, the allowed levels for holes in the valence band. In this equation m_e^* and m_h^* are the density of states effective masses of the electron and hole, respectively, in the crystal and are different from the electron rest mass. m_e^* and m_h^* account for the fact that the electrons and holes are located in a crystal rather than in free space. $N(E)$ is of course zero within the bandgap of a pure semiconductor.

Given these expressions for the allowed energy levels and Eq. (1.6) which describes the probability that an allowed level will actually be occupied, we can now determine how many free electrons and holes are actually present in the crystal. Figure 1–23 illustrates graphically how we do this. $F(E)$ is the probability distribution for electrons, which, for an undoped crystal, has a value of 0.5 at the middle of the forbidden band. $N(E)$, the density of allowed states, is plotted from Eqs. (1.7) and (1.8). Note that there are no allowed energy levels in the forbidden band. Above E_C or below E_V, the densities increase as the square root of the energy. The multiple lines in this part of the figure are meant to schematically represent the discrete allowed states that exist at any energy E. For a crystal with an appreciable number of atoms, the discrete energy levels are so close together and so numerous they appear to be a continuous distribution as shown in Eqs. (1.7) and (1.8). The product of the $F(E)$ and $N(E)$ curves on the right represents the electron population at any energy. Since we are interested only in the free electrons, we have shown this population only in the conduction band. In an analogous way, the product of $N(E)$ and $1 - F(E)$ represents the hole population, which we have shown only in the valence band since this is where holes are mobile. Note that most of the free electrons are located fairly close to E_C and most of the free holes close to E_V, because the respective probability functions rapidly fall towards zero further away from

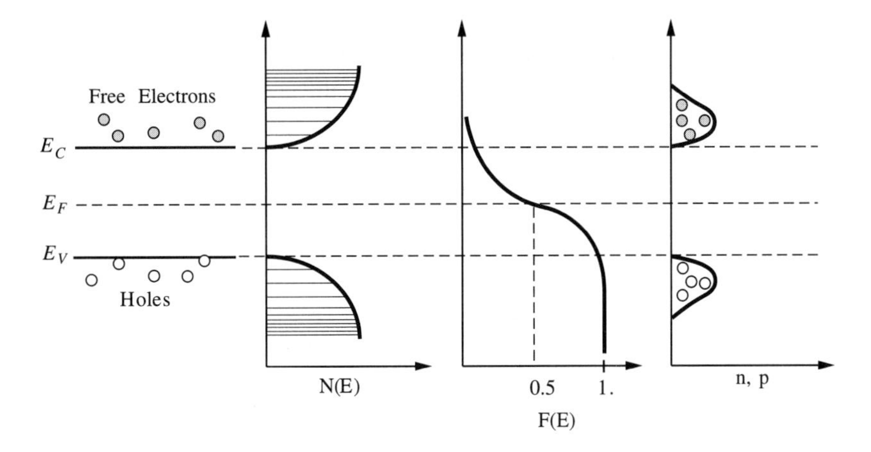

Figure 1–23 Density of allowed states, probability function, and resulting electron and hole populations in a semiconductor crystal.

the band edges. This is in spite of the fact that the number of allowed energy levels increases away from E_C or E_V.

Usually in device physics or in process physics, we are interested in the total number of electrons in the conduction band and the total number of holes in the valence band. These quantities are the areas under the right-hand curves in Figure 1–23 and can be calculated as follows:

$$n = \int_{E_C}^{\infty} F(E)N(E)dE \cong N_C \exp\left(-\frac{E_C - E_F}{kT}\right) \tag{1.9}$$

$$p = \int_{-\infty}^{E_V} [1 - F(E)]N(E)dE \cong N_V \exp\left(-\frac{E_F - E_V}{kT}\right) \tag{1.10}$$

where

$$N_C = 2\left(\frac{2\pi m_e^* kT}{h^2}\right)^{\frac{3}{2}}, N_V = 2\left(\frac{2\pi m_h^* kT}{h^2}\right)^{\frac{3}{2}} \tag{1.11}$$

N_C and N_V are often called the effective densities of states in the conduction and valence bands. They have values of 2.8×10^{19} cm^{-3} and 1.04×10^{19} cm^{-3}, respectively, in silicon at room temperature.

In integrating Eqs. (1.9) and (1.10), we have made use of the fact that the Fermi-Dirac probability function in Eq. (1.6) can be approximated by the Boltzmann distribution when the Fermi level is at least a few kT away from the conduction and valence bands and from any other allowed energy levels in the bandgap. When this is true, the $E - E_F$ term in Eq. (1.6) is much larger than kT and the 1 in the denominator may be dropped, resulting in the Boltzmann distribution function. Eqs. (1.9) and (1.10) apply only as long as this is true. When E_F approaches E_C, E_V, or other allowed energy levels in the bandgap, the full Fermi-Dirac distribution function must be used to describe the electrons populating the various energy levels. This may be required at low temperatures when not all donors or acceptors are ionized and E_F can approach E_D or E_A. Fermi-Dirac statistics are also generally required when doping levels exceed 10^{19} cm^{-3} in silicon, since then E_F moves up into the conduction band or down into the valence band, and allowed energy levels exist near E_F. Such heavily doped semiconductors are often called degenerate and act more like metals than semiconductors. We will in general use the simple results in Eqs. (1.9) and (1.10) in this text. However there will be cases where this is not valid. Generally when this is occurs, computer techniques are used to calculate n, p, and E_F. Such programs are widely available.

By combining Eq. (1.5) with Eqs. (1.9) and (1.10), we arrive at the result that

$$np = n_i^2 = N_C N_V \exp\left(-\frac{E_G}{kT}\right) = KT^3 \exp\left(-\frac{E_G}{kT}\right) \tag{1.12}$$

where $E_G = E_C - E_V$. Note the similarity of this result to Eq. (1.4). The exponential behavior of n_i with temperature is also apparent in Figure 1–16.

By combining Eqs. (1.9), (1.10) and (1.12), we obtain the following expressions

$$n = n_i \exp\left(\frac{E_F - E_i}{kT}\right) \tag{1.13}$$

$$p = n_i \exp\left(\frac{E_i - E_F}{kT}\right) \tag{1.14}$$

These forms of the equations are often convenient to use instead of Eqs. (1.9) and (1.10).

Eqs. (1.13) and (1.14) reflect the idea that as E_F moves above E_i, the electron population increases exponentially and the hole population decreases. Similarly, as E_F moves below E_i, n decreases and p increases, both exponentially with $|E_F - E_i|$. Eqs. (1.9) and (1.10) write this equivalently in terms of N_C or N_V. Figure 1–22 illustrates these ideas.

It is sometimes the case in semiconductors that N- and P-type doping concentrations are of the same order. Other situations may arise in which n and p are on the order of n_i. This latter case often occurs at high temperatures (such as those occurring during processing), as illustrated in Figure 1–21. In these cases a more general statement of overall charge neutrality can be used to calculate n and p. Overall charge neutrality requires that

$$N_D^+ + p = N_A^- + n \tag{1.15}$$

[Recall from Eqs. (1.2) and (1.3) that the dopants are charged, for example, As^+ or B^-, after they donate electrons or holes.]

Combining this equation with Eq. (1.5), results in the following general equations for electron and hole concentrations. Unless the donors or acceptors have energy levels deep in the forbidden band, or the temperature is very low, N_D^+ and N_A^- can generally be replaced in these expressions by N_D and N_A, respectively.

$$n = \frac{1}{2}\left[(N_D^+ - N_A^-) + \sqrt{(N_D^+ - N_A^-)^2 + 4n_i^2}\,\right] \tag{1.16}$$

$$p = \frac{1}{2}\left[(N_A^- - N_D^+) + \sqrt{(N_A^- - N_D^+)^2 + 4n_i^2}\,\right] \tag{1.17}$$

One additional piece of information is necessary in order to apply these concepts in the broadest sense. The bandgap in semiconductors changes as a function of temperature. Physically this occurs because the lattice constant (spacing between the atoms) changes with temperature and hence the energy needed to break bonds changes with temperature. Generally the lattice constant increases with temperature (the atoms move further apart). This weakens the bonds and the bandgap decreases. For silicon, this effect can be approximated with the following equation [1.9] where T is in °K. This effect is particularly important when we consider semiconductors at processing temperatures.

$$E_G(\text{eV}) = 1.17 - \frac{4.73 \times 10^{-4}T^2}{T + 636} \approx 1.16 - (3 \times 10^{-4})T \tag{1.18}$$

Figure 1–24 illustrates some of these concepts. The gray bands at the top and bottom represent the conduction and valence band edges. At higher temperatures, the bandgap narrows, as described by Eq. (1.18). The series of solid curves plot the position of the Fermi level for a specific doping concentration as temperature changes. Each of these

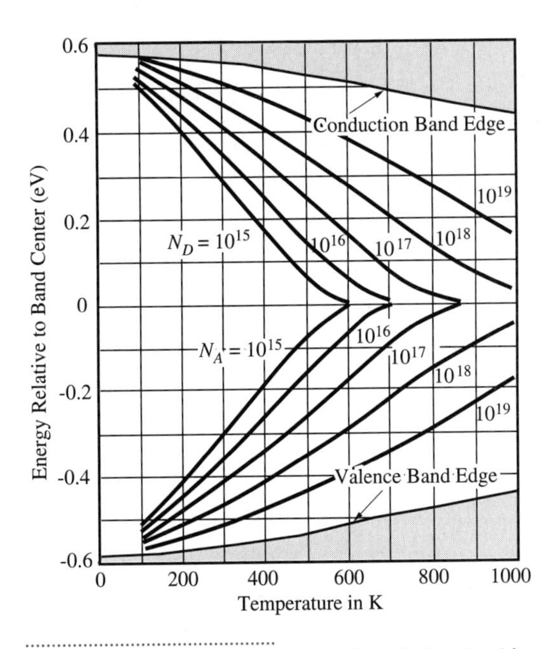

Figure 1–24 Fermi level position in the forbidden band for a given doping level, as a function of temperature. After [1.10].

curves moves closer to E_i as T increases, reflecting the fact that the material becomes more intrinsic at higher temperatures. Normally in studying semiconductor device physics, we are concerned with temperatures around 300K. In the processing world, however, temperatures are usually much higher. This means that in modeling process phenomena, we will use values of n_i which are much larger, values for E_G which are significantly smaller, and analyze materials which are more often intrinsic. In later chapters we will see the implications of these observations.

Example A sample of silicon which is doped with both N- and P-type dopants is shown in Figure 1–25. Calculate n, p, and E_F for (a) room temperature—a typical device operating condition; and (b) 1000°C—a typical processing temperature, which might be used during device fabrication.

Answer In general, in problems of this type, there are three unknowns, n, p, and E_F, assuming the dopants are fully ionized and $N_D = N_D^+$ and $N_A = N_A^-$. There are three independent equations taken from those presented above, which must be solved simultaneously. (There are actually four unknowns including n_i but it may be calculated directly from Eq. (1.4) since the temperature is known.) Generally we know N_D, N_A, and T, as in this problem. The three equations with three unknowns are as follows. Note that Eqs. (1.16) and (1.17) and (1.13) and (1.14) are pairs of equations, which are not independent but are related through Eq. (1.12).

$$\Rightarrow \quad \left\{ \begin{array}{l} n = \dfrac{1}{2}\left[(N_D^+ - N_A^-) + \sqrt{(N_D^+ - N_A^-)^2 + 4n_i^2}\right] \\ p = \dfrac{1}{2}\left[(N_A^- - N_D^+) + \sqrt{(N_A^- - N_D^+)^2 + 4n_i^2}\right] \end{array} \right\} \qquad (1.16, 1.17)$$

$$\Rightarrow \quad \left\{ \begin{array}{l} n = n_i \exp\left(\dfrac{E_F - E_i}{kT}\right) \\ p = n_i \exp\left(\dfrac{E_i - E_F}{kT}\right) \end{array} \right\} \qquad (1.13, 1.14)$$

$$\Rightarrow \quad np = n_i^2 \qquad (1.12)$$

In virtually every case of interest, physical insight can greatly simplify this situation, usually to the point where simultaneous equations do not have to be solved. In those cases in which simplifications cannot be made, there are computer programs available which efficiently calculate a solution. In solving this example, we will take the approach of first using physical insight to simplify the problem.

a. Room Temperature Solution At room temperature, it is reasonable to assume that all of the dopants are ionized. Both As (E_D = 0.049 eV) and B (E_A = 0.045 eV) are shal-

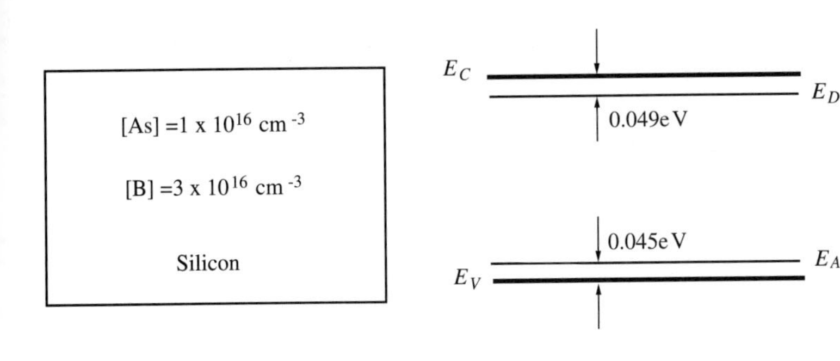

Figure 1–25 Silicon doped with both N- and P-type dopants.

low dopants. Furthermore, the net doping, $N_A - N_D$ is much greater than n_i so we have directly from Eqs. (1.16) and (1.12) that

$$p = N_A - N_D = 2 \times 10^{16}\text{cm}^{-3}$$

$$n = \frac{n_i^2}{p} = \frac{2.1 \times 10^{20}}{2 \times 10^{16}} = 1.05 \times 10^4\text{cm}^{-3}$$

The Fermi level position can now be calculated directly from Eq. (1.14):

$$p = n_i \exp\left(\frac{E_i - E_F}{kT}\right)$$

$$\therefore E_i - E_F = kT \ln \frac{p}{n_i} = (8.62 \times 10^{-5}\,\text{eVK}^{-1})(298K)\ln\frac{2 \times 10^{16}}{1.45 \times 10^{10}} = 0.36\text{ eV}$$

Another observation at this point may be helpful. To first order, it is the case that energy levels above E_F are not occupied by electrons, while levels below E_F are occupied. (Recall that E_F by definition is the level at which the probability of finding an electron is exactly 0.5. The probability drops rapidly toward 0 above E_F and approaches 1 below E_F as shown in Figure 1–23.) The result in Figure 1–26(a) shows E_F to be well below E_D which means that the donor levels are not occupied or have donated their electrons. E_F is also well above E_A which means that the acceptor levels are occupied or have accepted electrons. This is consistent with our assumption of complete ionization.

b. High Temperature Solution At 1000°C, we can calculate directly from Eq. (1.4) that n_i = 7.14 x 10^{18} cm^{-3}. This is much larger than the donor or acceptor concentrations so that the material will be intrinsic. Therefore, $n = p = n_i$ and the Fermi level will be essentially in the middle of the bandgap. Note that E_g is significantly smaller at this temperature than it is at room temperature [0.79 eV from the second expression in Eq. (1.18)]. This solution is shown in Figure 1–26(b). The solution is consistent with all the donors and acceptors being ionized since E_F is well below E_D and well above E_A.

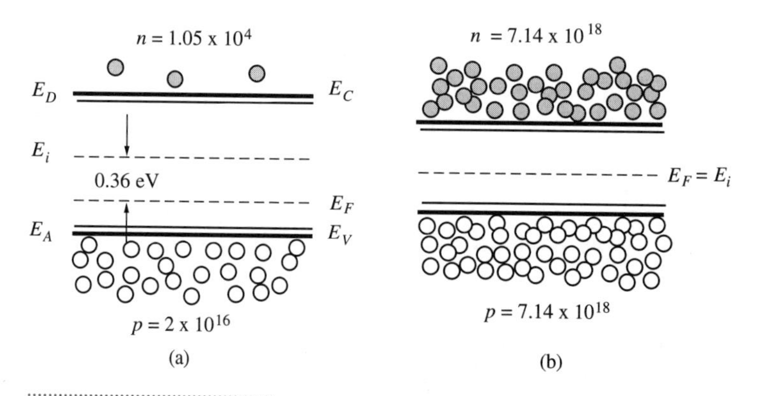

Figure 1–26 Solutions for the example at (a) room temperature, and (b) 1000°C.

The concepts we have been using to describe semiconductors and their band structure are not sufficient to describe many advanced aspects of device performance. For example, in all of our discussion of band diagrams, we have used one-dimensional pictures to represent the material properties. In actual fact, such pictures should be two-dimensional with the vertical axis being electron potential energy (as in our figures) and the horizontal axis being the crystal momentum (k). These more complete representations show that the maximum of the valence band and the minimum of the conduction band in general do not occur at the same value of momentum and are discussed in most device texts [1.11]. This means that in any electron transition from the valence to conduction band we must account for not only the energy change of the electron, but also its momentum change. This becomes important in some aspects of device operation. For example, efficient light emission such as in Light Emitting Diodes (LEDs) is generally only possible in semiconductors in which the conduction band minimum is at the same value of momentum as the valence band maximum. This is referred to as a direct bandgap semiconductor. In this case when an electron falls from the conduction band back to the valence band and recombines there with a hole, the resulting energy can be transferred to a photon (which has essentially no momentum). This occurs in many compound semiconductors such as GaAs.

In silicon, the same recombination process generally occurs through an intermediate energy level in the bandgap (such as a gold atom) which captures the electron and hole necessary for recombination and transfers the excess momentum to a phonon (lattice vibration). This sequence of events conserves both energy and momentum and is referred to as Shockley, Read, Hall or SRH recombination after the scientists who first developed a theoretical description of it.

We will need to understand the indirect recombination process through SRH traps a little more carefully in order to understand the role that impurities like Au, Cu, Fe, and other heavy metals play in silicon technology. These elements act as catalysts for recombination or "traps" in silicon. Consider the deep energy level in Figure 1–27 and assume that it represents an allowed energy level in the semiconductor bandgap. Elements like Au, Cu, and Fe introduce such levels in silicon as do lattice defects like vacancies and interstitials which we will discuss in more detail in Chapter 3. In indirect bandgap materials like silicon, the direct recombination of an electron and a hole is not a very probable process because of the need to conserve momentum. What is much more likely, and what generally occurs in silicon, is recombination through an intermediate trap level. The trap level first captures either a hole or an electron and then captures the other carrier, completing the recombination event. The excess momentum is given to the crystal through the trapping atom which generally sits on a lattice site.

These steps are illustrated in Figure 1–27 for the specific case of an N-type semiconductor. In N-type material, there are many electrons present, so the likelihood of one of them encountering the trap is much higher than for holes, which are few in number. The typical condition for the trap is therefore to have captured an electron and be waiting for a hole to come into close enough proximity to be captured. It is thus the minority carrier capture process that limits the overall recombination rate and we usually speak of the minority carrier lifetime as representing the time required for recombination to occur. This bulk lifetime to first order is given by

$$\tau_R = \frac{1}{\sigma\, v_{th} N_t} \tag{1.19}$$

where τ_R is the recombination lifetime, σ is the capture cross section of the trap (on the order of the atom cross sectional area or about 10^{-16} cm^2), v_{th} is the minority carrier thermal velocity (about 10^7 cm sec^{-1}), and N_t is the density of traps per cm^3. We will use

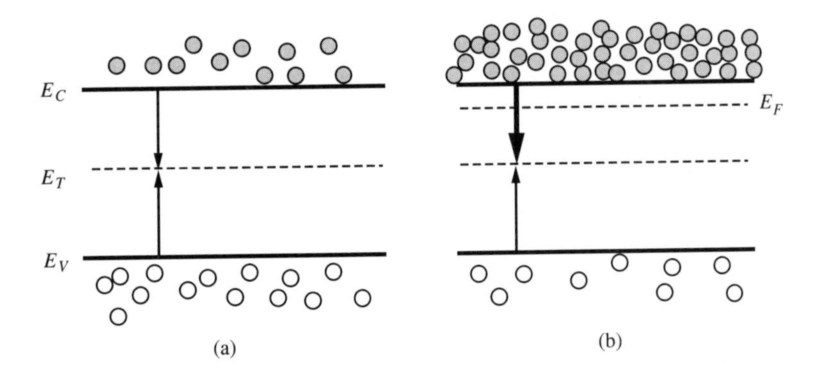

Figure 1–27 Shockley-Read-Hall recombination process. In (a) the trap level captures each carrier separately to accomplish recombination. In (b), the case of an N-type semiconductor is illustrated. The relative sizes of the arrows represent the easy capture of the majority carrier (electron) and the more difficult capture of the minority carrier (hole).

this equation in Chapter 4 to estimate the allowable contamination levels in silicon crystals (Section 4.2).

The band diagram on the right of Figure 1–27 illustrates another way of visualizing the recombination process. In N-type material, E_F will be in the upper half of the bandgap, above the trap level. Energy levels below E_F are normally occupied by electrons since the probability of finding an electron at a level below E_F is close to one. Thus we again conclude that the trap level will normally be occupied by an electron and the hole (minority carrier) capture will be the rate-limiting step. A similar argument in P-type material would show that the capture of the minority carrier electron is the rate-limiting step. This process of recombination is important in many types of devices, but especially in devices that depend on the behavior of minority carriers. Bipolar transistors are one example.

The inverse process—generation—through SRH traps is also possible and is often the dominant carrier generation process in indirect bandgap semiconductors like silicon. In this process, the trap level first generates an electron or hole and then generates the other species. These events can then be repeated to supply carriers to the semiconductor when they are needed. In this case, the material is characterized by a generation rather than a recombination lifetime. Depletion regions are a very common example in which such generation takes place. In general, the two lifetimes τ_R (recombination) and τ_G (generation) are not the same since the processes involved in each are somewhat different (capture of a free carrier versus emission of a carrier from a trap). In silicon τ_G is normally longer than τ_R. Eq. (1.19) provides a simple estimate of carrier lifetime and we will often not have to distinguish between τ_G and τ_R in this text.

SRH theory gives the rate of recombination (or generation) as

$$U = \frac{np - n_i^2}{\tau\left(p + n + 2n_i \cosh\left(\frac{E_T - E_i}{kT}\right)\right)} \tag{1.20}$$

where τ is the carrier lifetime. In equilibrium $np = n_i^2$ and U goes to zero. In this case, recombination and generation exactly balance each other. When excess carriers are present, $np > n_i^2$ and U is positive (net recombination). When $np < n_i^2$, U is negative (net generation). Note that the rate of recombination (or generation) is maximized when the trap level is near the middle of the bandgap.

At the surface of the semiconductor, the crystal structure terminates, usually at a thermally grown SiO_2 layer. Traps at such an interface can also act as SRH centers and can both generate and recombine carriers. The surface equivalent of Eq. (1.19) is

$$s = \sigma_S v_{th} N_{it} \tag{1.21}$$

where σ_s is the capture cross section of the surface trap (cm^2) and N_{it} is the density of traps per cm^2 at the surface. s has units of cm sec^{-1} and is called the surface recombination velocity. s is thus related to the rate at which carriers recombine at the surface. $1/\tau$ is the equivalent bulk recombination rate. When surface effects dominate, an analogous expression to Eq. (1.20) gives the net rate of recombination or generation.

$$U = \frac{s(np - n_i^2)}{p + n + 2n_i \cosh\left(\frac{E_T - E_i}{kT}\right)} \tag{1.22}$$

A final point is important to make. In direct bandgap materials like GaAs in which carriers can recombine without an intermediate trap level, minority carrier lifetimes are generally very short (on the order of nsec). In addition, these lifetimes are fundamental properties of the material and are not generally available to the process or device designer as design variables. In indirect bandgap materials like Si, the minority carrier lifetime is inversely proportional to the density of trapping centers. There is thus the possibility of designing a particular lifetime by controlling the concentration of these traps. In silicon technology, this generally means controlling the concentrations of impurities like Au, Cu, and Fe. Lattice defects created by ion implantation or electron beam radiation can also act as SRH centers. In many cases, it is simply important to minimize SRH centers, that is, to maximize the carrier lifetime. In other cases, it may be desirable to reduce the lifetime by the careful introduction of controlled concentrations of deep level traps.

1.4 Semiconductor Devices

This is, of course, a book on semiconductor technology and not semiconductor devices. However, a first-order understanding of how the basic devices used in ICs operate is useful, because it provides some understanding of the objectives we have for the technology. In this section we review the basic operation of PN junctions and MOS and bipolar transistors. Many excellent texts on these topics exist and the interested reader is referred to them for a more detailed description [1.11].

1.4.1 PN Diodes

The simplest semiconductor device is the PN junction, illustrated in Figure 1–28. Conceptually, simply bringing two pieces of semiconductor material, one N-type and the other P-type, into contact forms the device. In practice, such junctions are formed by starting with a wafer of one type and then doping the surface layer the opposite type. This results in a doping profile as shown on the right side of Figure 1–28.

With no applied bias, a PN junction will form a depletion region or a region in which there are no mobile carriers across the junction. It is easy to see why this happens by considering the fact that across the junction there are very high gradients of holes and electrons. If the doping on the N side is 10^{15} cm^{-3}, then the N side contains 10^{15} cm^{-3} electrons and 10^5 cm^{-3} holes. The P side contains carrier concentrations approximately the opposite of these. Across the junction then, an enormous gradient in each carrier type exists. If something did not happen, these enormous gradients would result in large currents flowing across the junction because the carriers would diffuse down the gradients. However, something does happen.

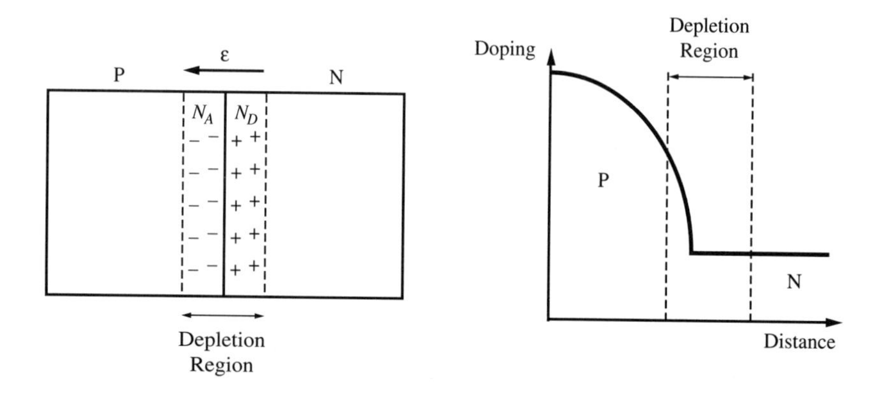

Figure 1–28 Schematic representation of a PN diode on the left. Typical doping profile on the right.

The free carriers in the vicinity of the junction do initially flow to the opposite side. This creates the depletion region and sets up an electric field. This field arises simply because once the free carriers move away, they leave behind the charged donor and acceptor ions N_D^+ and N_A^- bonded in substitutional sites in the silicon lattice. The dopant ions and the free carriers normally balance each other, resulting in a charge neutral material. Without the carriers, the field must exist as illustrated in Figure 1–28.

In the PN junction in equilibrium, drift and diffusion exactly balance, so that no net current flows. This actually results in rather large fields in the depletion region in order to "hold back" the large carrier gradients. Typical fields are on the order of a few volts per micron.

If we apply a positive voltage to the N side of the junction, the electric field across the junction will increase. This polarity adds to the built-in field that is already there. This added field creates additional positive charge on the N side and negative charge on the P side, widening the depletion region in Figure 1–28. We should not expect much current to flow under this bias condition since the internal field by itself is enough to stop carrier diffusion and we have simply made this field larger with this polarity of applied voltage. In fact, only very small leakage currents flow in a PN junction under such reverse bias.

If we now consider making the P side positive, exactly the opposite happens. The applied field partially cancels the built-in field, allowing majority carriers from both sides to diffuse across the junction. Under forward bias in a PN junction, large currents flow since the internal field holding back the diffusion of carriers is removed by this polarity of applied bias. The overall current-voltage relationship for a PN junction is expressed simply as

$$I = I_0\left(\exp\frac{qV}{kT} - 1\right) \tag{1.23}$$

where I_0 is the reverse leakage current. For positive voltages on the P side (forward bias), the current increases exponentially with applied bias. For reverse voltages, the current saturates at I_0 which is very small. Typically currents in the forward direction are on the order of mA; in the reverse direction, they are pA or smaller.

The built-in electric field across the junction produces a built-in voltage across the junction given by

$$\phi_i = \frac{kT}{q}\ln\left(\frac{N_D N_A}{n_i^2}\right) \tag{1.24}$$

For typical doping levels in silicon diodes this built-in voltage is about 0.7 eV, so an external forward bias on the order of 0.7 volts will therefore essentially eliminate this barrier, allowing large currents to flow. This is often referred to as the "turn-on" voltage of a silicon diode, although it is clear from Eq. (1.23) that there is no specific voltage at which the current turns on.

It is also easy to see physically why the *I-V* relationship should be exponential. Recall from Eq. (1.6) that the population of electrons falls off exponentially above the conduction band minimum. As forward bias is applied to the diode and the band bending is decreased, an exponentially increasing number of electrons are able to surmount the barrier and therefore I increases exponentially with voltage. The PN diode then really acts like a two-terminal switch. It is turned on (conducts) under forward bias and is turned off (blocks) under reverse bias.

One final property of PN diodes will be useful to us in later discussions. The depletion region associated with the diode may be thought of as a parallel plate capacitor. The insulating dielectric in the capacitor is of course the depleted silicon; the plates of the capacitor are formed by the conducting charge-neutral P and N regions adjacent to the depletion region. The capacitance of such a structure is given simply by

$$\frac{C}{A} = \frac{\epsilon_S}{x_d} = \left[\sqrt{\frac{q\epsilon_S}{2}\left(\frac{N_A N_D}{N_A + N_D}\right)\frac{1}{(\phi_i \pm V)}}\right] \tag{1.25}$$

Here ϵ_s is the permittivity of silicon and x_d is the width of the depletion region. ϕ_i and the applied voltage V add under reverse bias and subtract under forward bias. The capacitance decreases as reverse bias is applied to the junction because the depletion layer widens; it increases under forward bias as the width decreases. Eq. (1.25) is valid for a junction with uniform doping on the two sides of the junction and only as long as the forward current in the junction is small. Quite often junctions in semiconductor devices are asymmetrically doped (as in Figure 1–28). In this case only the doping on the more lightly doped side matters. Real diodes may also have both N_D and N_A as functions of position. In this case all of the above equations become more complex and generally computer techniques must be used to calculate ϕ_i, $C(V)$, and $I(V)$. Even in these more complex cases, however, the simple equations above usually provide good estimates.

1.4.2 MOS Transistors

All practical circuits today require three terminal switching devices as shown schematically on the left side of Figure 1–29. Circuits are much easier to design if the control terminal is electrically isolated from the output. In digital circuits, the simplest representation of the switching element is simply a switch which is closed and opened by an isolated control terminal. The two states, closed and open, represent digital 0 and 1 states. In analog circuits generally an input signal needs to be amplified. Again in simplified form, this is accomplished by a controlled current source whose current is proportional to an applied input or control signal.

There are two dominant types of such devices used in silicon ICs today, the MOS transistor and the bipolar junction or BJT device. Both of them operate to first order like the simple equivalent circuits in Figure 1–29. Historically, as we saw in Section 1.2, the MOS device was invented first, although it was not used in large-scale production until much later than the BJT because of problems in controlling its properties and in producing stable devices. The basic MOS device is shown in Figure 1–30, in this case an NMOS or N-type device. The device is a three-terminal structure with an input (source), output (drain), and a control terminal (gate).

The N^+ regions at the source and drain of the device provide a means of contacting the region under the gate, which is the active part of the device. The N^+ regions also provide a source of electrons in normal device operation, as we will see. Consider the central part of the device, under the gate electrode. The structure here is metal on top of an insulator (generally SiO_2) on top of silicon and thus provides the name for the device (MOS or Metal Oxide Semiconductor). The silicon is P-type and hence there are very few electrons normally present. Both PN junctions in the device are normally at zero bias or reversed biased, which means that very little current flows across these junctions. Thus with a negative or zero voltage on the gate, there is no connection between the input and output N^+ diffusions and the device operates as an open circuit. This condition is illustrated on the left of Figure 1–30. With negative bias on the gate, majority carrier holes are attracted to the surface, which makes the surface more strongly P-type. With two zero-biased or reverse-biased junctions in series, no current flows.

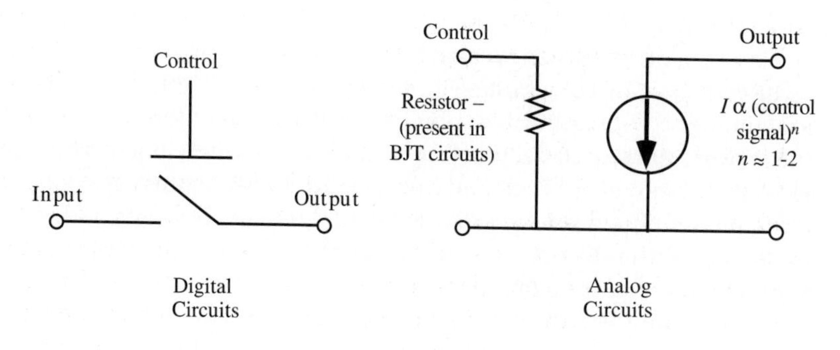

Figure 1–29 Simplified models for a three-terminal device used in digital and analog applications.

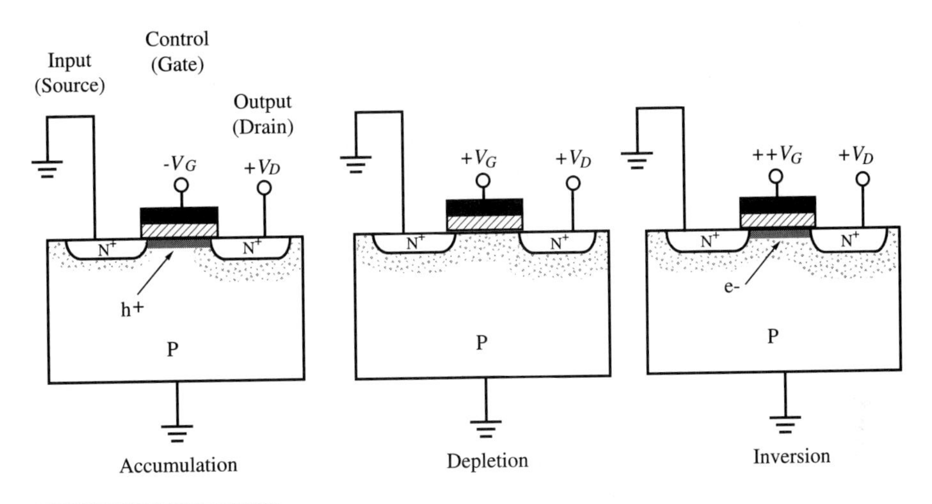

Figure 1–30 Simplified cross section of an MOS transistor biased in its OFF (accumulation), intermediate (depletion), and ON (inversion) states. The dotted areas are the depletion regions.

If we now apply a positive voltage to the gate electrode, the vertical electric field produced across the insulating gate oxide will attract electrons to the silicon surface and repel positively charged holes. Initially, this creates a depletion region in the central part of the device as shown in the middle of Figure 1–30. If a sufficiently positive voltage is applied to the gate, the electrons can actually become the dominant carrier in a narrow layer at the surface, effectively making the surface N-type as shown on the right of Figure 1–30. This process is called surface inversion and results in an inversion layer of electrons about 5 nm thick at the silicon surface. With this inversion layer present, the input and output N^+ diffusions are now effectively connected, resulting in a closed switch. The gate electrode thus allows the device to be turned on ($+V_G$) or turned off ($-$ or zero V_G). When the MOS transistor is turned on, the number of electrons in the inversion layer is proportional to the gate voltage. Thus the resistance of the inversion layer depends on the gate voltage and therefore the current that flows in the device depends on the gate voltage. The result is an equivalent circuit like that shown on the right of Figure 1–29, which allows the device to be used in analog as well as digital applications.

The process of turning the MOS device on or off would actually be very slow if it were not for the presence of the N^+ regions. Because the substrate is P-type, there are very few electrons present there and the only way for the substrate to provide the electrons needed for the inversion layer would be by actually generating them through breaking Si-Si bonds or through the Shockley-Read-Hall generation process described earlier. The only way for the substrate to get rid of the electrons in the inversion layer when the device is turned off is by electron hole recombination. These processes would limit the turn on and turn off times to msec or seconds, depending on the rates of generation and recombination and would certainly not allow the nsec or psec switching times that are common in today's ICs. The solution to this problem resides in the N^+

regions. These regions are rich in electrons and can provide a source or a sink for these carriers in the times required in modern circuits (psec). The inversion layer electrons thus flow out of the source and drain when the device is switched on, and back into these regions when it is switched off.

The depletion regions indicated in Figure 1–30 (the shaded areas) are the regions of the substrate in which there are essentially no mobile carriers. Beneath the gate, the holes in the P-type substrate are driven away by positive gate voltages. In the regions around the source and drain, the electric fields, due to reverse bias on the junctions or due to the built-in junction fields which are present even with zero applied external bias, also drive the mobile carriers away from the immediate vicinity of the junctions.

To fabricate the MOS transistor, we need techniques to dope the silicon N-type (for the NMOS transistor shown here) or P-type for PMOS devices. We will see that ion implantation followed by solid state diffusion provides this capability. We also need the ability to deposit or grow very thin insulating layers to produce the gate dielectric. Thermal growth or deposition of SiO_2 provide this capability and can also provide an Si/SiO_2 interface, which is almost perfect electrically. By this we mean that there are very few charges, electron or hole traps or other undesirable features of the interface that would degrade the operation of MOS devices. We also need to deposit and define thin films of polysilicon (and other materials) to build the gate electrode and thin metal films to provide a wiring capability on the chip. IC technology provides all these capabilities.

While the field effect mechanism to control semiconductor surfaces and convert them from P- to N-type, or vice versa, was known long before the invention of the IC, practical MOS devices were not manufactured until the mid 1960s. The principal reason for this was simply that attempts to build the devices earlier than this usually resulted in structures whose electrical characteristics were unstable or nonreproducible. Many laboratories investigated these problems during the 1960s and the problem was finally traced to charges (defects) present at the Si/SiO_2 interface and to minute (parts per million) concentrations of alkali ions in the MOS gate dielectrics. Charges at the Si/SiO_2 interface are sensitive to fabrication conditions and were gradually brought under control and minimized by better fabrication methods. Ions like Na^+ and K^+ are normally charged and mobile in SiO_2 even at room temperature and can drift around in the gate dielectric as the gate voltage is switched under normal device operating conditions. Charges moving inside the gate dielectric act exactly like a changing gate voltage because they change the vertical electric field in the active part of the MOS device. The result is an MOS device whose *I-V* characteristics change as the alkali ions drift around.

Many readers may have already drawn the conclusion that since the human body has large concentrations of Na^+ and K^+, the origin of the contamination problem may well have been handling of the IC wafers during device manufacturing. This is in fact correct, although other sources (chemicals and manufacturing equipment) were also identified. Strict attention to cleanliness in handling and processing the wafers largely solved the MOS stability problem by the end of the 1960s and made possible their large-scale manufacturing. Today's IC plants employ clean rooms with highly controlled environments to prevent a recurrence of these MOS stability problems, but even today, occasional MOS device instabilities arise because of improperly trained technicians or a batch of contaminated chemicals. We will discuss these issues in more detail in Chapter 4.

Charges present in the insulator layer, or at the Si/SiO_2 interface, affect the underlying semiconductor surface properties simply because these charges provide termination points for the electric field lines originating on the gate in MOS devices. If no such charges are present, then applying a voltage on the gate means that the electric field lines must penetrate through the insulator and into the underlying semiconductor where they can then terminate on mobile carriers or on ionized impurity atoms (n, p, N_D^+, and N_A^-). Thus depletion, inversion, and accumulation are possible. If large numbers of charges are present in the insulator or at the insulator/semiconductor interface, the field lines can terminate before they reach the underlying semiconductor and thus the field effect mechanism does not operate. Nature has provided us with only one superb insulator/semiconductor structure that we know of today, in which these charges are practically zero, the Si/SiO_2 interface. This is one of the main reasons why silicon is the material of choice for today's ICs.

1.4.3 Bipolar Junction Transistors

The other principal type of semiconductor device used in modern integrated circuits is the bipolar transistor, shown in Figure 1–31. In this device, the PN junctions play a more active role in the operation. There are three terminals just as there were in the case of the MOS device. The emitter forms the input, the collector is the output and the base is the control terminal. The simplest equivalent circuits for the device are similar to the MOS transistor (Figure 1–29).

In operation, the emitter is grounded, a small positive voltage is applied to the base, and a larger positive voltage is applied to the collector. The built-in electric field across the base-emitter junction is reduced, allowing the majority carriers on each side to diffuse across the junction. Electrons from the emitter flow into the base and holes from

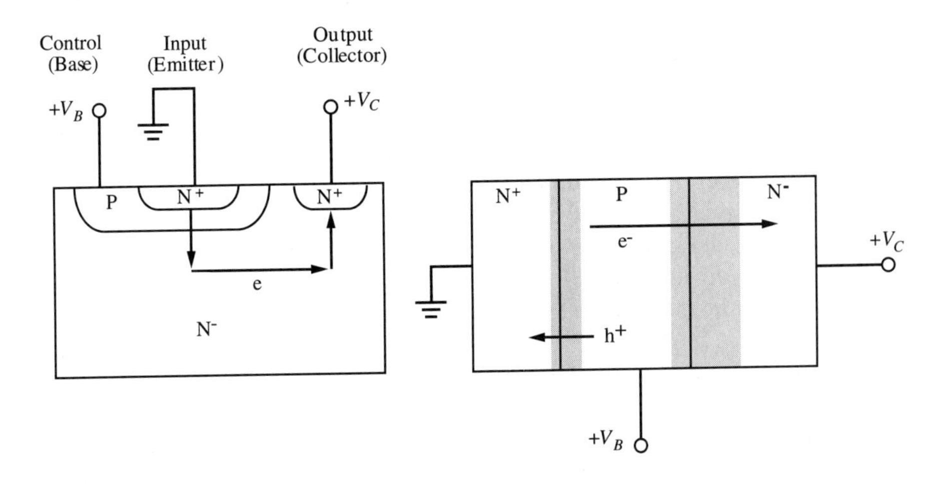

Figure 1–31 Simplified cross section (left) and 1D representation (right) of a bipolar transistor. The shaded areas are the depletion regions. The arrows indicate the path of carrier flow through the device.

the base flow into the emitter. In a well-designed BJT, the emitter doping is several orders of magnitude higher than the base doping, so that the electron population is much higher in the emitter than is the hole population in the base. As a result, when the electric field across the junction is reduced by applying an external V_{BE}, more electrons flow from the emitter into the base than do holes from the base into the emitter. (In other words, the injection of carriers across the junction is asymmetric because the doping is asymmetric.)

If there were no second PN junction present, then the structure would simply be the PN diode we discussed in Figure 1–28. In this case, the injected electrons and holes would diffuse away from the junction on both sides. Since they are minority carriers once they are injected across the junction (the electrons are injected into P-type material and the holes into N-type material), the injected carriers will tend to recombine with the majority carriers in each region. Each time such a recombination event takes place, a majority carrier must be supplied by the contacts to the P and N regions and hence a current flows into the device. From an external circuit point of view, then, we measure a current flowing into the device which is exactly equal to the current (electrons and holes) being injected across the junction. If the carriers injected across the junction do not fully recombine before they reach the ends of the structure, then they quickly recombine at the metal contacts where the rate of recombination is much higher than inside the device. Externally, it makes little difference where the recombination occurs. We simply measure a current going into the device.

The key additional idea that is needed to make the bipolar transistor is the second junction—the base collector junction. This junction is normally reverse biased so that it does not inject carriers itself. However, if carriers from the base emitter junction, particularly electrons from the emitter, diffuse to the collector junction, they will be swept across it by the electric field and "collected" by the collector. In fact, if the base is made narrow enough, virtually all of the electrons injected by the emitter will successfully diffuse through the base without recombining and be collected by the collector. From an external point of view then, we see a large number of electrons flowing in the emitter contact and collect almost all of them at the collector contact. This is the main current path through the device. A small current must be supplied at the control terminal (base) to account for holes that are injected from the base into the emitter and to provide holes for the few recombination events that take place in the base as the electrons flow through there on their way to the collector. The main current path from emitter to collector can easily and quickly be turned on and off by applying or removing V_{BE}. Conceptually, then, the device looks like a switch, which can be turned on and off, just like the MOS device, although the internal physics are quite different in the two cases. Since there is a nonzero input current from the control terminal in the BJT, a better equivalent circuit (Figure 1–29) would include a resistor to allow this current to flow.

Since most of the current in a BJT flows below the silicon surface, the device is much less sensitive to passivation problems than is the MOS transistor. For this reason, the BJT was used in the earliest ICs in the 1960s while researchers were trying to understand the stability problems of the Si/SiO_2 interface. Once these issues were resolved and stable manufacturing of MOS devices became routine, MOS devices became the switching devices of choice in most IC applications. Bipolar devices still find some uses in ICs today, but more than 90% of the ICs manufactured today rely on the MOS transistor for the basic switching element.

The fabrication of the bipolar device requires essentially the same technologies as in the MOS case. We need methods to locally dope the semiconductor N- and P-type. We need to be able to deposit or grow insulating layers and to deposit and define thin film layers on the semiconductor surface. All of these capabilities are provided in modern IC fabrication processes.

1.5 Semiconductor Technology Families

Active components are of course combined in circuits to implement complete systems on an IC chip. In digital systems, the basic circuit is an inverter, which simply converts a digital 0 to a 1, or vice versa. The implementation of this basic circuit has gone through a number of changes over the past 40 years as IC technology has changed.

In the 1960s, MOS transistors were not manufacturable, for the reasons briefly discussed earlier. As a result, the BJT was used as the basic switching device. Figure 1–32 illustrates the basic technology common in that decade. The NPN structure of the bipolar device is on the left side. The right side shows one implementation of a resistor, which was also needed to construct logic circuits. The basic technology used N^- layers grown epitaxially on P-type substrates. Deep P^+ diffusions were used to provide reverse biased PN junctions which laterally isolated between devices. Six to eight photolithography steps were commonly used. Figure 1–1 (left) illustrates an early example of such an IC.

By the 1970s, MOS technology became manufacturable because the contamination problems described earlier were brought under control. The technology typical of that decade is shown in Figure 1–33. N-type or NMOS devices were generally used because in silicon the electron mobility is about three times higher than the hole mobility,

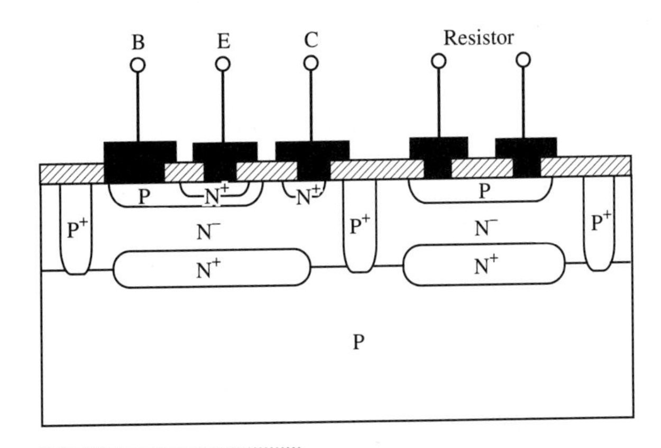

Figure 1–32 Technology typical of the 1960s. Bipolar transistors and resistors were the dominant components.

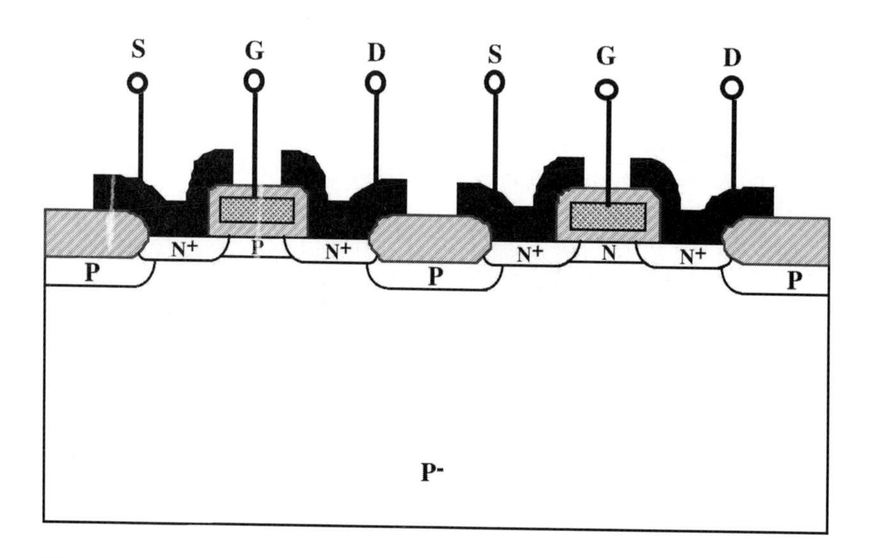

Figure 1–33 Technology typical of the 1970s. Enhancement mode and depletion mode NMOS transistors were the dominant components.

resulting in a 3X advantage in current capability for NMOS versus PMOS devices. The most common technology was Enhancement/Depletion or E/D illustrated in the figure. The device on the left has a P-type channel which requires positive gate voltage to invert or turn on. This is the enhancement device. The device on the right has an N-type channel and a negative threshold voltage. This is the depletion mode device. Although it may not be obvious, a depletion transistor can actually be implemented in a significantly smaller area than a resistor, resulting in denser circuits. NMOS E/D technology was built with about the same number of masks as the 1960s bipolar process.

The 1980s brought a further change in the basic technology. Complementary MOS or CMOS, illustrated in Figure 1–34, became the dominant technology. The basic change was to replace the depletion mode NMOS device in Figure 1–33, with a PMOS transistor. The basic CMOS inverter circuit is also shown in Figure 1–34. This circuit has a major advantage over earlier implementations. For positive input voltages, the NMOS transistor is turned on, pulling the output low. However, the PMOS device is turned off by positive inputs since its threshold voltage is negative. Thus no current flows through the NMOS/PMOS stack. If the input is zero, the PMOS turns on, pulling the output high, but the NMOS is off, so again no current flows in the inverter. Thus the CMOS inverter consumes no current in either state (no DC power). Only when the inverter is actually switching does a transient current flow. Other types of CMOS circuits have the same property. In large chips, with millions of components, this is a significant advantage in terms of overall power consumption and cooling requirements. CMOS technology increased the mask count to about 12–14 masks, depending on the particular technology.

The early 1990s brought a further change with the introduction of BICMOS technology. The structure basically combines bipolar and CMOS devices on the same chip.

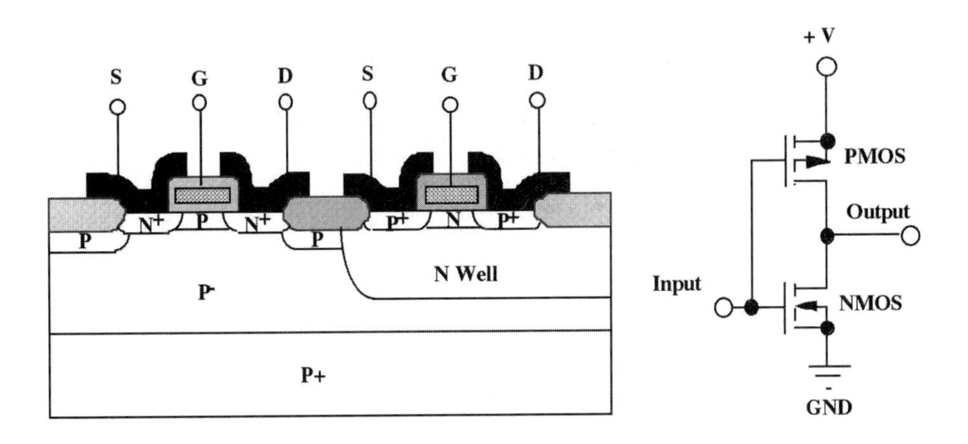

Figure 1–34 Technology typical of the 1980s. CMOS circuits with both NMOS and PMOS devices were dominant.

The penalty for doing this is, of course, additional masks. A BICMOS process typically requires more than 20 masking levels. This technology was used to implement many circuits in the early 1990s. Often much of the internal circuitry on a chip was implemented in CMOS, since this is a denser way to implement functions, with the output devices using bipolar drivers.

Today, technology is driven by the need for high performance, but also by the need for low power. Portable systems obviously need low power, but even in desktop systems, increasing integration levels have made chip and system cooling issues important. The simplest solution to these problems is to simply scale down the operating supply voltage of ICs, since power consumption generally reduces as the square of the supply voltage. These trends are apparent in the NTRS described earlier in this chapter. These trends also put a premium on circuit technologies, which work well at reduced supply voltages. CMOS technology excels at this and for this and other reasons, most workers today believe that it will be the dominant technology well into the next century. This is, in fact, what the NTRS assumes in its projections for the future. We will consider CMOS technology in detail in Chapter 2.

1.6 Modern Scientific Discovery—Experiments, Theory, and Computer Simulation

The history of scientific discovery has until quite recently usually been characterized by laboratory experiments followed by the development of physical models or theory. The invention of the integrated circuit described briefly in Section 1.2, is a good example. The basic contributions of Kilby, Noyce, Hoerni, and many others were largely based on experiments done in laboratories, and on insight gained from those experiments. In fact, as we shall see throughout this book, the basic physical mechanisms controlling IC technology are in many cases still not fully understood. This lack of full scientific understanding has obviously not prevented widespread industrial application of the technology, however! The invention of the transistor described by Shockley [1.5] is another classic example of experimental science preceding the development of a complete theoretical understanding. In his historical description of those events in the 1940s and 50s, Shockley wrote of the "creative failure methodology" by which he meant that experiments which produce unexpected or undesired results, often lead scientists down new paths to invention. There certainly are examples in science of theoretical predictions preceding and suggesting experiments. However, the reverse has more often been the case.

With the remarkable developments in computer capability in the past decade (due largely to IC technology) has come an opportunity to do experiments in a new way. In fields of science in which theories based on first principles are known, or in which models have been developed, it is quite common today to program those theories or those models in a computer. To the extent that such models are correct, it is then possible to do "computer experiments" or computer simulations. Chemicals can be mixed in a simulated beaker and the resulting reactions observed on a computer screen. Bridges can be constructed in a computer with stresses placed on them to determine failure points and failure mechanisms.

In the integrated circuit world, these tools have become useful adjuncts to real laboratory experiments in recent years. The basic equations, which describe electron and hole transport in semiconductors due to drift and diffusion, have been incorporated into powerful simulators which can today accurately predict the electrical characteristics of proposed device structures. In a similar way, models describing the steps used in fabricating ICs have also been incorporated into process simulators. It is therefore quite possible today to "build" new semiconductor structures and predict their performance using these computer tools.

The state of the art in such simulators today is that they are very useful, but they cannot completely replace real laboratory experiments. This is simply because the models used in the simulators are not complete in some cases, or are purely empirical in other cases. As the models are improved with additional research, the simulators will become more robust and therefore more generally useful. There is great motivation to do this because real laboratory experiments are very expensive and very time consuming, especially as chip technology continues to advance. In an industry as competitive as the semiconductor industry, the time required to get new products to market is a key indicator of a company's success. To the extent that simulators can decrease this time and the development costs, they can improve competitiveness.

We will make extensive use of process or Technology Computer-Aided Design (TCAD) simulators in this book. This is not only because they are becoming increasingly important as industrial tools, but also because we believe they can greatly enhance the learning process. Our experience with them is that they provide remarkable physical insight and intuition and we will use them throughout the book to illustrate physical principles and to provide accurate illustrations of what real integrated circuit structures look like. These tools also provide the ability to "look inside" structures or devices and to observe physical phenomena in action that often cannot be easily observed in the laboratory.

1.7 The Plan For This Book

Modern silicon integrated circuit processes are built from a number of what are often called unit process steps. Examples include oxidation, ion implantation, and lithography. Complete process flows are combinations of such steps, often with many hundreds of individual steps. Understanding such a complex fabrication sequence begins of course with understanding the individual steps.

There are generally four things that are required (or are at least highly desirable) in order to apply one of the unit process steps to integrated circuit fabrication:

- Reproducible fabrication techniques
- Measurement methods
- Models of the unit process
- Simulation capability

We will use these four criteria in describing the various unit processes throughout this book. We can take oxidation as a simple example to illustrate this approach. Oxidation simply involves placing a silicon wafer in a high temperature ambient (usually O_2 or H_2O). This results in a chemical reaction, which converts the silicon surface to SiO_2. To use such a process in building integrated circuits, we must first be able to accurately and reproducibly grow such layers (i.e., fabricate them). This will involve machines (in this case oxidation furnaces), controllers, and suitable recipes.

Once the SiO_2 layer is grown, we will need to measure its thickness and perhaps other properties like its dielectric constant or index of refraction. We need to be certain that the recipe worked and that the properties of the film are close to the desired values. Measuring generally involves instruments which are used after the process step is complete (ellipsometers or spectrophotometers in this case, which can measure the SiO_2 thickness).

The third requirement for a unit process to be incorporated into an overall IC manufacturing environment is that we understand it and be able to model it. We need to be able to predict the results of a given process sequence. In the case of oxidation, we need to know how the oxide properties (thickness, index of refraction, and perhaps defect density), depend on the process control parameters (time, temperature, etc.). There are many reasons why we need such a model. Clearly it is needed in designing new process conditions. If we desire a 1 μm oxide in a particular structure, we should be able to calculate a set of parameters that will give that thickness. We also often need to be able to estimate process sensitivities through our models. For example, we might like to know how sensitive our oxide thickness is to small changes in the furnace temperature. Such information would provide some indication of how robust our manufacturing process is. Finally, the existence of a model, particularly a physically based as opposed to an empirically based model, implies that we really do understand the unit process step. Such understanding is often crucial in solving problems that arise during manufacturing.

The last requirement is an ability to simulate the unit process. This is a fairly recent addition to the list and in fact is not always satisfied in silicon technology. However, if we have a model and we have incorporated that model in a computer simulation program, then we will have the ability to accurately and rapidly answer the kinds of questions posed in the preceding paragraph. Such simulators exist today for many, but not all, unit process steps and we will describe and use them throughout this book.

Many texts on silicon technology begin with a thorough discussion of each of the unit process steps. Only after this is done is the integration of these steps into an overall manufacturing sequence considered. Our experience is that considering the integration first has a significant advantage. That advantage is that the context for each of the unit processes is established first. The disadvantage, of course, is that a reader unfamiliar with silicon technology may not fully appreciate a description of a complete process flow before the individual steps have been discussed in detail. We devote Chapter 2 to such a process flow (a CMOS process) and recommend that it be read before the other chapters. Readers relatively new to silicon technology will likely not completely understand all the details of the CMOS process at first. A second reading of Chapter 2 after the others have been covered may provide additional insight.

1.8 Summary of Key Ideas

Integrated circuits are widely regarded as one of the key components of today's world. They are pervasive in their application. Modern CAD tools have enabled a wide variety of people from many different disciplines to design and use ICs in many different kinds of applications. Approximately every two years the complexity of ICs doubles; that is, the technology used to make them allows twice as many components to be integrated on a single chip, as was possible two years earlier. In addition, the performance of the chips improves every year through scaling down of device sizes. These trends are likely to continue through at least the first decade of the 21st century. Innovations and inventions are likely to continue to occur beyond that time, with the result that the complexity and performance of chips will continue to improve. Ultimately, the ability to turn ideas into useful products depends on the ability to actually build these chips. We will explore the technology that has enabled us to do this in detail in the remainder of this book.

1.9 References

[1.1]. Gordon Moore was one of the founders of Intel and first pointed out this "law" around 1970.

[1.2]. "National Technology Roadmap for Semiconductors," SIA, 1994.

[1.3]. "National Technology Roadmap for Semiconductors," SIA, 1997.

[1.4]. D. M. Eigler and E. K. Schweizer, "Positioning Single Atoms with a Scanning Tunneling Microscope," *Nature*, vol. 344, p. 524, 1990.

[1.5]. G. E. Moore, "Are We Really Ready for VLSI?" Keynote Address, 1979 ISSCC.

[1.6]. W. Shockley, "The Path to the Conception of the Junction Transistor," *IEEE Trans. Elec. Dev.*, vol. ED – 31, p. 1523, 1984.

[1.7]. J. S. Kilby, "Invention of the Integrated Circuit," *IEEE Trans. Elec. Dev.*, vol. ED – 23, p. 648, 1976.

[1.8]. E. H. Putley and W. H. Mitchell, "The Electrical Conductivity and Hall Effect of Silicon," *Proc. Phys. Soc.*, vol. 72, p. 193, 1958.

[1.9]. C. D. Thurmond, "The Standard Thermodynamic Function for the Formation of Electrons and Holes in Ge, Si, GaAs and GaP," *J. Electrochem. Soc.*, vol. 122, p. 1133, 1975.

[1.10]. W. E. Beadle, J. C. Tsai and R. D. Plummer, *Quick Reference Manual for Silicon Integrated Circuit Technology*, John Wiley & Sons, 1985.

[1.11]. See, for example, B. G. Streetman, *Solid State Electronic Devices*, Prentice Hall 1995, or R. F. Pierret, *Semiconductor Device Fundamentals*, Addison-Wesley, 1996.

1.10 Problems

1.1. Plot the NRTS roadmap data from Table 1–1 (feature size versus time) on an expanded scale version of Figure 1–2. Do all the points lie exactly on a straight line? If not, what reasons can you suggest for any deviations you observe?

1.2. Assuming dopant atoms are uniformly distributed in a silicon crystal, how far apart are these atoms when the doping concentration is (a) 10^{15} cm^{-3}, (b) 10^{18} cm^{-3}, (c) 5×10^{20} cm^{-3}?

1.3 Consider a piece of pure silicon 100 μm long with a cross sectional area of 1 μm^2. How much current would flow through this "resistor" at room temperature in response to an applied voltage of 1 volt?

1.4. Estimate the resistivity of pure silicon in Ω cm at (a) room temperature, (b) 77K, and (c) 1000°C. You may neglect the temperature dependence of the carrier mobility in making this estimate.

1.5. a. Show that the minimum conductivity of a semiconductor sample occurs when

$$n = n_i \sqrt{\frac{\mu_p}{\mu_n}}$$

b. What is the expression for the minimum conductivity?

c. Is this value greatly different than the value calculated in problem 1.4 for the intrinsic conductivity?

1.6. When a Au atom sits on a lattice site in a silicon crystal, it can act as either a donor or an acceptor. E_D and E_A levels both exist for the Au and both are close to the middle of the silicon bandgap. If a small concentration of Au is placed in an N-type silicon crystal, will the Au behave as a donor or an acceptor? Explain.

1.7. Show that E_F is approximately in the middle of the bandgap for intrinsic silicon.

1.8. Construct a diagram similar to Figure 1–27b for P-type material. Explain physically, using this diagram, why the capture of the minority carrier electrons in P-type material is the rate-limiting step in recombination.

1.9. A silicon diode has doping concentrations on the N and P sides of $N_D = 1 \times 10^{19}$ cm^{-3} and of $N_A = 1 \times 10^{15}$ cm^{-3}. Calculate the process temperature at which each of the two sides of the diode becomes intrinsic. (Intrinsic is defined as $n_i = N_D$ or N_A.)

1.10. A state-of-the-art NMOS transistor might have a drain junction area of 0.5×0.5 μm. Calculate the junction capacitance associated with this junction at an applied reverse bias of 2 volts. Assume the drain region is very heavily doped and the substrate doping is 1×10^{16} cm^{-3}.

Modern CMOS Technology

2

2.1 Introduction

In most of the remaining chapters in this book, we will discuss the process technologies used in silicon IC manufacturing individually. Individual technologies are clearly most useful when they are combined in a complete process flow sequence to produce chips. It is often the case that unit process steps are designed the way that they are because of the context in which those steps are used. For example, while a dopant may be diffused into a semiconductor to a desired final junction depth using many combinations of times and temperatures, the fact that the junction being formed might be diffused in the middle of a complex process flow may greatly restrict the possible choices of times and temperatures. In other words, the wafer's past history and the future process steps it may see can greatly influence how one chooses to perform a particular unit process step.

For this reason, and because we believe that understanding how complete process flows are put together aids understanding of individual process steps, we will describe in this chapter a complete modern Very Large Scale Integrated (VLSI) circuit process flow. The example we have chosen is typical of today's state of the art. CMOS technology has dominated silicon integrated circuits for the past 15 years and most people in the industry today believe that its dominance will continue for the foreseeable future for the reasons discussed in Chapter 1 (high performance, low power, supply voltage scalability, and circuit flexibility). In fact the SIA industry roadmap (NTRS) that we discussed in Chapter 1 assumes the continuation of CMOS technology through at least 2012.

For readers who are new to silicon technology, some of the ideas introduced in this chapter may not be fully appreciated until after later chapters on individual process steps have been read. However, we recommend that such people read this chapter before proceeding further because doing so will make the later material more understandable. A second reading of this chapter after the remainder of the book has been studied may also prove useful. In many cases, typical process conditions that might be used in a given step are presented in this chapter without full explanation. This is simply because we have not yet discussed the quantitative models and other tools at our disposal to calculate such parameters. As we do so in later chapters, we will revisit the CMOS process flow described here and discuss in more detail the reasons for particular process conditions used in this chapter.

2.2 CMOS Process Flow

Two typical CMOS circuits are shown in Figure 2–1. The simple inverter circuit on the left was described in Chapter 1. The NOR gate on the right illustrates how additional NMOS and PMOS devices can be added to the inverter circuit to realize more complex logic functions. In the NOR circuit, if either input 1 or input 2 or both of them are high, the output will be pulled to ground through one or both of the NMOS devices which will be turned on. Only if both inputs are low will the output be pulled high through the two series PMOS devices that are both turned on under this condition. The circuit thus implements the NOR function. To build these types of circuits, we need a technology that can integrate NMOS and PMOS devices on the same chip. In fact, many CMOS technologies also implement various types of resistors, capacitors, thin film transistors, and perhaps other types of devices as well. We will limit our discussion here to the two basic devices and describe a technology to build them. Extensions of this technology to include other components are reasonably straightforward and we will see some examples of such extensions in later chapters.

The end result of the process flow we will discuss is shown in Figure 2–2. To fabricate a structure like this, we will find that 16 photolithography steps and well over 100 individual process steps are required. The final integrated circuit may contain millions of components like those shown in the figure, each of which must work correctly.

There are two active device types shown in the figure, corresponding to those required to implement the circuits in Figure 2–1. The individual source, drain, and gate regions of the NMOS and PMOS devices are identifiable in the cross section. In addition to the active devices, there are many other parts to the overall structure. Some of this "overhead" is required to electrically isolate the active devices from each other. Other

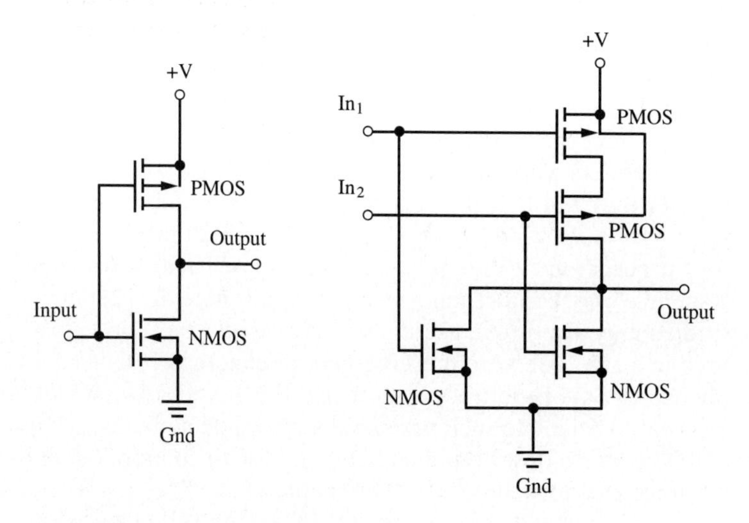

Figure 2–1 Simple CMOS circuits. An inverter is shown on the left and a NOR circuit on the right. The NOR circuit implements the function Output $= \overline{IN_1 + IN_2}$.

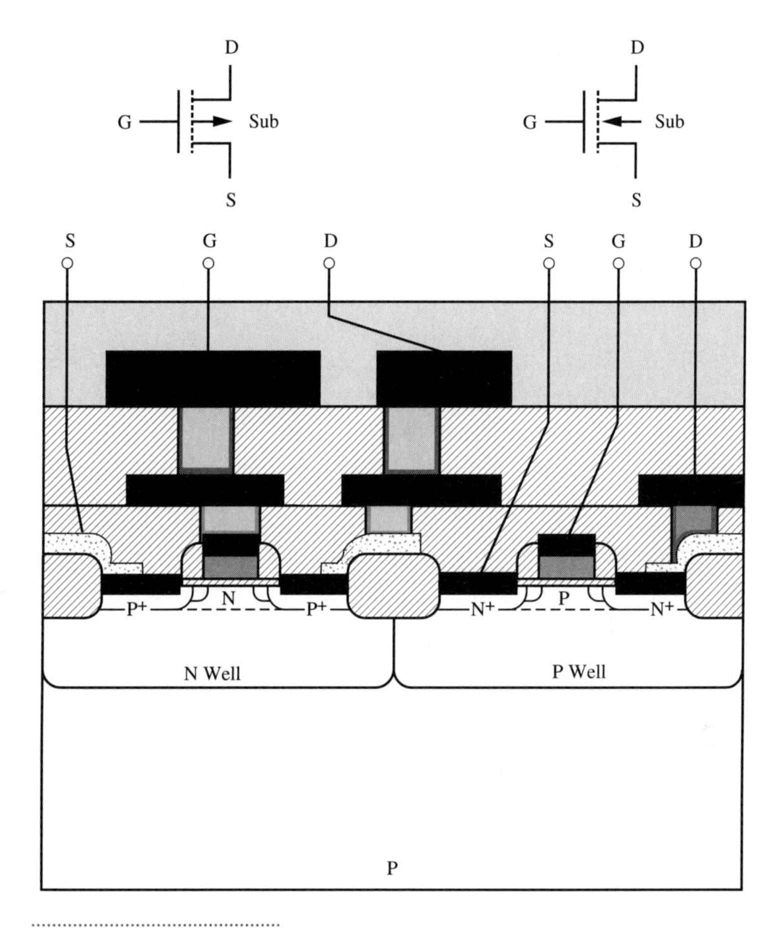

Figure 2–2 Cross section of the final CMOS integrated circuit. A PMOS transistor is shown on the left, an NMOS device on the right.

parts of the structure provide multiple wiring levels above the active devices to interconnect them to perform particular circuit functions. Finally, some regions are included simply to improve the performance of the individual devices by decreasing parasitic resistances or improving voltage ratings. As we proceed through the steps required to build this chip, we will discuss each of these points in greater detail.

2.2.1 The Beginning—Choosing a Substrate

Before we begin actual wafer fabrication, we must of course choose the starting wafers. In general this means specifying type (N or P), resistivity (doping level), crystal orientation, wafer size, and a number of other parameters having to do with wafer flatness, trace impurity levels, and so on. The major choices are the type, resistivity, and orientation.

Figure 2–2 indicates that the final structure has a P-type substrate. In most CMOS integrated circuits, the substrate has a moderately high resistivity (25–50 Ωcm) which corresponds to a doping level on the order of 10^{15} cm^{-3} (Figure 1–18). As is apparent from Figure 2–2, the active devices are actually built in wells diffused into the surface of the wafer. The doping levels in these wells are chosen to optimize the electrical properties of the active devices, as we will see later in this chapter. Typically the well doping levels are on the order of 10^{16} – 10^{17} cm^{-3} near the wafer surface. In order to reproducibly manufacture such wells, the background doping (the substrate doping in this case) needs to be significantly less than the well doping. Thus the substrate doping is normally chosen to be on the order of 10^{15} cm^{-3}.

The observant reader might notice that the NMOS device could actually be built directly in the P substrate without adding the P well near the surface. In fact this is exactly the way the structure was sketched in Figure 1–34 for simplicity. While some CMOS circuits are actually built this way today, the twin well process illustrated in Figure 2–2 is much more common because the doping process used to produce the P well (ion implantation) is much better controlled in manufacturing than is the substrate doping. Also, since the P well and N well doping concentrations are on the same order, it is easier to start with a much more lightly doped substrate and tailor the wells for the NMOS and PMOS devices individually.

The observant reader might also note in Figure 1–34 that a substrate consisting of a P layer on a P^+ substrate was illustrated. This is one of the technology options we will consider later in Section 2.2.5.

The only other major parameter we need to specify in the starting substrate is the crystal orientation. We will discuss crystal structure in more detail in Chapter 3. However, virtually all modern silicon integrated circuits are manufactured today from wafers with a (100) surface orientation. The principal reason for this is that the properties of the Si/SiO_2 interface are significantly better when a (100) crystal is used. We will discuss the reasons for this in detail in Chapter 6, but the key idea is that the electrical properties of this interface are intimately connected with the atomic bonding between Si and O that takes place when an SiO_2 layer is thermally grown on Si. It is found experimentally that there are fewer imperfections (unsatisfied bonds) on a (100) surface than is the case on other silicon surfaces. Primarily for this reason, we will choose a (100) surface orientation for our starting wafers.

We will also discuss in Chapter 4 some processing which is often done on the starting substrates before any actual device fabrication is begun. This processing is aimed at minimizing the sensitivity of the wafers to trace contaminants that can be introduced to the wafers during the many manufacturing steps they go through to build circuits. These preliminary processing steps are called gettering and the most common process today is known as "intrinsic gettering." Since these steps are not essential to the device fabrication process, we will defer discussion of them to Chapter 4.

2.2.2 Active Region Formation

Modern CMOS chips integrate millions of active devices (NMOS and PMOS) side by side in a common silicon substrate. Circuits are designed with these devices to implement complex logic or analog functions. In designing such circuits, it is usually assumed that the individual devices do not interact with each other except through their circuit interconnections. In other words, we need to make certain that the individual devices on the chip are electrically isolated from each other. This is accomplished most often by growing a fairly thick layer of SiO_2 in between each of the active devices. SiO_2 is essentially a perfect insulator and provides the needed isolation. This process of locally oxidizing the silicon substrate is known as the LOCOS process (LOCal Oxidation of Silicon). The regions between these thick SiO_2 layers, where transistors will be built, are called the "active" regions of the substrate.

We begin with the steps shown in Figure 2–3. The wafers are first cleaned in a combination of chemical baths that remove any impurities from the surface. A thermal SiO_2 layer is then grown on the Si surface by placing the wafers in a high-temperature furnace. A typical furnace cycle might be 15 minutes at 900°C in an H_2O atmosphere. Although the H_2O ambient could be produced by boiling water, it is more common today to actually react H_2 and O_2 in the back end of the furnace to produce H_2O. This is generally a cleaner method for generating the steam required for the oxidation. The furnace cycle described above would produce an oxide of about 40 nm (400 Å). Such an oxide could also be grown in a pure O_2 ambient using a cycle of about 45 min at 1000°C. The oxide growth rate is much slower in O_2 compared to H_2O (Chapter 6), so higher temperatures and/or longer times are required in O_2 to grow the same oxide thickness.

The wafers are then transferred to a second furnace, which is used to deposit a thin layer of Si_3N_4 (typically 80 nm). This deposition occurs when reactants like NH_3 and SiH_4 are introduced into the furnace at a temperature of about 800°C, forming Si_3N_4 through a simple chemical reaction such as

$$3SiH_4 + 4NH_3 \rightarrow Si_3N_4 + 12H_2 \tag{2.1}$$

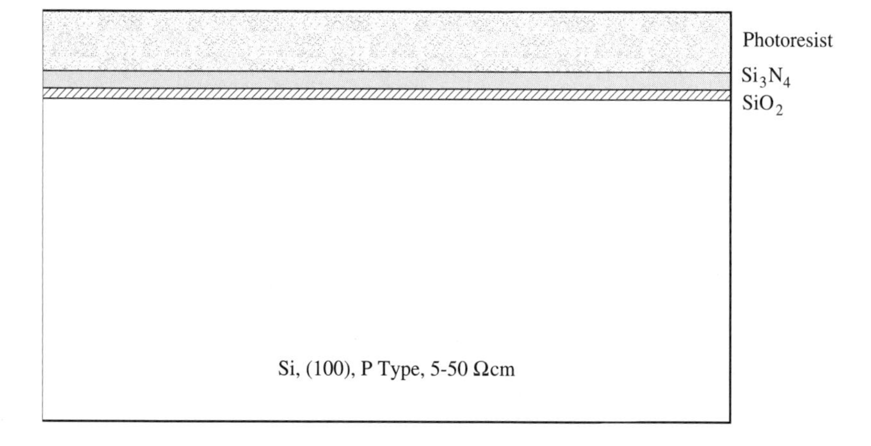

Figure 2–3 Following initial cleaning, an SiO_2 layer is thermally grown on the silicon substrate. A Si_3N_4 layer is then deposited by LPCVD. Photoresist is spun on the wafer to prepare for the first masking operation.

Generally this deposition is done below atmospheric pressure because this produces better uniformity over larger wafer lots in the deposited films. Pumps are normally used on the furnace exhaust to reduce the pressure. Systems in which such depositions are done are usually called Low-Pressure Chemical Vapor Deposition (LPCVD) systems. We will discuss them in more detail in Chapter 9.

The nitride layers deposited by such machines are normally highly stressed, with the Si_3N_4 under tensile stress. This produces a large compressive stress in the underlying Si substrate which can lead to defect generation if it is not carefully controlled. In fact, the major purpose of the SiO_2 layer under the Si_3N_4 is to help relieve this stress. SiO_2 layers are under compressive stress when they are thermally grown on Si and if the thicknesses of the SiO_2 and Si_3N_4 layers are properly chosen, the stresses in the two layers can partially compensate each other, reducing the stresses in the Si substrate. The thicknesses chosen above do this.

The final step in Figure 2–3 is the deposition of a photoresist layer in preparation for masking. Since photoresists are liquids at room temperature, they are normally simply spun onto the wafers. The resist viscosity and the spin speed determine the final resist thickness, which is typically about 1 μm. (Note that the dimensions in all the drawings in this book are not exactly to scale, since the photoresist layer in Figure 2–3 is really more than 10 times the thickness of the oxide or nitride layers, and the substrate is typically 500 times as thick as the photoresist layer. The liberties we take with scale in these drawings are intended to improve clarity.)

After the photoresist is spun onto the wafer, it is usually baked at about 100°C in order to drive off solvents from the layer. The resist is then exposed using a mask, which defines the pattern for the LOCOS regions. The photolithography process is both complex and expensive and was illustrated conceptually in Figure 1–9. We will describe it in much greater detail in Chapter 5. The machines which accomplish the exposure are often called "steppers" because they usually expose only a small area of the wafer during each exposure and then "step" to the next adjacent field to expose. Such machines must be capable today of printing lines on the order of 250 nm (0.25 μm) and placing these patterns on the wafer with an accuracy which is $<$ 100 nm. They typically cost several million dollars.

The photoresists themselves are complex hydrocarbon mixtures. The actual ultra violet (UV) light-sensitive part of the resist is only a portion of the total mixture. In the case of a positive resist, which is the most common type today, the molecule in the resist which is sensitive to light, absorbs UV photons and changes its chemical structure in response to the light. The result is that the molecule and the resist itself then dissolve in the developing solution. Negative resists also respond to UV light but become insoluble in the regions in which they are exposed. Figure 2–4 shows our CMOS wafer after the resist has been exposed and developed.

An additional step is also illustrated in Figure 2–4. After the pattern is defined in the resist, the Si_3N_4 is etched using dry etching, with the resist as a mask. This is usually accomplished in a fluorine plasma. We will discuss dry etching in Chapter 10, but a typical reaction might involve the generation of F atoms in a plasma, using a CF_4 or NF_3 gas source and a reaction of the following type:

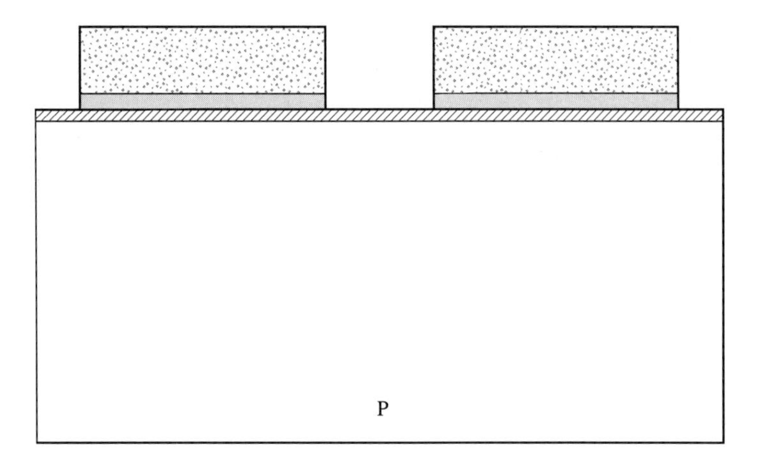

Figure 2–4 Mask 1 patterns the photoresist. The Si_3N_4 layer is removed where it is not protected by the photoresist by dry etching.

$$Si_3N_4 + 12F \rightarrow 3SiF_4 + 2N_2 \tag{2.2}$$

The most common type of etching system uses two parallel plates to confine the gas reactants. An RF voltage (usually 13.56 MHz) is applied across the electrodes to create a plasma and with it many neutral and charged molecules and atoms. It is important that the byproducts of the etching reaction be volatile at the etching temperature (usually room temperature), so that they can easily be pumped out of the reaction chamber.

Once the Si_3N_4 etching is completed, we are through with the resist and it can be chemically removed in sulfuric acid, or stripped in an O_2 plasma, neither of which significantly attacks the underlying Si_3N_4 and SiO_2 layers. Following cleaning, the wafers are then placed into a furnace in an oxidizing ambient. This grows a thick SiO_2 layer locally on the wafer surface. The Si_3N_4 layer on the surface prevents oxidation where it is present because Si_3N_4 is a very dense material and prevents the H_2O or O_2 from diffusing to the Si surface where oxidation takes place. This local oxidation or LOCOS process might be done at 1000°C for 90 min in H_2O to locally grow about 500 nm (0.5 μm) of SiO_2. The structure at this point is illustrated in Figure 2–5.

After the furnace operation, the Si_3N_4 layer can then be stripped. This is conveniently done in hot phosphoric acid, which is highly selective between Si_3N_4 and SiO_2. The Si_3N_4 could also be removed using dry (plasma) etching using a reaction like Eq. (2.2). However a process that gives good selectivity to SiO_2 would be required so that not very much of the LOCOS oxide is etched away during the stripping of the Si_3N_4. Selectivity is often a very important issue in etch steps throughout the wafer fabrication process. We will discuss this issue more carefully in Chapter 10.

An alternative to the SiO_2/Si_3N_4 stack used in Figure 2–3 is to use a three-layer stack of SiO_2, polysilicon, and Si_3N_4 to mask the oxidation process. This process is called the poly-buffered LOCOS process because of the incorporation of the polysilicon layer.

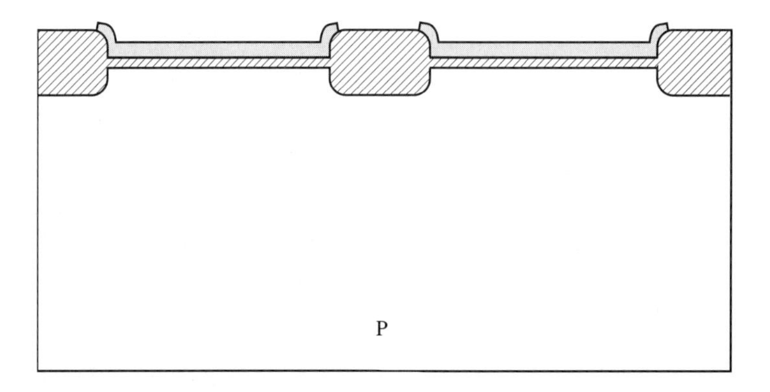

Figure 2–5 After photoresist stripping, the field oxide is grown in an oxidizing ambient.

As was the case in the LOCOS process, the function of the nitride layer is to block the oxidation from occurring wherever the Si_3N_4 is present. The underlying oxide and poly layers are both designed to help with the stress relief problem. Poly-buffered LOCOS uses a thicker Si_3N_4 layer than was the case in the LOCOS process (about 200 nm versus about 80 nm) and a thinner oxide layer (about 20 nm versus about 40 nm). The polysilicon layer permits these changes because it helps to relieve the large stresses, which would otherwise cause defects to form in the silicon substrate during the LOCOS oxidation. The polysilicon is deposited in an LPCVD machine similar to the one described for Si_3N_4 in connection with Eq. (2.1), except that only one reactant gas containing silicon is used (SiH_4 or SiH_2Cl_2, for example). A poly thickness of about 100 nm (0.1 μm) would be typical.

Why would we want to use a thicker nitride layer and a thinner pad oxide in the LOCOS process? The answer lies in a subtlety of LOCOS that we have not discussed to this point. Consider Figure 2–5 for example. The oxidation which takes place during LOCOS extends for some distance under the Si_3N_4 edge. The characteristic shape that this two-dimensional (2D) oxidation process produces is often called a bird's head or a bird's beak. This shape is only shown qualitatively in Figure 2–5; we will study this process in more detail in Chapter 6 and use numerical simulation tools to study the exact shape more carefully. The oxidation extends under the nitride edge because the oxidant (H_2O) can diffuse sideways as well as vertically through the pad oxide layer, to reach the silicon surface where it reacts to grow SiO_2. In fact, the nitride layer will bend up as oxide grows underneath it as Figure 2–5 qualitatively illustrates. This means that the oxide actually grows over a larger surface region than the mask pattern used to define the Si_3N_4. This is a major concern when we are defining very small active devices, because surface area that is lost to this encroachment of the oxide significantly decreases device density.

The answer to the question we posed then is that the combination of a thicker nitride, a thinner pad oxide which provides less of a pathway for lateral oxidant diffusion, and a polysilicon layer which itself can oxidize along its edges during LOCOS produces a much sharper transition between the oxidized and unoxidized regions. This allows for tighter design rules and higher device density.

2.2.3 Process Option for Device Isolation—Shallow Trench Isolation

We digress in our process flow description at this point to consider an alternative method for forming isolation regions between active devices. This alternative—Shallow Trench Isolation or STI—is beginning to be used in manufacturing today and will likely be the method of choice in the future. As we will see, STI actually etches trenches in the silicon substrate between active devices and then refills them with SiO_2. Such a process completely eliminates the bird's beak shape characteristic of LOCOS isolation and thus allows physically smaller isolation regions to be formed.

The process begins the same way as the LOCOS process. SiO_2 and Si_3N_4 layers are thermally grown and deposited respectively, as shown in Figure 2–3. The thicknesses of these layers are approximately the same as in the LOCOS process. However the stress-related issues, which tightly constrained these thicknesses in the LOCOS case, are relaxed somewhat in the STI process because there is no long high-temperature oxidation in STI, during which stresses can generate defects in the silicon substrate. Nevertheless, an SiO_2 thickness of about 10 – 20 nm and an Si_3N_4 thickness of about 50 – 100 nm would be typical. Photoresist is then applied, exposed, and developed as in Figure 2–4.

Figure 2–6 illustrates the next steps. The nitride and oxide layers are etched using the photoresist as a mask. This would typically be done as described above in Eq. (2.2), using a fluorine-based plasma chemistry for both materials. The next step is to etch the trenches in the silicon which are typically on the order of 0.5 μm deep. This can be done again using the photoresist as a mask, or the photoresists can be stripped and the nitride layer can then serve as the mask. The trench etching is a relatively critical step. It is important that the trench walls be relatively vertical so that there is little undercutting into the adjacent active device regions. However, the trench will later be filled with a deposited oxide and this filling process needs to completely fill the trenches without leaving voids. This often means that the trench walls should not be perfectly vertical but rather have a small slope. In addition, the top and bottom corners of the trenches ideally need to be slightly rounded in order to avoid problems later in oxidizing very sharp corners and to avoid electrical effects associated with very sharp corners. Thus the etch

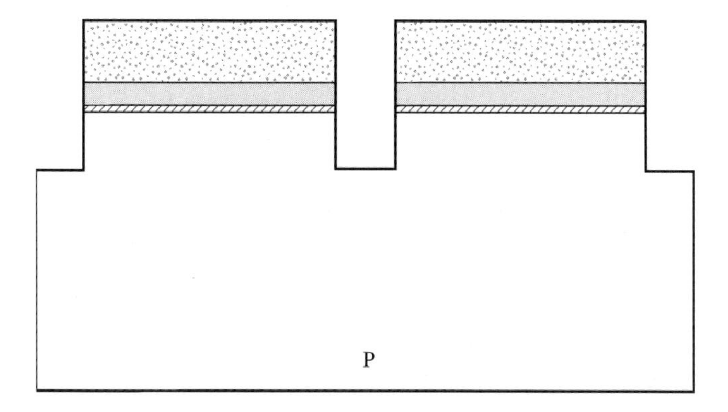

Figure 2–6 After mask 1 defines the photoresist, the Si_3N_4, SiO_2, and Si trenches are successively plasma etched to create the shallow trenches for isolation.

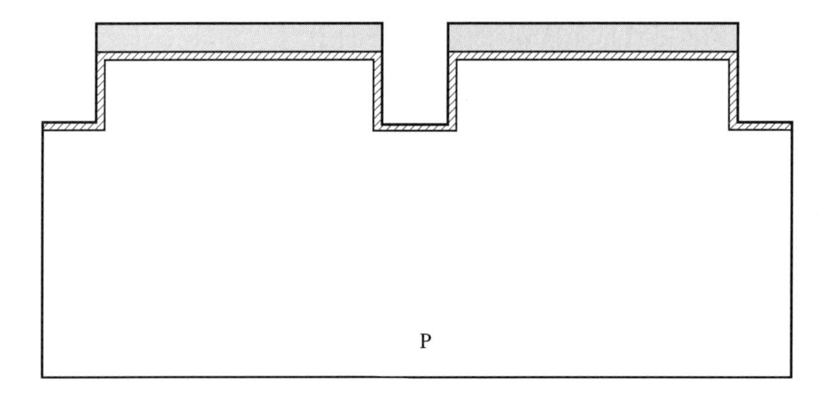

Figure 2–7 A thin "liner" oxide is thermally grown in the trenches. The nitride prevents any additional oxidation on the top surface of the wafer.

chemistry for this silicon etch must be very carefully chosen. Often a bromine-based plasma chemistry is used in this application, as discussed in more detail in Chapter 10.

The next step in the process is to thermally grow a thin (10 – 20-nm) "liner" oxide on the trench sidewalls and bottoms as shown in Figure 2–7. While most of the trench will be filled with a deposited oxide, thermally growing the first part produces a better Si/SiO_2 interface and if the oxidation is done at relatively high temperature ($\approx$ 1100°C), the process will also help to round the corners of the trenches as well. The better Si/SiO_2 interface results from the lower electrical charge densities that thermal oxidations can produce. The corner rounding results from the viscoelastic flow properties of SiO_2 at high temperatures. We will discuss these issues in Chapter 6.

The next step, illustrated in Figure 2–8, is the deposition of a thick SiO_2 layer by chemical vapor deposition. It is important here that the filling process not leave gaps or voids in the trenches, which could happen if the deposition closed the top part of the trench before the bottom parts were completely filled. A number of deposition systems exist which do a good job of filling structures like this. One example is a High-Density Plasma or HDP system, which could be used in this application. We will discuss these systems in Chapter 10.

The final step in the STI process is illustrated in Figure 2–9. This involves literally polishing the excess SiO_2 off the top surface of the wafer, leaving a planar substrate with SiO_2 filled trenches. This polishing process uses a technique known as Chemical-Mechanical Polishing or CMP, which we will discuss in Chapter 11 since the most common use of CMP today is in back-end processing. In this process, the wafer is placed face down in a polishing machine and the upper surface is literally polished flat using a high-pH silica slurry. While this process sounds crude compared to the sophisticated processing techniques generally used to fabricate chips, CMP has been found to work extremely well and it has found widespread application. The nitride layer serves as a polishing stop and once the CMP operation is complete, the Si_3N_4 can be chemically removed as in the LOCOS process described earlier.

At this stage, the wafers are ready for device fabrication in the active regions. A comparison of Figures 2–5 and 2–9 illustrates both the similarities and the differences

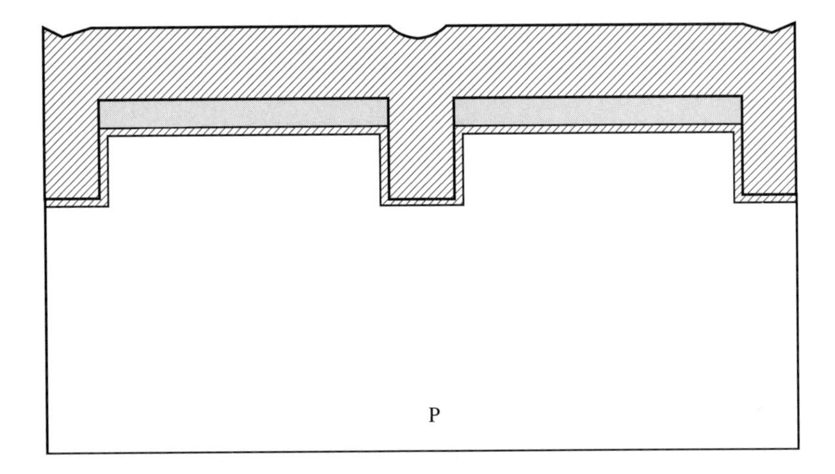

Figure 2–8 SiO_2 is deposited to completely fill the trenches. This would typically require 0.5 – 1 μm of SiO_2 to be deposited, depending on the trench depth and geometry.

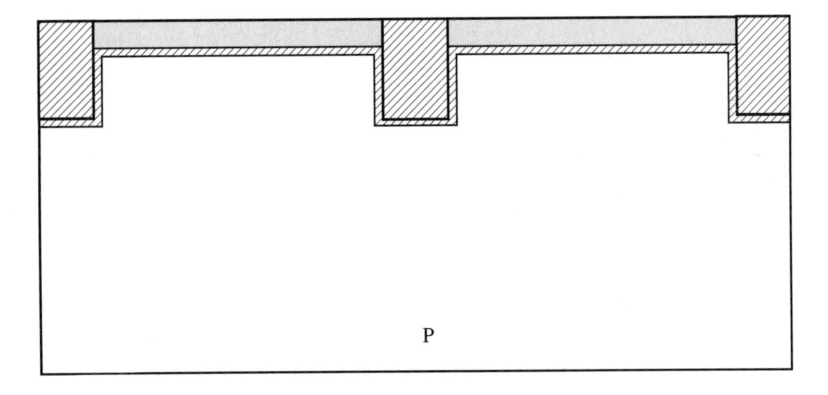

Figure 2–9 The deposited SiO_2 layer is polished back using CMP to produce a planar structure.

in LOCOS and STI. Both processes produce thick SiO_2 regions laterally isolating adjacent device structures. However the STI process produces more compact structures because there is very little lateral encroachment of the isolation structure into adjacent active regions.

One might ask why the STI process has not been used in manufacturing until quite recently since it seems like a simple process and it produces more compact isolation regions compared to LOCOS. There are really two answers to this question. The first is that when device geometries were larger, the small area loss due to lateral encroachment in the LOCOS process was not a significant factor in overall chip density. The second reason is perhaps more important. While STI seems like a simple process, there are actually a number of subtle issues associated with this technology which have proven difficult to solve in a manufacturing environment. These issues include filling the trenches with no gaps, using CMP to planarize the wafer, and avoiding subtle electrical effects associated with the corners of the trenches which can affect device isolation. These issues have now been largely solved with new processes and new manufacturing equipment, with the result that STI is now beginning to be used in manufacturing. Its inherent density advantage over LOCOS suggests that STI will dominate in the future.

2.2.4 N and P Well Formation

We now return to our CMOS process flow and we will pick up the LOCOS isolation technology where we left it in Figure 2–5. If STI were used as the isolation process, the steps below would be largely unchanged. We would simply use the cross section in Figure 2–9 rather than Figure 2–5 as our starting point to continue the process flow.

In the final device cross section in Figure 2–2, the active devices are shown in P- and N-type wells. These wells tailor the substrate doping locally to provide optimum device characteristics. The well doping affects device characteristics such as the MOS transistor threshold voltage and I-V characteristics and PN junction capacitances. For example, recall in Chapter 1, Eqs. (1.23) – (1.25) which describe the electrical properties of PN diodes and notice the presence of the doping levels N_D and N_A in these expressions. The steps required to form the P and N wells are illustrated in Figures 2–10 to 2–12.

In Figure 2–10, photoresist is spun onto the wafer and mask 2 is used to expose the resist and to define the regions where P wells are to be formed. The P regions are created by a process known as ion implantation, which we will discuss in Chapter 8. The machines which perform this step are really small linear accelerators. A source of the ion to be implanted (boron in this case) is provided, usually from a gas. Positively charged ions (B^+) are formed by exposing the source gas to an arc discharge. The ions

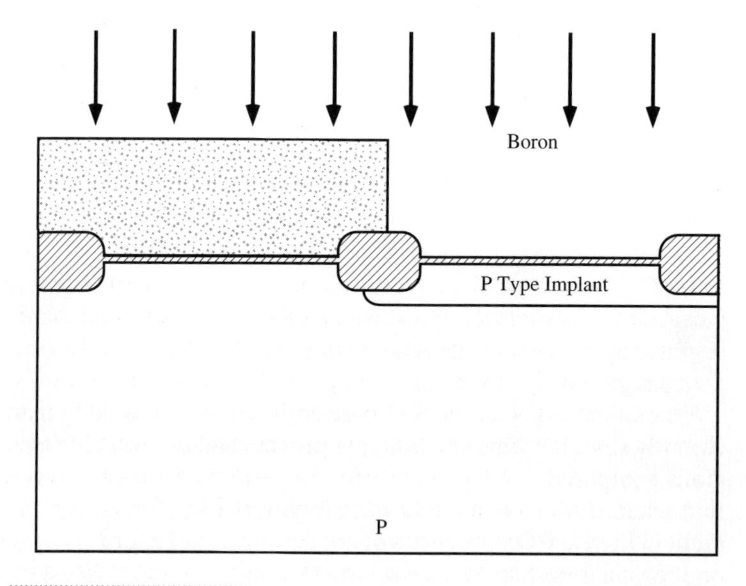

Figure 2–10 Photoresist is used to mask the regions where PMOS devices will be built using mask 2. A boron implant provides the doping for the P wells for the NMOS devices.

are then accelerated in an electric field to some final energy, usually expressed in keV. Since many types of ions may be formed in the source region, all ion implanters select the particular ion to be implanted by bending the ion beam through a magnetic field. Ions of different masses will bend at different rates in the magnetic field, allowing one type of ion to be selected at the output by adjustment of the field strength. Once the selection process is complete, final acceleration of the B^+ takes place along with either electrostatic scanning of the beam or mechanical scanning of the wafer to provide a uniform implant dose across the wafer.

In our case, we would need to pick an implant energy sufficiently large that the B^+ ions penetrated the thin and thick SiO_2 layers on the wafer surface, but not so large that the beam penetrated through the photoresist which must mask against the implant. This is possible in this case because the field oxide is on the order of 0.5 μm and the photoresist is at least twice this thick. The B^+ implant needs to penetrate through the thin SiO_2 layer in order to form the P well. It also needs to penetrate through the field oxide although the reason is not so obvious in this case. As was pointed out earlier, the purpose of the field oxide is to provide lateral isolation between adjacent MOS transistors. If the doping is too light under the field oxide, it is possible that surface inversion can occur in these regions, providing electrical connections between adjacent devices through parasitic MOS devices (field oxide transistors). By ensuring that the well implants penetrate through the field oxide, the doping is increased under the field oxide, preventing this parasitic inversion problem. We will study ion implantation in detail in Chapter 8 and see how to choose the accelerating energy for the B^+ ions, but for the situation described here, an energy of 150 – 200 keV would be typical.

The amount of B^+ we implant (or the dose), is determined by the device requirements. Here we are forming a P well whose concentration is required to be on the order of 5×10^{16} to 10^{17} cm^{-3} in order to provide correct device electrical characteristics. In Chapter 8 we will see how to calculate this dose, but a dose on the order of 10^{13} cm^{-2} would be typical. (Note that implant doses are expressed as an areal dose per cm^2, while doping concentrations are volume concentrations per cm^3.)

An important point about ion implantation has not been made to this point. Implantation of ions into a crystalline substrate causes damage. This is easy to visualize since an incoming ion with an energy of perhaps 100 keV can clearly collide with and dislodge silicon atoms in the substrate which have a binding energy of only 4 Si-Si bonds (about 12 eV). Visualize a billiard-ball-like collision between the incoming 100 keV B^+ ion and a stationary Si atom and you can easily imagine that the silicon atom will likely be recoiled a significant distance from its original lattice site. In fact many such recoils are produced as the B^+ ion gradually comes to rest. This damage must be somehow repaired since the devices we want to end up with require virtually perfect crystalline substrates. Fortunately, the repair process is not as difficult as it might initially seem. A simple furnace step usually suffices. Heating the wafers allows the dislodged silicon atoms to diffuse and find a vacant lattice site, thus repairing the damage. Such a high temperature step will soon occur in our process description and will accomplish this crystal repair function. This can be done in short times at high temperatures (e.g., 10 sec at 1000°C) or in longer times at lower temperatures (e.g., 30 min at 800°C). We will study implantation and damage annealing in greater detail in Chapter 8.

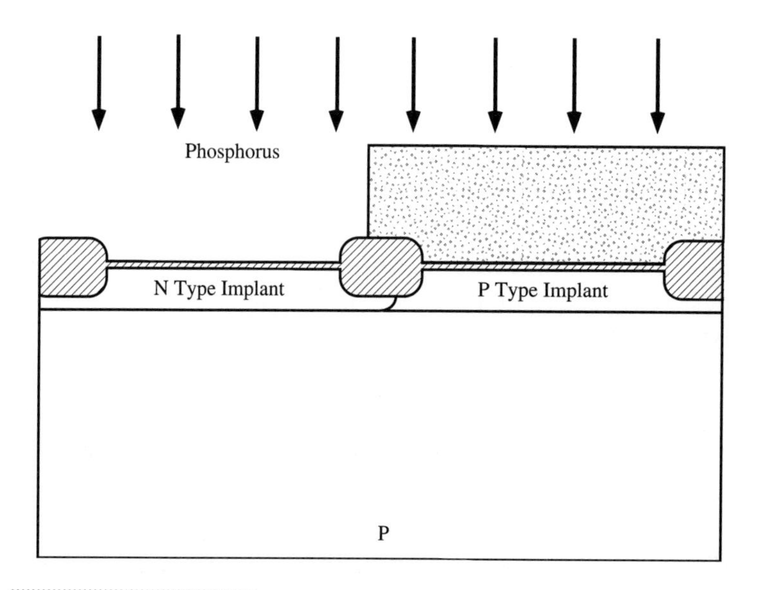

Figure 2–11 Photoresist is used to mask the regions where NMOS devices will be built using mask 3. A phosphorus implant provides the doping for the N wells for the PMOS devices.

Once the boron implant is complete, we are finished with the photoresist and it is then stripped either chemically or in an O_2 plasma. Photoresist and mask 3 are now used as shown in Figure 2–11 to define the regions where N wells will be placed in the silicon. The process is identical to that just described for the P wells except that in this case an N-type dopant, phosphorus, is implanted. The energy of the phosphorus implant is again chosen to penetrate the oxide layers but not the photoresist. Phosphorus is a heavier atom than boron (atomic mass = 31 versus 11), so a higher energy is required to obtain an implant to the same depth into the silicon. In this situation an energy of 300–400 keV would be chosen. The dose of the phosphorus implant would typically be on the same order as the boron P well implant since the purpose is similar in both cases.

There are several common N-type dopants available for use in silicon (phosphorus, arsenic, and antimony) and yet we specifically chose phosphorus in this case. The next step in the process is to diffuse the P and N wells to a junction depth of typically several microns, as illustrated in Figure 2–12. Boron and phosphorus have essentially matched diffusion coefficients and so they will produce wells with about the same junction depth when they are simultaneously diffused. The other N-type dopants, arsenic and antimony, both have much smaller diffusion coefficients and so for the process described here, the N well would be much shallower than the P well, which is not desired if we want matched NMOS and PMOS characteristics. Another issue with arsenic and antimony in this particular step in the process is that they are much heavier atoms than phosphorus and hence would require much higher implant energies.

After the phosphorus implant, the photoresist is removed and the wafers are cleaned. They are next placed in a drive-in furnace, which diffuses the wells to a junction depth of 2–3 microns (Figure 2–12). (Actually the depths they reach in this step will

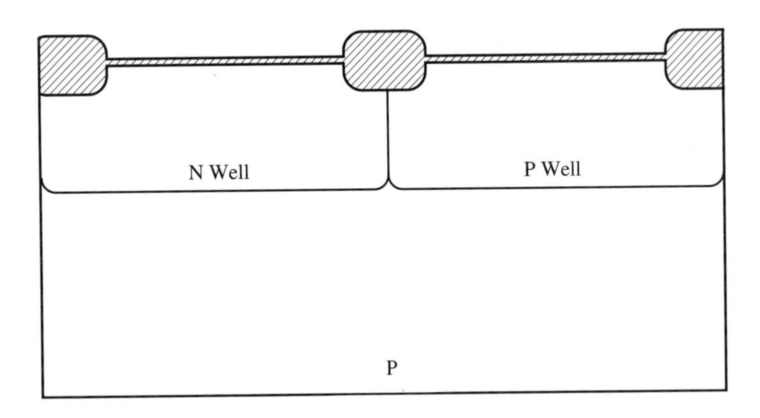

Figure 2–12 A high temperature drive-in completes the formation of the N and P wells.

not be their "final" depths because all subsequent high temperature steps will continue to diffuse the dopants. However, later high temperature steps will generally be either at lower temperatures or for shorter times, so that most of the well diffusion occurs during this drive-in process.) A typical thermal cycle might be 4 to 6 hours at 1000 to 1100°C. Diffusion coefficients increase exponentially with temperature as we will see in Chapter 7, so much shorter times are required at higher temperatures to achieve the same junction depth. This step could be performed in a largely inert ambient because no additional surface oxidation is needed at this point. The well drive-in step also repairs the damage from the implants, restoring the substrate crystallinity.

2.2.5 Process Options for Active Region and Well Formation

At this point we have completed the preparation of the substrate for the fabrication of the active devices. There are many process options which could be considered at almost every stage of our CMOS process. In general we will not consider very many of these options in this chapter, because there are simply too many to consider in a finite chapter. Also, our purpose here is not to explore all options but simply to give the reader a sense of what an integrated process flow looks like. However in addition to the STI option we considered earlier, there are several other options that are very commonly used in industrial manufacturing which will be useful for the reader to understand before reading later chapters. Two such options are explored briefly in this section before we return to our CMOS process flow as it is shown in Figure 2–12.

Option 1: Field Implants under LOCOS Regions

The first process option relates to the field oxide or LOCOS regions which provide lateral electrical isolation between adjacent devices. In the process flow we have described to this point, the implant energies of the P and N wells were carefully chosen to penetrate through the thick field oxide so that the substrate doping was increased under the

LOCOS regions. In practice this is not as simple to do as it might seem. Implanted ions are characterized by a range distribution not by a specific distance they travel. Since the stopping process is statistical in nature, we should expect such a range profile. Chapter 8 explores this idea in more detail, but for our purposes here we need only to understand that the entire implant dose cannot be placed in the silicon under the field oxide in Figures 2–10 and 2–11. If we tried to do this, the implant energy would have to be increased significantly to make certain that the shallowest ions went far enough to get through the field oxide. But the problem would then be that the deepest ions would likely penetrate through the masking photoresist layer. So the process as illustrated in Figures 2–10 and 2–11 is somewhat sensitive to layer thicknesses and to implant energy. This does not mean that it is too sensitive to be used in manufacturing, but it does mean that alternatives are often used.

One common alternative is illustrated in Figures 2–13 to 2–15. In this process flow, the field region doping is accomplished right after the steps shown in Figure 2–4, before the LOCOS oxide is grown. Thus a low-energy boron implant can be used which is easily masked by the photoresist/Si_3N_4/SiO_2 stack. This is illustrated in Figure 2–13. When the field oxide is then grown, most of the boron diffuses ahead of the growing SiO_2, creating the P regions shown in Figure 2–14. Some of the boron is actually incorporated into the growing SiO_2 and is therefore "lost" from the silicon. The fraction of the boron that is lost can be easily calculated, as we will see in later chapters. For obvious reasons, the implant in Figure 2–13 is often called the field implant. It increases the P-type doping in the substrate where we do not want to build active devices. A typical field implant might be 1×10^{13} cm^{-2} B^+ at 50 keV. This implant energy would easily pass through the

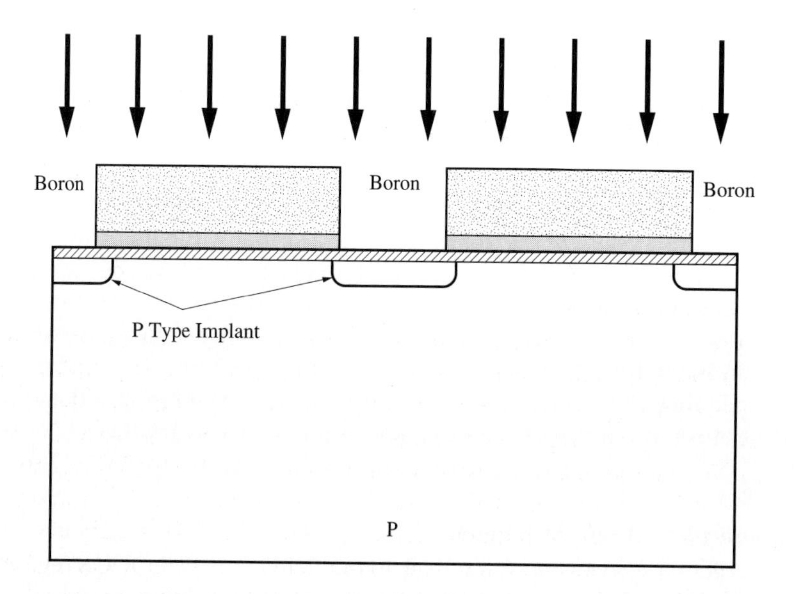

Figure 2–13 Process option for active region formation. A boron implant prior to LOCOS oxidation increases the substrate doping locally under the field oxide to minimize field inversion problems.

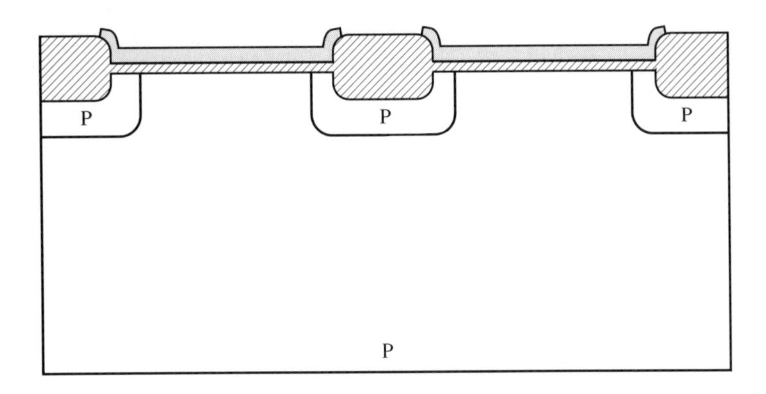

Figure 2–14 Process option for active region formation after LOCOS. The boron implanted regions diffuse ahead of the growing oxide producing the P-doped regions under the field oxide.

thin SiO_2 layer in Figure 2–13 and would also easily be completely masked by the photoresist/Si_3N_4/SiO_2 stack.

The P and N well formation in this process option would essentially follow the steps illustrated in Figures 2–10 and 2–11 except that the implant energies would be considerably lower to make sure that the phosphorus and boron did not penetrate through the field oxide. Implant energies on the order of 50 keV would be typical for the B^+ and P^+. The resulting structure is shown in Figure 2–15. Note that the P-type field implant regions continue to diffuse during the well drive-in. The wells are shown deeper than the field region in this example, but the exact geometry depends on the dopant concentrations in each region. Notice also that this process option does not require any more masking steps than the process we considered through Figure 2–12, since the field implant is done through the same mask that is used for the LOCOS process. As was the case in Figure 2–12, the substrate shown in Figure 2–15 is now ready for active device fabrication.

Option 2: Buried and Epitaxial Layers

Some CMOS circuits are built today in wafers that have buried heavily doped layers incorporated under the active devices. Alternatively, some CMOS circuits are built using heavily doped substrates such as the P on P^+ structure illustrated in Figure 1–34. Such heavily doped regions can help to minimize problems such as "latchup" in operating CMOS circuits. Latchup can occur because CMOS technology inherently contains parasitic PNPN structures. These structures have electrical I-V characteristics which, if triggered, can permit enough current to flow through the circuit that the chip may be destroyed. (Latchup is discussed in more detail in Chapter 8. See, for example, Figure 8–15.) One of the effective ways to prevent this from happening is to incorporate heavily doped buried layers or a heavily doped substrate beneath the active devices. These layers shunt the parasitic PNPN devices with low-value resistances, preventing the PNPN devices from turning on.

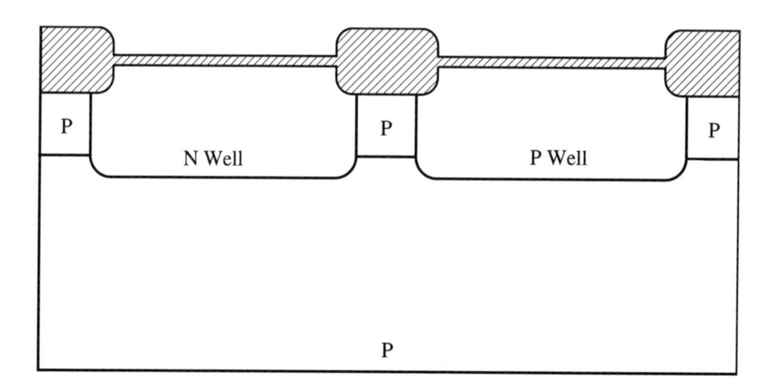

Figure 2–15 Process option for active region formation after the P and N wells are formed.

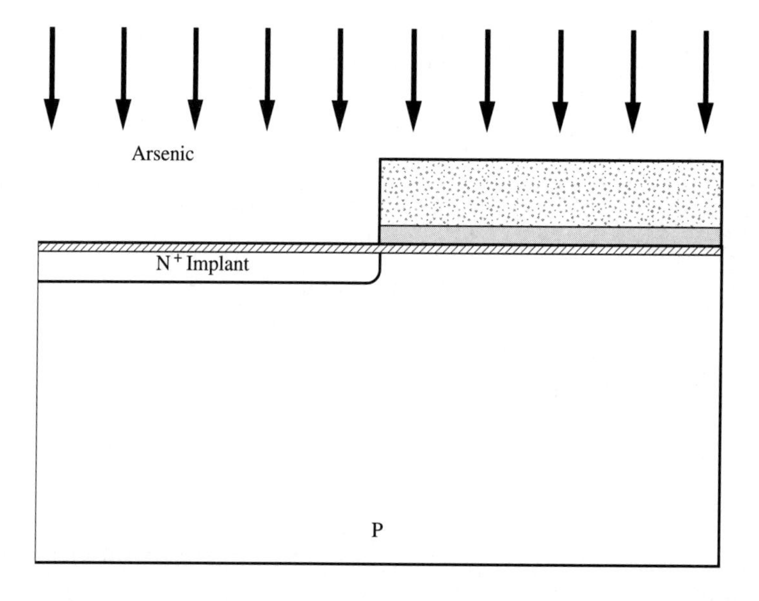

Figure 2–16 Process option incorporating buried and epitaxial layers. Mask 1 defines the regions for N^+ buried layers. An As^+ implant dopes the silicon locally.

The process steps needed to incorporate buried layers are shown in Figures 2–16 to 2–21. These steps are incorporated at the very beginning of the process flow, for reasons that will become obvious shortly.

We begin with the structure in Figure 2–3. The first mask is used as shown in Figure 2–16 to define the regions where an N^+ buried layer will be formed. An As^+ implant is then performed. Since the purpose here is to create a low-resistance region, we would want the N^+ layer to be fairly heavily doped and so a high-dose implant on the order of 10^{15} cm^{-2} would be used. The energy is not critical so long as it is sufficient to accelerate the As^+ through the thin SiO_2 layer. A reasonable energy would be 50 keV. Since the N^+ region we are forming will be buried below the surface (when we are finished), and we want it to stay there, we would want to pick an N-type dopant that diffuses slowly in silicon. As or Sb would thus be possible choices. Either could be used, but As is more common because of its higher solubility in silicon.

Once the implant is completed, we are through with the resist and it can be chemically removed in acid, or stripped in an O_2 plasma. Following cleaning, the wafers are then placed into a furnace. This high-temperature step accomplishes several things, as illustrated in Figure 2–17. First, it drives in the N^+ buried layer to a depth of about 1–2 μm. Second, part of the drive-in is done in an oxidizing ambient (H_2O). This grows a thick SiO_2 layer on the wafer surface, but only over the N^+ regions because of the masking provided by the Si_3N_4 layer. We will see that using a LOCOS process in this application allows both the N^+ and P^+ buried layers to be defined with a single mask, and it provides self-alignment between these two buried layers. By self-alignment, we mean that the two buried layers are correctly positioned with respect to each other automatically. Finally, the drive-in and oxidation create a step in the silicon surface at the edges of the N^+ buried layers because the oxidation consumes silicon. This step in the surface will be important later after the buried layers are truly buried by growing an epitaxial layer of silicon above them. We will need to know where the buried layers are located in order to align later masks to them and the step in the silicon surface will provide this information. The overall drive-in process might be done at 1000°C for 2 hours, with 60 min of this time in H_2O to locally grow about 0.4 μm of SiO_2. The structure at this point is illustrated in Figure 2–17.

After the furnace operation, the Si_3N_4 layer can then be stripped. The next step is ion implantation of the P^+ buried layer, illustrated in Figure 2–18. Here the self-aligning feature in the two buried layers becomes apparent. The thick oxide over the N^+ buried layers blocks the P^+ (boron) implant, while the original thin oxide layer elsewhere is transparent to the implant. Once again, we would choose the implant energy so that the boron penetrates the thin oxide and is stopped by the thick oxide (about 50 – 75 keV). The boron dose is determined by device constraints, as was the case for the N^+ buried

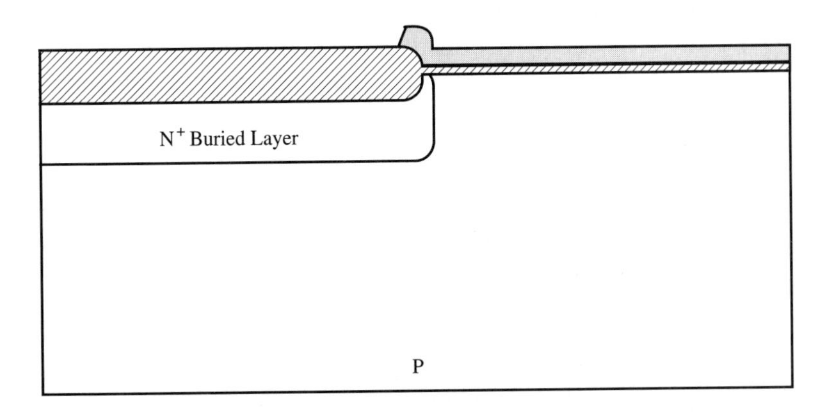

Figure 2–17 Process option incorporating buried and epitaxial layers. The N^+ buried layer is driven in in an oxidizing ambient after the photoresist is stripped. The LOCOS oxide forms only above the N^+ regions.

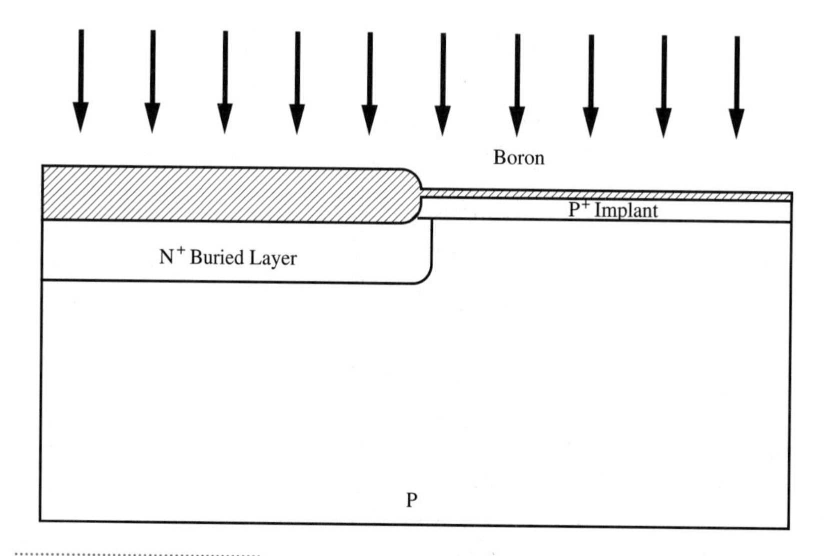

Figure 2–18 Process option incorporating buried and epitaxial layers. The P^+ buried layer is implanted using the thick SiO_2 layer as a mask.

layer. In the P^+ buried layer case, a lower dose is usually used, because boron has a much higher diffusivity than arsenic and in order to keep it from diffusing too far during subsequent processing the boron concentration needs to be kept lower than the arsenic concentration. A dose of about 10^{14} cm^{-2} might be typical. After the P^+ implant, a high-temperature drive-in would be done to diffuse the boron (and the arsenic) deeper into the substrate. No additional oxidation is required at this point so the drive-in could be done in an inert (N_2 or Ar) ambient. A typical furnace cycle at this point might be several hours at 1000 – 1100°C, resulting in the structure shown in Figure 2–19.

The active devices need to be fabricated in much more lightly doped wells than is provided by these buried layer regions in order to have the correct electrical properties. As a result, we require moderately doped P and N regions above the buried layers. These more lightly doped layers reduce the junction capacitances in the active transistors and are also important in setting device parameters such as MOS threshold or turn-on voltage. In principle we could counterdope the surface regions of the buried layers with opposite type dopants to produce these regions, but this is not a manufacturable technique. This is easy to see if we imagine trying to counterdope a 1.0×10^{19} cm^{-3} N^+ buried layer to form a 1.0×10^{16} cm^{-3} N layer. This would require 0.999×10^{19} cm^{-3} P-type counter doping. No doping technique available today provides this degree of precision.

Fortunately there is an alternative, a process called epitaxy. The oxide layer on the surface of the wafer in Figure 2–19 is first stripped in an HF solution. This acid is highly selective to SiO_2 over Si. After cleaning, the wafers are then placed into an epitaxial reactor which heats the wafers to temperatures on the order of 800 – 1000°C and exposes them to a gas ambient containing Si and a small concentration of dopant. SiH_4 or

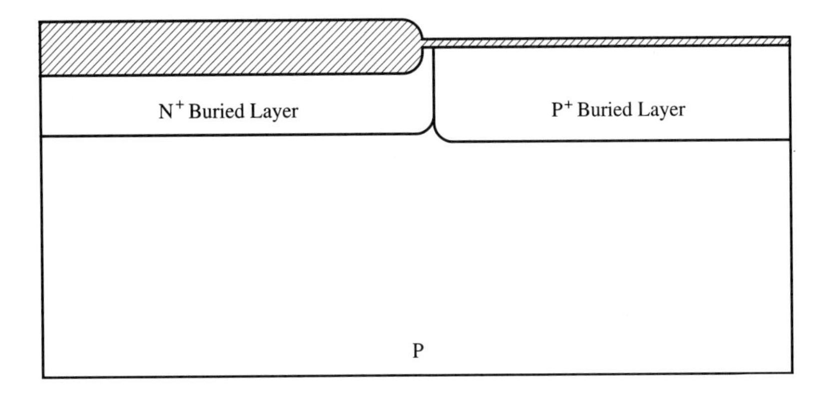

Figure 2–19 Process option incorporating buried and epitaxial layers. The P^+ and N^+ buried layers are driven in together.

SiH_2Cl_2 might be used as the silicon source and B_2H_6 or AsH_3 for the P- or N-type doping, for example. The process of epitaxy is conceptually simple. Si atoms fall on the wafer surface from the gas stream above it. At the high temperature in the reactor, the Si atoms are somewhat mobile on the surface and can diffuse via surface diffusion to a lattice site to which they can bond. Through this process, the crystal structure of the substrate is grown upward, atom by atom, and layer by layer, producing a perfect crystalline or "epitaxial" layer. The doping atoms in the gas stream are incorporated into the growing epitaxial layer in the same manner. This process allows us to grow single-crystal layers on single-crystal substrates at a rate of several tenths of a micron per minute and to dope those layers from 10^{14} cm^{-3} to 10^{20} cm^{-3} N- or P-type. We will study this process in more detail in Chapter 9. In fact, epitaxy is really a special case of CVD which we previously used to deposit Si_3N_4 and SiO_2 layers. In epitaxy, the substrate must be single crystal; in the more general CVD process, arbitrary substrates can be used because the films that are deposited are amorphous or polycrystalline.

Figure 2–20 illustrates our CMOS wafer after an epitaxial layer has been grown. The epilayer for our devices is grown undoped (intrinsic) since we will be doping various parts of it later in the process using ion implantation. The epilayer might typically be a few microns thick. Notice that the step in the silicon surface which we created by oxidation of the N^+ buried layers has propagated upward during epi growth, so that it now appears on the new wafer surface. This step is visible under an optical microscope and is necessary in order to align subsequent masks to the buried layer patterns.

The remaining steps in this process option would follow the LOCOS steps (Figures 2–3 to 2–5) and the P- and N-well steps (Figures 2–10 to 2–12). After the wells are driven in, they link up with the buried layers (which also diffuse upwards during all high temperature steps) as shown in Figure 2–21. Both downward and upward diffusion must be accounted for in order to determine the time and temperature needed to accomplish this linkup. A typical set of conditions might be several hours at 1000 – 1100°C depending on the exact epitaxial layer thickness. This could be performed in a

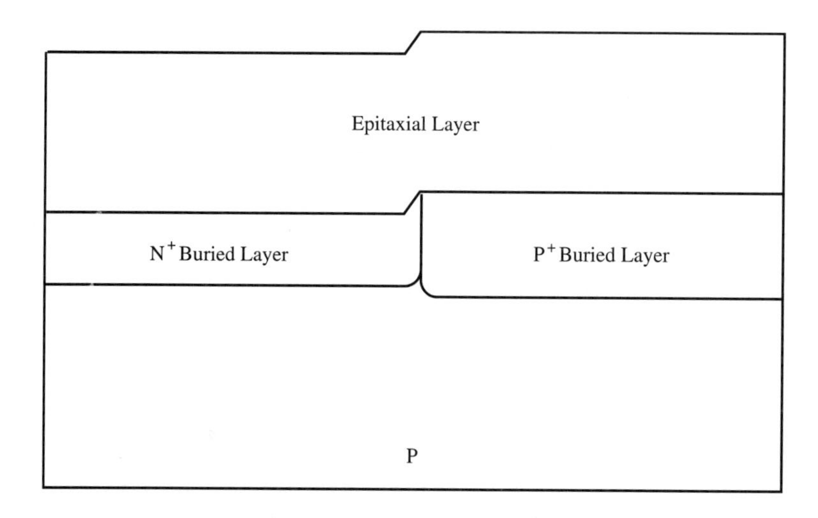

Figure 2–20 Process option incorporating buried and epitaxial layers. The surface SiO_2 layer is stripped off the wafer and an epitaxial layer is then grown.

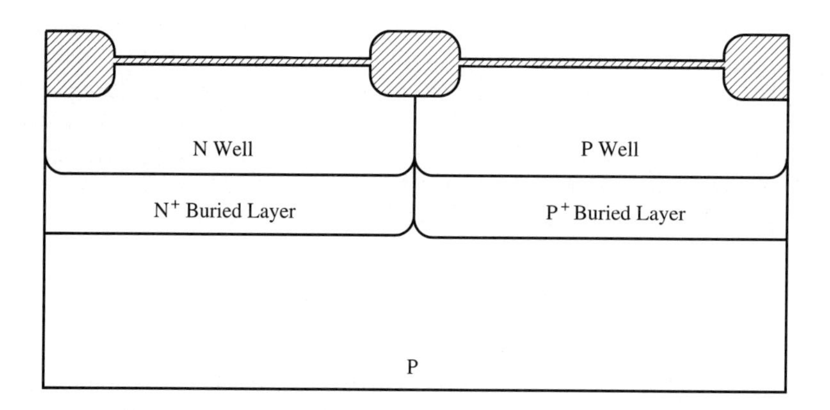

Figure 2–21 Process option incorporating buried and epitaxial layers.

largely inert ambient because no additional surface oxidation is needed at this point. Note that the incorporation of the buried and epitaxial layers into the structure has only required one additional mask (but many process steps!). As was the case in Figure 2–12, the substrate as shown in Figure 2–21 is now ready for active device fabrication. The step in the surface shown in Figure 2–20 would still be present in Figure 2–21 but is not explicitly shown.

Finally, the structure shown in Figure 1–34 is yet another variation on these process steps. This structure incorporates a P^- epitaxial layer and an N well using steps similar to those described above. The process flow in this case is left as an exercise for the reader. (See Problem 2.1.)

2.2.6 Gate Formation

We now return to the main process flow and Figure 2–12. If either of the process options described above were to be used, the substrate would appear as shown in Figure 2–15 or 2–21, but the process flow from this point on would be substantially the same. So for simplicity, we will continue the process description with Figure 2–12.

The next several steps, shown in Figures 2–22 to 2–26 are designed to form critical parts of the MOS devices. Probably the single most important parameter in both the NMOS and PMOS devices is the turn-on or threshold voltage, discussed in Chapter 1 and usually called V_{TH}. V_{TH} in its simplest form is given by

$$V_{TH} = V_{FB} + 2\phi_f + \frac{\sqrt{2\varepsilon_S q N_A (2\phi_f)}}{C_{OX}} \tag{2.3}$$

where V_{FB} is the gate voltage required to compensate for work function differences between the gate and substrate, and for any electrical charges that may be present in the gate oxide. ϕ_f is the position of the Fermi level in the bulk with respect to the intrinsic level and ε_s is the permittivity of silicon. For our present purposes, the two terms that are important are the doping concentration in the silicon N_A and the oxide capacitance C_{ox}. Since C_{ox} is inversely proportional to the gate oxide thickness, it is clear that we must control this thickness in order to control V_{TH}.

In writing the above expression, we have assumed that the doping in the silicon under the MOS gate is constant at N_A. This is usually not the case in modern devices because ion implantation is used to adjust the threshold voltage and this results in a nonuniform doping profile. Again to first order, we can include the effect of the implant on V_{TH} in the following way:

$$V_{TH} = V_{FB} + 2\phi_f + \frac{\sqrt{2\varepsilon_S q N_A (2\phi_f)}}{C_{OX}} + \frac{qQ_I}{C_{OX}} \tag{2.4}$$

where Q_I is the implant dose, in atoms per cm^2. This equation assumes that the entire implant dose is located in the near surface region, inside the MOS channel depletion region. This is often a reasonable approximation.

We are now ready to adjust the threshold voltages of both N- and P-channel MOS devices. In modern CMOS circuits, the target threshold voltage is generally around 0.5–0.8 volts for both the NMOS and PMOS devices. (The threshold voltage is positive for the NMOS devices and negative for the PMOS devices so that both transistors are normally off, enhancement mode devices.) Figure 2–22 illustrates the masking to adjust the NMOS V_{TH}. Photoresist is applied and mask 4 is used to open the areas where NMOS devices are located. After developing, a boron implant is used to adjust V_{TH}. A dose of $1–5 \times 10^{12}$ cm^{-2} at an energy of 50 – 75 keV might be used. We could estimate the necessary dose using Eq. (2.4) where N_A is the doping in the P well at the surface before the implant, and Q_I is the dose required to achieve a given V_{TH}. The energy is chosen to be high enough to get the implant dose through the thin oxide, but low enough to keep the boron near the silicon surface.

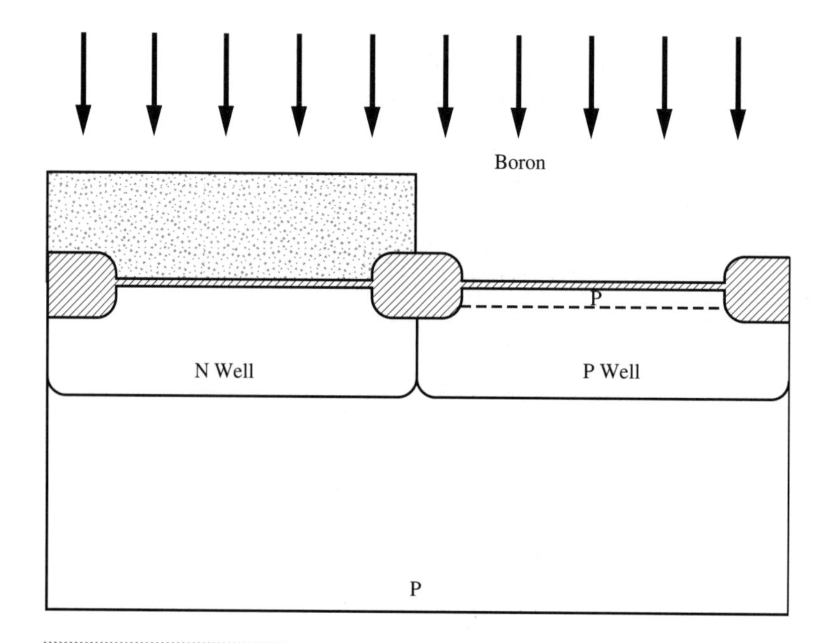

Figure 2–22 After spinning photoresist on the wafer, mask 4 is used to define the NMOS transistors. A boron implant adjusts the N-channel V_{TH}.

Figure 2–23 illustrates the same process sequence now applied to the PMOS device. Mask 5 is used. The required implant could be either N- or P-type depending on the doping level in the N well and the required PMOS V_{TH}. An N-type implant is illustrated in Figure 2–23. This would typically be arsenic with a dose of 1–5 $\times$ 10^{12} cm^{-2}. The energy would be somewhat higher than the NMOS channel implant in Figure 2–22 because of the heavier mass of arsenic.

If a P-type implant were needed, boron would be used with a dose and energy in the same range as for the NMOS device in Figure 2–22. In some cases, it might be possible to use only one mask to adjust both NMOS and PMOS V_{TH} if both require P-type implants. One possible process might be to implant boron unmasked into both devices at the smaller of the two doses required for the MOS devices. A mask would then be used along with a second implant to increase the dose in the device requiring more boron.

Figure 2–24 illustrates the next steps. We are now ready to grow the gate oxides for the MOS transistors. The thin oxide, which is present over the active areas of each transistor, is first stripped in a dilute HF solution. HF is a highly selective etchant and will stop etching when the underlying silicon is reached. Note however that we will etch a small portion of the field oxide during this step because the HF etch is unmasked. Since we are etching only 10 or 20 nm of oxide, this is usually not a problem, although the etch needs to be timed so that it does not etch too much of the field oxide.

The reason that the thin oxide is stripped and then regrown to form the MOS gate oxide is that the oxide on the silicon surface prior to stripping is too thick to serve as the device gate oxide. Stripping and regrowing this oxide results in a well-controlled final

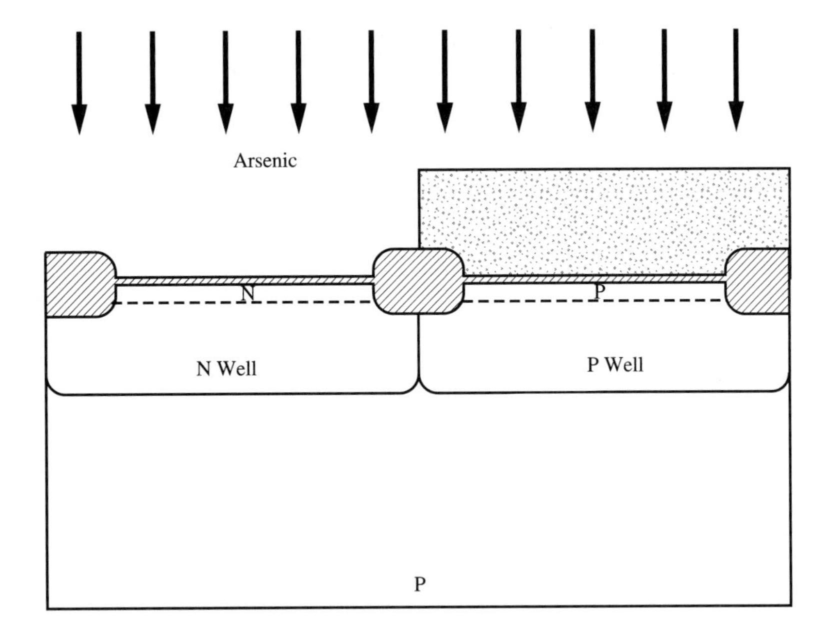

Figure 2–23 After spinning photoresist on the wafer, mask 5 is used to define the PMOS transistors. An arsenic implant adjusts the P-channel V_{TH}.

oxide thickness. The original thin oxide on the wafer surface has also been exposed to several implants at this stage in the process, which create damage in the SiO_2, so stripping and regrowing a new oxide produces a higher quality gate oxide. In state-of-the-art MOS devices today, the gate oxide is typically thinner than 10 nm. This oxide could be formed by a variety of processes (times and temperatures). For example, oxidation in O_2 at 800°C for 2 hours would produce about 10 nm of oxide. Similarly, oxidation in H_2O at 800°C for 25 min would produce a similar thickness oxide. Figure 2–24 illustrates the devices after the gate oxide has been grown.

The next steps deposit and define the polysilicon gate electrodes for the MOS devices. Using LPCVD, a layer of polysilicon is deposited over the entire wafer surface as illustrated in Figure 2–25. This process is similar to that described in Eq. (2.1) except that only a silicon source such as silane is needed. Thermal decomposition of the silane produces a silicon deposition with H_2 as a byproduct, as shown in Eq. (2.5). The deposited layer will be either amorphous or polycrystalline depending on the deposition temperature because it is deposited on an amorphous "substrate," the underlying SiO_2 regions. Typically a polysilicon layer 0.3 – 0.5 μm thick would be deposited in an LPCVD system operating at about 600°C.

$$SiH_4 \rightarrow Si + 2H_2 \tag{2.5}$$

The polysilicon is then doped N-type by an unmasked ion implant. Either phosphorus or arsenic could be used here since both are highly soluble in silicon (and polysilicon) and thus can produce low-sheet-resistance poly layers. The implant energy is not

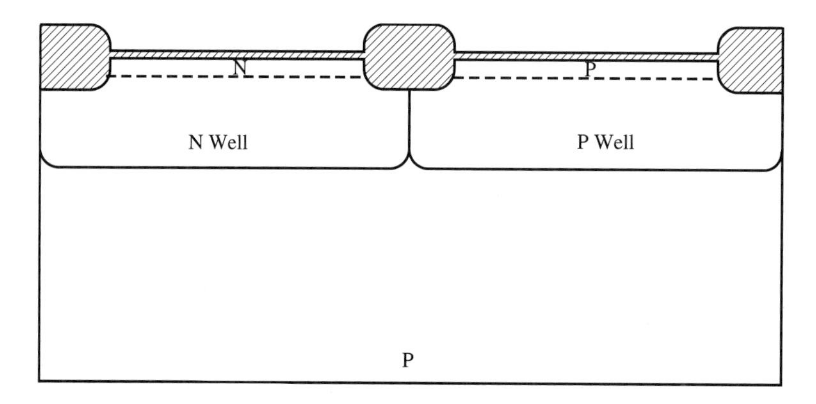

Figure 2–24 After etching back the thin oxide to bare silicon, the gate oxide is grown for the MOS transistors.

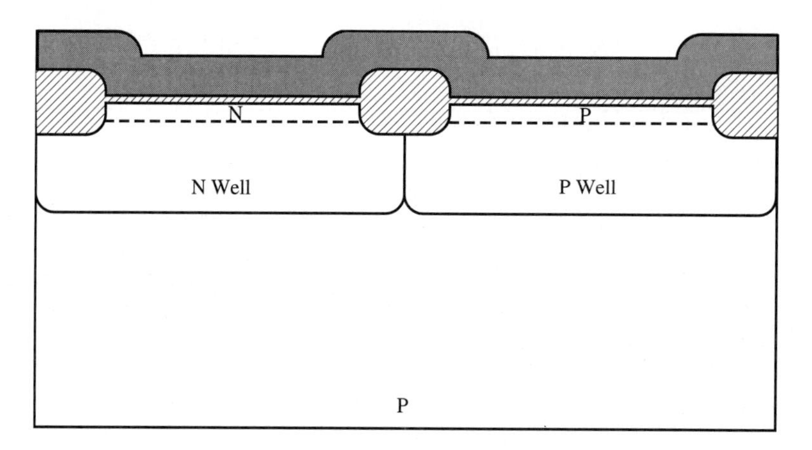

Figure 2–25 A layer of polysilicon is deposited. Ion implantation of phosphorus follows the deposition to heavily dope the poly.

very critical here, provided the phosphorus or arsenic do not penetrate through the poly and into the underlying gate oxide and substrate. Both dopants rapidly redistribute in poly at elevated temperatures because diffusion is rapid along the grain boundaries in poly, so uniform doping of the poly will occur later in the process when the wafers are next heated in a furnace. The N^+ dose is not critical for the MOS gates other than the fact that we would like it to be as high as possible in order to obtain low poly sheet resistivity and hence low gate resistance. A dose of about 5×10^{15} cm^{-2} would be typical. In some polysilicon deposition systems, the poly can be doped while it is being deposited. This is referred to as "in situ" doped poly. In this case, the ion implantation doping step would not be necessary.

The final step, illustrated in Figure 2–26 uses resist and mask 6 to etch the poly away in regions where it is not needed. Photoresist is spun onto the wafer, baked, and then exposed and developed. The poly etching would again be done in a plasma etcher. Typically a chlorine- or bromine-based plasma chemistry would be used in order to achieve

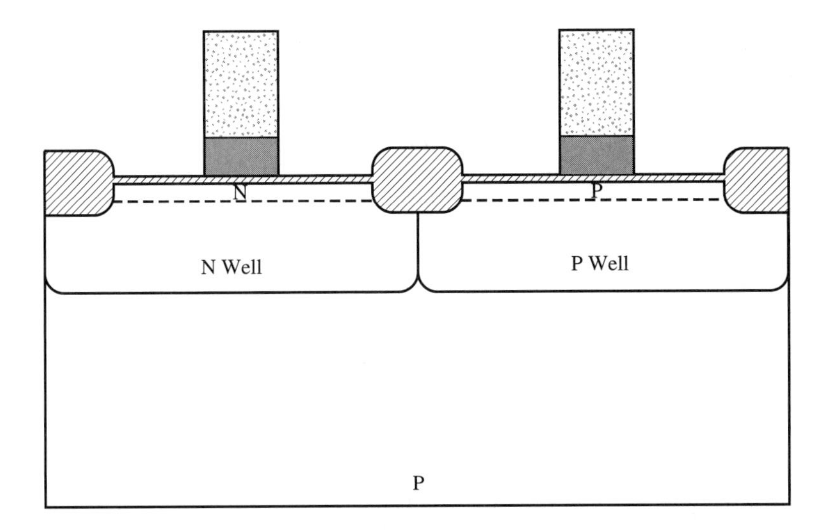

Figure 2–26 Photoresist is applied and mask 6 is used to define the regions where MOS gates are located. The polysilicon layer is then etched using plasma etching.

good selectivity to SiO_2. Although it is not shown in Figure 2–26, the polysilicon layer can also be used to provide wiring between active devices on the chip (for example to connect the NMOS and PMOS poly gates). In this sense it can serve as the first level of interconnect. Since the poly sheet resistance is relatively high compared to later metal layers that will be deposited ($\approx 10\ \Omega$/sq versus $< 0.1\ \Omega$/sq), long interconnects are not made with the polysilicon. The RC delays associated with long poly lines would have a significant effect on circuit performance, hence the term "local interconnects" for these relatively short polysilicon wires.

A final point with regard to all these etching steps is worth making at this point, although we will discuss it in much more detail in Chapter 10. In general there are two key parameters that must be understood and controlled in any etching step. The first is selectivity and the second is the degree of anisotropy the etch provides. Selectivity is a key issue because we nearly always find ourselves in the situation where we wish to etch one material but stop etching when we hit an underlying material. For example, in Figure 2–26, we wanted to etch the poly layer, but we of course did not want to etch through the gate oxide and into the underlying silicon substrate. This means that we would need to select an etching process during the poly etch that was highly selective between SiO_2 and Si, so that the etch would in essence stop when it reached the SiO_2 layer. Techniques exist to detect the endpoint of an etching process, but usually some amount of overetching is necessary to make certain that all areas on a wafer or wafers have completed etching, so selectivity is usually very important.

Anisotropy is a key issue because we are usually very concerned about the shape of edges on etched regions. We are often required to etch through materials whose thicknesses are on the same order as the lines we are trying to etch or define. Ideally we would like the edges of the etched materials to be nearly vertical to preserve the mask dimensions in the etched layers. Anisotropic etches approach this ideal; isotropic etches produce about as much undercutting as the vertical depth they etch and so are generally unsuitable for small geometry devices. So in general, we want highly selective, anisotropic etches. Unfortunately, it is often the case that anisotropy comes at the expense of selectivity and vice versa. Plasma etching often means a search for the best trade-off between the two that can be achieved in a given system. We will return to these issues in Chapter 10.

2.2.7 Tip or Extension (LDD) Formation

The next several steps are illustrated in Figures 2–27 to 2–30. Our objective in these steps is twofold. First, we want to introduce the N^- and P^- implants shown in the NMOS and PMOS devices in Figures 2–27 and 2–28 and second, we want to place along the edges of the polysilicon gates, a thin oxide layer usually called a "sidewall spacer." Both of these steps are required because of scaling trends that have taken place in the semiconductor industry over the past decade.

Ten years ago, MOS devices used in ICs were built with minimum dimensions well above one micron and were operated in circuits with supply voltages of 5 volts. Today, device dimensions have been reduced to 0.25 μm or smaller in order to improve performance. However, supply voltages in circuits have not been proportionally reduced. Many ICs still use 5-volt power supplies, although many chips are now being designed with 3.3- and 2.5-volt supplies. There is great benefit at the system level to maintaining a standard power supply level because then new ICs are compatible with older parts,

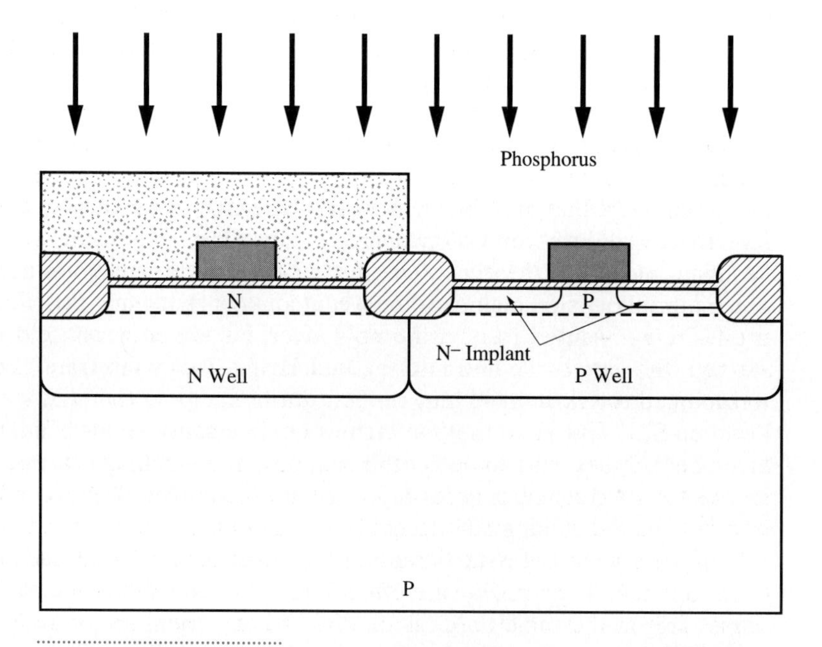

Figure 2–27 Mask 7 is used to cover the PMOS devices. A phosphorus implant is used to form the tip or extension (LDD) regions in the NMOS devices.

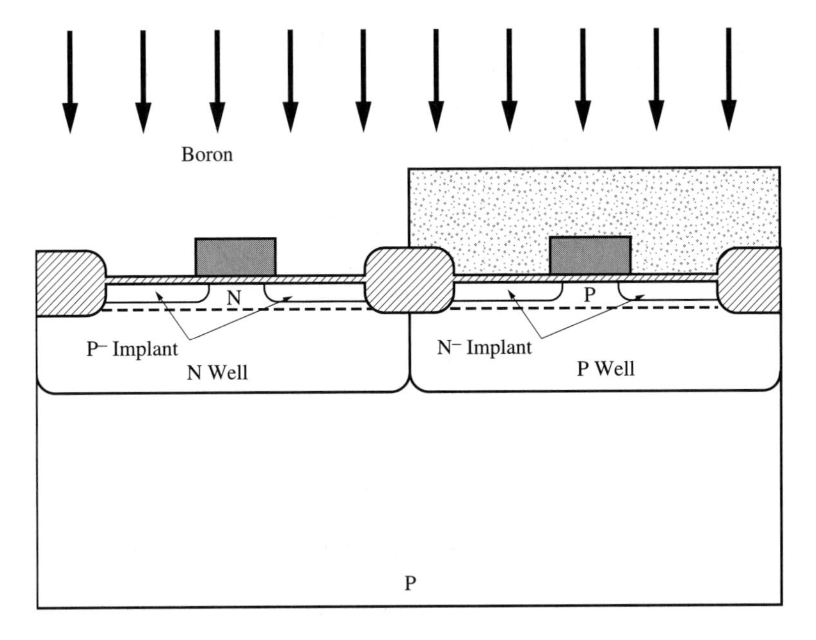

Figure 2–28 Mask 8 is used to cover the NMOS devices. A boron implant is used to form the tip or extension (LDD) regions in the PMOS devices.

system power supplies do not have to be redesigned and circuit noise margins remain adequate. However, if device dimensions are reduced and voltage levels are not correspondingly scaled, electric fields inside the devices necessarily rise. Five volts applied across a 2-μm channel length MOS device implies an average electric field in the channel of about 2.5×10^4 V cm^{-1}. Decreasing the channel length in the device to 0.5 μm without reducing the supply voltage increases this average field to about 10^5 V cm^{-1}. Fields this high are large enough to cause problems in semiconductor devices. Such problems are often called "hot electron" problems because most of them are due to the high energies that electrons (or holes) can reach in high electric fields. Carriers at high energies can cause impact ionization which creates additional hole-electron pairs by breaking Si-Si bonds. Such carriers can also sometimes gain sufficient energy to surmount large energy barriers such as the 3.2 eV barrier between the Si conduction band and the SiO_2 conduction band. The result can be carriers injected into gate dielectrics which may become trapped and cause device reliability problems.

Because of these larger fields in scaled devices, considerable effort has gone into designing MOS device structures that can withstand high electric fields. One of the innovations that is almost universally used is the Lightly Doped Drain or LDD device. The idea behind this structure is to grade the doping in the drain region to produce an N^+N^-P profile between the drain and channel in the NMOS devices and a corresponding P^+P^-N profile in the PMOS devices. This allows the drain voltage to be dropped over a larger distance than would be the case if an abrupt N^+P junction were formed. This reduces the peak value of the electric field in the near drain region. Since many of the deleterious effects of high electric fields in modern MOS devices depend exponentially on the electric field, modest reductions in the field strength obtained through the LDD structure can make a significant difference in device reliability.

A final point regarding these N^- and P^- implants is also important to make. As device geometries have become smaller, "short channel effects" have become very important in MOS transistors. These effects result when the drain electric field penetrates through the channel region and begins to affect the potential barrier between the source and channel regions. The result is drain current that is not controlled effectively by the gate. An important strategy for minimizing these effects is the use of shallow junctions. Such junctions are less susceptible to short channel effects essentially because their geometry minimizes the junction areas adjacent to the channel. The LDD structure also provides these shallow junctions which in this context are often called the "tip" or "extension" regions since they must be combined with deeper source and drain junctions away from the channel in order to make reliable contacts to the device. The N^- and P^- implants in Figures 2–27 and 2–28 and the sidewall spacers in Figure 2–30 are used to construct these tip or extension or LDD regions.

In Figure 2–27, photoresist is spun on the wafer and mask 7 is then used to protect all the devices except the NMOS transistors. A phosphorus implant is done to form the N^- region. The dose and the energy are carefully controlled in this implant to ultimately produce the desired graded drain junction. Typically, a dose of about 5×10^{13} to 5×10^{14} cm^{-2} at a low energy might be used. A similar sequence of steps is used for the PMOS devices in Figure 2–28 to produce the LDD regions in these devices. A similar implant would be performed although boron would be used in this case. In some modern MOS device structures, the "LDD" implants may actually consist of several implants at different energies and doses. Some of these implants may even be done at angles tilted with respect to the wafer surface in order to get the implant further under the edge of the gate. The objective is to carefully tailor the doping profile near the drain junction (and the source junction) in order to minimize short channel effects. The exact 2D shape of the resulting profile is crucial in obtaining the correct device characteristics and computer simulation is often very useful in understanding and predicting the structure and properties of these critical regions. We will consider these issues more carefully in later chapters.

The next step is the LPCVD deposition of a conformal spacer dielectric layer (SiO_2 or Si_3N_4) on the wafer surface, shown in Figure 2–29. The thickness of this layer will determine the width of the sidewall spacer region and would be chosen to optimize device characteristics. Typically this might be a few hundred nm. If SiO_2 is used, it could be deposited by a $SiH_4 + O_2$ reaction at about 400°C or by a $SiH_2Cl_2 + N_2O$ reaction at about 900°C or other similar reactions, in a standard furnace configured as a CVD or LPCVD system.

$$SiH_4 + O_2 \rightarrow SiO_2 + 2H_2 \quad (2.6)$$

$$SiH_2Cl_2 + N_2O \rightarrow SiO_2 + 2N_2 + 2HCl \quad (2.7)$$

We now make use of a technique to form the sidewall spacers that really is a result of the efforts that have gone into developing anisotropic plasma etching capabilities in

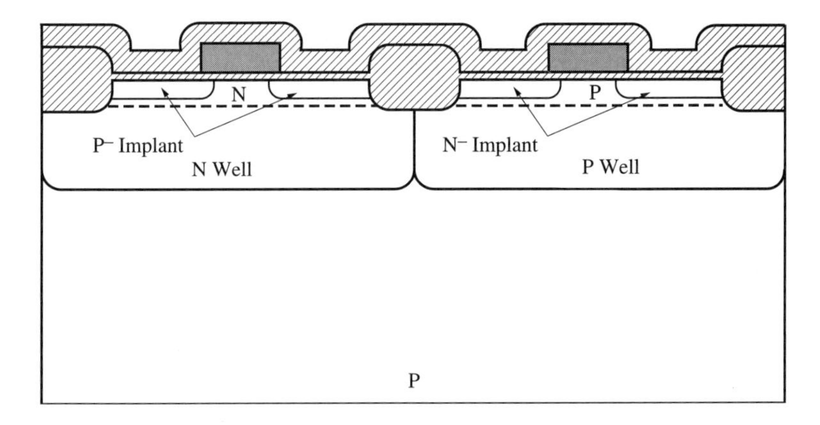

Figure 2–29 A conformal layer of SiO_2 is deposited on the wafer in preparation for sidewall spacer formation.

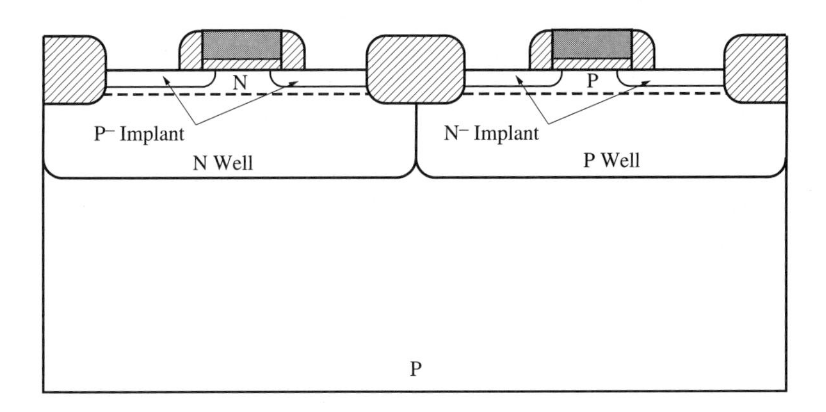

Figure 2–30 The deposited SiO_2 layer is etched back anisotropically, leaving sidewall spacers along the edges of the polysilicon.

recent years. Notice in Figure 2–29 that the deposited SiO_2 layer is much thicker along the edges of the polysilicon than it is above flat regions of the wafer surface. This is because of the vertical edges of the polysilicon regions, and the conformal deposition of the oxide. If we now etch back the deposited SiO_2 layer using an etching technique that is highly anisotropic (etches vertically but not horizontally) then we will be left with the structure shown in Figure 2–30. Typically this would be done in a fluorine-based plasma.

The deposited oxide is removed everywhere except along the edges of vertical steps in the underlying structures. Simply by a deposition and then an etchback, we have formed the sidewall spacers. We have also created lateral features on the chip surface that are smaller than the minimum feature size of the lithographic process. In fact the width of the spacers is determined largely by the thickness of the deposited oxide. It should also be noted that there is nothing magic about the use of SiO_2 in this application. We could form such spacers using almost any deposited thin film. In this particular case we need an insulating material for reasons that will become apparent shortly, so SiO_2 is a convenient choice.

2.2.8 Source/Drain Formation

At this point, most of the doped regions in the structure have been formed except for the MOS transistor source and drain regions. Note however that in Figure 2–30 the oxide was etched off the source and drain regions as part of the sidewall spacer formation process. Generally implants are done through a thin "screen" oxide, whose purpose is both to help avoid channeling and to minimize the incorporation of trace impurities into the silicon from the implanter. Channeling is a result of the fact the silicon is crystalline. If the implanted ions have a velocity vector that lines up with the crystal structure of the substrate, ions can go down "channels" between lattice sites for long distances without encountering silicon atoms which slow the implanted atoms down via collisions. If this happens, the range of the implanted ions can be significantly larger than expected. This is generally undesirable and the thin screen oxide (which is amorphous) helps to randomize the directions of the implanted ions and therefore minimize channeling. We will discuss these effects in more detail in Chapter 8. Prior to doing the source drain implants then, a thin screen oxide of perhaps 10 nm is grown. Note that this also produces a thin oxide on the top exposed surface of the polysilicon.

The first source drain implant is illustrated in Figure 2–31. Photoresist and mask 9 are used to define the regions where NMOS source/drain implants will be done. Arsenic

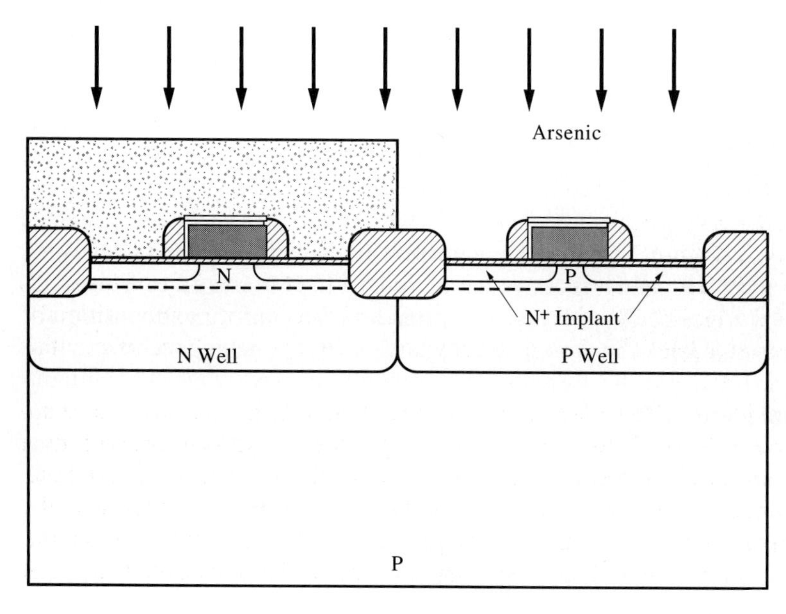

Figure 2–31 After growing a thin "screen" oxide, photoresist is applied and mask 9 is used to protect the PMOS transistors. An arsenic implant then forms the NMOS source and drain regions.

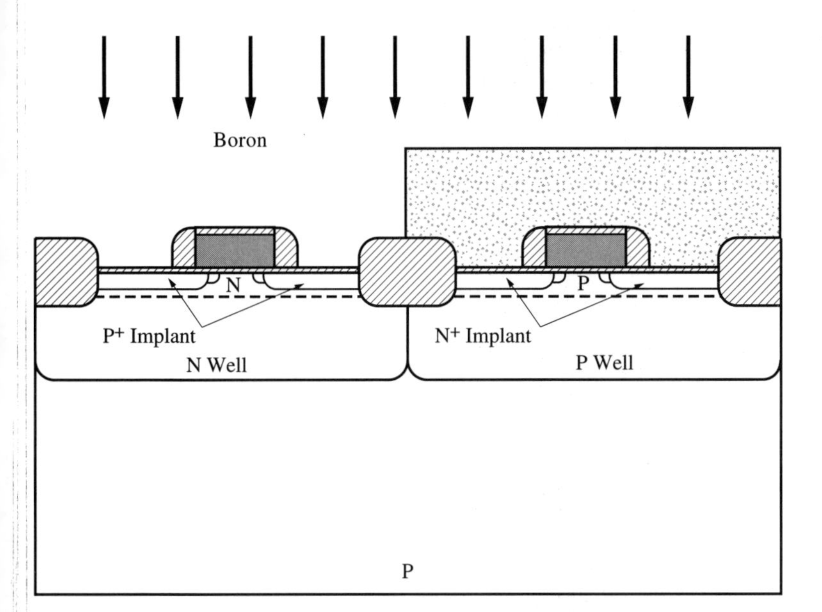

Figure 2–32 After applying photoresist, mask 10 is used to protect the NMOS transistors. A boron implant then forms the PMOS source and drain regions.

would be the dopant of choice in modern processes, because of the need to keep junctions shallow in small geometry devices. An implant of $2 - 4 \times 10^{15}$ cm^{-2} at an energy of 75 keV might be typical. This would allow the arsenic to penetrate the screen oxide in the implanted areas but still be easily masked by the photoresist.

The final mask used for doping is illustrated in Figure 2–32. Photoresist and mask 10 allow a boron implant to form the PMOS source/drain regions. This implant would also be a high-dose implant, on the order of $1–3 \times 10^{15}$ cm^{-2}, but at a lower energy of about 50 – 75 keV because boron is much lighter than arsenic and therefore requires less energy to reach the same range. High-dose implants minimize the parasitic resistances associated with the source and drain regions in the MOS transistors. It is also interesting to notice that the polysilicon gate regions receive at least two high-dose implants in the process flow we have described. The first, which was N^+, occurred in connection with Figure 2–27 and initially heavily doped the poly N type. In the NMOS devices, a second N^+ implant goes into the poly in Figure 2–31. In the PMOS device a P^+ implant dopes the poly in Figure 2–32. In most processes today both the PMOS and NMOS gates are N type. If this is the case, then the P^+ dose in Figure 2–32 needs to be smaller than the N^+ dose implanted in Figure 2–27. This is the case for the numbers we have used in this process flow.

The final step in active device formation is illustrated in Figure 2–33. A furnace anneal, typically at $\approx$ 900°C for 30 min, or perhaps a rapid thermal anneal for $\approx$ 1 min at 1000 – 1050°C activates all the implants, anneals implant damage, and drives the junctions to their final depths. The many implants that have been done to form the N and P regions in the transistors create significant damage to the crystal structure of the silicon. This damage is generally repairable as was pointed out earlier. However the repair

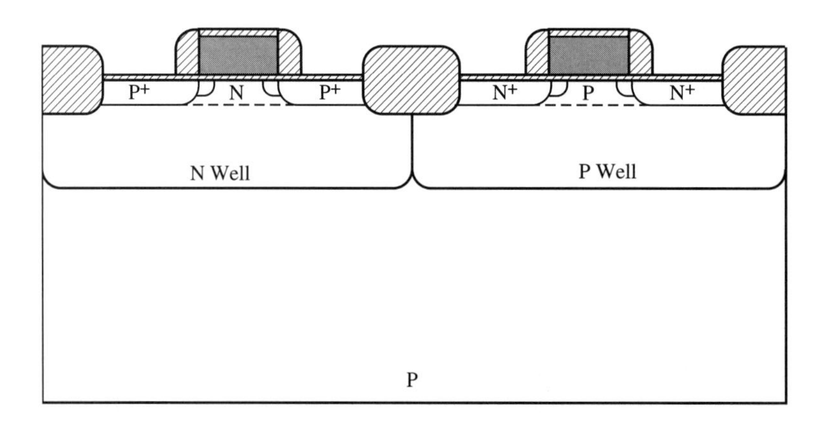

Figure 2–33 A final high-temperature drive-in activates all the implanted dopants and diffuses junctions to their final depth.

process takes some time (< 1 min at 1000°C or several hours at very low temperatures like 700°C). While this repair is occurring, dopants diffuse with anomalously high diffusivities because the damage enhances their diffusion coefficients. This phenomenon in known as Transient Enhanced Diffusion, or TED, and is a very important issue in keeping junctions shallow in scaled devices. We will discuss this in more detail in Chapter 8.

2.2.9 Contact and Local Interconnect Formation

All of the steps needed to form the active devices have now been completed. However, we obviously need to provide a means of interconnecting them on the wafer to form circuits, and a means to bring the input and output connections off the chip for packaging. The CMOS process we are describing will actually provide three levels of wiring to accomplish these objectives. The first or lowest level is often called the "local interconnect" and the steps needed to form it are shown in Figures 2–34 to 2–37. (Actually as we pointed out earlier, the polysilicon gate level itself can also be used as a local interconnect.)

The first step, illustrated in Figure 2–34, removes the oxide from the areas the interconnect is to contact. Since this is the bottom level of the interconnect structure, it will provide the connections to essentially all doped regions in the silicon and to all polysilicon regions. This oxide etch can actually be unmasked because the oxide is quite thin over the regions we wish to contact (the ≈ 10 nm screen oxide we grew just prior to source drain formation). A short dip in a buffered HF etching solution will remove these oxide layers, without significantly reducing the thickness of the oxide layers elsewhere.

The next step (Figure 2–35) involves the deposition of a thin layer (50 – 100 nm) of Ti on the wafer surface. This is usually done by sputtering from a Ti target. In a sputtering system, atoms of the desired material (Ti in this case) are physically knocked off a solid target by bombarding the Ti target with Ar^+ ions. The Ti atoms then deposit on

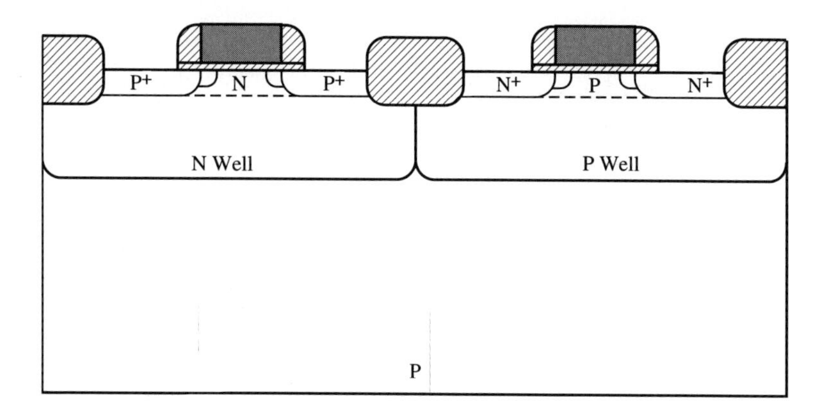

Figure 2–34 An unmasked oxide etch removes the SiO_2 from the device source drain regions and from the top surface of the polysilicon.

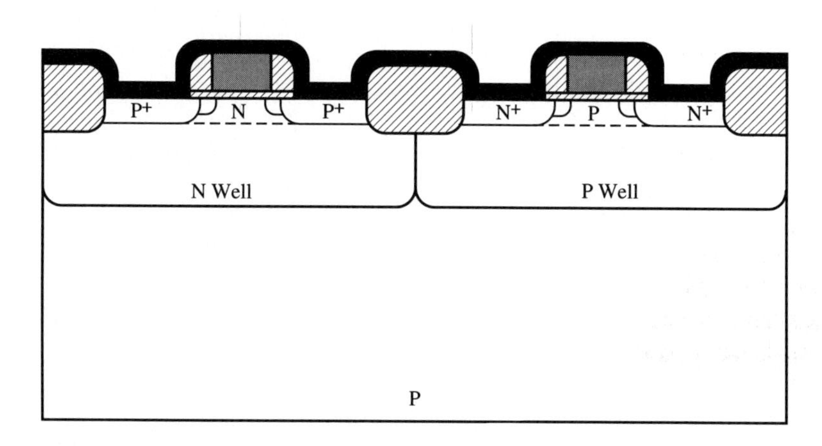

Figure 2–35 Titanium is deposited on the wafer surface by sputtering.

any substrates that are located nearby. This produces a continuous coating of Ti on the wafer as shown in Figure 2–35.

The next step, shown in Figure 2–36, makes use of two chemical reactions. The wafers are heated in an N_2 ambient at about 600 – 700°C for a short time (about 1 minute). At this temperature, the Ti reacts with Si where they are in contact to form $TiSi_2$, consuming some silicon in the process. This is why deeper source and drain junctions are required outside the tip or extension regions. $TiSi_2$ is an excellent conductor and forms low resistance contacts to both N^+ and P^+ silicon or polysilicon. This material is shown in black in Figure 2–36. The Ti also reacts with N_2 to form TiN (the dotted top layer in Figure 2–36). This material is also a conductor, although its conductivity is not as high as most metals. For this reason, it is used only for "local" or short-distance interconnects.

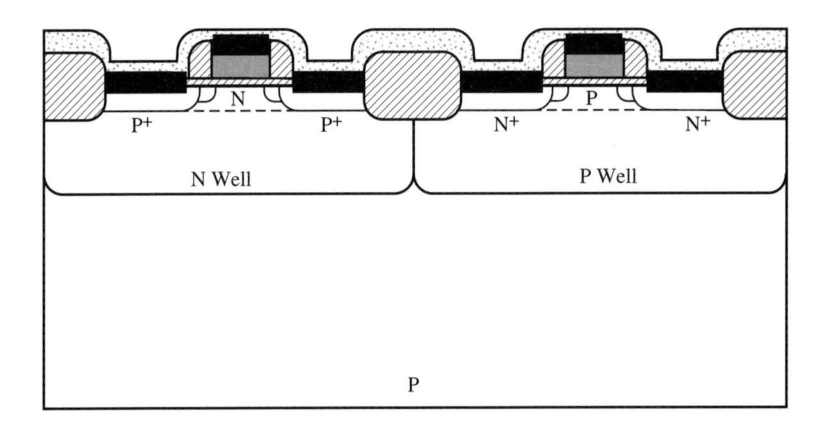

Figure 2–36 The titanium is reacted in an N_2 ambient, forming $TiSi_2$ where it contacts silicon or polysilicon (black regions in the figure) and TiN elsewhere.

The resistance of long lines made from TiN would cause unacceptable RC delays in most circuits.

Figure 2–37 illustrates the patterning of the TiN layer. Photoresist is applied and mask 11 protects the TiN where we want it to remain on the wafer. The remaining TiN is etched in $NH_4OH:H_2O_2:H_2O$ (1:1:5) to remove it. It is interesting to note at this point that the sidewall spacers we used earlier to provide graded N^+N^- or P^+P^- drain junctions also serve the function here of separating the $TiSi_2$ on the poly gates from contacting the silicon doped regions. After photoresist removal, the wafer would typically be heated in a furnace in an Ar ambient at about 800°C for about 1 minute to reduce the resistivity of the TiN and $TiSi_2$ layers to their final values (about 10 Ω/sq and 1 Ω/sq, respectively). The photoresist would be removed prior to this last high temperature anneal in an O_2 plasma or through chemical stripping, since photoresist cannot tolerate temperatures much above 100°C.

2.2.10 Multilevel Metal Formation

The final steps in our CMOS process involve the deposition and patterning of the two layers of metal interconnect. These steps are illustrated in Figures 2–38 to 2–44.

At this stage in the process, the surface of the wafer is highly nonplanar. We have grown and deposited many thin films on the surface and after these films are patterned, they leave numerous hills and valleys on the surface. It is not desirable to deposit the metal interconnect layers directly on such topography because there are potential problems with metal discontinuities (opens) at steps on the surface. There are also potential reliability problems even if the metal does not break at such steps, because it will likely be thinner where it crosses the steps. In addition, and perhaps most importantly, photolithography is very difficult with highly nonplanar substrates, especially when metal patterning is involved.

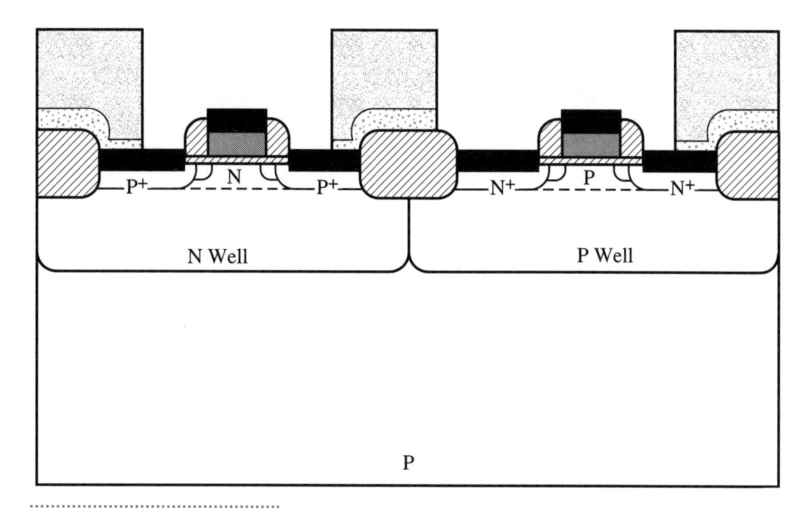

Figure 2–37 Photoresist is applied and mask 11 is used to define the regions where TiN local interconnects will be used. The TiN is then etched.

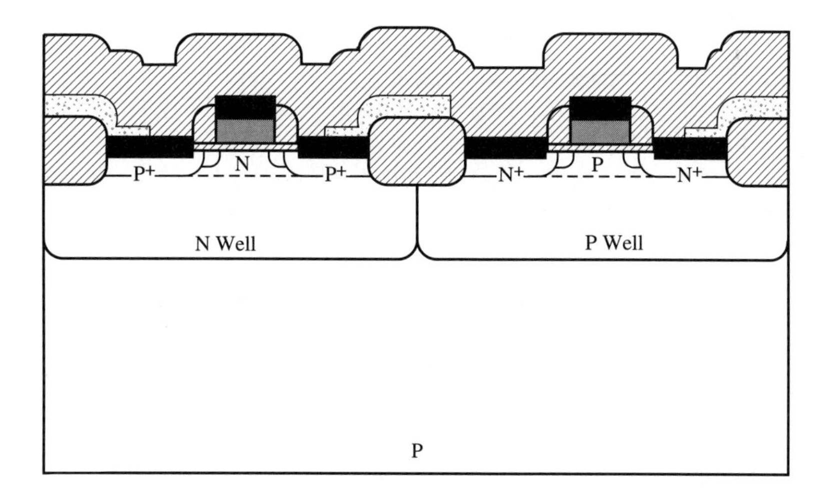

Figure 2–38 After stripping the photoresist, a conformal SiO_2 layer is deposited by LPCVD.

In an effort to circumvent these problems, many techniques have been devised to "planarize" or flatten the surface topography. One such method that is widely used is illustrated in Figures 2–38 and 2–39. A fairly thick SiO_2 layer is first deposited on the wafer surface by CVD or LPCVD. This layer is deposited thicker than the largest steps which exist on the surface and would typically be about 1 μm. This SiO_2 layer is often doped with phosphorus and sometimes with boron as well, in which cases the deposited oxide is known as PSG (phosphosilcate glass) or BPSG (borophosphosilicate glass), respectively. In some cases an undoped SiO_2 layer is added on top of the PSG or BPSG

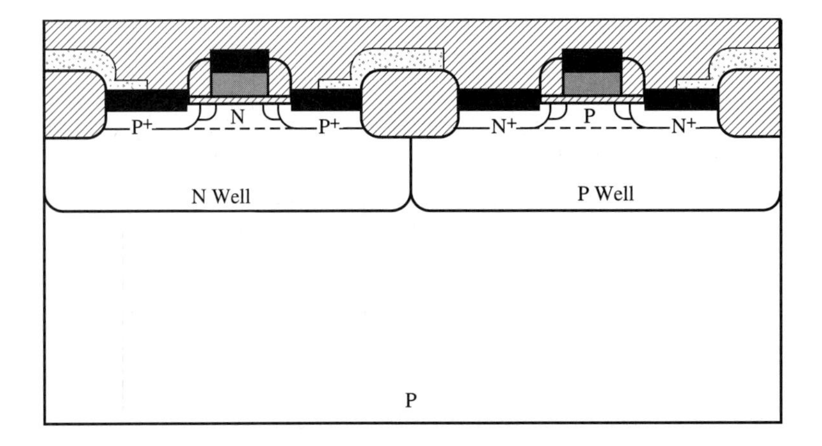

Figure 2–39 Chemical-Mechanical Polishing (CMP) or resist etchback is used to polish or etchback the deposited SiO_2 layer. This planarizes the wafer surface.

layer. The phosphorus provides some protection against mobile ions like Na^+ which can cause instabilities in MOS devices as was briefly mentioned in Chapter 1. The addition of the boron reduces the temperature at which the deposited glass layer "flows." This is important because following the deposition, the wafer is often heated to a temperature of 800 – 900°C which allows the glass to flow and to smooth the surface topography. Adding the boron minimizes the heat treatment required to accomplish this reflow, which is an issue because of the limited temperature tolerance of some of the underlying films at this point in the process. We will discuss these issues in more detail in Chapter 4 (Na^+ problems) and in Chapter 11 (glass reflow issues).

Reflowing the deposited PSG or BPSG layer is not sufficient to completely planarize the surface topography, so generally additional steps are required. For many years, this was commonly done by next spinning a layer of photoresist on to the wafer. Since the resist is a liquid, it will fill in the hills and valleys on the surface and produce a fairly flat upper surface. (We have actually drawn all the resist layers in earlier drawings this way, although without any explanation until this point.) The "trick" to accomplish planarization now takes place. It is possible to find a set of plasma etch conditions in which both resist and SiO_2 are etched at about the same rate. If we use such a plasma and etch the structure with no mask, then Figure 2–39 will result. We simply etch through the resist and down into the underlying oxide and stop when we have etched into the oxide everywhere. The 1:1 etch rate of resist and oxide preserves the originally flat resist upper surface as we etch.

Within the past few years, a replacement for this resist etchback technique has been commonly adopted in the semiconductor industry. This replacement is Chemical-Mechanical Polishing or CMP which we previously described in connection with the STI process option (Figures 2–8 and 2–9). In this process, the wafer is placed face down in a polishing machine and the upper surface is literally polished flat using a high-pH sil-

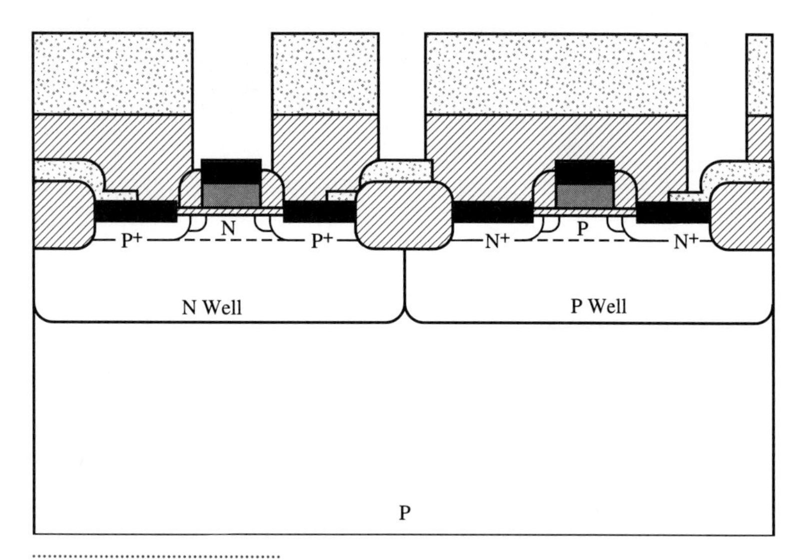

Figure 2–40 Photoresist is spun onto the wafer. Mask 12 is used to define the contact holes. The deposited SiO_2 layer is then etched to allow connections to the silicon, polysilicon and local interconnect regions.

ica slurry. The polishing process also results in the structure shown in Figure 2–39. CMP is discussed in more detail in Chapter 11.

The next step is again application of photoresist. We use mask 12 to define the regions where we want contact to be made between metal level 1 and underlying structures. This is shown in Figure 2–40. The SiO_2 layer would be etched in a plasma. After etching the contact holes, the photoresist would be stripped off the wafer.

We wish to maintain the planar surface as we add metal layers to the structure. While there are a number of process flows which can achieve this, the particular process we will describe here (Figure 2–41) is one of the more common. The first step is a blanket deposition of a thin TiN layer or Ti/TiN bilayer by sputtering or CVD. This layer is typically only a few tens of nm thick. It provides good adhesion to the SiO_2 and other underlying materials present in the structure at this point. The TiN also acts as an effective barrier layer between the upper metal layers and the lower local interconnect layers which connect to the active devices. The next step is deposition of a blanket W layer by CVD as illustrated in Figure 2–41. A typical reaction might be

$$WF_6 + 3H_2 \rightarrow W + 6HF \tag{2.10}$$

The next step, illustrated in Figure 2–42, again involves CMP to planarize the wafer. The polishing in this case removes the W and the TiN everywhere except in the contact holes and provides a planar surface on which the first level metal can be deposited. This process flow we have described, in which contact holes are etched, filled, and planarized, is known as the damascene process. It is very common in back-end processing in silicon chips today and will be discussed in more detail in Chapter 11.

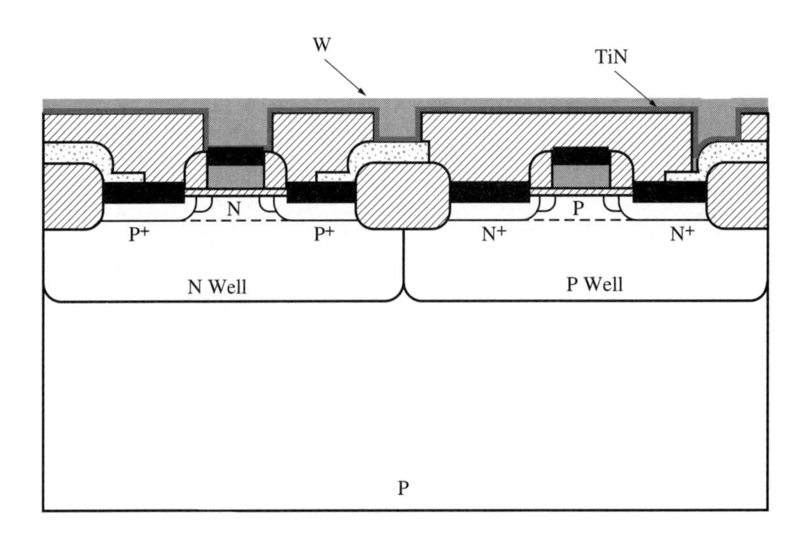

Figure 2–41 A thin TiN barrier/adhesion layer is deposited on the wafer by sputtering, followed by deposition of a W layer by CVD.

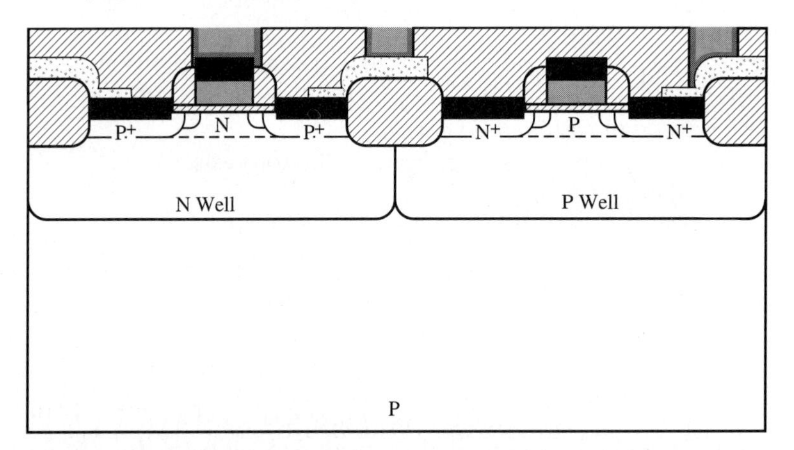

Figure 2–42 CMP is used to polish back the W and TiN layers, leaving a planar surface on which the first level of metal can be deposited.

Metal 1 is then deposited, usually by sputtering, and defined using resist and mask 13, as shown in Figure 2–43. The metal is commonly Al with a small percentage of Si and Cu in it. The Si is used because Si is soluble in Al up to a few percent and if the silicon is not already present in the Al, it may by absorbed by the Al from underlying silicon rich layers. This can cause problems with contact resistance and contact reliability. (Si absorption from underlying layers is less of a problem when barrier layers like TiN are used.) The Cu is added because it helps to prevent a reliability problem known as electromigration in Al thin films. This phenomenon causes open circuits in Al interconnects

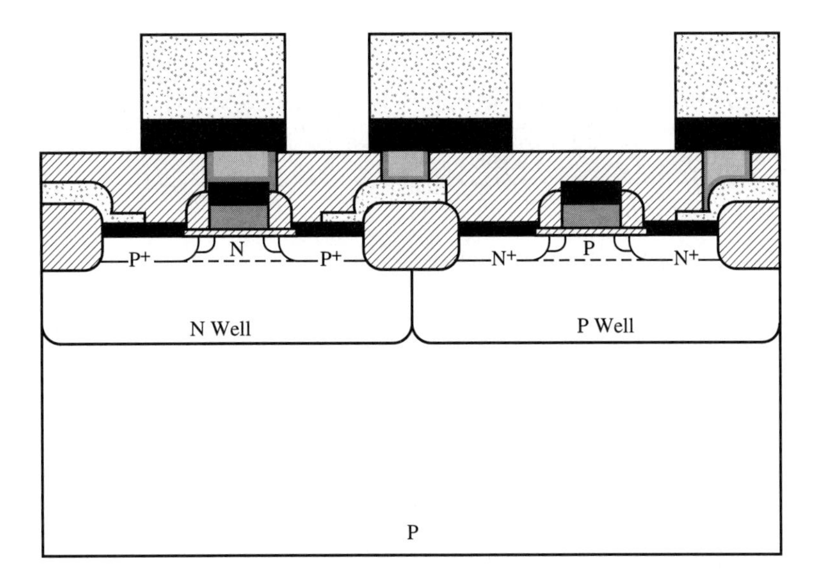

Figure 2–43 Aluminum is deposited on the wafer by sputtering. Photoresist is spun on the wafer and mask 13 is used to define the first level of metal. The A1 is then plasma etched.

after many hours of circuit operation, especially at elevated temperatures and high current densities, and is due to the formation of voids in the Al lines caused by diffusion of Al atoms. The Cu helps to prevent this from occurring.

Because of its better electrical conductivity, Cu is now beginning to replace Al as the interconnect metal. Cu is deposited using electroplating. Because Cu is quite difficult to etch using plasma etching, a somewhat different process flow is required than that described here for Al-based interconnects. Chapter 11 discusses these issues in more detail.

Most modern VLSI processes use more than one level of wiring on the wafer surface because in complex circuits it is usually very difficult to completely interconnect all the devices in the circuit without multiple levels. The processes that are used to deposit and define each level are similar to those we described for level 1 and usually involve a planarization step. Figure 2–44 illustrates this for the dielectric between metal 1 and metal 2. The process would again involve depositing an oxide layer and using CMP to planarize the deposited oxide. Figure 2–44 also illustrates the filling of the via holes between metal 1 and metal 2 with TiN and W, deposition and etching of metal 2, and the final deposition of a top dielectric to protect the finished chip. This top layer could be either SiO_2 or Si_3N_4 and is designed to provide some protection for the chip during the mechanical handling it will receive during packaging, as well as to provide a final passivation layer to protect the chip against ambient contamination (Na^+ or K^+). After the final processing steps are completed, an anneal and alloy step at a relatively low temperature (400 – 450°C) for about 30 minutes in forming gas (10% H_2 in N_2) is used to alloy the metal contacts in the structure and to reduce some of the electrical charges associated with the Si/SiO_2 interface. We will discuss these charges in more detail in

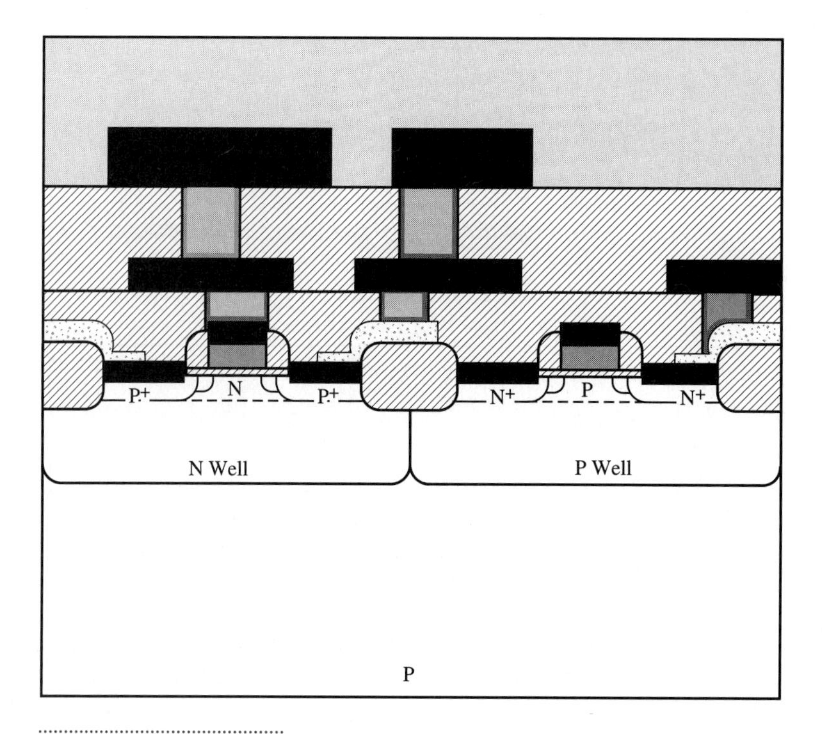

Figure 2–44 The steps to form the second level of Al interconnect follow those in Figures 2–38 to 2–43. Mask 14 is used to define via holes between metal 2 and metal 1. Mask 15 is used to define metal 2. The last step in the process is deposition of a final passivation layer, usually Si_3N_4 deposited by PECVD. The last mask (16) is used to open holes in this mask over the bonding pads.

Chapter 6. This finally brings us back to Figure 2–2 which is the completed CMOS chip that we started out to build.

2.3 Summary of Key Ideas

The purpose of this chapter was to describe in some detail a complete CMOS process flow. For readers relatively new to silicon technology, many new ideas were presented, often without full explanation or justification. All of these will be described in later chapters as we deal with the individual process steps. At this point, the context in which such processes are used should be clear.

A final point which is important to make is that the process we have described is not a unique way of achieving the final result shown in Figure 2–2. Many commercial companies and research laboratories today build chips with final cross sections similar to this figure, with however, quite different process details. As an example of the differences between commercially available CMOS process flows, the process described here required 16 masks through two levels of metal. Commercial processes range from simple CMOS with one level of metal and perhaps 10 masks, to very complex processes with five to six levels of metal and 20–25 masks. The reasons for these differences from one process to another may have to do with specific types of equipment a particular laboratory or plant has, or they may have to do with the applications targeted for the technology. Trade-offs in technology complexity and device performance may lead an individual company to a process flow quite different than the one we have described. Some of these trade-offs will become clearer as we discuss the individual process steps in later chapters.

Many of the process steps described in this chapter could be simulated with modern Technology Computer-Aided Design (TCAD) tools. We have not chosen to include such simulations in this chapter because the objective here was simply a qualitative description of a CMOS process flow. As we discuss the various technology steps in detail in subsequent chapters, we will also introduce simulation tools for those process steps.

2.4 Problems

2.1 Sketch a process flow that would result in the structure shown in Figure 1–34 by drawing a series of drawings similar to those in this chapter. You only need to describe the flow up through the stage at which active device formation starts since from that point on, the process is similar to that described in this chapter.

2.2. During the 1970s, the dominant logic technology was NMOS as described briefly in Chapter 1. A cross sectional view of this technology is shown below (see also Figure 1–33). The depletion mode device is identical to the enhancement mode device except that a separate channel implant is done to create a negative threshold voltage. Design a plausible process flow to fabricate such a structure, following the ideas of the CMOS process flow in this chapter. You do not have to include any quantitative process parameters (times, temperatures, doses, etc.) Your answer should be given in terms of a series of sketches of the structure after each major process step, like the figures in this chapter. Briefly explain your reasoning for each step and the order you choose to do things.

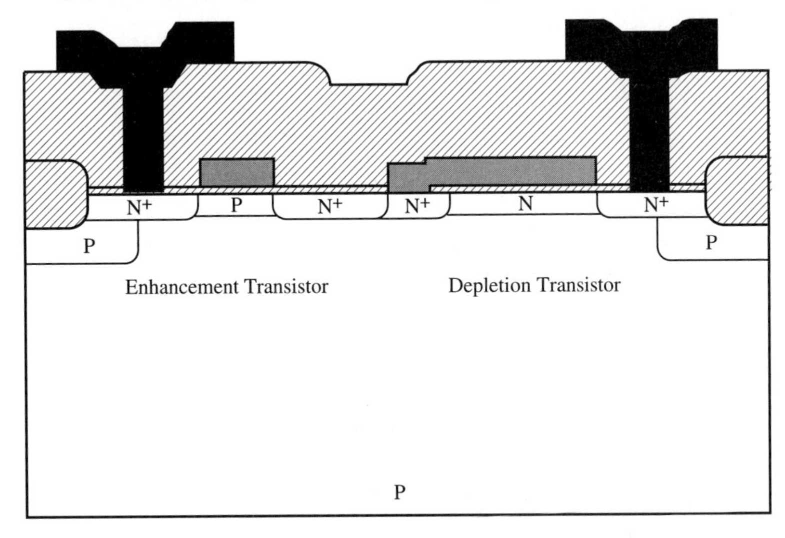

2.3. The cross section below illustrates a simple bipolar transistor fabricated as part of a silicon IC. (See also Figure 1–32.) Design a plausible process flow to fabricate such a structure, following the ideas of the CMOS process flow in this chapter. You do not have to include any quantitative process parameters (times, temperatures, doses, etc.) Your answer should be given in terms of a series of sketches of the structure after each major process step, like the figures in this chapter. Briefly explain your reasoning for each step and the order you choose to do things.

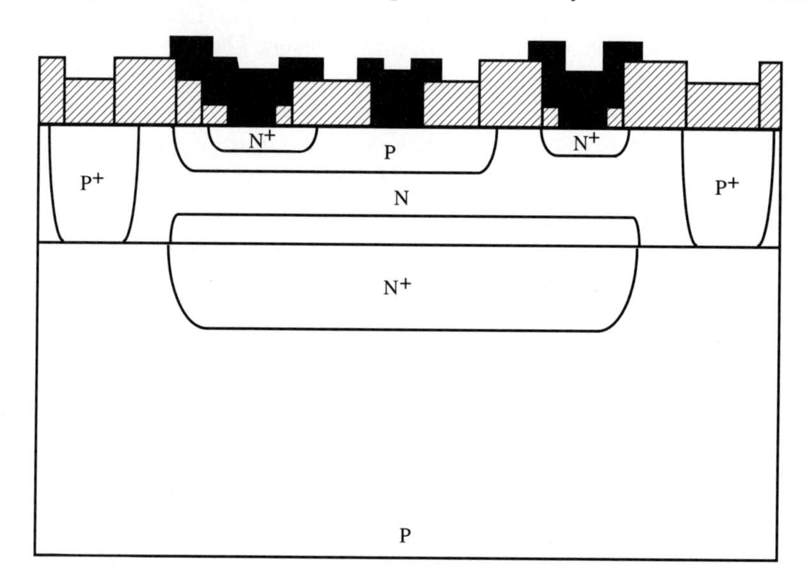

Crystal Growth, Wafer Fabrication and Basic Properties of Silicon Wafers

3

3.1 Introduction

In Chapter 1 we traced some of the important historical developments that led to the silicon IC industry as we know it today. Almost from the very beginning, it was clear that silicon was the best choice for the material on which to base this industry. The abundance of silicon, the availability of simple techniques for refining it and growing single crystals, the essentially ideal properties of the Si/SiO_2 interface, and the invention of manufacturing techniques based on the planar process, all led to the dominance of silicon based devices by the early 1960s.

The silicon industry depends on a ready supply of inexpensive, high-quality single-crystal wafers. In this chapter we will discuss the methods by which such wafers are prepared and some of the basic properties of these wafers. Integrated circuit manufacturers typically specify physical parameters (diameter, thickness, flatness, mechanical defects like scratches, crystallographic defects like dislocation density, etc.), electrical parameters (N or P type, dopant, resistivity, etc.), and finally, impurity levels (oxygen and carbon in particular) when purchasing wafers. All these parameters must be tightly controlled in order to use the wafers in the high-volume manufacturing of complex chips. We saw a specific example of this type of specification in Chapter 2 in the CMOS process. In that example, we specified a starting substrate which was P type (boron doped), (100) orientation, with a resistivity between 25 and 50 Ωcm. This resistivity corresponds to a doping concentration of about 10^{15} cm^{-3} or about 20 parts per billion boron. Although these are the principal parameters that need to be specified, a more complete wafer description would actually include many additional parameters as outlined above.

3.2 Historical Development and Basic Concepts

Although the first transistors were built in polycrystalline germanium, all modern integrated circuits depend on single-crystal material for optimum device operation. Polycrystalline or even amorphous materials can be used to build semiconductor devices, but the defects present in these materials act as generation and recombination centers and have significant effects on basic device properties like mobility and minority carrier lifetime. The result is poor performance in the devices—lower output currents for a given applied voltage, higher leakage currents in junctions, and poor reproducibility from one device to another. We begin this chapter with a discussion of some of the basic properties of crystals.

3.2.1 Crystal Structure

In crystalline materials, the atoms are arranged spatially in a periodic fashion. A basic unit cell can be defined which repeats in all three dimensions. A standard terminology is used to describe crystal directions and planes, which we will briefly describe here. In some cases, the electrical properties of devices fabricated in silicon depend on the particular crystal orientation used for the starting wafer. [Recall that in Chapter 2 in our discussion of the CMOS process, we chose a (100) crystal.] Quite often, these orientation-dependent effects are associated with wafer surfaces or material interfaces, where the crystal terminates. Here, atoms may be incompletely bonded and the exact atomic arrangement can make a difference in the electrical properties. Bulk properties in silicon are generally isotropic (independent of direction) because of the cubic symmetry of the silicon crystal.

Figure 3–1 illustrates three simple crystal unit cells. All are based on a cubic structure. The Body-Centered Cubic or BCC cell has an extra atom in the center of the cube; the Face-Centered Cubic or FCC cell has as extra atom in the center of each face of the cube. Silicon and other semiconductors have more complex unit cells than these simple examples, but we can illustrate all of the basic ideas about crystal directions and planes with these simpler structures. An *xyz* coordinate system defines the directions in the crystal. The dimension a is called the lattice constant and is the basic distance over which the unit cell repeats in the cubic crystal. Directions in crystals are expressed in terms of three integers, which are the same as the components of a vector in that direction. For example, to get from atom A in the cubic crystal to atom B, we move 1 unit in each (x, y, and z) direction. This is then the [111] direction in this crystal. To get from

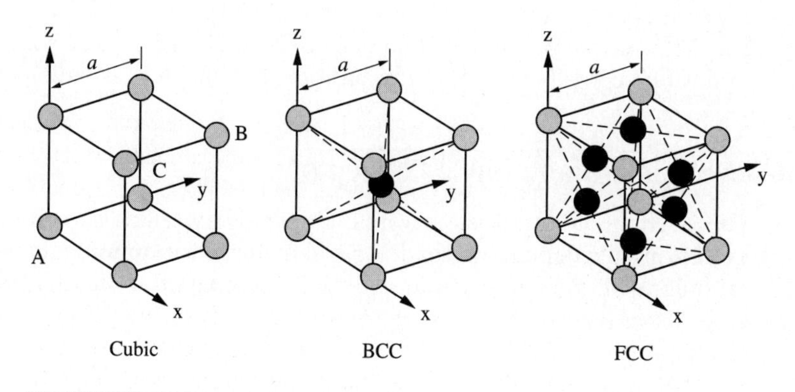

Figure 3–1 Unit cells in simple cubic crystals.

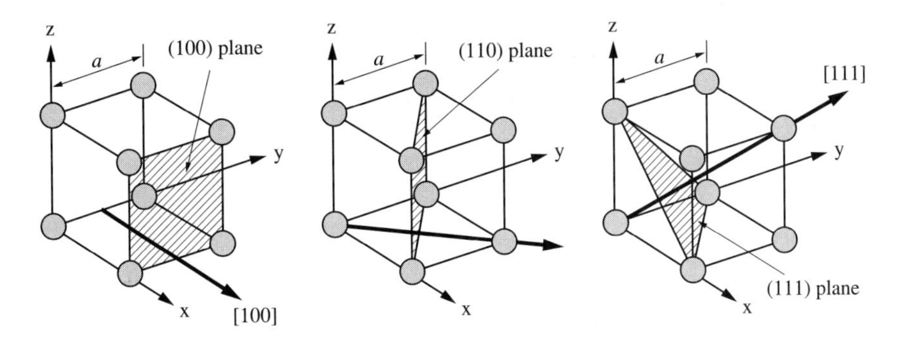

Figure 3–2 Crystal planes and major directions for a cubic lattice. The heavy arrows in each case illustrate crystal directions, designated [hkl]. The cross-hatched areas are the corresponding crystal planes, designated (hkl).

atom A to atom C, we would move in the [010] direction. By symmetry, many directions in a crystal are often equivalent, simply depending on our choice of reference. For example, the [100], [010], and [001] directions are all equivalent in this example and by convention, are referred to as <100> directions.

It is also useful to describe planes in a crystal and a convention has been adopted for doing this. Figure 3–2 illustrates three simple planes in a cubic crystal. Such planes are described by Miller indices, which are a set of three integers calculated as follows. For a particular plane, the intercepts of that plane with the three crystal axes are determined. In the middle example in Figure 3–2, the intercepts of the (110) plane with the x-, y-, and z-axes are 1, 1, and ∞, respectively. The reciprocals of these three intercepts are then taken, which gives 1/1 , 1/1 , and $1/\infty$ or simply the (110) plane. (The reciprocals eliminate infinities in the notation.) A minor complication can arise in this procedure if we pick a plane with intercepts outside the basic unit cell. For example, if we picked a plane with xyz intercepts of 3, 4, and 2, respectively, the reciprocals would be 1/3 , 1/4 , and 1/2 . In this case the smallest set of integers that have the same relative values are chosen for the Miller indices, which would result in the (436) plane in this case. There is also no reason why we could not pick a plane with a negative intercept, for example 1, −1, 2. In this case the reciprocals are 1/1 , 1/−1, and 1/2, respectively. The nomenclature in this case places a bar over the corresponding Miller indice, so that this plane becomes the $(2\bar{2}1)$ plane. Finally, as was the case for crystal directions, many crystal planes are also equivalent. The (100), (010), and $(0\bar{1}0)$ planes are all equivalent and are designated as {100} planes. Note that there are conventions which are used here for the style of bracket used to describe crystal directions and planes.

It should be noted that in cubic lattices, the direction [hkl] is perpendicular to a plane with the identical three integers (hkl), as illustrated in Figure 3–2. This is sometimes helpful in visualizing directions and planes in these crystals.

Silicon has a diamond cubic lattice structure, shown in Figure 3–3. This structure is most easily visualized as two merged FCC lattices with the origin of the second lattice offset from the first by $a/4$ in all three directions. Equivalently, one could think of the structure as an FCC lattice with two atoms at each lattice point, with the two offset from each other by $a/4$ in all three directions. Each atom is individually covalently bonded to four nearest neighbors, providing the electrical properties that we described in Chapter

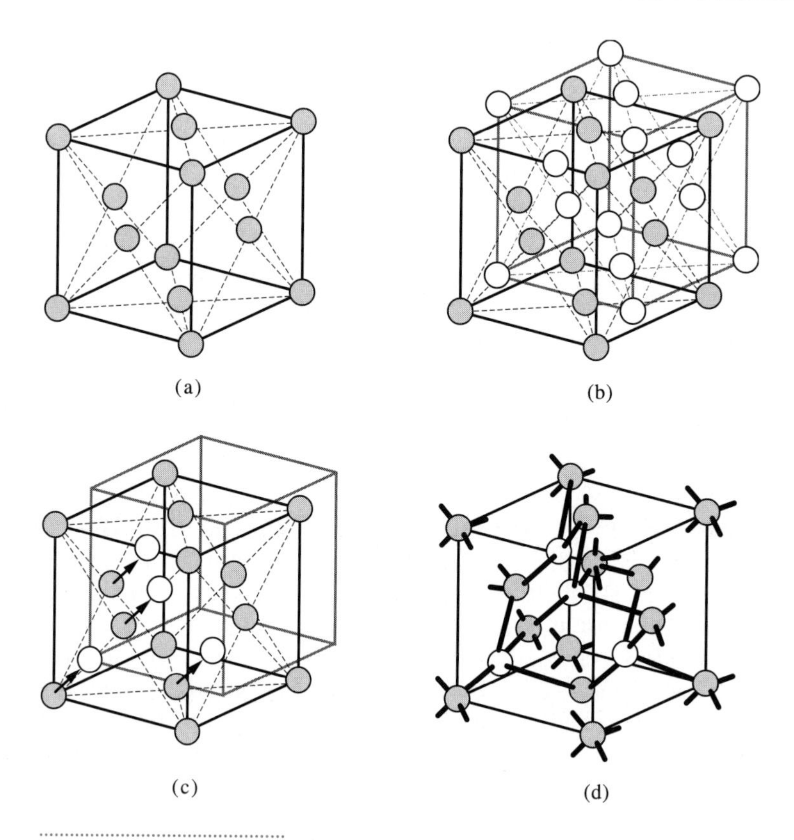

Figure 3–3 Diamond crystal structure of silicon. The unit cell may be visualized as two merged FCC cells, offset from each other by $a/4$ in all three directions. (a) shows the basic FCC unit cell. (b) shows two merged cells, offset by $a/4$. In (c), only the four atoms in the second FCC cell that lie within the first FCC cell are shown. The arrows show the corresponding $a/4$ displacement of these four atoms. In (d), the actual tetragonal bonding between the atoms in the diamond cell is shown.

1. Figure 3–3 illustrates the construction of the diamond lattice from the two merged FCC lattices.

There are two principal silicon crystal orientations that are used in manufacturing integrated circuits, (111) and (100) (meaning that the crystal terminates at the wafer surface on {111} or {100} planes respectively). As mentioned earlier, bulk properties of silicon are generally isotropic since the cubic crystal is symmetric. Thus we find, for example, that dopant diffusion coefficients are independent of the direction in which the dopant is diffusing as long as surfaces play no role in the process (Chapter 7). However, real devices are always built near surfaces and which crystal plane the surface terminates on can make a difference in the surface electrical and physical properties. {111} planes in silicon have the largest number of silicon atoms per cm^2, {100} planes the lowest. This results in a number of differences in properties. {111} planes oxidize faster than {100} because the oxidation rate is proportional to the number of silicon atoms available for reaction (Chapter 6). {111} surfaces have higher densities of electrical defects (interface states) because at least some of these defects are believed to be associated with dangling silicon bonds (Chapter 6). Finally, dopant diffusion coefficients and other properties in bulk silicon usually do depend on the surface orientation of the crystal because surfaces are often active interfaces and can perturb bulk properties large distances away from the surface (Chapter 6). Primarily because of the superior electrical properties of the (100) Si/SiO_2 interface, (100) silicon is dominant in manufacturing today. Virtually all MOS-based technologies use crystals with this orientation (like the CMOS process in Chapter 2). Historically many bipolar technologies used (111) crystals because this orientation is somewhat easier to grow by the Czochralski method described later in this chapter; however as bipolar devices have shrunk in size in recent years, they have become more sensitive to surface properties and increasingly also use (100) wafers.

A final point should be made regarding surface effects on device and process parameters. The CMOS process flow described in Chapter 2 illustrated the fact that many etching, oxidation, and deposition steps are used in modern processes. Such steps can end up producing a very nonplanar surface. In other words, the shaping and patterning of the silicon inherent to device fabrication will produce a device surface, which contains {100} surface regions along with almost every other possible crystal orientation. Physical or electrical parameters, which vary with surface orientation, will therefore vary with position in modern ICs. Modeling such effects is only possible with modern computer simulation tools which need to first predict the structure accurately enough to know the surface orientation as a function of position, and then predict the resulting orientation effects on device parameters.

3.2.2 Defects in Crystals

There are several types of defects which are commonly found in crystals. It is useful to classify these into four categories, depending on their dimensionality. The usual categories are point defects, line defects, area defects, and volume defects. Figure 3–4 illustrates some of the more common defects in a simple two-dimensional representation. We will find in later chapters that a number of these defects play important roles in various aspects of silicon technology.

Point defects are the simplest to visualize and they play crucial roles in impurity diffusion (Chapter 7), in ion implantation damage (Chapter 8), and lesser roles in oxidation kinetics (Chapter 6) and other phenomena. In general, anything other than a silicon atom on a lattice site constitutes a point defect. By this definition, for example, a substitutional doping atom is a point defect and might be referred to as an impurity-related defect. However, there are two principal types of point defects we shall be primarily concerned with which are often referred to as native point defects. The first is simply a missing silicon lattice atom or vacancy, which we shall designate simply as V. The other is an extra silicon atom which we shall designate simply as I. Figure 3–4 illustrates two possible arrangements of such an extra atom in the lattice. The upper case illustrates a purely interstitial atom, that is, an atom sitting unbonded in one of the available sites between silicon atoms. The second illustrates two atoms sharing one lattice

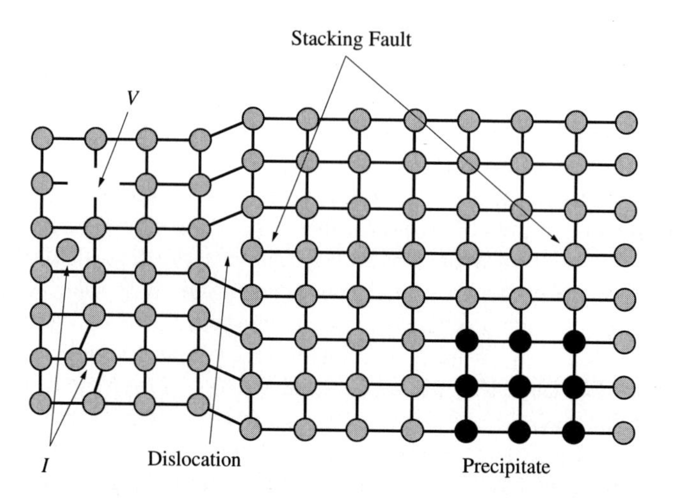

Figure 3–4 Simple 2D representation of some of the common defects found in crystals. *V* and *I* are point defects, the edge dislocation represents a typical line defect, the stacking fault is an area defect, and the precipitate is a volume defect.

site, a defect usually referred to as an interstitialcy. Most of the literature on silicon technology does not distinguish between these two defects, designating both of them as simply a silicon interstitial or *I*. Since the distinction is not usually important in modeling processes in silicon, we shall adopt this strategy in this book and simply use the symbol *I* to refer to an excess silicon atom. Most workers in the field today believe that the interstitialcy is likely the defect that is important in silicon processes, because of the lower energies required to create this defect compared to a pure interstitial. In general, the concentrations of both *V* and *I* increase as temperature increases. The equilibrium concentrations of these defects are essentially zero at room temperature, but they are much higher at process temperatures (10^{12}—10^{15} cm^{-3} at 1000°C). Quantitative models have been developed which describe the equilibrium concentrations of these defects in silicon. We will discuss these models later in this chapter.

One-dimensional defects in crystals are known as dislocations. An example is illustrated in Figure 3–4. The right-hand part of the crystal contains an extra plane of atoms, which terminates at a dislocation. The dislocation itself, then, is a linear defect in the direction into the paper. Dislocations either terminate at the edge of the crystal (edge dislocation), or they form a closed loop within the crystal (dislocation loops). Macroscopic edge dislocations are never present in silicon wafers at the start of IC manufacturing; such wafers are normally specified as "dislocation free." However, such defects can be generated during the high-temperature steps normally used in wafer fabrication, particularly if thin films present on the wafer surface generate high stresses. We saw one example of such a process in Chapter 2 when we considered the LOCOS method of forming SiO_2 locally on the wafer surface. The Si_3N_4 layer used in Figures 2–3 to 2–5 as a mask against oxidation is usually under large tensile stress, resulting in corresponding compressive stress in the silicon substrate. If these stresses are large enough, they can result in dislocation formation during the high-temperature LOCOS oxidation.

Another way in which such stresses can be generated is through temperature gradients. These can occur during crystal growth, when the seed is first inserted into the melt and the outside of the seed heats up more rapidly than the inside, or during wafer processing if a heating system is used which is nonuniform. In the crystal growth case, dislocation formation is inevitable when the seed is first inserted into the liquid silicon, but such dislocations can be grown out to the edge of the crystal during the initial stages of growth as discussed in Section 3.3. In the wafer heating case, large temperature gradients are not normally a problem during gradual heating or cooling cycles such as those encountered in furnaces. However, they can be a problem in newer rapid thermal processing systems, which use high-intensity lamps to heat wafers at a rate of hundreds of °C per second. Such systems are finding increased use for Rapid Thermal Annealing (RTA) of implant damage (Chapter 7), Rapid Thermal Oxidation (RTO) described in Chapter 6 and for other types of Rapid Thermal Processing (RTP). If the lamps in such systems are not configured to maintain a uniform temperature across the wafer, temperature gradients can result. Note that maintaining a uniform temperature is not necessarily the same thing as maintaining uniform energy input into the wafer because heat loss due to radiation or conduction may vary with position across a wafer, especially at the edges. If temperature gradients exist, the resulting thermal stresses are given approximately by

$$\sigma = \alpha Y \Delta T \tag{3.1}$$

where α is the thermal expansion coefficient of silicon, Y is Young's modulus and ΔT is the temperature difference across the wafer. The yield strength of silicon is on the order of 0.5×10^9 dyne cm^{-2} at process temperatures. Such stress levels can be reached, and dislocations therefore generated, with ΔT values on the order of 100°C.

Microscopic dislocation loops usually are present in silicon starting wafers. At the high temperatures associated with crystal growth, point defect concentrations are quite high. As the crystal is pulled from the melt and cools, there may not be sufficient time for the populations of these defects to reduce to the much lower equilibrium populations associated with lower temperatures. (The V and I concentrations could be reduced by recombination of the two defects with each other, or diffusion of the individual defects to the crystal surface.) Small dislocation loops can form during the cooling process as a result of the agglomeration of excess V or I. If, for example, the extra half-plane of atoms on the right of Figure 3–4 extended only over a small number of lattice sites, the dislocation bounding the extra plane would form a closed loop, often a circle, since a circle has the shortest dislocation length and lowest energy. Such a defect could be formed by a group of I forming the extra half-plane on the right of Figure 3–4, or by a group of V forming the missing half-plane on the left.

Dislocations are active defects in crystals, that is they can move when subjected to stresses or when excess point defects are present. The process of "climb" occurs when excess point defects are absorbed by the dislocation. It is easy to visualize in Figure 3–4, for example, the dislocation moving one lattice plane to the left by absorbing an I, or

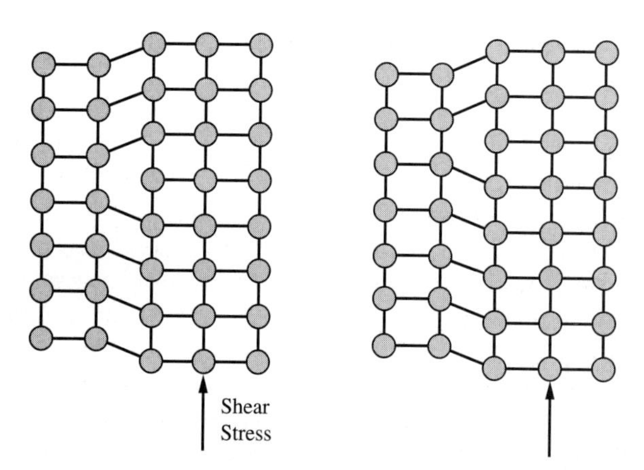

Figure 3–5 Movement of a dislocation by glide in response to shear stress.

moving one lattice plane to the right by absorbing a V. In fact these kinds of processes are often useful in determining whether a particular processing step increases or decreases V or I concentrations, by observing whether dislocations move during that step. We will discuss this idea more carefully in connection with stacking faults below. It is also possible for dislocations to move by "gliding" in response to shear stresses. Figure 3–5 illustrates this process. In silicon, the glide planes are {111} planes, the most densely packed planes. The fact that dislocations prefer to propagate along these planes also makes it possible to "grow out" such defects during the initial stages of crystal growth.

The most common kind of 2D or area defect found in silicon is the stacking fault. Such a defect is schematically shown in Figure 3–4. Stacking faults always form along {111} planes and are simply the insertion or removal of an extra {111} plane. In the silicon crystal structure shown in Figure 3–3, there are actually 3 parallel {111} planes in each unit cell commonly referred to as A, B, and C. In a perfect crystal, the stacking order is ABCABC, and so on. When a stacking fault is present, either an extra plane is inserted (ABCACBC, etc.) or a plane is missing (ABCABABC, etc.). Such faults are referred to as "extrinsic" if there is an extra plane of atoms, or "intrinsic" if a plane is missing. Stacking faults are bounded by dislocations and, when they intersect the wafer surface, are usually referred to as surface stacking faults. It is relatively easy to measure the density and the size of stacking faults in silicon using chemical etchants, which preferentially attack the highly stressed regions associated with the dislocations that bound the faults. This is discussed in more detail in Section 3.4.

Most of the stacking faults observed in silicon have been determined to be of the extrinsic type, implying that they formed in an environment of excess interstitials. Since the size of the faults can be determined experimentally, this measurement can be used as a means of determining whether a particular process increases or decreases point defect concentrations. If the faults are extrinsic, then they will grow by absorbing more I, or shrink by absorbing V. Experiments like this have been used to determine that oxidation injects excess interstitials into the underlying substrate, since stacking faults are observed to grow during oxidation. Stacking faults which are used as markers in such experiments are sometimes called Oxidation Induced Stacking Faults or OISF. We will discuss these experiments in more detail in Chapters 6 and 7 when we examine point defect based models for oxidation and diffusion.

Volume defects in crystals can include agglomerations of point defects such as a void caused by a collection of vacancies, precipitates of dopants or impurities, which may be crystalline or amorphous, or other 3D defects. One example is shown in Figure 3–4 where a cluster of doping atoms is shown, in this case as a crystalline precipitate (presumed in this example to extend into the third dimension). "Crystalline precipitate" is used in this case because each of the precipitated atoms occupies a lattice site. Such defects may nucleate either heterogeneously because of an existing crystal defect such as a dislocation, or homogeneously when through random diffusion, several of the species involved come close enough together to form a critical size nucleus for the precipitate. There are several such situations of importance in silicon technology. When doping concentrations are pushed too high (beyond the solubility of the dopant in the crystal), precipitation of dopant atoms in amorphous or crystalline clusters is often observed. The doping atoms in these clusters are usually not electrically active. Another example occurs in CZ silicon because of the relatively high oxygen impurity level. The oxygen is usually incorporated at a level corresponding to its solubility at the crystal growth temperature ($\approx 10^{18}$ cm^{-3}). This is far higher than oxygen's solubility at normal device fabrication temperatures, with the result that oxygen precipitation and clustering can occur during normal device fabrication. In some situations, this can actually be a useful event, since if the resulting dislocations and damage are kept away from active device regions, these heavily faulted regions can actually preferentially getter or collect unwanted impurities like heavy metals, keeping them away from device active regions. This is usually accomplished by precipitating the oxygen in the bulk of the wafer, away from the surface where the active devices are located. We will discuss this process in more detail later in this chapter in Section 3.5.5.

We will find many examples throughout this book in which crystalline defects play important roles in process steps. In some cases the role is very beneficial; in others the defects are minimized as much as possible to prevent unwanted effects. In both cases, it has become very important in recent years to both understand and control these defects. We will deal with specific cases of how this is done as the need arises for specific technology steps throughout the book.

3.2.3 Raw Materials and Purification

Fortunately, silicon is a very abundant material, representing about 25.7% of the earth's crust. Naturally occurring minerals containing silicon are very impure, however, which means that the silicon must be refined as well as be converted into the crystalline form. This is usually a multistage process, beginning with quartzite, a type of sand. Chemically quartzite is SiO_2. The first step in the refining process is to convert the quartzite to Metallurgical Grade Silicon or MGS. This process usually takes place in a furnace in which a mixture of the quartzite and a carbon source (usually coal or coke) is heated to temperatures approaching 2000°C. The power source is electric, provided by submerged electrodes, which arc and heat the charge. A number of reactions take place in the furnace, the overall result of which is that liquid silicon is drawn off and CO is given off as a gas, as shown below.

$$2C(solid) + SiO_2(solid) \rightarrow Si(liquid) + 2CO \tag{3.2}$$

Significant amounts of electric power are required to drive this process (about 13 kWh kg^{-1}). The MGS grade silicon that results is about 98% pure, with aluminum and iron being two of the dominant impurities. Interestingly, most of the silicon that is used each year in industry is of the MGS form. A small portion of this is used for electronic applications (low-efficiency solar cells, for example), but the vast majority is used in the manufacturing of aluminum or for silicone polymers.

To convert the MGS to Electronic Grade Silicon (EGS), several steps are required. In the first of these the MGS reacts with gaseous HCl, usually by grinding the MGS to a fine powder and then reacting it in the presence of a catalyst at elevated temperatures. This process can form any of a number of SiHCl compounds (SiH_4—silane; SiH_3Cl—chlorosilane; SiH_2Cl_2—dichlorosilane; $SiHCl_3$—trichlorosilane; or $SiCl_4$—silicon tetrachloride). The formation of $SiHCl_3$ is most commonly used today. $SiHCl_3$ is a liquid at room temperature, so it can be purified by fractional distillation. In this process, the $SiHCl_3$ is boiled along with the impurities it contains and separated by its boiling point. After this process, the $SiHCl_3$ is extremely pure and is ready to be converted back to purified polysilicon. This is accomplished in a large Chemical Vapor Deposition (CVD) reactor using the following reaction:

$$2SiHCl_3(gas) + 2H_2(gas) \rightarrow 2Si(solid) + 6HCl(gas) \tag{3.3}$$

A thin silicon rod is used as the nucleation surface, on which the silicon deposits. Since the rod is not a single-crystal, polysilicon is deposited. Typically the rod is heated by passing an electric current through it. The polysilicon, which is deposited, may be several meters long and several hundred mm in diameter. The overall deposition can take many days. Finally, the resulting polysilicon is broken up into pieces to load into crucibles for Czochralski crystal growth, or the poly rod itself could be used as the starting material for float-zone crystal growth. Both are described later in this chapter. The overall result of these purification steps is that the final product (polysilicon) has only parts per billion (ppb) or on the order of $10^{13} - 10^{14}$ cm^{-3} impurities. This represents about an eight order of magnitude improvement from the starting quartzite and makes EGS the purest material routinely available on earth.

It is interesting to note that the CVD process represented by Eq. (3.3) is conceptually similar to the polysilicon CVD process we described in Chapter 2 in the CMOS process. However, the constraints are different in the two cases. In the CMOS application, a well-controlled, smooth layer was needed so the deposition was done at relatively low temperatures and at a fairly slow rate. In the MGS applications these issues are unimportant so the deposition can be done at a much higher temperature and in a much less controlled manner. The only thing that matters in the latter case is depositing the poly as economically as possible.

3.2.4 Czochralski and Float-Zone Crystal Growth Methods

The two methods used to grow silicon crystals today are the Czochralski (CZ) and the Float-Zone (FZ) techniques. CZ is much more common because it is capable of easily producing large diameter crystals, from which large diameter wafers can be cut. The only significant drawback to the CZ method is that the silicon is contained in liquid form in a crucible during growth and as a result, impurities from the crucible are incorporated in the growing crystal. Oxygen and carbon are the two most significant contaminants. These impurities are not always a drawback, however. Oxygen in particular can be very useful in mechanically strengthening the silicon crystal and in providing a means for gettering other unwanted impurities during device fabrication. We will return to these issues later in this chapter.

The CZ growth technique is illustrated conceptually in Figure 3–6. Pieces of EGS are placed in a silica (SiO_2) crucible along with a small amount of doped silicon and melted. The melt temperature is stabilized at just above the silicon melting point (1417°C). In a typical modern crystal CZ crystal puller, a silicon charge of about 100 kg is placed in a 50-cm diameter crucible. This results in a 20-cm diameter crystal about 1 meter long after growth. A small single-crystal seed is then lowered into the melt. The crystal orientation of this seed will determine the orientation of the resulting pulled crystal and

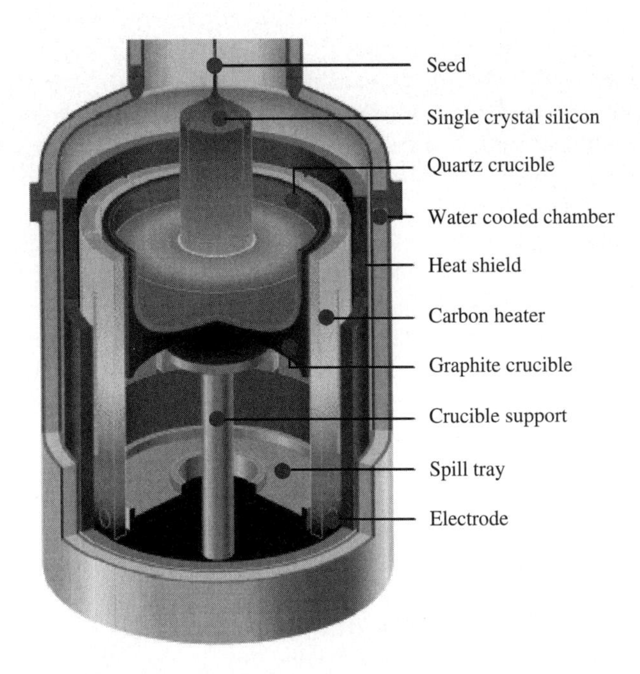

Figure 3–6 Basic Czochralski (CZ) crystal growing apparatus. This figure was taken directly from the Silicon Database on the Mitsubishi Materials Silicon Corporation web site at www.egg.or.jp/MSIL/english/index-e.html.

wafers. The amount of dopant placed in the crucible with the silicon charge will determine the doping concentration in the resulting crystal. The seed is then slowly pulled out of the melt. Silicon atoms from the melt bond to the atoms in the seed, lattice plane by lattice plane, forming a single crystal as the seed is pulled upwards. The diameter of the resulting crystal is controlled primarily by the rate at which the crystal is pulled. Faster pulling results in a smaller diameter crystal, an intuitive result that we will quantify later in the chapter.

During CZ crystal growth, the seed and the crucible are normally rotated in opposite directions to promote mixing in the liquid and more uniform growth. Unfortunately, this also has the effect of increasing the corrosion of the crucible by the melt. Very few options are available in terms of crucible materials that are relatively inert to molten silicon. The dominant choice today is quartz, but such crucibles are slowly dissolved by the silicon, resulting in both silicon and oxygen being incorporated into the melt. Much of the oxygen evaporates as SiO, but some is incorporated into the growing crystal, producing oxygen levels of $10^{17} - 10^{18}$ cm^{-3}. (The solid solubility of oxygen in silicon is $\approx 10^{18}$ cm^{-3} at melt growth temperatures.) The quartz crucible requires a graphite susceptor for mechanical support. During crystal growth, carbon evaporation from this source and carbon from the EGS charge itself, result in carbon incorporation in the crystal, typically at levels of $10^{15} - 10^{16}$ cm^{-3}. To avoid additional impurities from the ambient, the growth is normally performed in an argon ambient.

The basic CZ process has not changed very much since it was first applied to silicon and germanium in the early 1950s by Teal [3.1]. Crystal diameters are continuing to increase in size as wafer suppliers and IC manufacturers are able to process larger wafers. Impurity levels are generally lower and better controlled today than they were in the past and mechanical and crystallographic defects are virtually nonexistent today. It is really quite remarkable that large diameter silicon wafers (up to 200 mm or 8″ today) with essentially ideal properties can be routinely purchased today at a cost of about $50 which is a small fraction of the total wafer fabrication costs associated with IC manufacturing.

The FZ process is illustrated conceptually in Figure 3–7. The principal difference between this process and the CZ process is that no crucible is used. This markedly reduces impurity levels in the resulting crystal, particularly oxygen, and makes it easier to grow high-resistivity material. FZ material is used primarily today in applications which require high resistivities, low oxygen content, or both, such as in some types of detectors and power devices. These applications represent a small fraction of the silicon market.

In the FZ process, a rod of EGS polysilicon is clamped at both ends, with the bottom in contact with a single-crystal seed. A small RF coil provides power, which generates large currents in the silicon and locally melts it through I^2R heating. Usually the molten zone is about 2 cm long. Surface tension and levitation due to the RF field keep the system stable. If the melting is initiated in a zone at the seed end and slowly moved up the rod, a single crystal results. As was the case in the CZ process, atoms from the liquid phase bond to the single-crystal solid material atomic plane by atomic plane as the zone slowly moves up the rod (or as the rod is translated downwards through a stationary coil). Doping of the crystal can be accomplished either by starting with a doped polysilicon rod, a doped seed, or by maintaining a gas ambient during the FZ process that

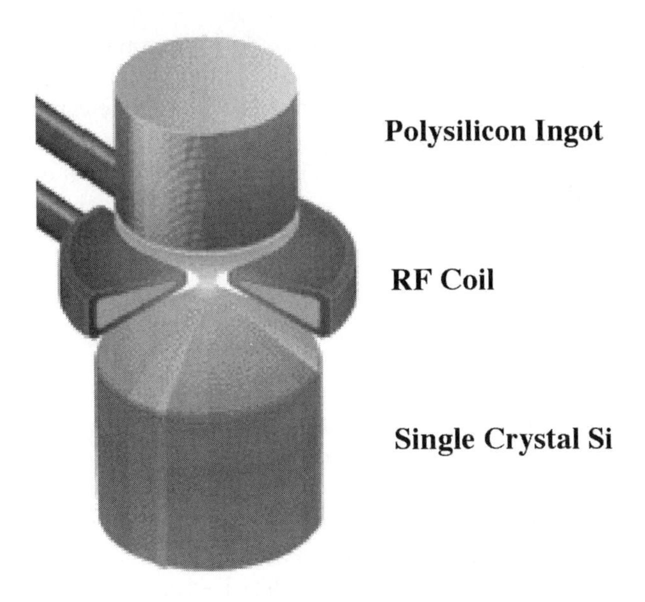

Figure 3–7 Basic Float-Zone (FZ) crystal growth or zone refining apparatus. This figure was taken directly from the Silicon Database on the Mitsubishi Materials Silicon Corporation web site at www.egg.or.jp/MSIL/english/index-e.html.

contains a dilute concentration of the desired dopant. These processes are described and modeled in more detail later in this chapter.

It is not as straightforward to scale up the crystal diameter using the FZ process because of stability problems associated with the liquid zone in a gravity environment. For these same reasons, FZ wafers usually have greater microscopic resistivity variations than do CZ wafers. It is thus likely that the CZ technique will remain the dominant growth method for large diameter silicon crystals.

3.2.5 Wafer Preparation and Specification

After a crystal is grown by either the CZ or FZ method, individual wafers must then be prepared for IC manufacturing. This involves a series of mechanical steps, which result in wafers that are almost perfectly flat, polished to a mirror finish on the topside and free of any mechanical defects from the sawing and other operations. Silicon is a hard and fairly brittle material. The most convenient method to shape and cut it is with industrial diamonds, although other materials like SiC and Al_2O_3 have been used and even materials like SiO_2 are used as part of the polishing operation.

The process of creating the individual wafers begins with shaping the grown crystal or boule to a uniform diameter. Modern crystal growers cannot maintain perfect control over the crystal diameter during growth so the crystal is normally grown slightly oversized and then trimmed to the desired final diameter. This shaping operation involves placing the boule in a lathelike machine and grinding it with a diamond wheel. In modern IC manufacturing facilities wafer diameters are usually about 150 – 200 mm (6″ – 8″). The boule is ground to a diameter slightly larger than this to allow for etching, which is done after the grinding to remove mechanical damage, and edge rounding and other operations that occur subsequently which further reduce the diameter. After the boule is ground to an appropriate diameter, one or more "flats" are normally ground along its length. These will end up as straight edges on otherwise circular wafers. They serve several purposes. The first is as a reference plane for many types of automatic equipment that handle wafers during manufacturing. The second purpose is to indicate the type and crystal orientation of the wafers. The flats are normally ground along a major crystal axis. The longest ("primary") flat is, by convention, oriented perpendicular to the <110> direction. In manufacturing, the integrated circuits that are later built on these wafers are normally rectangular and are lined up parallel and perpendicular to the (110) flats on the wafers. This means that the edges of the chips are on {110} crystal planes. When the completed chips are ready to be separated for packaging, a dicing operation is performed in which the scribe lines between adjacent chips are partially sawn through. The individual chips can then be separated by simply breaking the wafer mechanically along these scribe lines. Silicon actually cleaves naturally along {111} planes. In (100) crystals, the {111} planes meet the surface at an angle of 54.7° along the <110> directions which are at right angles to each other. Thus placing the scribe lines parallel and perpendicular to the wafer flat results in easy cleaving.

The next step in wafer preparation is the actual sawing of the boule into individual wafers. This is usually accomplished with a diamond-tipped blade that cuts on its inside edge. Using an inside edge cutting procedure allows the outer part of the saw blade to be thicker and hence more rigid, without wasting large amounts of the boule in the saw cut regions. As we saw earlier in the chapter, the two common surface orientations for wafers today are (100) and (111). Wafers with these surface orientations are usually produced using seeds of the appropriate orientation, which then allows cutting of the individual wafers perpendicular to the boule.

As the diameter of silicon wafers has increased over the years, so has the thickness of the wafers required to provide adequate mechanical support during IC manufacturing. 200-mm-diameter wafers today are usually about 725 μm thick in their final finished form. They must be sawed somewhat thicker than this, however, in order to allow for losses that will occur during subsequent lapping, etching, and polishing. Typically, sawn wafer thickness would be about 850 μm. The saw blade itself is about 400 μm thick and so this thickness is lost from the boule as silicon dust every time a wafer is cut. Thus, including losses at the seed and tail end of the crystal, only about 50% of the boule ends up in wafer form.

Two additional mechanical steps are performed on the individual wafers at this point. The first is a mechanical lapping operation that removes about 50 μm of silicon using pressure and a mixture of Al_2O_3, water and glycerine. This step serves to improve the flatness of the wafers to about ± 2 μm, removing most of the taper and bow that results from the sawing operation. The lapping also removes much of the saw damage from the wafer surfaces. A sequence of successively finer-grit Al_2O_3 powders are used in the lapping to produce the final uniform wafer. It is important that the wafers be flat because later in the IC manufacturing process, high-resolution printing processes will be used to produce the patterns needed for the various device structures. Lithography is typically performed with steppers which can achieve submicron resolution, but which also have a very limited depth of field (Chapter 5). Hence the need for very flat wafers. The final purely mechanical process normally performed on the wafers produces rounded edges. This is again performed on a tool with diamond cutting edges and grinds a radius on the wafer edges. This greatly decreases chipping and the introduction of dislocations and other defects at the wafer edges during IC manufacturing.

At this stage, the wafers are ready for the final few steps that produce a mirror finish on one surface. A two-step process is used, chemical etching, followed by chemical-mechanical polishing. The chemical etching is done as a batch process, with the wafers loaded into cassettes and immersed in a mixture of nitric, hydrofluoric, and acetic acids. The acetic acid serves to dilute the mixture and control the etch rate. The actual etching takes place with the nitric acid oxidizing the silicon and the HF dissolving the resulting oxide. Overall the reaction that takes place is the following:

$$3Si + 4HNO_3 + 18HF \rightarrow 3H_2SiF_6 + 4NO + 8H_2O \tag{3.4}$$

Generally about 20 – 25 μm of silicon is etched off each side of the wafer. The process removes the surface layers containing damage from the various mechanical operations performed earlier. It is important that the wafer flatness be maintained during this operation through a uniform etch rate across the wafer. This can accomplished by agitation during the etch. An alternative is to use an alkali etch based on KOH or NaOH. In these cases, the etching reaction is limited by the chemistry occurring on the wafer surface and as a result, mixing of the bath is not as crucial.

The final step in preparing the wafers is Chemical-Mechanical Polishing (CMP). This process is illustrated in Figure 3–8. The wafers are polished under pressures on the order of 20 psi. The wafers are rotated in the polishing machine in a slurry consisting of a suspension of fine (10 nm) SiO_2 particles in an aqueous solution of NaOH. The rotation and pressure generate heat that drives a chemical reaction in which OH^- radicals from the NaOH oxidize the silicon. The SiO_2 particles abrade the oxide away. The overall process is thus a combination of chemical and mechanical polishing. Typically about 25 μm of silicon is polished away, producing a surface which is defect free and with a mirror finish suitable for IC fabrication. The CMP technology described here represents the origin of the now more broadly used CMP processes used by chip manufacturers. (See Figure 2–39 in the CMOS process flow in Chapter 2, for example.)

Integrated circuit manufacturers purchasing these wafers would typically specify a long list of parameters including basic electrical quantities like type and resistivity, mechanical properties like wafer thickness, bow, taper, and edge rounding, and crystallographic parameters like orientation, dislocation density, flat location, and so forth. Many of these quantities are standardized in the industry and all of them are specified with appropriate tolerances.

A final point regarding wafer preparation should be mentioned. It is often important in IC manufacturing to track individual wafers through the fabrication process. This

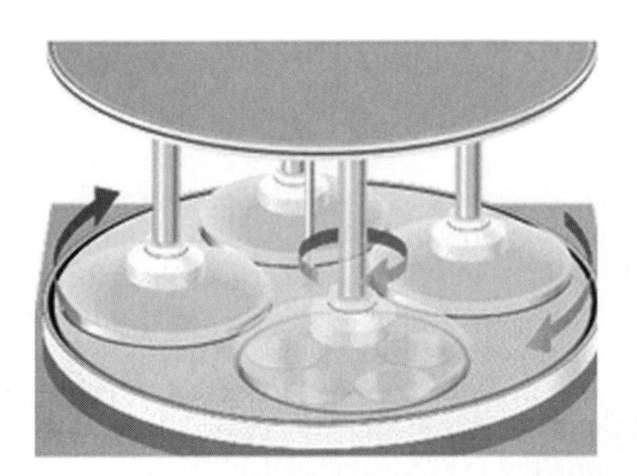

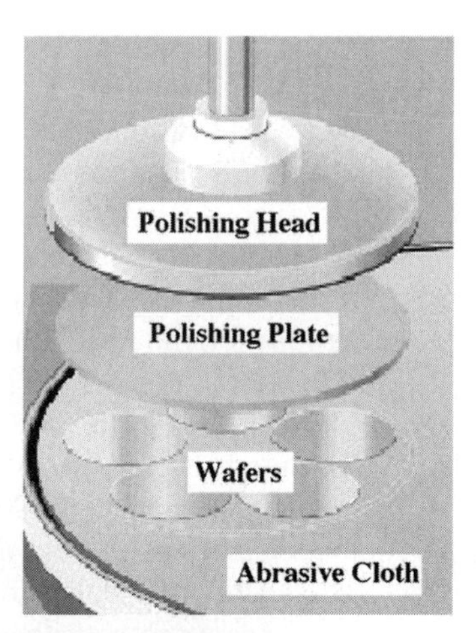

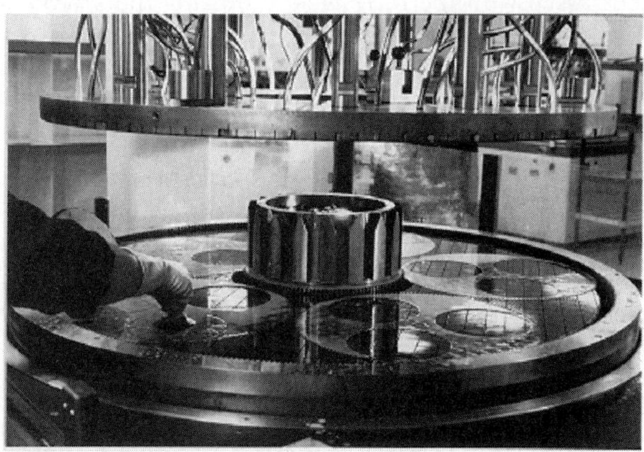

Figure 3–8 The upper figures were taken directly from the Silicon Database on the Mitsubishi Materials Silicon Corporation web site at www.egg.or.jp/MSIL/english/index-e.html. They conceptually illustrate the wafer polishing operation. An actual machine is shown below. Photo courtesy of R. Carranza.

might be important, for example, if yields began to decrease at some point in time and it became important to know exactly which machines were used, which process steps were performed, who did them, and when they were done on a particular set of wafers. Lot tracking and individual wafer tracking require that the wafers carry some identification. Generally either an alphanumeric code or a bar code is used, which is unique to each wafer. Typically the code is written with a laser on the wafer near the primary flat. This operation could be performed either by the wafer or the IC manufacturer. Since the laser process does damage the wafer surface and may create particle contamination of the surface, this step is often performed by the wafer supplier and is done before some of the final etching and polishing steps described above.

3.3 Manufacturing Methods and Equipment

Actual manufacturing of CZ or FZ crystals is, of course, more complicated than the simple conceptual description given earlier. Since the CZ process is dominant today, and likely to remain so, we will discuss some of these manufacturing issues in the context of the CZ process. Figure 3–6 showed an idealized version of a CZ growth apparatus whereas Figure 3–9 shows an actual machine used in manufacturing.

The crucible is a crucial issue in CZ growth, because it is in intimate contact with the molten silicon. There really are few choices for materials in this application because of the high temperatures involved and the fact that molten silicon is highly reactive. Quartz is the universal choice today. Silicon nitride has been considered as an alternative because it is a fairly stable, high-temperature material. However, the molten silicon

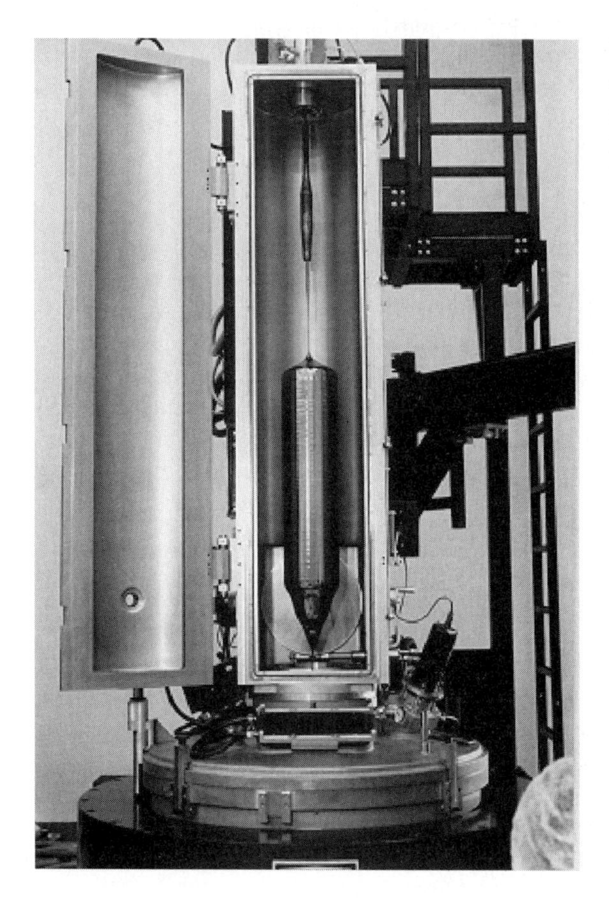

Figure 3–9 Modern CZ crystal growing machine. The crucible containing the liquid silicon is in the round housing at the bottom. The small seed and the pulled crystal are visible with the upper part of the machine open. Photo courtesy of R. Carranza.

slowly dissolves it and the nitrogen that is then incorporated into the growing crystal is a weak N-type dopant. Quartz is a glass and softens at high temperatures and therefore requires the use of a supporting susceptor. Graphite is the best choice here since it is a fairly inert, high-temperature material. Graphite is also generally used for the heating elements that are resistors through which a DC current is passed. This is an energy intensive process because of the high temperatures involved, typically requiring tens of kW of power. All these hot graphite elements contribute carbon to the melt, with the result that CZ crystals usually contain $10^{15} - 10^{16}$ cm^{-3} carbon along with the $10^{17} - 10^{18}$ cm^{-3} oxygen from the crucible. Since the carbon and oxygen impurities evolve from time-dependent sources, they are usually not incorporated into the growing crystal uniformly along the length of the crystal. Often the seed end of the crystal will contain higher oxygen concentrations than the tail end because as the level of silicon in the melt reduces, there is less dissolution of the crucible by the molten silicon. It is possible to control more precisely the oxygen and carbon concentrations in the crystal using more advanced growth methods. The rotation (mixing) of the melt is an important variable. Magnetic fields can be added with external magnets to help control the mixing processes in the crucible. (See Section 3.6.)

The crystal pulling apparatus itself is a mechanical assembly that must both pull the crystal and rotate it during growth. This must be done with great precision and with minimal vibration if uniform crystals with few defects are to be grown. Both lead screws and cable systems can be used to pull the crystal; the primary design constraint is mechanical stability. Figure 3–10 shows the sequence of events occurring in a modern CZ crystal grower.

We will derive a relationship in Section 3.5 that shows the coupling between pull rate and crystal diameter. Intuitively one would expect that faster pulling would produce a smaller diameter crystal, and this is in fact the case. The control parameters during the process are temperature and pull rate, and modern crystal pullers use computer control, usually in a feedback system, to monitor temperature and crystal diameter and to control both the pull rate and the power into the heater. Secondary parameters that influence the growth rate are the gas flows in the system and crystal and crucible rotation. Typically, an infrared temperature sensor is focused on the melt/crystal interface and lasers may be used to monitor the crystal diameter and the level of liquid in the melt. These inputs to the control system are used to adjust the pull rate and power levels to the heater. Such systems operate with little human intervention.

When the cold seed is first inserted into the molten silicon, very large temperature gradients exist through the seed volume. This results in high stresses and the generation of dislocations in the crystal. As discussed in Section 3.2, dislocations are active defects in a crystal. They can grow or shrink during high-temperature processing and are very detrimental to device electrical characteristics. Fortunately, it is possible to eliminate them from the crystal during the growth process. Dash first demonstrated these ideas [3.2]. By beginning the growth at a high pull rate, a thin neck is produced just below the seed. This grows out the dislocations to the crystal (neck) surface where they terminate. The growth is then slowed down, the diameter increases, and a dislocation free, large diameter crystal is grown, provided of course, that the rest of the growth is done under conditions which do not introduce large stresses or growth perturbations.

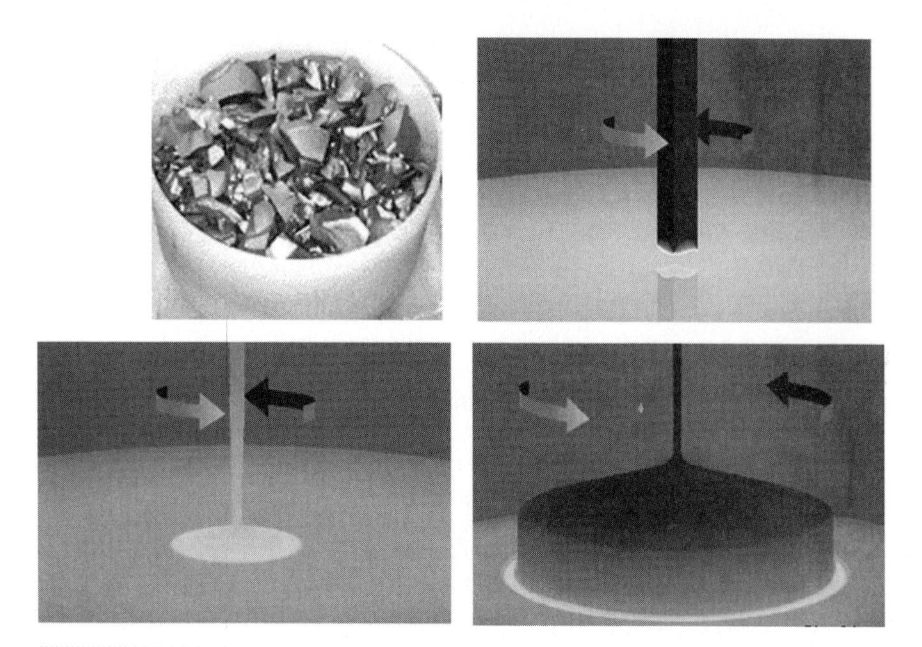

Figure 3–10 Sequence of photographs and drawings illustrating CZ crystal growth. The charge is melted, the seed is inserted, the neck region is grown at a high rate to remove dislocations and finally the growth is slowed down to produce a uniform crystal. These figures were taken directly from the Silicon Database on the Mitsubishi Materials Silicon Corporation web site at www.egg.or.jp/MSIL/english/index-e.html

3.4 Measurement Methods

We have seen in earlier sections of this chapter that a variety of electrical and physical parameters are typically specified in starting wafers that are used for IC manufacturing. All of these parameters need to be measurable of course; otherwise, there is little point in specifying them. In this section we will describe some of the principal methods that are used to measure wafer parameters. Some of these methods will have other applications in later chapters as well, for measuring other specific features of the IC fabrication process. Generally we can divide the techniques into two categories: electrical measurements and physical measurements.

3.4.1 Electrical Measurements

Simple electrical measurements of silicon wafers basically measure the concentration of electrons or holes in the material. Such methods can tell us directly the resistivity of the material and thus the electrically active doping concentration. In some cases, we can also easily determine whether the dominant carrier is holes or electrons and thus whether the material is N or P type. There are several measurement methods that we will discuss in this section that are widely used in the semiconductor industry to characterize starting wafers. The techniques described here generally do not have good spatial resolution. That is, they are designed to measure parameters averaged over a large area, which are assumed to be uniform over that area. This is generally a good assumption for starting wafers. However, doped regions in device structures require more sophisticated techniques, which we discuss in Chapter 7.

3.4.1.1 Hot Point Probe

The simplest method of determining whether a wafer is N or P type is, of course, to simply look at the flat designations which by convention give the crystal orientation and type. However, if the flats are not present, or if an independent check is needed, the hot point probe is a simple and reliable means to answer this question. The basic operation of this probe is illustrated in Figure 3–11. Two probes make ohmic contact with the wafer surface. One is heated 25 – 100°C hotter than the other. A voltmeter placed across the probes will measure a potential difference whose polarity indicates whether the material is N or P type.

Consider the case illustrated for an N-type sample. The majority carriers are electrons in this case. At the hot probe, the thermal energy of the electrons is higher than at the cold probe so the electrons will tend to diffuse away from the hot probe, driven by the temperature gradient. If a wire were connected between the hot and cold probes, this would result in a measurable current, whose direction would correspond to the electrons moving right to left in Figure 3–11. (The current by definition would be in the opposite direction.) If instead we place a high-impedance voltmeter between the probes, no current flows, but a potential difference is measured as illustrated. As the electrons diffuse away from the hot probe, they leave behind the positively charged, immobile donor atoms that provided the electrons in the first place. The negatively charged mobile electrons tend to build up near the cold probe. This results in the hot probe becoming positive with respect to the cold probe. By a similar set of arguments, if the material were P type, positively charged holes would be the majority carriers and

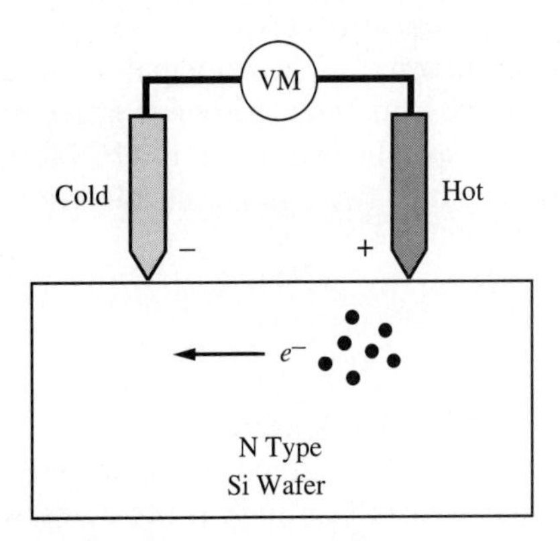

Figure 3–11 Basic principle of the hot probe, illustrated for an N-type sample, for determining N- or P-type behavior in semiconductors.

the polarity of the induced voltage would be reversed. The direction of the current between the two probes would also be reversed in P-type material, if they were shorted with a wire. Thus a measurement of either the short-circuit current or the open circuit voltage tells us the type of the material. The current that flows due to the majority carriers is given by

$$J_n = qn\mu_n P_n \frac{dT}{dx} \tag{3.5}$$

where P_n is the thermoelectric power, which is negative for electrons and positive for holes. A similar expression holds for holes in P-type material. The voltage measured by the hot probe method is known as the thermal emf or Seebeck voltage. This technique is generally used only to indicate the type of the material; other methods are used to accurately determine the doping level in the semiconductor.

3.4.1.2 Sheet Resistance

Once the type of the wafer is known either from the flat information or by a hot probe measurement, the next quantity of interest is usually the resistivity, which is related to the free electron or hole concentration as described in Chapter 1.

$$\rho = \frac{1}{q\mu_n n + q\mu_p p} \ \Omega\text{cm} \tag{3.6}$$

Generally only one of the two terms is important because $n >> p$ or $p >>$ n under most conditions. The resistivity is thus a measure of the product of the mobility and the majority carrier concentration. A measurement of ρ thus provides n or p, provided the mobility is known. (See Figure 1–18.)

The most common method of measuring the wafer resistivity is with the four-point probe illustrated in Figure 3–12. We basically want to measure the sample resistance by measuring the current that flows for a given applied voltage. This could be done with

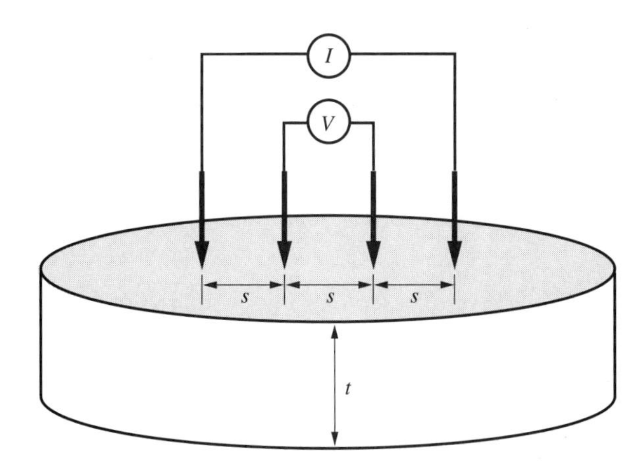

Figure 3–12 Four-point probe measurement method. The outer two probes force a current through the sample; the inner two probes measure the voltage drop.

just two probes. However, in that case, contact resistances associated with the probes and current spreading problems around the probes are important and are not easily accounted for in the analysis. Using four probes allows us to force the current through the two outer probes, where there will still be contact resistance and current spreading problems, but measure the voltage drop with the two inner probes using a high-impedance voltmeter. Problems with probe contacts are thus eliminated in the voltage measurement since no current flows through these contacts.

If we assume that the semiconductor dimensions are large compared to the probe spacings, then the potential measured at a distance r from a probe carrying a current I in a material with resistivity ρ is simply

$$V = \frac{\rho I}{2\pi r} \tag{3.7}$$

For the geometry of Figure 3–12, in which the probe spacings are uniform, this reduces simply to

$$\rho = 2\pi s \frac{V}{I} \ \Omega\text{cm} \tag{3.8}$$

where I is the current driven through the two outer probes and V is the potential difference measured between the inner two. In most instruments of this type, s is on the order of 0.5 to 1.5 mm. In fact if s is chosen to be 1.588 mm, $2\pi s = 1$ cm and the conversion is particularly simple. V is measured in volts and I in amps. It should be emphasized that in order for Eq. (3.8) to be valid, the wafer diameter and the wafer thickness must both be $>> s$. This is usually a reasonable assumption for the wafer diameter, but it is often not valid for the wafer thickness since wafers are generally less than a mm thick. In cases in which t is not $>> s$, the thickness must be accurately known in order to determine ρ.

A variety of correction factors have been derived for Eq. (3.8) to account for different geometries. Van der Pauw, for example, showed that the resistivity can be measured for an arbitrary shape provided that a few conditions are met. A more complete discussion of many types of correction factors is given in [3.3]. One limiting case which is of practical interest, is the case where $t << s$, that is for thin samples. This situation often arises when a surface diffusion or implant is performed in the wafer and the junction depth that results is much less than s. In this case, the thickness t is simply the junction depth x_j and the measured resistivity is

$$\rho = \frac{\pi t}{\ln(2)} \frac{V}{I} = 4.532 \frac{V}{I} x_j \ \Omega\text{cm} \tag{3.9}$$

Note that in the case of an implanted or diffused region, the doping varies with depth and ρ in this case is the average resistivity of the diffused region. In such thin layers, another common quantity often used is the sheet resistance ρ_s that is defined as

$$\rho_S = \frac{\rho}{x_j} = \frac{\pi}{\ln(2)} \frac{V}{I} = 4.532 \frac{V}{I} \ \Omega/\text{square} \tag{3.10}$$

Often the correction factors like the 4.532 are built into instruments that measure ρ and ρ_s automatically. In the semiconductor industry today, it is common to produce "wafer maps" of resistivity or sheet resistance through the use of a four-point probe that steps and repeats across a wafer to produce a map of the measured parameter.

We will make extensive use of ρ_s throughout this book, especially in Chapters 7 and 8, to characterize not only diffused and implanted layers, but also thin film materials like polysilicon. We saw a number of examples of the use of this parameter in Chapter 2 in describing the CMOS process.

3.4.1.3 Hall Effect Measurements

The Hall effect was discovered more than 100 years ago when Hall observed a transverse voltage across a conductor subjected to a magnetic field. The technique is more powerful than the sheet resistance method described above because it can determine the material type, carrier concentration and carrier mobility separately. The basic method is illustrated in Figure 3–13. The left part of the figure defines the reference directions and the various currents, fields and voltages; the right part of the figure illustrates a top view of a practical geometry that is often used in semiconductor applications.

Consider the left part of Figure 3–13 first. A current I_X is forced through the sample. This results in a measurable voltage drop V_X from which the material resistivity may be determined just as in the four-point probe method described above.

$$\rho = \frac{wt}{s}\frac{V_X}{I_X} \tag{3.11}$$

In the example in the figure, the majority carriers are electrons (N type). If we now apply a magnetic field in the Z direction (B_Z), the total force acting on the electrons is given by

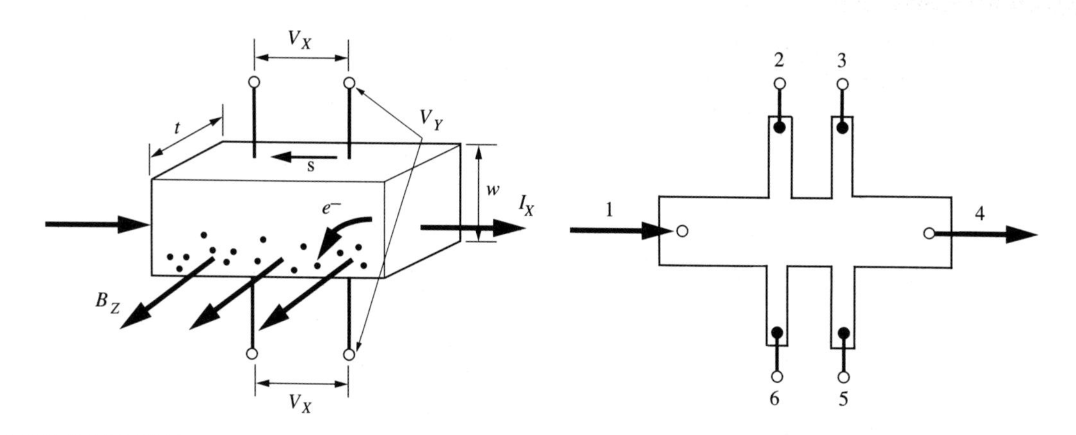

Figure 3–13 Conceptual representation of Hall effect measurement. The right sketch is a top view of a more practical implementation.

$$\text{Force} = Q(\varepsilon + v \times B) \tag{3.12}$$

where v is the electron velocity and all of the quantities in the equation are vectors. A magnetic field in the Z direction will force the electrons to the bottom of the slab where they will tend to build up in concentration. Since no current flows in the Y direction, an ε field must build up to exactly balance the magnetic force. Thus

$$F_Y = q(\varepsilon_Y + v_X B_Z) = 0 \tag{3.13}$$

so that the transverse ε field is

$$\varepsilon_Y = -B_Z v_X = B_Z \frac{I_X}{qwtn} \tag{3.14}$$

In writing this expression, we have made use of the fact that $I_X = qwtnv_X$ since in general the current is given by the number of carriers times their velocity.

In the experiment, we actually measure V_Y which is simply the integral of ε_Y from 0 to w, so that

$$V_Y = B_Z \frac{I_X}{qtn} \tag{3.15}$$

Since B_Z will force either electrons or holes (whichever is the majority carrier) to the bottom of the sample, the sign of V_Y changes depending on the material type. The Hall coefficient R_H is defined as

$$R_H = \frac{tV_Y}{B_Z I_X} \tag{3.16}$$

The sign of R_H will also change with the material type. All of the quantities in R_H are measured experimentally, so that we have finally that

$$p,n = \pm \frac{1}{qR_H} \tag{3.17}$$

where the + sign applies for holes and the − sign for electrons.

Thus the Hall experiment provides the material type through the polarity of V_Y, and the electron (or hole) concentration through Eq. (3.17). A consistent set of units would measure dimensions in meters, voltages in volts, currents in amperes, and magnetic fields in Teslas ($1\text{T} = 10^4$ Gauss $= 10^4$ G $= 1$ V sec m^{-2}). The units of R_H are then m^3 coul^{-1}. B_Z values are commonly in the range of 0.5 – 10 kG.

Combining Eqs. (3.6) and (3.17), we have

$$\mu_H = \frac{|R_H|}{\rho} = |R_H|\sigma \tag{3.18}$$

The quantity μ_H is called the Hall mobility to distinguish it from μ_e or μ_h which we have simply called the mobility to this point, but which are more properly called the conductivity mobilities. In general $\mu_{e,h} \neq \mu_H$ although they are usually less than a factor of two different. The reason for this is that as we saw in Chapter 1, mobility is a measure of the carrier scattering mechanisms at work in the semiconductor. Applying a strong magnetic field can affect the scattering processes. This is written as $\mu_H = r\,\mu_{e,h}$ where r is the Hall scattering factor. In most cases, $r > 1$. It depends on the strength of B_Z, on temperature, and on the particular semiconductor material. For silicon, r values are generally close to unity and are often taken as 1 in Hall measurements. A more detailed discussion of many of these issues is given in a number of texts such as [3.3].

The right side of Figure 3–13 shows a top view of a geometry that is often used in practice. Current is forced between terminals 1 and 4. Resistivity is measured from the voltage drop between terminals 2 and 3 or between 5 and 6 in the absence of a magnetic field. The Hall voltage is measured between terminals 2 and 6 or between 3 and 5 with a magnetic field applied perpendicular to the paper. For bulk samples, structures with the shape of this bridge are cut using ultrasonic tools. When implants or diffusions are to be measured, they can be patterned using normal photolithography techniques so that the diffusion or implant is in the shape of the bridge structure in the wafer. However in this case, a Hall measurement will measure an average resistivity and mobility in the layer since the doping will typically vary with depth in such a structure. It is possible to profile diffused or implanted regions using the Hall method, but this generally requires multiple measurements with a thin portion of the layer removed by etching between each measurement. This is a fairly tedious measurement and other methods involving CV profiling, spreading resistance or Secondary Ion Mass Spectrometry (SIMS), are usually used instead. We will discuss these methods in Chapter 7 since they are most often used to profile diffused or implanted regions.

3.4.2 Physical Measurements

A variety of physical techniques have been applied to the characterization of silicon wafers. Entire texts have been written on this topic [for example, 3.4, 3.5] so that we will only briefly describe some of the more important techniques here. Generally these techniques are aimed at understanding various types of defects that may be present in the crystal (dislocations, stacking faults, etc.) or at determining impurity levels (oxygen and carbon in particular).

3.4.2.1 Defect Etches

Silicon wafers delivered to IC manufacturers today are typically free of macroscopic crystallographic defects like dislocations and stacking faults. However, such defects can be introduced into the crystal during subsequent high-temperature processing. They may be nucleated by oxygen precipitation in CZ crystals (Section 3.5.5), by stresses due to thin films deposited on the wafer surface, or by processes like oxidation (Chapter 6). A number of chemical etchants have been developed to delineate these defects so that their density, size, and physical location can be determined. Other types of defects such as "swirl defects," which are believed to be due to an agglomeration of excess interstitial point defects (Section 3.5.4), and "saucer pits," which are thought to be due to metal precipitates, can also be exposed by these etches. Generally the etchants work by preferentially attacking the strained or faulted regions in the silicon associated with the various defects using an oxidation followed by a dissolution process. This produces pits in the surface whose shape depends on the specific defect and the crystal orientation. The pits are typically easily visible under an optical microscope. These etchants can be used either on the wafer surface to expose surface defects or on cross sections of the wafer to investigate defects through the wafer. Three of the more common defect etches are listed in Table 3–1.

Table 3–1 Composition of three common etchants used to delineate defects in silicon wafers

Etch	Composition
Sirtl	Cr_2O_3 (5M):HF 1:1
Secco	$K_2Cr_2O_7$ (0.15M):HF or Cr_2O_3 (0.15M):HF 1:2
Dash	HF:HNO_3:acetic acid 1:3:10

3.4.2.2 Fourier Transform Infrared Spectroscopy (FTIR)

As we have seen, the CZ crystal growth process introduces oxygen and to a lesser extent, carbon, into the silicon. In recent years, it has become apparent that these elements are not inert in the crystal (Section 3.5.5). It is not necessarily desirable to eliminate these impurities; what is important is to be able to measure them and to control them. The most common method for measuring them is Fourier Transform Infrared Spectroscopy or FTIR. The basic method is illustrated in Figure 3–14.

FTIR measures the absorption of infrared energy by the molecules that are present in a given sample. Many molecules have vibrational modes that absorb specific wavelengths when they are excited. By sweeping the wavelength of the incident energy and detecting which wavelengths are absorbed, a characteristic signature of the molecules present is obtained. Grown-in oxygen in CZ crystals is located in interstitial sites in the silicon lattice, bonded to two silicon atoms. Low concentrations of carbon are substitutional in silicon since carbon is located in the same column of the periodic table as silicon and easily replaces a silicon atom. In these positions, oxygen exhibits a vibrational mode that absorbs energy at 1106 cm^{-1} (wavenumber), that is, at a wavelength of about 9 microns; carbon absorbs energy at 607 cm^{-1}. There are, of course, many other wavelengths of IR light that are absorbed by the silicon atoms themselves. By measuring the

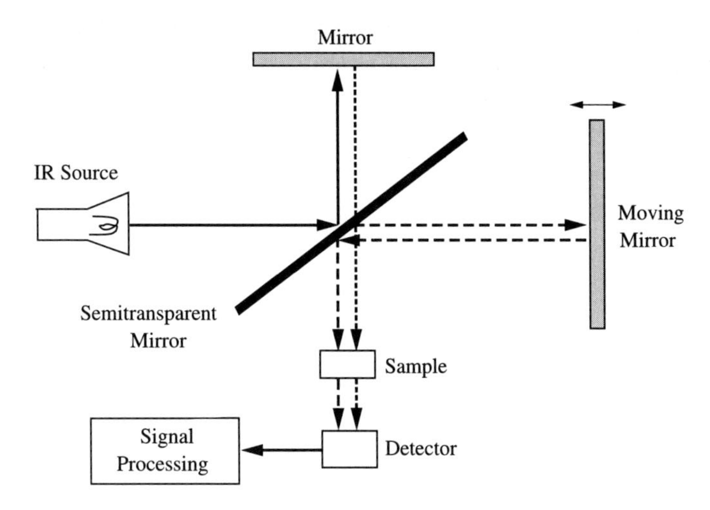

Figure 3–14 FTIR experimental apparatus.

absorption of a particular wafer at 1106 or 607 cm^{-1}, and comparing this absorption with an oxygen or carbon free reference, the FTIR technique can be made quantitative.

As shown in Figure 3–14, an IR beam is split by a partially reflecting mirror and then follows two separate paths to the sample and the detector. In the simplest case, without the sample present, the two beams will interfere with each other at the detector producing a signal whose amplitude will depend on the phase of the two signals with respect to each other. If the movable mirror is translated back and forth at constant speed, the detected signal will be sinusoidal as the two beams go in and out of phase. The Fourier transform of this signal will simply be a delta function proportional to the incident intensity. If the frequency of the source is swept, the Fourier transform of the resulting signal will produce an intensity spectrum. If we now insert the sample, the resulting intensity spectrum will change because of absorption of specific wavelengths by the sample. The benefit of using the Fourier transform method as opposed to simply directly measuring the intensity spectrum is simply that the signal to noise ratio is improved and as a result, the detection limit is reduced. With modern instruments, the detection limit for interstitial oxygen in silicon is about 2×10^{15} cm^{-3}. Carbon can be detected down to about 5×10^{15} cm^{-3}. We will describe in Section 3.5.5 how thermal processing of CZ wafers can cause the oxygen to precipitate into small SiO_2 clusters. This process can be detected by FTIR because in the SiO_2 form, the oxygen does not absorb at 1106 cm^{-1}. As the precipitation occurs, the IR absorption at this wavenumber decreases.

3.4.2.3 Electron Microscopy

Optical microscopes are well known and are widely used for inspection purposes in the integrated circuit industry. However as device sizes have decreased, higher-resolution imaging methods have become necessary in order to see not only the device structures themselves clearly, but also many of the defects that can affect device performance. This higher resolution has been provided by a variety of electron based imaging instruments.

The higher resolution is possible simply because electron wavelengths at energies commonly used in these instruments are usually less than 0.1 nm, compared to the hundreds of nm typical of visible light. DeBroglie first demonstrated that particle beams can have wavelike properties, with a wavelength given by

$$\lambda = \frac{h}{\sqrt{2qmV}} \tag{3.19}$$

where h is Plank's constant, m is the mass of the particle, and V is the potential difference through which the particle is accelerated. The resolution of an optical system is given to first order [see Eq. (5.4) in Chapter 5] by

$$\text{Resolution} = \frac{k_1\lambda}{NA} \tag{3.20}$$

where k_1 is on the order of unity and depends on the parameters of the imaging system. NA is the numerical aperture of the lens system that is defined in Chapter 5. In optical systems, NA is on the order of unity whereas in electron imaging systems, it is more typically 0.01. However, the electron wavelength is $10^4 - 10^5$ times smaller than that of optical photons, so the electron microscope has much better resolution.

We will find many examples throughout this text in which SEM (Scanning Electron Microscope) and TEM (Transmission Electron Microscope) images are used to identify and understand material and device properties. In this chapter we will briefly discuss the basis on which these instruments operate and show their utility in imaging crystalline defects such as dislocations and stacking faults in silicon.

The principle of the SEM is straightforward. A beam of typically 1 – 40 keV electrons is focused using electrostatic or magnetic lenses onto the sample to be imaged. The beam is rastered in an XY pattern, similar to a television screen, to scan the region of interest. When the electrons strike the sample, a number of interactions occur. Some of the electrons may be backscattered from the sample. Other electrons in the beam transfer energy to electrons in the sample. These excited electrons may be emitted from the sample as secondary electrons, or they may give off photons or X-rays as they decay back to their equilibrium energy levels. We will discuss these processes more carefully in Chapter 4. (See Figures 4–16 to 4–18.) The SEM collects one or more of the electrons, photons, or X-rays coming off the sample and displays the intensity of this signal on a CRT that is rastered along with the electron beam in the SEM. Thus a scanned image is built up from the sample. Most often, the SEM uses secondary electrons to form the image, but other modes are used as well. Magnification in the SEM is obtained simply by rastering the display CRT beam over a much larger area than the corresponding electron beam on the sample. SEMs are capable of magnification up to 300,000X, have a resolution below 5 nm and a large depth of focus. Figure 1–12 showed an example of an SEM image, in this case of a chip cross section.

The TEM, as the name implies, operates by passing electrons completely through a sample. Higher energies are used than in an SEM (typically 100 – 300 keV), but even so, samples must be thinned to less than 1 μm in order to obtain sufficient transmission of the beam for high-quality imaging. Such thinning is a nontrivial task and is usually done through a combination of lapping and ion milling. The image that is formed in a TEM comes from the transmitted electrons after they pass through the sample and impinge on a photographic plate or phosphor screen. The variations in intensity of the transmitted beam that form the image may be due to diffraction effects in crystalline samples, or they may be due to abrupt thickness changes, composition changes, or crystallographic orientation changes in amorphous or polycrystalline samples. The resolution capability of the TEM is about 0.2 nm, on the order of atomic dimensions. In recent years, quite remarkable images have been obtained with this technique. We will see a number of examples of these images throughout this book. Figure 3–15 shows an example of a TEM image of the Si/SiO_2 interface. Further information on these techniques is available in a number of texts devoted to measurement methods, such as [3.3, 3.4].

3.5 Models and Simulation

From a device fabrication point of view, the most important things we need to know about the starting wafers used in fabrication are the doping concentration, the crystal orientation, what impurities are present and whether there are mechanical defects in the crystal. The crystal orientation, of course, is determined simply by the seed used during growth and by the sawing operation that cuts the boule into individual wafers. The other important parameters, are largely determined by the crystal growth process itself. In this section we will consider a number of models for crystal growth, dopant incorporation during growth, and some of the important defects which are intrinsic to silicon crystals. These models allow, at least to first order, calculation of many of the important properties of the silicon wafers produced by CZ or FZ growth processes.

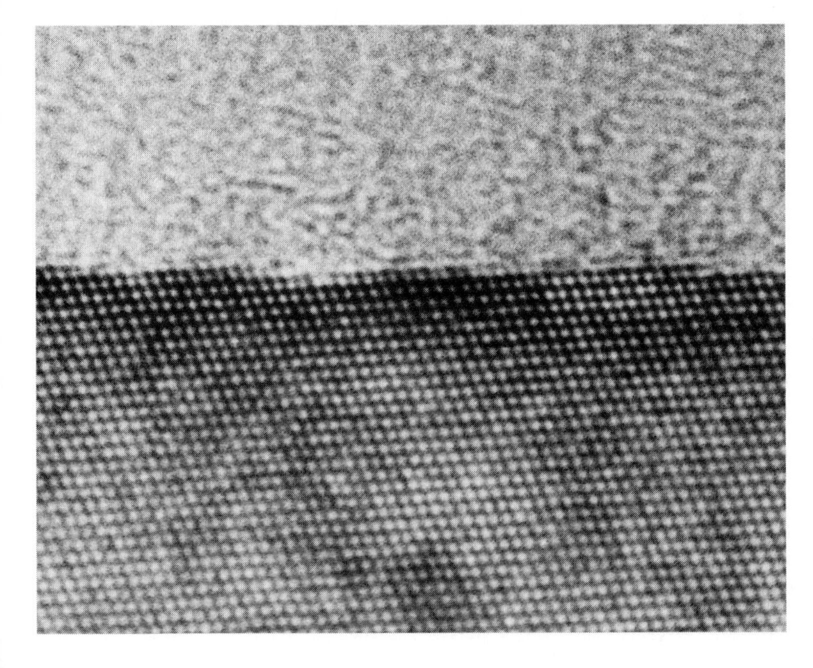

Figure 3–15 TEM image of the Si/SiO_2 interface. The crystalline structure of the silicon is visible on the bottom. The thermally grown SiO_2 is amorphous. Photo courtesy of John Bravman, Stanford University.

3.5.1 Czochralski Crystal Growth

The CZ growth process that we described qualitatively earlier in this chapter has been the dominant method used to produce silicon wafers from the inception of the IC industry in the 1950s. It is capable of producing very high-purity wafers with well-controlled properties, very inexpensively. The basic process has not changed fundamentally since the early work of Teal [3.1] and others.

We seek initially an expression that will tell us something about the rate at which a CZ crystal can be pulled from the melt. Intuitively, we would expect that this pull rate should be slower for larger diameter crystals. In fact, we will find that the pull rate is inversely proportional to the square root of the crystal diameter. This result can be derived and the growth process itself can be understood to first order by considering a heat balance equation, which represents the dominant heat fluxes present during the freezing process. Consider Figure 3–16. x_1 is a constant temperature surface (isotherm) just inside the liquid. x_2 is an isotherm just inside the solid. During the freezing process, which occurs between these two isotherms, heat is released to allow the silicon to transform from the liquid to solid state (the heat of fusion). This heat must be removed from the freezing interface, a process that occurs primarily by heat conduction up the solid crystal. Thus we may write

$$L\frac{dm}{dt} + k_L\frac{dT}{dx_1}A_1 = k_S\frac{dT}{dx_2}A_2 \tag{3.21}$$

where L is the latent heat of fusion, dm/dt is the amount of silicon freezing per unit time, k_L is the thermal conductivity of the liquid, dT/dx_1 is the temperature gradient across the isotherm x_1, k_S is the thermal conductivity of the solid, dT/dx_2 is the temperature gradient across the isotherm x_2, and A_1 and A_2 are the respective cross-sectional

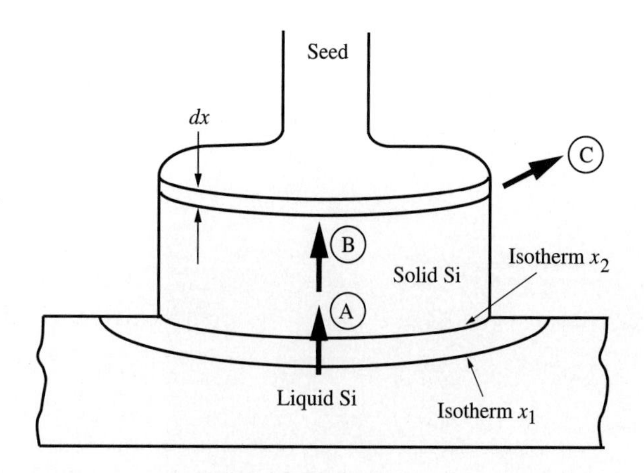

Figure 3–16 Freezing process occurring during CZ crystal growth. x_1 is an isotherm in the liquid adjacent to the solid crystal. x_2 is an isotherm in the solid adjacent to the liquid phase. The heat fluxes *A*, *B* and *C* are described in the text.

areas. The middle term, which we will drop from this point on, represents any additional heat that may flow from the liquid to the solid because of temperature gradients between the two. By neglecting it we will include only the absolute minimum heat which must be transported away from the freezing interface. The effect of this on our final result will be that the crystal pull rate we calculate will be an upper bound. We will also assume that $A_1 \approx A_2 \approx A$.

The rate at which the crystal is pulled out of the melt is simply

$$\frac{dm}{dt} = v_P A N \tag{3.22}$$

where v_P is the pull rate of the crystal and N is the density of silicon. Neglecting the middle term in Eq. (3.21) and substituting, we find that

$$v_{PMAX} = \frac{k_S}{LN}\frac{dT}{dx_2} \tag{3.23}$$

v_{PMAX} should represent an upper bound on how fast we can pull the crystal from the melt.

In order to eliminate the temperature gradient term from Eq. (3.23), we need to consider how the heat is conducted up the solid crystal and how it is eliminated from the solid. Consider Figure 3–16 again. The latent heat of crystallization (A) is transferred from the liquid to the solid. This heat is then transported away from the freezing interface primarily by conduction up the solid crystal (B). The heat is lost from the crystal by radiation (C) and by convection, although we will consider only radiation to keep the analysis simple.

The Stefan-Boltzmann law describes heat loss due to radiation (C):

$$dQ = (2\pi r dx)(\sigma \varepsilon T^4) \tag{3.24}$$

The $2\pi r dx$ term represents the radiating surface area of an incremental length of the crystal. σ is the Stefan-Boltzmann constant and ε is the emissivity of the silicon.

The heat conducted up the crystal (B) is given by

$$Q = k_S(\pi r^2)\frac{dT}{dx} \tag{3.25}$$

where the πr^2 term is the cross sectional area of the crystal conducting the heat and dT/dx is the temperature gradient. Differentiating Eq. (3.25) we have

$$\frac{dQ}{dx} = k_S(\pi r^2)\frac{d^2T}{dx^2} + (\pi r^2)\frac{dT}{dx}\frac{dk_S}{dx} \cong k_S(\pi r^2)\frac{d^2T}{dX^2} \tag{3.26}$$

The second term in the derivative is normally neglected in comparison to the first term. Substituting (3.26) into (3.24), we have

$$\frac{d^2T}{dx^2} - \frac{2\sigma\varepsilon}{k_S r}T^4 = 0 \tag{3.27}$$

which is now a differential equation describing the temperature profile up the solid crystal. [Recall that we need dT/dx_2 in Eq. (3.23).]

The thermal conductivity of silicon k_S varies approximately as $1/T$, at least for temperatures below about 1000°C. Using

$$k_S = k_M \frac{T_M}{T} \tag{3.28}$$

where k_M is the thermal conductivity at the melting temperature T_M, we find that

$$\frac{d^2T}{dx^2} - \frac{2\sigma\varepsilon}{k_M r T_M} T^5 = 0 \tag{3.29}$$

This differential equation has a solution given by

$$T = \left(\frac{3k_M r T_M}{8\sigma\varepsilon}\right)^{\frac{1}{4}} \frac{1}{\sqrt{x + \left(\frac{3k_M r T_M}{2\sigma\varepsilon}\right)^{\frac{1}{2}}}} \tag{3.30}$$

Differentiating this expression to find dT/dx, evaluating the result at $x = 0$ (the freezing interface) and substituting the result into (3.23), we have finally that

$$v_{PMAX} = \frac{1}{LN}\sqrt{\frac{2\sigma\varepsilon k_M T_M^5}{3r}} \tag{3.31}$$

which is the desired result, showing that the maximum crystal pull rate is inversely proportional to the square root of the crystal radius.

Example Calculate the maximum pull rate for a 6″-diameter CZ crystal.

Answer Numerical values to substitute into Eq. (3.31) are contained in the appendix.

$$v_{PMAX} = \frac{1}{LN}\sqrt{\frac{2\sigma\varepsilon k_M T_M^5}{3r}}$$

$$= \frac{1}{(430 \text{ cal gm}^{-1})(2.328 \text{ gm cm}^{-3})} \cdot$$

$$\sqrt{\frac{2\left(5.67 \times 10^{-5} \frac{\text{erg}}{\text{cm}^2 \text{ sec K}^4}\right)(0.55)\left(0.048 \frac{\text{cal}}{\text{sec cm K}}\right)(1690 \text{ K})^5\left(2.39 \times 10^{-8} \frac{\text{cal}}{\text{erg}}\right)}{3(7.62 \text{ cm})}}$$

$$= 0.00656 \text{ cm sec}^{-1} \text{ or } 23.6 \text{ cm hr}^{-1}$$

Actual pull rates are typically less than this number, primarily because the analysis we did neglected many factors which are important in real crystal pullers. We considered only one source of heat going into the crystal, for example, the heat of fusion. We also considered only one sink for removing heat from the solid silicon, radiation, when in fact convection plays a role as does conduction heat loss to the mechanical support holding the seed end of the crystal, particularly during the early stages of growth when the crystal is relatively short. Finally, temperature fluctuations and gradients in the melt itself occur because of convection currents in the liquid silicon and because the melt volume changes during the crystal growth. All of these factors make more accurate modeling very difficult, with the result that actual crystal pulling machines use feedback techniques to monitor and control the crystal diameter. Optical techniques are used to monitor the crystal diameter during growth and to adjust the pull rate in real time as needed to maintain a uniform diameter. Infrared temperature sensors that observe the melt surface during growth, and thermocouples close to the liquid silicon container, monitor the melt temperature and control the power input to the crucible. In modern machines, the whole process is completely automatic with computer control used during the growth.

3.5.2 Dopant Incorporation during CZ Crystal Growth

Doping is required in virtually all silicon wafers. In the CMOS process we discussed in Chapter 2, we started with P-type, boron-doped, 25–50 Ωcm wafers. The boron or other dopants that are required by IC manufacturers are incorporated into the crystal during growth simply by adding dopants to the melt. This is typically done by adding a small amount of doped silicon to the charge placed in the crucible before melting.

It is important, of course, to be able to predict the dopant concentration in the pulled crystal. This is not as straightforward as might be first thought because of a process called segregation. All impurities, whether they are intentional dopants or unwanted trace elements, segregate between the liquid and solid phases when the two phases are in intimate contact. By this we mean that if the concentrations of the impurity are C_S in the solid and C_L in the liquid, then in general $C_S \neq C_L$. In fact we can define a segregation coefficient k_O as follows

$$k_O = \frac{C_S}{C_L} \tag{3.32}$$

C_S and C_L are the concentrations just on either side of the solid/liquid interface and k_O is usually referred to as the equilibrium segregation coefficient. If $C_S > C_L$, the impurity prefers to be in the solid phase; if $C_S < C_L$, the reverse is true. Physically, segregation occurs because impurities have different solubilities in the two phases. Stated differently, the chemical potential of an impurity must be the same in the two phases across the interface and this results in segregation. k_O values are normally experimentally measured quantities for a particular impurity in a particular system at a particular temperature. If the experimental conditions are far from equilibrium, then an effective value different from k_O may be measured. This might happen, for example, if the freezing process occurred so rapidly that the impurities did not have time to adjust their concentrations across the interface before they were frozen into the solid. Segregation will also be important in later chapters when we deal with oxidation and diffusion of impurities since in those cases we generally have an SiO_2/Si interface across which dopants will also partition themselves.

For most impurities in silicon CZ growth, $k_O < 1$. This means that these impurities prefer to be in the liquid phase. If we start with a certain concentration C_L in the melt at the beginning of growth, then as the crystal grows, C_L will increase over time as the silicon from the melt is incorporated into the growing crystal faster than the impurity is. The result will be a crystal that is doped more heavily toward the end of growth than it is at the beginning. In other words, both C_L and C_S will be functions of time during the growth and both will increase if $k_O < 1$. Table 3–2 contains equilibrium segregation coefficients for many of the impurities of interest in Si CZ growth.

Table 3–2 Equilibrium segregation coefficients during CZ crystal growth for Si

Impurity	Segregation Coefficient
As	0.3
Bi	7×10^{-4}
C	0.07
Li	10^{-2}
O	0.5
P	0.35
Sb	0.023
Al	2.8×10^{-3}
Ga	8×10^{-3}
B	0.8
Au	2.5×10^{-5}

We can model the incorporation of dopants into growing crystals with the help of Figure 3–17. We define V_O, I_O, and C_O to be, respectively, the initial volume, number of impurities and impurity concentration in the melt, V_L, I_L, and C_L to be, respectively, the volume, number, and concentration of impurities in the melt during growth, and finally V_S and C_S to be the corresponding quantities in the solid crystal. Note that V_L, I_L, C_L, V_S and C_S will all be functions of time (or alternatively functions of position along the crystal) if $k_O \neq 1$.

If during the growth process, an additional volume of melt dV freezes, it will remove from the melt a number of impurities given by

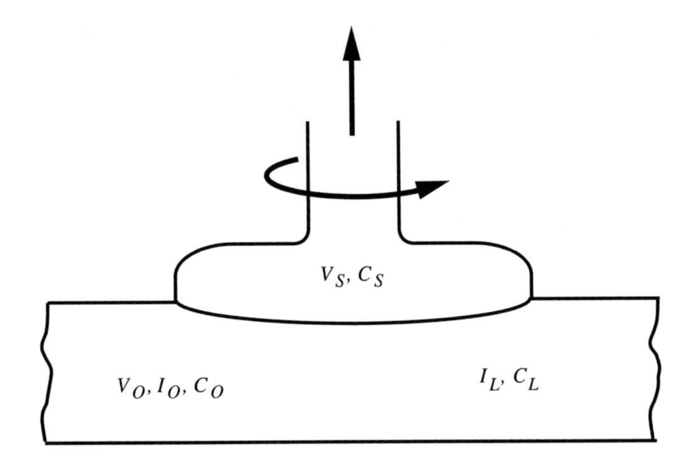

Figure 3–17 Dopant behavior during CZ crystal growth.

$$dI = -k_O C_L dV = -k_O \frac{I_L}{V_O - V_S} dV \tag{3.33}$$

$$\therefore \int_{I_O}^{I_L} \frac{dI}{I_L} = -k_O \int_0^{V_S} \frac{dV}{V_O - V_S} \tag{3.34}$$

$$\therefore \log\left(\frac{I_L}{I_O}\right) = \log\left(1 - \frac{V_S}{V_O}\right)^{k_O} \tag{3.35}$$

$$\therefore I_L = I_O \left(1 - \frac{V_S}{V_O}\right)^{k_O} \tag{3.36}$$

which gives the number of impurities in the melt as a function of how much of the melt has been frozen. We are really interested, of course, in C_S, the impurity concentration in the solid crystal. When an incremental volume of the liquid freezes,

$$C_S = -\frac{dI_L}{dV_S} \tag{3.37}$$

$$\therefore C_S = C_O k_O (1 - f)^{k_O - 1} \tag{3.38}$$

which is the desired result, expressing C_S in terms of $f = V_S/V_O$, the fraction frozen.

Eq. (3.38) is plotted in Figure 3–18 for the common dopants used in silicon technology. For dopants like antimony where $k_O << 1$, the doping concentration increases dramatically along the length of the pulled crystal. The common P-type dopant, boron, produces a much flatter profile because k_O is closer to 1. In actual pulled crystals, Eq. (3.38) is not exactly followed because of nonidealities that we did not model in the derivation above. These include inhomogeneities in the impurity concentration in the melt, small temperature gradients in the melt, convection currents in the melt, and

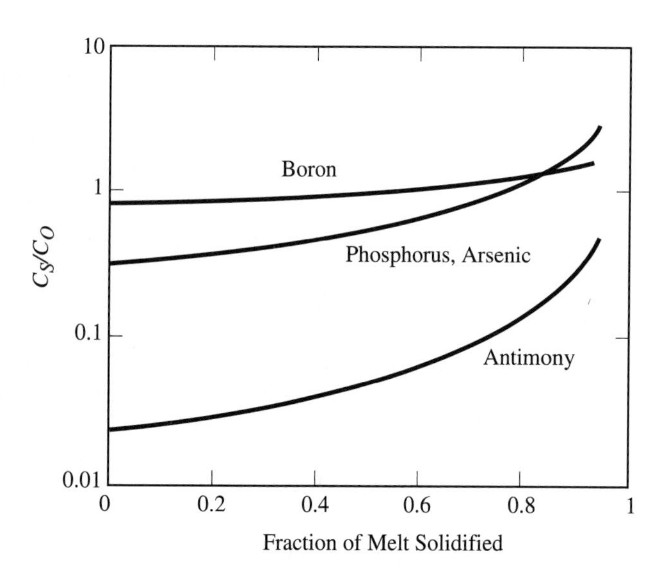

Figure 3–18 Doping concentration versus position along the grown CZ crystal for common dopants in silicon.

boundary layers that form at the freezing interface. The rotation of the crystal and the crucible during growth help to minimize all these effects, but in real crystals, there are doping variations both radially and axially on microscopic and more macroscopic scales due to these nonidealities. Radial doping variations also result from the fact that the freezing interface is actually concave into the melt, as illustrated conceptually in Figure 3–16, with the result that freezing at each radial point on a wafer occurs at a different time in the crystal growth process. Section 3.6 describes some recent developments in crystal growth that help to minimize these nonuniformities.

3.5.3 Zone Refining and FZ Growth

One of the drawbacks to the Czochralski growth process is that a crucible must be used to hold the molten silicon. At the melting temperature of 1417°C, there are few inert choices for materials in which to contain the silicon. As a result, silica is normally used, and oxygen from the crucible is incorporated into the silicon crystal, typically at concentrations of $10^{17} - 10^{18}$ cm^{-3}. This is often actually advantageous as we saw earlier in this chapter because the oxygen provides mechanical strength and it may be used as part of an intrinsic gettering procedure (Chapter 4). However, there are applications in which silicon wafers with much lower oxygen concentrations are needed. One example is in power control devices in which a single high-current, high-voltage device may be built on a wafer and the current flow is through the wafer, from the top to the bottom. High-resistivity, high-purity starting silicon is required. For these and other applications, silicon wafers are often prepared by the float-zone growth process. Since this same process can also be used to refine silicon, it is also sometimes referred to as zone refining.

The basic technique was illustrated in Figure 3–7. A rod of polycrystalline silicon obtained by the purification techniques described earlier in this chapter is mechanically supported at its top and bottom and held vertically. An RF power source is used to locally melt a small section of the rod, typically about 2 cm. The RF source and the liquid zone are then swept slowly along the length of the rod (or the rod is passed slowly through the coil). If a single-crystal seed is used at the beginning of the process, then the freezing liquid will form a single crystal. The "floating zone" thus moves up the polycrystalline rod, leaving behind a single crystal. Since no crucible is used in the process, very little oxygen is incorporated into the growing crystal.

Segregation effects also play an important role in the float-zone process, just as they did in the CZ method we discussed earlier. For most impurities in the liquid/solid silicon system, $k_O < 1$. As we saw in the CZ case earlier, this means that most impurities prefer to be in the liquid phase. We can now see what is meant by zone refining. As the liquid zone sweeps up the polycrystalline rod, impurities will tend to stay in the liquid and be swept to the top of the rod. The resulting single crystal will have lower impurity levels than the starting rod. The process thus refines the material or improves its purity.

Consider this process a little more carefully. Referring to the idealized geometry in Figure 3–19, the zone length is L. Assume that the rod has an initial uniform impurity concentration of C_O. If the molten zone moves upwards by a distance dx, the number of impurities in the liquid zone will change since some will be dissolved into the melting liquid at the top and some will be lost to the freezing solid on the bottom. Thus

$$dI = (C_O - k_O C_L)dx \tag{3.39}$$

where I is the number of impurities in the liquid. But $C_L = I/L$. Substituting and integrating, we find that

$$\int_0^x dx = \int_{I_O}^{I} \frac{dI}{C_O - \frac{k_O I}{L}} \tag{3.40}$$

where I_O is the number of impurities in the zone when it is first formed at the bottom. Carrying out the integration and noting that $I_O = C_O L$ and $C_S = k_O I/L$, we have finally that

$$C_S(x) = C_O\left\{1 - (1 - k_O)e^{-\frac{k_O x}{L}}\right\} \tag{3.41}$$

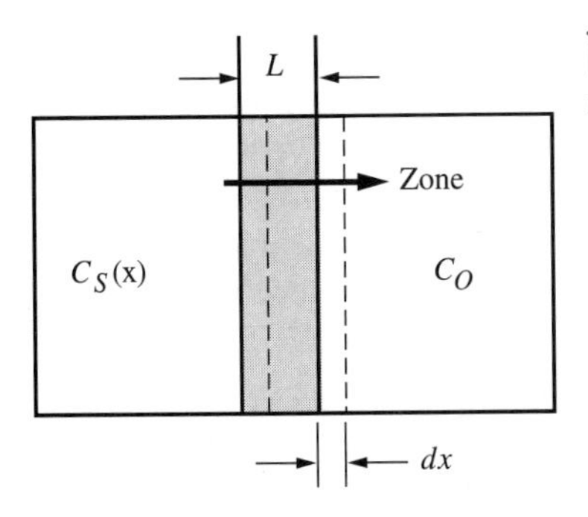

Figure 3–19 Float-zone crystal growth process. The liquid zone moves left to right.

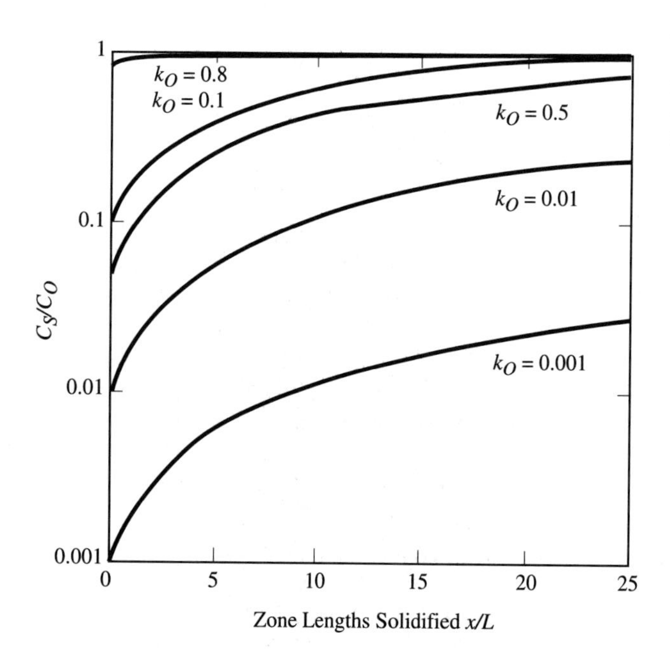

Figure 3–20 Behavior of impurities during float-zone growth or zone refining. The solid is assumed to start with a uniform doping concentration C_O. The curves correspond to one pass of the molten zone through the solid.

This result is plotted in Figure 3–20. Note that the initial single-crystal material will have an impurity level of $k_O C_O$ which is generally much less than C_O. Thus the single-crystal material is purified and the impurities are swept up toward the top of the rod. The simple solution given by Eq. (3.41) applies only for a single pass through the solid rod because C_O is assumed constant in the derivation. C_S/C_O asymptotically approaches 1 as the concentration in the liquid zone rises during refining.

The refining process can be repeated using multiple passes of the zone up the rod. In this case, C_O is not constant (after the first pass). This problem can be modeled using a simple spreadsheet analysis. (See problem 3.5). The resulting impurity profile is illustrated in Figure 3–21 for the particular case in which $k_O = 0.1$. In practice, to reduce the refining time, multiple zones can be melted and moved along a horizontal boat. This does create the problem of finding a boat material that will not contaminate the molten silicon and to which the freezing silicon will not stick. Orienting the silicon vertically eliminates the need for a boat since the liquid zone can be supported by surface tension and electromagnetic forces, but only a single liquid zone can be used in this case.

In most applications, the silicon wafers that result from the float-zone process are required to be doped, usually very lightly since high-resistivity material is needed for most float-zone-based devices. It is clear from the analysis above that starting with uniform doping in the polycrystalline rod will not produce uniform doping along the length of the single-crystal ingot. Several approaches can be used to solve this problem. In some cases, the float-zone process is carried out in a gas ambient that contains the dopant species. Dilute concentrations of PH_3 or B_2H_6 could be used for example. In this case the dopants are incorporated into the liquid zone, in which they diffuse rapidly, producing a reasonably uniform doping profile. Another alternative is to dope only the seed end of the polysilicon rod. In this case, no additional dopant is added as the liquid zone moves up the rod and a fairly uniform doping profile can be obtained.

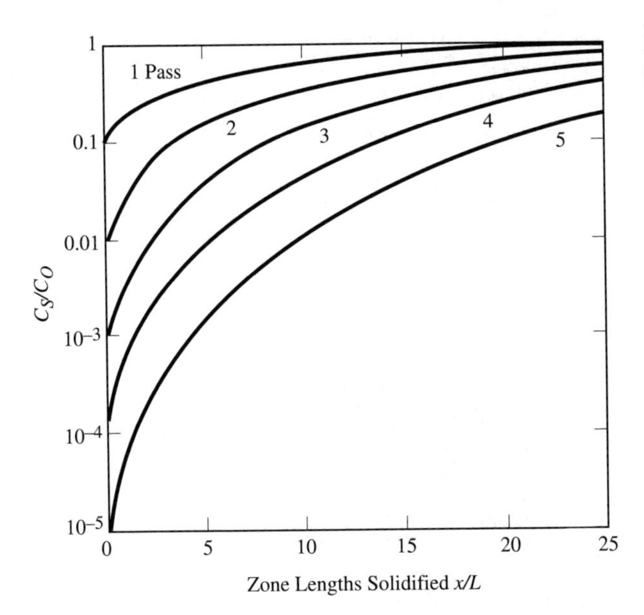

Figure 3–21 Zone refining with multiple passes. $k_O = 0.1$ in this example.

The final possibility is to grow the float-zone crystal undoped and then to use a process known as Neutron Transmutation Doping (NTD) to uniformly dope the ingot. In this process, the FZ ingot is placed inside a nuclear reactor and exposed to thermal neutrons. Silicon naturally occurs in three isotopes ^{28}Si, ^{29}Si and ^{30}Si with relative abundances of approximately 91%, 6%, and 3%, respectively. The neutrons in the reactor react with the ^{30}Si atoms to produce an unstable isotope ^{31}Si, which then decays to a stable phosphorus isotope ^{31}P, with a half-life of about 2.6 hours. The overall reaction is

$$^{30}\text{Si} + (\text{n},\gamma) \rightarrow {}^{31}\text{Si} \rightarrow {}^{31}\text{P} + \beta^- \tag{3.42}$$

Since the neutron absorption depth is large compared to the ingot diameter, very uniform doping tends to result from this process. The ingot must be shielded during the radioactive decay process that produces the ^{31}P. Radiation damage does result from this technique, but it can be annealed at modest temperatures after the process is complete. NTD silicon can generally be purchased only with resistivities greater than about 5 Ωcm because more heavily doped ingots would require excessive times to become safe to handle.

3.5.4 Point Defects

Earlier in this chapter, we identified several types of defects commonly found in crystals. The simplest of these were the native point defects, vacancies, and interstitials, illustrated in Figure 3–4. Thermodynamics predicts from fundamental principles that such defects will exist in equilibrium at all temperatures above 0K because the presence of such defects minimizes the free energy of the crystal. The concentrations of both V and I increase with temperature and are given by [3.5, 3.6]

$$C^*_{V^0}, C^*_{I^0} = N_S \exp\left(\frac{S^f}{k}\right) \exp\left(\frac{-H^f}{kT}\right) \tag{3.43}$$

where $C^*_{V^0}$ and $C^*_{I^0}$ are the equilibrium concentrations (denoted by *) of the vacancies and interstitials in their neutral charge states, N_S is the number of lattice sites, S^f is the formation entropy of the defect, and H^f is the enthalpy of formation of the defect. There is no requirement from thermodynamics that these two concentrations be equal, so in general the S^f and H^f values for the two are different. We should consider this issue a little more carefully because it will be important in later chapters. V and I can be generated in the interior of a crystal by simply moving a silicon atom off a lattice site. This is known as the Frenkel process and it necessarily creates equal numbers of V and I. However, other processes are possible which can affect the two concentrations. Generation processes at crystal surfaces can create only one type of defect. For example, an I is created if a silicon atom at the surface moves into the bulk. Recombination events can also take place between V and I in the bulk (which eliminates one defect of each type), or at the surface (which eliminates only one type of defect). There may also be generation or recombination events that take place at other types of defects in crystals. Stacking faults may capture either type of defect, for example, and grow or shrink by one lattice site in doing so. The net result of all these processes is that the crystal has a number of means to achieve different, yet equilibrium populations of V and I. Whenever a change is made in the temperature of the crystal, the equilibrium population of the native point defects will change through a combination of the processes described above.

The time required for the crystal to achieve new equilibrium populations is not specified by thermodynamics and depends on the kinetics of the processes taking place (i.e., generation and recombination rates). An important assumption which is usually made in modeling processes in silicon is that temperature changes instantaneously change $C^*_{V^0}$ and $C^*_{I^0}$. This assumption really says that the generation and recombination rates are fast compared to times of interest in process steps like oxidation and diffusion. The actual generation and recombination rates for V and I are not known with any accuracy in silicon; however, the assumption of instantaneously achieved equilibrium populations at the start of any process step generally seems to produce reasonable models of silicon processes. One clear exception to this statement occurs when ion implantation is used to introduce impurities into silicon. The resulting damage introduces large excess concentrations of V and I and other types of defects, which do not disappear immediately upon heating the crystal. Thus large, nonequilibrium populations of the defects may be present in the crystal for extended periods of time, with important implications for process phenomena like diffusion. Other situations can also arise which produce nonequilibrium point defect concentrations. We will pursue these issues further in later chapters.

The equilibrium concentrations of V and I have never been measured directly in silicon at process temperatures, primarily because they are very small. Most of the estimates of $C^*_{V^0}$ and $C^*_{I^0}$ come from fitting impurity diffusion data with models which involve the native point defect concentrations (Chapter 7). Since such estimates are subject to the particular model used, and since there is still considerable controversy over such models, exact values for the parameters in Eq. (3.43) are still in question. However, reasonable estimates today give the following values [3.6].

$$C_{I^0}^* \cong 1 \times 10^{27} \exp\left(\frac{-3.8 \text{ eV}}{kT}\right) \quad (3.44)$$

$$C_{V^0}^* \cong 9 \times 10^{23} \exp\left(\frac{-2.6 \text{ eV}}{kT}\right) \quad (3.45)$$

These expressions give numbers at 1000°C on the order of 10^{12} cm^{-3} for $C_{I^0}^*$ and 5 × 10^{13} cm^{-3} for $C_{V^0}^*$. At this temperature, the intrinsic carrier concentration n_i is about 7.14 × 10^{18} cm^{-3}. Normal doping concentrations in silicon devices are 10^{15} – 10^{20} cm^{-3}. It is easy to see then why it is so difficult to measure the point defect concentrations directly. They are much smaller than the impurity concentrations, much smaller than electron or hole concentrations, and since they represent only about 1 in 10^{10} lattice sites, they are well below the detection limit of physical techniques.

There are a few conditions under which point defect concentrations are large enough to be measurable. At crystal growth temperatures, equilibrium point defect concentrations are high. If the crystal is cooled rapidly as it is pulled from the melt, there may not be time for these point defects to recombine or outdiffuse, with the result that non-equilibrium, excess concentrations may be frozen into the crystal. This often results in what are referred to as swirl defects in silicon crystals, which are believed to be condensed I defects. Such macroscopic defects can be delineated in silicon by etchants and rough estimates can be made of defect populations. Annealing of the crystal for extended periods at lower temperatures can dissolve such defect precipitates by allowing time for recombination and diffusion processes to eliminate the excess point defects. A second example relates to the ion implantation process mentioned earlier. Ion implantation damage often results in very large concentrations of point defects, large enough to completely destroy the crystalline nature of the silicon in many cases. Such concentrations are easily measurable by physical techniques like Rutherford Backscattering. We will discuss this particular case in more detail in Chapter 8.

Point defects are extremely mobile in the silicon lattice. While their diffusivity cannot be directly measured experimentally (because of their small concentrations), it can be inferred from other experimental measurements of dopant diffusivities (Chapter 7). Point defect diffusivities can also be "measured" by doing a computer simulation of an interstitial or vacancy in the silicon lattice at different lattice temperatures and following their migration path. The diffusivity can be estimated this way at different temperatures and can then be expressed in Arrhenius form. Current estimates for the effective diffusivities of intersititials and vacancies are [3.6], [3.7]

$$d_I = 51 \exp\left(-\frac{1.8}{kT}\right) \text{cm}^2 \text{ sec}^{-1} \quad (3.46)$$

$$d_V = 3.65 \times 10^{-1} \exp\left(-\frac{1.58}{kT}\right) \text{cm}^2 \text{ sec}^{-1} \quad (3.47)$$

These equations give numbers for d_I and d_V that are orders of magnitude larger than dopant diffusivites. This will have significant implications in Chapter 4 when we discuss gettering, and in Chapters 7 and 8 when we discuss dopant diffusion and ion implantation.

It is well established that native point defects in silicon can exist in charged as well as neutral states [3.6, 3.8]. Singly charged $(+, -)$ and doubly charged $(++, =)$ vacancies have been identified experimentally using electronic techniques after excess point defects were introduced by high-energy electron bombardment. Similar charge states for Si_I are assumed to exist, although they have not been measured experimentally, probably because of the fast diffusion of these defects in silicon.

Charged point defects have energy levels in the silicon bandgap. That is, the defects can take on various charge states depending on the location of the Fermi level E_F. In Chapter 1 we saw that shallow donors and acceptors are usually ionized, at least at room temperature, while impurity levels lying deeper in the bandgap are ionized only when E_F is above them (acceptors) or below them (donors). The charged point defect levels behave very much like deep donors and acceptors.

The positions of the vacancy energy levels are illustrated qualitatively in Figure 3–22 at a particular temperature. E_F will be at the E_i position for intrinsic conditions and would be higher in the bandgap as illustrated, for N-type doping. We saw in Chapter 1, that $n_i = 7.14 \times 10^{18}$ cm^{-3} at 1000°C, so that at this temperature, for all doping levels below this value, $E_F \approx E_i$. For higher doping levels, the material will be extrinsic and E_F will move up or down in the bandgap for N- or P-type doping, respectively. Consider first the intrinsic case for which $E_F = E_i$. In this situation, E_F is below the vacancy acceptor levels V^- and $V^=$. It is also above the vacancy donor levels V^+ and V^{++}. Thus, none of these levels will ionized and the dominant vacancy charge state in the silicon will be the neutral vacancy V^0.

If the silicon is extrinsic, the dominant vacancy charge state will be different. Consider the case illustrated in Figure 3–22 for extrinsic N-type doping. E_F is now above the V^- level. Thus this level will be populated by an electron; that is, the vacancy will be acting as an acceptor and will be charged negatively. Since the background material is N type in this example, there will be many electrons available from the shallow donors to charge the vacancy. It is therefore likely that the dominant vacancy charge state will be V^- and not the neutral vacancy. Similarly in P-type material, the dominant vacancy charge state will be V^+ or V^{++} since E_F will be in the lower half of the bandgap, below one or both of these levels.

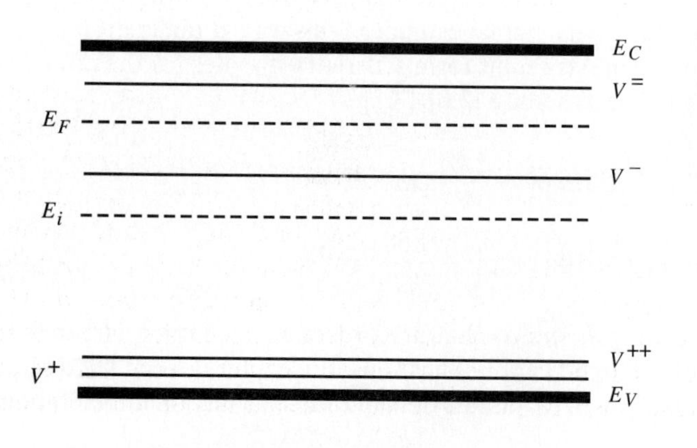

Figure 3–22 Approximate location of charged vacancy energy levels in the silicon bandgap. E_i is the intrinsic Fermi level. E_F is the Fermi level in N-type material.

The same statistics that we used in Chapter 1 to describe donors and acceptors can also be used to describe the equilibrium populations of V and I in their various charge states. Shockley and Last [3.9] first presented the results in the following equations.

$$C^*_{V^+} = C^*_{V^0}\exp\left(\frac{E_{V^+} - E_F}{kT}\right) \tag{3.48}$$

$$C^*_{V^{++}} = C^*_{V^0}\exp\left(\frac{E_{V^+} + E^{V++} - 2E_F}{kT}\right) \tag{3.49}$$

$$C^*_{V^-} = C^*_{V^0}\exp\frac{(E_F - E_{V^-})}{kT} \tag{3.50}$$

$$C^*_{V^=} = C^*_{V^0}\exp\left(\frac{2E_F - E_{V^-} - E_{V^=}}{kT}\right) \tag{3.51}$$

Similar equations can be written for I defects.

There are several important observations that need to be made regarding these equations and the populations of charged point defects in silicon. The first is that the equilibrium populations of the neutral and charged defects are always small compared to either n_i or dopant concentrations. This is important because it means that the number of electrons or holes bound to V and I is always a negligible number compared to the total number of electrons or holes present in the material (at least in equilibrium). This greatly simplifies calculations involving the charged point defects. To find the charged defect populations, we simply

1. Calculate the position of E_F in the usual way (described in Chapter 1), ignoring the point defects.
2. Calculate the concentrations of the charged point defects using this value of E_F and Eqs. (3.48) to (3.51). The resulting numbers for the charged point defect populations will always be much smaller than either n_i or n or p (whichever is dominant). Because of this, there is no need to take the charged defects into account when calculating the position of E_F. If the numbers of charged point defects were comparable to n or p, then the charging of the defects would necessarily reduce the free electron or hole population and hence change E_F.

A second point that turns out to be very important is that as the doping in the silicon changes and hence E_F changes, not only does the dominant charge state of the V and I change, but so also does the total number of each type of defect. This is not an obvious result at first glance but can be explained as follows. The neutral vacancy and interstitial concentrations are only a function of temperature, not of doping. Eqs. (3.44) and (3.45) depend only on temperature. If we change the population of charged defects by doping the material and moving E_F, $C^*_{V^0}$ and $C^*_{I^0}$ do not change. So where do the charged vacancies and interstitial comes from? Our initial guess would likely have been that we get the charged defects simply by adding an electron or hole to a neutral defect. That cannot be correct, however, because that would decrease the population of neutral defects. The correct answer, therefore, must be that new V and I are created by the crystal to supply the need for charged defects. This, of course, can occur through the generation processes described earlier. Thus in doped material, we should expect to find not only more charged point defects than in intrinsic material, but also more total V and I. In fact, at the same temperature, the $C^*_{V^0}$ and $C^*_{I^0}$ will be identical in extrinsic and intrinsic silicon. The difference will be that the extrinsic material will have many more charged defects—V^-, $V^=$, I^-, and $I^=$ in N-type material and V^+, V^{++}, I^+, and I^{++} in P-type material. These points are discussed in more detail by Shockley and Last [3.9]. Actual energy levels for the various charged defects are only partially established in silicon. Current values are summarized in Table 3–3 [3.6].

Table 3–3 Estimated energy levels of V and I energy levels in the silicon bandgap [3.6]. The question marks indicate values that are unknown or uncertain.

	V		I
$E_C - E_{V^-}$	0.57 eV	$E_C - E_{I^-}$	0.3 eV ??
$E_C - E_{V^=}$	0.11 eV	$E_C - E_{I^=}$	??
$E_{V^+} - E_V$	0.05 eV	$E_{I^+} - E_V$	0.4 eV ??
$E_{V^{++}} - E_V$	0.13 eV	$E_{I^{++}} - E_V$	??

In general, the V levels are better established than the I levels. The positions in the bandgap of these levels are generally given with respect to the conduction band E_C for the defect acceptor levels and with respect to the valence band E_V for the defect donor levels as is done in Table 3–3. The reason for this is that it is believed that the energy levels expressed this way, are not a function of temperature. We saw in Chapter 1 that the bandgap of semiconductors decreases as temperature increases. Thus the energy levels of the point defects must change with respect to at least one of the band edges as temperature changes. Since it is thought that the point defect acceptor levels track E_C as T changes, and the donor levels track E_V, then the values in the table are temperature independent and can be used directly in Eqs. (3.48) to (3.51) at any temperature.

Example Consider the structure illustrated in Figure 3–23. Suppose this structure is placed in a furnace at a temperature of 1000°C. What are the equilibrium point defect concentrations in the N and P regions of the sample?

Answer We first need to determine the basic properties of silicon at 1000°C. Using Eqs. (1.18) and (1.4) from Chapter 1, we find that $E_g = 0.778$ eV and $n_i = 7.14 \times 10^{18}$ cm^{-3}. Given the energy levels in Table 3–3, we can now construct the band diagrams shown in Figure 3–24. The Fermi level in the P region will be at the midband position since $p << n_i$. In the N region, it is reasonable to assume that all

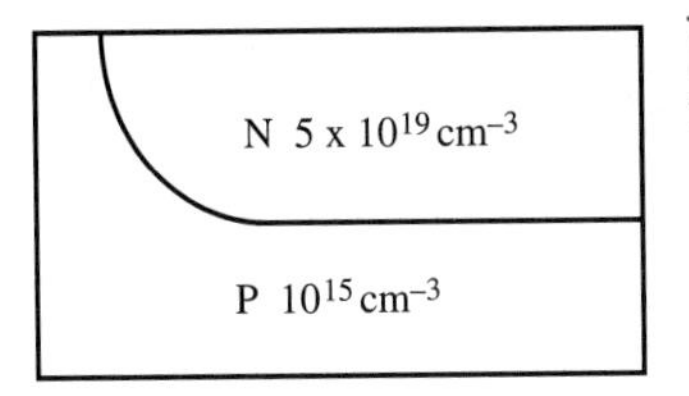

Figure 3–23 Silicon structure with two different doping levels. The structure is assumed to be in a furnace at 1000°C.

the dopants are ionized and therefore that n is much larger than n_i. Thus $n \approx N_D = 5 \times 10^{19}\ \mathrm{cm}^{-3}$. The Fermi level may now be calculated directly from Eq. (1.15), which gives $E_F - E_i = 0.21$ eV, placing E_F in the upper half of the bandgap.

Next, we will need to calculate the neutral vacancy and interstitial concentrations in the silicon. These concentrations will be the same in the N and P regions since they do not depend on doping. From Eqs. (3.44) and (3.45),

$$C^*_{I^0} = 9.13 \times 10^{11}\ \mathrm{cm}^{-3} \qquad C^*_{V^0} = 4.6 \times 10^{13}\ \mathrm{cm}^{-3} \tag{3.52}$$

To find the charged point defect concentrations, we could now substitute directly into Eqs. (3.48) to (3.51) and similar equations for the I. However, a few observations regarding the band diagrams in Figure 3–24 can save us some time. In the P region of the semiconductor, E_F is at the midband position since $p << n_i$ at 1000°C. Thus the V^+ and V^{++} energy levels will not be ionized and there will be few vacancies in these charge states. (In other words, these levels are well below E_F so they will be occupied by electrons and will not be acting as donors.) Similarly, the $V^=$ energy level is well above E_F so there will not be many vacancies in that charge state. (Few electrons will occupy the $V^=$ level so the vacancies will not be acting as acceptors.) Thus we conclude that in the P region, only V^0 and V^- will be important. By similar reasoning, we can conclude that I^0, I^+ and I^- may all be important in the P region. In the N region, E_F is in the upper half of the bandgap since the silicon is extrinsic in this region. Here, V^0, V^-, $V^=$, I^0, and I^- may all be significant. Substituting numbers into Eqs. (3.48) to (3.51) and similar equations for the interstitials, we find the results in Table 3–4. In this table we have included calculated values for all the vacancy and interstitial charge states. Note that the qualitative reasoning we used above to determine which charge states should dominate in the P and N regions is in agreement with the calculations. However, some of the charge states we qualitatively thought should be negligible are actually not a lot smaller than those we thought would dominate. The $V^=$ concentration in the P region, for example, is not a lot smaller than the V^0 concentration. The reason for this is that arguments that assume energy levels below E_F are all occupied by electrons and all those above E_F are empty, are fairly accurate at room temperature where the Fermi function is a fairly abrupt function. At higher temperatures, the transition from empty to occupied occurs over a much wider energy range, with the result that qualitative arguments like those above must be considered more carefully. In other words, kT that describes the transition is much larger at higher T! Note also that the total V and I concentrations in each region are much larger than

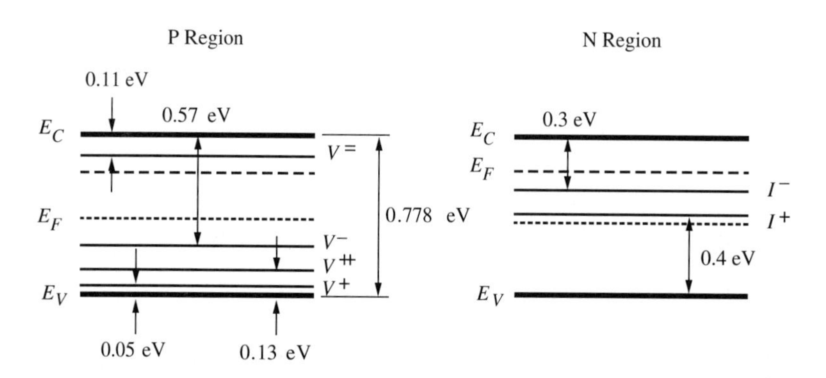

Figure 3–24 Calculated bandgap, point defect energy levels and Fermi levels at 1000°C.

Table 3–4 Point defect concentrations at 1000°C in the structure of Figure 3–23

	P Region	N Region
Doping	1×10^{15} cm^{-3}	5×10^{19} cm^{-3}
n_i	7.14×10^{18} cm^{-3}	7.14×10^{18} cm^{-3}
V^0	4.6×10^{13} cm^{-3}	4.6×10^{13} cm^{-3}
V^-	2.37×10^{14} cm^{-3}	1.61×10^{15} cm^{-3}
$V^=$	1.85×10^{13} cm^{-3}	8.50×10^{14} cm^{-3}
V^+	2.08×10^{12} cm^{-3}	3.06×10^{11} cm^{-3}
V^{++}	1.94×10^{11} cm^{-3}	4.23×10^{9} cm^{-3}
I^0	9.13×10^{11} cm^{-3}	9.13×10^{11} cm^{-3}
I^-	4.02×10^{11} cm^{-3}	2.73×10^{12} cm^{-3}
I^+	8.32×10^{10} cm^{-3}	1.48×10^{11} cm^{-3}

$C_{I^0}^*$ and $C_{V^0}^*$. Many of the models we will describe and use in later chapters will build on these point defect concepts and will use the equations presented here to calculate point defect concentrations.

3.5.5 Oxygen in Silicon

Oxygen is the most important impurity found in silicon wafers. As we saw earlier in this chapter, it is incorporated in silicon during the CZ growth process as a result of dissolution of the quartz crucible in which the molten silicon is contained. The oxygen is typically at a level of about 10^{18} cm^{-3} although the actual concentration depends on the particular growth conditions used. Earlier we modeled dopant incorporation in the growing silicon crystal based on a simple equilibrium segregation coefficient. Usually the incorporation of oxygen in the growing silicon cannot be described in such terms because the oxygen is being continuously injected into the melt and the transport dynamics in the molten silicon are often important. As a result, empirical means are usually used to characterize and control the oxygen concentration. It has recently become possible to use a magnetic field during CZ growth to control thermal convection currents in the melt. This slows down the transport of oxygen from the crucible walls to the growing silicon interface and thus reduces the oxygen concentration in the resulting crystal. Magnetic CZ growth or MCZ is discussed in more detail in Section 3.6.

It is important to understand the behavior of oxygen in silicon because it is always present at concentrations of 10 – 20 ppm ($5 \times 10^{17} - 10^{18}$ cm^{-3}) in CZ silicon. The oxygen is not inert in silicon and can affect processes used in wafer fabrication such as impurity diffusion (Chapter 7). Over the past 20 years, much effort has gone into understanding the behavior of oxygen in silicon and much has been learned. However, even today, much of what is known is qualitative. There are few quantitative models available that can accurately predict effects which occur. We will summarize in this section what is known qualitatively and attempt to quantify things where possible.

Oxygen is usually characterized as having three principal effects in the silicon crystal. The first is beneficial. In an as-grown crystal, the oxygen is believed to be incorporated primarily as dispersed single atoms designated O_I occupying interstitial positions in the silicon lattice, but covalently bonded to two silicon atoms. The oxygen atoms thus replace one of the normal Si-Si covalent bonds with a Si-O-Si structure. The oxygen atom is neutral in this configuration and can be detected with the FTIR method described earlier in Section 3.4. Such interstitial oxygen atoms improve the yield strength of silicon by as much as 25% [3.10, 3.11], making the silicon wafers more robust in a manufacturing facility. The improvement, due to solution hardening, increases with oxygen concentration, as long as the oxygen stays on interstitial sites and does not precipitate.

The second principal effect of oxygen in silicon is the formation of oxygen donors. A small amount of the oxygen in the crystal forms what are thought to be SiO_4 complexes which act as donors. They can be detected by changes in the silicon resistivity corresponding to the free electrons donated by the oxygen complexes. As many as 10^{16} cm^{-3} donors can be formed in this way, which is sufficient to dramatically increase the resistivity of lightly doped P-type wafers under extreme conditions. The donors form most readily at temperatures around 400 – 500°C at a rate proportional to $[C_{O_I}]^4$. During the CZ growth process, the crystal cools slowly through this temperature range and oxygen donors normally form. The SiO_4 complexes are unstable at temperatures above 500°C and so usually wafer manufacturers anneal the grown crystal or the wafers themselves after sawing and polishing, to remove the oxygen complexes. These donors can reform, however, during normal IC manufacturing, if a thermal step around 400 – 500°C is used. Such steps are not uncommon, particularly at the end of a process flow. In the CMOS process in Chapter 2, for example, the last thermal step was a 30-minute 400 – 450°C anneal to alloy the metal contacts and to minimize some of the charges associated with the Si/SiO_2 interface.

The third effect of oxygen in silicon is the tendency of the oxygen to precipitate under normal device processing conditions, forming SiO_2 regions inside the wafer. This process has been studied in detail over the past 20 years, although parts of the process are still only qualitatively understood today. The precipitation arises because the oxygen was incorporated at the melt temperature and is therefore supersaturated in the silicon at process temperatures. The solubility of oxygen in silicon increases at higher temperatures and is given by [3.12]

$$C_O^* = 5.5 \times 10^{20} \exp\left(-\frac{0.89 \text{ eV}}{kT}\right) \text{cm}^{-3} \tag{3.53}$$

where C_O^* is the equilibrium solubility. This gives a value of about 1.2×10^{18} cm^{-3} at the melting point of 1417°C. At normal processing temperatures of about 1000°C, the solubility is much lower, about 1×10^{17} cm^{-3}. There is thus a strong driving force for the grown-in oxygen to precipitate during wafer processing.

If a wafer containing oxygen in this form is heated as part of a normal IC fabrication process, precipitation of the oxygen can occur. The oxygen is believed to precipitate as SiO_2 although the exact structure has not been determined. The process can really be thought of as an internal oxidation, occurring in the bulk of the wafer, with the oxidant provided by the grown in oxygen. Precipitates can be nucleated either by heterogeneous or homogeneous means. Heterogeneous nucleation occurs when there is a particular lattice site (perhaps a defect or impurity cluster) which provides a disturbance in the otherwise perfect lattice at which precipitation can take place. Homogeneous nucleation occurs when enough oxygen atoms come together through random diffusion, to form a cluster of critical size. The distinction between the two is often not important. From a more macroscopic point of view, small SiO_2 precipitates are constantly forming and either growing or shrinking as oxygen atoms are either added or escape. The growth process is controlled by the in-diffusion of the oxygen atoms. These ideas are illustrated in Figure 3–25. Oxygen's diffusivity in silicon is well characterized and is given by [3.13]

$$D_O = 0.13 \exp\left(-\frac{2.53 \text{ eV}}{kT}\right) \text{cm}^2 \text{ sec}^{-1} \tag{3.54}$$

Qualitatively, what occurs is the following. At any temperature, small SiO_2 precipitates or embryos are constantly forming as diffusing oxygen atoms randomly encounter each other. Normally these embryos dissolve because when they are small, there is a strong tendency for them to shrink. This occurs simply because in-diffusing oxygen atoms do not arrive at a rate sufficient to overcome the flow of oxygen atoms that leave the embryo due to normal thermal bond breaking and diffusion processes. If the embryo manages to reach a critical size of something like 1 nm, then it is stable. That is, it will only grow beyond that point and is considered to have nucleated. Because all of these processes are temperature dependent, there is an optimum temperature at which SiO_2 precipitates can be nucleated. That temperature is around 700°C in silicon. At lower temperatures the diffusivity of oxygen is too low to provide an appreciable probability of nuclei forming; at higher temperatures, the embryos tend to break up before they reach the critical size.

Once the nuclei are formed, they continue to grow as long as the wafer is at process temperatures. In fact, they grow faster at higher temperatures because the growth rate

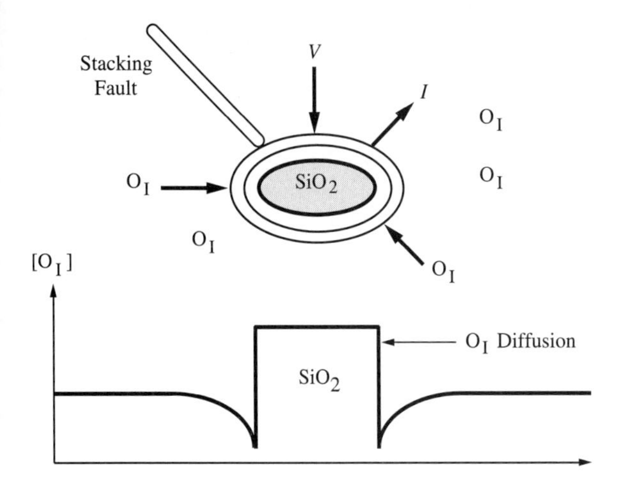

Figure 3–25 Illustration of point defect and diffusion mechanisms that contribute to the growth or shrinkage of SiO_2 precipitates in silicon. After Kennel [3.14].

is limited by the in-diffusing oxygen and D_O is higher at higher temperatures. In processes in which it is desirable to have these SiO_2 precipitates, then, it is common to follow a two-step thermal cycle. First, a low-temperature ($\approx$ 700°C) nucleation step is used, followed by a higher-temperature ($\approx$ 1000°C) growth step. All other thermal process steps that might be part of the normal IC manufacturing sequence can also nucleate and/or grow these SiO_2 precipitates. One common example of the importance of these SiO_2 precipitates is their use in intrinsic gettering that we will discuss in more detail in Chapter 4.

The growth of these SiO_2 precipitates can be described in a slightly different way, which will also prove to be useful in later chapters. An important observation regarding their growth, is that volume must be provided for the SiO_2 to form. The volume occupied by the SiO_2 precipitates is larger by about a factor of two than the volume occupied by the silicon atoms used to form the SiO_2. The oxygen atoms which help to form the SiO_2 were originally located on interstitial sites, not lattice sites. In the SiO_2 precipitates, however, the oxygen atoms take up a lattice site, requiring the volume expansion. Another way to appreciate this is to recall that in Chapter 2 when we discussed surface oxidation in the CMOS process, we observed that a volume expansion was part of the oxidation process. (Recall Figure 2–5.) The same thing happens here during the "internal" oxidation.

Because of the need for volume during the precipitation process, we can consider the roles that point defects present in the crystal might play. Vacancies can be thought of as microscopic empty sites in the crystal or, in other words, they could provide some of the volume or lattice sites needed for the SiO_2 precipitates to form. Stated another way, if a V happened to be present at a precipitate, an in-diffusing oxygen atom could occupy the site of the V. Thus the V could provide the volume required. Growing precipitates should thus consume V. By a similar argument, precipitates should also be able to obtain the needed volume by ejecting an I that is by removing a silicon atom from the perimeter of the precipitate. This I would then diffuse off into the crystal. Figure 3–25 also illustrates these ideas. We can express the precipitate growth process as follows [3.14]:

$$(1 + 2\gamma)\text{Si} + 2\text{O}_\text{I} + 2\beta V \leftrightarrow \text{SiO}_2 + 2\gamma I + \text{stress} \tag{3.55}$$

where γ is the number of I that contribute to the precipitation process per O_I atom joining the SiO_2, and β is a similar fraction for V. O_I represents the interstitial oxygen atom and Si is simply a lattice site in the crystal. We have included a stress term on the right-hand side because it is unlikely that the point defects could provide all the necessary volume and so it is likely that the region surrounding the SiO_2 precipitates will be under stress with the precipitate and the surrounding silicon under compression. From Eq. (3.55) we can observe that process environments which enhance the V population should promote precipitate growth, while those which enhance the I population should retard growth. We can also observe that when precipitates are growing, they themselves should produce an excess of I and a deficiency of V in the surrounding crystal. We will see examples of these effects in later chapters when we see how point defect populations affect diffusion (Chapter 7) and other processes. A final point worth noting in connection with Figure 3–25 is that a stacking fault is shown associated with the SiO_2 precipitate. Such faults along with dislocation loops are often found in connection with such precipitates. They occur as a result of the high compressive stresses generated around the SiO_2 region because of volume expansion. In most cases, then, it is undesirable to have these SiO_2 precipitates form near the wafer surface where devices are to be built. The intrinsic gettering process described in Chapter 4 ensures that the precipitates and the resulting faults form only in the bulk of the wafer, away from the surface regions.

3.5.6 Carbon in Silicon

Carbon is normally present in CZ grown silicon crystals at concentrations on the order of $1 \times 10^{16}\ \text{cm}^{-3}$. The carbon comes from the graphite components in the crystal pulling machine (see Figure 3–6). The actual mechanism of incorporation is believed to be the following. The melt contains silicon and modest concentrations of oxygen as was discussed above. This results in the formation of SiO that evaporates from the melt surface. Generally the ambient in the crystal puller is Ar flowing at reduced pressure, and the SiO can be transported in the gas phase to the graphite crucible and other support fixtures. SiO reacts with graphite (carbon) to produce CO that again transports through the gas phase back to the melt. From the melt, the carbon is incorporated into the growing crystal.

At the low concentrations in which it is normally present in CZ crystals, carbon is mostly substitutional in the silicon lattice. Since it is a column IV element, it does not act as a donor or acceptor in silicon and one might think that at 1 ppm, it might be relatively benign. This is not necessarily the case however. Carbon is known to affect the precipitation kinetics of oxygen in silicon even at such very small concentrations [3.15]. This is likely because there is a volume expansion when oxygen precipitates and a volume contraction when carbon precipitates because of the relative sizes of O and C. There is thus a tendency for precipitates that are complexes of C and O to form to minimize stresses in the crystal. Since precipitated SiO_2 is crucial in intrinsic gettering, this can have an effect on gettering efficiency. Carbon is also known to interact with point defects in silicon. Silicon interstitials tend to displace carbon atoms from lattice sites, presumably because this can help to compensate the volume contraction present when there is carbon in the crystal. Finally, the thermal donors described above (in Section 3.5.5) normally form around 450°C. There is also evidence that if C is present at > 1 ppm, these donors may also form at higher temperatures (650 – 1000°C). Much is still unknown or poorly understood about the roles of carbon in silicon, but it is clear today that it is important to control the C concentration during CZ crystal growth.

The carbon concentration is typically measured by FTIR as is the oxygen concentration. The relevant wavenumber is 607 cm^{-1} for C versus 1107 and 515 cm^{-1} for O. Typically the C concentration is less than 0.5 ppm ($\approx 2.5 \times 10^{16}$ cm^{-3}), that is, smaller than the O concentration by 25 – 50×. Both these concentrations are higher than the equilibrium bulk solubilities at typical IC fabrication temperatures however. Therefore the Si is in nonequilibrium during processing and there is a driving force to precipitate both C and O.

It is likely that there will be considerably more work in the future aimed at understanding the roles of carbon in silicon. This will be partly driven by the important interactions between carbon and oxygen. In addition, adding higher concentrations of C to Si (a few percent) can change the bandgap of the silicon and may allow the fabrication of new types of semiconductor devices in the future.

3.5.7 Simulation

Computer simulation tools would be useful in the context of this chapter to predict the properties of starting silicon wafers that would result from a particular CZ or FZ growth process. These properties might include doping concentration, oxygen and carbon impurity levels, defect concentrations, and perhaps most importantly, how all these parameters might vary across a wafer and along the length of the grown crystal. Unfortunately, such computer simulation tools are not generally available, in some cases because the appropriate physical models have not been developed or because the programs have simply not been written and widely distributed at this point in time.

Modeling and simulating the growth process in a CZ crystal puller is a tremendously difficult task. Realistic modeling would have to first calculate the temperature distribution inside the melt and crystal at all points. In order to do this, a finite element model for much of the crystal pulling machine would have to be implemented. Heat transfer and heat loss by conduction, convection, and radiation would have to be included. This challenge is as much equipment modeling as it is process modeling. As we will see in later chapters when we discuss process models for various steps in chip manufacturing, much of what has been done to this point in process modeling is really wafer scale or feature scale modeling, not equipment modeling. Thus the modeling and simulation of crystal growth is a broader problem than has been tackled for most other aspects of chip fabrication. In spite of the complexity of the problem, however, considerable progress has been made in the research community [3.16 – 3.18]. These codes can calculate the temperature distribution inside a crystal pulling machine and as a result in the melt and crystal itself. Very recently there have also been attempts to extend these models to calculate things like the carbon concentration profile inside a CZ grown silicon crystal [3.19]. Other proprietary codes that simulate some of the parameters of interest have been developed in specific companies that manufacture silicon wafers. One example of such a program is a computer model of the crystal growth process itself that is often used in the control system for the crystal growing machine to help maintain uniform diameter.

Another computer tool which would be very useful, but which does not exist today, would be a simulator that models oxygen precipitation effects in CZ crystals. It would be of great benefit to be able to predict the rate of oxygen precipitation based on the thermal cycling a wafer is subjected to and to be able to predict the resulting changes in point defect concentrations in CZ wafers. Some progress has been made toward this objective [3.14]. Since the simulation tools related to crystal growth and silicon wafer properties are at this point not complete and are not widely available, we will not discuss them in more detail here.

3.6 Limits and Future Trends in Technologies and Models

In some respects the future direction of silicon wafer technology is straightforward to predict. Silicon will be the dominant material used for ICs for as far into the future as we can reliably see. There will be increasing demand for larger diameter wafers since manufacturing economics favor larger wafers and the resulting larger numbers of chips they can carry. It is also easy to predict that as device dimensions continue to shrink, increasing demands will be made on wafer suppliers to reduce impurity levels in the starting wafers or to tightly control these levels as in the case of oxygen.

Two recent changes in the CZ growth process should help in controlling wafer properties. The first of these is the use of a magnetic field during CZ growth, resulting in MCZ or magnetic CZ ingots and wafers. The principle is simple. Surrounding the crucible containing the molten silicon with a magnetic field results in suppression of the thermal convection currents in the melt. This occurs because according to Lenz's law, currents are induced in a conductor whenever that conductor crosses magnetic field lines. The direction of the magnetic force tends to reduce the currents flowing in the silicon conductor due to thermal convection. This produces a more uniform ingot diameter and resistivity because the temperature fluctuations are smaller, and it produces lower and more uniform oxygen concentrations in the crystal because there is less dissolution of the crucible walls. MCZ silicon is now commercially available and may be a dominant method of growing crystals in the future.

Another method that is also being investigated to improve the uniformity of crystal properties, is the double crucible method. In this process, there are actually two crucibles of molten silicon. Growth occurs in one of them; the second is a reservoir of additional molten silicon. The two crucibles may sit side by side or be concentric with the inner one used for growth. The feed mechanism is usually a capillary tube between the two. The advantage of this approach is that the melt conditions in the growth crucible can be held more nearly constant. Silicon can be supplied during growth to maintain a more uniform liquid level in the growth crucible. The reservoir can also help to maintain a more nearly constant doping concentration in the growth chamber as well. The result is better control and uniformity of doping and oxygen concentration. This process may also find increased use in the future.

Two other possible changes may occur in at least some of the silicon wafers supplied to the IC industry. The first involves the use of epitaxial layers (Chapter 9). Many ICs today use such layers as the first step in device fabrication. P epi layers on P^+ substrates or N/N^+ combinations are common. Provided there are no buried layers in the process, these wafers are not specific to a particular circuit and so the wafer vendors could provide the epi layers. In fact vendors could even provide oxidized epi wafers to IC manufacturers since this would passivate the wafer surfaces for shipping. Note that this strategy would not be very attractive in the CMOS process flow we discussed in Chapter 2 because the epi layer option in that process was grown after a masking step and the introduction of both N- and P-type buried layers. IC manufacturers using such a process would likely do all the processing themselves and would simply purchase P-type starting wafers.

The final change that may impact starting wafers in the future is the current interest in Silicon On Insulator (SOI) structures. An example of such a starting wafer is shown in Figure 3–26. The advantages of such a structure come about because the devices are built in a thin silicon film on an insulator (SiO_2 in this case). This can reduce parasitic capacitances and as a result, speed up circuits. Several approaches are being used to produce such wafers. The first involves starting with a normal CZ or FZ wafer and ion implanting a large dose ($\approx 10^{18}$ cm^{-2}) of oxygen. Subsequent annealing of the implanted oxygen at high-temperature forms a buried SiO_2 layer [3.20]. The silicon above the buried SiO_2 can be of reasonable crystal quality if the structure is properly annealed, although the quality is generally not as good as the starting wafer. This process is know as SIMOX for "separation by implanted oxygen" and such wafers are now commercially available and are being investigated by a number of wafer manufacturers for IC applications.

A second approach to realizing "wafers" like Figure 3–26 is called the BESOI or "bonded and etch-back technology." It starts with two oxidized conventional CZ wafers. If these wafers are placed face to face after proper surface treatment, they will "stick" together. After annealing in a high-temperature furnace, an intimate bond is formed between the two wafers which is about as strong as the original wafers. One of the two wafers can then be etched or lapped away to leave a thin silicon film on an insulating SiO_2 substrate. A combination of lapping and chemical-mechanical polishing not unlike that described in Section 3.2.5 for conventional wafers, is often used. The ad-

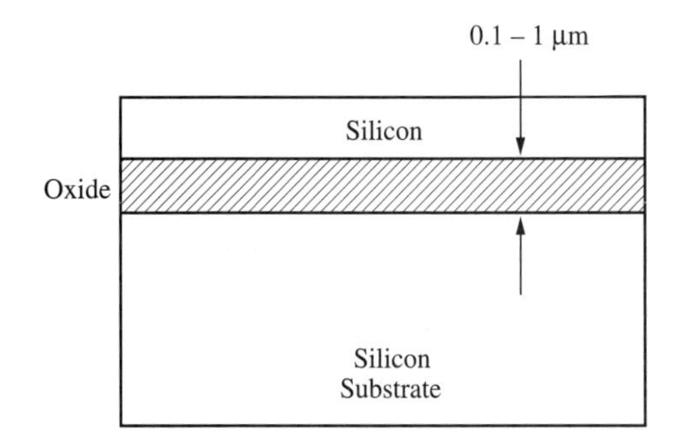

Figure 3–26 Silicon On Insulator (SOI) wafer technology. The buried oxide layer is typically several hundred nm thick.

vantage of the bonded wafer approach is that the resulting silicon should be of the same quality as the starting wafer. The disadvantage is that it is difficult to control the etch-back process well enough to leave a very uniform thin silicon film on the underlying SiO_2. Devices today may require submicron silicon films and it is very difficult to etch-back a wafer which starts at about 600 μm and leave a thin layer that is, for example, 0.5 μm ± 10%. A number of techniques are being investigated today to achieve the required tolerances.

Another approach to SOI substrates that has recently created great interest is the "Smart-Cut" process [3.21]. In this approach, a high-dose hydrogen implant is done into an oxidized silicon wafer. The energy of the implant is chosen to place the peak of the hydrogen implant at a depth below the silicon surface corresponding to slightly more than the desired final silicon thickness in the SOI structure. This wafer is then "stuck" to a second oxidized silicon wafer as in the BESOI process. The two wafers are then annealed in a two-step process. During the first, low temperature anneal (400 – 600°C) the first wafer splits apart at the location of the hydrogen implant. This leaves a thin and very uniform silicon layer from the first wafer sitting on an oxide, on the second wafer. The second high-temperature anneal (> 1000°C) strengthens the bond between the two wafers. A final polish of the thin silicon layer produces the SOI structure. This process has two significant advantages. First, it produces a thin, well-controlled and high-quality silicon layer in the SOI material. Second, it uses only one starting wafer per SOI substrate (unlike the two wafers in the BESOI process), because after the wafers split apart, the first wafer can be reused.

As a final comment, there are also approaches being pursued today involving epitaxial growth of silicon layers out of seed holes in an oxide coated wafer. The silicon can be made to grow out of the seedholes and then laterally over the SiO_2 layer. This results in a structure somewhat like Figure 3–26 as well, although the silicon layer is connected to the underlying substrate in isolated areas. This process is called Epitaxial Lateral Overgrowth (ELO).

3.7 Summary of Key Ideas

In this chapter we have described the techniques by which silicon wafers are produced. Through a process of refining, raw materials like quartzite (SiO_2) are turned into silicon with a purity unmatched by any other routinely available material on earth. This raw material is then used to grow single crystals, principally using the Czochralski method. Today the resulting boules may be 150 – 200 mm in diameter and up to a meter long. They are essentially defect free and the only significant impurities in the crystals, aside from dopants, are usually oxygen and carbon which come form the machines used to grow the crystals. A series of sawing, mechanical lapping, and chemical-mechanical polishing steps finally produce the individual wafers that are supplied to IC manufacturers. These wafers are 150 – 200 mm in diameter, mirror polished on one side, flat to within about ± 2 μm, and defect free. They contain dopants typically in the ppm range with tight tolerances, controlled oxygen concentrations in the $10^{17} – 10^{18}$ cm^{-3}, controlled carbon concentrations in the 10^{16} cm^{-3} range, and levels of all other undesirable impurities in the ppb range or lower. These wafers then form the starting material for IC manufacturers. It is remarkable that such wafers can be manufactured in enormous volumes and sold for about $50.

3.8 References

[3.1]. G. K. Teal, "Single Crystals of Germanium and Silicon—Basic to the Transistor and Integrated Circuit," *IEEE Trans. Elec. Dev.*, vol. ED-23, p. 621, 1976.

[3.2]. W. C. Dash, "Evidence of Dislocation Jogs in Deformed Silicon," *J. Appl. Phys.*, vol. 29, p. 705, 1958.

[3.3]. D. K. Schroder, *Semiconductor Material and Device Characterization*, John Wiley & Sons, 1990.

[3.4]. *Characterization of Solid Surfaces*, edited by P. F. Kane and G. B. Larrabee, Plenum Press, 1974.

[3.5]. M. Lannoo and J. Bourgoin, in *Point Defects in Semiconductors I: Theoretical Aspects*, Springer Series in Solid State Sciences, No. 22, Springer, 1981.

[3.6]. P. M. Fahey, P. B. Griffin, and J. D. Plummer, "Point Defects and Dopant Diffusion in Silicon," *Reviews of Modern Physics*, vol. 61, p. 289, 1989.

[3.7]. M. Tang, L. Colombo, J. Zhu, and T. Diaz de la Rubia, "Intrinsic Point Defects in Crystalline Silicon: Tight-binding Molecular Dynamics Studies of Self-diffusion, Interstitial-Vacancy Recombination, and Formation Volumes," *Phys. Rev. B (Condensed Matter)*, vol. 55, p.14279, 1997.

[3.8]. G. D. Watkins, in *Lattice Defects in Semiconductors, 1974*, Institute of Physics Conference Series No. 23, edited by F. A. Huntley, Institute of Physics, London, p. 1, 1975.

[3.9]. W. Shockley and J. Last, "Statistics of the Charge Distribution for a Localized Flaw in a Semiconductor," *Phys. Rev.*, vol. 107, p. 392, 1957.

[3.10]. J. Doerschel and F. G. Kirscht, "Differences in Plastic Deformation Behavior of CZ and FZ Grown Silicon Crystals," *Phys. Stat. Solidi A,* vol. 64, p. K85, 1981.

[3.11]. K. Sumino, H. Harada, and I. Yonenaga, "The Origin of the Difference in the Mechanical Strengths of Czochralski Silicon," *Jpn. J. Appl. Phys.*, vol. 19, p. L49, 1980.

[3.12]. W. Wijaranakula, "Solubility of Interstitial Oxygen in Silicon," *Appl. Phys. Lett.*, vol. 59, 1991.

[3.13]. J. C. Mikkelsen Jr., "The Diffusivity and Solubility of Oxygen in Silicon," *Mat. Res. Symp. Proc.*, vol. 59, p. 19, 1986.

[3.14]. H. W. Kennel, "Physical Modeling of Oxygen Precipitation, Defect Formation and Diffusion in Silicon," Ph.D. Thesis, Stanford University, TR No. G710-2, Feb. 1991.

[3.15]. Y. Shimanuki, H. Furuya, and I. Suzuki, "The Role of Carbon in Nucleation of Oxygen Precipitates in CZ Silicon Crystals," *J. Electrochem. Soc.*, vol. 136, p. 2058, 1989.

[3.16]. T. A. Kinney, D. E. Bornside, and R. A. Brown, "Qualitative Assessment of an Integrated Hydrodynamic Thermal-Capillary Model for Large-scale Czochralski Growth of Silicon: Comparison of Predicted Temperature Field with Experiments," *J. Crystal Growth*, vol. 126, p. 413, 1993.

[3.17]. T. A. Kinney, "Quantitative Modeling for Optimization of the Czochralski Growth of Silicon," Ph.D. Thesis, Massachusetts Institute of Technology, Cambridge, MA, 1992.

[3.18]. Some examples of proprietary commercial simulations can be found on the Mitsubishi Semiconductor Web site at http://www.egg.or.jp/MSIL/english/semicon/image-e.html/.

[3.19]. D. E. Bornside, R. A. Brown, T. Fujiwara, H. Fujiwara, and T. Kubo, "The Effects of Gas-Phase Convection on Carbon Contamination of Czochralski-Grown Silicon," *J. Electrochem. Soc.*, vol. 142, p. 2790, 1995.

[3.20]. K. Izumi, "Current Status of SIMOX Technology—High Quality ITOX-SIMOX Wafers and Their Application to Quarter-Micron CMOS LSIs," *Proc. Sixth International Symp. on Ultralarge Scale Integration Science and Technology, ECS Proceedings*, vol. 97, p. 221, 1997.

[3.21]. M. Bruel, "Silicon on Insulator Material Technology," *Electronics Lett.*, vol. 31, July 6, 1995.

3.9 Problems

3.1. Calculate the temperature difference across a (100) silicon wafer necessary for the silicon to reach its yield strength. This gradient sets an upper bound on the temperature nonuniformity that is acceptable in an RTA heating system.

3.2. A boron-doped crystal pulled by the Czochralski technique is required to have a resistivity of 10 Ωcm when half the crystal is grown. Assuming that a 100-gm pure silicon charge is used, how much 0.01 Ωcm boron-doped silicon must be added to the melt? For this crystal, plot resistivity as a function of the fraction of the melt solidified. Assume $k_O = 0.8$ and the hole mobility $\mu_p = 550$ cm^2 volt^{-1} sec^{-1}.

3.3. A Czochralski crystal is pulled from a melt containing 10^{15} cm^{-3} boron and 2×10^{14} cm^{-3} phosphorus. Initially the crystal will be P-type but as it is pulled, more and more phosphorus will build up in the liquid because of segregation. At some point the crystal will become N-type. Assuming $k_O = 0.32$ for phosphorus and 0.8 for boron, calculate the distance along the pulled crystal at which the transition from P- to N-type takes place.

3.4. A Czochralski crystal is grown with an initial Sb concentration in the melt of 1×10^{16} cm^{-3}. After 80% of the melt has been used up in pulling the crystal, pure silicon is added to return the melt to its original volume. Growth is then resumed. What will the Sb concentration be in the crystal after 50% of the new melt has been consumed by growth? Assume $k_o = 0.02$ for Sb.

3.5. Consider the zone refining process illustrated in Figures 3–7 and 3–19. Set up a simple spreadsheet to analyze this problem and use it to generate plots like those shown in Figure 3–21. Divide the crystal up into n segments as shown below. Consider a zone length dx which steps in increments dx up the crystal during refining. As the zone moves an amount dx, it incorporates an impurity concentration given by $C_S^p(n+1)$ where $n + 1$ is the next zone to be melted and $C_S^p(n)$is the impurity concentration in that zone from the previous pass. The liquid zone also leaves behind an impurity concentration given by $k_O C_L$ where C_L is the concentration in the liquid during the current pass. Note that the impurity concentration in the liquid consists of $C_S^p(n)$ plus all the impurities "swept up" by the liquid during the current pass. Note that the final zone at the end simply solidifies and can be neglected.

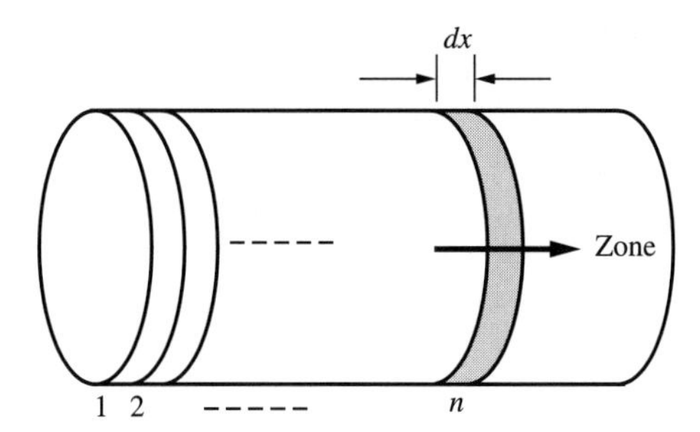

3.6. Suppose your company was in the business of producing silicon wafers for the semiconductor industry by the CZ growth process. Suppose you had to produce the maximum number of wafers per boule that met a fairly tight resistivity specification.
a. Would you prefer to grow N-type or P-type crystals? Why?
b. What dopant would you use in growing N-type crystals? What dopant would you use in growing P-type crystals? Explain.

Semiconductor Manufacturing—Clean Rooms, Wafer Cleaning, and Gettering

4

4.1 Introduction

In describing the CMOS process in Chapter 2, the sentence "The wafers are first cleaned in a combination of chemical baths that remove any impurities from the surface" was used many times. As we have seen in previous chapters, semiconductor devices are fabricated by introducing dopants, often at concentrations of parts per million, and by depositing and patterning thin films on the wafer surface, often with a thickness control of a few nm. Such processes are manufacturable only if stray contaminants can be held to levels below those that affect device characteristics or chip yield. In practice, this means that unwanted impurities must be kept below the ppm or ppb range and stray particles must be essentially eliminated.

Modern IC factories employ a three-tiered approach to control unwanted impurities—clean rooms, wafer cleaning, and gettering. The first level is implemented by building the chips in a clean environment. The air is highly filtered. Machines are designed to minimize particle production. Ultra-pure chemicals and gases are used in wafer processing. The second line of defense is to chemically clean the wafers often and thoroughly. This removes particles and contaminant films from the wafer surface before they can get into the thin films on the wafer or into the silicon itself. The final line of defense is called gettering and is a method whereby those unwanted impurities that do get into the wafer are made to collect in noncritical parts of the wafer, typically the wafer backside or the wafer bulk, far away from the active devices on the top wafer surface.

We described in Chapter 1 the great strides that have been made in shrinking device geometries and in improving manufacturing so that larger chips can be economically built. This progress requires that defect control associated with the manufacturing process also dramatically improve. Consider the SIA roadmap data summarized in Table 4–1 [4.1]. The entries in bold are new entries from those we previously discussed in Chapter 1.

The critical defect size in the table is an indication of how large a random particle needs to be in order to create a malfunctioning chip. For example, if a particle is present on the wafer surface when photoresist is being exposed, then that particle will likely prevent exposure beneath it. If such a defect is a significant fraction of the feature size being printed and it is located in a "critical area" of the chip, it will likely lead to a malfunctioning device. What constitutes a "critical area" on the chip depends on the particular manufacturing step. For example, at the gate oxidation stage, a particle located in the gate oxide region of a MOSFET will likely cause a malfunctioning device (gate short). It has been estimated that about 75% of the yield loss in a modern silicon IC manufacturing plant is due directly to defects caused by particles on the wafer. Note that the projected critical defect size in 2012 is only 0.025 μm (25 nm) or about 100 atoms across.

The defect density numbers in Table 4–1 arise from the fact that economic manufacturing of complex chips requires that most of the ICs on a wafer work at the end of the process. The roadmap numbers are driven by the desire to achieve chip yields on the order of 90% at the end of the manufacturing process. This implies that the yield on each individual step must be far higher (>99%) since so many steps are performed

Table 4–1 Semiconductor industry projected progress in chip size and feature size and the implications of this progress for defect size, density and contamination levels [4.1]

Year of First DRAM Shipment	1997	1999	2003	2006	2009	2012
Minimum Feature Size	250 nm	180 nm	130 nm	100 nm	70 nm	50 nm
Wafer Diameter (mm)	200	300	300	300	450	450
DRAM Bits/Chip	256M	1G	4G	16G	64G	256G
DRAM Chip Size (mm^2)	280	400	560	790	1120	1580
Microprocessor Transistors/chip	11M	21M	76M	200M	520M	1.40B
Maximum Wiring Levels	6	6–7	7	7–8	8–9	9
Minimum Mask Count	22	22/24	24	24/26	26/28	28
Critical Defect Size	**125 nm**	**90 nm**	**65 nm**	**50 nm**	**35 nm**	**25 nm**
Starting Wafer Total LLS (cm^{-2})	**0.60**	**0.29**	**0.14**	**0.06**	**0.03**	**0.015**
DRAM GOI Defect Density (cm^{-2})	**0.06**	**0.03**	**0.014**	**0.006**	**0.003**	**0.001**
Logic GOI Defect Density (cm^{-2})	**0.15**	**0.15**	**0.08**	**0.05**	**0.04**	**0.03**
Starting Wafer Total Bulk Fe (cm^{-3})	**3×10^{10}**	**1×10^{10}**	**Under 1×10^{10}**	**Under 1×10^{10}**	**Under 1×10^{10}**	**Under 1×10^{10}**
Critical Metals on Wafer Surface After Cleaning (cm^{-2})	**5×10^9**	**4×10^9**	**2×10^9**	**1×10^9**	**$< 10^9$**	**$< 10^9$**
Starting Material Recombination Lifetime (μsec)	**≥ 300**	**≥ 325**	**≥ 325**	**≥ 325**	**≥ 450**	**≥ 450**

in series in a manufacturing process. Fortunately, not all steps are critical and so optimizing the yield of chips requires identifying the critical steps, understanding the types of defects or contaminants that affect the yield in each step, and then setting upper bounds on those types of defects for each step. We will discuss yield issues more fully in Section 4.5.

The critical particle size is on the order of half of the minimum feature size. Particles larger than this have a high probability of causing a manufacturing defect. In starting wafers, the particle density is defined in terms of Localized Light Scatterers (LLS). Laser-based systems are often used to detect such particles and can produce automated counts (Section 4.4). At the gate insulator stage of the process, the issue is the electrical integrity of the gate dielectric and so the specification is in terms of Gate Oxide Integrity (GOI). This measurement is usually made by applying electric fields to test MOS structures and measuring the maximum field they can withstand before dielectric breakdown. The amount of charge trapping that occurs in the dielectric when current flows under high fields is also often measured as part of a GOI evaluation (Section 4.4). Note that the allowable particle density is much higher on starting wafers than it is at the critical gate insulator step. This is because the wafers are cleaned by the wafer manufacturer immediately before gate insulator processing. This step, when done properly, removes many particles as we will see later in this chapter. Notice also in Table 4–1 that the requirements are different for DRAM and logic chips, because of the greater gate insulator area on DRAM chips.

Table 4–1 also contains representative data from the SIA NTRS regarding contamination levels. The numbers for starting wafers are expressed in terms of volume concentrations in the wafer and are the contamination levels resulting from the crystal growth and wafer preparation processes. These numbers (on the order of $1 \times 10^{10}\ cm^{-3}$) are well below 1 ppb. While the numbers are specifically given for Fe contamination, similar specifications apply to other metals and to elements like Na and Ca. We will see why these elements are important later in this chapter. Following a wafer cleaning step during chip manufacturing, the specification of metal contamination is expressed as a surface "dose" per cm^2 because the chemical cleaning procedures are surface cleaning steps. These specifications (metal contamination levels on the order of $10^9\ cm^{-2}$) represent only about 0.0001% of a monolayer. We will see later in this chapter how modern cleaning procedures can consistently achieve such remarkably clean surfaces.

It is obvious that great care must be taken in making sure that the factories in which chips are manufactured are as clean as possible. Even with such ultra-clean environments, and even with procedures which clean wafers thoroughly and often, it is not realistic to expect that all impurities can be kept out of silicon wafers. There is simply too much processing and handling of the wafers during IC fabrication. As a result, some means of removing these impurities from active device regions—gettering—is normally incorporated into the manufacturing process. We will discuss in this chapter how this three-tiered approach—clean factories, wafer cleaning, and gettering—combine to make possible the economical manufacturing of today's integrated circuits.

4.2 Historical Development and Basic Concepts

If workers from one of todays modern IC manufacturing facilities were suddenly transported to a 1960s semiconductor plant, they would probably be amazed that chips could be successfully manufactured in such a place. Such factories were "dirty" by today's standards, wafer cleaning procedures were poorly understood, and gettering was an art rather than a science if it was used at all. Of course chips were manufacturable even in those days, but they were very small and contained very few components by today's standards. Since defects on a chip tend to reduce yields exponentially as chip size increases, small chips can be manufactured even in quite dirty environments. (We will discuss yield issues in more detail in Section 4.5.) However all of the progress that has been made in the past three decades in shrinking device sizes and designing very complex chips would have been for naught if similar advances had not been made in manufacturing capability, specifically in defect density.

Figure 4–1 illustrates the problem. Silicon wafers ready for cleaning may have a variety of surface films (SiO_2, polysilicon, silicides, metals, etc.) and doped regions, which generally must not be significantly attacked by the cleaning chemicals. Photoresists are commonly on the surface since photolithography is such a frequent step in IC manufacturing. Particles may well be present from the room air or from process steps the wafers have been exposed to; these must be removed. Finally, small concentrations of undesirable elements such as metals (Fe, Au, Cu, etc.) and alkali ions (Na, K, etc.) may be present from machines, chemicals, or the people the wafers have been exposed to; these must also be removed. Several examples may help to illustrate both the importance of removing these particles and undesirable contaminants, and also the deleterious effects they can have on device performance.

In Section 1.4.2 in Chapter 1 we described the sensitivity of modern MOS devices to trace levels of alkali ion contamination in gate oxides (Na^+, K^+ in particular). The threshold voltage of an MOS transistor (see Section 2.2.5 in Chapter 2) is to first order given by

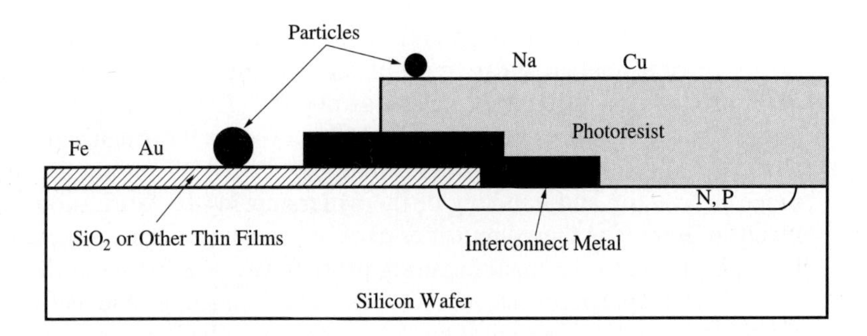

Figure 4–1 Example of a silicon wafer ready for cleaning. Contaminants include photoresist films, particles (usually 0.01 – 100 μm in size) and small concentrations of atoms or small clusters of metals, alkali ions, and other species.

$$V_{TH} = V_{FB} + 2\phi_f + \frac{\sqrt{2\varepsilon_S q N_A(2\phi_f)}}{C_{OX}} + \frac{qQ_M}{C_{OX}} \tag{4.1}$$

where Q_M is the mobile charge density (number of charges per cm^2) associated with Na^+ or K^+ in the gate oxide. The other terms are defined in Chapters 1 and 2. If we consider a typical gate oxide thickness of 10 nm, then a Q_M value of 6.5×10^{11} ions cm^{-2} is sufficient to cause a 0.1-volt shift in V_{TH}. Such a shift is an upper bound on what is acceptable today. 6.5×10^{11} ions cm^{-2} corresponds to less than 0.1% of a monolayer of surface Na^+ or K^+ contamination. Equivalently, it corresponds to a volume concentration of 6.7×10^{17} cm^{-3} or $\approx$ 10 ppm contamination in the gate oxide. Identifying the sources of Na^+ or K^+ contamination and learning to control them dominated research on the MOS system in the 1960s and largely prevented MOS technologies from being important commercially until toward the end of that decade. Wafer cleaning procedures today effectively remove alkali ions as we will see, and clean facilities largely prevent their introduction into wafers.

As a second example, consider the Dynamic Random Access Memory or DRAM. DRAMs are the highest-volume product manufactured by the semiconductor industry. Chips containing up to 256 million memory bits are now commercially available (256-MBit DRAMs). The basic memory cell structure is shown in Figure 4–2. Charge stored on an MOS capacitor represents the "1" or "0" state. The MOS transistor is used to write information onto the capacitor and to access the stored information. Most of the time, information stored on any particular capacitor simply waits to be read. During this time, the stored charge will decay because of leakage currents that discharge the capacitor. (The drain-substrate junction of the MOS transistor is electrically in parallel with the capacitor and the junction leakage will discharge it.) Periodically, circuitry on the DRAM chip must refresh the stored charge so that the data are not permanently lost. This typically happens automatically every few msec (the "refresh" time in a DRAM).

In silicon devices, junction leakage currents are often dominated by SRH recombination as described in Chapter 1. To provide a refresh time of a few msec, the minority carrier lifetime in the silicon must typically be greater than approximately 25 μsec. In fact numbers much larger than this are specified in the SIA NTRS (Table 4–1). From Chapter 1,

$$\tau_G = \frac{1}{\sigma v_{th} N_t} \tag{4.2}$$

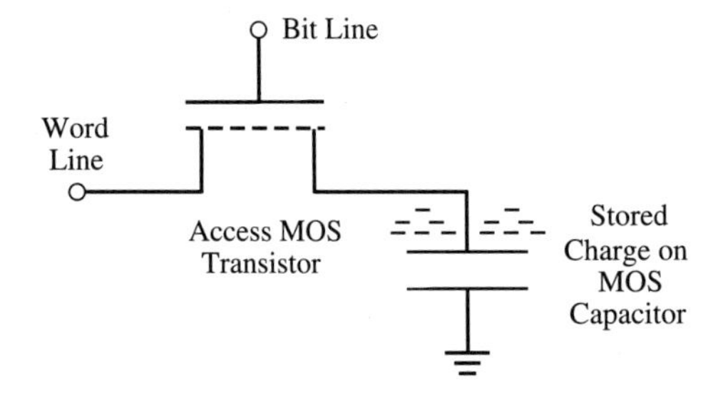

Figure 4–2 Equivalent circuit of a DRAM memory cell. Charge is stored on a MOS capacitor and the stored information is accessed through the MOS transistor switch.

where τ_G is the generation lifetime, σ is the capture cross section of the trap (on the order of the atom cross section or about 10^{-15} cm^2), v_{th} is the minority carrier thermal velocity (about 10^7 cm sec^{-1}) and N_t is the density of traps per cm^3. If $\tau_G = 100$ μsec, then using typical values for σ and v_{th}, gives $N_t \approx 10^{12}$ cm^{-3}. We saw in Chapter 1 that in silicon, these traps are normally associated with deep-level impurities like Au, Cu, Fe, and other elements. This simple calculation therefore suggests that proper DRAM operation requires impurity levels of these elements in the parts per billion range or lower. In fact the requirements may be even more severe than this calculation would suggest because deep level traps like Au, Cu, and Fe preferentially tend to accumulate at wafer surfaces and in junction regions of devices. (These elements segregate to defects or imperfections or simply regions of the crystal that are different from the normal perfect periodic lattice.) It is really quite difficult to keep the levels of these impurities below the ppb range simply by purifying the starting wafers and by excluding metal contaminants from manufacturing environments. The cost of doing this is usually simply too high. Fortunately, however, an alternative exists. Gettering, a process we will discuss in this chapter, provides a means of removing these unwanted elements from the regions of wafers where active devices are located. Normal manufacturing practice then simply recognizes that small amounts of deep-level impurities will inevitably be present and includes a gettering operation as part of the IC fabrication process to eliminate them.

A final example will illustrate a very different effect of "contaminants" and the importance of cleaning procedures. In an interesting set of experiments in 1978, Schwettman and colleagues cleaned silicon wafers with several different chemical cleaning procedures and then oxidized the wafers together in an oxidation furnace [4.2]. They measured the resulting oxide growth kinetics, with the results shown in Figure 4–3. The cleaning procedures that were used were chosen because they are variations on the industry standard "RCA clean" that we will discuss in detail later in this chapter. It is clear from this data that the cleaning procedure has a significant effect on the oxide

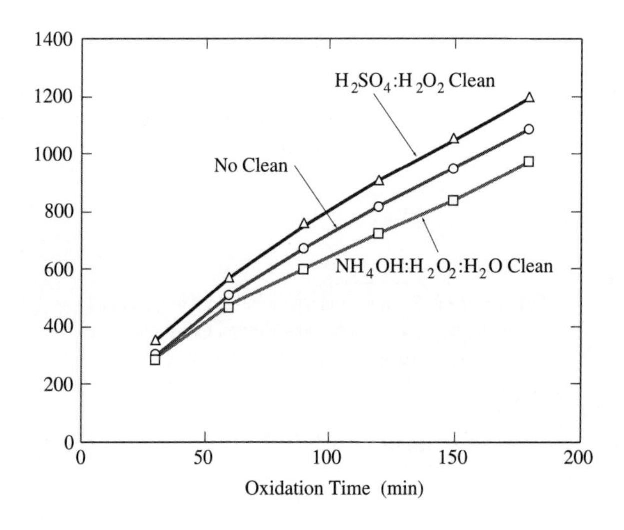

Figure 4–3 Effect of preoxidation cleaning procedure on oxide growth kinetics. (After [4.2]).

growth rate, presumably because of residual chemicals or surface oxides left on the wafers following cleaning. At the time these experiments were done, there was no understanding of the basic mechanism responsible for the results. Only in recent years with careful studies of surface chemistry have the reasons become clear.

We now turn to a more specific discussion of the three levels of contamination control used in modern IC manufacturing—clean factories, wafer cleaning, and gettering.

4.2.1 Level 1 Contamination Reduction: Clean Factories

The laboratories in which ICs are manufactured today clearly must be clean facilities. Particles that might deposit on a silicon wafer and cause a defect may originate from many sources including people, machines, chemicals, and process gases. Such particles may be airborne or may be suspended in liquids or gases. It is common to characterize the cleanliness of the air in IC facilities by the designation "class 10" or "class 100." Figure 4–4 illustrates the meaning of these terms. Class X simply means that in each cubic foot of air in the factory, there are less than X total particles greater than 0.5 μm in size. A typical office building is about class 100,000, while room air in state-of-the-art manufacturing facilities today is typically class 1 in critical areas. This level of cleanliness is obtained through a combination of air filtration and circulation, clean room design, and through careful elimination of particulate sources.

Particles are always present in a distribution of sizes and shapes. Those that are of most concern in semiconductor plants are between about 10 nm and 10 μm in size. In room air, particles smaller than 10 nm tend to coagulate into larger sizes; those larger than 10 μm tend to be heavy enough to precipitate fairly quickly. Particles between 10 nm and 10 μm can remain suspended in the air for very long periods of time. Such particles deposit on surfaces primarily through two mechanisms: Brownian motion and

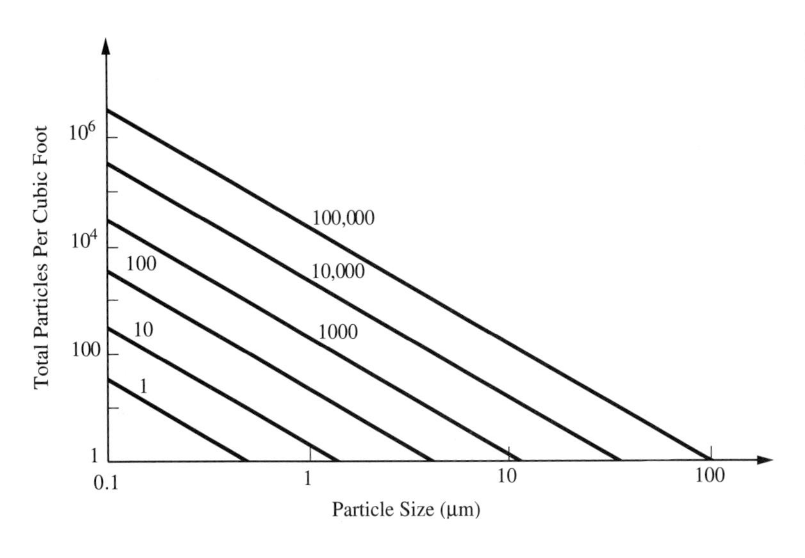

Figure 4–4 Particle size distribution curves for various classes of clean rooms (Federal Standard 209D, U.S. GSA 1989). The vertical axis is the total number of particles larger than a given particle size.

gravitational sedimentation. The first is the random motion of the particles in the air that occasionally brings them into contact with surfaces; the second is the gravitational force acting on the particles. Assuming a clean room environment in which the airflow is laminar at 50 cm sec^{-1}, Hu has estimated the rate of particle deposition on horizontal surfaces [4.3]. He finds that Brownian motion dominates for particles smaller than about 0.5 μm and gravitational effects dominate for larger particles. The net result is that in a class 100 clean room, about 5 particles larger than 0.1 μm will deposit on each square cm of surface area per hour. Comparing this estimate with the requirements in Table 4–1 illustrates why class 10 or class 1 clean rooms are now required.

Particles in the air in a manufacturing plant generally come from several main sources. These include the people who work in the plant, machines that operate in the plant, and supplies that are brought into the plant. Many studies have been done to identify particle sources and the relative importance of various sources. For example, people typically emit several hundred particles per minute from each cm^2 of surface area. The actual rate is different for clothing versus skin versus hair, but the net result is that a typical person emits 5 – 10 million particles per minute. This rate also varies with activity level, ranging from less than 10^6 to more than 10^7 particles min^{-1} for sitting versus running. Most modern IC manufacturing plants make extensive use of robots for wafer handling in an effort to minimize human handling and therefore particle contamination.

The first step in reducing particles is to minimize these sources. People in the plant wear "bunny suits" which cover their bodies and clothing and which block particle emission from these sources. Often face masks and individual air filters are worn to prevent exhaling particles into the room air. Air showers at the entrance to the clean room blow loose particles off people before they enter and clean room protocols are enforced to minimize particle generation. Machines that handle the wafers in the plant are specifically designed to minimize particle generation and materials are chosen for use inside the plant which minimize particle emission.

Since the sources of particles can never be completely eliminated, constant air filtration is used to remove particles as they are generated. This is accomplished by recirculating the factory air through High Efficiency Particulate Air (HEPA) filters. Interestingly, these filters were developed during World War II for the removal of airborne fissionable particulates. HEPA filters are composed of thin porous sheets of ultrafine glass fibers (< 1 μm diameter). Room air is forced through the filters with a velocity of about 50 cm sec^{-1}. Large particles are trapped by the filters; small particles impact the fibers as they pass through the filter and "stick" to these fibers primarily through electrostatic forces. The airborne particles may be charged when they impact the filter. Even if they are neutral, differences in the electron work function between the particle and the filter material can result in charge transfer and electrostatic forces. The net result is that HEPA filters are 99.97% efficient at removing particles from the air. With careful attention to leaks and sealing around the filter edges, the exit air is typically better than class 1.

Particles can also be introduced to wafer surfaces during chemical cleaning steps. Filtration of these chemicals is the normal method used to minimize this source of contamination. A special case is the water which is used in wafer rinsing, a common step in wafer cleaning procedures. Most IC manufacturing facilities produce their own clean water on site, starting with water from the local water supply. This water is filtered to remove dissolved particles and organics. Dissolved ionic species are removed by ion exchange or reverse osmosis. The result is high-purity water that is used in large quantities in the plant.

4.2.2 Level 2 Contamination Reduction: Wafer Cleaning

Contamination on wafers consists of particles, which we discussed in the last section, films such as photoresist which must be removed after they serve their purpose in lithography, and trace levels of any element which has not been purposely introduced. The latter category is perhaps the most difficult to measure and to control. The second level of contamination reduction is wafer cleaning. There is probably no step that is used more often in IC manufacturing. Cleaning must remove particles, films such as photoresist, and it must remove trace concentrations of any other elements present on the wafer surface.

Figure 4–5 illustrates the general strategy used in cleaning wafers. Most cleaning procedures begin with photoresist removal since photolithography normally precedes each processing step. Photoresists are organic compounds and can be stripped in a variety of chemicals. For front-end processing (no metals on the wafers), two methods are common. The first uses an acid (usually H_2SO_4) and a strong oxidant (usually H_2O_2) to decompose the resist into CO_2 and H_2O. The second method uses an oxygen plasma to convert the resist to gaseous byproducts (again CO_2 and H_2O). The oxygen plasma method offers the advantages of reduced pollution problems and very good selectivity to almost all underlying materials. For removal of photoresists in back-end processes the oxygen plasma approach can be used as can a variety of phenol-based organic strippers that do not significantly attack metals.

The most important aspects of wafer cleaning are the steps that are used following photoresist removal for front-end processes. Front-end processes often involve high temperatures (oxidations, anneals, film deposition etc.) and it is these steps which can allow diffusion of contaminants into thin films on the silicon or into the silicon itself. It is thus essential that the cleaning procedure remove contaminants from the wafer surface prior to these steps. Back-end processes are normally low temperature, so the

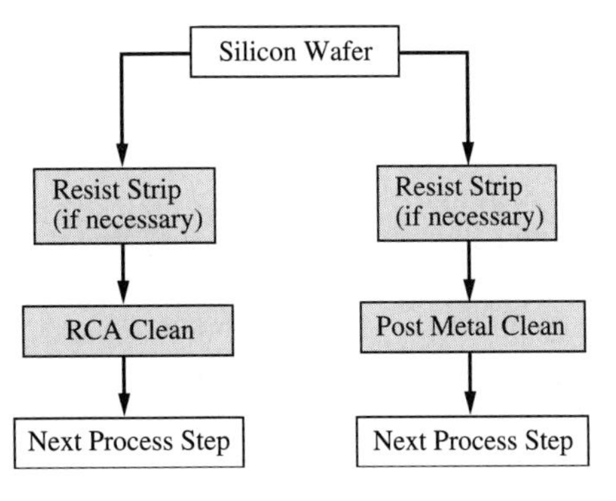

Figure 4–5 Typical cleaning strategies in a modern IC fabrication process. Left, front-end cleaning; right, back-end cleaning.

wafer cleaning, while important, is not as critical. (Both front-end and back-end cleaning procedures must remove particles from the wafers however since these translate directly into defects.)

Prior to about 1970, a variety of front-end chemical cleaning procedures were used in the semiconductor industry. In that year, however, a classic paper was published [4.4] which provided both a "standard" cleaning procedure and the beginnings of a scientific basis for wafer cleaning. This paper by Kern and Puotinen described work done at RCA over the previous several years in which detailed measurements were made of the effectiveness of various cleaning procedures in removing contaminants from silicon wafers. The resulting cleaning procedure became known as the "RCA clean" and has been the mainstay of the industry since that time. An excellent general reference on wafer cleaning issues is [4.5].

The original RCA clean is based on a two-step oxidizing and complexing treatment using hydrogen peroxide solutions. The first solution (called SC-1 in the literature) is a high-pH solution consisting of 5 H_2O:1 H_2O_2:1 NH_4OH in which the wafers are placed at 70 – 80°C for 10 minutes. This solution oxidizes organic films and complexes Group IB and IIB metals as well as other metals like Au, Ag, Cu, Ni, Zn, Cd, Co, and Cr. The SC-1 solution slowly dissolves the thin native oxide layer on silicon and continuously grows a new oxide layer by oxidation. This combination of etching and reoxidation helps to dislodge particles from the wafer surface. NH_4OH etches silicon and this solution can produce microroughening of the silicon. In recent years, the concentration of NH_4OH in the SC-1 solution has generally been reduced to minimize these effects. This improves the quality of very thin gate oxides grown in modern devices on these cleaned surfaces.

The second solution (called SC-2 in the literature) is a low-pH solution consisting of 6 H_2O:1 H_2O_2:1 HCl in which the wafers are placed at 70 – 80°C for 10 minutes. This solution removes alkali ions and cations like Al^{+3}, Fe^{+3}, and Mg^{+2} that form NH_4OH insoluble hydroxides in basic solutions like SC-1. These metals precipitate onto the wafer surface in the SC-1 solution. In the SC-2 solution, they form soluble complexes. The SC-2 solution also completes the removal of metallic contaminates such as Au that may not have been completely removed by the SC-1 step. The scientific basis for the SC-1 and SC-2 solutions comes from reaction chemistry and oxidation potentials; we will discuss these issues more carefully in Section 4.5.

Particles may sometimes adhere tenaciously to surfaces primarily due to electrostatic forces, so additional steps may be necessary to remove them. We depend on these forces in HEPA filters which clean the room air in IC plants. On wafer surfaces, however, we need to fully remove such particles. The original RCA cleaning procedure was really designed for removing contaminant films and atomic elements rather than particles, so additional strategies have evolved for dealing with particles. Ultrasonic scrubbing works well and can be combined with the RCA cleaning chemicals. Ultrasonic agitation is produced usually with piezoelectric transducers operating at 20 – 50 KHz. The sound waves in an appropriate liquid cause the generation, expansion, and violent collapse of tiny vapor bubbles under the alternating tensile and compressive stresses of the ultrasound. The bubble collapsing is known as cavitation and it literally knocks particles off the wafers or loosens them. Ultrasonic cleaning generally becomes less efficient as the frequency increases because at higher frequencies only very small bubbles can collapse in the compressive portion of the sound cycle. However, it has been found that very high frequencies ($\approx$ 1 MHz) are also quite effective for wafer cleaning and some commercial systems use these frequencies (megasonic cleaning).

The second approach to particle removal literally involves scrubbing the wafers with a brush in a liquid. The liquid allows the brush to hydroplane over the wafer surface, minimizing scratching while the rapidly rotating brush loosens particles from the surface.

4.2.3 Level 3 Contamination Reduction: Gettering

The term gettering has its origins in the vacuum tube industry where it referred to the use of materials like cesium which were used to remove trace gases from vacuum tubes. The basic idea of gettering in silicon manufacturing is simple. It is very difficult to reduce the concentration of undesirable elements such as metals (Fe, Au, Cu, etc.) and alkali ions (Na^+, K^+, etc.) in silicon materials to levels where they would have no effect on device performance. Clean factories and wafer cleaning are crucial as we have seen, but they are generally not sufficient. Gettering is the third tier defense and is a means of collecting these unwanted elements in regions of the chip where they do minimal harm. This is not as difficult as it might seem because the active devices in chips occupy a very small fraction of the wafer volume. In addition, the undesirable elements tend to have very high diffusivities (which is part of the reason why they are so "bad") and they tend to be easily captured either in regions with mechanical defects or in regions which chemically trap them. The elements we are most concerned about are highlighted on the periodic table in Figure 4–6.

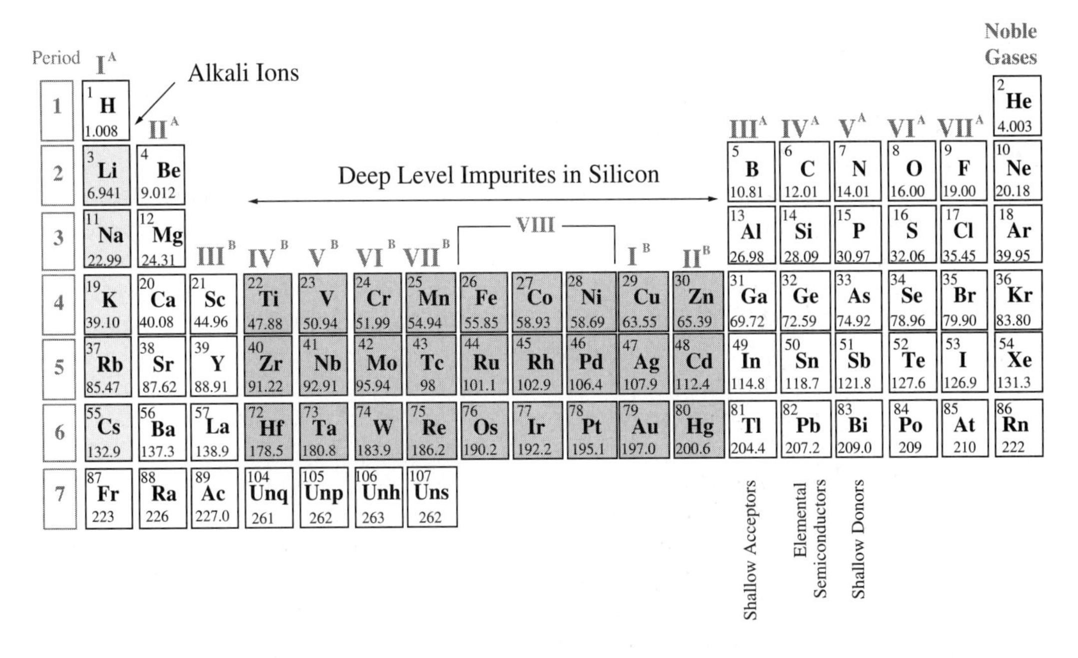

Figure 4–6 Periodic table indicating the elements that are of most concern in gettering. The alkali ions are in column 1 of the table; the metal ions that form deep level SRH centers are largely in the central portion of the table.

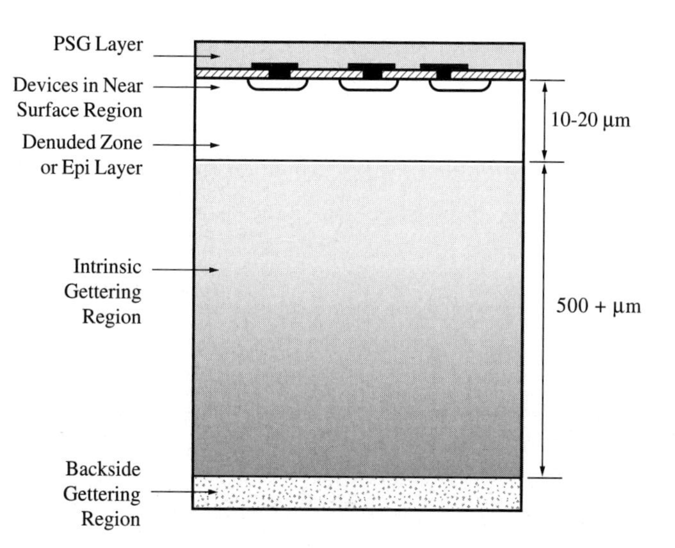

Figure 4–7 Wafer gettering strategies showing a surface denuded zone, intrinsic or bulk gettering regions and backside gettering.

Gettering therefore consists of three steps. First, the elements to be gettered must be "freed" from any trapping sites they may currently occupy and made mobile. Second, they must diffuse to the gettering site. Finally, they must be trapped. Figure 4–7 illustrates some of the key points.

Gettering strategies differ for the alkali ions (Na^+, K^+, etc.) and metals. The alkali ions are of most concern in the thin dielectrics on the top surface of ICs as the example earlier on MOS V_{TH} stability showed. Several approaches to gettering such elements have been explored, beginning in the 1960s [4.6 – 4.9]. The PSG (phosphosilicate glass) layer on the top of the wafer in Figure 4–7 is a common example. PSG is a P_2O_5/SiO_2 glass that is normally deposited by CVD or LPCVD. Usually it is about 5% by weight phosphorus. This glass has been found to be a very efficient trap for alkali ions, forming a stable complex that binds Na^+ or K^+ ions. Depositing such a glass as one of the upper thin film layers on a chip can thus effectively keep such ions from penetrating down to sensitive gate oxides or field oxides which are adjacent to the silicon surface. PSG layers are also effective getters for such ions. Na^+ and K^+ are very mobile at temperatures above room temperature and they will easily diffuse to and be trapped by a PSG layer. Effective gettering of these ions from dielectric layers below the PSG can thus take place. We used such a layer in the CMOS process in Chapter 2 (see Figure 2–34).

There are some drawbacks to PSG layers however. These layers contain charge dipoles that can affect surface electric fields [4.9], they are susceptible to absorbing water vapor and they can cause Al corrosion problems. These effects can be minimized by keeping the P concentration to a few percent. An alternative is to use a deposited Si_3N_4 layer as the top dielectric layer on a chip. These layers are impermeable to alkali ions and can form effective barriers to indiffusion. Using a barrier layer like this requires that earlier processing steps be free from significant alkali ion contamination since if Na^+ or K^+ ions were introduced earlier in the process, they would simply be locked into the IC structure by the surface nitride layer and could therefore cause instability problems. This strategy—clean processing plus a nitride cap layer—has been found to be workable by many VLSI manufacturers.

Trace metal atoms in the silicon bulk are gettered in a different fashion. Two basic methods are widely used. Extrinsic gettering makes use of a layer, usually on the wafer backside, which is created explicitly to trap such atoms. Intrinsic gettering makes use of a property of CZ silicon, namely that it contains oxygen. The oxygen can be made to precipitate and create traps for metal atoms within the wafer bulk.

Two basic properties of metal atoms, which act as deep level traps, have been well established for many years. The first is that these atoms have very high diffusion coefficients in silicon. Figure 4–8 shows some representative data [4.10, 4.11]. Note that the metals have diffusivities many orders of magnitude larger than the common dopants like P, B and As in silicon. Most of these metals diffuse as interstitials in silicon whereas dopants are substitutional and diffuse by interacting with point defects (see Chapter 7). Because of this, in the same time that standard dopants are diffusing to produce a PN junction 1 μm below the silicon surface, metals such as Au can easily diffuse completely through a silicon wafer. From a positive perspective, this makes it easy to getter these elements to regions away from active devices. From a negative perspective, metal contamination anywhere on a wafer can redistribute throughout an entire wafer.

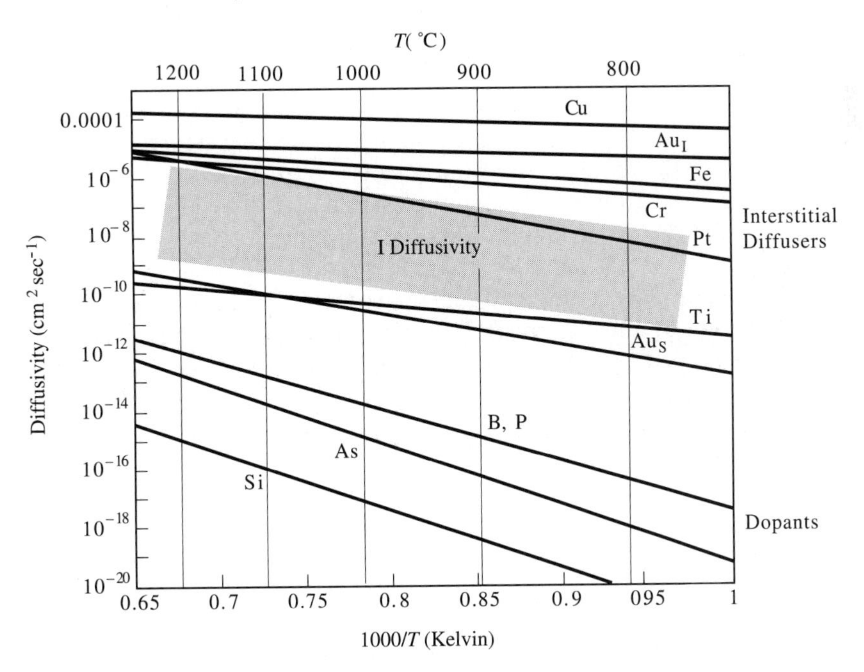

Figure 4–8 Diffusivities of various species in silicon. Au_S refers to gold in substitutional form (on a lattice site); Au_I to gold in an interstitial site. The silicon interstitial (I) diffusivity is also shown and will be discussed later. The gray area representing the I diffusivity indicates the uncertainty in this parameter. (After [4.10, 4.11].)

The second important property of these metals is the fact that they preferentially reside at sites in the silicon lattice where "imperfections" exist. Simply stated, these elements do not "fit" in the silicon lattice easily because of their very different atomic size. Thus if there are regions where faults or disorder exist, it is easier for these elements to find a suitable home. If we can create such regions in noncritical areas of the wafer, then we can getter these elements to those regions. Figure 3–4 illustrated some of the simple types of defects that can exist in a silicon crystal. Dislocations and stacking faults are well known sites for metals like Au, Cu, and Fe to "decorate." If such regions exist near or in device structures, metals can decorate them and this will result in significant degradation in device performance. The trick is to form such defects in the silicon, but away from the devices.

Extrinsic gettering sites have been formed in silicon by a wide variety of methods. Normally they are created on the wafer backside, which is an accessible surface far away from the devices on the top surface. Methods that have been used range from grinding and sandpaper abrasion, to ion implantation, laser melting, depositing amorphous or polycrystalline films (usually polysilicon), or high-concentration backside diffusions (usually phosphorous). Whatever the method, the objective is to create extended defects—dislocation loops, grain boundaries, precipitates—or other traps that are stable through subsequent high-temperature processing and hence can trap and hold metal atoms. Modern processes tend to use the "cleaner" methods from this list to produce backside damage (ion implantation, deposited polysilicon films, or backside phosphorus diffusions), since it is clearly not desirable to introduce additional contamination into the wafer during the gettering step. Once the backside damage sites are created, any subsequent high-temperature processing step will allow the metal atoms to diffuse to the backside where they can be trapped.

Intrinsic gettering relies on the ideas we described in Chapter 3 in connection with Figure 3–25. Oxygen in CZ silicon is normally supersaturated at processing temperatures because it is incorporated during growth at 1417°C. As we saw in Chapter 3, CZ silicon normally contains 10 – 20 ppm ($\approx 10^{18}$ cm^{-3}) oxygen. SiO_2 precipitates can form in the silicon under appropriate processing conditions. These precipitates are normally accompanied by stacking faults and other extended defects because of the volume mismatch of the SiO_2 and the host silicon lattice. Such sites are ideal trapping sites for unwanted metal ions. The trick here is to cause this precipitation to occur in the bulk of the Si wafer, but not in the near surface region where the devices are located. This turns out to be quite possible. In many cases, an epitaxial layer is grown on the silicon substrate as part of normal device fabrication (this was an option in the CMOS process we considered in Chapter 2). If this is the case, epitaxial silicon is normally very low in oxygen and so no precipitation would occur in the epilayer. Alternatively, the oxygen in the near surface region can be outdiffused from the wafer as one of the first steps in wafer processing, creating the denuded zone shown in Figure 4–7. In either case, SiO_2 precipitation can then take place only in the wafer bulk, away from the active devices.

4.3 Manufacturing Methods and Equipment

In this section we will discuss how the three levels of contamination control are actually implemented in modern IC manufacturing.

4.3.1 Level 1 Contamination Reduction: Clean Factories

Modern IC manufacturing plants are designed to continuously recirculate the room air through HEPA filters to maintain a class 10 or class 1 environment. A typical clean room is shown in Figure 4–9. All of the mechanical support equipment (pumps, etc.) is located beneath the clean room to minimize contamination from those sources. The HEPA filters are located in the ceiling of the clean room and the fans that recirculate the air are normally above these filters. Within the clean room, fingerwalls or chases provide a path for air return as well as a means to bring in electrical power, DI water, and process gases. Notice in the photo in Figure 4–9 the clean room clothing being worn. These "bunny suits" are designed to minimize particle emission from the people in the clean room.

The chemicals, gases, and DI water used in the plant are also potential sources of contamination. Normally electronic grade chemicals and gases are supplied by vendors to the plant. These may be further filtered on-site. DI water is usually generated at the plant site using filtering and deionization. The resulting water is extremely pure and is used in large quantities for cleaning wafers.

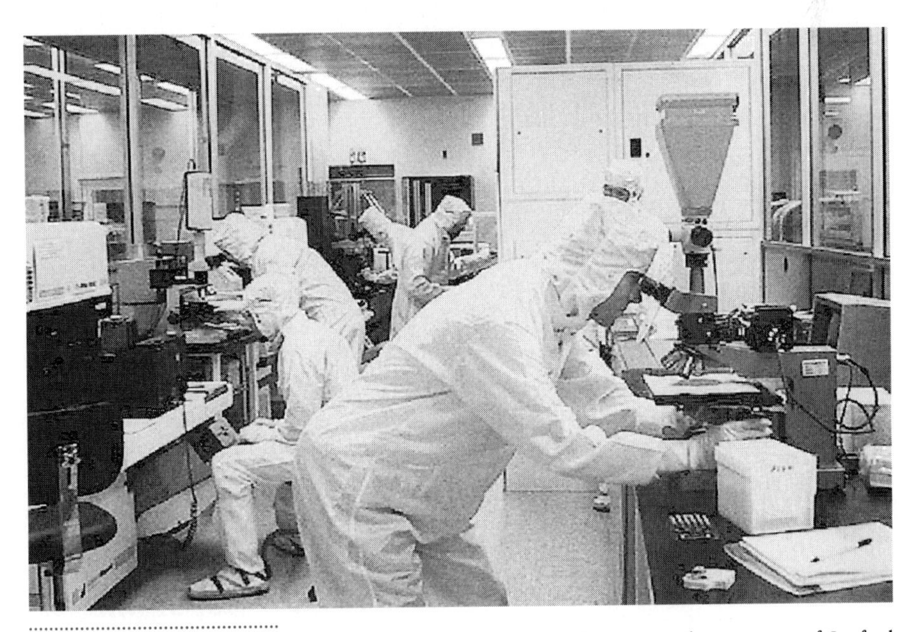

Figure 4–9 Configuration of typical modern cleanroom for IC fabrication. Photo courtesy of Stanford Nanofabrication Facility.

4.3.2 Level 2 Contamination Reduction: Wafer Cleaning

Wafer cleaning is usually accomplished today either using immersion of cassettes of wafers into cleaning baths or through chemical sprays. A typical wet bench for immersion cleaning is shown in Figure 4–10. Such baths may use recirculating filter systems and ultrasonic or megasonic agitation to enhance particle removal. Note the robot arm that is used to transfer the wafer cassettes from bath to bath. In spray systems, the wafers are generally mounted on a spinning drum and rotated past nozzles that spray the cleaning chemicals.

The standard implementation of the RCA cleaning procedure is shown in Figure 4–11. Options include the addition of ultrasonic agitation to the SC-1 or SC-2 solutions, using heated DI water for the rinses, the addition of a 50:1 H_2O/HF step between the SC-1 and SC-2 solutions (with DI H_2O rinses before and after the HF step), or the addition of a 50:1 H_2O/HF step at the end of the cleaning procedure (followed by another DI H_2O rinse). The ultrasonic agitation is designed to help particle removal as we have previously discussed. The additional 50:1 H_2O/HF steps are designed to remove the chemical oxide layers that are grown during the RCA cleaning steps. Removing these oxides remains a controversial option. The advantage is that any impurities contained in the oxide are stripped by the 50:1 H_2O/HF step. However this step leaves the silicon surface hydrogen terminated which is not particularly stable, which makes it more susceptible to absorbing additional contaminants during subsequent processing.

Other cleaning solutions are used during back-end processing as described earlier in this chapter. Generally the equipment used is similar to that described here for front-end cleaning. The cleaning solutions themselves are usually purchased and used as is from suppliers.

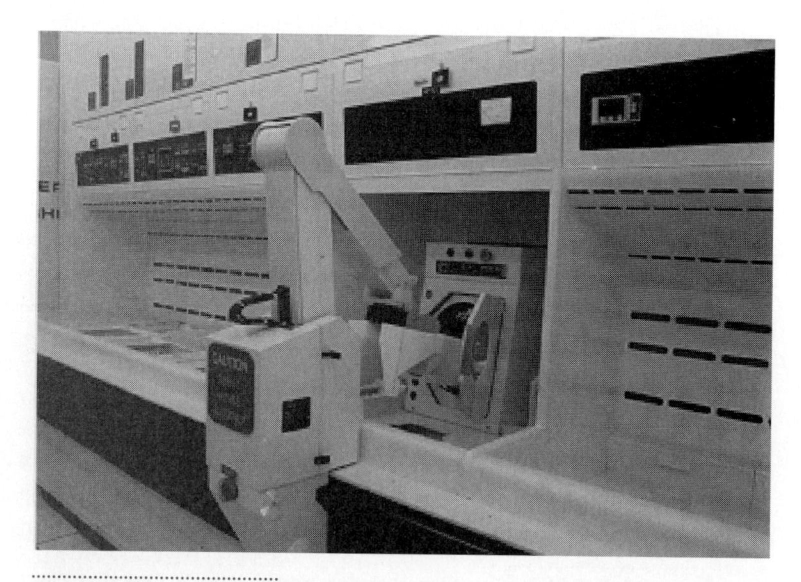

Figure 4–10 A typical cleaning station in a modern IC manufacturing facility. Wet chemical cleaning baths are in the sinks. The robot is loading a cassette of wafers into a spin dryer. Photo courtesy of Ruth Carranza.

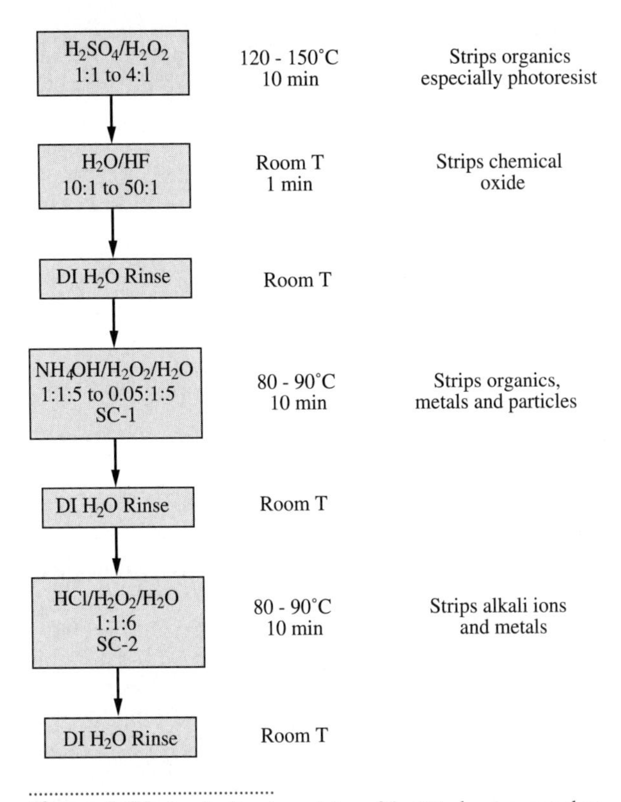

Figure 4–11 Standard implementation of the RCA cleaning procedure.

4.3.3 Level 3 Contamination Reduction: Gettering

Both extrinsic and intrinsic gettering processes are common in the semiconductor industry and sometimes both are used for added insurance. Often an extrinsic gettering process is used in which backside damage or a backside polysilicon layer is created at some convenient time during the normal process flow and then simply left in place during subsequent high-temperature steps. Gettering then takes place automatically without any special high-temperature step. This approach requires that the backside damage or the polysilicon layer be thermally stable during all the remaining high-temperature steps. If the damage anneals out, or the polysilicon recrystallizes, the gettered metal ions can be released and recontaminate the device regions on the wafer topside.

Intrinsic gettering is more popular because it tends to be a better controlled process. The damaged region is much larger than simply the wafer backside, is closer to the devices than the backside, and is thermally stable once it is created. As described conceptually earlier, intrinsic gettering consists of creating SiO_2 precipitates in the wafer bulk by appropriate thermal cycling of the wafer. Because of the volume mismatch between these precipitates and the silicon lattice, defects such as dislocations are generated as a result of the precipitation. These defects provide trapping sites for the gettered species, well away from the device region on the wafer surface.

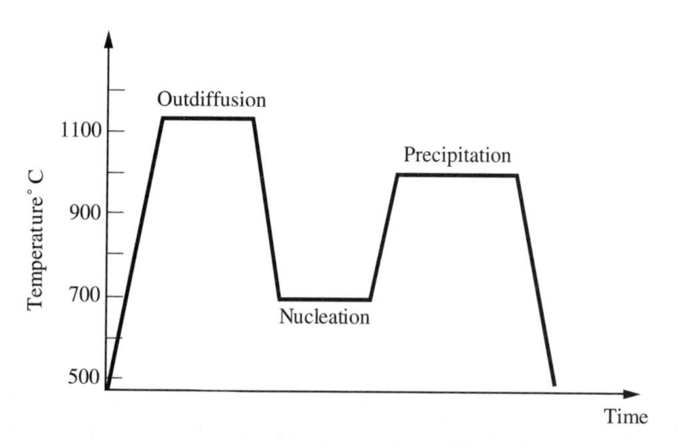

Figure 4–12 Processes and time/temperature cycle for a typical intrinsic gettering process.

The SiO_2 precipitates and the resulting damage are created using a thermal cycle like that illustrated in Figure 4–12. This is normally done near the beginning of the wafer fabrication process flow. If there is no epi layer on the wafer surface, an initial high-temperature step is used to outdiffuse the oxygen in the near surface region. This creates the denuded zone shown in Figure 4–7. As we saw in Chapter 3, oxygen diffuses interstitially in silicon with a diffusivity given by [4.12]

$$D_O = 0.13 \exp\left(-\frac{2.53 \text{ eV}}{kT}\right) \text{cm}^2 \text{sec}^{-1} \tag{4.3}$$

The time required to create an "oxygen free" surface region can thus be easily calculated. The surface region does not actually have to be oxygen free. What is required is that the oxygen concentration is reduced below the level at which precipitation will occur in the next part of the cycle. Normal oxygen concentrations in CZ silicon are 15–20 ppm ($\approx 10^{18}$ cm^{-3}). If the concentration is much higher than 20 ppm, too much precipitation will take place and there may be problems with wafer warpage or excessive defect formation. Precipitation does not readily occur below concentrations of about 10 ppm. A temperature cycle of several hours at 1100 – 1200°C is sufficient to create a denuded zone several tens of μm deep.

The next step in the process is precipitation of the oxygen to form small SiO_2 precipitates or embryos. We described this process in some detail in Chapter 3 (Section 3.5.5). The optimum temperature for precipitation is around 700°C [4.13]. Precipitation usually takes place over several hours. The embryos must be grown to a minimum critical size during this step so that during the subsequent higher temperature growth step they will grow and not shrink. This critical size depends on process conditions (especially temperature), but is on the order of 1 – 3 nm. The density of embryos created also depends strongly on process conditions, but is on the order of 10^{11} cm^{-3}.

The final step in creating the intrinsic gettering region is growth of the embryo precipitates. This is accomplished by raising the temperature to approximately 1000°C for several hours, which allows them to grow to 50 – 100 nm in size. It may be necessary to carefully control the temperature ramp rate at the start of the growth cycle, because the critical embryo size increases with temperature. If the temperature is ramped up too quickly, the embryos may be below the critical size at the growth temperature and therefore shrink rather than grow. Slow ramping gives them a chance to grow during the ramp up in temperature. The net result of these process steps is shown in Figure 4–13 [4.14]. In this series of experiments, an initial outdiffusion for 10 hours at 1100°C was used, followed by nucleation at 750°C for 6 – 24 hours and growth (precipitation) at 1000°C for 8 – 48 hours. A denuded zone about 25 μm deep is visible at the surface of the wafers. Notice that longer precipitation and growth times result in a higher density and larger precipitates in the wafer bulk.

4.4 Measurement Methods

Accurate measurement methods are critical if contamination sources are to be identified and controlled. Instruments are needed for particle detection and for identification and measurement of the concentrations of contaminating species. As IC manufacturing processes have become cleaner, sensitivity requirements on measurement methods have become correspondingly higher. We will describe in this section some of the common methods used to detect and measure such contaminants.

4.4.1 Level 1 Contamination Reduction: Clean Factories

As we have seen, the biggest issue in clean factories is particle control. We need methods to accurately detect particle concentrations of < 10 particles per wafer, with a critical particle size well below 0.1 μm (see Table 4–1). The simplest approach is optical microscopy, which can routinely detect particles down to about 1 μm in size. Manual inspection can be used to search for particles but this is a very time consuming and inefficient process.

Particle detection is simplest on blank wafers since there is no pattern present to scatter the light. One common method of particle detection involves running a blank wafer through a process and then counting the particles to assess the cleanliness of that process. Automated systems generally rely on lasers and the scattering of laser light that takes place when the light strikes a particle on the wafer. The laser beam is scanned over the surface of the wafer. The light is reflected at a predictable angle unless the light strikes a particle. Light that is scattered off particles is collected by an optical system, amplified by a photodetector, and used to produce a wafer map of the particles present. This process can reliably detect particles down to ≈ 0.2 μm in size and can produce a wafer map in a few seconds. Shorter wavelength lasers can reduce the detected particle size. The process is simple and reliable, but it is restricted to unpatterned wafers. Several commercial systems are available to make this measurement.

While the data from blank wafers are useful, the real interest of course is in defect densities on product wafers. Since these wafers are necessarily patterned, simple laser scanning systems are not a solution. Two approaches to this problem are used. The first uses an optical system and comparison of the image with a "known good reference." The reference can be either an adjacent die or a database from the chip design of what the pattern is supposed to look like. When an adjacent die is used as the reference, any differences in the images from the two die are "interesting events" and are usually shown to a technician for evaluation. In more advanced systems, image processing and

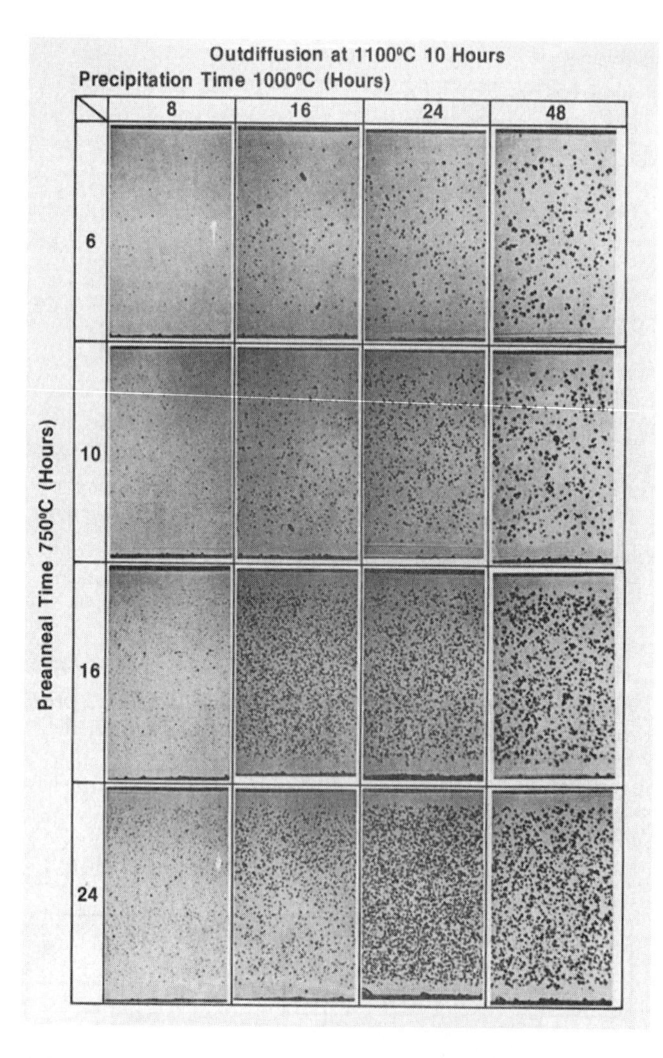

Figure 4–13 Cross-sectional SEM images of a wafer utilizing intrinsic gettering under various process conditions. All samples were initially outdiffused at 1100°C for 10 hrs. The SiO_2 precipitates are clearly visible in the wafer bulk, as is the denuded zone at the surface. Reprinted with permission of Solid State Technology [4.14].

pattern recognition software can be used to help identify defects. This approach is much more time consuming than the simple laser scanning systems (5 – 10 minutes per wafer), but it does provide information on real product wafers. The particle sizes that can be observed in this way are limited by the optical system used, but the principle of image comparison can be extended to very small particle sizes through the use of Scanning Electron Beam (SEM) systems. There are, however, throughput issues associated with the SEM systems in a manufacturing environment.

The second approach to measuring defect densities on product wafers involves test structures specifically designed to detect defects. These test structures may occupy a few test sites on a product wafer or they may occupy a full wafer processed alongside the product wafer. A simple example is shown in Figure 4–14 in which a mask level for an interconnect layer is shown (metal or polysilicon layer for example). Simple electrical

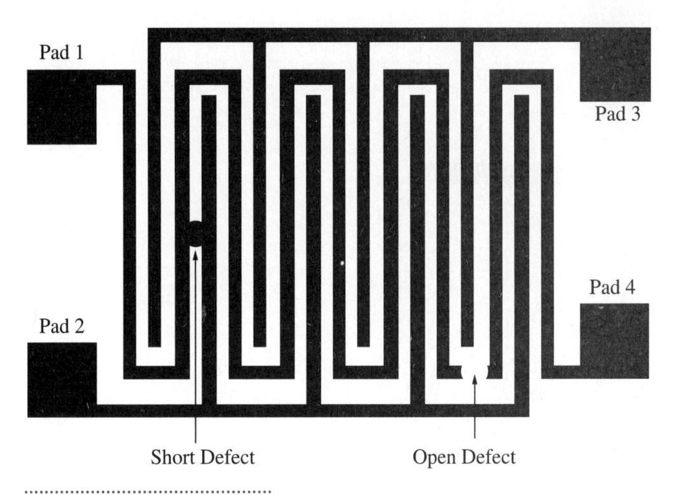

Figure 4–14 Layout (top view) of a typical electrical test structure designed to detect defects in an interconnect layer. Typical open and short defects are illustrated.

measurements of connectivity at the end of the process can give information on defect densities. For example, an open between pads 1 and 4 would indicate a break in what should be a continuous line, probably caused by a particle defect during the deposition or etching of that line. A short between pads 1 and 2 would indicate bridging between two metal lines, again, probably caused by a particle during deposition or etching of the metal lines. A significant amount of research in recent years has investigated the design of such defect monitors [4.15 – 4.17]. They are widely used, especially during the development of a new process or technology. Obviously, the lower the defect density, the larger such structures must be to reliably detect the defects. Once a product is in high-volume manufacturing, it is generally undesirable to "waste" wafer area on such monitors since a chip that is used for monitoring could also be a product chip.

It is also common to use electrical methods to detect defects in insulating layers, particularly gate insulators. Here the simplest test structure is a MOS capacitor, illustrated in Figure 4–15. In the simplest case a thin insulator is grown on a silicon wafer and then metal gates are patterned. A voltage is then applied to each capacitor structure and ramped up until dielectric breakdown occurs. The field at which this occurs is recorded and a histogram plot generated as shown. Ideally, all the capacitors would break down at the same field, corresponding to the maximum field the insulator can sustain. In practice, some capacitors break down prematurely, because of defects in the insulator, often caused by particles present on the surface when the dielectric was grown.

More sophisticated measurements are also possible with this simple MOS structure. For example, a high field (below breakdown) can be applied to the capacitor for a fixed time period. Some current will flow through the insulator due to tunneling or other conduction mechanisms. Traps or defects in the insulator can capture some of the electrons or holes while this current is flowing, resulting in charge accumulation in the insulator. This charge trapping can be measured through a change in the threshold voltage of the

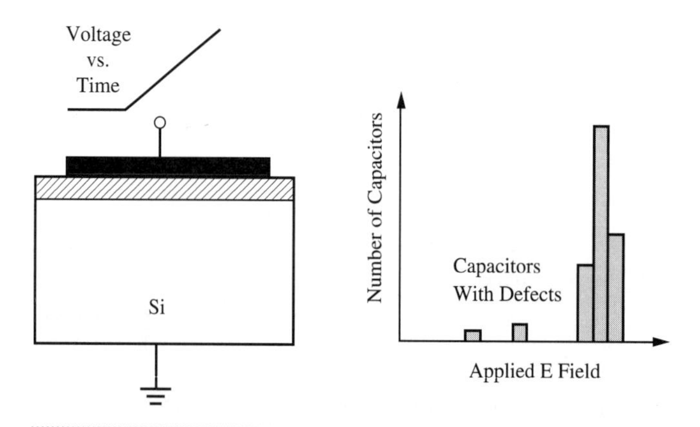

Figure 4–15 MOS capacitor test structure. The voltage applied to the gate is ramped up until significant current flows through the gate dielectric. The electric field at which this breakdown occurs is plotted on the right.

capacitor [trapped charge Q_T replaces mobile charge Q_M in Eq. (4.1)]. The amount of trapped charge is a measure of the quality of the dielectric layer (generally the smaller the better). Capacitors with defects due to particles or contaminants would show up as outliers as in Figure 4–15.

The most common chemical used in IC manufacturing is water. As we have seen, this water is filtered and deionized and is usually referred to simply as DI water. The most common impurities in DI water are ions. A simple measurement of water resistivity is often used to assess the "quality" of DI water. In pure water the resistivity is not infinite because the following reaction, at equilibrium, provides finite concentrations of H^+ and OH^- ions

$$H_2O \leftrightarrow H^+ + OH^- \tag{4.4}$$

Example At room temperature in equilibrium, $[H^+] = [OH^-] \approx 6 \times 10^{13}\ \text{cm}^{-3}$ in water. The diffusivities of the H^+ and OH^- ions are $9.3 \times 10^{-5}\ \text{cm}^2\ \text{sec}^{-1}$ and $5.3 \times 10^{-5}\ \text{cm}^2\ \text{sec}^{-1}$, respectively. Using the Nerst-Einstein relationship $\mu = zqD/kT$, where z is the charge on the ion, calculate the ion mobilities, and the DI water resistivity.

Answer

$$\mu_{H^+} = \frac{qD}{kT} = \frac{9.3 \times 10^{-5}\ \text{cm}^2\ \text{sec}^{-1}}{25.9 \times 10^{-3}\ \text{V}} = 3.59\ \text{cm}^2\ \text{volt}^{-1}\ \text{sec}^{-1}$$

$$\mu_{OH^-} = \frac{qD}{kT} = \frac{5.3 \times 10^{-5}\ \text{cm}^2\ \text{sec}^{-1}}{25.9 \times 10^{-3}\ \text{V}} = 2.04\ \text{cm}^2\ \text{volt}^{-1}\ \text{sec}^{-1}$$

Using Eq. (1.1) for the resistivity, we finally have

$$\rho = \frac{1}{1.6 \times 10^{-19}[(3.59)(6 \times 10^{13}) + (2.04)(6 \times 10^{13})]} \cong 18.5\ \text{M}\Omega\text{cm}$$

DI water in an IC manufacturing facility is normally monitored to make certain its resistivity is at least 18 MΩcm. When DI water is used for rinsing at the end of cleaning procedures, its resistivity can also be easily monitored to determine when the rinsing is complete.

4.4.2 Level 2 Contamination Reduction: Wafer Cleaning

The purpose of wafer cleaning is to remove particles and contaminants from the surface of wafers. Measurement techniques associated with cleaning thus focus on identifying and measuring the concentration of any residual contaminants left on the wafer after the cleaning process. Particles can be measured with the methods described in the previous section, so we will focus here on measuring and quantifying the concentrations of impurities left on the surface or introduced onto the surface by cleaning procedures. These techniques are basically surface analysis techniques. We will describe the more useful techniques here. More details on these and other methods are available in a number of excellent texts on this topic such as [4.18].

Surface analysis generally involves exciting the surface atoms of the material (using electron beams, X-rays, or ions) and then measuring a characteristic emission (of electrons, X-rays, or ions) from the surface atoms. Identification relies on the fact that the emitted species carry a unique atomic signature. Quantitative measurement relies on the fact that the magnitude of the signal is generally proportional to the concentration of the particular atomic species present in the sample. Figure 4–16 illustrates many of the commonly used measurement techniques.

When a high-energy electron beam strikes a solid, the incoming electrons give up their energy through a variety of physical processes, some of which result in electrons being emitted from the solid. Figure 4–17 illustrates the energy spectrum of these emitted electrons. Secondary electrons have the lowest energies (typically peaking at about 5 eV). They result from processes in which the incoming electrons collide inelastically with electrons in the solid and transfer enough energy to the target electrons to allow them to escape from the solid. These are the electrons that are normally collected and used to form the images in Scanning Electron Micrographs (SEMs) as described in Section 3.4.2.3 in Chapter 3. At the highest energies we find backscattered electrons which result from elastic collisions between the incoming electrons and atoms in the solid. (The incoming electrons "bounce" off atoms and are reflected back out of the sample, with energies similar to their initial energy.)

At intermediate energies, we find the Auger electrons, which are released through a process illustrated in Figure 4–18. This figure extends the band diagrams we introduced in Chapter 1 over a wider energy spectrum. The core electron energy levels (E_K, E_{L1} and

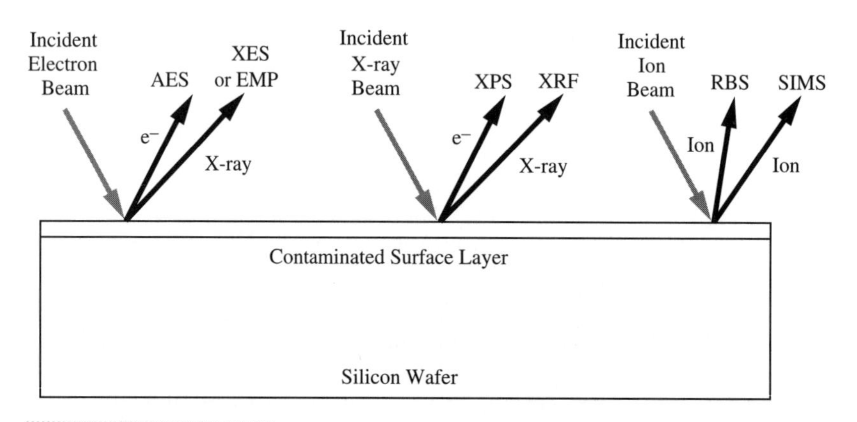

Figure 4–16 Surface analysis techniques used to identify and quantify contamination in IC manufacturing.

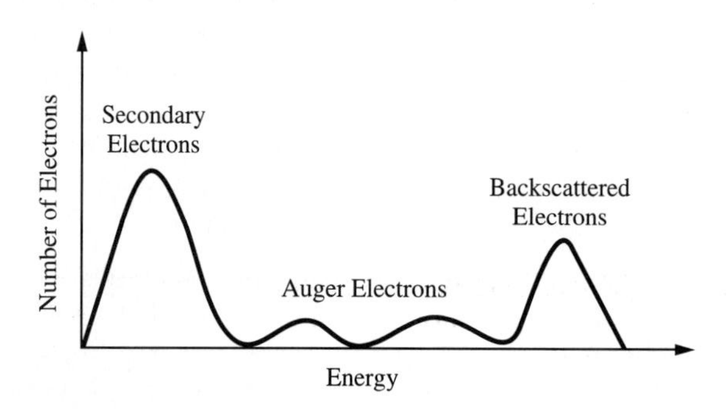

Figure 4–17 Energy distribution of electrons emitted from a solid under electron bombardment.

E_{L2}) represent those electrons nearer the nucleus which are more tightly bound. In this example, the incident (primary) electron with an energy of several keV enters the sample and "kicks out" a core electron from the E_K level (the secondary electron). A higher energy electron from the E_{L1} level drops into the vacant E_K level. The energy released in this process may be given off as an X-ray as illustrated on the right side of the figure. In this case the analysis method is called XES (X-ray Electron Spectroscopy) or EMP (Electron Microprobe). The released energy from the E_{L1} to E_K transition may also be given to a third electron as shown on the left of the figure. In this case this electron is ejected from the E_{L2} level and is known as an Auger electron. The analysis method in this case is AES (Auger Electron Spectroscopy). The transition in this example is called a KLL transition and involves three electrons as do all Auger processes. The Auger electron in AES or the X-ray in XES carry a unique signature of the element from which they were emitted because transitions between specific atomic energy levels are involved. Thus these techniques can be used for compositional analysis. Since the ejection of an Auger electron or an X-ray are competitive processes, the relative probabilities of the two events determine which is more likely. In general the lighter elements produce

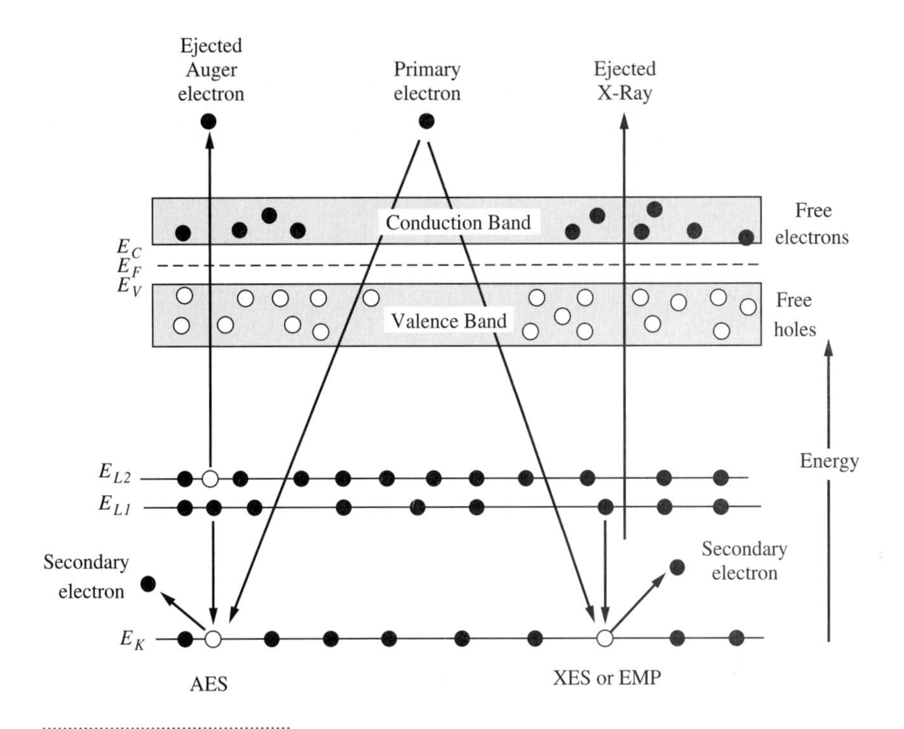

Figure 4–18 Band diagram representation of some of the processes used in surface analytical methods.

Auger electrons; the heavier elements X-rays. The crossover in probability between the two processes occurs around Z = 33 (arsenic).

The incident energy can also be provided by an X-ray as illustrated in Figure 4–16. The emitted particle can be either an electron or an X-ray, providing atom specific information as do the electron beam techniques described above. With an X-ray input, the analysis methods are known as XPS (X-ray Photoelectron Spectroscopy) when an electron is emitted or XRF (X-ray Fluorescence) when an X-ray is emitted.

Two other analysis methods are also conceptually shown in Figure 4–16. RBS (Rutherford Backscattering) detects ions which are elastically scattered by collisions with atomic nuclei in the substrate. Typically He ions with an energy of 1 to 3 MeV are used. This technique also provides compositional information because the backscattered ions have an energy equal to their incident energy minus an energy characteristic of the atom with which they collided and the depth in the sample at which the collision occurred.

The final analytic technique illustrated in Figure 4–16 is SIMS (Secondary Ion Mass Spectrometry). In this case, ions (usually O^+ or Cs^+) are used to bombard the sample. Collisions of these ions with sample atoms cause ejection (sputtering) of the sample atoms. The sputtered atoms are mass analyzed to provide compositional information on the sample. SIMS is the dominant method used today for dopant profiling and will be discussed in greater detail in Chapter 7 on dopant diffusion.

All of these techniques can be used to identify and measure the concentration of residual contaminants left on the wafer after cleaning. Each technique has advantages and disadvantages related to elemental sensitivity, spatial resolution, and depth resolution. In general, the techniques that use a primary electron beam (left side of Figure 4–16), can produce good lateral resolution because electron beams can be easily focused. Techniques that detect ejected electrons (AES and XPS) provide good depth resolution and surface sensitivity since the ejected electrons can escape only from the near surface region. Techniques that detect emitted X-rays (XES and XRF) are not surface sensitive and do not provide good depth resolution because X-rays can escape from significant depths inside the sample. XES is particularly easy to use in practice because it is implemented as a simple add-on to an SEM. SIMS provides superb sensitivity (often ppm), is surface sensitive, and has excellent depth resolution but is a destructive technique because the sample is physically sputtered. RBS provides good depth resolution, reasonable sensitivity (0.1 atomic %), but poor lateral resolution because the incident ion beam is usually not well focused. In practice all of these methods (and others) have been used to evaluate the effectiveness of cleaning procedures.

Finally, it should be pointed out that less direct methods of evaluating cleaning effectiveness and particle densities can also be used. As we saw in Section 4.2, oxidation kinetics are sensitive to cleaning procedures. So are many other processes used in fabricating chips. For example the quality of an epitaxial layer grown on silicon is very sensitive to trace contaminants or particles left on the surface prior to epitaxial growth. Thus the next process step after cleaning may often serve as a very real measure of how well the wafers were cleaned.

4.4.3 Level 3 Contamination Reduction: Gettering

Measuring the concentration and location of the metal atoms that gettering steps try to remove is a difficult task because the metal concentrations are normally very low. IC manufacturers, therefore, usually focus on measuring what they are really interested in—device properties and carrier lifetime.

Many studies of gettering have measured device characteristics directly, usually with large sample sizes to improve the statistical significance. Histograms of diode leakage currents, refresh time in DRAM cells, breakdown voltage in PN diodes, breakdown voltage in thin dielectric layers (as in Figure 4–15), low current BJT current gain, and other similar parameters have been widely used. Typically the mean value of a particular parameter and its standard deviation are measured in comparing various gettering procedures.

In some studies, more fundamental material parameters are measured, the most common of which is simply carrier lifetime. The hypothesis is that better carrier lifetimes correspond to better gettering treatments. Both carrier generation and recombination processes are important in semiconductor devices and so both the generation lifetime and the recombination lifetime are of interest. As we saw in Chapter 1, the two lifetimes are not equal in general. τ_G is usually much longer than τ_R. Different experimental approaches measure one or the other. We will describe in this section several of the more common methods for measuring carrier lifetime. More details on these and other methods are available in a number of excellent texts on this topic such as [4.18]. The carrier lifetimes that are extracted by these various methods may be dominated by bulk carrier lifetimes or by surface recombination or by both, depending on the measurement method.

Perhaps the oldest and one of the simplest methods for measuring lifetime involves the use of photoconductive decay. If light is shined on a semiconductor sample with an energy greater than the bandgap, excess hole electron pairs are generated when the photons break Si-Si covalent bonds. The concentrations of excess holes and electrons are equal since each photon interaction generates one of each. If the light is shut off at some time $t = 0$, the excess carriers will recombine with a time constant equal to the carrier lifetime. Thus

$$\Delta n(t) = \Delta n(0) \exp\left(-\frac{t}{\tau_R}\right) \tag{4.6}$$

If the light intensity is high enough to change the majority carrier concentration, the excess carriers change the conductivity of the sample, which can be measured in a variety of ways. The simplest, of course, is a measurement of resistance, but this involves placing contacts on the sample. Contactless methods have been developed which use either an RF circuit in which the semiconductor resistance is part of an RF bridge [4.19], or a microwave circuit in which the power reflected by the wafer depends on its conductivity [4.20]. Eq. (4.6) is not strictly correct under these high level injection conditions, but it can be modified to extract an effective carrier lifetime [4.18]. The extracted τ_R usually reflects both bulk and surface recombination although it is possible to design the experiment to maximize one or the other. For example, the depth at which the photons are absorbed depends on their wavelength with higher energy photons being absorbed closer to the surface. Thus choosing a high photon energy would maximize surface recombination effects.

One of the most common methods for extracting carrier lifetime is the use of MOS Capacitance-Voltage measurements (MOS CV). The attraction of this technique is that it measures exactly what is important in MOS devices and these devices, of course, dominate modern ICs. We will discuss this method in much more detail in Chapter 6 (Section 6.4), because it is widely used to measure the properties of the Si/SiO_2 interface. Readers interested in a more complete description of the technique may wish to read that material at this point. Here we will focus only on a specific application, the extraction of carrier lifetime.

Figure 4–19 again shows the basic MOS capacitor structure—a metal or doped polysilicon electrode on an insulator (usually thermally grown SiO_2) on a silicon substrate. This is of course the basic gate structure of the MOS transistor and the capacitor is fabricated identically to the transistor. If the gate electrode is stepped to $+V_G$ (typically + 5 volts) at $t = 0$, the vertical electric field produced in the silicon will push the mobile carriers (holes since this example is P type), away from the surface. This creates a depleted region near the surface in which the depletion region charge (due to the acceptor doping ions) exactly balances the positive charge on the gate electrode. $Q_G = Q_D$. This is not the final equilibrium state of the structure, however. After some time, an inversion layer of electrons forms. We described this process qualitatively in Chapter 1 in

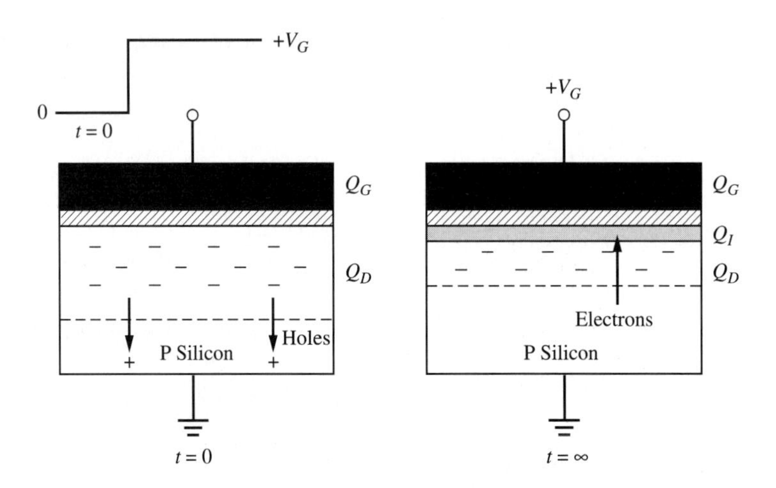

Figure 4–19 MOS CV measurement to extract the carrier generation lifetime. At $t = 0$ the gate voltage is stepped to $+V_G$. The capacitor goes into deep depletion. As carriers are generated to form the inversion layer, the depletion region shrinks.

Section 1.4.2 in connection with MOS transistors. Once the inversion layer forms, the gate charge is balanced by the sum of the depletion region charge and the inversion layer charge. $Q_G = Q_D + Q_I$. To satisfy this balance, the depletion layer shrinks as the inversion layer forms.

The electrons needed for the inversion layer are generated in the silicon through SRH generation. Thus if we can measure the time dependence of this process, we can extract the carrier generation lifetime. The simplest way to do this is to measure the capacitance of the structure. The MOS structure behaves very much like a simple parallel plate capacitor with the upper plate being the metal electrode and the lower plate being the undepleted silicon substrate. As the depletion layer shrinks, the distance between these plates decreases and therefore the capacitance rises. The time required for the capacitance to reach its final equilibrium value is given by [4.21]

$$t = 10\left(\frac{N_A}{n_i}\right)\tau_G \tag{4.7}$$

where τ_G is the generation lifetime and N_A is the doping concentration in the substrate. For typical lifetime values of 10 μsec to 1 msec, the measured capacitor response time is thus in the range of seconds to minutes. The extracted τ_G value is an effective value that reflects the contributions of bulk and surface generation.

Another very simple electrical measurement that can be made to estimate carrier lifetime makes use of a PN diode and is called the open circuit voltage decay method. Figure 4–20 illustrates this method. A power supply and resistor are used to establish a DC forward current through the diode. At $t = 0$, the switch is opened, forcing the circuit current to 0. We saw in Chapter 1 (Section 1.4.1), that when a diode is forward biased ($V_D \approx 0.7$ volts), minority carriers are injected across the diode. When the switch

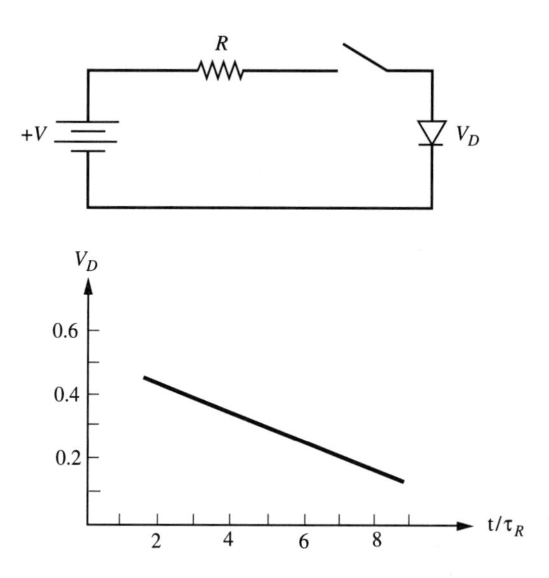

Figure 4–20 Diode open circuit voltage decay to extract the carrier recombination lifetime. The switch is opened at $t = 0$. The diode voltage decays due to carrier recombination.

is opened, these carriers are gradually eliminated in the diode by recombination and the diode voltage gradually returns to 0. The simplest analysis of this process leads to the following equation:

$$V_D(t) = V_D(0) - \frac{kT}{q}\ln\left(\text{erfc}\sqrt{\frac{t}{\tau_R}}\right) \tag{4.8}$$

where erfc is the complementary error function (tabulated in the appendix). This equation can be derived from the ideal diode current voltage relationship described in Chapter 1 [Eq. (1.23)] [4.18]. For t/τ larger than ≈ 4, this produces a straight line as shown in Figure 4–20. The slope of the line gives the recombination lifetime from

$$\tau_R = \frac{kT/q}{dV_D/dt} \tag{4.9}$$

Since PN diodes are always part of any integrated circuit, this simple measurement is usually straightforward to make. As was the case in the MOS CV method described above, the extracted τ_R value is usually an effective value that reflects the contributions of bulk and surface recombination.

The experimental methods we have described for extracting carrier lifetime do not give detailed information on the spatial distribution of the SRH centers or on the species (Au, Cu, Fe, etc.) responsible for the lifetime degradation. Nonetheless, they are simple measurements and do provide a clear indication of whether carrier lifetime is good or bad. They thus are very useful in evaluating the effectiveness of gettering procedures. If more detailed information is required, more sophisticated measurement methods are available such as neutron activation which can provide information on the specific SRH species involved, and DLTS (Deep Level Transient Spectroscopy) which can identify the species and give information on the spatial location of the contaminants [4.18].

4.5 Models and Simulation

Integrated circuit manufacturing is among the most complex industrial processes practiced today. Because of this, there is a great need for computer tools for monitoring, controlling, simulating, and analyzing manufacturing steps. Most modern IC manufacturing facilities employ sophisticated CIM (Computer Integrated Manufacturing) tools to monitor and control the status of machines, to download process recipes from central computer databases, to control wafer throughput in the fab, to store information about factory performance, and to improve operating efficiency. These topics are generally outside the scope of this book, but there are extensive references in the literature on these topics. See for example [4.22, 4.23].

One issue with respect to these kinds of CIM tools that is insightful is the use of these tools and the information they provide to quickly ramp up high yield manufacturing on new products in new factories. Table 4–2, taken from the 1997 NTRS, illustrates this point.

The last two rows (in bold) are the new information in this table, compared to Table 4–1 which we previously discussed. Notice that today it is common to introduce a new product into manufacturing with a yield less than 50%. Projections for the future suggest that it will be necessary for new products to achieve much higher yields right from the start. The reason for this is that it is often the case that the largest profits on a new product are made when the product is new (higher prices can often be charged for new, better products and there is usually less competition when a product is new). Today it takes several years before a new product achieves a mature level. That time is also projected to decrease dramatically in the future. The only way in which these dramatic improvements will be achieved is through better understanding and control of the manufacturing process.

Table 4–2 Semiconductor industry projected progress and the implications of this progress for chip yield and manufacturing yield ramp-up [4.1].

Year of First DRAM Shipment	**1997**	**1999**	**2003**	**2006**	**2009**	**2012**
Minimum Feature Size	250 nm	180 nm	130 nm	100 nm	70 nm	50 nm
Wafer Diameter (mm)	200	300	300	300	450	450
DRAM Bits/Chip	256M	1G	4G	16G	64G	256G
Initial Yield Level (%)	**25**	**50**	**80**	**85**	**88**	**90**
Time to Mature Yield Level (years)	**4**	**3**	**1**	**0.8**	**0.6**	**0.5**

Simulation and modeling have begun to be applied to the manufacturing related topics discussed in this chapter, although the level of sophistication of these simulation tools is generally rudimentary in comparison to the TCAD tools discussed in other chapters of this book. We will describe in this section some of the current modeling and simulation efforts and also point out where future work is needed.

4.5.1 Level 1 Contamination Reduction: Clean Factories

As we have seen, contamination reduction at the factory level is primarily associated with particle control. Since it has been estimated that 75% of the yield loss in modern IC manufacturing facilities is due to particle contamination, there has been a considerable effort to develop models relating particles to wafer yield. There are no computer simulation tools in widespread use today to predict particle deposition rates on wafers in factories. However given a defect density (usually measured), yield models are commonly used.

A number of empirical relationships have been used to describe the distribution of particle sizes in air. As we saw earlier, we are mostly concerned with particles with sizes between 10 nm and 10 μm. The actual size distribution of particles has been described with a power law function where $N(d_p)$, the number of particles larger than some diameter d_p, is given by

$$N(d_p) = K(d_p)^{-3} \tag{4.10}$$

where K is a constant [4.24]. This formula must fail for very small particles and so in practice, the distribution function, which cannot be easily measured at small sizes, is assumed to also fall off at small sizes as illustrated in Figure 4–21.

The second issue with respect to particles and yield is how large a particle needs to be to cause a defect. Generally, particles on the order of the technology minimum feature size or larger will cause defects unless they happen to occur in a noncritical area of

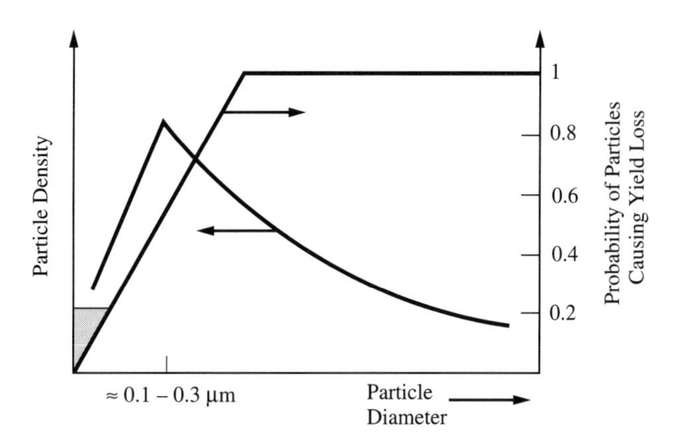

Figure 4–21 Left axis: Empirical particle size distribution in room air. Right axis: Probability of a particle causing a chip defect.

the chip. For example, an unintended isolated area of metal due to a photolithography defect during the metal etching may not cause a yield problem if it is well away from other metal lines. If the particle is in a critical area, then the probability it will cause a defect behaves empirically as shown in Figure 4–21. The probability is 1 for large particles and falls off as the particle or defect size decreases. Note that the probability may not be zero for very small particles, depending on the type of process involved (gray area near the origin in Figure 4–21). For example, a pinhole in a gate oxide is a catastrophic failure no matter how small the pinhole is.

A wide variety of yield models have been developed to describe IC manufacturing [4.24 – 4.26]. The simplest of these assumes Poisson statistics and independent randomly distributed defects each large enough to cause a chip defect. Thus,

$$Y = \exp^{-A_C D_O} \tag{4.11}$$

where Y is the yield, A_C is the critical area of the chip and D_O is the defect density. A_C may be less than the total chip area because not all of the area may be sensitive to particular defects. If some fraction of the wafer always produces zero yield (around the edges for example), or if some die sites are occupied by test devices, then

$$Y = (1 - G)\exp^{-A_C D_O} \tag{4.12}$$

where G is the fraction of the wafer where all the ICs fail. If information on particle size distribution and/or the probability of a particular size defect causing a fault (i.e., the information in Figure 4–21) is available, it can be used in defining A_C and/or D_O.

A variety of more sophisticated yield models have been investigated in recent years mainly driven by the inadequate predictions of the simple Poisson model. This model tends to underpredict the yield of large chips because of its assumptions about independent and randomly distributed defects. A somewhat better model is the negative binomial model that recognizes the fact that defects may not be completely randomly distributed and independent. In this model,

$$Y = \frac{1}{\left(1 + \frac{A_C D_O}{C}\right)^C} \tag{4.13}$$

where C is a measure of the particle spatial distribution called the clustering factor. When $C \to \infty$, the particles become independent and Eq. (4.13) reduces to Eq. (4.11). Figure 4–22 plots these yield functions. Note that the Poisson distribution predicts much lower yields for large chips than does the binomial distribution.

Figure 4–23 plots the negative binomial distribution ($C = 2$) for various defect levels. The value of $C = 2$ is suggested by the SIA NTRS [4.1]. Superimposed on this plot are the expected DRAM chip areas from the SIA NTRS through 2012. It is apparent from this plot that defect densities will have to be around 0.01 cm^{-2} to achieve manufacturable yields after the turn of the century. This number is consistent with the projections in Table 4–1 earlier in this chapter.

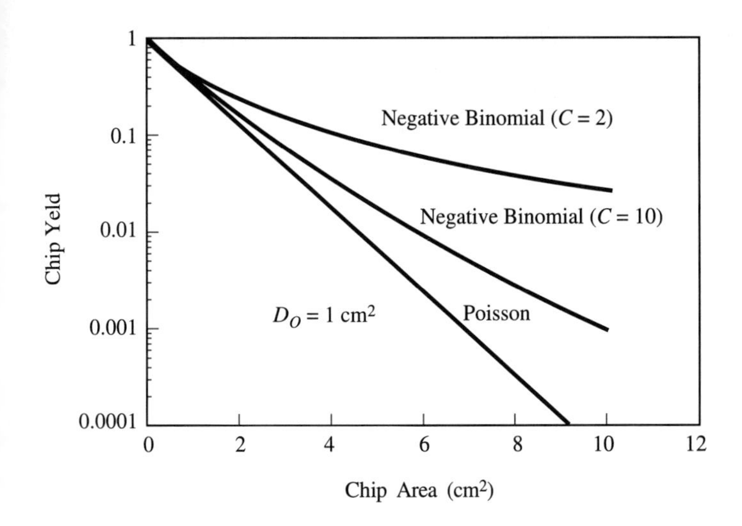

Figure 4–22 Plots of various yield functions assuming $D_O = 1$ defect/cm^{-2}.

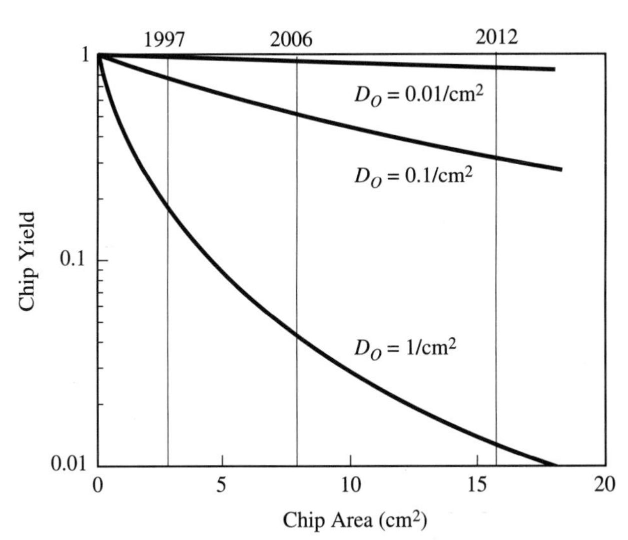

Figure 4–23 Plots of the negative binomial yield function versus chip area for various defect densities. $C = 2$ in all plots. The vertical lines correspond to DRAM chip areas in specific years from the SIA NTRS [4.1].

In manufacturing environments, it is generally very useful to monitor defect levels for as many of the individual process steps or process modules as possible. This can be done as described in Section 4.4.1 by running blank wafers through a particular process step or series of process steps and then using a particle counter to estimate the particles introduced by that particular step. If data like this are available, then the overall yield associated with a manufacturing process flow is simply the product of the individual module yields, assuming that the individual yields are independent. Any of the yield distribution functions described above can be used to describe the overall yield. For example, for the negative binomial distribution, the overall yield would be given by

$$Y = \prod_{i=1}^{\text{levels}} \left(1 + \frac{A_{Ci} D_{Oi}}{C_i}\right)^{-C_i}$$

$$\cong \left\{1 + \left(\sum_{i=1}^{\text{levels}} A_{Ci} D_{Oi}\right) / C_i\right\}^{-C_i} \tag{4.14}$$

Note that the defect density numbers in Table 4–1 and in Figures 4–22 and 4–23 are the total defect densities at the end of the manufacturing cycle. Obviously in order to achieve these overall defect densities, individual process modules must be considerably better.

4.5.2 Level 2 Contamination Reduction: Wafer Cleaning

As was the case with particle counts in manufacturing facilities, there are no computer simulation tools today which are used to predict the efficiency or effectiveness of wafer cleaning procedures. However, there is a solid scientific base of understanding about how and why cleaning procedures work, so the potential does exist to develop simulation tools should they be needed in the future.

Wafer cleaning is aimed at removing particles, organics, and metals from the surface of wafers. Particles are best dealt with by adding ultrasonic or megasonic agitation to the cleaning baths as was discussed earlier. Major organic contaminants like photoresist are removed in an oxygen plasma or in H_2SO_4/H_2O_2 solutions prior to the main RCA clean. Any remaining trace organics are removed in the RCA clean along with the metals.

To remove metal atoms from the surface of a silicon wafer, they need to be converted into ions that are soluble in the cleaning solution. This process involves oxidizing the metal atoms. Oxidation is defined as a process that removes electrons from an atom, while reduction is the opposite process in which an atom gains electrons. We can understand the various processes through the use of chemical reactions and oxidation potentials. Consider the following reactions, which could take place on a silicon wafer in an aqueous solution:

$$Si + 2H_2O \leftrightarrow SiO_2 + 4H^+ + 4e^- \tag{4.15}$$

$$M \leftrightarrow M^{Z+} + ze^- \tag{4.16}$$

where M represents a metal atom and z is the charge on the metal ion. Oxidation reactions go to the right, reduction reactions to the left. If electrons are available to drive reactions, the stronger oxidant will consume them. Table 4–3 summarizes the standard oxidation potentials of a number of reactions of interest in silicon cleaning (Cu, Ni, and Fe are usually the dominant impurities in silicon). These potentials are the open circuit voltages that would be measured in an electrochemical cell operating with the given reaction, referenced to a standard hydrogen cell. In this table, stronger oxidants have more negative oxidation potentials. In the chemical reactions, oxidants are on the right side of the equations, reductants are on the left side. Standard chemistry references discuss these concepts in more detail. (See for example [4.27].)

Suppose we now have a water solution containing a silicon wafer and metal atoms (dissolved in the liquid or on the wafer surface). Consider the SiO_2/Si and Fe^{3+}/Fe reactions as examples. Here the Fe^{3+}/Fe reaction has the stronger oxidation potential and

Table 4–3 Oxidation-reduction reactions for a number of species of interest in silicon wafer cleaning

Oxidant/ Reductant	Standard Oxidation Potential (volts)	Oxidation-Reduction Reaction
Mn^{2+}/Mn	1.05	$Mn \leftrightarrow Mn^{2+} + 2e^-$
SiO_2/Si	0.84	$Si + 2H_2O \leftrightarrow SiO_2 + 4H^+ + 4e^-$
Cr^{3+}/Cr	0.71	$Cr \leftrightarrow Cr^{3+} + 3e^-$
Ni^{2+}/Ni	0.25	$Ni \leftrightarrow Ni^{2+} + 2e^-$
Fe^{3+}/Fe	0.17	$Fe \leftrightarrow Fe^{3+} + 3e^-$
H_2SO_4/H_2SO_3	−0.20	$H_2O + H_2SO_3 \leftrightarrow H_2SO_4 + 2H^+ + 2e^-$
Cu^{2+}/Cu	−0.34	$Cu \leftrightarrow Cu^{2+} + 2e^-$
O_2/H_2O	−1.23	$2H_2O \leftrightarrow O_2 + 4H^+ + 2e^-$
Au^{3+}/Au	−1.42	$Au \leftrightarrow Au^{3+} + 3e^-$
H_2O_2/H_2O	−1.77	$2H_2O \leftrightarrow H_2O_2 + 2H^+ + 2e^-$
O_3/O_2	−2.07	$O_2 + H_2O \leftrightarrow O_3 + 2H^+ + 2e^-$

hence this reaction will go to the left, plating out Fe atoms on the wafer surface. The SiO_2/Si reaction will go to the right, oxidizing the silicon.

If we now consider adding H_2O_2 to the solution, the H_2O_2/H_2O reaction near the bottom of the table will dominate the Fe^{3+}/Fe reaction because of its stronger oxidation potential. Thus the H_2O_2 will take electrons from the metal atoms, creating ions which are soluble in aqueous solutions. This is the basis for the use of H_2O_2 in the RCA cleaning procedure. At the same time, the silicon will also be oxidized by the H_2O_2 since the SiO_2/Si reaction is also dominated by the H_2O_2/H_2O reaction. The general rule is that the lowest reaction in Table 4–3 dominates, going to the left and driving all reactions above it to the right. Only ozone (O_3) has a stronger oxidation potential than H_2O_2. Some recent work has suggested that cleaning procedures based on O_3 may actually be superior to the standard RCA clean [4.28]. We will discuss these possibilities in Section 4.6.

We can now see on a more fundamental level how the RCA cleaning procedure works. The first solution (SC − 1) is a high-pH solution consisting of 5 H_2O:1 H_2O_2: 1 NH_4OH in which the wafers are placed at 70 – 80°C for 10 minutes. This solution oxidizes organic films into water soluble compounds (CO_2, H_2O, etc.) and complexes Group IB and IIB metals as well as other metals like Au, Ag, Cu, Ni, Zn, Cd, Zn, Co, and Cr. For example, Cu forms a soluble $Cu(NH_3)_4{}^{+2}$ amino-complex.

The second solution (SC − 2) is a low-pH solution consisting of 6 H_2O:1 H_2O_2:1 HCl in which the wafers are placed at 70 – 80°C for 10 minutes. This solution removes alkali ions and cations like Al^{+3}, Fe^{+3}, and Mg^{+2} that form NH_4OH insoluble hydroxides in basic solutions like SC − 1. The SC − 2 solution also completes the removal of metallic contaminates such as Au through reactions like Eq. (4.16) that may not have been completely removed by the SC − 1 step. Both SC − 1 and SC − 2 solutions depend on the strong oxidation potential of H_2O_2 to remove metal atoms from the wafer surface. The kinetics of the cleaning process depend of course on the reaction rate constants associated with reactions like Eq. (4.16). These are temperature dependent so that the necessary cleaning time is reduced at elevated temperatures.

4.5.3 Level 3 Contamination Reduction: Gettering

Many models have been developed in recent years for metal gettering. The process seems conceptually simple as illustrated in Figure 4–24. If metal atoms are present throughout the wafer, three steps need to occur to getter them. First they need to be freed from whatever sites they presently occupy. Second, they need to migrate to the gettering sites, either the wafer bulk or the wafer backside. Third, they need to be trapped at the gettering sites. Models that have been developed for these processes attempt to treat all three parts of this process. There is still considerable uncertainty about the exact mechanisms responsible for gettering and as a result, the models that we will discuss are not universally accepted. Nevertheless, they do provide a coherent physical picture of how gettering probably operates.

4.5.3.1 Step 1: Making the Metal Atoms Mobile

Most of the metals of interest in gettering (those that create deep levels in silicon), exist in two states in the silicon crystal, either occupying a substitutional lattice site M_S, or an interstitial site M_i. These metals are pure interstitials in the latter case, and generally do not occupy interstitialcy sites (see Section 3.2.2 in Chapter 3). Metals can diffuse in silicon in either state, but their diffusivities are generally orders of magnitude higher in the interstitial form. We will discuss diffusion mechanisms in much more detail in Chapter 7, but it should be easy to imagine that substitutional diffusion involves hopping from lattice site to lattice site, a process that involves breaking bonds. Interstitial diffusion simply involves moving through the interstitial spaces between lattice atoms with no bond breaking. In general the interstitial process is much faster. The data in Figure 4–8 illustrate this. Interstitial diffusers like Au and Cu have orders of magnitude higher diffusivities than substitutional dopants like P or even Si itself. Thus step 1—

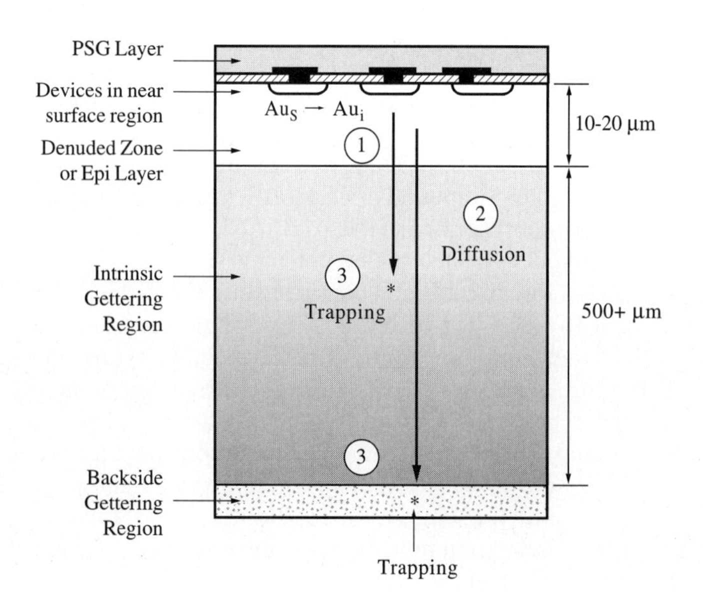

Figure 4–24 Three-step gettering process: release, diffusion, and trapping. Au is used as a specific example.

making the metal atoms mobile—generally involves getting the metal atoms into their interstitial form.

The importance of this first step depends on the specific metal atom being considered. Some metals (Cu and Ni, for example) have much higher solubilities in their interstitial form and so most such atoms are in the interstitial form naturally. The release step is therefore unnecessary unless these atoms have formed precipitates due to very high concentrations. A second category of metals (Au and Pt are examples) have much higher solubilities in their substitutional form but diffuse rapidly once they become interstitials. For these elements, the release process is very important. Finally, there are some elements (Ti and Mo, for example) that are primarily substitutional, but which have relative slow diffusion rates in either interstitial or substitutional form (see Figure 4–8). These elements are the most difficult to getter effectively because they will not diffuse over long distances (to the wafer backside for example), unless very long thermal cycles are used.

Metals such as Au and Pt are the most interesting case, because they need to be converted from substitutional to interstitial sites to be gettered effectively. This can happen through one of two reactions, where we have taken Au as a specific example:

$$Au_S + I \leftrightarrow Au_i \tag{4.17}$$

$$Au_S \leftrightarrow Au_i + V \tag{4.18}$$

In Eq. (4.17), a silicon interstitial exchanges places with the Au atom on a lattice site, creating a Au interstitial. This is called the "kick-out" mechanism. In Eq. (4.18), the Au atom jumps off its lattice site, creating a silicon vacancy. This is known as the dissociative or Frank-Turnbull mechanism [4.29]. Process conditions that create excess concentrations of I should be useful in driving Au_S to Au_i and thus help the gettering process. Similarly, processes that create excess V should hinder the gettering process by driving Au_i back on to substitutional sites. It has been proposed that many of the effective gettering procedures inject excess concentrations of I and thus drive Eq. (4.17) to the right [4.30]. For example, we will see in Chapter 7 that high-concentration phosphorus diffusions produce very large supersaturations of I. Backside P diffusions are known to be among the most effective gettering treatments and such diffusions are thought to inject large quantities of I. Similarly, ion implantation damage creates excess I as we will see in Chapter 8. Such damage is also effective at backside gettering. Internal gettering involves oxidation (SiO_2 formation) and this process also injects I (see Figure 3–25).

4.5.3.2 Step 2: Metal Diffusion to the Gettering Site

Once the metal atoms are in their interstitial (fast diffusing) form, they can diffuse through the wafer to the backside sink, or to the trap sites associated with SiO_2 precipitates if internal gettering is being used. Obviously the diffusion distance is a lot smaller for the intrinsic gettering case, which is one of the reasons why it is more popular today.

The expected general shape of the Au profiles as they outdiffuse is illustrated in Figure 4–25. The Au concentration goes to zero at the wafer backside where the Au atoms are trapped. We will see in Chapter 7 how to calculate the actual detailed shape of such profiles, but the general shape should be intuitive. As time increases, the depth over

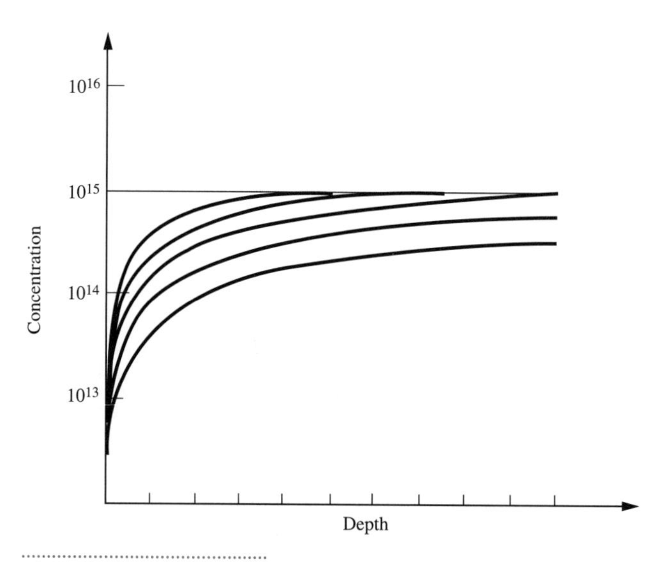

Figure 4–25 General shape of Au outdiffusion profiles if simple outdiffusion dominates the gettering process. Starting with a flat profile (10^{15} cm^{-3}), the concentration drops off with time through the wafer as the Au diffuses to the back surface (left side). This simulation was done with Silvaco's SSUPREM IV, a process simulator we will discuss in more detail in later chapters.

which the Au is gettered increases away from the wafer backside, until at long enough times, the Au is removed entirely from the wafer.

Some actual experimental measurements of Au profiles are shown in Figure 4–26 [4.31]. Note that the shape is quite different from the expected simple outdiffusion profile in Figure 4–25. The experimental data can be understood in connection with the model in Figure 4–27 and the diffusivity of the I species indicated in Figure 4–8 [4.30]. There is still great uncertainty about the value of the diffusion coefficient of the silicon interstitial (see Chapter 7), so we have indicated a region in which it likely lies in Figure 4–8. Note that this diffusion coefficient is much faster than dopant diffusivities, but significantly slower than metal atom diffusivities. Thus if the gettering process depends on the backside gettering region for injection of I to drive reaction (4.17), then the slowest (rate limiting) part of the process will be the indiffusion of the I from the backside. As quickly as silicon interstitials reach a particular depth from the backside, the Au_S in that region are driven to Au_i which then quickly diffuse to the wafer backside where they are trapped. This qualitative explanation leads to Au profiles like those in Figure 4–26. The sharp drop in the Au profile which moves away from the backside as time goes on, occurs at the depth corresponding to how far the silicon interstitials have diffused in from the backside at that particular time.

Other types of gettering processes also often lead to Au profiles like Figure 4–26, so it is quite possible that the process described here operates in many common gettering methods. When gettering is performed at higher temperatures, the equilibrium concentration of I may be high enough that reaction (4.17) can proceed without the excess I

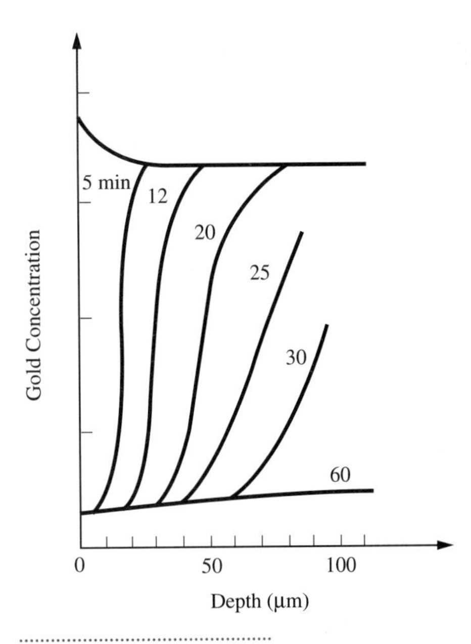

Figure 4–26 Experimental 1000°C Au outdiffusion profiles during gettering to the wafer backside. (After [4.31].)

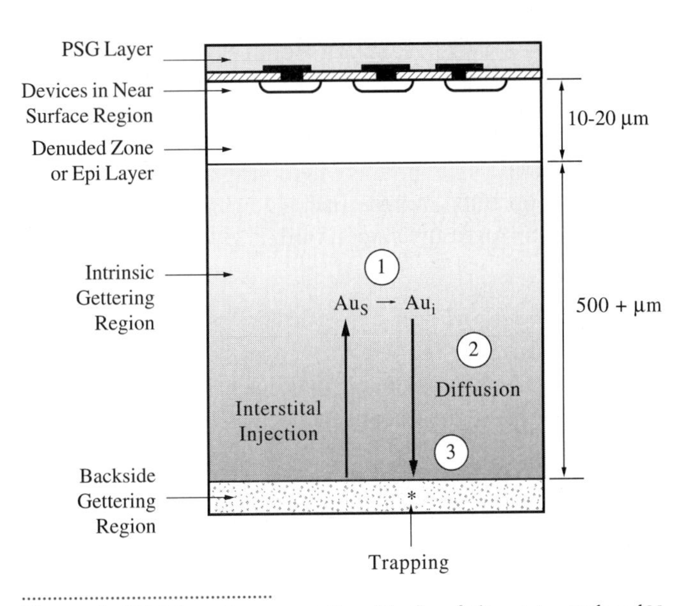

Figure 4–27 Schematic representation of the flux of silicon interstitials and M_I during back surface gettering. (After [4.30].)

provided by the backside. In that case the metal outdiffusion profiles should be more like Figure 4–25 and the rate limiting process should be simply the metal atom diffusivity. The few metals which have diffusivities smaller than I (Ti for example in Figure 4–8) should also show outdiffusion profiles similar to Figure 4–25 since the rate limiting step in this case is also metal diffusion at all temperatures.

4.5.3.3 Step 3: Trapping the Metal Atoms at the Gettering Site

For extrinsic gettering, the trapping process at the wafer backside (process 3 in Figure 4–27) has been modeled in a variety of ways and in fact, different models may be appropriate depending on the type of backside treatment used. Backside treatments that have been used include ion implantation damage, phosphorus diffusion, laser damage, polysilicon films, mechanical damage, and a number of others. It is quite clear that any of these methods can "trap" metal atoms. Many studies have used physical measurements like RBS, SIMS, and others described in connection with Figure 4–16, to directly measure the trapped metals. Many other studies have used measurements of bulk generation lifetime to show that gettering removes the metal atoms (SRH centers) from the wafer bulk regions. The question of how they are trapped, however, is less clear. Physical damage to the wafer backside (ion implantation, laser or mechanical damage, or polysilicon films containing many grain boundaries), is generally believed to trap the metal atoms at defect sites. This trapping process is most simply characterized by some binding energy E_B of the metal atom to the trap site. In that case, the metal atoms are kept trapped at low temperatures. As T increases, more and more of them are able to escape the traps. Clearly we would want E_B as large as possible.

$$\text{Fraction Bound} = (1 - K_1 \exp^{-E_B/kT}) \tag{4.19}$$

Another approach to modeling the trapping process uses a segregation model [4.32, 4.33]. Segregation is a process that we used in Chapter 3 to describe dopant behavior between liquid and solid phases in growing crystals. The same concept applies here, between the silicon bulk and the backside gettering region. The solubility of a substitutional metal like Au in the silicon bulk is given by

$$C_{\text{Au,Si}} = N_{\text{Si}} \exp\left(-\frac{E_{A1}}{kT}\right) \tag{4.20}$$

where $C_{\text{Au,Si}}$ is the substitutional Au concentration in the silicon, N_{si} is the density of silicon atoms and E_A is an activation energy. Similarly, the solubility of Au in the gettering region is given by

$$C_{\text{Au,G}} = N_G \exp\left(-\frac{E_{A2}}{kT}\right) \tag{4.21}$$

where N_G is the density of gettering sites. The segregation coefficient of the Au between the two regions is now defined as

$$k_O = \frac{C_{\mathrm{Au,G}} + C_{\mathrm{Au,Si}}}{C_{\mathrm{Au,Si}}} = 1 + K_2 \exp - \left(\frac{E_{A1} - E_{A2}}{kT}\right) \tag{4.22}$$

If $E_{A1} - E_{A2}$ is a positive number, then k_O decreases as temperature goes up, providing the same qualitative behavior as Eq. (4.19). For the specific case of phosphorus gettering in which a backside phosphorus diffusion is used, Baldi [4.32] estimate that k_O is given by

$$k_O = 1 + \frac{N_G}{5 \times 10^{22}} \exp\left(\frac{0.82\ \mathrm{eV}}{kT}\right) \tag{4.23}$$

which indicates that the phosphorus concentration should be as high as possible (to maximize N_G since the phosphorus atoms are believed to provide the N_G sites) and the temperature should be as low as possible to provide the best trapping.

Other proposals have also been made to explain the trapping. Enhanced solubility of metals in heavily doped silicon can be understood by taking Au again as an example. In its substitutional form, Au introduces deep levels (both acceptor and donor) which are near the middle of the bandgap in silicon. Thus in N-type silicon, in which the Fermi level is close to the conduction band, Au tends to be an acceptor. (The acceptor level is below E_F and hence is filled.) In P-type silicon, Au tends to be a donor. If we consider the reaction

$$\mathrm{Au} + \mathrm{e}^- \leftrightarrow \mathrm{Au}^- \tag{4.24}$$

then we can write from the definition of the equilibrium constant that

$$K_{eq} = \frac{[\mathrm{Au}^-]}{[\mathrm{Au}][\mathrm{e}^-]} = \text{constant} \tag{4.25}$$

where [ ] denotes equilibrium concentrations of the various species. Since Eq. (4.25) holds both in intrinsic and in doped silicon where $[\mathrm{e}^-] = n_i$ and $[\mathrm{e}^-] = n$, respectively, we have that

$$\frac{[\mathrm{Au}_i^-]}{[\mathrm{Au}]n_i} = \frac{[\mathrm{Au}_n^-]}{[\mathrm{Au}]n} \quad or \quad \frac{[\mathrm{Au}_n^-]}{[\mathrm{Au}_i^-]} = \frac{n}{n_i} \tag{4.26}$$

Thus the solubility of the Au acceptor is much higher in N-type silicon. For example, we saw in Chapter 1 that $n_i = 7.14 \times 10^{18}\ \mathrm{cm}^{-3}$ at 1000°C. If the gettering step is carried out at this temperature, with an N-type doping level of $10^{21}\ \mathrm{cm}^{-3}$, the solubility is over 100 times greater in the N-doped region than in the wafer bulk. This model has been used to explain why phosphorus-doped regions are effective getters.

The ion pairing model [4.34] suggests that a large atom like Au prefers to pair with a small atom like P, forming AuP complexes, because this minimizes the strain in the crystal. There would also be coulombic interactions between the Au and P because $\mathrm{Au}^-\mathrm{P}^+$ complexes could form. The solubility of such complexes would be higher in N-type Si than in lightly doped silicon because of the higher P concentration.

Finally, we saw in Chapter 3 that the point defect concentrations are much higher in doped silicon than in intrinsic silicon. Au diffuses primarily by an interstitial mechanism as we have seen, so when it arrives at the gettering site at the wafer backside, it needs to find a lattice site on which to sit since in equilibrium, the Au prefers to be predominantly on substitutional sites. One possible reaction is

$$Au_i + V^- \leftrightarrow Au_S^- \tag{4.27}$$

The much higher V^- population in N^+ silicon would drive this reaction to the right, with the vacancies essentially providing lattice sites for the Au atoms.

Intrinsic gettering relies on trapping the metal atoms at defects in the wafer bulk. These defects are generally dislocations and/or stacking faults that are caused by the precipitation of oxygen while forming SiO_2 precipitates in CZ silicon. We discussed the process of precipitate formation in some detail in Chapter 3 (Figure 3–25) and again briefly earlier in this chapter. As the SiO_2 precipitates form, a net volume expansion takes place because the oxide occupies more volume than the silicon crystal. We modeled this process in Chapter 3 with the following equation:

$$(1 + 2\gamma)Si + 2O_I + 2\beta V \leftrightarrow SiO_2 + 2\delta I + \text{stress} \tag{4.28}$$

where γ is the number of I that contribute to the precipitation process per O_I atom joining the SiO_2, and β is a similar fraction for V. O_I represents the interstitial oxygen atom and Si is simply a lattice site in the crystal. The terms involving point defects model the fact that the volume needed for formation of the SiO_2 can come partly by consuming vacancies or ejecting interstitials. We have included a stress term on the right-hand side because it is unlikely that the point defects could provide all the necessary volume and so it is likely that the region surrounding the SiO_2 precipitates will be under stress with the precipitate and the surrounding silicon under compression. The dislocations and stacking faults that form around the precipitates are natural sites for metal atoms to be trapped. Dislocations have regions of both compressive and tensile stress, so they provide "homes" for metal atoms that are smaller and larger, respectively, than silicon atoms [4.33]. Many studies have shown the metal atoms located around these dislocations. These trapping processes can be qualitatively modeled by expressions similar to Eqs. (4.19) or (4.22) since the metal trapping at dislocations in intrinsic gettering is similar to what occurs at the wafer backside in extrinsic gettering processes that produce similar damage.

It is interesting to note that the reaction given by Eq. (4.28) injects I. In fact, surface oxidation of silicon does the same thing (Chapter 6). These injected I coalesce to form the dislocations and stacking faults around the precipitates. They can also help to drive reaction (4.17) to the right, freeing up substitutional metal atoms so they can diffuse to the gettering sites. Finally, we would expect that intrinsic gettering would be a better approach for gettering metals which have relatively small diffusion coefficients (like Ni), because they would not have to diffuse nearly as far as they would if extrinsic gettering were being used.

The variety of models described in this section should give some indication of the ways in which gettering is understood today. There is still considerable controversy about many of the ideas described in this section. However, it is likely that the qualitative concepts described here do play important roles in the gettering process.

4.6 Limits and Future Trends in Technologies and Models

The goals for the future are fairly clear—cleaner environments in which to process wafers, better cleaning procedures that remove particles and trace contaminants more reliably, and better gettering procedures for eliminating contaminants from device regions of wafers. In each of these areas, there is considerable ongoing research that we will briefly describe in this section.

Traditionally, semiconductor manufacturing facilities have used the approach of providing clean rooms in which to manufacture the chips. While this has been very successful, it is in some sense a wasteful approach because the volume of the clean room is far larger than the wafers that are being processed. There are approaches to minimizing the actual volume of "clean room" which must be maintained. These approaches keep the wafers in sealed minienvironments in which they are transported from one machine or process to another. This approach was proposed many years ago and has been implemented by providing sealed cassettes to transport the wafers from machine to machine. This approach is becoming popular today and some newer factories employ these SMIF (standard mechanical interface) boxes extensively to provide a cleaner environment for the wafers as shown in Figure 4–28. This alternative approach to "mini-clean rooms" may be more common in the future than it is today [4.1]. Economics may play a significant role in determining how extensively such minienvironments are used in the future, since the costs associated with constructing and operating large clean rooms are very high.

Wafer cleaning has remained largely unchanged for the past 25 years, because of the success of the RCA clean. Yet there are reasons to investigate improved methods. The RCA cleaning method uses large quantities of chemicals and DI water at high

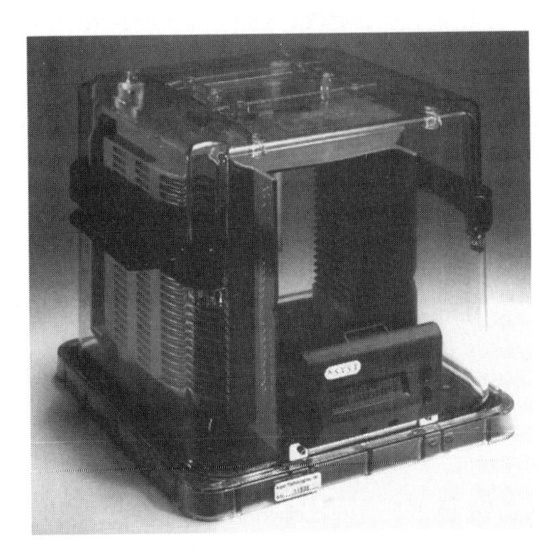

Figure 4–28 Example of a SMIF box or pod for transporting wafers in an IC manufacturing facility. These carriers connect directly to manufacturing machines so that the wafers are not exposed to room air. This figure was taken directly from the Asyst Technologies Corp. web site at http://www.asyst.com/.

temperatures. This generates large amounts of chemical vapors that must be exhausted from the clean rooms and then treated. The chemicals themselves must also be treated before disposal. These environmental issues are becoming increasingly important as the scale of IC manufacturing plants increases. One simple change which is being used by some wafer manufacturers is to simply use SC−1 and SC−2 solutions that are more dilute. These have been found to be as effective as the original concentrations and they reduce the environmental issues associated with chemical disposal. In addition, H_2O_2 is unstable at the temperatures used in the SC−1 and SC−2 solutions, especially in acidic solutions, decomposing into H_2O and O_2. As a result, the composition of the solutions can change with time, resulting in less effective cleaning. In the SC−1 solution, if the concentration of H_2O_2 drops too much, the NH_4OH will attack silicon.

A number of replacement cleaning procedures have been proposed [4.35]. A particularly interesting procedure is that proposed by Ohmi [4.28]. In Table 4–3 the only oxidant stronger than H_2O_2 is O_3. Ohmi's process uses ozonized ultrapure water as shown in Figure 4–29. This process is all at room temperature, uses far fewer chemicals than the standard RCA clean, and is claimed to be as effective in cleaning wafers. The principles behind Ohmi's cleaning procedure are similar to the RCA clean. A strong oxidant is used to oxidize organics and metals. Megasonic agitation is used to loosen particles that may have adhered to the wafers. The final steps in Ohmi's process involve an HF etch of the surface. This strips away the chemical oxide that naturally grows as part of the

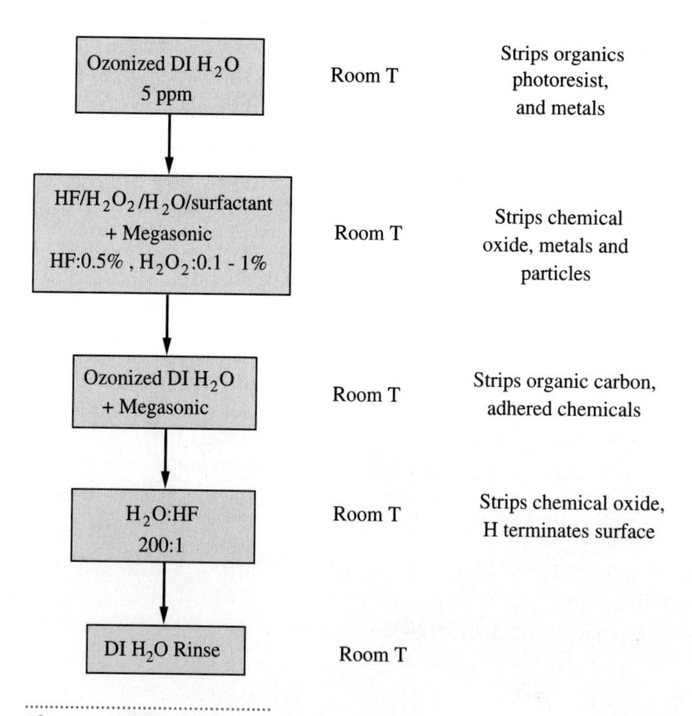

Figure 4–29 Possible room temperature cleaning procedure replacement for the RCA clean [4.28].

cleaning procedure. The silicon surface atoms are left with dangling (incomplete bonds) which are highly reactive and which form hydrogen bonds with H atoms from the HF solution [4.36]. The hydrogen-passivated surface that results is ready for immediate further processing, such as epitaxial layer growth. There are some concerns with using a final HF step for wafers whose next processing step is oxidation. The hydrogen passivated Si (100) surface is roughened by the H passivation process and this may lead to poorer quality thin oxides grown on these surfaces [4.37]. In addition, the hydrogen passivated surface is very sensitive to ambient effects between the time the cleaning ends and the next process step begins, so special care may have to be taken in transporting and handling such wafers.

There has also been considerable recent work on "dry" or vapor phase cleaning procedures [4.5]. This work has been motivated both by the environmental issues associated with wet chemistries and by the increasing use of cluster tools in IC manufacturing. In these tools, multiple-process steps, often on single wafers, are performed in a single machine by moving wafers from one chamber to another. There is great interest in accomplishing the cleaning process in one of these chambers because the wafers would then move directly to the process step under well-controlled ambient conditions, minimizing contamination between cleaning and the next step. "Dry" cleaning methods which are under investigation include the use of gas vapors, plasmas, low-energy physical processes like sputtering, and photochemically enhanced cleaning in which UV energy is used to help break surface bonds and release contaminants on the wafer surface. None of these techniques is currently in widespread use in manufacturing.

Gettering methods have remained relatively unchanged for the past decade. The scientific knowledge providing our understanding of how gettering actually works has certainly improved in recent years, primarily because of improved understanding of point defect properties in silicon. It is likely that intrinsic gettering will dominate in the future because with smaller devices, thermal budgets for IC processing will have to decrease. The closeness of the gettering traps to the active devices in intrinsic gettering gives this process a distinct advantage over extrinsic gettering. It is likely that tighter controls on oxygen concentration in CZ wafers will be required in the future, because this is an essential element of the intrinsic gettering process and is also required in order to control warpage and the mechanical strength of the wafers. Better understanding is also needed of the role of carbon in the oxygen precipitation process. The SIA NTRS [4.1] lists two primary future needs in the gettering area. The first of these emphasizes low-temperature gettering, for the reasons just described. Intrinsic gettering is the best hope at this point, but alternatives may be needed for very low thermal budget processes. The second priority is a high-quality simulation tool for gettering. Such a tool will have to be based on the ideas we have discussed in this chapter—the role of point defects and the three gettering steps of release, diffusion, and trapping.

Some workers believe that gettering will be unnecessary in the future, because the level of cleanliness in factories and wafer cleaning procedures will be sufficient to keep metal atom concentrations to levels that will not affect device performance and chip yield. This approach is no doubt possible but the cost of such manufacturing practices may be very high and the alternative of providing some safety margin through gettering will remain the cost-effective solution in many cases.

4.7 Summary of Key Ideas

In this chapter, we have considered some of the "nuts and bolts" of IC manufacturing. Particle control, wafer cleaning, and gettering sometimes do not receive the attention in the scientific community that more "high-tech" processes such as ion implantation, etching, and lithography do. However, the topics we have discussed in this chapter are crucial for the successful manufacturing of complex chips. In fact it is likely the case that the economic success of any company in this business depends as much on its attention to particles, cleaning, and gettering as it does on the design features of a particular product. High yields, which come from attention to these issues, are the mark of successful manufacturers.

We have seen that a three-tiered approach is used to minimize contaminants in silicon wafer processing. The first step is to clean the environment around the wafers. Most commonly this is done through advanced air filtration systems to remove particles, careful protocols for workers in the plant, and the use of highly purified, filtered chemicals and gases. The second tier of contamination control is careful wafer cleaning. This is probably the most common step performed in wafer manufacturing. Cleaning needs to remove particlulates that adhere to wafer surfaces, and it needs to strip trace levels of organic and metal contaminants. The RCA clean, which is most commonly used, is based on a solid scientific understanding of the processes occurring in cleaning. Finally, gettering is the third level of contamination control. This process collects metal atoms in regions of the wafer away from the active devices. Gettering occurs by releasing the metal atoms from whatever their current position is, allowing them to diffuse to the gettering site, and then trapping them at those sites. While both extrinsic and intrinsic gettering are used in wafer manufacturing today, it is likely that intrinsic gettering will be the most common in the future because the gettering sites are physically closer to the devices, minimizing the thermal cycling needed for gettering.

The bottom line is yield. A difference of a few % in good die from each wafer can make a tremendous difference in the profitability of a company. Because of the batch fabrication processes used in IC manufacturing, with hundreds of die per wafer, the bad die are inherently manufactured along with the good die. There is generally no additional manufacturing cost when the yield goes up, so the incremental good die are essentially pure profit for the manufacturer. This fact should provide strong motivation for careful attention to the topics discussed in this chapter.

4.8 References

[4.1]. "National Technology Roadmap for Semiconductors," SIA, 1997.

[4.2]. F. Schwettman, K. Chiang, and W. Brown, "Variation of Silicon Dioxide Growth Rate with Pre-Oxidation Clean," *Electrochem. Soc. Abstracts*, vol. 78–1, p. 689, 1978.

[4.3]. S, M. Hu, private communication.

[4.4]. W. Kern and D. A. Puotinen, "Cleaning Solutions Based on Hydrogen Peroxide for Use in Silicon Semiconductor Technology," *RCA Review*, vol. 31, p. 187, 1970.

[4.5]. W. Kern, editor, *Handbook of Semiconductor Wafer Cleaning Technology*, Noyes Publications, 1993.

[4.6]. C. W. Pearce, J. L. Moore, and F. A. Stevie, "Removal of Alkaline Impurities in a Polysilicon Gate Structure by Phosphorus Diffusion," *J. Electrochem. Soc.*, vol. 140, p. 1409, 1993.

[4.7]. P. Balk and J. M. Eldridge, "Phosphosilicate Glass Stabilization of FET Devices," *Proc. IEEE*, vol. 57, p. 1558, 1969.

[4.8]. G. Masetti and M. Severi, "Dependence of Flat-band Voltage of MOS Structures on Phosphosilicate-glass Growing Conditions," *Appl. Phys. Lett.*, vol. 37, p. 226, 1980.

[4.9]. E. Snow and B. E. Deal, "Polarization Effects in Insulating Films on Silicon—a Review," *Trans. Metall. Soc. of AIME*, vol. 242, p. 512, 1966.

[4.10]. E. R. Weber, "Transition Metals in Silicon," *Appl. Phys.*, vol. A30, p. 1, 1983.

[4.11]. W. E. Beadle, J. C. C. Tsai and R. D. Plummer, *Quick Reference Manual for Silicon Integrated Circuit Technologies*, John Wiley & Sons, 1985.

[4.12]. J. C. Mikkelsen Jr., "The Diffusivity and Solubility of Oxygen in Silicon," *Mat. Res. Symp. Proc.*, vol. 59, p. 19, 1986.

[4.13]. H. W. Kennel, "Physical Modeling of Oxygen Precipitation, Defect Formation and Diffusion in Silicon," Ph.D. Thesis, Stanford University, TR. No. G710–2, Feb. 1991.

[4.14]. D. Huber and J. Reffle, "Precipitation Process Design for Denuded Zone Formation in CZ-Silicon Wafers," *Solid State Tech.*, p. 137, Aug., 1983.

[4.15]. M. Buehler, "Microelectronic Test Chips for VLSI Electronics," in *VLSI Electronics, Microstructure Science*, vol. 6, p. 529, Academic Press, 1983.

[4.16]. W. Lukaszek, K. G. Grambow, and W. J. Yarbrough, "Test Chip Based Approach to Automatic Diagnosis of CMOS Yield Problems," *IEEE Trans. on Semi. Manufac.*, vol. 3, 1990.

[4.17]. C. Weber, "Generic Test Chip Formats for ASIC-Oriented Semiconductor Process Development," *Proc. IEEE Int. Conf. on Microelectronic Test Structures*, p. 247, March 1993.

[4.18]. D. K. Schroder, *Semiconductor Material and Device Characterization*, John Wiley & Sons, 1990.

[4.19]. T. Tiedje, J. I. Haberman, R. W. Francis, and A. K. Ghosh, "An RF Bridge Technique for Contactless Measurement of the Carrier Lifetime in Silicon Wafers," *J. Appl. Phys.*, vol. 54, p. 2499, 1983.

[4.20]. Y. Mada, "A Nondestructive Method for Measuring the Spatial Distribution on Minority Carrier Lifetime in Si Wafer," *Jpn. J. Appl. Phys.*, vol. 18, p. 2171, 1979.

[4.21]. D. K. Schroder and J. Guldberg, "Interpretation of Surface and Bulk Effects Using the Pulsed MIS Capacitor," *Solid State Electronics*, vol. 14, p. 1285, 1971.

[4.22]. Y. Mizokami, "The Total CIM System for Semiconductor Manufacturing," *Proc. 1990 IEEE International Semiconductor Manufacturing Science Symposium*, p. 24, 1990.

[4.23]. J. McGehee, J. Hebley, and J. Mahaffey, "The MMST Computer-Integrated Manufacturing Framework," *IEEE Trans. Semi. Manufac.*, vol. 7, p. 107, 1994.

[4.24]. C. H. Stapper, "Fact and Fiction in Yield Modeling," *Microelectronics Journal*, vol. 20, 1989.

[4.25]. D. Dance and K. Gildersleeve, "Estimating Semiconductor Yield From Equipment particle Measurements," *1992 IEEE/SEMI International Semiconductor Manufacturing Science Symposium.*

[4.26]. G. Check and G. O'Donoghue, "Yield Models in a Design for Manufacturability Environment: A Bibliography," *1993 IEEE/SEMI International Semiconductor Manufacturing Science Symposium.*

[4.27]. J.W. Hill and R.H. Petrucci, *General Chemistry, An Integrated Approach*, Prentice Hall, 1999.

[4.28]. T. Ohmi, "Total Room Temperature Wet Cleaning of Silicon Surfaces," *Semiconductor International*, p. 323, July 1996.

[4.29]. F. C. Frank and D. Turnbull, "Mechanism of Diffusion of Copper in Germanium," *Phys. Rev.*, vol. 104, p. 617, 1956.

[4.30]. G. B. Bronner and J. D. Plummer, "Gettering of Gold in Silicon: a Tool for Understanding the Properties of Silicon Interstitials," *J. Appl. Phys.*, vol. 61, p. 5286, 1987.

[4.31]. H. Higuchi and S. Nakamura, "Gettering of Electrically Active Gold in Silicon," *Extended Abstracts of the Electrochem. Soc. Meeting, Spring 1975*, vol. 75–1, p. 412, 1975.

[4.32]. L. Baldi, G. F. Cerofolini, G. Ferla, and G. Frigerio, "Gold Solubility in Silicon and Gettering by Phosphorus," *Phys. Status Solidi A*, vol. 48, p. 523, 1978.

[4.33]. J. S. Kang and D. K. Schroder, "Gettering in Silicon," *J. Appl. Phys.*, vol. 65, p. 2974, 1989.

[4.34]. R. L. Meek and T. E. Seidel, "Enhanced Solubility and Ion Pairing of Cu and Au in Heavily Doped Silicon at high Temperatures," *J. Phys. Chem. Solids*, vol. 36, p. 731, 1975.

[4.35]. W. A. Cady and M. Varadarajan, "RCA Clean Replacement," *J. Electrochem. Soc.*, vol. 143, p. 2064, 1996.

[4.36]. Y. J. Chabal, G. S. Higashi and K. Raghavachari, "Infrared Spectroscopy of Si (111) and Si (100) Surfaces After HF Treatment: Hydrogen Termination and Surface Morphology," *J. Vac. Science and Tech. a,* vol. 7, p. 2104, 1989.

[4.37]. M Offenberg, M. Liehr, and G. W. Rubloff, "Ultraclean Integrated Processing of Thermal Silicon (111) and (100) Surfaces," *Appl. Phys. Lett.*, vol. 57, p. 1254, 1990.

4.9 Problems

4.1. An IC manufacturing plant produces 1000 wafers per week. Assume that each wafer contains 100 die, each of which can be sold for $50 if it works. The yield on these chips is currently running at 50%. If the yield can be increased, the incremental income is almost pure profit because all 100 chips on each wafer are manufactured whether they work or not. How much would the yield have to be increased to produce an annual profit increase of $10,000,000?

4.2. Calculate and plot the total number of allowable LLS (Localized Light Scatterers) on an 8″ wafer, through 2012, according to the NTRS. Generate a similar plot of the total number of allowed gate oxide defects in DRAMs. What conclusions do you draw about these requirements?

4.3. As MOS devices are scaled to smaller dimensions, gate oxides must be reduced in thickness.

a. As the gate oxide thickness decreases, do MOS devices become more or less sensitive to sodium contamination? Explain.

b. As the gate oxide thickness decreases, what must be done to the substrate doping (or alternatively the channel V_{TH} implant, to maintain the same V_{TH}? Explain.

4.4. A new cleaning procedure has been proposed which is based on H_2O saturated with O_2 as an oxidant. This has been suggested as a replacement for the H_2O_2 oxidizing solution used in the RCA clean. Suppose a Si wafer, contaminated with trace amounts of Au, Fe, and Cu is cleaned in the new H_2O/O_2 solution. Will this clean the wafer effectively? Why or why not? Explain.

4.5. Explain why it is important that the generation lifetime measurement illustrated in Figure 4–19 is done in the dark.

4.6. If you wanted to look for trace levels of contaminants left on a wafer surface after cleaning, would XRF or XPS be a better choice? Explain.

4.7. In the discussion in the text related to Figure 4–12 the importance of the temperature ramp rate between the nucleation and precipitation stages is described. Is the ramp rate coming back down to room temperature after the precipitation stage important in terms of gettering? Explain.

Lithography

5

5.1 Introduction

Lithography is the cornerstone of modern IC manufacturing. The ability to print patterns with submicron features and to place those patterns on a silicon substrate with better than 0.1-μm precision is what makes today's chips possible. Virtually all ICs are manufactured today with optical lithography, the basic process introduced in Figure 1–9 in Chapter 1. The concept is simple. A light sensitive photoresist is spun onto the wafer forming a thin layer on the surface. The resist is then selectively exposed by shining light through a mask which contains the pattern information for the particular layer being fabricated. The resist is then developed which completes the pattern transfer from the mask to the wafer. As we saw in the process flow in Chapter 2, the resist may then be used as a mask to etch underlying films or it may be used as a mask for an ion implantation doping step.

While the concept is simple, the actual implementation is very expensive and very complex, primarily because of the demands placed on this process for resolution, exposure field, placement accuracy, throughput, and defect density. Resolution requirements result from the ever-increasing demand for smaller device structures. Exposure field requirements result from ever-increasing chip sizes and the need to expose at least one full chip (preferably more) with each exposure. Placement accuracy is an issue because generally each mask layer needs to be carefully aligned with respect to the existing patterns already on the wafer. Throughput and defect density are of course issues because of the competitive nature of the semiconductor industry. Throughput translates directly into manufacturing cost. Defects translate directly into yield loss and therefore higher costs for the finished chips. Defects introduced during the lithographic process are a significant contributor to final chip yields.

The SIA NTRS defines the needs for future generations of silicon technologies. A portion of this roadmap relating to lithography is shown in Table 5–1 [5.1]. There are a number of interesting observations that can be made from this chart. First, as we saw in Chapter 1, the principal driving force behind this roadmap is the steady reduction in device dimensions or minimum feature size. The feature size reduction corresponds to a factor of 0.7X in linear dimension or a decrease in the area required per transistor by 50% approximately every three years. It is also interesting to note in the table that the most commonly cited minimum feature sizes in the NTRS (the bold entries in the table corresponding to the dense lines and spaces in DRAM chips) are actually not as small as the isolated lines (MOS gates) required on microprocessor (MPU) chips. These features are generally 20% – 30% smaller than the usually cited "minimum feature size."

Table 5–1 Lithography requirements for future generations of silicon technology [5.1]

Year of first DRAM Shipment	1997	1999	2003	2006	2009	2012
DRAM Bits/Chip	256M	1G	4G	16G	64G	256G
Minimum Feature Size nm						
Isolated Lines (MPU)	200	140	100	70	50	35
Dense Lines (DRAM)	**250**	**180**	**130**	**100**	**70**	**50**
Contacts	280	200	140	110	80	60
Gate CD Control 3σ (nm)	20	14	10	7	5	4
Alignment (mean + 3σ) (nm)	85	65	45	35	25	20
Depth of Focus (μm)	0.8	0.7	0.6	0.5	0.5	0.5
Defect Density (per layer/m^2)	100	80	60	50	40	30
@ Defect Size (nm)	@ 80	@ 60	@ 40	@ 30	@ 20	@ 15
DRAM Chip Size (mm^2)	280	400	560	790	1120	1580
MPU Chip Size (mm^2)	300	360	430	520	620	750
Field Size (mm)	22x22	25x32	25x36	25x40	25x44	25x52
Exposure Technology	248 nm DUV	248 nm DUV	248 nm or 193 nm DUV	193 nm DUV or ?	193 nm DUV or ?	?
Minimum Mask Count	22	22/24	24	24/26	26/28	28

Minimum features must not only decrease in average size with each technology generation, but the variation of these feature sizes must also decrease with time. Generally the CD (Critical Dimension) control is required to be about 10% of the smallest feature size. This requirement is usually expressed in terms of the 3σ control (three standard deviations of the feature size population need to be within the specified 10% of the mean).

The corresponding placement or alignment accuracy for these features (overlay) remains at about one-third of the minimum feature size for each generation of technology. The size of chips is projected in the NTRS to increase significantly over time. The corresponding lithographic printing area (field size) therefore also needs to increase in order to be able to print at least one chip with each exposed field. Typically about one-third of the total wafer manufacturing costs are consumed by lithography. Thus with a wafer manufacturing cost of about $1000 for an 8″ wafer, only a few hundred dollars can be spent on lithography. Wafer exposure tools today cost about $10 million and thus must be capable of printing on the order of 50 wafers per hour in order to meet these cost objectives.

Optical lithography will certainly be used through the 0.18- and 0.13-μm generations, and it is likely that it will be extendible to the 0.1-μm generation as well. Beyond that point, there is considerable uncertainty, for reasons that we will discuss in detail in this chapter. Potential candidates to replace optical lithography include X-ray, e-beam direct write, projection e-beam, and Extreme Ultraviolet (EUV), each of which is being explored in a variety of approaches. The last two are currently the most likely "winners," but there is still considerable debate as to which (if any) of these techniques will prove to be successful in manufacturing beyond 0.1 μm. This uncertainty is perhaps the greatest single challenge facing the semiconductor industry today in terms of continuing the historic trends represented by the NTRS.

In this chapter we will explore two major areas associated with the lithographic process. The first of these is the exposure system used to print the patterns on the wafer. We will focus on optical exposure systems because these dominate the industry today. Typical systems today use "step and repeat" or "step and scan" reducing projection printing with complex lens systems. The second major area we will explore is the photoresist material itself. Here the primary issues are sensitivity, resolution, and ruggedness. Typical resists today are carbon-based organic materials that have been engineered for optimum performance in IC manufacturing.

5.2 Historical Development and Basic Concepts

The overall lithography process is conceptually illustrated in Figure 5–1. The patterns that comprise the various layers in an integrated circuit are designed using Computer-Aided Design (CAD) systems. Today these systems contain many advanced capabilities that greatly improve the efficiency of designing chips with many millions of components. Libraries of previous designs that are known to work are usually available, from which basic functions or circuits can be cut and pasted into new designs. Software tools are used to help route or wire the connections between functional blocks. Additional tools check the design to make sure that there are no violations of design rules. And finally, circuit- and system-level simulation tools are available to predict the performance of the new design.

Once the design is complete and ready to transfer to the fabrication facility, the information for each mask level is transferred to a mask making machine that is either an

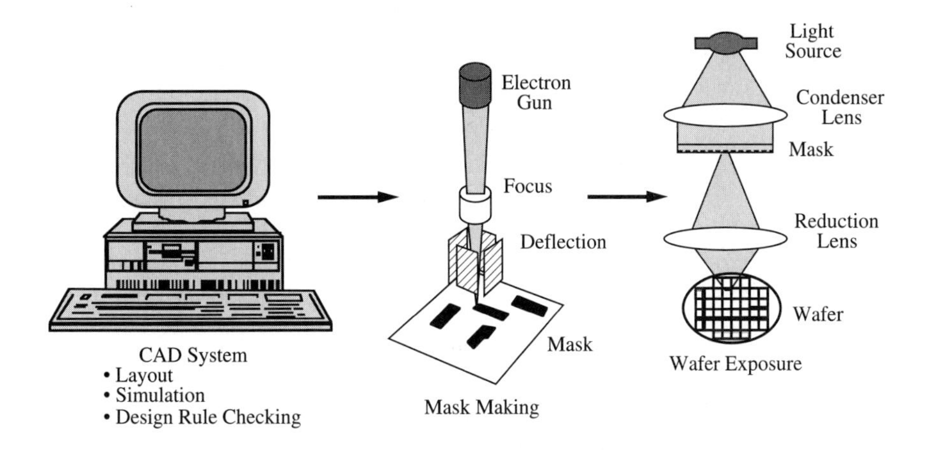

Figure 5–1 Lithography process from mask design to wafer printing.

electron beam or laser pattern generator. The pattern for each mask is literally written on a mask blank using a scanning electron or laser beam. The mask itself is usually a fused silica plate covered with a thin layer (≈ 80 nm) of chromium and a layer of photoresist. A thin antireflection coating (ARC) layer (10 – 15 nm) is also often used between the chrome and the resist to prevent reflections from the chrome layer which can degrade pattern resolution. The electron or laser beam exposes the resist which is then developed and used as an etch mask to transfer the mask pattern into the chrome. The chrome layer is usually wet etched because the process is simple although dry etching may be more widely used in the future as dimensions continue to decrease. Tight dimensional control can be maintained because the chrome layer is so thin. Once the chrome is etched, the photoresist is removed. The fused silica substrate has highly polished surfaces so that light is not scattered as it passes through the mask and ideally has a small thermal expansion coefficient so that mask dimensions are stable over small temperature changes. It is also obviously important that the clear areas of the mask where the chrome has been etched away have high transparency at the wavelength of light used in the wafer exposure system. This is becoming more difficult to achieve in practice as the exposing wavelength moves deeper into the UV region to achieve higher resolution. Even though the mask material (basically SiO_2) has a large bandgap (≈ 9 eV), trace impurities in the glass can degrade optical transparency because they can absorb light at these short wavelengths.

Usually the mask is fabricated with pattern dimensions 4X to 5X larger than the features actually desired on the wafer because the wafer exposure system reduces the image by the same factor. Demagnification in the wafer exposure system makes the mask easier to fabricate and easier to check for imperfections. This is a crucial step because any defects on the mask will be directly imaged on every wafer exposed with the mask and contribute to yield loss. Since step and repeat exposure systems typically expose only a one- or two-chip area at a time, a mask defect which prints on the wafer can easily make the yield zero. Mask inspection is performed by comparing the mask chrome pattern with another identical pattern when there are two or more chip patterns on the mask. If the mask pattern is so large that only one chip pattern is present, the comparison can be with the database in the CAD system used to produce the mask. Defects can usually be repaired at this stage either by removing unwanted chrome areas with laser ablation or ion beams, or by depositing additional chrome to fill in pinholes. Once the mask is checked, and repaired if necessary, it is usually protected from later contamination by dust particles with a thin transparent membrane (pellicle) stretched over a metal frame above the chrome side of the mask. Pellicles are usually made from nitrocellulose a few microns thick. Since the pellicles are offset from the mask, dust particles that fall on the pellicle during use will be out of focus on the wafer and therefore will usually not print. Typically the pellicle might be mounted a few mm above the mask. Since the depth of focus of modern exposure systems is only a few μm, dust particles as large as 100 μm will not print on the wafer during exposure.

The actual mask writing is usually done with a laser or an electron beam pattern generator, as shown in Figure 5–1. These machines raster a laser beam or a beam of electrons in an X-Y pattern across the mask with the beam blanked on and off as necessary to generate the appropriate mask pattern. Generally the beam size is on the order of 0.1 – 0.5 μm for e-beam systems and slightly larger for laser-based systems, which is adequate for writing 4X or 5X masks for today's steppers. As minimum feature sizes continue to decrease, the beam size will have to shrink as well in order to produce masks with adequate resolution. It is perhaps obvious that the e-beam system could be used directly to write images on a wafer simply by putting the electron sensitive resist on the wafer rather than on the mask. The reason this is not done in high-volume manufacturing is simply because the wafer throughput would be too slow. Typical e-beam pattern generators would require tens of minutes to expose a full wafer. This is much slower than optical steppers that typically have throughputs on the order of 50 wafers per hour. However, as device dimensions continue to shrink, e-beam approaches to wafer exposure at least offer the required resolution, if means could be found to improve throughput. We will return to this issue later in the chapter.

The pattern information is transferred to the wafer by printing the mask pattern in a layer of photoresist on the wafer surface. Generally today this is done with a projection exposure system as also illustrated in Figure 5–1. Light from a high-intensity source is collimated and passed through the mask. Each clear area on the mask transmits the light which is then collected and focused by a second lens system. This second lens system also serves to reduce the image size by 4X – 5X. The field of view of such systems is typically only a few cm on a side, so that only a few chips are printed during each exposure. The wafer is physically moved ("stepped") to the next exposure field and the process repeated so these systems are commonly called step and repeat tools or simply steppers. In some systems ("scanners") a narrow slit of light is produced by the light source system and the mask and wafer are simultaneously scanned mechanically so that the mask image is scanned across the wafer. Note that in systems of this type, the mechanical system must scan the mask 4X or 5X times faster than the wafer, corresponding to the optical reduction factor. Scanners greatly increase the field size up to the limit of the mask dimension, at least in the scanning direction.

It is convenient to separate the lithography process into three parts. The first, which is the most straightforward, is the light source used to generate the photons which ultimately expose the resist. While this might seem to be a simple task, higher-resolution lithography demands shorter wavelength photons and this makes the source issue more complex. The second part of the lithography process is the exposure system that images the mask on the wafer surface. This system produces what is known as the aerial image (Figure 5–2) at the top surface of the resist. This image is basically the pattern of optical radiation striking the top surface of the resist. In the example in Figure 5–2, a positive resist is illustrated since this polarity of resist represents the vast majority of manufacturing applications today. The incoming photons strike the resist in the light areas, changing its properties in those regions. The three-dimensional optical intensity pattern through the photoresist layer produces a 3D latent image of the mask pattern that can then be developed. The exposed positive resist in this example would dissolve in the resist developer. After developing, the resist in this example is used as an etch mask so that the TiN local interconnect level can be etched away where it is not desired (see Figure 2–37 in the process flow in Chapter 2). The third part of the lithography process contains all the issues associated with the resist itself: exposure, developing, baking, and so on.

The aerial image thus serves as the dividing line between the major parts of the lithography system (the exposure tool and the resist). The job of the exposure tool is to produce the best aerial image possible. Best is defined in terms of resolution, exposure

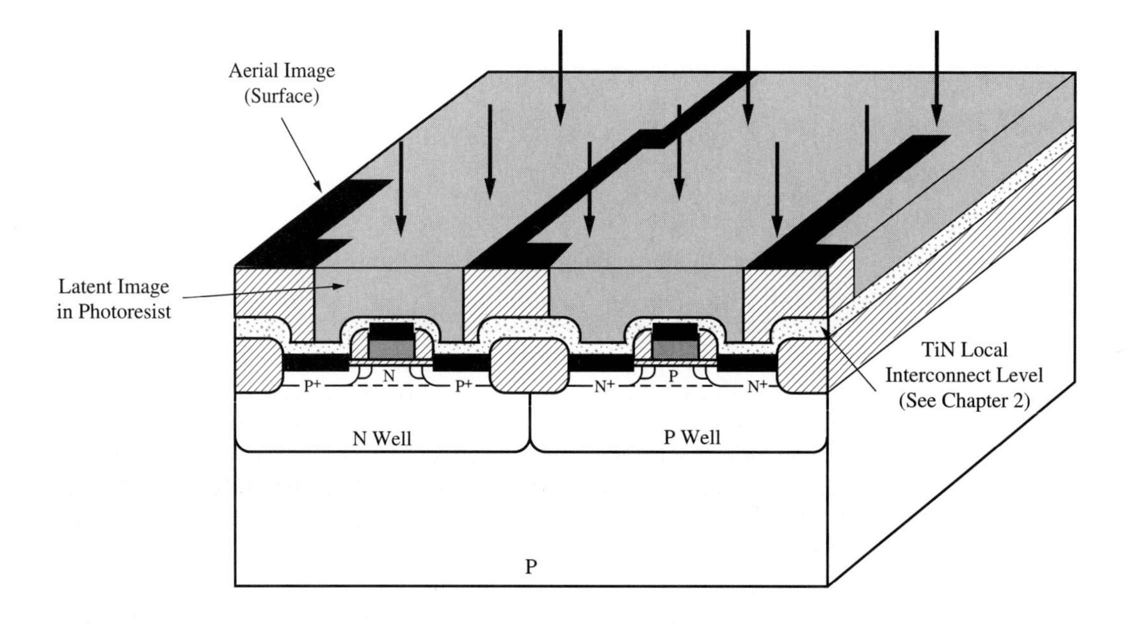

Figure 5–2 Separation of the lithography process into exposure and wafer features. The dividing line is the aerial image of the mask, which is the pattern of radiation that strikes the surface of the photoresist. This example corresponds to Figures 2–36 and 2–37 in Chapter 2.

field, depth of focus, uniformity, and lack of aberrations across the field, photon intensity, and so forth. The job of the photoresist is to translate this aerial image into the best thin film 3D replica of the aerial image possible. Here best is defined in terms of geometric accuracy, exposure speed, and resist resistance to subsequent processing (ruggedness). In the following sections we will consider many of the basic concepts associated with exposure tools and resists and also briefly consider the issues associated with the light source itself.

5.2.1 Light Sources

It is probably obvious to most readers that higher-resolution lithography requires shorter wavelength photons. Modern exposure systems produce diffraction limited images and diffraction effects are strongly related to the wavelength of the exposing radiation. We will discuss this issue in more detail shortly, but in this section we consider first the issues associated with generating the light in modern lithography systems. Historically, most lithography systems have used arc lamps as the primary light source. These lamps usually contain Hg vapor inside a sealed glass envelope. Two conducting electrodes inside the envelope are separated by several mm. An arc is struck between the electrodes by applying a high enough voltage to ionize the gas (typically several kV). Once the gas is ionized, it behaves like a plasma, conceptually similar to the plasmas used in the deposition and etching systems described in Chapters 9 and 10. In the arc lamp, the plasma is conducting and consists of ions, electrons, and neutral species. Typical lamps used for photolithography consume about one kW of power. At room temperature, the Hg vapor pressure is on the order of 1 atm, but once the lamp is operating, power dissipation quickly raises the temperature and therefore the internal pressure to $\approx 20 - 40$ atm.

Light emission occurs through two processes. The free electrons in the plasma have an effective temperature on the order of 40,000K and emit black body radiation according to Planck's law. The wavelength corresponding to this temperature is very deep in the ultraviolet and is above the bandgap of the fused silica used to form the glass envelope of the lamp. Thus this radiation is mostly absorbed before it exits the lamp.

The second source of emitted light comes from the Hg atoms themselves. Collisions in the gas between the free electrons and the Hg atoms provide energy to some of the electrons in the Hg atoms, raising them to higher energy levels. When these electrons drop back to their lower energy states, they radiate photons at specific energies (frequencies) characteristic of the allowed energy levels in the Hg atom. This process is very much like that shown in Figure 4–18 in Chapter 4, where we discussed the use of these energy transitions in identifying the specific elements from which photons are emitted. In the case of Hg, there is strong emission at a number of UV wavelengths. Most steppers use a single wavelength by simply filtering out the unwanted emissions. The complex optical systems in these exposure tools are much easier to design if they need to focus only a single wavelength. Two that are commonly used are 436 nm (g-line) and 365 nm (i-line). Most exposure tools in the early 1990s used the g-line. However, as linewidths shrunk, use of the i-line became dominant because of the better resolution it provides. Some exposure tools, particularly simple contact and proximity printers, sometimes use broader wavelength light (several lines from the Hg source) for exposure since there are no focusing optics in these systems.

i-line steppers dominated production for the 0.35-μm generation of technology. Generations beyond 0.35 μm require shorter exposure wavelengths and new light sources. The brightest sources in the deep UV part of the spectrum are excimer lasers. Two that are of specific interest for lithography are KrF (248 nm) and ArF (193 nm). In excimer lasers two elements are present which do not normally react in their unexcited state (often a noble gas and a halogen containing compound). However if these elements (Kr and NF_3, for example) are excited, a chemical reaction forming, for example, KrF, is possible. When the excited molecule returns to its ground state, a photon is emitted in the deep UV and the molecule breaks up. Energy must be continually provided, therefore, usually from an internal pulsed discharge, to replenish the population of the excited species. Usually the laser source is strobed at a frequency of several hundred Hz and generally about 100 flashes are used at each exposure site on the wafer to minimize speckle noise. A total energy of several hundred mJ is provided to each exposure site. In steppers, this energy is focused on a wafer area of a few cm^2, providing reasonable exposure times. A number of problems exist with these exposure sources, including reliability and longevity of the laser, transparency of optical components in the lens systems at these wavelengths, and finding suitable resists. These problems have been solved at 248 nm (KrF) and this source is now being used in commercial production for the 0.25-μm and 0.18-μm generations. ArF is the most likely source for the 0.13-μm and 0.10-μm technology generations. The picture is much less clear beyond the 0.1-μm generation.

5.2.2 Wafer Exposure Systems

We now consider in more detail one of the critical elements in modern lithography, the system used to create the aerial image at the photoresist surface. There are three general classes of optical wafer exposure tools, contact, proximity, and projection systems, although only the last is in widespread high-volume manufacturing use today. These are conceptually illustrated in Figure 5–3.

Contact printing is the oldest and the simplest printing process. The mask is placed chrome side down in direct contact with the resist layer on the wafer. The exposure of the resist then takes place by shining light through the mask. The aligning of the mask to patterns already on the wafer takes place prior to exposure, by observing both the mask and wafer patterns through a microscope with the mask slightly separated from the wafer. Contact printing systems are actually capable of high-resolution printing because with the mask and wafer in contact, diffraction effects are minimized. In addition, the machines to perform contact printing are relatively inexpensive. However these types of systems cannot be used in high-volume manufacturing of complex chips for one very simple reason. The hard contact between the mask and the wafer results in damage to both the mask and the resist layer and therefore results in high defect densities. The resulting chip yields are not compatible with economic manufacturing of today's chips. However, contact printing systems are used in some manufacturing applications where low volumes or small chip sizes make the economics of these systems more attractive.

Proximity printing largely solves the defect issues associated with contact printing, because the mask and wafer are kept separated by 5 – 25 μm. However, these systems are also not suitable for manufacturing most of today's chips because the separation of the mask and wafer degrades the resolution of the printed patterns due to diffraction effects. We will quantify these effects shortly, but in practice it is not possible to print features smaller than a few μm with UV exposure and gaps on the order of 20 μm. Interestingly, the resolution of these systems improves as the exposure wavelength de-

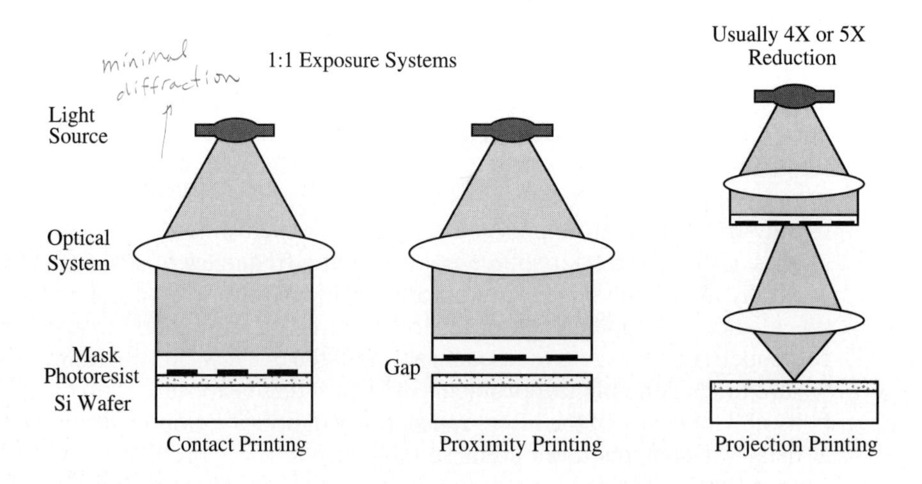

Figure 5–3 Three basic methods of wafer exposure.

creases and X-ray lithography systems can use proximity printing and achieve high resolution because of the very short exposure wavelength (1 – 2 nm). We will return to X-ray systems at the end of this chapter. Both contact and proximity systems require 1X masks, which are more difficult to produce than masks for reduction systems.

The dominant method of wafer exposure today is projection printing. These systems provide high resolution but without the defect problems of contact printing. In projection exposure tools, the mask is physically separated from the wafer and an optical system is used to image the mask on the wafer. This obviously solves the defect issues associated with contact printing. The resolution of projection printers is generally limited by diffraction effects that we will describe in detail. Generally the optical system reduces the mask image by 4X to 5X which means that only a small portion of the wafer is printed during each exposure. Typically such steppers today are capable of printing 0.25-μm or smaller features over an exposure field of several cm^2 and have a throughput of 25 – 50 wafers per hour. They also cost many millions of dollars.

5.2.2.1 Optics Basics—Ray Tracing and Diffraction

In order to understand and quantify the capabilities of modern wafer exposure systems we will need to review some basic concepts about light and optical systems. Many standard references exist on these topics (see, for example, [5.2]) and the reader is referred to these texts for a more detailed treatment of the concepts described here. The application of basic optical principles to lithography systems is also described in detail in a number of books, for example [5.3, 5.4]. In this section we will introduce the basic ideas in a somewhat qualitative way. In Section 5.5, we will be more quantitative.

Light travels as an electromagnetic wave through space. When one is interested in the behavior of an optical system in which all of the dimensions are very large compared to the wavelength of light, the light can usually be treated as particles traveling in straight lines between the optical components. This simplifies the problem to one of "ray tracing." In projection lithography systems, for example, this approach can often be used in describing the optical source and condenser lens, but it fails when the light passes through the mask because the feature dimensions on the mask are comparable to the wavelength of the light. To understand the behavior of the light as it passes through the mask, the objective lens, and on to the wafer, we must include the wave nature of light. The single most important effect that we must account for is diffraction.

Diffraction effects occur because light does not in fact travel in straight lines. Many simple experiments can demonstrate this fact. Figure 5–4 illustrates the passage of light through a small aperture. The light pattern which strikes the screen (image plane) covers a much larger area than can be accounted for by simply drawing straight lines (ray tracing) to describe the light propagation. In fact the smaller the aperture becomes, the more spread out the screen image becomes. This is very much like the situation we find in modern lithography where light passes through a mask with apertures (clear regions) with dimensions on the order of the light wavelength. (We actually illustrated these effects in Figures 5–1 and 5–3 by showing the light spreading out after passing through the mask, but did not explain why this happens in connection with those figures.)

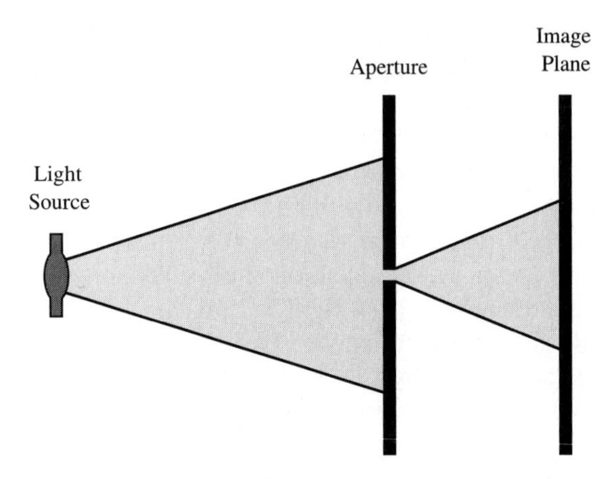

Figure 5–4 Simple example of diffraction effects. Light passes through a narrow aperture. The image formed covers a much larger area than can be explained based on simple straight line ray tracing.

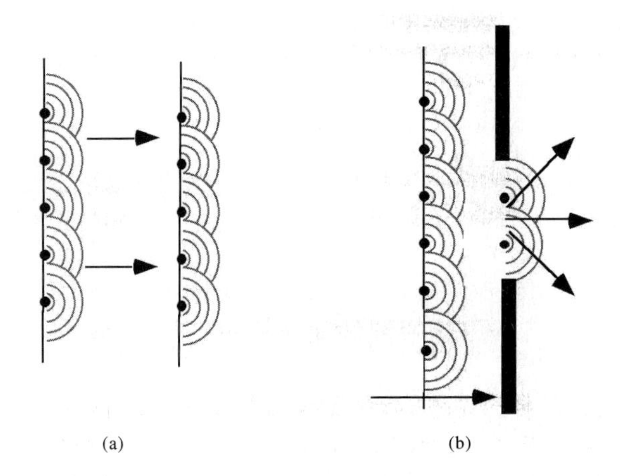

Figure 5–5 Propagation of a plane wave in (a) free space and (b) through a small aperture, illustrating the use of the Huygens-Fresnel principle to construct the wavefront as it propagates.

Consider Figure 5–5. A plane wave is shown propagating through space, unobstructed in (a) and passing through an aperture in (b). The Huygens-Fresnel principle can be used to construct the wavefront versus position as it propagates. This principle states that every unobstructed point of a wavefront at a given instant in time acts as a source of a spherical secondary wavelet of the same frequency as the primary wave. The amplitude of the optical field can be found by superimposing all these wavelets, considering their relative magnitudes and phases. In (a) this superposition simply results in a propagating plane wave. In (b), only the source points in the aperture serve as sources of Huygens wavelets and the resulting propagating pattern beyond the aperture involves diffraction. As the arrows in (b) illustrate, the light spreads out beyond the aperture. In fact the smaller the aperture becomes, the more the light spreads out because there are fewer wavelets able to pass through the aperture and thus more spherical propagation results beyond the aperture.

Diffraction can be thought of simply as the "bending" of light when it passes through an aperture. The light that passes through the aperture carries with it the information on the size and shape of that aperture. If, for example, the aperture were part of a mask that we wished to print on a wafer, then the information about the aperture size and shape needs to be carried by the light to the photoresist on the wafer. The problem is that this information spreads out in space because of diffraction and it must all be collected to convey perfect information about the aperture to the resist on the wafer. Figure 5–6 illustrates this in a qualitative way. Because of its finite size, the focusing lens collects only part of the total diffraction pattern associated with the light passing through the aperture. The light diffracted to wider angles carries the information about the finer details of the aperture, so it is those details that are lost first when a lens of finite size is used to collect and focus the light.

The actual image produced in this simple example is shown in Figure 5–7 for a small circular aperture and is known as Airy's disk after Sir George Biddell Airy who first derived the expression describing the central intensity maximum. The central maximum approximates the image of the circular aperture. Because of diffraction effects, the image is composed of a bright center disk surrounded by a series of faint rings. The image intensity can be described mathematically by Bessel functions, and the approximate size of the image is given by

$$\text{Diameter of central maximum} = \frac{1.22\lambda f}{d} \tag{5.1}$$

where d is the focusing lens diameter, f is the focal length, and λ is the wavelength of the light. Note that a point source only produces a point image if $d \to \infty$ (or if λ or $f \to 0$).

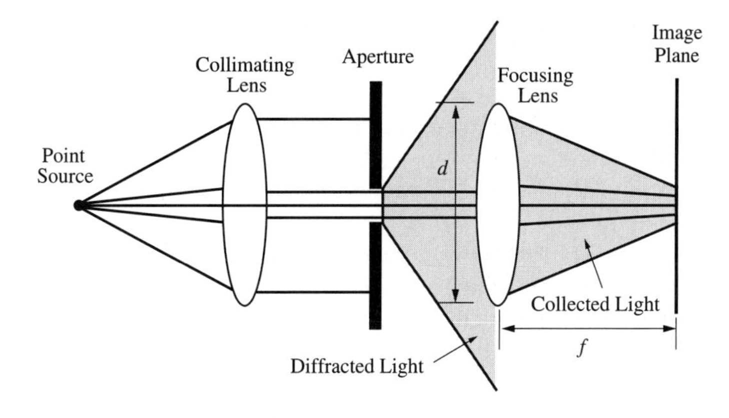

Figure 5–6 Qualitative example of a small aperture being imaged.

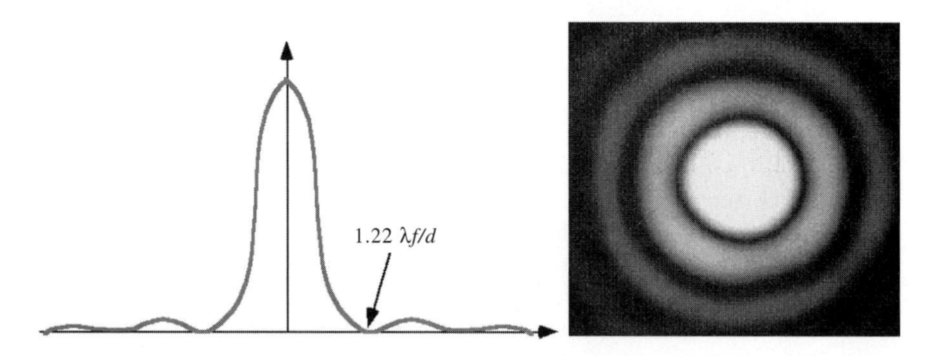

Figure 5–7 Image intensity of a circular aperture in the image plane (Fraunhofer diffraction pattern). The intensity is sketched along any diameter on the left. The pattern on the right illustrates the 2D image. Photo courtesy of J. Goodman. Reprinted with permission of McGraw-Hill [5.2].

Two types of diffraction are usually distinguished: Fresnel or near field diffraction and Fraunhofer or far field diffraction. Both are fundamentally due to the same effect—the wave nature of light. In Fresnel diffraction, the image plane is close to the aperture. The light travels directly from the aperture to the plane where the image is formed, as in Figure 5–4 with no intervening lens system. In Fraunhofer diffraction, the image is far from the aperture and a lens is normally placed between the aperture and the image plane to capture and focus the image, as in Figure 5–6. In modern lithography systems, Fresnel diffraction applies to contact and proximity exposure systems and Fraunhofer diffraction applies to projection systems as should be apparent by considering Figure 5–3. Mathematical descriptions and detailed models have been developed for both of these regimes. Powerful simulation tools based on these models have also been developed, which allow the calculation of the aerial image formed by the wafer exposure system. We will discuss these issues in more detail in Section 5.5.

5.2.2.2 Projection Systems (Fraunhofer Diffraction)

The performance of projection printers is usually specified in terms of a number of basic parameters such as resolution, depth of focus, field of view, Modulation Transfer Function (*MTF*), alignment accuracy, throughput, and so on. At least the first four of these are directly related to the basic properties of optical systems, which we will discuss in this section. The last two issues are more associated with the mechanical design of the system.

Consider Figure 5–8 where we now imagine that we have two point sources close together that we are trying to image. These could be, for example, two small adjacent features on a mask we are trying to print in resist on a wafer. How close together can they be and still be resolved in the image plane? The images produced by the two point sources will each be an Airy disk as shown in Figure 5–7. Rayleigh suggested that a reasonable criterion for resolution was that the central maximums of each point image lie at the first minima of the adjacent point image, the distance given by Eq. (5.1). While

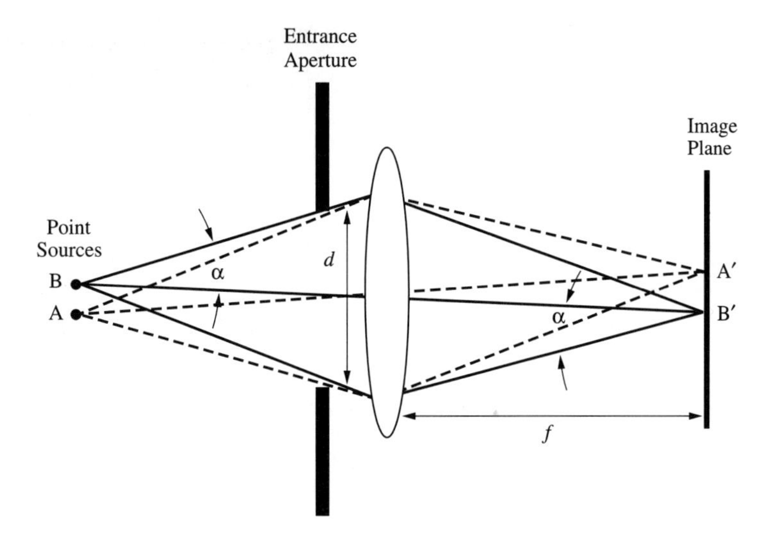

Figure 5–8 Illustration of the resolving power of a lens when two point sources are to be separated in the image.

this definition is somewhat arbitrary, it is useful and has been widely adopted. With this definition, the resolution R of the lens is given by [5.5]

$$R = \frac{1.22\lambda f}{d} = \frac{1.22\lambda f}{n(2f\sin\alpha)} = \frac{0.61\lambda}{n\sin\alpha} \tag{5.2}$$

where n has been included for generality and is the index of refraction of the material between the object and the lens (usually air with $n = 1$ in lithography systems). α is the maximum half-angle of the diffracted light that can enter the lens or the acceptance angle of the lens. α may be limited by the physical size of the lens itself, or by an entrance aperture or pupil in front of the lens. α is really a measure of the ability of the lens to collect diffracted light. This property was named the Numerical Aperture (NA) by Ernst Abbe.

$$NA \equiv n\sin\alpha \tag{5.3}$$

$$\therefore\ R = \frac{0.61\lambda}{NA} = k_1\frac{\lambda}{NA} \tag{5.4}$$

Eq. (5.2) was derived from the Fraunhofer diffraction pattern for an Airy disk and as such strictly applies only to point sources. Because of this the 0.61 factor is often replaced by k_1 in Eq. (5.4). In real lithography systems the mask contains a variety of shapes. k_1 also depends in practice on the ability of the resist chemistry to distinguish closely spaced features on the wafer structure below the resist (topography, reflectivity, etc.) and on defocusing at the image plane. Actual k_1 values achieved in practical optical lithography systems are 0.6 to 0.8.

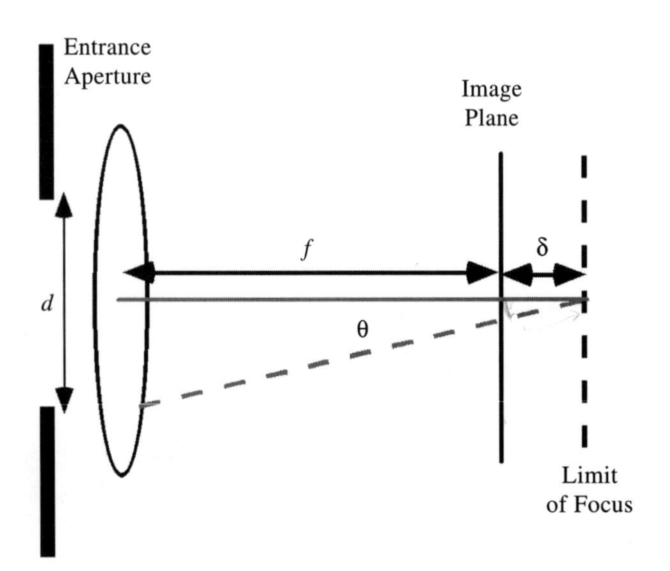

Figure 5–9 Geometry for estimating the depth of focus of an imaging system.

It is obvious from Eq. (5.4) that shorter exposure wavelengths lead to better image resolution. It is also clear that lenses with higher numerical apertures also achieve better resolution, basically because they are able to capture more of the diffracted light and therefore construct a better image. Aside from the difficulty of building larger (higher *NA*) lenses, there is also a significant drawback to using higher *NA* lenses. This is the depth of focus of the lens, which can be estimated as shown in Figure 5–9.

If δ is the on-axis path length difference at the limit of focus, then the path length difference for a ray from the edge of the entrance aperture is simply δcosθ. The Rayleigh criteria for depth of focus is simply that these two lengths not differ by more than λ/4. Thus

$$\lambda/4 = \delta - \delta\cos\Theta \tag{5.5}$$

Assuming θ is small,

$$\lambda/4 = \delta\left[1 - \left(1 - \frac{\Theta^2}{2}\right)\right] \cong \delta\frac{\Theta^2}{2} \tag{5.6}$$

$$\Theta \cong \sin\Theta = \frac{d}{2f} = NA \tag{5.7}$$

$$\therefore\ DOF = \delta = \pm\frac{\lambda}{2(NA)^2} = \pm k_2\frac{\lambda}{(NA)^2} \tag{5.8}$$

The factor of $^1/_2$ is often replaced by k_2 in Eq. (5.8) because the $^1/_2$ value is appropriate at the Rayleigh resolution limit but does not take into account the increase in depth of focus for larger features nor the dependence in practice on other parameters like the resist process.

Example Estimate the resolution and depth of focus of a state-of-the-art excimer laser stepper using a KrF light source ($\lambda = 248$ nm) with a $NA = 0.6$. Assume $k_1 = 0.75$ and $k_2 = 0.5$.

Answer

$$R = k_1 \frac{\lambda}{NA} = 0.75 \left(\frac{0.248\ \mu m}{0.6} \right) = 0.31\ \mu m$$

$$DOF = \pm k_2 \frac{\lambda}{(NA)^2} = \pm 0.5 \left[\frac{0.248\ \mu m}{(0.6)^2} \right] = \pm 0.34\ \mu m$$

Using additional technical "tricks" like off-axis illumination, the resolution can be pushed below 0.25 μm, suitable for the SIA NTRS 0.25-μm generation. Further improvements can be obtained through more sophisticated mask designs using concepts like optical proximity correction and phase shift masks, which we will describe later. The depth of focus is on the same order as the resist layer thickness itself and therefore requires very flat topography and careful attention in the stepper to keeping the image plane focused by adjusting the height of the wafer with respect to the lens.

There is an additional basic concept regarding optical exposure systems that will be useful to us. This is the Modulation Transfer Function or *MTF* illustrated in Figure 5–10. This concept strictly applies only to coherent illumination and as a result is not really applicable to modern steppers, which generally use partially coherent illumination. However the basic idea is a useful one in understanding lithography issues.

Figure 5–10 shows a generic projection lithography system in which a reducing lens system is used to image a mask pattern in resist. Since diffraction effects are only important after the light passes through the mask, the optical intensity pattern as the light exits the mask will be almost an ideal representation of the mask. Because of diffraction effects and other nonidealities in the optical system however, the aerial image produced at the resist plane will not be perfectly black and white. If the features are widely separated, the aerial image may approach the ideal shown on the left in the Figure 5–10, but as the features move closer together, the aerial image will look more like that sketched on the right. As a simple example, imagine two Airy disks (Figure 5–7) partially overlapping. A useful measure of the quality of the aerial image is the *MTF* that can be defined as

$$MTF = \frac{I_{MAX} - I_{MIN}}{I_{MAX} + I_{MIN}} \tag{5.9}$$

where I is the intensity of the light.

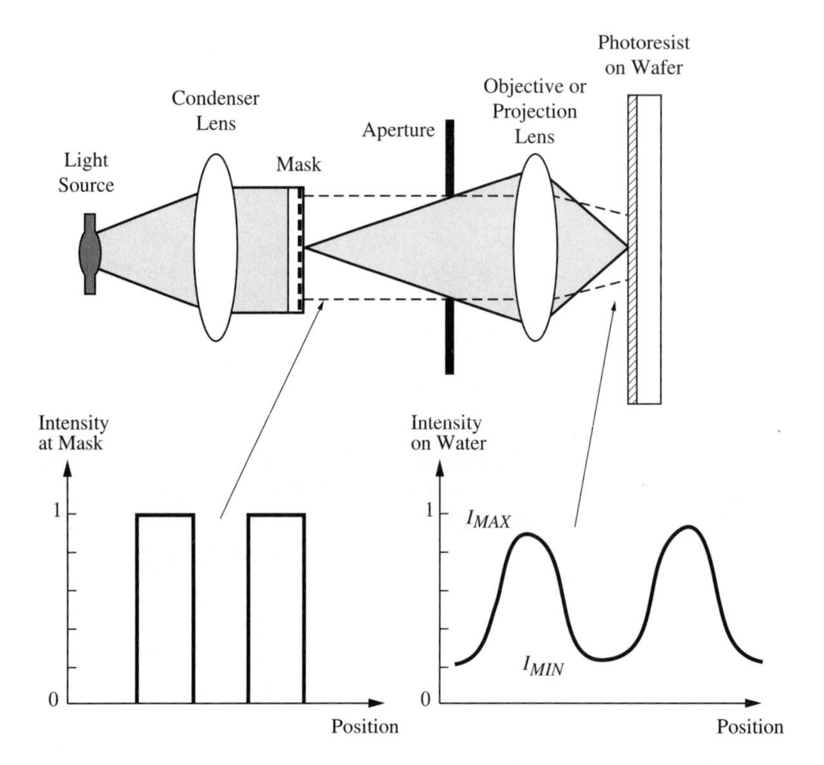

Figure 5–10 Modulation Transfer Function (*MTF*) concept. A generic lithography system is shown at the top with a mask being imaged on photoresist on a wafer. The mask *MTF* is almost ideal ($MTF = 1$) since the feature sizes are 4 – 5 X larger than those imaged in the resist and diffraction effects are minimal. The aerial image *MTF* is much lower ($MTF \approx 0.6$) because of diffraction effects in the optical system.

The *MTF* is really a measure of the contrast in the aerial image produced by the exposure system. Generally an exposure system needs to achieve a *MTF* value of 0.5 or larger in order for the resist to properly resolve the features. Recently developed Deep UV (DUV) resists can work with somewhat smaller *MTF* values.

The *MTF* obviously depends on the feature size in the image and generally has the behavior illustrated in Figure 5–11. For large features, the resulting aerial image produced by the exposure system has excellent contrast and the *MTF* is unity. As the feature size decreases, diffraction effects cause the *MTF* to degrade and to finally reach zero when the features are so closely spaced that there is no remaining contrast in the aerial image.

The *MTF* is also affected by a parameter known as the spatial coherence of the light source. Figure 5–12 illustrates the concept of spatial coherency. An ideal point source produces light in which the waves are in phase at all points along the emitted wavefronts. A condenser lens can then convert these waves to plane waves, all of which strike

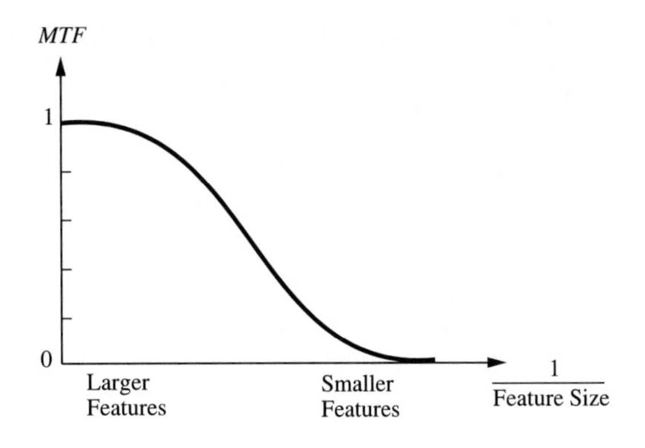

Figure 5–11 Modulation Transfer Function (*MTF*) versus feature size in the image.

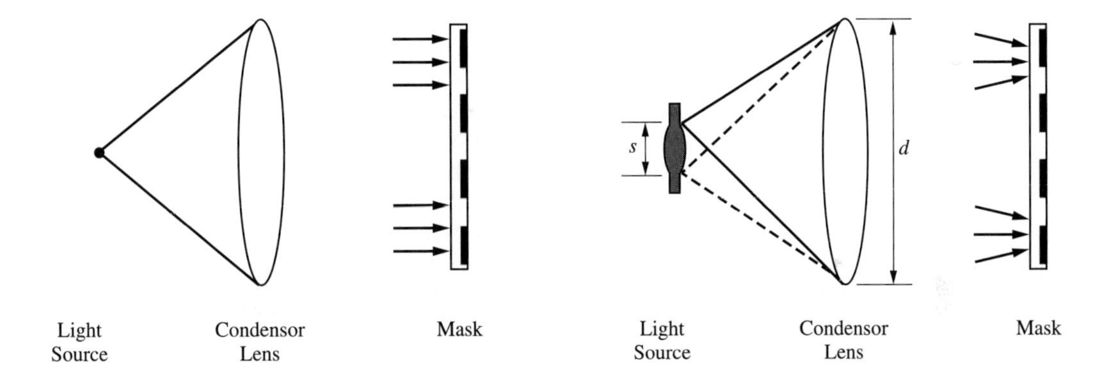

Figure 5–12 Examples of spatially coherent (left) and partially coherent (right) light sources.

the mask at exactly the same angle as illustrated in the left of the figure. Such a source is an ideal coherent source. As the physical size of the source increases as shown in the right of Figure 5–12, light is emitted from a volume rather than a point and the waves will not be perfectly in phase everywhere. If the same condenser lens is used to convert the light to plane waves, the result will be light arriving at the mask from a variety of angles as illustrated. Such a source is a partially coherent source. In the limit, if the size of the source became infinite (and the condenser lens were also infinite to collect all the light), the source would become completely incoherent. A useful definition of the spatial coherence of practical light sources for lithography is simply

$$S = \frac{\text{light source diameter}}{\text{condenser lens diameter}} = \frac{s}{d} \tag{5.10a}$$

Alternatively, S is defined in terms of the NA of the condenser and projection optics in the exposure tool,

$$S = \frac{NA_{condenser\ optics}}{NA_{projection\ optics}} \tag{5.10b}$$

It might appear at first glance that we would choose to have an ideal coherent source ($s = 0$) for optical lithography. However this is not the case for the following reasons. First, as $s \to 0$, the optical intensity also goes to zero, resulting in infinite exposure times to print the mask pattern in the resist. Second, the MTF is also affected by the value of s and having $s = 0$ in not the optimum choice.

To understand this latter point, we need to consider diffraction effects once again. If the light passing through the mask is partially coherent (i.e., coming in at a variety of angles), then the diffraction patterns resulting from mask features will be smeared out. If we refer again to Figure 5–6, this means that the diffraction pattern for a given feature will be spread over an angle larger than α. This initially seems like a bad thing, because it means that some information will be lost because the finite aperture of the objective lens will not collect it. However, this smearing also means that information from closely spaced features that would have been completely lost outside the aperture of the focusing lens is now partially collected because it is smeared inside the lens aperture. The result of these effects is that the MTF behavior with feature size is modified, as shown in Figure 5–13. As s increases, the source becomes more incoherent, and the MTF is somewhat degraded for large features. However, it is improved for the smallest features and this is usually a good trade-off in projection imaging systems that are being pushed toward their resolution limits. In practice, a spatial coherence of 0.5 to 0.7 is often used in chip manufacturing, using the definition in Eq. (5.10b).

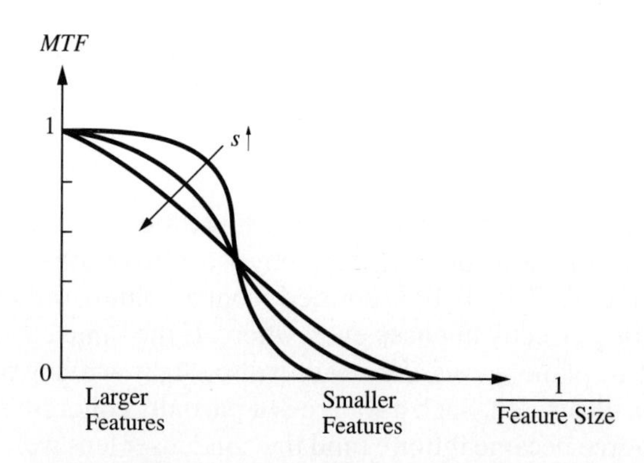

Figure 5–13 Modulation Transfer Function (MTF) versus feature size in the image. As s increases (more incoherent source), the MTF degrades for larger features but improves for very small features.

5.2.2.3 Contact and Proximity Systems (Fresnel Diffraction)

Contact and proximity exposure systems (Figure 5–3) operate in the near field or Fresnel diffraction regime. There is no lens between the mask and the resist on the wafer, so the diffraction pattern resulting from the light passing through the mask directly impinges on the resist surface. The aerial image that is created therefore depends on the near field diffraction pattern.

Figure 5–14 illustrates the situation conceptually. We assume for the moment that the mask and the wafer are separated by some small gap g. A plane wave is assumed to be incident on an aperture in a mask. The diffraction pattern on the opposite side of the mask can be constructed by imagining Huygens wavelets emanating from each point in the aperture. The resulting light intensity distribution striking the top surface of the resist is also illustrated in Figure 5–14. There are several features in the light distribution of interest. First, notice that the intensity rises gradually near the edges of the mask aperture. Because of diffraction effects, the light "bends" away from the aperture edges, producing some resist exposure outside the aperture edges. Second, note the "ringing" in the intensity distribution within the aperture dimension. This arises because of constructive and destructive interference between the Huygens wavelets emanating from the aperture. Contact and proximity printers often use multiple wavelengths for exposure and also do not use light sources with perfect spatial coherence. Both of these approaches minimize the ringing effects illustrated in Figure 5–14, but of course do not eliminate diffraction effects.

As the separation g increases between the mask and the resist, the quality of the aerial image produced at the resist surface will degrade because diffraction effects will

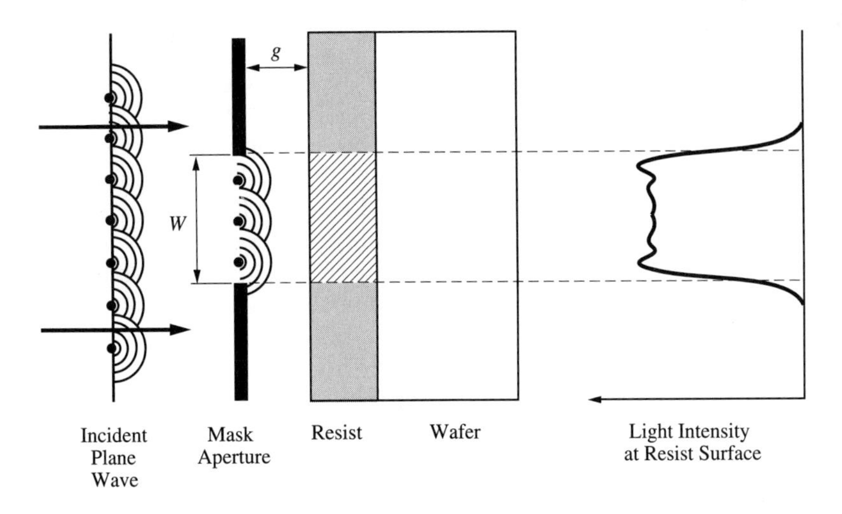

Figure 5–14 Basic contact or near field exposure system illustrating the use of Huygen's wavelets emanating from an aperture in the mask. A mask feature size of W is assumed, along with a mask to resist separation of g. The resulting light intensity distribution (aerial image) at the resist surface is shown on the right.

become even more important. Contact printers minimize these effects by attempting to reduce g to zero, but in most practical systems g is not strictly zero because the top surface of the resist is not perfectly flat due to topography on the wafer surface. In the limit when the mask and wafer are pressed into hard contact, the resolution of such systems can be very good (well below 0.1 μm). However, even in this case, the resist itself still has a finite thickness and the resolution will still be limited by light scattering in the resist and by light reflection from surface features on the underlying wafer which scatter the light laterally into regions adjacent to the mask apertures. We will discuss some of these scattering issues more carefully in the next section on resist exposure.

Generally the aerial image can be calculated using Fresnel diffraction theory whenever the gap g falls within the limits

$$\lambda < g < \frac{W^2}{\lambda} \tag{5.11}$$

where W is the size of the mask aperture (feature size). The lower limit on g is certainly satisfied by proximity printing systems and is often satisfied by contact printing systems unless hard contact is used. If g falls below the wavelength of the light used for the exposure, the resulting light intensity distribution can still be calculated but only by a full numerical solution to Maxwell's equations. Such solutions are very complex, but fortunately are rarely needed [5.6]. The upper bound on g arises because when g increases, Fresnel diffraction theory must be replaced by far field (Fraunhofer) diffraction theory in order to calculate the aerial image.

Within the Fresnel diffraction range, the minimum resolvable feature size is on the order of

$$W_{min} \approx \sqrt{\lambda g} \tag{5.12}$$

Thus a proximity exposure system operating with a 10-μm gap and an i-line light source ($\lambda = 365$ nm) can resolve features slightly smaller than 2 μm. This is much larger than the dimensions used in modern VLSI chips, so these systems are not useful for manufacturing such chips. However proximity printers are much less expensive than the projection systems described earlier, so for applications in which features sizes are compatible with them, proximity printers are an economical solution.

Figure 5–15 attempts to conceptually summarize the discussion in the previous two sections. We imagine a plane wave passing through a mask aperture. The aperture is imaged on the resist on a wafer through one of the three types of exposure systems. In the contact printing case, a very high resolution image is produced because the mask and resist are assumed to be in hard contact. If the wafer and mask are separated slightly as in a proximity printing system, the resolution degrades because of near field Fresnel diffraction effects. Finally, if we place a lens between the mask and wafer and focus the aperture on the wafer, an image characterized by Fraunhofer diffraction is produced. In the example in this figure, the resolution of the proximity system image is illustrated as inferior to both of the other systems. This is usually the case in actual systems, as we saw

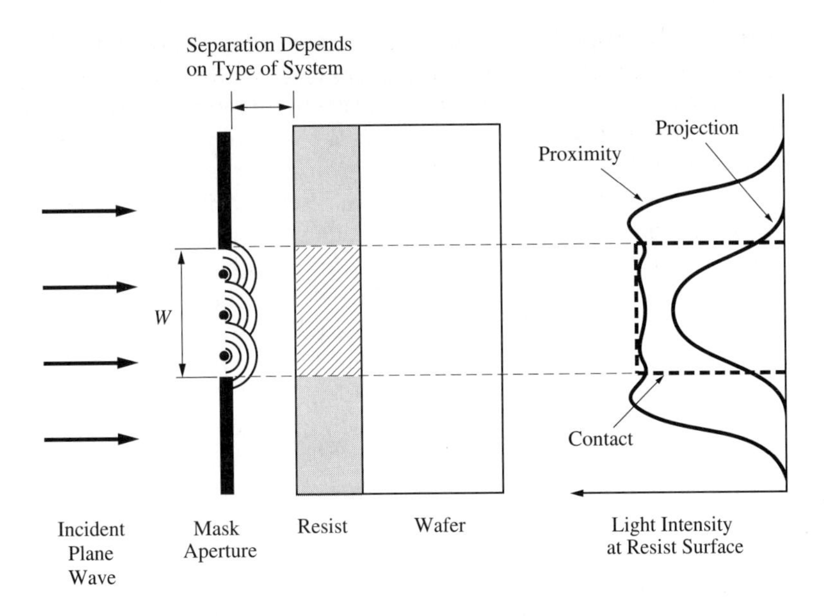

Figure 5–15 Aerial images produced by the three types of optical lithography tools. The mask and wafer would be in hard contact in a contact aligner, separated by a gap g in a proximity aligner, and far apart with an intervening focusing lens in a projection system.

in the numerical example earlier and is the reason why projection systems are used in manufacturing today.

5.2.3 Photoresists

Photoresist materials are designed to respond to incident photons by changing their properties when they are exposed to light. Many materials of course absorb light, but often the absorption results in electronic processes rather than chemical changes. Semiconductors, for example, absorb photons and the energy is given to electrons and holes. As we have seen in earlier chapters, the free carriers will dissipate the absorbed energy through recombination or through phonon interactions (transferring the energy to heat). In some cases the energy can actually be collected as in solar cells. None of these processes are useful in lithography because in photoresists we require a material that maintains a latent image of the impinging photons at least until the resist is developed. A long-lived response to light generally requires a chemical change in the material.

Almost all resists today are fabricated from hydrocarbon-based materials. When these materials absorb light, the energy from the photons generally breaks chemical bonds. After this happens, the resist material chemically restructures itself into a new stable form. Positive resists respond to light by becoming more soluble in the developer solution. Negative resists do the opposite. They become less soluble where they are exposed. Current practice in the semiconductor industry relies primarily on positive resists because they generally have better resolution than do negative resists.

Photoresists in use today are liquids at room temperature and are applied to the surface of wafers by placing the liquid on the wafer and then spinning the wafer at several thousand RPM. The spin speed and the viscosity of the resist determine the final resist thickness, which is usually $\approx 0.6 - 1$ μm. The viscosity of the resist is controlled by a solvent, which is a constituent of the resist. Once the resist is spun on to the wafer, a baking step (prebake) is generally used to drive off the remaining solvent. The resist is then exposed. Developing is done using liquid developers either by immersion of the wafer in the liquid, by spraying the developer on the wafer or, most commonly, by placing a "puddle" of the developer on the wafer. After developing is complete, the resist is generally baked again (postbaked) to harden it and to improve its ability to act as an etch mask or ion implantation mask, depending on the particular step in the process flow. Finally, after the etching or implantation process, the resist is removed, usually in an oxygen plasma, although chemical stripping can also be used.

A number of important parameters determine the usefulness of a particular resist. Sensitivity is a measure of how much light is required to expose the resist. This is usually measured in mJ cm^{-2} and for g-line and i-line resists is typically 100 mJ cm^{-2}. Newer Deep UV (DUV) resists often achieve sensitivities of 20–40 mJ cm^{-2} because they use chemical amplification, a process we will describe later. Generally, high sensitivity is desired because this decreases the exposure time of the resist and therefore improves throughput in the lithography process. However, extremely high sensitivity is usually not desired because this tends to make the resist material unstable, makes it very sensitive to temperature, and can also create problems with statistical variations due to shot noise during the exposure. Usually higher contrast and more process latitude are achieved at lower sensitivities. However, DUV chemically amplified resists achieve both higher sensitivity and higher contrast than the older g-line and i-line resists. Since the light used to expose the resist is at a specific wavelength, it is also important that the sensitivity of the resist be optimized for the exposure wavelength.

Resolution is obviously important in resists. The quality of resist patterns today is generally limited by the exposure system (aerial image) and not by the resist itself. However the resist materials and the process steps (exposure dose, baking, and developing cycles) must be carefully controlled to achieve diffraction limited resolution in the resist images.

The third parameter of importance has to do with the "resist" function of photoresists. The term "resist" describes the need for the photoresist to withstand etching or ion implantation after the mask pattern is transferred to the resist. Practical resists need to have reasonable robustness with respect to these processes. In practice this means that resists must be able to resolve small features even when the resist is of reasonable thickness.

g-line and i-line photoresists generally consist of three components, an inactive resin which is usually a hydrocarbon which forms the base of the material, a photoactive compound (*PAC*) which is also a hydrocarbon, and a solvent which is used to adjust the viscosity of the resist. DUV resists replace the *PAC* component with a Photo-Acid Generator (*PAG*) which acts as a chemical amplifier or catalyst, and often add other components as well for stability. Most of the solvent in resists evaporates during spinning on to the wafer and during prebake processes before the resist is exposed, leaving a material that is about 1:1 base and active components.

5.2.3.1 g-line and i-line Resists

The most commonly used g-line and i-line resists today are diazonaphthoquinones or DNQ materials. A base resin is added which is generally novolac, with the structure shown in Figure 5–16. Novolac is a polymer material consisting of basic hydrocarbon rings with 2 methyl groups and 1 OH group attached. The basic ring structure which is shown in the figure may be repeated many times to form a long chain polymer material. Novolac by itself will readily dissolve in the developer solution at a typical dissolution rate of about 15 nm sec^{-1}.

The *PACs* in these resists are often diazoquinones. The basic structure of these compounds is shown in Figure 5–17. The photoactive part of the structure is the portion

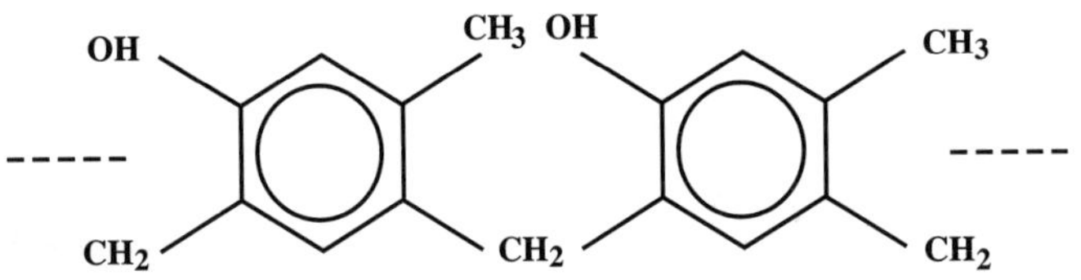

Figure 5–16 Basic structure of novolac, a thick resin used as the base material in positive photoresists.

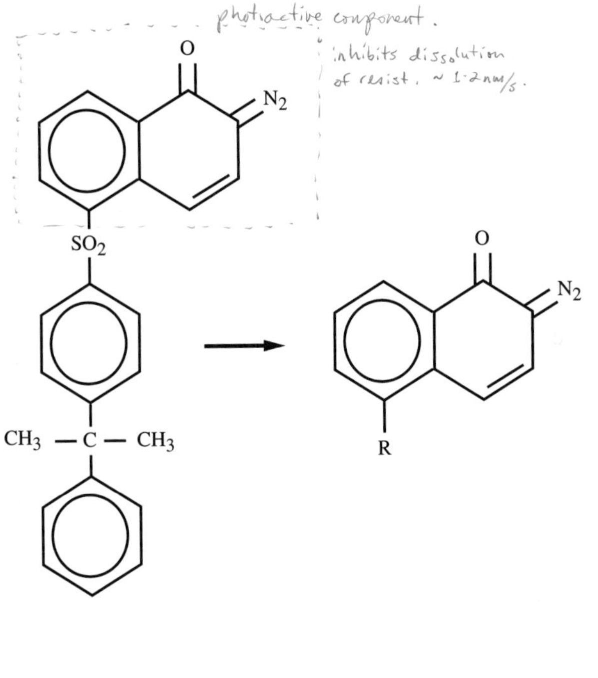

Figure 5–17 Basic structure of diazoquinone, a commonly used photoactive compound in positive photoresists. R represents the bottom part of the molecule.

above the SO_2. The remainder of the molecule is often abbreviated as shown in the figure. The role of the *PAC* is to inhibit the dissolution of the resist material in the developer. Diazoquinones are insoluble in typical developers and they reduce the overall dissolution rate of the resist to approximately 1–2 nm sec^{-1}. Thus the DNQ material is essentially insoluble in the resist developer before it is exposed to light.

When the resist is exposed to light, the diazoquinone molecules chemically change as illustrated in Figure 5–18. The N_2 molecule is weakly bonded in the *PAC* and the first part of the photochemical reaction involves the light breaking this bond. This leaves behind a highly reactive carbon site. The *PAC* structure can stabilize itself by moving a carbon atom outside the ring with the oxygen atom covalently bonded to it. This is known as the Wolff rearrangement. The resulting ketene molecule finally transforms into carboxylic acid (lower left in Figure 5–18) in the presence of water. The carboxylic acid is now readily soluble in a basic developer [typically TMAH (tetramethyl ammonium hydroxide), KOH, or NaOH dissolved in H_2O]. The novolac matrix material is also readily soluble in this solution. The exposed resist material thus dissolves at a rate of 100 – 200 nm sec^{-1}. The unexposed regions of the resist are essentially unaffected by the developer and so if the exposed pattern accurately reproduces the mask pattern, the photoresist can produce a high resolution image of the mask.

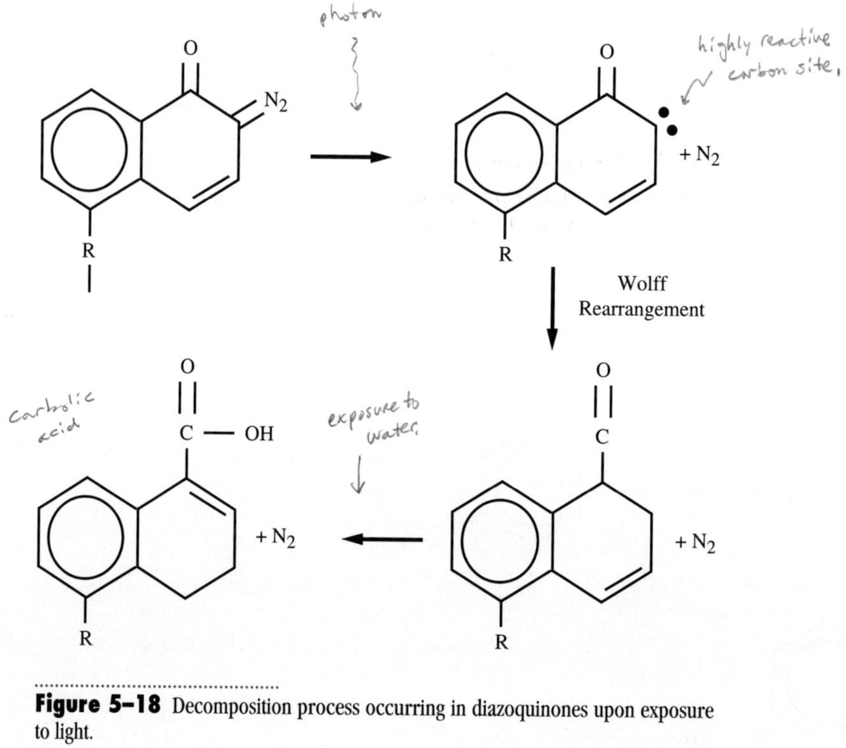

Figure 5–18 Decomposition process occurring in diazoquinones upon exposure to light.

5.2.3.2 Deep Ultraviolet (DUV) Resists

Conventional DNQ resist materials have two significant problems when shorter exposure wavelengths are used. The first is that for wavelengths below i-line (365 nm), these resists strongly absorb the incident photons. Thus the incident radiation cannot penetrate through the full thickness of the resist. This is a significant issue at 248 nm (KrF) which is the wavelength used for the 0.25-μm and 0.18-μm generations. The second problem has to do with resist sensitivity. Some years ago when resists suitable for DUV applications were first being explored, the only viable light source was the Hg arc lamp. These sources work well for g-line and i-line systems, but the intensity of their output in the DUV is much lower than at i-line. Thus it was believed at that time that whatever resist was used for DUV applications, it would have to have improved sensitivity over the standard DNQ resists, in order to maintain manufacturing throughput. Of course bright excimer laser sources are now available and are reliable at 248 nm and so the sensitivity issue is not as crucial. As a result, DNQ-type resists are being revisited today with modified *PAC* compounds that work more effectively at 248 nm.

DUV resists that are in use today, however, are not modified DNQ resists. They are based on a completely new chemistry and make use of chemical amplification (CA resists) [5.7 – 5.9]. Standard DNQ resists achieve quantum efficiencies of about 0.3. This means that about 30% of the incoming photons interact with *PAC* molecules and are effective in exposing the resist. Thus the sensitivity improvement possible with these resists is at most a factor of about 3. CA resists use a different exposure process in which the incoming photons react with a Photo-Acid Generator (*PAG*) molecule, creating an acid molecule. These acid molecules then act as catalysts during a subsequent resist bake to change the resist properties in the exposed regions. Both positive and negative resist versions are possible. In the positive resist case, the *PAG* initiates a chemical reaction that makes the resist soluble in the developer; in a negative resist, the opposite happens. The key point in either case is that the reactions are catalytic; the acid molecule is regenerated after each chemical reaction and may thus participate in tens or hundreds of further reactions. Thus the overall quantum efficiency in a CA resist is the product of the initial efficiency of the light/*PAG* reaction, times the number of subsequent reactions that are catalyzed. This product can be much larger than 1 and is responsible for the improvement in sensitivity of DUV resists compared to DNQ resists (20–40 mJ cm^{-2} compared to 100 mJ cm^{-2}).

Chemical amplification is a very powerful new approach to create resists. Since the number of possible acid catalyzed reactions is very much larger than the number of photochemical reactions, an explosion of new resist possibilities has occurred in recent years. Figure 5–19 illustrates the basic principle behind these resists. Positive resists consist of a *PAG* and a blocked or protected polymer, which is insoluble in the developer because of attached molecules (labeled INSOL in Figure 5–19). A typical example would be a polyhydroxystyrene polymer with attached acid labile groups [5.10, 5.11]. The incident DUV photons react with the *PAG* molecules to create an acid molecule. The spatial pattern of acid molecules in the resist after the exposure is thus a "stored" or latent acid 3D image of the mask pattern. After exposure, the wafer is baked at a temperature on the order of 120°C for a few minutes (Postexposure Bake or PEB). The

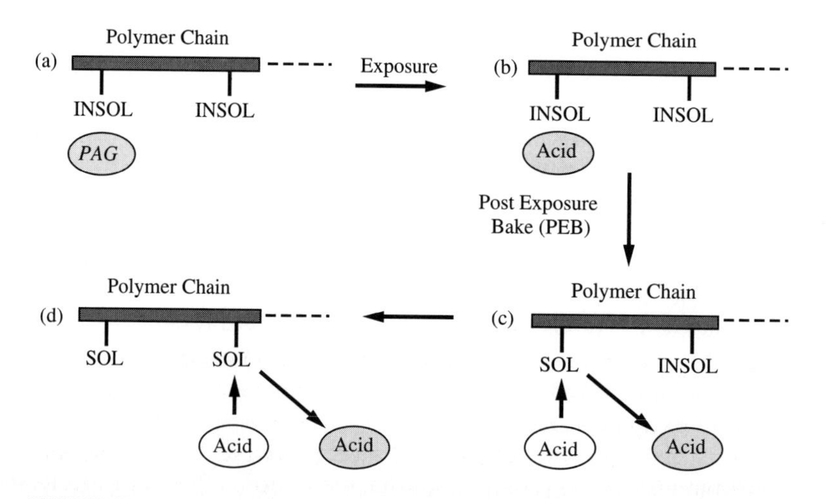

Figure 5–19 Basic operation of a Chemically Amplified (CA) resist. *PAG* is the photo-acid generator; INSOL and SOL are the insoluble and soluble portions of the polymer base. Steps (c) and (d) may repeat tens or hundreds of times during the PEB.

heat provides the energy needed for the reaction between the acid molecules and the insoluble fragments on the polymer chains to take place. It also provides mobility (through diffusion) for the acid molecules to find the insoluble fragments and to react with tens or hundreds of such fragments during the PEB. Thus during the PEB, the insoluble blocked polymer is converted into an unblocked polymer that is soluble in an aqueous alkaline developer. In negative working DUV resists, the *PAG* catalyzes a reaction which crosslinks the polymer chains, making the resist insoluble in the developer. The key mechanism in either process is the catalytic behavior of the acid molecules that are regenerated after each reaction.

While these new resists offer superb sensitivity and resolution more than adequate for today's device structures, they also require very careful manufacturing control. Because there is a time delay between the light exposure and the acid reaction with the polymer chain fragments, poisoning (contamination) of the acid molecules is a concern. Some early DUV resists were very sensitive to very small concentrations of airborne contaminants that reacted with the acid molecules before they could catalyze the resist reactions during the PEB. This resulted in a surface layer on the resist where the acid was neutralized and the resist effectively unexposed. These kinds of problems have been largely solved by adding additional components to DUV resists, by adding protective surface layers, and by careful environmental and manufacturing control. DUV resists also require very careful control of the PEB conditions because that bake is used to drive the chemical reaction that completes the resist exposure. Chemical reactions and the diffusion associated with the acid molecules during the PEB generally depend exponentially on temperature, requiring temperature control on the order of a fraction of a °C during the PEB.

5.2.3.3 Basic Properties and Characterization of Resists

Two basic parameters are often used to describe the properties of photoresists: contrast and the Critical Modulation Transfer Function (*CMTF*). We will define these terms and explain their importance in the following paragraphs. Contrast is really a measure of the resist's ability to distinguish light from dark areas in the aerial image the exposure system produces. As we have seen, diffraction effects and perhaps other imperfections in the exposure system result in an aerial image that does not have abrupt transitions from dark to light. An important question is how the resist responds to the "gray" region at the edges of features in the aerial image.

Contrast is an experimentally determined parameter for each resist and its value is extracted from plots like that shown in Figure 5–20. The data from which these plots can be derived are obtained by exposing resist layers to a variety of exposure doses. Each of the samples is then developed for a fixed period of time and the thickness of the photoresist remaining after developing is measured. For positive resists, samples receiving small exposure doses will not be attacked by the developer to any appreciable extent; those receiving large doses will completely dissolve in the developer. Intermediate doses will result in partial dissolution of the resist. For negative resists, the opposite behavior occurs. Given data like those shown in the figure, the contrast is simply the slope of the steep part of the curve, defined as

$$\gamma = \frac{1}{\log_{10}\frac{Q_f}{Q_O}} \tag{5.13}$$

where Q_O is the dose at which the exposure first begins to have an effect and Q_f is the dose at which exposure is complete.

Typical g-line and i-line resists achieve contrasts of 2–3 and Q_f values of about 100 mJ cm^{-2}. DUV resists achieve significantly better contrast and better sensitivities than this.

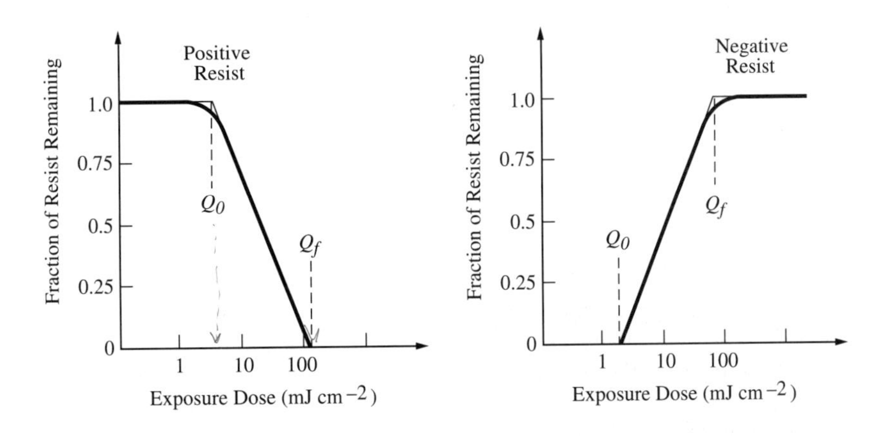

Figure 5–20 Idealized contrast curves for positive and negative resists.

This is basically because the chemical amplification that occurs in DUV resists steepens the transition from the unexposed to the exposed condition. (Once the reaction is begun, the catalytic nature of the process carries it to completion unlike DNQ resists where the *PAC* molecules in the resist must be exposed one by one by incoming photons during the exposure.) Thus DUV resists typically achieve γ values of 5 – 10 and Q_f values of about 20 – 40 mJ cm^{-2}.

It is important to note, however, that γ is not a constant for a particular resist composition. Rather, the experimentally extracted value of γ depends on process parameters like the development chemistry, bake times, temperatures before and after exposure, the wavelength of the exposing light, and the underlying structure of the wafer on which the resist is spun. In general it is desirable to have a resist with a high contrast because this produces better (steeper) edge profiles in the developed resist patterns. (See Figure 5–21.) Intuitively, this arises because a high contrast implies that the resist sharply distinguishes between dark and light areas in the aerial image. Thus resists with high contrast can actually "sharpen up" a poor aerial image.

The Modulation Transfer Function (*MTF*) of the aerial image was defined in Eq. (5.9) and in Figure 5–10. The *MTF* is simply a measure of the "dark" versus "light" intensities in the aerial image produced by the exposure system. It is often useful to define a similar quantity for the resist, in this case called the Critical *MTF* or *CMTF*. The CMTF is roughly the minimum optical transfer function necessary to resolve a pattern in the resist.

$$CMTF_{resist} = \frac{Q_f - Q_O}{Q_f + Q_O} = \frac{10^{1/\gamma} - 1}{10^{1/\gamma} + 1} \tag{5.14}$$

Typical *CMTF* values for g-line and i-line resists are around 0.4. With their higher γ values, chemically amplified DUV resists achieve significantly smaller *CMTF* values ($\approx$ 0.1 – 0.2). The significance of this number is that the *CMTF* must be less than the aerial image *MTF* if the resist is going to resolve the aerial image.

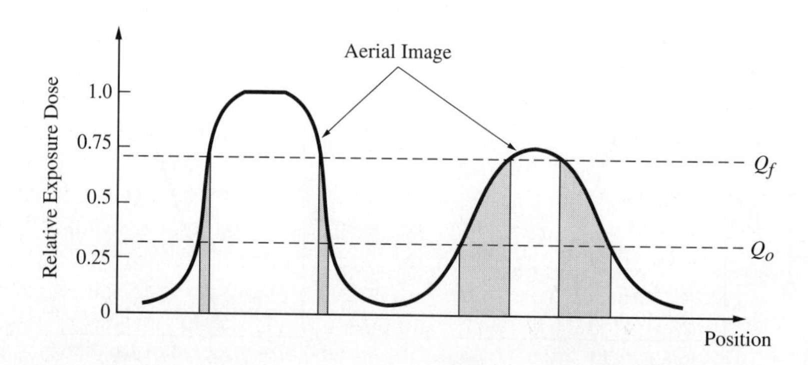

Figure 5–21 Example of how the quality of the aerial image and the resist contrast combine to produce the resist edge profile. The left side shows a sharp aerial image and steep resist edges (gray area). The example on the right shows a poorer aerial image and the resulting gradual edges on the resist profile.

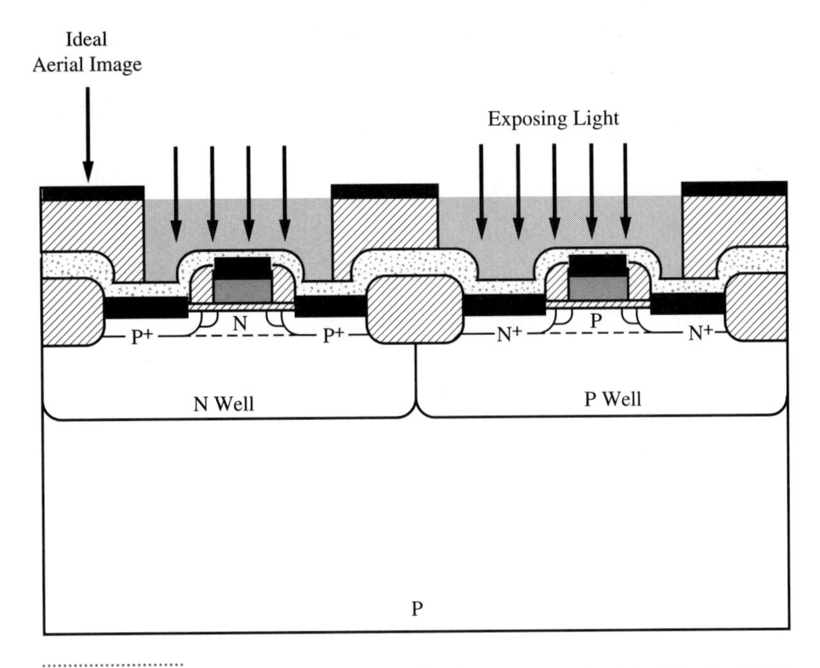

Figure 5–22 Exposure process associated with Figures 2–36 and 2–37 in the CMOS process in Chapter 2. The black bars in the aerial image represent areas on the mask that are opaque and hence ideally no photons strike the resist in these areas.

To this point in our discussion of resists we have effectively treated them as having uniform thickness and we have also treated the exposure process as occurring simultaneously throughout the volume of the resist material. In fact, neither of these is a very good assumption in many cases. Figure 5–22 illustrates some of these issues. Notice in that figure that the resist thickness tends to be nonuniform across the wafer because it is spun on as a liquid and therefore tends to fill in the "hills and valleys" of the underlying topography. The exposure process therefore often has to contend with exposing different regions with different thicknesses of resist. Effectively the resist is thinner on top of high structures and thicker over low lying structures. This may be a particular problem at the edges of underlying thin films where the resist thickness can change abruptly. The result of these effects is that the resist can be effectively underexposed where it is thicker and overexposed where it is thinner. This can result in linewidth variations, particularly where the photoresist features cross steps in the underlying structures.

A second issue is that the light absorption by the resist varies with depth below the surface of the resist and it also changes with time during the exposure process. Again imagine in connection with Figure 5–22 that the exposure process has just begun. The *PAC* concentration is assumed uniform throughout the resist. As *PAC* molecules near the resist surface absorb light photons, those photons are not available for exposing the deeper layers of the resist. Thus the light concentration falls off with depth. We will model this more carefully in Section 5.5, but to first order, the light intensity falls off exponentially with distance into the resist.

$$I = I_0 E^{-\alpha z} \tag{5.15}$$

where z is the depth below the surface, I_0 is the intensity at the surface, and α is the optical absorption coefficient in the resist. Thus the resist is first exposed near the top surface.

Fortunately a process known as "bleaching" occurs in g-line and i-line DNQ resists. As the resist is exposed, the *PAC* is altered, absorbing less and less light, and therefore it becomes more and more transparent. Thus as the top layers of the resist are exposed, they transmit more of the light to the deeper layers which are subsequently exposed. This results in a more uniform exposure. The bleaching process is not surprising since as the *PAC* component of these resists reacts and converts to carboxylic acid, more of the light will pass through to the deeper layers. Detailed modeling of these effects also has to include the light absorption by the novolac base component of the resist, as we will see in Section 5.5. Bleaching typically does not occur in DUV resists. This is a problem with these materials because the light can reflect off surfaces below the resist during the entire exposure. This can be mitigated by using antireflection coatings below the DUV resist (see below) and dyes in the resist itself to minimize reflections.

If there are highly reflective layers below the photoresist, light which passes all the way through the resist without being absorbed will be reflected by these underlying layers and pass back up through the resist again. While this may speed up the exposure process, it also has the potential for setting up standing wave light patterns in the resist because of constructive and destructive interference between the incoming and outgoing waves. Furthermore, if the light is scattered sideways, image resolution can be degraded. Figures 5–23 and 5–24 illustrate these issues. In some cases an Antireflective Coating (ARC) is deposited on the wafer prior to spinning on the resist. This can greatly help in minimizing standing wave effects, but of course increases process complexity. Another approach that is often used in g-line and i-line resists is to add dyes to the resist, which absorb light and minimize reflections.

The "scalloped edges" illustrated in Figure 5–24 are also strongly affected by post-baking of the resist after exposure but before development, since this heat treatment allows diffusion of the *PAC* in g-line and i-line resists or the *PAG* in DUV resists on a limited basis. This smoothes out the standing wave pattern. It is quite possible to model these standing wave effects and to predict the resulting resist edge patterns that result. We will consider these issues more carefully in Section 5.5.

5.2.4 Mask Engineering—Optical Proximity Correction and Phase Shifting

In our discussion to this point, we have considered the mask to be simply a digital device. That is, it has clear areas and dark areas and the patterns of these areas represent exactly the pattern that we wish to print in the resist on the wafer. It is actually possible to do better than this in designing the mask if the objective is to produce the highest quality aerial image. We will briefly discuss two approaches to doing this: Optical Proximity Correction (OPC) and Phase Shift Masks (PSMs). These approaches might be considered "mask engineering." These methods are also sometimes called "wavefront engineering" [5.12].

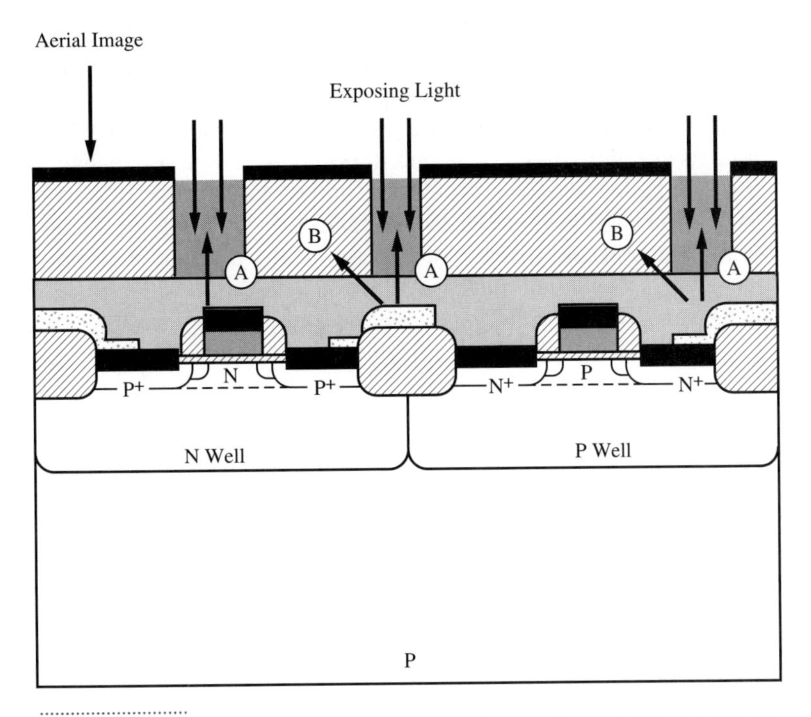

Figure 5–23 Photolithography exposure occurring between Figures 2–39 and 2–40 in the CMOS process described in Chapter 2. The A and B symbols indicate examples of standing wave patterns and sideways light scattering, respectively.

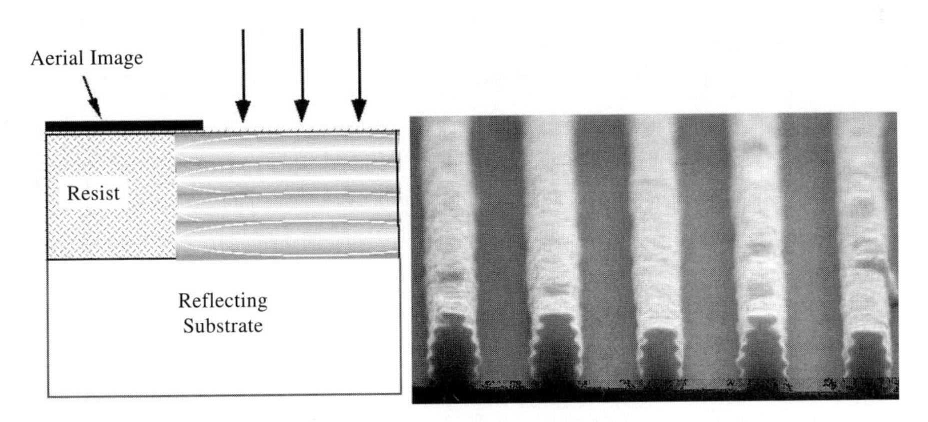

Figure 5–24 The light intensity pattern resulting from a standing wave is sketched on the left. A photoresist image that illustrates these effects after developing is shown on the right. Courtesy of A. Vladar and P. Rissman, Hewlett Packard.

We saw in our discussion of exposure systems that the finite aperture of projection systems results in a loss of some of the light diffracted from the mask features. In addition to their finite size, apertures and lenses in projection systems are generally circular, not square or rectangular like most of the features on masks. What are lost are the high-frequency components of the diffraction pattern. This lost information results in an aerial image which has rounded rather than square corners, changes in linewidth between isolated and grouped lines, and shortening of the ends of narrow linear features. These effects are quite predictable and in principle can be somewhat compensated for by adjusting the feature dimensions and shapes on the mask. In principle, this could be done purely through software once the mask design is complete. The problem is very difficult in the general case because of the complexity of modern masks. An example of what is possible is shown in Figure 5–25 [5.13].

A second approach to mask engineering involves actually changing the transmission characteristics of the mask in selected areas. In 1982, Levenson and colleagues suggested the use of phase shifting techniques to improve the resolution of the printed aer-

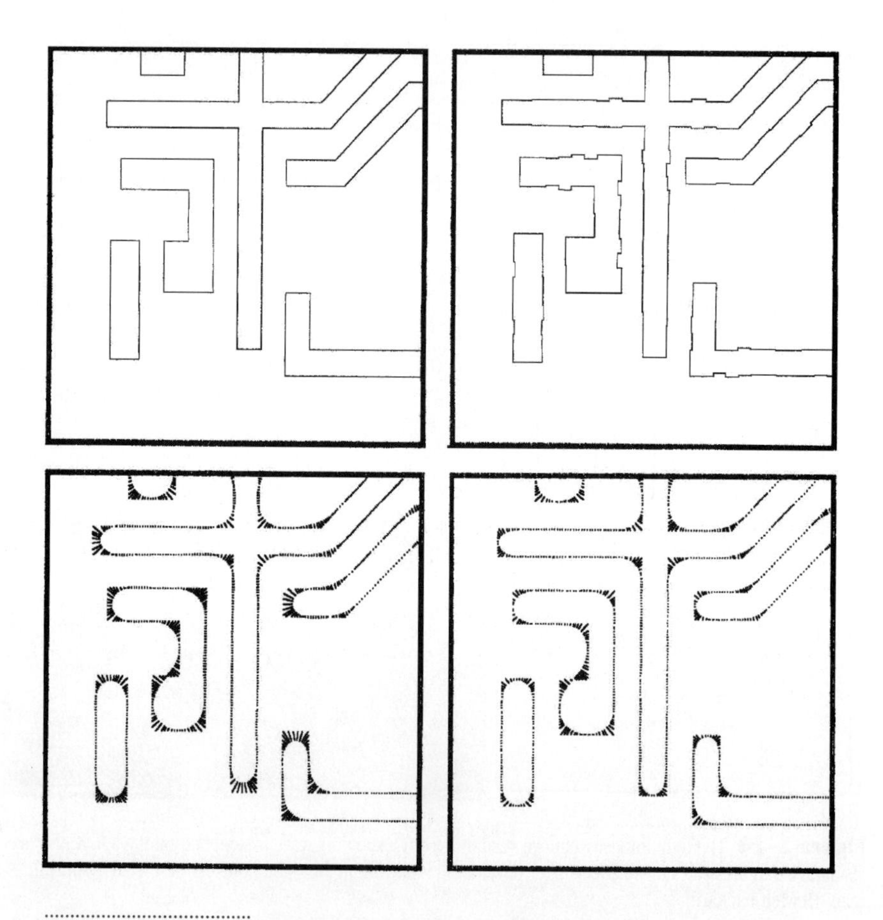

Figure 5–25 Mask patterns with (right) and without (left) OPC are shown on the top. The corresponding aerial images (calculated) are shown on the bottom. Note the improvement in the quality of the aerial image when OPC is used. The dark lines in the bottom patterns indicate the difference between the mask and aerial image in each case [5.13]. Reprinted with permission of SPIE.

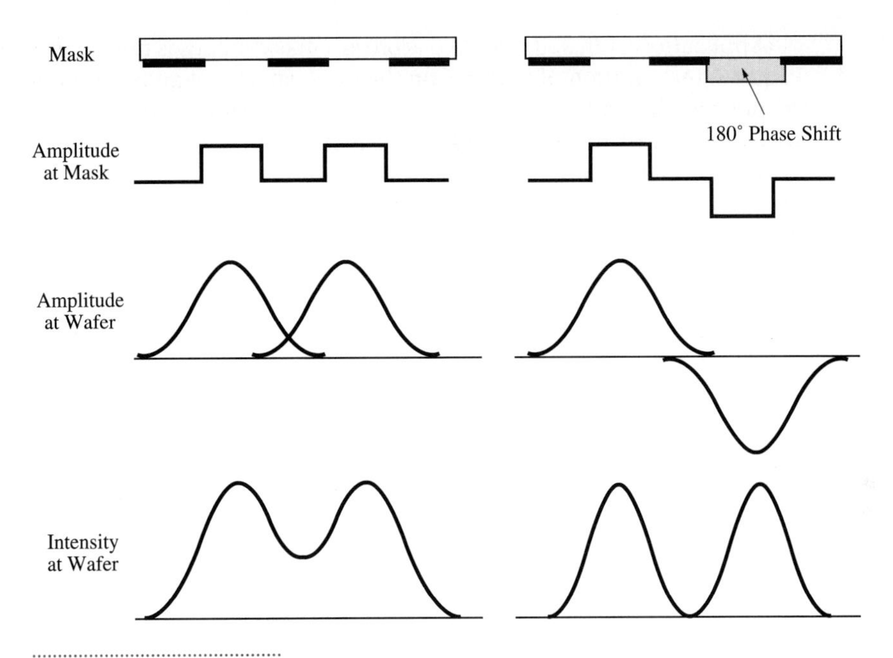

Figure 5–26 Example of the use of phase shifting techniques on masks to improve the resolution of the aerial image. (After Levenson et al. [5.32].)

ial image [5.14]. A simple example of the principle is illustrated in Figure 5–26. In this example a periodic mask with equal lines and spaces (diffraction grating) is used as the mask. The left side shows the electric field, ε, associated with the light just after it passes through the mask and also at the wafer (far field diffraction pattern), without any phase shifting in the mask. The period of the grating is chosen in this case so that the lines on the mask are barely resolved on the wafer. The photoresist responds to the intensity of the light or $(\varepsilon \text{ field})^2$ and hence the intensity pattern on the bottom left is barely sufficient to resolve the two lines.

In the example on the right, a material whose thickness and index of refraction are chosen to phase shift the light by exactly 180° is added to the mask. The thickness of this layer is given by

$$d = \frac{\lambda}{2(n-1)} \tag{5.16}$$

where n is the index of refraction of the phase shift material. The period of this added pattern is half the period of the original grating. The corresponding ε fields at the mask and wafer are also shown. Since the light intensity at the aerial image is the square of the ε field intensity, the quality of the resulting aerial image is significantly improved as illustrated. Such phase shifting techniques can either be used to improve the quality of the aerial image or to improve the depth of focus of the exposure system at a constant resolution by using a lower NA system.

Application of this principle to arbitrary mask shapes is quite complex and generally requires the addition of features on the mask smaller than the minimum feature size to be printed. Simulation tools provide a very powerful approach to exploring the benefits of phase shifting masks and they can also help in the optimum design of mask patterns. We will look at an example later in Section 5.5.

One final point with respect to masks is worth making. We have assumed in our discussion that a simple digital mask (without OPC or phase shifting) is an exact replica of the desired pattern designed in the CAD system. As geometries get smaller, this is less true because the mask making systems themselves have resolution limits. Even at 4X or 5X compared to the patterns on wafers, the mask patterns may have rounded corners or other "imperfections" that degrade the quality of the aerial image produced on the wafer.

5.3 Manufacturing Methods and Equipment

The lithography process dominates the cost and the throughput of modern IC manufacturing. Since the SIA NTRS is driven by constant reductions in linewidth, lithography is expected to remain in this key position in the future. In this section we will examine typical industrial processes and equipment for lithography. While contact and proximity printers played a major role in the early days of the silicon industry, they no longer do so because of unacceptable defect levels and/or limited resolution. As a result, we will restrict our discussion in this section to projection aligners. Also, since DNQ positive resists and DUV resists for 248-nm systems dominate industrial use today, we will restrict our discussion to these materials.

5.3.1 Wafer Exposure Systems

Projection aligners have been the dominant exposure tools in the silicon industry for more than 20 years. Perkin-Elmer Corp. pioneered the earliest systems of this type under the name Micralign. These systems were scanning projection aligners, which used 1:1 masks. The principle behind such scanning systems is illustrated in Figure 5–27. The basic idea in these systems is that it is easier to correct optics for aberrations in a small area rather than a large area. Thus the illumination source produces a slit of light which is mechanically scanned across the mask. The wafer is simultaneously scanned so that the mask pattern is printed across the wafer. The system that is illustrated in Figure 5–27 is a purely reflective system, using mirrors. Systems of this general type are also used which have a combination of mirrors and lenses (both reflecting and refracting optics). Such optical systems are known as catadioptic optical systems.

While scanning systems of the type illustrated in Figure 5–27 are very cost effective and have high throughput, they require 1X masks that contain the pattern information for all the chips to be printed on each wafer. Linewidth control on such masks becomes more difficult as geometries shrink. Also, as chips became more complex and as wafers became larger in the late 1970s, it became increasingly difficult to produce perfect full

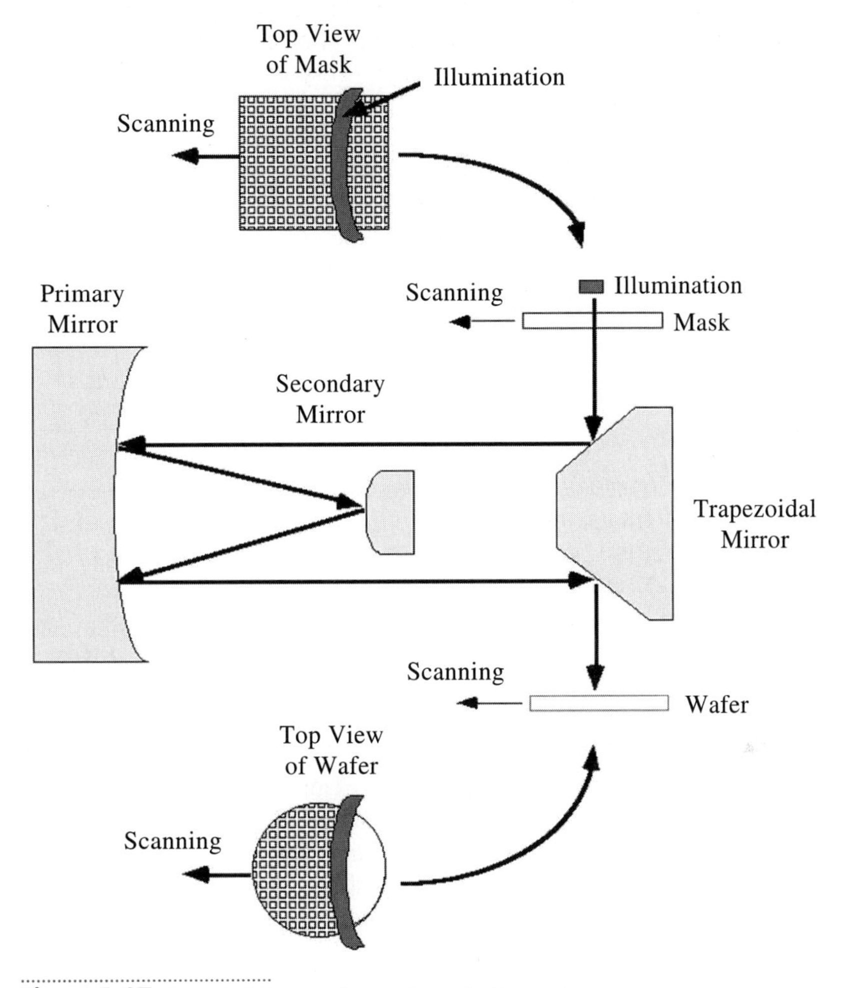

Figure 5–27 Conceptual diagram of a scanning projection printer.

wafer masks and to make optical systems which could scan entire wafers with the required resolution. Scanning systems also generally only allow global alignment of the mask and the wafer patterns, that is, alignment at the wafer level before the scanning begins. With tighter dimensions and the corresponding need for better placement accuracy, local alignment on a die by die or similar scale is often highly desirable. The solution to these issues was to replace the scanning systems with steppers that exposed a limited portion of the wafer (typically a few cm^2) at a time. This eliminates wafer size as a major issue. The mask problem is also addressed in these systems by making the steppers reduce the image by 4X or 5X. Thus the masks use much larger dimensions which makes them more easily repairable and they contain only a few die rather than a full wafer pattern. Steppers also allow alignment on an exposure field by exposure field ba-

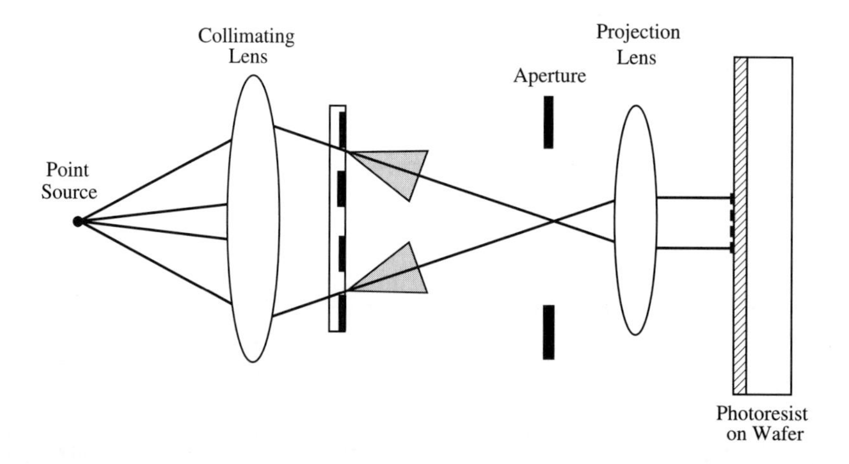

Figure 5–28 Kohler illumination system. The triangles emanating from the mask regions represent the diffracted light pattern.

sis and hence improve overlay accuracy compared to full wafer scanners. (This capability is often not used in manufacturing, however, because of throughput issues.) Such step and repeat projection aligners have dominated the industry for the past decade. Most often, these systems use purely refractive optical systems. In concept they are very much like the system shown in Figure 5–3.

While we described the basic features and performance of these projection steppers earlier in this chapter, there are several key additional ideas that are used in practice to improve the performance of these systems. These include the use of Kohler illumination and off-axis illumination, which we will briefly describe here.

Figure 5–28 illustrates the idea behind a Kohler illumination source. The light passing through the mask is focused at the entrance pupil of the projection lens, rather than having collimated light pass through the mask as illustrated conceptually in Figure 5–3. The reason for using a Kohler source arrangement is so that the projection lens can capture the diffracted light from any of the features on the mask equally well. This is illustrated in Figure 5–28 by the triangles emanating from the mask apertures that represent the angular spread of the diffracted light. If collimated light were used though the mask, it is apparent that much of the diffracted light would be lost from mask features near the outside edge of the mask.

The second "trick" which is often used in modern projection aligners is off-axis illumination. The idea behind this technique can be understood in connection with Figure 5–29. If the light from a coherent source is incident at an angle to the mask, rather than normal to the mask, this illumination is called off-axis illumination. Such illumination obviously changes the angle of the light passing through the mask and changes the angle of the diffracted light as well. While some of the diffracted light will be lost through the use of off-axis illumination because it will be outside the projection lens aperture, some of the higher-order diffracted light which would be lost through nor-

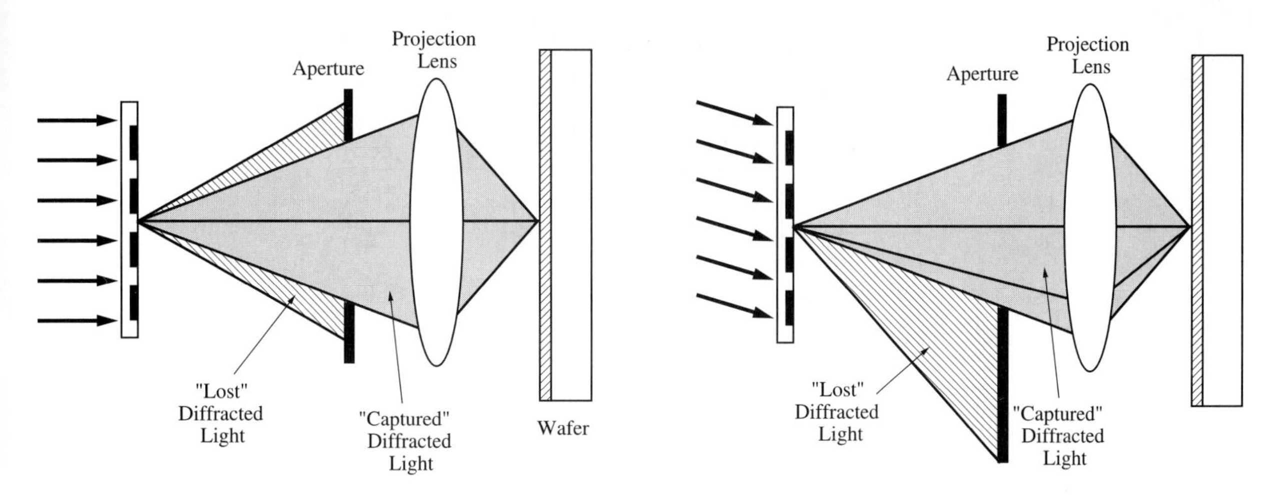

Figure 5–29 Illustration of the idea of on-axis illumination (left) and off-axis illumination (right). The shaded areas emanating from the mask regions represent the diffracted light pattern. Practical implementations generally use a light source producing several angles of incident light (+ and −). Some of the higher order diffracted information is captured in the off-axis scheme.

mally incident radiation will also be captured in the off-axis system. The net result is that the resolution can be somewhat improved. The basic idea is similar to the arguments presented earlier for using partially coherent illumination rather than coherent illumination. It is apparent then, that considerable attention must be paid to the illumination part of the optical system as performance in projection aligners is pushed toward physical limits.

Within the past few years, it has become increasingly difficult to build steppers that have the resolution required by the SIA NTRS and also the field of view required by this roadmap. Because of this, a hybrid type of system which uses both stepping and scanning has recently come into use. Figure 5–30 illustrates the principle. Stepping is used to move the wafer between major exposure fields. Within each exposure field, the mask pattern is scanned across the wafer. This type of system has some of the advantages of scanners (the optical system needs to be "perfect" in a smaller area). It also has some of the advantages of the stepper systems (4X or 5X reduction can be used to simplify mask fabrication, and the total field printed at each exposure is much smaller than the wafer, eliminating wafer size as a major issue and simplifying lens design). However, the mechanical system does need to scan the mask 4X or 5X times faster than the wafer and keep them synchronized. These hybrid systems also allow local alignment of the mask pattern with the wafer at each exposure field, which is one of the inherent advantages of stepper systems. At the same time, however, these systems are very complex and very expensive because they have some of the disadvantages of each type of system (the synchronized mechanical motion of scanners, and the costly refractive lens design of steppers). Nevertheless, it is likely that these hybrid systems will find widespread use through the next several technology generations.

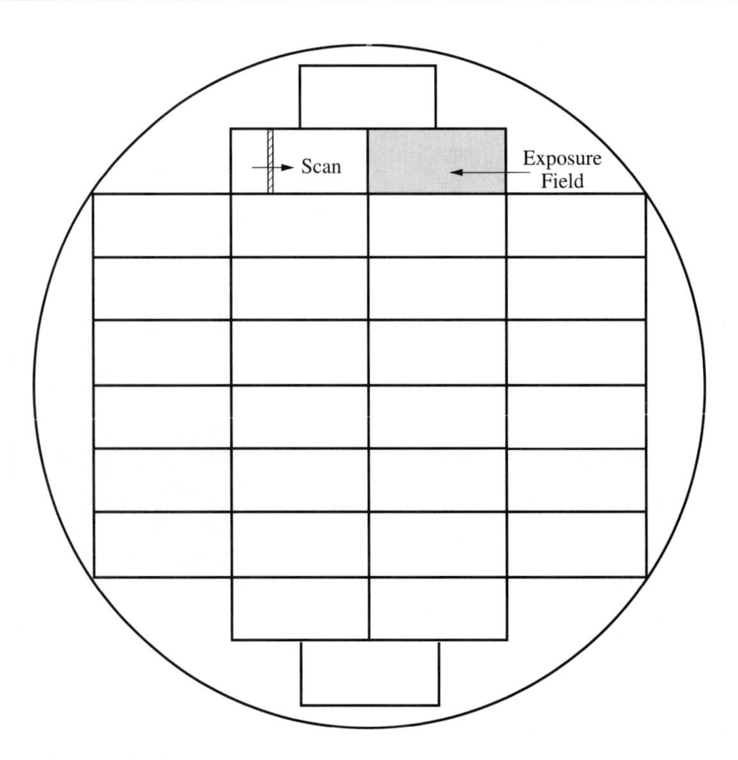

Figure 5–30 Step and scan system. Stepping accomplishes the major moves from one exposure field to another. Within each exposure field, the mask pattern is scanned across the field.

5.3.2 Photoresists

The actual details associated with photoresist exposure and processing are, not surprisingly, considerably more complicated than the qualitative description given earlier might indicate. The additional details that we will consider here are generally designed to make the whole process more manufacturable. Figure 5–31 illustrates a typical process flow associated with photolithography. The specific numbers refer to typical conditions for DNQ g-line or i-line resists. DUV resists generally utilize a similar process flow with some changes in the process details.

The first step in the lithography process is ensuring that the resist will adhere well to the wafer. Depending on the stage in the process flow, this may involve one or more operations. Normally the wafer is clean just before resist application since resist is commonly deposited on wafers just after thin film deposition or just after some other high-temperature process step. If this is not the case, the wafer may need to be chemically cleaned, using the procedures described in Chapter 4. It may also be necessary to heat the wafer to several hundred °C to drive off any water vapor on the surface. These steps are represented by the first box in Figure 5–31.

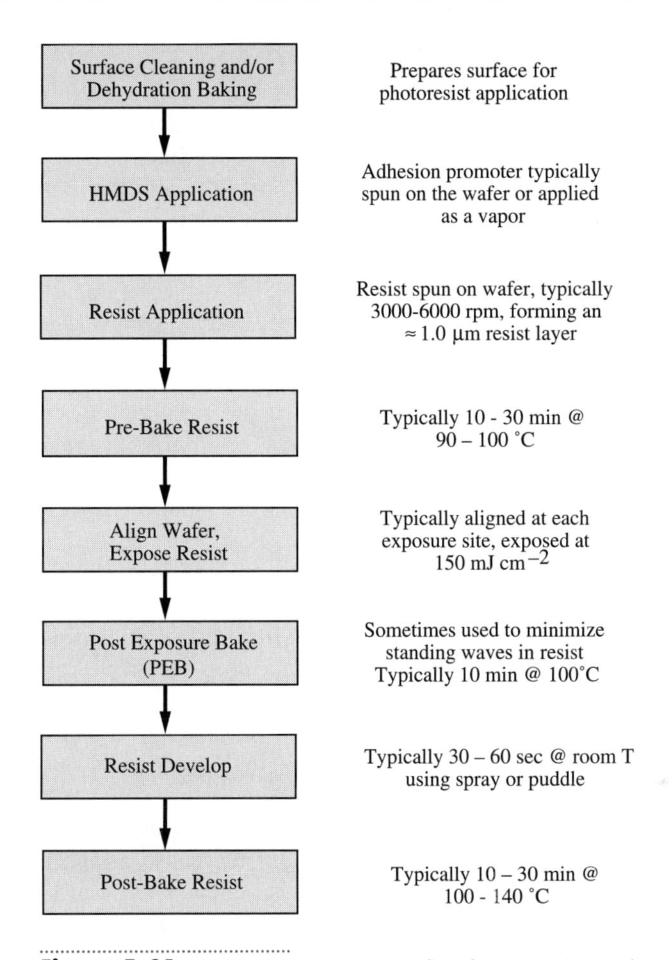

Figure 5–31 Typical photoresist process flow for DNQ g-line and i-line positive resists.

Even with a clean, dry surface, adhesion of resists to silicon ICs may not be as good as desired and so it is common practice to use an adhesion promoter. Hexamethyldisilane (HMDS) is the most common substance used for this purpose. HMDS can be applied to the wafer in liquid form at room temperature by spinning under conditions similar to resist spinning (3000 – 6000 RPM for $\approx$ 30 sec). However, in most cases it is applied in vapor form with the HMDS being introduced as a vapor into a chamber containing the wafers since this more easily produces the desired single monolayer on the wafers. In either case, one end of the HMDS molecule bonds readily with SiO_2 surfaces and the other bonds with the resist. Thus the HMDS acts an adhesion promoter. For surfaces other than SiO_2, other adhesion treatments may be used in addition to or instead of HMDS (Chapter 6 of [5.4]).

The next step is spinning the resist itself onto the wafer and this should normally be done immediately after the HMDS application. The resist is dispensed onto the wafer and then the wafer is spun (3000 – 6000 RPM for ≈ 30 sec) to produce a thin (≈ 0.6 – 1-μm) uniform layer. If the resist is going to be used to mask an implant, it may be thicker than these values. While the procedure sounds simple, there are some subtleties associated with it. The dispensing of the resist can be done while the wafer is stationary or while it is spinning at slow speed to produce a uniform liquid layer on the wafer. The acceleration of the wafer to its final spin speed is also important and is typically done rapidly (in a fraction of a second). The solvent in the resist begins to evaporate rapidly after the resist is dispensed and while it is being accelerated. Generally more uniform films are obtained if the acceleration is as rapid as possible. During the first few seconds the wafer spends at high spin rates, the film levels to a uniform thickness. During the remainder of the ≈ 30-sec spin, the solvent continues to evaporate to produce the final resist thickness. The fluid dynamics of the spin coating process have been studied in some detail [5.4], but the exact process for a particular resist is usually determined experimentally. The viscosity of the resist in its liquid state (solvent content) and the spin speed are the primary factors affecting the final resist thickness. The spinning process produces an "edge bead," that is, a thicker resist at the very edge of the wafer, which generally needs to be removed before proceeding further.

The next step in the lithography process is the prebake. This is normally accomplished on a hot plate at 90 – 100°C. Infrared or microwave heating can also be used, which are faster processes. The prebake step accomplishes several things. First, the remaining solvent in the resist is largely evaporated, reduced from ≈ 25% to ≈ 5% of the resist content. Second, adhesion of the resist is improved since the heating strengthens the bonds between the resist and the HMDS and substrate. Finally, stresses present in the resist as a result of the spinning process are relieved through thermal relaxation. Chemical changes do take place in the resist during this high temperature bake with the result that required exposure times are increased as the bake temperature increases. The mechanism responsible for this is believed to be a decomposition of the *PAC* at high temperature with the result that the resist sensitivity is degraded. We will discuss these effects more quantitatively in Section 5.5.

The exposure process creates a latent image in the resist that can be developed later. Most resists exhibit reciprocity, which means that light intensity and exposure time can be directly traded off with each other. Thus increases in the exposure system aerial intensity directly reduce exposure times. The required exposure time is also affected by the prebake thermal cycle as was just discussed and by the thickness of the resist. All of these parameters must therefore be carefully controlled. Exposure doses are normally designed to be well above Q_f (Figure 5–20) since this produces latent images in the resist that have the sharpest edges (limited of course by the quality of the aerial image). For typical DNQ resists, this corresponds to a dose > 100 mJ cm^{-2}. For DUV resists, which use chemical amplification, the dose is typically 20 – 40 mJ cm^{-2}. Detailed models of the exposure process have been developed, including the effects of the quality of the aerial image, standing waves in the resist, and so forth. We will consider these in Section 5.5.

The next step illustrated in Figure 5–31 is a Postexposure Bake (PEB). In g-line and i-line resists, this step is sometimes performed before development of the resist latent image, in order to minimize standing wave effects in the resist. The mechanism is straightforward. At elevated temperatures, the *PAC* in these resists can diffuse. If the temperature and time are well controlled in this bake, the *PAC* molecules can diffuse far enough to "smear out" the standing wave effects along the edge of the resist features, but not diffuse far enough to significantly distort the image features themselves. A typical bake cycle might be $\approx$ 10 min at 100°C. If antireflective coatings are used under the resist, this postexposure bake may not be necessary because the standing wave problem is less severe.

In DUV resists, the PEB is a necessary and critical step in the process. This is the step in which the *PAG* reacts with the polymer chain to complete the exposure process. The time and especially the temperature must be very tightly controlled because chemical reaction rates and diffusion typically depend exponentially on temperature.

DNQ resists are developed in basic solutions (normally TMAH—tetramethyl ammonium hydroxide—solutions diluted with H_2O, but NaOH or KOH solutions can also be used). The developer can be applied in a number of ways. The wafers may be immersed in the developer, the developer may be sprayed on a batch of wafers or on a single wafer at a time, or a puddle of the developer may be placed on the wafer. In each case, rinsing the wafers with H_2O stops the developing process. The rate at which developing proceeds is highly dependent on temperature, on developer concentration, and on all the exposure and bake procedures used before developing. In DNQ resists, the developing proceeds by dissolving the carboxylic acid that results from the exposed *PAC* in the alkaline solution. The rate of developing is dependent on the local carboxylic acid concentration, which is proportional to the local exposure intensity in the resist. In positive working DUV resists, developing takes place in a similar fashion since the unblocked polymer chains are soluble in the basic developer. We will consider detailed models in Section 5.5.

The final step in the photolithography process is the postbake. This step is done at higher temperature than the earlier bakes (typically 10 – 30 min at 100 – 140°C), and is designed to harden the resist and improve its etch resistance. This bake process causes the resist to flow slightly and hence may also modify edge profiles. Any remaining solvents in the resist are driven off by this bake and the adhesion of the resist to the underlying substrate is also improved. In some cases when the resist must withstand a particularly harsh etching process or a high current ion implantation which may raise its temperature considerably, a further hardening and crosslinking of the resist with a blanket deep UV exposure at elevated temperatures can improve the robustness of the resist layer.

In modern lithography processes, many of the steps we have described above are accomplished in a single integrated machine known as a wafer track system. These machines cost $>$ $1 million and are usually tightly integrated with the exposure tool so that easy wafer transfer can occur between the two systems.

5.4 Measurement Methods

Measurement issues associated with lithography can be divided into several areas. The first is the mask itself. Here we need to know the dimensions of the features on the mask and to verify that they correspond to the intended design. It is generally also important to ensure that there are no defects on the mask which are large enough to print on the wafer during the exposure process.

As we have seen in our earlier discussion, it is convenient to divide the exposure process into the optical system that produces the aerial image, and the resist processing which transfers the aerial image into a resist profile. The aerial image itself is not normally directly measurable, so that measurement issues associated with lithography normally focus on the resist pattern after it is developed. This is the second major area where measurement methods are needed. In many process steps, of course, the resist pattern is transferred into underlying thin films or into the silicon substrate itself by etching and in these cases, there is also a need to measure the etched pattern.

The final issue associated with the lithographic process is alignment of patterns with respect to underlying features on the wafer (earlier mask layers). As we saw earlier in this chapter, generally layers must be aligned with a tolerance on the order of one-fifth to one-third of the minimum feature size. We will discuss a number of these issues in this section. An excellent reference on many of these topics is [5.15].

5.4.1 Measurement of Mask Features and Defects

Virtually all exposure systems used today in high-volume manufacturing are reducing steppers or reducing step and scan projection systems. This means that the mask contains the features for only a few die and this pattern is exposed multiple times on each wafer. If there is a defect on such a mask, it will affect a large fraction of all chips on every wafer the mask is used to print. This would result in intolerable yield loses and so it is absolutely crucial that the mask be "perfect." What this really means is that there are no printable defects on the mask. Since the mask has 4X to 5X larger feature sizes than the wafer patterns, mask defects below some critical size will not print on the wafer. Nevertheless, the two issues with respect to the mask are the following: Does the mask pattern correspond to the design for that mask level? And are there any defects large enough to print on the wafer?

While mask inspection was accomplished many years ago simply by using a microscope, such an approach is unworkable today because of the complexity of today's chips. As a result, highly automated systems have been developed to accomplish this inspection. The principle of operation is illustrated in Figure 5–32. Light is passed through the mask and collected by an imaging system. Generally a solid-state image sensor is used to detect the pattern of the transmitted light. This information can be compared either with the design database used to generate the mask, or with a second identical mask pattern, if the mask contains the patterns for more than one chip. Scanning the inspection system over the mask thus provides full information on defects due either to errors in transmitting data from the database or due to random defects on the mask. If the mask incorporates Optical Proximity Correction (OPC) or advanced techniques like phase shifting, the inspection process is often more difficult because these techniques introduce structures on the mask that may be smaller than the minimum feature size and therefore might be interpreted as "defects" by the inspection system.

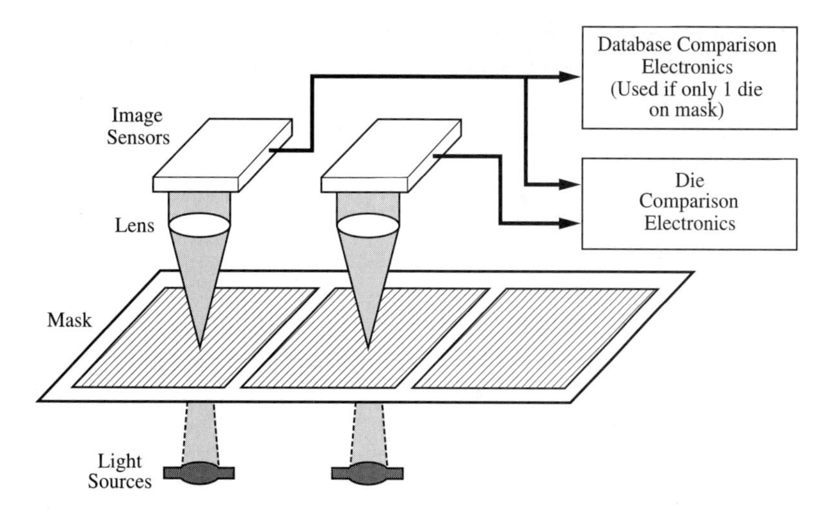

Figure 5–32 Mask inspection system. Such systems operate by comparing the feature information on the mask either with the original design database or with an identical feature on an adjacent mask site. In this example three identical die are shown on the mask.

If defects are detected by this approach, they can often be corrected. Opaque defects, in which chrome is present on the mask in areas where it should not be, can be corrected with lasers or ion beams which are focused on the defect area and which evaporate the excess chrome. Clear defects, in which chrome is not present where it should be, are often more difficult to correct because they require a deposition of an opaque material to cover the clear area. Laser-assisted deposition from a chromium bearing gas which is introduced above the mask can be used, as can ion beam deposition.

The final crucial issue with respect to the mask is the actual size of the features on the mask. There are a number of issues associated with e-beam mask making that can lead to disparities in feature size between the design database and the mask. The spot size of the e-beam is finite (usually 0.125 to 0.5 μm) and this can be important in writing very small features. Also, when small features are being written, "proximity effects" can be an issue when such features are closely spaced. Proximity effects arise from electron backscattering in the resist on the mask and can result in pattern distortion.

Many masks today are made with laser-based systems instead of e-beam systems because the laser-based systems are less expensive. However, laser-based systems have the same kinds of resolution limits as do the steppers used in projecting images onto the wafer. Thus the features printed on the mask itself can suffer from rounded corners and other diffraction effects just as is the case in aerial images projected onto the wafer.

The feature sizes on the mask can be measured with a system very similar to that shown in Figure 5–32. Alternatively, a video camera and microscope can be used on the top side of the mask. In either case, edge detection techniques are used on the signal that is received to determine the feature dimension. This is a relatively straightforward procedure on masks because the thin chrome layer on masks provides a high contrast image with good edge definition. In addition, the linewidths are 4X to 5X larger than the final wafer feature sizes, so optical methods generally work well for mask features. The National Bureau of Standards has linewidth standards available that can be used as references in accurately measuring the feature dimensions on masks. Linewidth measurement is not as simple when the feature is on the wafer and resist or other thin film structures are being measured, as we will see in the next section.

5.4.2 Measurement of Resist Patterns

Once the exposed resist is developed, the structure is really three dimensional, as was graphically illustrated in Figure 5–24. The resist edges may be sloped and they may contain standing wave patterns. The definition and the measurement of the "linewidth" in the resist is thus not straightforward. When linewidths in chips were larger than about 1 μm, optical methods using a microscope and edge detection were commonly used to measure resist feature sizes. However these methods are not extendible to the small features on today's chips and as a result, SEM measurements have largely replaced optical methods for accurate linewidth measurements.

We discussed the basic operation of electron microscopes in Chapters 3 and 4 (Sections 3.4 and 4.4). SEM methods have the potential for very high resolution. The electron wavelength is < 1 nm at typical accelerating voltages, so diffraction effects are negligible. SEMs designed for inspection and metrology applications usually have to operate nondestructively because the wafers that are used for the inspections are product wafers. Thus ideally the SEM operates in an in-line fashion as part of the manufacturing line. Such tools are widely available today. They generally operate with a small beam size (≈ 10 nm) and at fairly low voltage (a few keV) to minimize damage to the wafer structures, to minimize charging problems, and to allow imaging of the resist surface. They generally are designed to handle full 6″ or 8″ wafers. Low-voltage operation also minimizes the depth to which the electrons penctrate in the resist or other thin films and thus confines the interactions of the electrons to the near surface region. This improves the ability of the SEM to image surface features and topography.

Figure 5–33 shows examples of SEM images of a resist pattern after development. The resolution capability of the technique is apparent, but these photos and Figure 5–24 also illustrate some of the difficulties in "measuring" linewidths in such structures. The possibility of sloped edges, standing wave patterns, and variations in the linewidth along photoresist lines all create difficulties in defining exactly what is meant by the linewidth. Generally, the linewidth is defined as the width of the photoresist material at a specific height above the resist-substrate interface. Often sophisticated algorithms are used to translate an SEM line scan into a "number" representing the linewidth.

5.4.3 Measurement of Etched Features

Photoresist patterns are often transferred into underlying thin films by etching, a process described in detail in Chapter 10. The quality of this pattern transfer process is obviously just as important as the quality of the photoresist pattern itself. The same

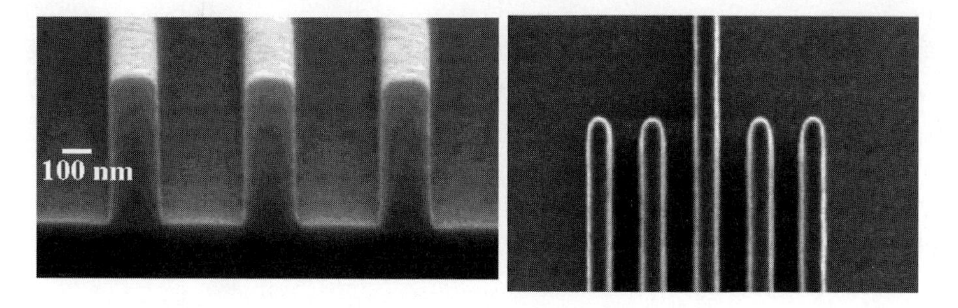

Figure 5–33 Cross section (left) and top (right) view SEM images of developed photoresist features showing well-developed lines with sub 0.25-μm lines and spaces. Courtesy of A. Vladar and P. Rissman, Hewlett Packard.

linewidth measuring methods, primarily based on SEMs, are used to measure the etched patterns in oxide, polysilicon, Al, or other materials.

Unlike the photoresist patterns, which are removed from the wafer after they are used, the etched thin film patterns remain as part of the final chip. Because of this, it is possible in many cases to make measurements on these thin film layers after wafer processing is complete. In addition to SEM methods, it is often convenient to make such measurements electrically during wafer testing. A significant amount of work has been done in recent years to develop electrical test structures which measure parameters like linewidth and alignment accuracy, in addition to the more usual device electrical parameters [5.15 – 5.19]. Complete test chips have been developed which provide detailed information about the process. These chips are very useful during the development stages of new processes. Specific test structures are also sometimes incorporated onto product chips once a process is in manufacturing in order to provide ongoing information about manufacturing tolerances. Usually these test structures are placed in the scribe lines between chips so they do not consume chip area.

Figure 5–34 illustrates the basic idea behind many of these test structures. The overall structure is assumed to be a conducting material (polysilicon, silicide, aluminum, etc.). The right-hand part of this structure (pads 3–6) is a van der Pauw structure designed to extract the sheet resistance of the material making up the test structure. The geometry is chosen to define one square of the material (labeled with the ρ_s symbol in the figure). If a current I_{5-6} is forced between terminals 5 and 6, and the voltage V_{3-4} is measured between terminals 3 and 4, then the sheet resistance is given simply by [see Eq. (3.10) in Chapter 3].

$$\rho_S = \frac{\pi}{\ln(2)} \frac{V_{3-4}}{I_{5-6}} \tag{5.17}$$

Once the sheet resistance is measured, then the linewidth W can be extracted from the rest of the structure through an additional electrical measurement. In this case, a current I_{1-5} is forced between terminals 1 and 5, and a voltage V_{2-3} is measured between terminals 2 and 3. The linewidth W is then given by

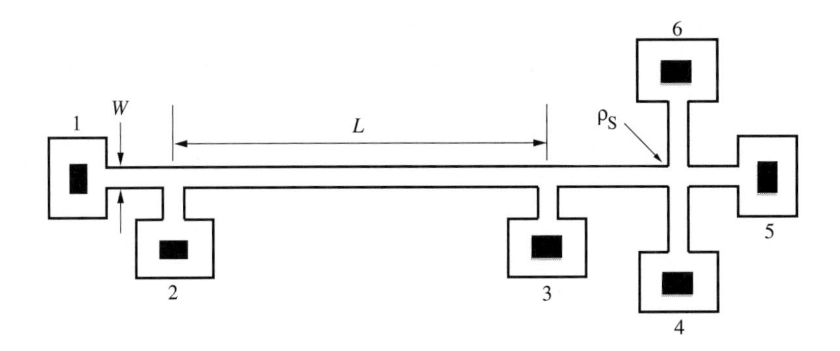

Figure 5–34 Test structure designed to electrically extract sheet resistance and linewidth *W*.

$$W = \rho_S L \frac{I_{1-5}}{V_{2-3}} \tag{5.18}$$

It should be noted that the linewidth extracted from test structures such as this may be different than the linewidth measured optically or with an SEM. This is because the electrical linewidth really measures the effective cross sectional area through which current flows in the material. If the edges of the material are sloped, or if the surfaces affect the conductivity, the electrical width may be slightly different than the physical width extracted from an image of the line.

Finally, modifications to the basic test structure shown in Figure 5–34 can allow similar structures to extract information about alignment between levels on a chip. In this case, parts of the structure are fabricated in different levels of the circuit and measurements of resistances in the completed test structure provide the alignment information [5.17, 5.18].

5.5 Models and Simulation

Lithography simulation relies on two principal areas of science. The first of these is optics, which provides a mathematical description of the behavior of light in the exposure systems used in modern lithographic tools. The second is chemistry which provides the tools to treat exposure, baking, and developing of the resists that are used to convert the aerial image created by the exposure system into a three-dimensional replica of the mask patterns. Many of the basic ideas and models that optics provides about light propagation and diffraction effects have their origins in work done more than 100 years ago by Maxwell, Kirchoff, and others. And of course the basic ideas from chemistry regarding the rates of chemical reactions, catalysts, and the like are equally old ideas.

Applying these concepts to lithography, however, is a relatively recent venture, dating back only to the mid 1970s. The pioneering work in this area began at IBM and resulted in a series of widely referenced papers written by Dill and his co-workers [5.20

– 5.23]. Following that work, a number of other groups began work on lithography simulation [5.24, 5.25]. Within the past 10 years, a number of simulation tools for optical lithography have become commercially available. Representative examples include PROLITH (Finle Technologies) [5.3], DEPICT (Avant!) [5.26], and ATHENA (Silvaco) [5.27]. The basic models used in each of these simulation tools are similar. In the following sections we will describe these models in a general way and show specific examples of the use of these simulators in optical lithography. As we did earlier in this chapter, we will divide the discussion into the formation of the aerial image (exposure system) and the resist processing.

5.5.1 Wafer Exposure Systems

Since projection exposure systems dominate industrial practice today, most of the simulation tools that are currently available apply to these kinds of systems. They thus model far field or Fraunhofer diffraction. Some simulators do have the ability to simulate contact or proximity printing (PROLITH, for example), but because these systems are not used for VLSI manufacturing, we will not consider near field (Fresnel diffraction) simulation tools in this book. The interested reader is referred to [5.25] for issues related to simulation of proximity or contact lithography simulation.

For the purposes of this discussion, we will consider a generic projection lithography system as illustrated in Figure 5–35. Mathematically modeling such a system requires a mathematical description of how light behaves. We begin with a basic description of light waves and their propagation.

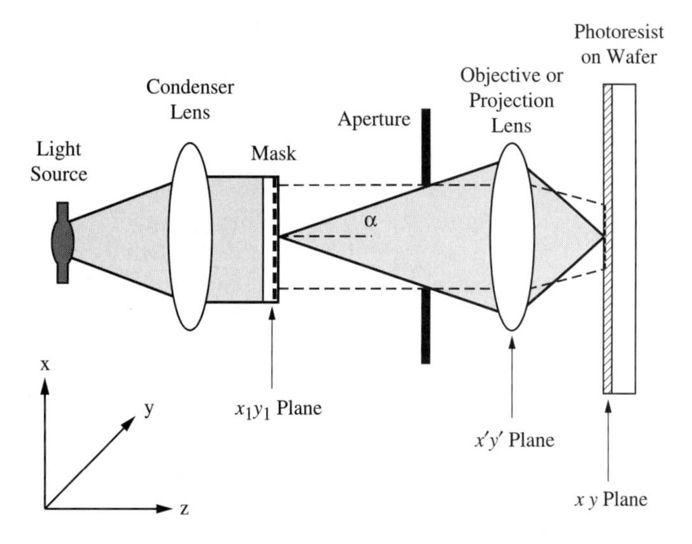

Figure 5–35 Generic projection lithography system. The shaded area to the right of the mask illustrates the portion of the diffraction pattern that is collected by the projection lens and used to form the aerial image of the mask feature.

Light travels as an electromagnetic wave. The electric and magnetic fields are perpendicular to each other and both are perpendicular to the direction of wave propagation. However, the materials that photons interact with in lithography are generally nonmagnetic, so we can treat the light waves in such systems simply in terms of a traveling electric field ε. Thus a general description of a propagating monochromatic light wave at a point W in space is simply

$$\varepsilon(W,t) = C(W)\cos(\omega t + \phi(t)) \tag{5.19}$$

where C is the amplitude, ω is the frequency and ϕ is the phase. We can also write this in the form of a complex exponential function.

$$\varepsilon(W,t) = Re\{U(W)e^{-j\omega t}\} \text{ where } U(W) = C(W)e^{-j\phi(W)} \tag{5.20}$$

The generic projection lithography system in Figure 5–35 consists of several components, each of which we have discussed in earlier sections of this chapter. The light source and condenser lens form the illumination system which needs to deliver light to the mask with the specified intensity, uniformity, spectral characteristics, and spatial coherency. Once the light passes through the mask, diffraction effects come into play. The objective or projection lens is required to collect as much of the diffracted light as possible and focus it onto the resist layer on the wafer. Generally demagnification also takes place through the objective lens.

We will consider the mask to be transparent in some areas and completely opaque in others. For the chrome masks that are typically used today, this is a very good approximation since the mask contrast is very high. Thus in the x_1y_1 plane, we can represent the transmission of the mask with a simple digital function.

$$t(x_1,y_1) = \begin{Bmatrix} 1 \text{ in clear areas} \\ 0 \text{ in opaque areas} \end{Bmatrix} \tag{5.21}$$

where $t(x_1,y_1)$ is the mask transmittance. If more advanced mask techniques such as phase shifting are used, then $t(x_1,y_1)$ will vary both in magnitude and phase and will obviously be more complex than a simple digital function. We will consider such an example later. After the mask diffracts the light, it is described by the Fraunhofer diffraction integral in the far field region. Thus at the entrance to the objective lens, the electric field intensity pattern of the light is given by [5.2, 5.3]

$$\varepsilon(x',y') = \int_{-\infty}^{+\infty}\int_{-\infty}^{+\infty} t(x_1,y_1)e^{-2\pi j(f_x x + f_y y)}dxdy \tag{5.22}$$

In this expression, the terms f_x and f_y are known as the spatial frequencies of the diffraction pattern and are defined as

$$f_x = \frac{x'}{z\lambda} \text{ and } f_y = \frac{y'}{z\lambda} \tag{5.23}$$

where z is the distance from the mask to the lens. Eq. (5.22) is simply the Fourier transform of the mask pattern. The light intensity pattern entering the objective lens can thus be calculated using well-known methods from the field of Fourier optics. In the shorthand of the Fourier transform, we can rewrite Eq. (5.22) as

$$\varepsilon(f_x, f_y) = F\{t(x_1, y_1)\} \tag{5.24}$$

where F represents the Fourier transform. f_x and f_y are simply scaled spatial coordinates in the x', y' plane. The intensity distribution of the light is the square of the magnitude of the electric field, so that

$$I(f_x, f_y) = |\varepsilon(f_x, f_y)|^2 = |F\{t(x_1, y_1)\}|^2 \tag{5.25}$$

Example Consider a mask pattern, which is simply a long rectangular slit of width $w/2$ (Figure 5–36). Find the resulting optical intensity pattern in the far field (Fraunhofer) region.

Answer The Fourier transform of the function $t(x)$ is found in standard textbooks [5.2] and is given by

$$\varepsilon(x') = F\{t(x)\} = \frac{\sin(\pi w f_x)}{\pi f_x} \tag{5.26}$$

The resulting optical intensity distribution is the square of this function and is also shown plotted in Figure 5–36. The first zero of the intensity occurs at

$$f_x = \frac{1}{w} \text{ or } x' = \frac{z\lambda}{w} \tag{5.27}$$

Thus the image of the slit spreads out the further away we move from the mask (z increases). The image also spreads out more when longer wavelengths of light are used. Both of these results are to be expected based on our previous discussion of diffraction. Perhaps counterintuitively, the image spreads out more the smaller the slit is (as w decreases). This was discussed in connection with Figure 5–5 earlier.

We now return to our generic lithography system in Figure 5–35. When the diffracted light passes the $x'y'$ plane, it enters the objective lens. Note that only a portion of the diffracted light is captured by the lens because of its finite size. We characterized this through the $NA = \sin\alpha$ in our earlier discussion. The function of the objective lens is to reconstruct the diffraction pattern and to focus it on the wafer. Since the intensity pattern of the light at the $x'y'$ plane is simply the Fourier transform of the mask pattern, the objective lens effectively needs to perform an inverse Fourier transform. This is in

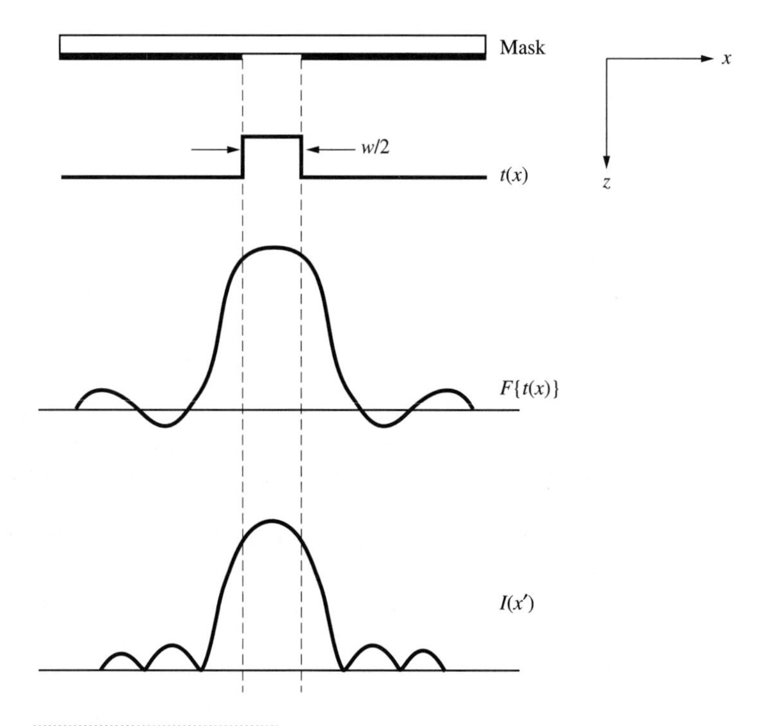

Figure 5–36 Rectangular aperture in a mask and the resulting far field Fraunhofer diffraction pattern and optical intensity pattern.

fact exactly what spherical lenses do. The lens can perform this operation only on the portion of the diffracted light that enters the lens and in this sense we speak of the image that the lens forms as being "diffraction limited."

We can characterize the portion of the diffracted light that the objective lens captures with a "pupil function P" defined as

$$P(f_x, f_y) = \begin{Bmatrix} 1 \text{ if } \sqrt{f_x^2 + f_y^2} < NA/\lambda \\ 0 \text{ if } \sqrt{f_x^2 + f_y^2} > NA/\lambda \end{Bmatrix} \tag{5.28}$$

since for small angles the spatial frequencies f_x and f_y are given by,

$$f_x = \frac{x'}{z\lambda} \cong \frac{\sin\alpha}{\lambda} = \frac{NA}{\lambda} \tag{5.29}$$

P may be limited by the physical size of the objective lens, or by an aperture placed in front of the lens. Either way, the information passing through the objective lens is effectively low pass filtered by the pupil function P. Spatial frequencies higher than NA/λ are simply not passed on to the image on the wafer. The analogy in electric circuits, a sharp pulse passed through a low-pass filter which then ends up with rounded edges, may help to explain the optical degradation in the aerial image caused by P. A sharply defined object on the mask is imaged on the wafer with "smeared" edges, and sharp corners become rounded.

The objective lens now performs the inverse Fourier transform function on the portion of the diffracted light that it captures. Thus at the image plane on the wafer (resist surface), the electric field associated with the light pattern is given by

$$\varepsilon(x,y) = F^{-1}\{\varepsilon(f_x,f_y)P(f_x,f_y)\} = F^{-1}\{F\{t(x_1,y_1)\}P(f_x,f_y)\} \tag{5.30}$$

Finally, the intensity of the light distribution at the resist surface $I_i(x,y)$ is simply given by

$$I_i(x,y) = |\varepsilon(x,y)|^2 \tag{5.31}$$

Eq. (5.31) now represents the aerial image produced by the exposure system. Figure 5–37 summarizes the mathematical models that are used to describe the exposure system.

In real projection lithography systems, there are some additional issues that must be considered in calculating the aerial image. We discussed these issues qualitatively earlier in this chapter, but we now need to quantify them to enable simulation in real systems. The issues which are often important in real imaging systems include off-axis illumination, the use of a partially coherent light source, aberrations in the lens system, depth of focus issues, and the finite thickness of the photoresist, which means that the aerial image must be determined over some volume, not just at the resist surface. We will describe in the following paragraphs the modifications we need to make to Eq. (5.31) in order to deal with these issues.

The first issues are off-axis illumination and partially coherent light sources. In both cases, the light that enters the mask does not have a direction normal to the mask. The result of this (Figure 5–30) is that the position of the diffraction pattern is shifted in the x' y' plane at the entrance to the objective lens. If the light enters the mask at an angle

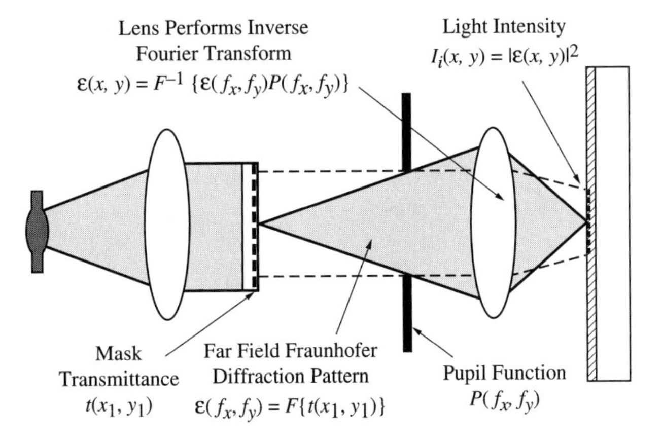

Figure 5–37 Mathematical models used to describe the projection exposure system at each point in space.

θ, then in terms of the spatial frequencies f_x and f_y, the diffraction pattern is shifted by an amount $\sin\theta/\lambda$. The result then is that the electric field associated with the light pattern in the image plane is expressed as [5.3]

$$\varepsilon(x,y,f'_x,f'_y) = F^{-1}\{\varepsilon(f_x - f'_x, f_y - f'_y)P(f_x,f_y)\} \tag{5.32}$$

and

$$I_i(x,y,f'_x,f'_y) = |(x,y,f'_x,f'_y)|^2 \tag{5.33}$$

In the case of a partially coherent source, light enters the mask from a variety of angles. This is usually treated by superposition [5.27]. The source is divided up into individual point sources and the intensities of the light at the image plane due to each point source are added. Expressed mathematically, if $S(f'_x, f'_y)$ is the function describing the source intensity versus position or angle, then [5.3]

$$I_{total}(x,y) = \frac{\iint_{source} I(x,y,f'_x,f'_y)S(f'_x,f'_y)df'_x df'_y}{\iint_{source} S(f'_x,f'_y)df'_x df'_y} \tag{5.34}$$

where I_{total} is the total light flux falling on the resist surface. Eq. (5.34) thus allows the calculation of the aerial image for an arbitrary source illumination.

Aberrations or defects are always present in practical lens systems. They arise from manufacturing tolerances, mechanical changes in a system during use (lenses out of alignment with each other), and from the fact that it is impossible to design a perfect lens which is completely free of aberrations. While such issues could be modeled in a number of ways, the most common method is to treat the wavefront emerging from the lens as having an error in phase or path difference, compared to an ideal aberration free lens. The error in a practical lens will be a function of position along the wavefront and is usually expressed in polar coordinates since lenses are generally circular. The phase error is often expressed as a Zernike polynomial $W(R,\theta)$, which may have many terms [5.3]. $W(R,\theta)$ is the path length difference between an ideal lens and one with aberrations. The effect of these aberrations on the aerial image is included by modifying the pupil function

$$P(f_x,f_y) = P_{ideal}(f_x,f_y)e^{2\pi jW(R,\Theta)} \tag{5.35}$$

Thus if $W(R,\theta)$ is known, the aerial image can be calculated including the effects of lens aberrations.

If the resist is not physically located in the plane of focus of the objective lens, further image degradation will occur. These effects can also be treated as a phase error in the wavefront emerging from the objective lens [5.2, 5.26]. Thus they can be treated mathematically in the same manner as lens aberrations [Eq. (5.35)]. In the defocus case, the path length error can be calculated as illustrated in Figure 5–38. Here we imagine that if the image were properly focused at the resist surface, the light would have originated from an objective lens with a larger radius of curvature (dashed lines) rather than from the actual lens. The Optical Path Difference (*OPD*) is zero at the center of the lens and maximum at the outside radius of the lens. If $R >> \delta$, then

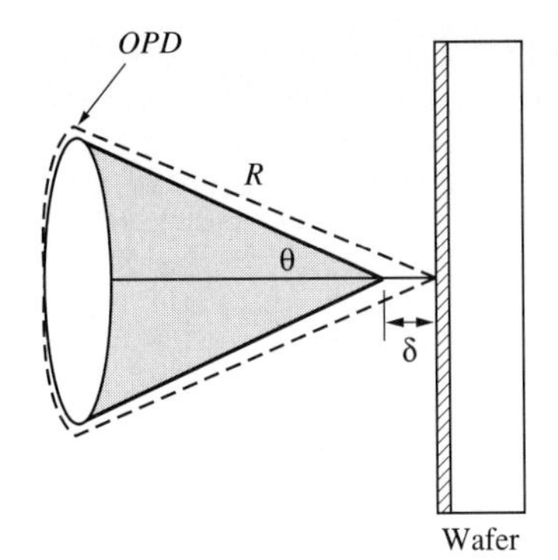

Figure 5–38 Representation of defocusing (δ) as an error in optical path length (optical path difference = *OPD*).

$$OPD \cong \delta(1 - \cos\Theta) \tag{5.36}$$

This expression can then be used in Eq. (5.35) to calculate the effect on the aerial image due to defocusing. Notice that the *OPD* is greatest at the edges of the lens where the higher order diffracted light passes through. This is the light that contains the detailed information about the mask shape, so defocusing will clearly degrade the quality of the aerial image.

There are a number of commercially available simulation tools that implement the models we have just described. Generally the mask is described either as a combination of rectangles or as an arbitrary geometrical structure. In some cases, mask information directly from a design database can be downloaded into the lithography simulation tool. However it is accomplished, a transmittance function $t(x_1, y_1)$ must be specified by the user. The exposure tool is described in terms of its *NA*, the illumination wavelength λ the degree of coherence of the source, any defocusing present, and any aberrations in the lens. The simulation tools then calculate the aerial image using the equations from Fourier optics that we have described. Figures 5–39 to 5–41 show examples of the kinds of simulations that can be done with these tools. Especially as linewidths shrink and lithography tools operate closer to their physical limits, simulators become essential to understand and to predict the details of the aerial images produced during exposure.

5.5.2 Optical Intensity Pattern in the Photoresist

The aerial image calculated above is the optical intensity in the air immediately above the surface of the photoresist. The second step in simulating the performance of lithography tools is to calculate the optical intensity pattern through the photoresist layer as illustrated in Figure 5–42. Once this is done, we can then calculate the chemical response of the resist and therefore the three-dimensional structure of the resist after its pattern is developed.

The optical intensity pattern through the resist layer will be different than the aerial image for a number of reasons. First, the resist has a finite thickness and hence the image produced by the optical system cannot be in perfect focus everywhere in the resist. Another potential issue is the presence of standing waves in the resist, caused by light

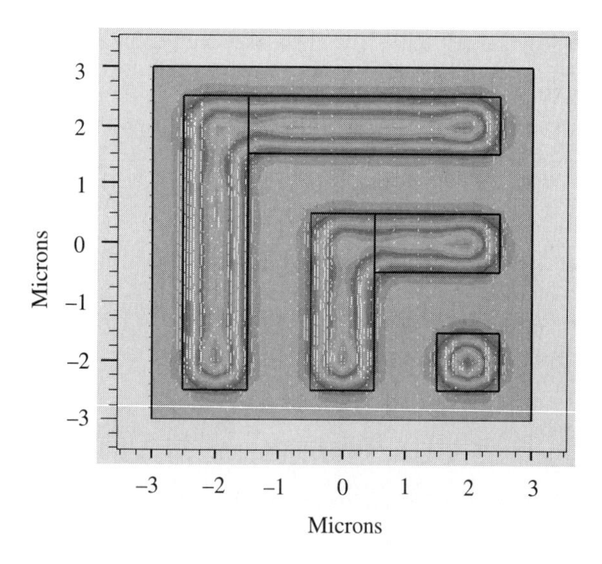

Figure 5–39 Example of aerial image calculation using the ATHENA simulator by Silvaco. The shading corresponds to optical intensity in the aerial image. The black borders correspond to the mask image that is being printed. The exposure system simulated had a $NA = 0.43$, partially coherent g-line illumination ($\lambda = 436$ nm) and no other aberrations or defocusing. The minimum feature size is 1 μm.

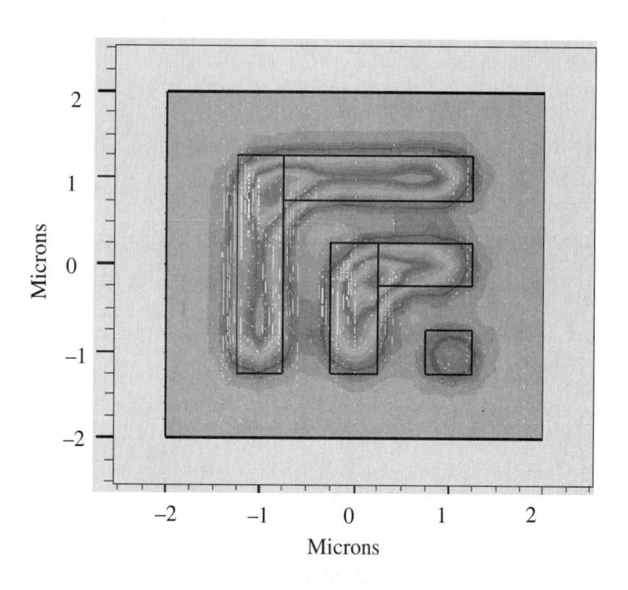

Figure 5–40 Same example as in Figure 5–39 except that the feature size has been reduced to 0.5 μm. Note the much poorer image quality.

reflections from underlying structures. We illustrated this problem in Figures 5–23 and 5–24. In addition, as we also discussed in connection with Figure 5–22, how absorption of light in typical DNQ resists changes with exposure time due to bleaching. This results in a light intensity that varies with depth and with time in the resist. Finally, in high NA exposure systems, the light striking the resist is not all vertically incident. This complicates the calculation of any standing wave patterns that may be present in the resist and generally requires that an integration over the total angle of the incoming light be performed. This procedure can also include the effects of partial coherency in the light source because this also results in light striking the resist at nonnormal angles.

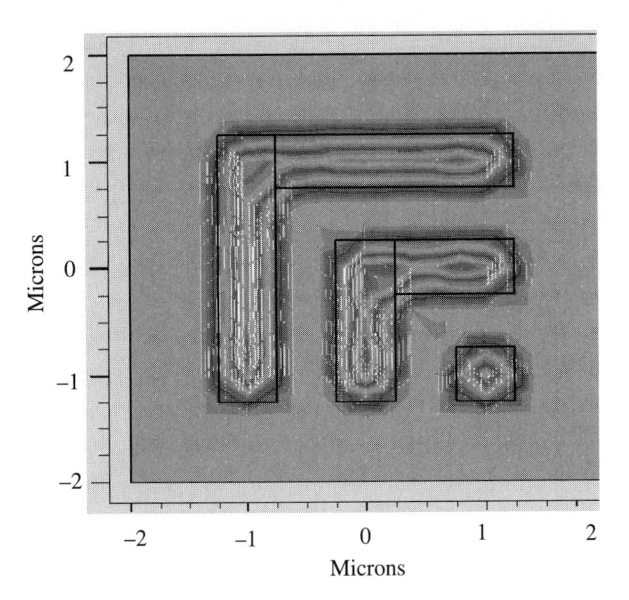

Figure 5–41 Same example as in Figure 5–40 except that the illumination wavelength has now been changed to i-line illumination ($\lambda = 365$ nm) and the *NA* has been increased to 0.5. Note the improvement in image quality resulting from the shorter exposure wavelength and higher *NA* system.

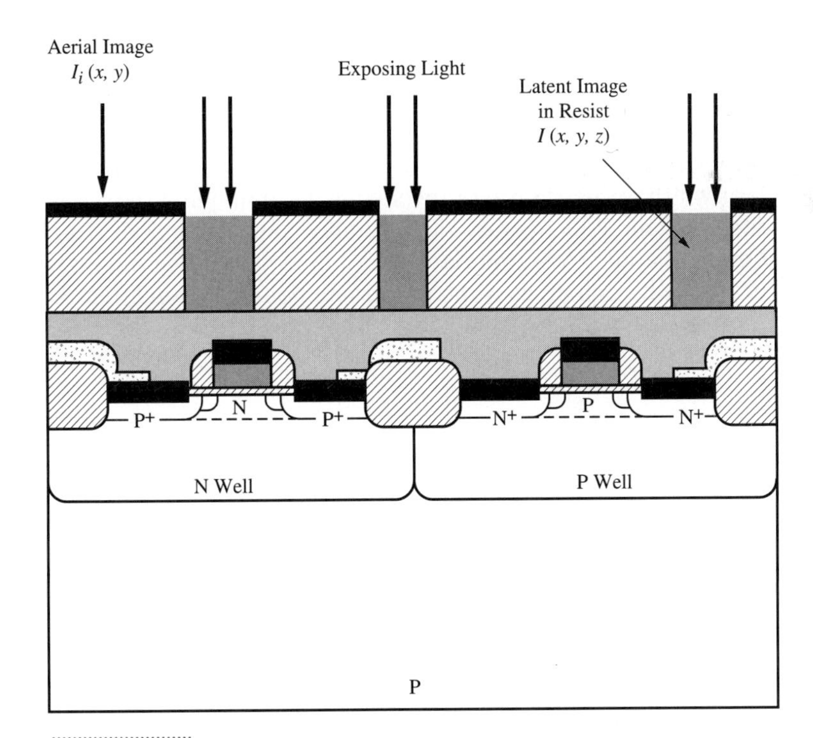

Figure 5–42 Translation of the aerial image into light intensity through the resist layer. This is the latent image produced in the photoresist by the exposing photons. Standing waves, defocusing, and bleaching effects all contribute to make $I(x,y,z)$ different from $I_i(x,y)$.

The simplest way to deal with many of these issues is to modify Eq. (5.31) as follows:

$$I(x,y,z) = I_i(x,y)I_r(x,y,z) \tag{5.37}$$

$I_i(x,y)$ is again the light intensity pattern incident on the top surface of the resist [aerial image given by Eq. (5.31)] and $I_r(x,y,z)$ is a correction factor which includes the effects of defocus, standing waves, and resist bleaching.

Defocusing of the image through the resist layer can be dealt with through Eqs. (5.35) and (5.36). If the aerial image is in focus at the top surface of the resist, then the defocusing that occurs through the resist thickness is given by

$$\delta(z) = \frac{z}{n} \tag{5.38}$$

where z is the depth into the resist and n is the index of refraction of the resist material. This factor can then be included in Eq. (5.37) through the use of the pupil function [Eq. (5.35)]. Eq. (5.38) does assume normally incident light. However a similar approach can be used to account for nonnormally incident light.

Standing waves in the resist can also be dealt with in a simple conceptual fashion. Consider Figure 5–43 in which n is the index of refraction of each of the layers, and ε is the electric field in each layer due to a monochromatic, normally incident electromagnetic plane wave. Reflection from the resist substrate interface results in a reflected wave and the total electric field in the resist is then the sum of the two plane waves traveling in opposite directions. If there is no attenuation of the wave amplitude as it passes through layer 2 (the resist) in the two directions, then the resulting standing wave pattern will have nodes where the summed amplitude is zero and antinodes where the summed amplitude is twice the incoming wave amplitude. More generally, accounting for attenuation in the resist layer, the resulting standing wave is described by a solution of Maxwell's equations with appropriate boundary conditions at each interface. Mack showed that in this system, the standing wave could be described by [5.22]

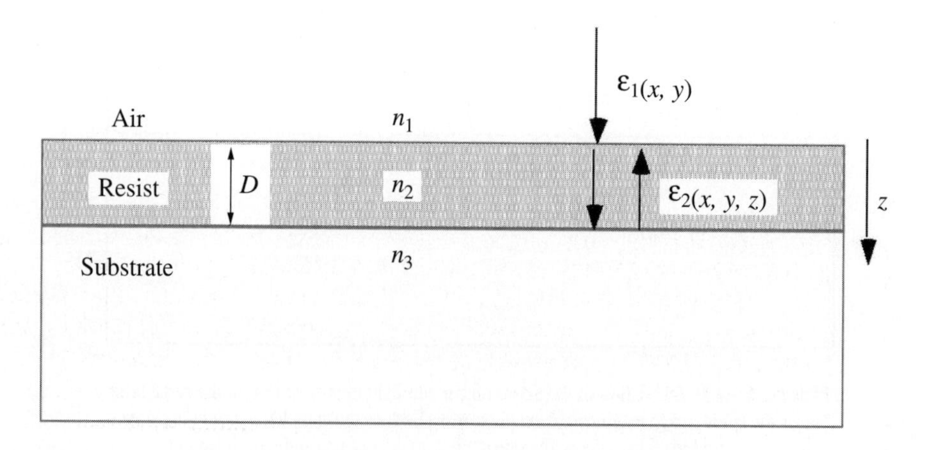

Figure 5–43 Simple example of the formation of standing waves in a resist layer.

$$\varepsilon_2(x,y,z) = \varepsilon_1(x,y)\frac{\tau_{12}\left(e^{-2\pi j n_2 z/\lambda} + \rho_{23}\tau_D^2 e^{2\pi j n_2 z/\lambda}\right)}{1 + \rho_{12}\rho_{23}\tau_D^2} \tag{5.39}$$

where $\varepsilon_1(x,y)$ is the incident electromagnetic plane wave, $\varepsilon_1(x,y)$ is the plane wave in the resist, n_j is the complex index of refraction of layer j, λ is the wavelength of the incident light, and

$$\rho_{ij} = \frac{n_i - n_j}{n_i + n_j}, \text{ the reflection coefficient at interface } ij$$

$$\tau_{ij} = \frac{2n_i}{n_i + n_j}, \text{ the transmission coefficient across interface } ij$$

$$\tau_D = \exp(-jk_2D), \text{ the transmittance of the resist film}$$

$$k_j = \frac{2\pi n_j}{\lambda}, \text{ the propagation constant of layer } j$$

The light intensity in the resist is simply the square of the magnitude of $\varepsilon_2(x,y,z)$.

The actual calculation of the standing wave pattern in a real IC structure is considerably more complicated than Eq. (5.39) might indicate. In general there will be multiple layers (some optically transparent like SiO_2 and some opaque like Al) below the resist, and the resist thickness itself will usually vary with position. Furthermore, the incident light is often not normally incident and it may not even be monochromatic in some exposure systems. Nevertheless, basic optical theory can be used to calculate $\varepsilon_2(x,y,z)$ at each point in the resist even with all these additional complications [5.3, 5.26, 5.27].

An example of such a simulation is shown in Figure 5–44. A relatively simple structure is defined with a silicon substrate etched to form a sloped step. The photoresist layer is deposited so it has a flat upper surface and hence its thickness varies over the structure. A mask is defined which allows light to enter in the center part of the structure ($x = 1$ to $x = 2$ μm). The lower part of Figure 5–44 illustrates the calculated DNQ resist *PAC* concentration after the exposure. As we will see in the next section on resist exposure kinetics, this 2D concentration profile corresponds to the integrated light intensity profile through the exposure process. There are a number of interesting features that can be observed from this simulation.

First, notice at the left-hand side of the exposed region the effects of standing waves in the light intensity. The silicon substrate in this example is a reflecting substrate and so standing waves will be set up. Nodes of maximum light intensity correspond to minimums in the *PAC* (maximum exposure). These are the dark bands on the left side. They occur at $\lambda/2n_2$ distance intervals. The nodes of minimum light intensity (maximum *PAC* concentration) also occur with a period of $\lambda/2n_2$ and are the light gray bands. Notice also the effect of the sloped sidewall in the center part of the structure. Here the incoming light waves are reflected to the right, setting up a standing wave pattern parallel to the

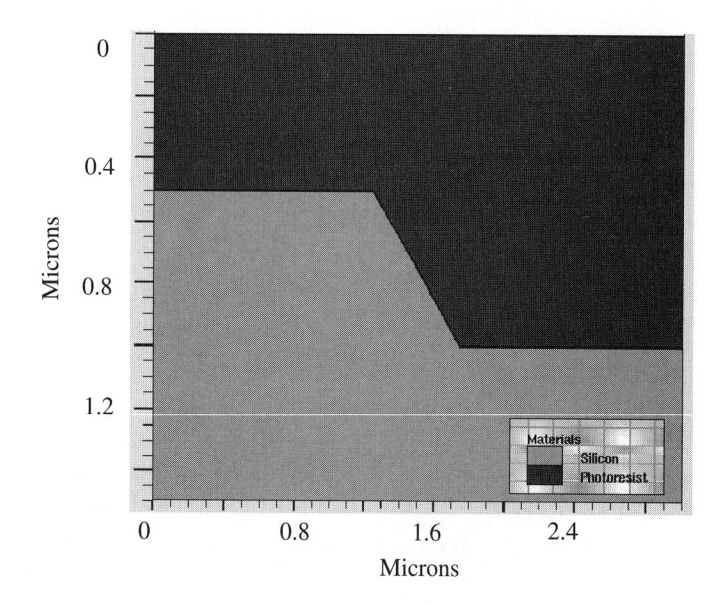

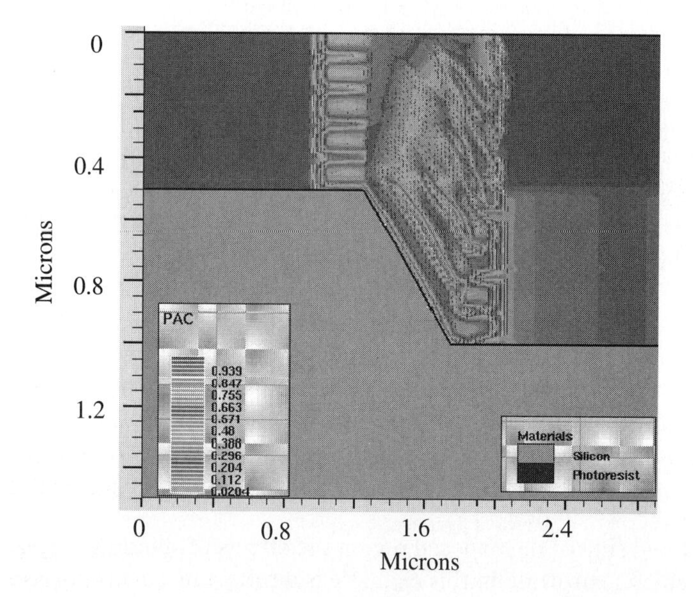

Figure 5–44 Example of calculation of light intensity distribution in a photoresist layer during exposure using the ATHENA simulator by Silvaco. A simple structure is defined at the top with a photoresist layer covering a silicon substrate, which has two flat regions and a sloped sidewall. The exposure takes place between $x = 1$ and $x = 2$ μm. The bottom simulation shows the calculated DNQ resist *PAC* concentration after an exposure of 200 mJ cm^{-2}. Lower *PAC* values correspond to more exposure. The gray-scale contours thus correspond to the integrated light intensity from the exposure.

sloped sidewall. In addition to this standing wave pattern, the reflected light waves will cause the exposed region to extend into the masked region on the right. This will result in image degradation. We will return to this example later to see the effects of postbaking and resist development on the final resist structure. For now, it should be apparent that numerical simulation tools are required to deal with the complexity of structures encountered in modern ICs.

The final issue with respect to the light intensity distribution through the photoresist is resist bleaching. As we saw earlier, this occurs in DNQ resists because the *PAC* in these resists initially absorbs photons while it is being exposed, and then becomes more transmissive as the *PAC* component is converted to carboxylic acid. Thus the top layers of the resist initially absorb the incoming photons and later in the exposure allow more light to penetrate to the deeper layers of the resist. This results in a time-dependent light intensity throughout the resist. Because this issue is directly related to the resist exposure chemistry, we will discuss models for it in the next section on resist exposure. Qualitatively, the effects of this bleaching process can be observed in the bottom of Figure 5–44 which shows, on average, a gradual increase in the *PAC* concentration with depth into the resist.

5.5.3 Photoresist Exposure

In this section until its end, we will neglect any standing waves that might be present in the resist. These effects can easily be included in the exposure model using Eq. (5.39) and we will include such effects in the simulation examples at the end of the section. However, the principle ideas of photoresist exposure can be understood without the complexity of standing waves, and that is the approach we will initially take here. We will also, for the moment, simply consider a one-dimensional structure with a uniform resist layer being exposed.

5.5.3.1 g-line and i-line DNQ Resists

The light incident on the photoresist is primarily absorbed by the *PAC* component of the resist. The *PAC* is assumed to be uniformly distributed throughout the resist. As we have seen, bleaching occurs from the top layers of the resist downward as the *PAC* is exposed. The basic equation describing the light absorption is given by

$$\frac{dI}{dz} = -\alpha I \tag{5.40}$$

where z is the direction into the resist. This equation basically says that the probability that a photon will be absorbed is proportional to the light intensity with alpha, the absorption coefficient, as the proportionality constant. If alpha is a constant, integration of this equation results in Eq. (5.15), which we presented earlier as a simple description of how the light intensity falls off in the photoresist with depth.

Alpha will turn out to be related to the concentration of the *PAC*, which is unexposed in the resist at a particular time and location. Thus alpha is not a constant but rather is a function of position and time. At any time during the exposure, the light intensity profile in the resist will be given by

$$I(z) = I_0 \exp\left(\int_0^z \alpha(z')dz'\right) \tag{5.41}$$

where the integral in the exponent is the absorbance of the resist down to a depth z.

We now need to relate α to the material properties of the resist. If the *PAC* component of the resist is dilute, then the absorption coefficient of the resist is simply

$$\alpha_{resist} = \alpha_{PAC}[PAC] \tag{5.42}$$

where $[PAC]$ is the concentration of the PAC constituent in the resist and α_{PAC} is the absorption coefficient of the PAC material. Eq. (5.42) simply says that the resist absorption is determined by the amount of PAC in the resist. The dilute approximation required for Eq. (5.42) has been shown to hold for practical resist formulations [5.29].

DNQ resists consist of several constituents as we saw earlier in this chapter. In general, such resists will have a resin R (usually novolac), a photoactive component PAC, a solvent S, and as the exposure proceeds, exposure products P (principally the carboxylic acid produced by the PAC). More generally, then, Eq. (5.42) can be written as

$$\alpha_{resist} = \alpha_{PAC}[PAC] + \alpha_R[R] + \alpha_S[S] + \alpha_P[P] \tag{5.43}$$

Since the exposure products result from the PAC, we may write that

$$P = [PAC]_0 - [PAC] \tag{5.44}$$

Following the approach of [5.21], we rewrite Eq. (5.43) in the following form

$$\alpha_{resist} = Am + B \tag{5.45}$$

where

$$A = (\alpha_{PAC} - \alpha_P)[PAC]_0$$
$$B = \alpha_P[PAC]_0 + \alpha_R[R] + \alpha_S[S]$$
$$m = \frac{[PAC]}{[PAC]_0}$$

A and B in Eq. (5.45) are experimentally measurable parameters for a given photoresist and are known as the first two Dill parameters [5.21]. A is the absorption coefficient of the bleachable components of the resist and B is the absorption coefficient of the nonbleachable components of the resist. We will describe how these parameters can be measured for a given resist shortly. Note that when the resist is unexposed, $m = 1$ and $\alpha_{resist} = A + B$. When the resist is fully exposed, $m = 0$ and $\alpha_{resist} = B$.

We can now substitute Eq. (5.45) into Eq. (5.40) and express the light intensity through the resist layer as

$$\frac{dI}{dz} = -(Am + B)I \tag{5.46}$$

Unfortunately, solving this equation is complicated by the fact that m is a function of time and position so that Eq. (5.46) really should be written

$$\frac{dI}{dz} = -[Am(z,t) + B]I \tag{5.47}$$

m is the fraction of the PAC component of the resist that is unexposed at time t. If we again assume first order reaction kinetics, then

$$\frac{dm}{dt} = -CIm \tag{5.48}$$

This equation states that the exposure rate of the PAC is proportional to the remaining unexposed PAC concentration and to the light intensity. The constant of proportionality is C, which is the third Dill resist parameter.

Eqs. (5.47) and (5.48) are coupled equations that must be solved simultaneously. The third equation that must be included is Eq. (5.39), which accounts for any standing wave patterns in the resist. Simulators which are available today [5.3, 5.26, 5.27] solve this system of equations to calculate the time evolution of the exposure of the resist. An iterative procedure is used which basically operates as follows.

At $t = 0, m = 1$ and the light intensity pattern can be calculated in the resist using Eq. (5.39). This intensity distribution is then used in Eq. (5.48) to calculate the exposure versus position. The result is $m(x,y,z,t_0)$ in the general three-dimensional case. The result is then used in Eqs. (5.47) and (5.39) to calculate the light intensity at $t = 0 + \Delta t$. This result is again used in Eq. (5.48) to calculate the new light intensity after the next time step. Through this iterative procedure, the time evolution of the exposure process is simulated. The overall result is that the aerial image produced by the optical system is converted into a latent 3D image in the photoresist. Figure 5–44 showed an example of such a simulation in which the output shown in the bottom of the figure is the [PAC] as a function of position at the end of the exposure.

Calculation of the latent image in the resist requires knowledge of the Dill resist parameters A, B, and C. These parameters can be measured experimentally for a particular resist material as illustrated in Figure 5–45. In their series of classic papers in 1975, Dill and his co-workers showed that a simple measurement of the time dependent light transmission through an exposing resist film could be used to extract the A, B, and C parameters. As illustrated in Figure 5–45, light at the exposing wavelength is used to illuminate a resist coated substrate. In the simplest case, a transparent substrate is chosen to have the same index of refraction as the resist, so that there are no reflections at the resist/substrate interface. An antireflection coating is used on the backside of the substrate to avoid reflections at that interface. A typical measurement result is shown schematically in Figure 5–46. For this simple case, Dill and colleagues showed that [5.21]

$$A = \frac{1}{D}\ln\left(\frac{T_\infty}{T_0}\right) \tag{5.49}$$

$$B = -\frac{1}{D}\ln(T_\infty) \tag{5.50}$$

$$C = \frac{A + B}{AT_0(1 - T_0)T_{12}}\left.\frac{dT}{dE}\right|_{E=0} \tag{5.51}$$

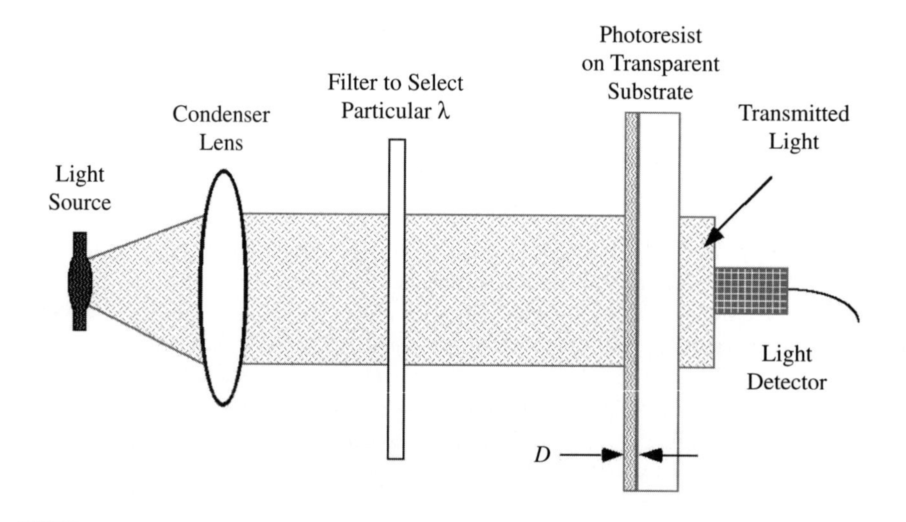

Figure 5–45 Conceptual experimental setup for measuring the Dill parameters characterizing a particular resist.

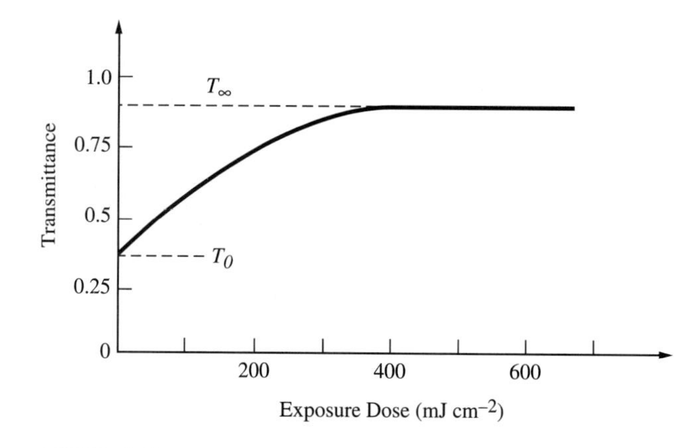

Figure 5–46 Typical experimental result from a measurement like that shown in Figure 5–48.

where
$$T_{12} = 1 - \left(\frac{n_{resist} - 1}{n_{resist} + 1}\right)^2 \tag{5.52}$$

T_0 is the transmitted light intensity at the start of the exposure, T_∞ is the transmitted light intensity at the end of the exposure, D is the resist thickness, and T_{12} is the transmittance through the air/resist interface, with n_{resist} the index of refraction of the resist. More sophisticated parameter extraction methods can be used if the experimental situation is not quite as ideal as Figure 5–45 [5.3, 5.21].

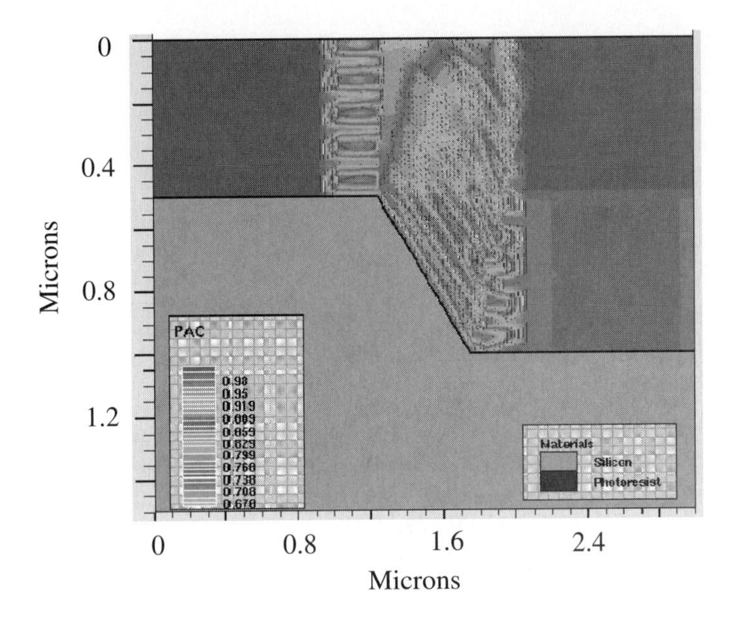

Figure 5–47 Same simulation example as in Figure 5–44 except that the exposure dose has been reduced to 10% of the value used in Figure 5–44. The deeper regions of the photoresist are not as exposed as the near surface regions because of the effects of bleaching.

Figure 5–47 shows an additional simulation with the same structure as was used in Figure 5–44. The exposure dose in Figure 5–47 has been reduced to 10% of the previous value to illustrate the effects of bleaching during resist exposure. With only 10% of the exposure dose, it is apparent that the upper layers of the resist are still exposed but the lower regions have not received sufficient photon flux to fully expose the resist.

5.5.3.2 DUV Resists

Chemically amplified DUV resists consist of a polymer resin (blocked to make it insoluble in the developer in the case of a positive resist), a *PAG*, and other additives. The kinetics of the exposure reaction are assumed to be first order, that is,

$$\frac{d[PAG]}{dt} = -CI[PAG] \tag{5.53}$$

where $[PAG]$ is the time-dependent *PAG* concentration, I is the exposure intensity, and C is the exposure rate. Note the similarity to Eq. (5.48). If I is constant during the exposure,

$$[PAG] = [PAG]_0 e^{-CIt} \tag{5.54}$$

Since the acid concentration $[H]$ results directly from the *PAG* exposure, $[H]$ is given by

$$[H] = [PAG]_0(1 - e^{-CIt}) \tag{5.55}$$

where in general, $[H]$ and I will be $f(x,y,z)$. If the light intensity is also a function of time, then an iterative technique like that described in the previous section can be used to calculate $H(x,y,z,t)$.

The aerial image is thus converted into a latent 3D image in the resist which is "stored" as $H(x,y,z)$ at the end of the exposure. Simulation results would look much like the examples shown earlier in Figures 5–44 and 5–47.

5.5.4 Postexposure Bake (PEB)

Once the exposure of the resist is complete, the next step is often a postexposure thermal bake (PEB). There are actually several bake steps that are normally employed in photoresist processing and each of these steps can have an impact on the final resist pattern.

As was indicated in Figure 5–31, the first bake step is usually a prebake step before the resist is exposed. This step is designed to evaporate most of the remaining solvent in the resist. However this step can also have an impact on the photoresist chemistry. At the prebake temperature (typically 90 – 100°C), the *PAC* in DNQ resists begins to decompose into a nonphotosensitive product [5.30]. The qualitative result of this is that the concentration of the *PAC* at the start of the exposure, $[PAC]_0$, is smaller than the original concentration in the resist. Standard prebake conditions usually result in 10% or less of the *PAC* being decomposed. There has been some work on quantitative modeling of these effects [5.3, 5.31], but in many cases the resist parameters needed for such models are not well known and the chemical processes taking place are not fully understood. Most lithography simulators that are available today do not model the effects of resist prebake at all, so we will not deal with this particular bake step further.

5.5.4.1 g-line and i-line DNQ Resists

The postexposure bake is sometimes incorporated into DNQ resist process flows in order to reduce the effects of standing waves. We saw examples of these effects in the simulations in the last section. If nothing is done to mitigate the standing wave effects, the developed resist image will have distinctly scalloped edges (recall Figure 5–24). This is generally undesirable because it degrades linewidth control and resolution. Fortunately, it has been found that a simple thermal bake between exposure and development can have a dramatic effect on the standing wave effects [5.32]. Typically this bake is 10–30 minutes at about 100°C (similar to the resist prebake step).

The effect of the postexposure bake on DNQ resist chemistry is usually modeled as a simple diffusion process. The exposed *PAC* (*P* in our terminology), is assumed to be able to diffuse in the resist with some diffusivity given by

$$D_P = D_0 \, e^{-E_A/kT} \tag{5.56}$$

This is of the same form as dopant diffusion coefficients that we will discuss in Chapter 7. The effect of the *PAC* diffusion is simply to "smear out" the standing wave effects.

Such a diffusion process can be modeled in lithography simulators. However, this is more complicated than might appear at first glance, first because D_P has not been measured for most resists, and second, because it is likely that the diffusivity is not as simple as Eq. (5.56) might suggest. For example, it is believed that D_P is concentration dependent.

In some lithography simulators, default or user specified values for D_P are used along with Eq. (5.56). The postexposure bake is then modeled as a diffusion process. In other simulators, a simpler approach is taken because of the lack of D_P data. These simulators model the postexposure bake with a simple diffusion length model. The distance over which the *PAC* "smearing" occurs during the bake is simply given by

$$\sigma = \sqrt{2D_P t_{bake}} \tag{5.57}$$

where t_{bake} is the bake time. σ has units of distance and is generally a user-supplied parameter in simulators. A typical value might be $\approx 0.05\ \mu m$ (50 nm) or about $^1/_4\ \lambda$.

Figure 5–48 illustrates the effect of such a postexposure bake on the simulation previously shown in Figure 5–44. The smearing out of the standing wave pattern is apparent in the calculated [*PAC*].

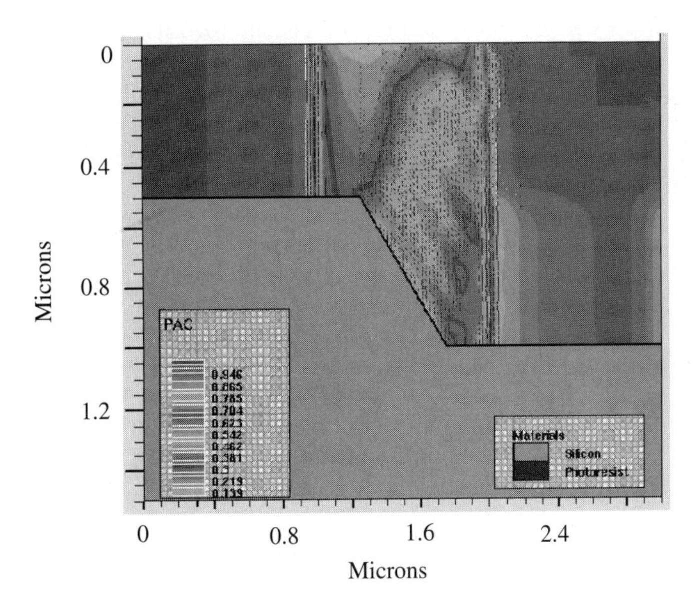

Figure 5–48 Same simulation example as in Figure 5–44 except that a postexposure bake of 45 minutes at 115°C has now been included. The gray-scale contours again correspond to the [*PAC*] after exposure. Note that the standing wave effects apparent in Figure 5–46 have been "smeared out" by this bake, producing a more uniform [*PAC*] distribution.

5.5.4.2 DUV Resists

In DUV resists, the PEB is a critical step because it completes the exposure process by driving the reaction between the *PAG* molecules and the polymer chains. In positive DUV resists this reaction unblocks the polymer chain, making it soluble in the developer. In negative resists, the *PAG* drives a crosslinking reaction that makes the resist insoluble in the developer. In either case, the acid molecules are not consumed by the reactions and hence to first order, $[H]$, given by Eq. (5.55), remains constant during the PEB.

If $[M]$ represents the concentration of the reactive sites on the resist polymer chains, then

$$\frac{d[M]}{dt} = -C[M][H] \tag{5.58}$$

where C is the reaction rate constant. This expression assumes that the reaction between the acid H and the reactive sites M is first order. During the PEB, M begins with a starting concentration $[M_0]$ and decreases with time.

$$[M_0] - [M] = [M_0](1 - e^{-C[H]t}) \tag{5.59}$$

In general $[H]$ and therefore $[M]$ are $f(x,y,z,t)$.

The PEB provides the thermal energy for this reaction to take place because C in Eq. (5.58) is generally exponentially dependent on temperature. The second process driven by temperature is the diffusion of the acid molecules, since they must physically move from reactive site to reactive site to complete the resist exposure (recall Figure 5–19). This diffusion process is described by a standard diffusion equation, which in one dimension is

$$\frac{\partial[H]}{\partial t} = \frac{\partial}{\partial x}\left(D_H \frac{\partial[H]}{\partial x}\right) \tag{5.60}$$

We will discuss diffusion and this equation in much more detail in Chapter 7.

The diffusivity D_H of the acid molecules generally depends exponentially on temperature as in Eq. (5.56). But it may also depend on the acid concentration, making the modeling problem more difficult. Simulation of the PEB process in a DUV resist thus depends on simultaneously solving Eqs. (5.58) and (5.60), a system of equations known as reaction-diffusion equations. This is straightforward to implement although a number of parameters including D_H, M_0, C and of course $H(x,y,z)$ are required. A final complication that can arise in such simulations is that the acid concentration $[H]$ may not be time independent because of various loss mechanisms that can occur during the PEB. These mechanisms include poisoning by atmospheric base contaminants, evaporation of the acid molecules, or simply trapping of the acid molecules at sites in the photoresist. All of these mechanisms can be modeled and included in simulations if specific models and parameters are available. Generally such effects are not included in simulators today. Simulation of the PEB effects on DUV resists would look similar to Figure 5–48.

5.5.5 Photoresist Developing

A number of models have been used to describe photoresist developing. The earliest models came from Dill and his co-workers and were empirically based [5.21]. Some more recent models have attempted to use a more physical basis [5.33]. In all cases, the process is basically described as a surface controlled etching process. The developer solution is assumed to etch the surface of the resist isotropically at a point (x,y,z) at a rate that is determined by the resist inhibitor concentration at that point. The photoactive compound (*PAC*) in DNQ resists or the blocked polymers in DUV resists are insoluble in the developer whereas when the *PAC* is converted to carboxylic acid (*P*) in DNQ resists, or when the *PAG* unblocks the polymer chains in DUV resists in the exposure process, the resist becomes quite soluble in the developer. We will describe the developing process below in terms of DNQ resist parameters. However, the same models apply to DUV resists.

The development or etching rate at point (x,y,z), thus depends on the $[P]$ or $[PAC]$ at that point. This is exactly what is calculated by the exposure models we previously described, and what is shown in the examples in Figures 5–44, 5–47 and 5–48. What is needed then, is a mathematical relationship between $[P]$ or $[PAC]$ and the development rate.

The first such relationship was described by Dill and colleagues [5.21] and is implemented in simulators today typically in a form like the following [5.26]:

$$R(x,y,z) = \begin{cases} 0.006 \exp(E_1 + E_2 m + E_3 m^2) & \text{if } m > -0.5\dfrac{E_2}{E_3} \\ 0.006 \exp\left(E_1 + \dfrac{E_2}{E_3}(E_2 - 1)\right) & \text{otherwise} \end{cases} \tag{5.61}$$

$R(x,y,z)$ is the local development or etching rate in μm min^{-1}, m [actually $m(x,y,z)$] was defined in Eq. (5.45) and is the local $[PAC]$ after exposure, and E_1, E_2 and E_3 are empirical parameters obtained from fitting Eq. (5.61) to experimental data.

A more physically based model for resist development has been proposed by Mack [5.33]. This model has many similarities to the Deal-Grove oxidation model that we will discuss in Chapter 6. Mack's model is illustrated in Figure 5–49. In this model, three fluxes are used to describe the development process. F_1 represents the diffusion of developer from the bulk of the liquid to the resist surface. F_2 represents the reaction of the developer with the resist, and F_3 represents the diffusion of the reaction products back into the developer solution. F_3 is assumed to be very fast (not rate limiting) and hence is neglected in Mack's analysis.

F_1 is assumed to be driven by the concentration gradient between the liquid developer and the resist surface and is given by

$$F_1 = k_D(C_D - C_S) \tag{5.62}$$

where k_D is the mass transfer coefficient associated with developer diffusion (cm sec^{-1}), C_D is the bulk developer concentration and C_S is the developer concentration at the re-

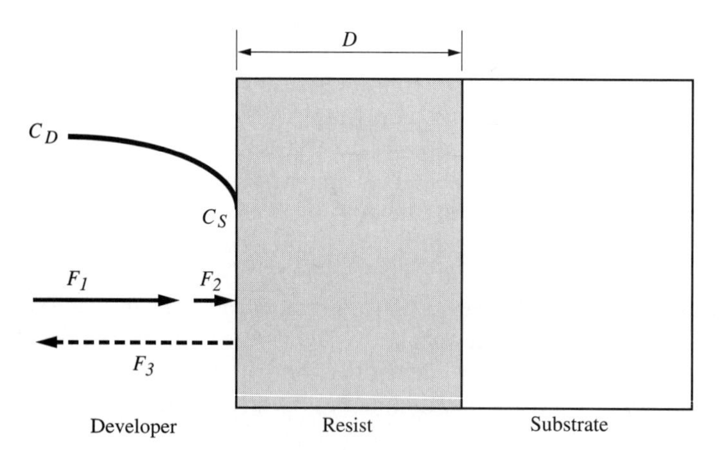

Figure 5–49 Mack's model for photoresist development.

sist surface. F_2 is assumed to depend on the concentrations of the two reacting species at the resist surface and is given by

$$F_2 = k_R C_S [P]^n \tag{5.63}$$

where k_R is the rate constant associated with the developer-resist reaction (cm sec^{-1}) and $[P]$ is the local concentration of the reacted PAC as defined earlier. Here it is assumed that the reaction is proportional to some power of $[P]$, that is, that some number of molecules n of product P react with the developer to dissolve a resin molecule in the resist.

F_1 and F_2 are in series and so we let $F_1 = F_2$ in steady state. Thus

$$F_1 = F_2 = \frac{k_D k_R C_D [P]^n}{k_D + k_R [P]^n} \tag{5.64}$$

Recalling the definition of $[P]$ and m in Eqs. (5.44) and (5.45), we have finally that the development rate $r = F_1 = F_2$ is

$$r = \frac{k_D C_D (1 - m)^n}{\dfrac{k_D}{k_R [PAC]_0^n} + (1 - m)^n} \tag{5.65}$$

When $m = 1$, the resist is unexposed and $r \to 0$. This is not physically correct because conventional DNQ resists do dissolve in the developer at a nonzero rate even if they are unexposed. Eq. (5.65) can be corrected to account for this as follows:

$$r = \frac{k_D C_D (1 - m)^n}{\dfrac{k_D}{k_R [PAC]_0^n} + (1 - m)^n} + r_{min} \tag{5.66}$$

where r_{min} is the dissolving rate in unexposed resist. When $m = 0$, the resist is fully exposed and $r \rightarrow r_{max}$ where

$$r_{max} = \frac{k_D C_D}{\dfrac{k_D}{k_R[PAC]_0^n} + 1} + r_{min} \tag{5.67}$$

We can consider two limiting cases of this model. If the diffusion process in the liquid developer is fast, the overall reaction will be limited by the reaction at the surface (surface reaction rate limited). On the other hand, if the surface reaction rate is the faster of the two processes, the overall reaction will be "diffusion limited."

$$r \approx \begin{Bmatrix} k_R C_D [P]^n + r_{min} & \text{Surface Reaction Rate Limited} \\ k_D C_D + r_{min} & \text{Diffusion Rate Limited} \end{Bmatrix} \tag{5.68}$$

Eq. (5.66) is often written in the following form:

$$r = r_{max} \frac{(a + 1)(1 - m)^n}{a + (1 - m)^n} + r_{min} \tag{5.69}$$

where

$$a = \frac{k_D}{k_R[PAC]_0^n} \tag{5.70}$$

The parameter a is really a measure of the relative rates of diffusion and the surface reaction.

To use this model, there are four parameters that must be determined experimentally, a, m, r_{max} and r_{min} although r_{min} is often negligible so there may be only three parameters. Dill's original model also contained three parameters. However Mack's model attempts to use parameters which have some physical basis as opposed to the purely empirical parameters in Dill's model.

Commercially available simulators generally implement a number of models for resist development, including the two described here. The time evolution of the developing resist profile is calculated by setting up a two- or three-dimensional grid in which each grid point in the resist has a specific value of $m(x,y,z)$. The developing pattern is then allowed to evolve over time with the developer moving into the resist at a local rate determined by the development model.

Figure 5–50 shows an example of a simulation of the development process. In this example the simplest development model (the Dill model) was used. Normal parameters were used in the simulation for exposure time and development time, and a postexposure bake was included to minimize standing wave effects. The resulting developed resist pattern shows good resolution and fairly sharp sidewalls. The simulation on the bottom left shows the resist profile partway through the development. Note how the shape of the remaining resist at this point mirrors the *PAC* concentration in the resist pattern.

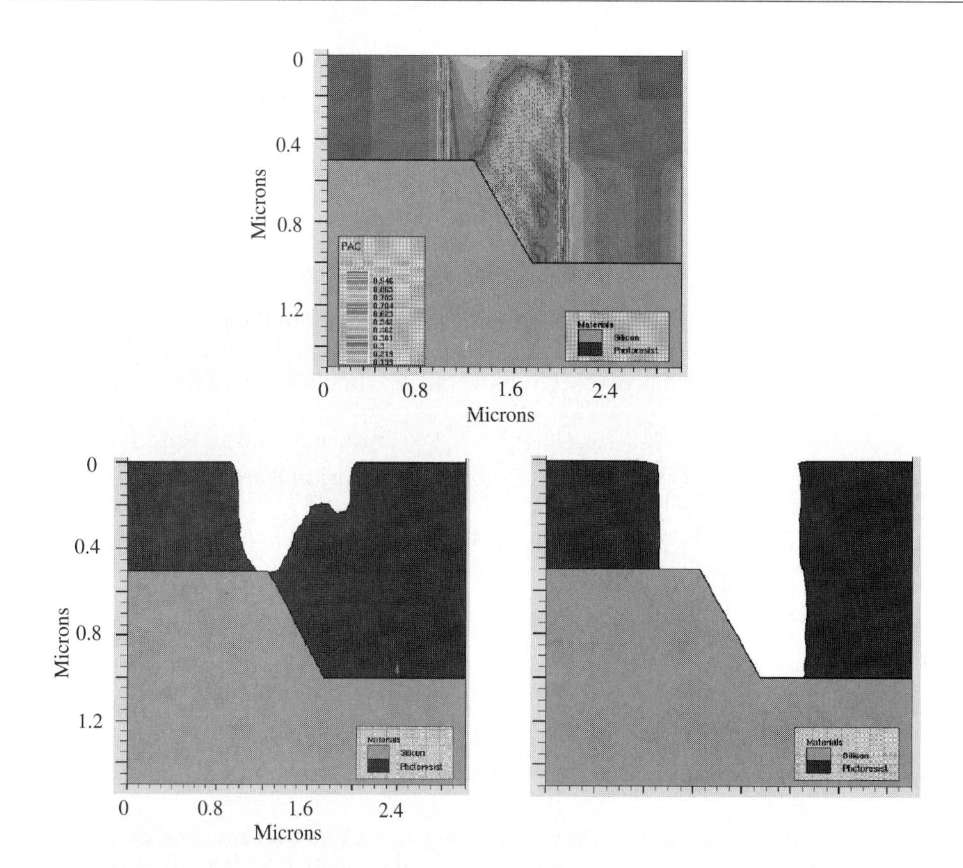

Figure 5–50 Example of the calculation of a developed photoresist layer using the ATHENA simulator by Silvaco. The resist was exposed with a dose of 200 mJ cm^{-2}, a postexposure bake of 45 min at 115°C was used, and the pattern was developed for 60 seconds, all normal parameters. The Dill development model was used. The top image shows the *PAC* concentration after exposure and postbake. The bottom simulations show the developed resist pattern partway through the development (left) and after complete development (right). The resist pattern is well defined in this simulation.

5.5.6 Photoresist Postbake

As shown in Figure 5–31, the final step in a typical photoresist process is a postbake, typically done at 100 – 140°C for 10 – 30 minutes. This step hardens the resist by evaporating any remaining solvents and also improves adhesion to underlying materials. Since the resist is generally used to mask a plasma etching step, or to block an ion implantation step, this hardening process is important in improving the robustness of the resist. The resist will generally flow somewhat during this postbake, rounding the edges of the profile. Obviously the degree of flowing depends on the time and temperature of the postbake, as well as on the resist material properties.

Most lithography simulators do not model this postbake process. However some of these tools have implemented a flow simulator using models which are similar to the

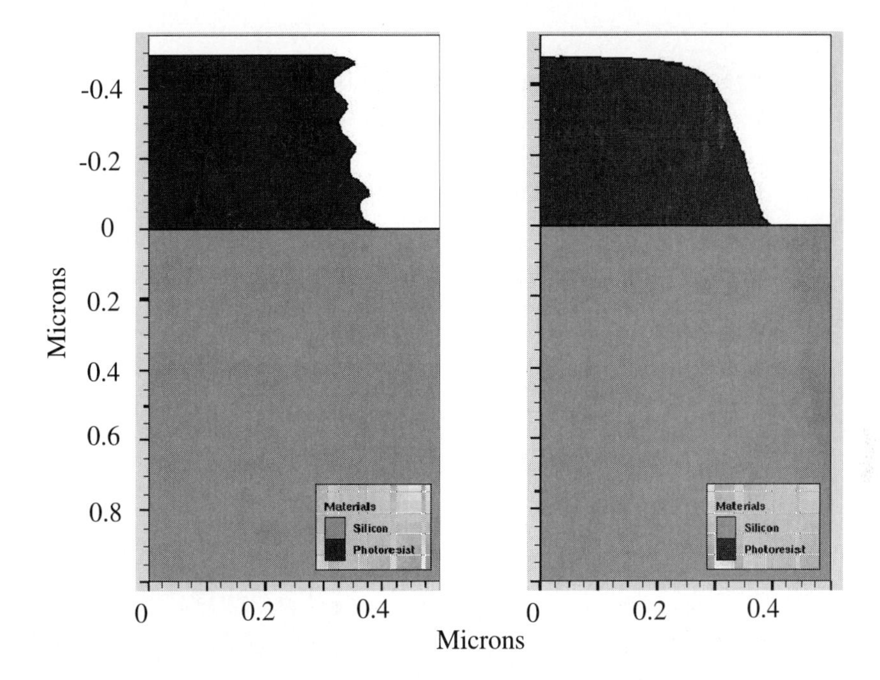

Figure 5–51 Example of the simulation of the reflow process using the ATHENA simulator by Silvaco. The initial developed resist pattern is shown on the left. A 10-min 130°C postbake results in the structure on the right. Note the standing wave effects present in the developed resist profile, which disappear after the reflow.

glass reflow models discussed in Chapter 11. A detailed discussion of such models is included in Chapter 11, so it will not be repeated here. Figure 5–51 shows an example of the simulated effects of the postbake on the resist profile.

5.5.7 Advanced Mask Engineering

In Section 5.2.4, we described some of the advanced mask engineering concepts that are being applied to masks to improve the resolution of optical projection systems. These methods include Optical Proximity Correction (OPC) and phase shift masks. These techniques basically change the description of the mask transmission function [Eq. (5.21)]. Modern simulators include these possibilities simply by changing the mask description in the simulator input. An example of such a simulation is shown in Figure 5–52 in which a small contact hole is printed in resist using a mask with and without phase shifting. The higher quality of the developed image in the resist is apparent in the case with a phase shifted mask.

Simulation tools will probably play an increasingly important role as more mask designs incorporate these advanced features. The design of such mask patterns is not straightforward and the use of computers to both help in the design and to "check" the design using simulation tools is likely to become very common in the future.

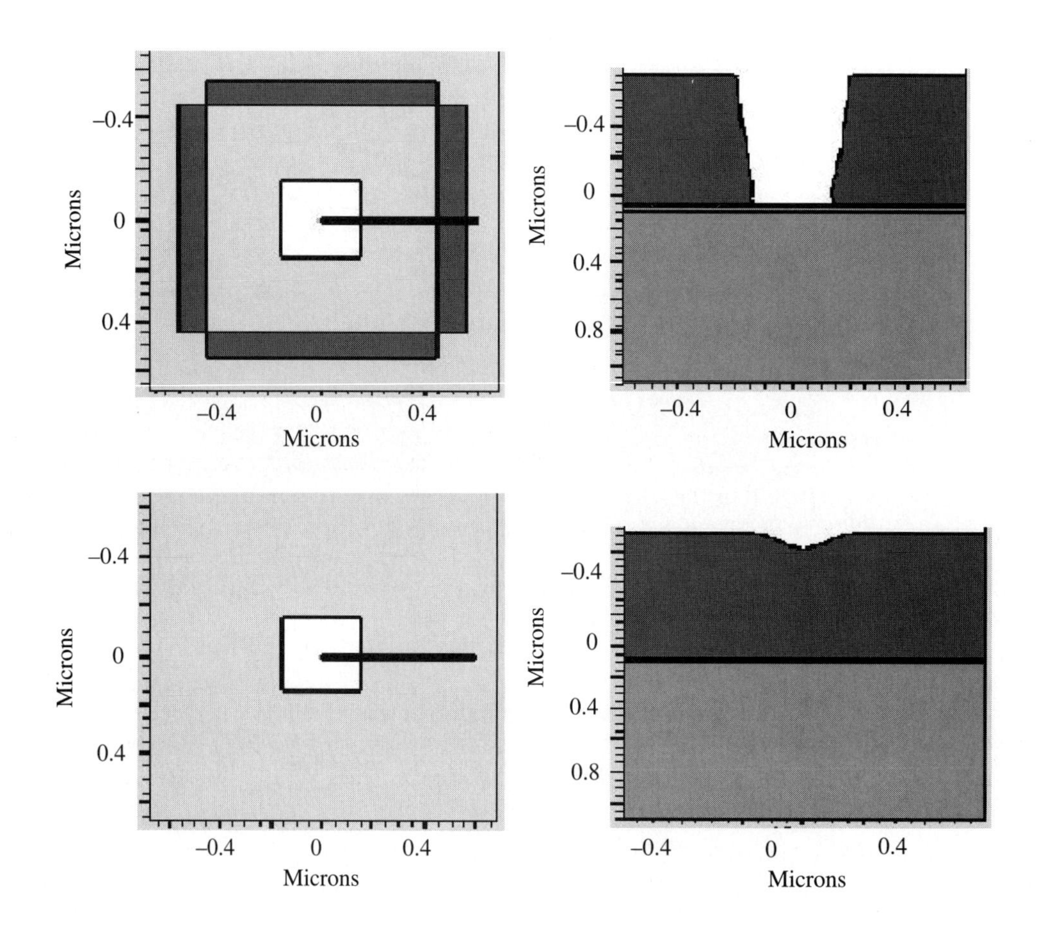

Figure 5–52 Example of the simulation of an developed photoresist image with a phase shifting mask using the ATHENA simulator by Silvaco. In the top example, the mask design on the left is a 0.3-μm contact hole (central area) with 0.1-μm phase shifting features outside the border of the contact hole ("outriggers"). These features are absent in the bottom example. The difference in the developed contact hole features is apparent. In this case an i-line stepper with a 0.54 *NA* was used in the simulation along with normal postexposure bake and development cycles.

5.6 Limits and Future Trends in Technologies and Models

The demise of optical lithography has been predicted many times over the past decade. Yet continued innovations in optical exposure systems have kept pace with manufacturing needs. The SIA NTRS described at the beginning of this chapter projects the need for 0.13-μm features in 2003, and 0.1-μm features in 2006. It now appears likely that optical exposure systems can provide the tools needed for the 0.13-μm generation and perhaps even the 0.1-μm generation, using 193 nm excimer laser sources and step and scan systems. There is even some work today on a 157-nm (F_2) excimer laser source. Somewhere beyond the 0.1-μm generation, however, the actual demise of optical lithography probably will occur. Diffraction limits will require much shorter wavelength sources, and exposure systems likely will not use refracting optics because of the difficulty in finding transparent materials at these shorter wavelengths.

There is no consensus on lithography approaches for manufacturing < 0.1-μm integrated circuits. There is obviously a significant amount of research currently underway to evaluate various alternatives, because if a solution is not found, this problem will be a show stopper for the continued evolution of ICs. We will briefly mention here some of the significant alternatives for lithography in the future.

5.6.1 Electron Beam Lithography

Electron beam systems have been used for many years to make the masks needed for optical lithography, as was illustrated in Figure 5–1. There is no conceptual reason why such a system cannot be used to directly write patterns in photoresist on wafers rather than in photoresist on mask substrates. In fact for many years, this technique has been the method of choice for advanced device research because of the superb resolution offered by e-beam tools. While electrons do have wavelike properties, the wavelength of the electrons used in these exposure tools is less than 0.1 nm, so diffraction effects and the limits they impose on optical exposure systems are not an issue in e-beam systems. Even 20 years ago, feature sizes smaller than 10 nm had been demonstrated [5.34]. Thus there is no question about the ability of e-beam tools to provide the resolution required for feature sizes through the end of the current SIA NTRS.

The major drawback of e-beam tools is the very small throughput compared to current optical steppers. The simplest e-beam tools essentially expose the resist pixel by pixel, a serial process. Optical steppers on the other hand expose the pixels on an area of the wafer in parallel. This is a major difference and results in e-beam lithography tools having a throughput on the order of one wafer per hour compared with >50 wafers per hour for modern optical steppers. The manufacturing cost differences associated with the two technologies are such that e-beam tools have not found application to date in mainstream manufacturing plants. e-beam tools are used today for fabricating small quantities of experimental devices and circuits and for small-scale manufacturing of special-purpose chips, which require small features or fast turnaround. (Since no masks have to be made, the time required to go from design to a fabricated chip can be shorter using e-beam lithography, although only for small quantities of chips.)

The throughput limitation on e-beam systems arises from a number of considerations. First, the electron source can provide only a finite current density. Since a minimum number of electrons are required to expose each pixel in the resist, this sets an upper bound on how fast the beam can be scanned on the wafer. If the resist sensitivity is S, then the minimum number of electrons needed to expose each pixel is simply

$$N = \frac{S I_P^2}{q} \tag{5.71}$$

where I_P is the pixel dimension. Second, at high-beam intensities, resolution can be degraded because of defocusing caused by the coulomb repulsion of the charged electrons in the beam. Approaches to overcoming these limitations include using multiple-electron sources so that parallel writing can be accomplished, shaping the beam into rectangles large enough to expose full features on the wafer rather than individual pixels, improving the sensitivity of e-beam resists, and using e-beam projection lithography in which a stencil mask containing complex patterns is focused on the wafer. This latter approach is most useful when the IC contains repetitive patterns, such as in memory chips.

Proximity effects are an additional significant issue associated with e-beam direct writing. The electrons striking the resist typically have an energy of 10 – 20 keV and travel distances greater than a micron before coming to rest. They give up their energy to the resist and substrate materials through a variety of interactions including elastic scattering off nuclei and inelastic interactions like those illustrated in Figure 4–18. In fact the overall stopping process is not unlike the ion implantation process described in detail in Chapter 8. Because the electrons have such a long range and because they scatter so readily, exposure of regions adjacent to the desired exposure areas does occur. This is known as the proximity effect. It is possible to model this effect since the overall mask pattern is known and to correct the exposure process for this effect. The procedure basically is to calculate how much exposure takes place in adjacent regions because of scattering and then to adjust the electron dose spatially to compensate for such effects. Sophisticated algorithms have been developed to accomplish this [5.35].

Perhaps the most promising approach to high-throughput e-beam lithography is the SCALPEL® (SCattering with Angular Limitation Projection Electron-beam Lithography), invented at Bell Laboratories in 1989 [5.36]. This invention was motivated by two observations about e-beam projection systems. The first observation was that existing stencil mask systems which basically absorb the electron beam in the parts of the mask intended to be opaque are subject to heating problems because of the energy absorbed from the e-beam. This limits the accelerating voltage that can be used in these systems. The second observation was that full field electron optics systems require small numerical apertures as die sizes increase and feature sizes decrease. As a result, the beam current densities needed for reasonable throughput in these systems result in significant space-charge effects that destroy the system resolution.

The solution to these problems proposed in the SCALPEL® system basically involves a new mask design. The principle is illustrated in Figure 5–53. The mask consists of a low atomic number membrane (typically Si_3N_4) and a thin high atomic number pattern (typically a few tens of nm of Cr or W). Both regions are essentially transparent to the collimated, incoherent 100-KeV electron beam that is used in the system. However the electrons interact differently with the two mask regions. In the membrane areas, the electrons are only weakly scattered to small angles. In the Cr/W regions, the electrons are strongly scattered to large angles. An electron lens system focuses the scattered electrons on the wafer. However, an aperture in the back focal plane of the projection system blocks the strongly scattered electrons. Thus a high-contrast, high-resolution image is produced on the wafer. This concept has been demonstrated experimentally and has both the resolution and the potential throughput to meet the SIA NTRS requirements through all the technology generations currently in the roadmap [5.37]. The system reduces the mask image typically by 4:1, requires no exotic mask patterning (OPC or phase shift masks), utilizes a step and scan approach very similar to modern optical exposure systems, achieves a large depth of focus, and works with the same chemically amplified DUV resists currently used for 248-nm lithography. This approach has not yet

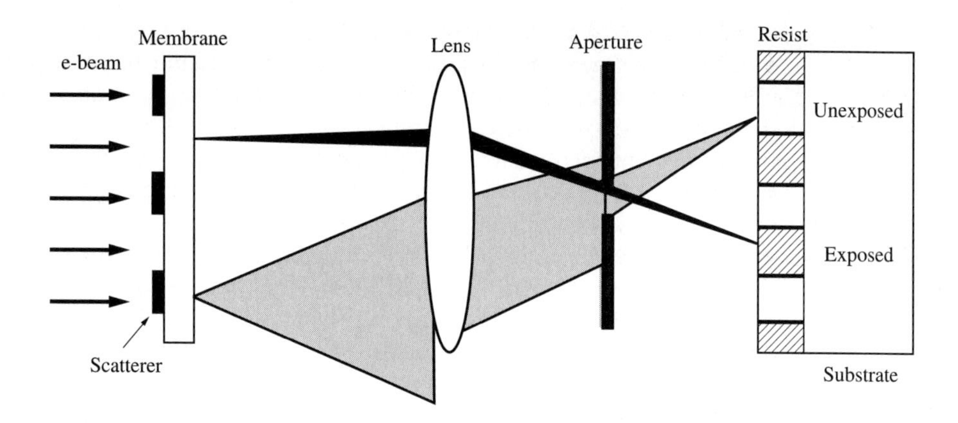

Figure 5–53 SCALPEL® e-beam projection lithography system. The resist is "exposed" in areas where the e-beam has not been widely scattered (mask areas where there is no scatterer). When the e-beam is widely scattered, the intensity reaching the resist is insufficient for exposure.

been demonstrated in a full-scale manufacturing environment, but it appears to have significant promise for future lithography needs.

5.6.2 X-ray Lithography

X-ray lithography systems use X-rays (photons) with energies in the 1 – 10 keV region, corresponding to wavelengths on the order of 1 nm. Thus diffraction effects are negligible as was the case with e-beam lithography. Focusing of X-rays is a very difficult problem so X-ray systems today are generally proximity printing systems. They have the basic configuration illustrated in Figure 5–3 except that an X-ray source is used rather than an optical source. The system is normally operated in a vacuum environment, although the wafer itself is usually in an air ambient. The X-rays emerge from the exposure tool through a thin Be window.

The discussion of near field (Fresnel) diffraction earlier in the Chapter (Section 5.2.2.3), would suggest that very good resolution could be achieved with a system operating with an exposure wavelength of about 1 nm. This is indeed the case with X-ray systems. A number of such systems are in use today in research laboratories and they have achieved < 0.1-μm feature sizes. These systems also have throughputs comparable to optical exposure systems because they expose a significant area on the wafer during each exposure. The systems often use a step and repeat system approach like optical steppers because of the limitations in making large area 1:1 X-ray masks.

The principal issues limiting the adoption of X-ray systems in manufacturing have to do with the masks and the X-ray source. The "clear" areas on the mask must be transparent to 1-nm X-rays and the "dark" areas must stop them. No materials transmit X-rays easily, so the clear areas need to be made from thin layers of low mass materials. Si, Si_3N_4, SiC, and BN a few microns thick are common choices. The dark areas need to be made from materials like Au or W which absorb X-rays, with W likely being the dominant choice in the future because of concerns with Au contamination in fabrication facilities. Thus a typical mask structure is a thin Si_3N_4 membrane with a deposited Au or W film etched to define the mask pattern. Such a mask is a mechanically fragile and requires very careful manufacturing to control stresses in the thin membrane. The actual writing of the pattern on the X-ray mask is usually accomplished using photoresist spun on to the Au or W absorber and direct write e-beam lithography.

There are several options for X-ray sources. The simplest approach is to bombard a metal target with high energy electrons. The incident electrons excite core level electrons in the target, which emit X-rays when they fall back to their normal states. (Recall Figure 4–17.) The wavelengths of the emitted X-ray photons are characteristic of the target material. The intensity of these sources can be increased by water cooling and rotating the target. It is also possible to use laser-heated plasma sources. In these sources, an intense laser pulse is applied to a thin metal film, causing vaporization of the metal. The energy is high enough that the superheated metal vapor radiates X-rays with a wavelength of 0.5 – 2 nm. The most intense X-ray sources are synchrotron storage rings. In these systems, electrons are circulated around a ring at energies of $10^6 - 10^9$ eV. At each bending magnet around such a ring, an intense X-ray beam is emitted, each of which is suitable as the source for an X-ray exposure system. Thus one storage ring can support many aligners. Several such rings have been built in recent years for lithography research and ICs have been fabricated with them. The major drawback to synchrotron storage rings is their very high cost. However, any lithography approach for < 0.1-μm feature sizes is likely going to be very expensive and synchrotron sources are the likely choice if X-ray systems are widely used in the future. Figure 5–54 illustrates a modern proximity X-ray system with a synchrotron source.

Another area of current research involves lenses and mirrors for reflecting and focusing X-rays. Most such lenses use reflection from glancing incidence mirrors or multilayer mirrors with layer thicknesses designed to make use of constructive interference

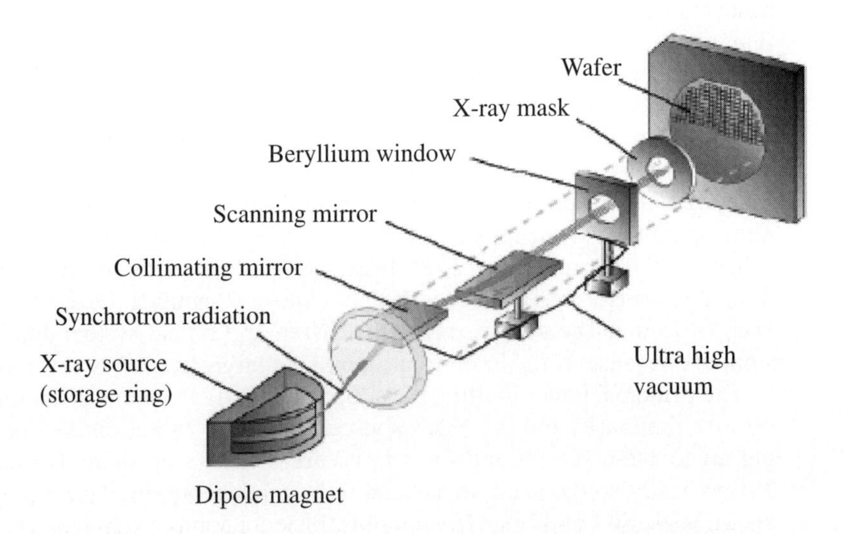

Figure 5–54 Proximity X-ray exposure system. This figure was taken from the Sematech Web site at http://www.sematech.org/public/.

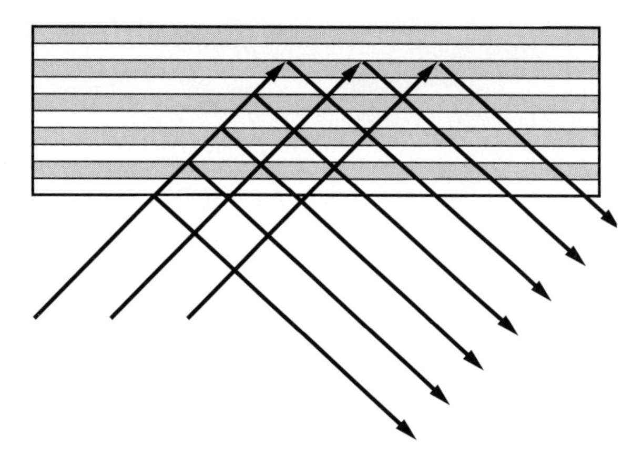

Figure 5–55 Multilayer mirror suitable for X-ray reflection.

effects. If such lenses could be sufficiently developed, they hold out the promise of making X-ray masks on reflecting substrates, a development that would have a significant impact on the potential for X-ray exposure systems.

The most promising approach for X-ray mirrors uses the concept illustrated in Figure 5–55. These mirrors use alternating layers of two materials with widely different electron concentrations (often Mo and Si). The high-mass layer acts as a scatterer and the low-mass layer acts as a spacer. The thicknesses are chosen so that constructive interference occurs between the partially reflected waves at each layer. These mirrors were originally developed for X-ray astronomy [5.38] and in recent years have achieved reflectivities above 60%. They require extraordinary manufacturing tolerances on the layer thicknesses (typically 0.1 nm) because of the short wavelengths the mirrors are designed to reflect. If such mirrors can be developed for lithography applications, designs have been proposed for complete exposure systems that use them both for masks and for reducing optics [5.39]. In the latter case, the mirrors would have to be constructed on curved surfaces. Such systems have been termed EUVs or Extreme Ultraviolet lithography systems. Figure 5–56 conceptually illustrates what an EUV lithography system might look like.

The throughput capability and the potential resolution of X-ray lithography systems will likely drive continued research on these systems. If the mask problems can be solved for either proximity or EUV systems, such systems may provide a viable manufacturing option for < 0.1-μm features.

5.6.3 Advanced Mask Engineering

Efforts to continue to improve the resolution of lithography systems must focus on the entire system, not just the exposure tool. Powerful approaches to designing masks with a more sophisticated pattern than simply a binary, exact representation of the desired pattern are beginning to be used. These methods include optical proximity correction

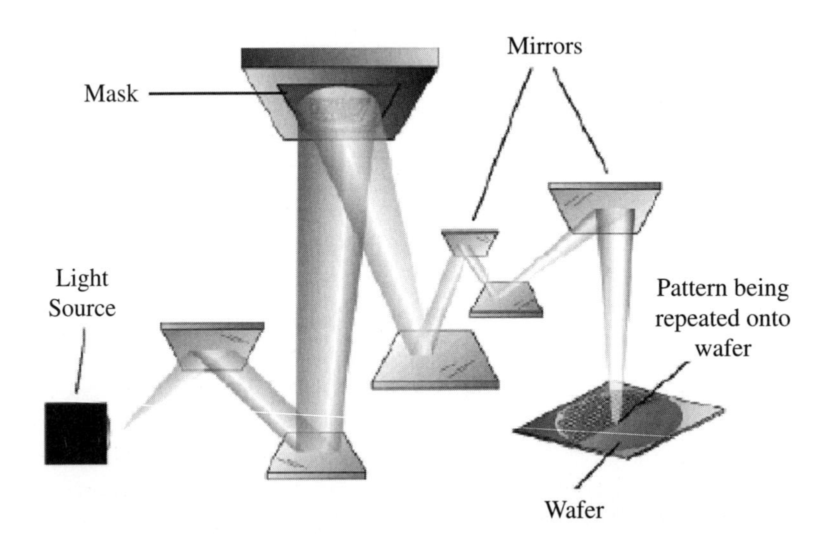

Figure 5–56 Conceptual drawing of an EUV imaging system. The mirrors reduce the projected image by about 4X. This figure was taken directly from the Sematech Web site at http://www.sematech.org/public/.

and phase shift masks. It is likely that these methods will be more widely used in the future. The major barriers to more widespread use include the sophisticated software tools that are needed to help in designing such masks, and of course, the higher cost of the mask fabrication itself. Since many of these techniques involve placing features on the mask that are smaller than the minimum feature size, mask inspection and defect detection are also more difficult with such masks. Nevertheless, these methods do provide a significant improvement in resolution and hence the motivation for using them is strong.

Many of the proposed replacements for optical lithography require innovation or invention in the masks used with the exposure tool. It is likely that these issues will have a significant impact on which of the postoptical exposure systems actually reach manufacturing maturity.

5.6.4 New Resists

DNQ resists that have been the mainstay of the semiconductor industry for many years are now being replaced with new materials and new chemistries more suitable for DUV exposure systems. The basic resin (Novolac) in DNQ resists begins to strongly absorb UV radiation below 250-nm wavelengths. Thus these resists cannot be used for 248-nm KrF or 193-nm ArF excimer laser-based exposure systems.

The concept of chemical amplification has proven to be a powerful idea for new resists and many new materials have been developed in recent years. Resists of this type are now used in manufacturing in 0.25-μm and 0.18-μm technology generations and will likely dominate the industry for some years to come. Many alternative material systems have been and are being explored, including inorganic resists (Ag-doped Se-Ge) [5.40], organosilanes which form SiO_2 when exposed [5.41], and polysilanes [5.42]. Standard e-beam resists like PMMA are also available, of course. While it is not clear at this point which of these approaches will ultimately be successful, it does seem likely that suitable resists will be found with adequate sensitivity, resolution, defect density, and process robustness for technology generations beyond 0.1 μm.

Before concluding this section, there are several other topics we will briefly consider. These include planarization and multilayer resists. These improvements to the basic lithography process are aimed at improving the resolution of the image produced in the resist or improving the resist sensitivity. Some of these techniques are currently beginning to find use in manufacturing.

The need for planarization in resist processing was briefly discussed earlier in connection with Figure 5–22. The issue is that surface topography under the resist will cause thickness variations in the spun on resist. The result of this will be changes in the exposure process in thin versus thick regions. The thick resist regions will be underexposed, or the thin regions will be overexposed and therefore there will be linewidth variations in the latent image produced in the resist. From a practical perspective, these issues become most important at steps in the underlying topography because that is where there are abrupt changes in resist thickness. Generally what is observed is a narrowing of the resist image right at the step and a broadening of the image just off the step. These effects become very important when the height of the step is on the order of the feature size being printed, a criterion which is increasingly being met in silicon technology as linewidths shrink.

A solution to this problem is to planarize the wafer surface before the resist is applied. In back-end processing, it is common today to use Chemical Mechanical Polishing (CMP) to do this, as discussed in Chapters 2 and 11. CMP is also beginning to find application in front-end processing as well. (See Figure 2–9 in the CMOS process flow in Chapter 2.) Alternatives include the use of multilayer resists, which we will discuss below.

Figure 5–57 illustrates the basic idea behind multilayer resists. A two- or three-layer structure is used, whose purpose is to first planarize the underlying topography and then to form a relatively thin photoresist layer on top, which is the imaging layer. The intermediate layer may be needed as an etch stop in some particular cases. While there are a number of variations to this structure, the basic idea is as follows. First a relatively thick layer is spun onto the wafer to planarize the surface. Often this is simply a photoresist layer that is not sensitive to the particular wavelength of light being used in the exposure system. For example, PMMA, which is an electron beam resist that is not sensitive in the near UV, might be used in connection with a g-line or i-line exposure system. In the simplest mutlilayer resist systems, this layer would then be baked and a second thin layer of resist spun directly on top of it. This upper resist layer is sensitive to the exposure wavelength and after appropriate prebaking, this resist layer would then be exposed. Because the imaging resist layer is thin and uniform in thickness, a high-resolution latent image can be generated. The upper imaging layer is then developed.

Using this layer now as a mask, the lower planarizing layer is now flood exposed with a DUV source. Here it is important that the upper imaging layer not be transparent to the DUV, so that the lower planarizing layer is exposed only in the regions where the upper layer has been developed away. With a PMMA lower-layer DUV exposure would work since this resist is sensitive to DUV wavelengths. In essence, the thin imaging layer is being used as a contact mask for the exposure of the lower layer. As we saw earlier,

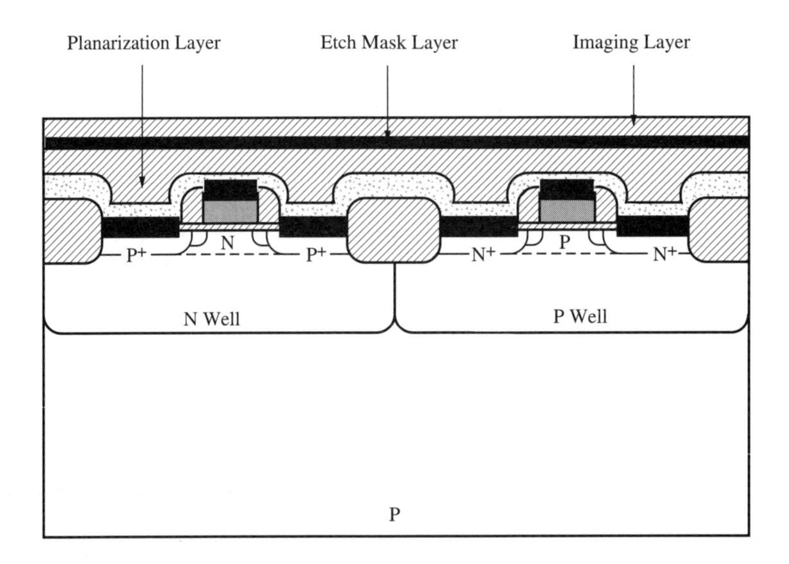

Figure 5–57 Multilayer resist structure designed to create a thin, uniform imaging layer suitable for high-resolution imaging.

contact printing can produce high-resolution images because it minimizes diffraction effects. The lower resist latent image is now developed, producing a patterned resist layer that can then be used to etch underlying layers or as an ion implantation mask.

An alternative to the above process uses the intermediate etch stop layer also shown in Figure 5–57. Here this additional layer is deposited between the planarizing and imaging layers. Typically this might be a layer of SiO_2 deposited from a spun on glass source, or it could be deposited by PECVD at a low temperature that could be tolerated by the planarizing layer. The exposure and developing of the upper imaging layer proceeds as described previously. However, etching is now used to transfer the pattern into the bottom planarizing layer. First Reactive Ion Etching (RIE) is used to etch the intermediate etch stop layer using the imaging resist as a mask. Since the imaging resist layer is thin, it likely would not be possible to use this layer as a mask during RIE etching all the way through the underlying thick planarization layer. Thus the etch stop layer is used as an intermediate pattern transfer layer. Once the pattern is etched in the etch stop layer, RIE etching of the bottom planarization layer then transfers the pattern to that layer. If PMMA or another organic material is used for the bottom layer, an O_2 RIE process can be used to etch this layer. This process has high selectivity to the intermediate layer (SiO_2, for example) and hence a relatively thin etch stop layer can be used. Whether a two- or three-layer process flow is used, the key ideas are planarization of the underlying topography followed by exposure of a thin high-resolution imaging resist layer.

Multilayer resists have not found widespread use in manufacturing at this point in time, primarily because the more complex process has not been economically viable because of high defect densities. However as minimum feature sizes continue to shrink, the concept of a thin and uniform imaging layer becomes increasingly attractive and this approach may be used in the future [5.43].

Another variation in these mutlilayer resist structures is to make the lower planarizing layer act as an Antireflection Coating (ARC) as well as a planarizing layer. In this case, the material chosen for the planarizing layer is highly absorbing at the exposure wavelength and does not bleach appreciably. Thus photons that pass through the upper thin imaging resist layer will be absorbed by the planarizing layer and will not reflect off underlying substrate features. Hence the term antireflection coating that is applied to such layers. Once the latent image is formed in the upper imaging layer, it can be transferred through the lower planarizing layer (ARC) by dry etching following development. ARC layers are useful in DNQ resists to minimize standing wave effects (Figure 5–24). They are essential in DUV resists because these resists do not bleach and hence reflections are more of an issue throughout the exposure.

5.7 Summary of Key Ideas

Lithography is one of the fundamental technologies on which modern ICs are based. The two key elements of modern optical lithography systems are the exposure tool and the photoresist. Exposure tools today generally use projection optics with diffraction-limited refracting lenses. These systems can print an area on the order of a few cm^2 on the wafer so that a step and repeat or step and scan approach must be used to print an entire wafer. g-line and i-line resists today are largely based on DNQ materials, which are used for manufacturing down to the 0.35-μm generation. DUV resists that use chemical amplification are used in the 0.25-μm and 0.18-μm technology generations and should be suitable for several future generations. Lithography simulation tools are based on two scientific fields: Fourier optics to describe the performance of exposure tools and resist chemistry to describe the formation of the mask pattern in the resist. These tools are very useful today in understanding and optimizing the performance of lithographic systems. A major change in the way in which patterns are printed on wafers will likely have to occur within the next 10 years. It does not seem possible to extend today's optical lithography techniques to the end of the SIA NTRS. Options do exist to replace optical lithography, but none are clearly viable today. If history is any guide, however, solutions will be found to the lithography problem, allowing continued shrinkage in semiconductor feature sizes.

5.8 References

[5.1]. "National Technology Roadmap for Semiconductors," SIA, 1997.

[5.2]. J. W. Goodman, *Introduction to Fourier Optics*, McGraw-Hill, 1968.

[5.3]. C. A. Mack, *Inside Prolith, a Comprehensive Guide to Optical Lithography Simulation*, Finle Technologies, Austin TX, 1997.

[5.4]. W. M. Moreau, *Semiconductor Lithography Principles, Practices and Materials*, Plenum Press, 1988.

[5.5]. W. Waldo, "Techniques and Tools for Optical Lithography" in *Handbook of VLSI Microlithography Principles, Technology and Applications*, edited by W. B. Glendinning and J. N. Helbert, Noyes Publications, 1991.

[5.6]. B. J. Lin, "Electromagnetic Near-Field Diffraction Pattern of a Medium Slit," *J. Opt. Soc. of Amer.*, vol. 62, p. 976, 1972.

[5.7]. H. Ito and C. G. Willson, "Polymers in Electronics," T. Davidson, ed., *Symposium Series 242*, American Chemical Society, Washington DC, p. 11, 1984.

[5.8]. D. Seeger, "Chemically Amplified Resists for Advanced Lithography: Road to Success or Detour?" *Solid State Tech.*, p. 115, June 1997.

[5.9]. D. Wallraff et al. "Single Layer Chemically Amplified Photoresists for 193 nm Lithography," *J. Vac. Sci. Tech.*, vol. B11, p. 2783, 1993.

[5.10]. H. Ito, "Deep-UV Resists: Evolution and Status," *Solid State Tech.*, p. 164, July 1996.

[5.11]. H. Ito, "Chemical Amplification Resists: History and Development Within IBM," *IBM J. Res. and Dev.*, vol. 41, p. 69, 1997.

[5.12]. M. D. Levenson, "Extending the Lifetime of Optical Lithography Technologies with Wavefront Engineering," *Jpn. J. Appl. Phys.*, vol. 33, p. 6765, 1994.

[5.13]. J. P. Stirniman and M. L. Rieger, *Proc. SPIE*, vol. 2197, 294, 1994.

[5.14]. M. D. Levenson, N. S. Visnwathen, and R. A. Simpson, "Improving Resolution in Photolithography with a Phase Shifting Mask," *IEEE Trans. Elec. Dev.*, vol. ED-29, p. 1828, 1982.

[5.15]. R. Larrabee, L. Linholm, and M. T. Postek, "Microlithography Metrology" in *Handbook of VLSI Microlithography Principles, Technology and Applications*, edited by W. B. Glendinning and J. N. Helbert, Noyes Publications, 1991.

[5.16]. D. Nyyssonen and R. D. Larrabee, "Submicrometer Linewidth Metrology in the Optical Microscope," *J. Res. Natl. Bur. Stand.,* vol. 92, p. 187, 1987.

[5.17]. M. G. Buehler, "Microelectronic Test Chips for VLSI Electronics," in *VLSI Electronics: Microstructure Science*, vol. 6, p. 529, Academic Press, 1983.

[5.18]. T. F. Hasan and D. S. Perloff, "Automated Electrical Measurement Techniques to Control VLSI Linewidth, Resistivity and Registration," *Test and Measurement World*, vol. 5, p. 78, 1985.

[5.19]. D. K. Schroder, *Semiconductor Material and Device Characterization*, John Wiley & Sons, 1990.

[5.20]. F. H. Dill, "Optical Lithography," *IEEE Trans. Elec. Dev.*, vol. ED-22, p. 440, 1975.

[5.21]. F. H. Dill, W. P. Hornberger, P. S. Hauge, and J. M. Shaw, "Characterization of Positive Photoresist," *IEEE Trans. Elec. Dev.*, vol. ED-22, p. 445, 1975.

[5.22]. K. L. Konnerth and F. H.Dill, "In-Situ Measurement of Dielectric Thickness During Etching of Developing Processes," *IEEE Trans. Elec. Dev.*, vol. ED-22, p. 452, 1975.

[5.23]. F. H.Dill, A. R. Neureuther, J. A. Tuttle, and E. J. Walker, "Modeling Projection Printing of Positive Photoresists," *IEEE Trans. Elec. Dev.*, vol. ED-22, p. 456, 1975.

[5.24]. W. G. Oldham, S. N. Nandgaonkar, A. R. Neureuther, and M. O'Toole, "A General Simulator for VLSI Lithography and Etching Processes: Part 1—Application to Projection Lithography," *IEEE Trans. Elec. Dev.*, vol. ED-26, p. 717, 1979.

[5.25]. C. A. Mack, "PROLITH: A Comprehensive Optical Lithography Model," *Optical Microlithography IV, Proc. SPIE,* vol. 538, p. 207, 1985.

[5.26]. DEPICT User's manual, Dec. 1996, Avant! Inc.

[5.27]. ATHENA User's Manual, Oct. 1996, Silvaco Inc.

[5.28]. C. A. Mack, "Analytical Expression for the Standing Wave Intensity in Photoresist," *Appl. Optics*, vol. 25, p. 1958, 1986.

[5.29]. C. A. Mack, "Absorption and Exposure in Positive Photoresists," *Appl. Optics*, vol. 27, p. 4913, 1988.

[5.30]. F. H. Dill and J. M. Shaw, "Thermal Effects on the Photoresist AZ1350J," *IBM Journal Res. and Dev.*, vol. 21, p. 210, 1977.

[5.31]. C. A. Mack and R. T. Carback, "Modeling the Effects of Prebake on Positive Resist Processing," *Proc. of Kodak Microelectronics Seminar*, p. 155, 1985.

[5.32]. E. J. Walker, "Reduction of Photoresist Standing-Wave Effects by Postexposure Bake," *IEEE Trans. Elec. Dev.*, vol. ED-22, p. 464, 1975.

[5.33]. C. A. Mack, "New Kinetic Model for Resist Dissolution," *J. Electrochem. Soc.*, vol. 139, p. L35, 1992.

[5.34]. A. N. Broers, W. W. Molzen, J. J. Cuomo, and N. D. Wittels, "Electron Beam Fabrication of 80 Å Metal Structures," *Appl. Phys. Lett.*, vol. 29, 1976.

[5.35]. C. Y. Chang, G. Owen, R. F. Pease, and T. Kailath, "A Computational Method for the Correction of Proximity Effects in Electron-Beam Lithography, Electron-Beam, X-ray and Ion Beam Submicron Lithographies," *Proc. SPIE*, vol. 1671, p. 208, 1992.

[5.36]. S. D. Berger and J. M. Gibson, "New Approach to Projection-Electron Lithography with Demonstrated 0.1 μm Linewidth," *Appl. Phys. Lett.*, vol. 57, p. 153, 1990.

[5.37]. L. R. Harriott, "Preliminary Results From a Prototype Projection Electron-Beam Stepper —SCALPEL Proof-of-Concept System," *J. Vac. Sci. Tech.*, vol. B14, p. 3825, 1996.

[5.38]. E. Spiller, "Reflective Multilayer Coatings for the Far UV Region," *Appl. Optics*, vol. 15, p. 2333, 1975.

[5.39]. A. M. Hawryluk, N. M. Ceglio, and D. A. Markle, "EUV Lithography," *Solid State Tech.*, p. 151, 1997.

[5.40]. Y. Yoshikawa, O.Ochi, H. Nagai, and Y. Mizushima, "A Novel Inorganic Photoresist Utilizing Ag Photodoping in Se-Ge Glass Films," *Appl. Phys. Lett.*, vol. 29, p. 677, 1977.

[5.41]. D. C. Hofer, R. D. Miller, and C. G. Willson, "Polysilane Bilayer UV Lithography," *SPIE Proc.*, vol. 469, p. 16, 1984.

[5.42]. R. R. Kunz, P. A. Bianconi, M. W. Horn, R. R. Paladuga, D. C. Shaver, D. A. Smith, and C. A. Freed, "Polsilyne Resists for 193 nm Excimer Laser Lithography," *Advances in Resist Technology and Processing VIII, SPIE Proc.*, vol. 1446, p. 218, 1991.

[5.43]. D. E. Seeger, D. C. La Turlipe Jr., R. R. Kunz, C. M. Garza, and M. A. Hanratty, "Thin-Film Imaging: Past, Present, Prognosis," *IBM J. Res. and Dev.*, vol. 41, p. 105, 1997.

5.9 Problems

5.1. Calculate and plot versus exposure wavelength the theoretical resolution and depth of focus for a projection exposure system with an *NA* of 0.6 (about the best that can be done today). Assume $k_1 = 0.6$ and $k_2 = 0.5$ (both typical values). Consider wavelengths between 100 nm and 1000 nm (DUV and visible light). Indicate the common exposure wavelengths being used or considered today on your plot (g-line, i-line, KrF, and ArF). Will an ArF source be adequate for the 0.13-μm and 0.1-μm technology generations according to these simple calculations?

5.2. In a particular positive resist process it is sometimes noticed that there is difficulty developing away the last few hundred angstroms of resist in exposed areas. This sometimes causes etching problems because the resist remains in the areas to be etched. Suggest a possible cause of this problem and therefore propose a solution.

5.3. An X-ray exposure system uses photons with an energy of 1 keV. If the separation between the mask and wafer is 20 μm, estimate the diffraction-limited resolution that is achievable by this system.

5.4. Estimate the exposure wavelength that was used in the simulation example in Figure 5–44 in the text. Assume that the index of refraction of the photoresist is 1.68 (typical value).

5.5. In this chapter, we considered an example of an isolated space on a mask and saw that the Fourier transform of this pattern is the $\sin(x)/x$ function. This function describes the spatial variation of the light intensity that the objective lens must capture. An even more illustrative example of the effects of diffraction is given by a mask pattern consisting of a periodic pattern of lines and spaces as shown below.

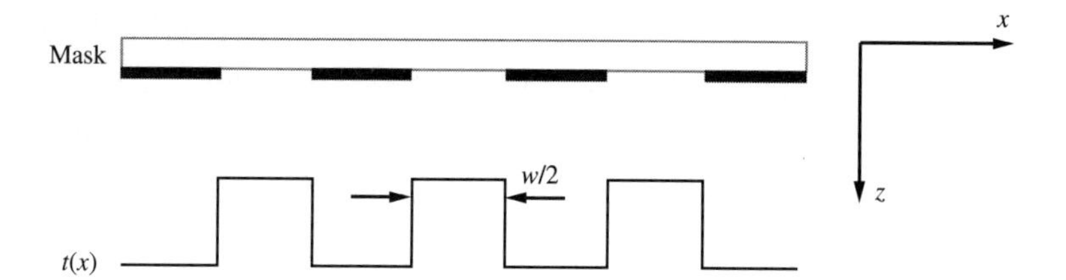

Find the Fourier transform for this mask function and plot it as was done in the example in the chapter. The objective lens must capture at least the first diffraction order if it is going to resolve features with a pitch p. Use this criterion to derive an equation like Eq. (5.2) for the resolution of such a system.

5.6. Assume that Figure 5–46 in the text was experimentally determined for a 0.6-μm-thick resist with an index of refraction of 1.68. Estimate the Dill resist parameters from the data in this figure.

5.7. Lithography often has to be done over underlying topography on a silicon chip. This can result in variations in the resist thickness as the underlying topography goes up and down. This can sometimes cause some parts of the photoresist image to be underexposed and/or other regions to be overexposed. Explain in terms of the chemistry of the resist exposure process why these underexposure and overexposure problems occur.

5.8. As described in this chapter, there are no clear choices for lithography systems beyond optical projection tools based on 193-nm ArF eximer lasers. One possibility is an optical projection system using a 157-nm F_2 excimer laser.

a. Assuming a numerical aperture of 0.8 and $k_1 = 0.75$, what is the expected resolution of such a system using a first order estimate of resolution?

b. Actual projections for such systems suggest that they might be capable of resolving features suitable for the 2009 0.07-μm generation. Suggest three approaches to actually achieving this resolution with these systems.

5.9. Current optical projection lithography tools produce diffraction-limited aerial images. A typical aerial image produced by such a system is shown in the simulation below where a square and rectangular mask regions produce the image shown. (The mask features are the black outlines, the calculated aerial image is the gray scale inside the black rectangles.) The major feature of the aerial image is its rounded corners compared to the sharp square corners of the desired pattern. Explain physically why these features look the way they do, using diffraction theory and the physical properties of modern projection optical lithography tools.

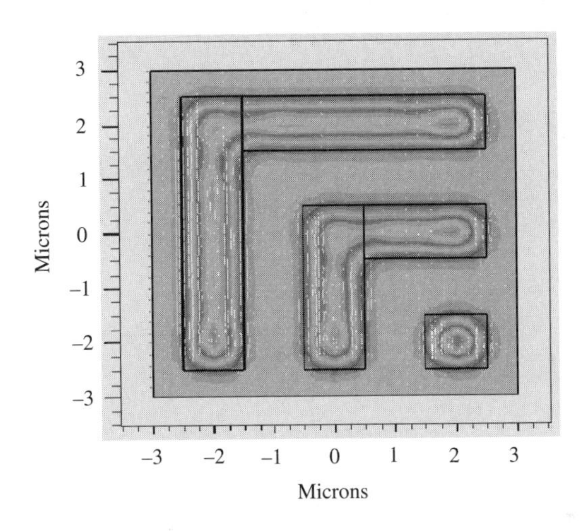

5.10. Future optical lithography systems will likely use shorter exposure wavelengths to achieve higher resolution and they will also likely use planarization techniques to provide "flat" substrates on which to expose the resist layers. Explain why "flat" substrates will be more important in the future than they have been in the past.

Thermal Oxidation and the Si/SiO$_2$ Interface

6

6.1 Introduction

Silicon is unique among semiconductor materials in that its surface can be easily passivated with an oxide layer. The interface between Si and SiO$_2$ is perhaps the most carefully studied of all material interfaces and its electrical and mechanical properties as well as those of the oxide layer itself are almost ideal. SiO$_2$ layers are easily grown thermally on silicon or deposited on many substrates. They adhere well, they block the diffusion of dopants and many other unwanted impurities, they are resistant to most of the chemicals used in silicon processing and yet can be easily patterned and etched with specific chemicals or dry etched with plasmas, they are excellent insulators, and they have stable and reproducible bulk properties. The interface that forms between Si and SiO$_2$ has very few mechanical or electrical defects and is stable over time. These properties make MOS structures easy to build in silicon and they imply that silicon devices of all types are generally reliable and stable. Virtually all other semiconductor/insulator combinations suffer from one or more problems that significantly limit their applicability.

We saw a number of applications of SiO$_2$ layers in the CMOS technology example in Chapter 2. These included use as the gate dielectric layer in MOS devices, as a mask against implantation, as an isolation region laterally between adjacent devices, and as an insulator between metal layers in back-end processing. These and some other uses are illustrated in Figure 6–1.

The SIA NTRS provides a roadmap for SiO$_2$ and other insulating layers as part of its general technology requirements. Some of the key issues are summarized in Table 6–1 [6.1]. Most of these requirements relate to oxides < 10 nm since these are the critical gate insulators and tunneling oxides in modern MOS structures. The last two rows in the table relate to thicker insulators used primarily for masking and in back-end processing. These insulating layers are normally deposited rather than thermally grown and will be discussed in more detail in Chapters 9 and 11.

Even at room temperature, silicon exposed to an oxygen or air ambient will form a thin native oxide layer on its surface. This oxide rapidly covers the surface to a thickness of 0.5–1 nm (5–10 Å). Growth then slows down and effectively stops after a few hours, with a final thickness on the order of 1–2 nm. Both the growth rate and the final native oxide thickness depend on the surface preparation and in particular on the presence or absence of chemical residues from cleaning procedures. For example, the SC-1 and SC-2 cleaning procedures we discussed in Chapter 4 create chemical oxides on the silicon surface which are typically 1–2 nm thick.

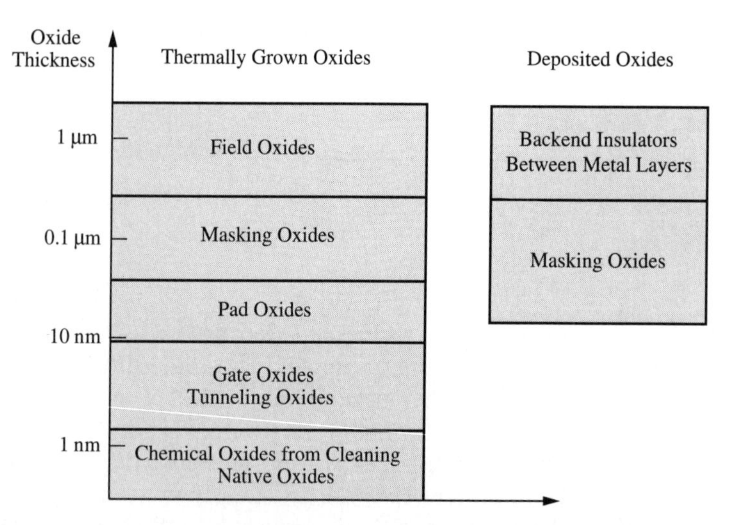

Figure 6–1 Uses of SiO_2 in silicon technology.

Table 6–1 Future projections for silicon technology taken from the SIA NTRS [6.1]

Year of First DRAM Shipment	1997	1999	2003	2006	2009	2012
Minimum Feature Size (nm)	250	180	130	100	70	50
DRAM Bits/Chip	256M	1G	4G	16G	64G	256G
Minimum Supply Voltage (volts)	1.8–2.5	1.5–1.8	1.2–1.5	0.9–1.2	0.6–0.9	0.5–0.6
Gate Oxide T_{ox} Equivalent (nm)	4–5	3–4	2–3	1.5–2	<1.5	<1.0
Thickness Control (% 3 σ)	± 4	± 4	± 4–6	± 4–8	± 4–8	± 4–8
Equivalent Maximum E-field (MV cm^{-1})	4–5	5	5	>5	>5	>5
Gate Oxide Leakage (DRAM) (pA μm^{-2})	<0.01	<0.01	<0.01	<0.01	<0.01	<0.01
Tunnel Oxide (nm)	8.5	8	7.5	7	6.5	6
Maximum Wiring Levels	6	6–7	7	7–8	8–9	9
Dielectric Constant, K for Intermetal Insulator	3.0–4.1	2.5–3.0	1.5–2.0	1.5–2.0	<1.5	<1.5

The most critical application of insulators in CMOS technology is as the gate insulator. As shown in Table 6–1, these layers are typically 3–5 nm thick in current state-of-the-art technology and are projected to be < 1 nm in another 10–15 years. Even today, these layers are only about 25—50 atomic layers thick. It is quite remarkable that VLSI chips can be manufactured today with tens of millions of such oxides, each defect free and capable of reliably sustaining electric fields within a factor of about two of the material limit of SiO_2 which is about 10–15 MV cm^{-1}. Notice also in Table 6–1 that gate insulators must be controlled in thickness to essentially single atomic distances. Continued scaling will make it very difficult for SiO_2 films to meet all these requirements. As a result, it is very likely that the very thin gate insulators projected for the future will not be pure SiO_2 films. Oxynitride films (SiO_2 with nitrogen incorporated through a variety of processes) are the most likely near-term solution.

With films as thin as those projected in the NTRS, the term "insulator" begins to lose some of its meaning because such thin films will conduct finite amounts of current due to quantum mechanical tunneling of electrons or holes. This process occurs because of the wave nature of electrons and basically allows electrons to pass through an otherwise impenetrable barrier such as SiO_2, if the barrier is thin enough. The probability of such an event happening decreases exponentially with oxide thickness, so tunneling oxides must be quite thin for significant currents to flow. If a polysilicon gate is deposited on top of such an oxide and electrically isolated by surrounding it with SiO_2 on all sides, then the electrons which tunnel through the thin oxide underneath the polysilicon can be trapped in the poly layer, allowing it to take on a negative charge. This can be used as the basis for a nonvolatile memory element. In fact, oxide layers between 4 and 10 nm are often used in electrically programmable memories and are referred to as tunneling oxides in these applications.

In gate dielectrics, tunneling is undesirable and in some applications like DRAM pass transistors is a major problem since it directly affects data retention. The specifications on leakage current shown in Table 6–1 for DRAMs are likely not achievable in SiO_2 layers thinner than about 4 nm and so it is likely that thicker gate dielectrics will be used in these applications. For more general-purpose logic applications, higher levels of gate leakage current can be tolerated.

Many of the other applications listed in Figure 6–1 were discussed in detail in Chapter 2. Thermal oxides in the range of 10–30 nm are often used under Si_3N_4 layers as stress relief or "pad" oxides during LOCOS type processes. We saw several examples of this application in the CMOS process in Chapter 2. Thicker thermal oxides often serve as masks for ion implantation or gas-phase doping steps. Here it is usually only important that the oxide layer be thick enough to block dopant penetration into the underlying silicon substrate. We will consider these applications more carefully in Chapters 7 and 8. Thick oxides may also serve as "field" or isolation oxides in many technologies. In this case they provide lateral isolation between adjacent components on the wafer surface.

It is also quite possible to deposit SiO_2 layers using CVD or LPCVD techniques. For back-end applications, after the wafers have metal on them, deposition is the only option. In fact for any application in which the oxide must be placed on top of underlying films, deposition is generally the only option since silicon may not be available from the underlying films for SiO_2 thermal growth. Deposition usually involves a much smaller "thermal budget" compared to thermal oxidation and hence is preferred even in front-end processes whenever it is important to limit the temperature cycle the wafers are subjected to. Deposited oxides are usually not used for layers thinner than about 10 nm because control of the deposition process is not as good as the thermal oxidation process. The interface between a deposited oxide and the underlying silicon is not as perfect electrically as that formed by a thermal oxide either, so thermal oxides are usually used for gate dielectrics and other critical oxides in device structures. It is possible to anneal a deposited oxide/Si interface, however, to produce electrical properties close to those of a thermally grown oxide. The simplest way to "anneal" such an interface is simply to grow a thin thermal oxide underneath the deposited oxide. This is straightforward to do because new SiO_2 always grows at the Si/SiO_2 interface, as we will see in the next section.

Finally, note that the NTRS in Table 6–1 specifies a dielectric constant less than 3.9 (SiO_2) for intermetal dielectrics in technology generations in the future. This is required in order to improve the speed of interconnects (RC delay) and implies that deposited films will not be SiO_2 in back-end processes in the future. We will discuss so-called "low K" deposited dielectrics in Chapter 11. In contrast to back-end "low K" dielectrics, gate oxides are likely to use "high K" dielectrics in the future. Thus the equivalent electrical gate oxide thicknesses in Table 6–1 may be achieved with higher K materials physically thicker than the values in the table.

This chapter will focus primarily on the thermal oxidation process and the properties of the Si/SiO_2 interface. Deposited oxides and other deposited thin films are described in detail in Chapter 9.

6.2 Historical Development and Basic Concepts

A number of experiments done in the past 30 years [6.2–6.5] have conclusively shown that when silicon is oxidized, the oxidation process occurs at the Si/SiO_2 interface as illustrated in Figure 6–2. Because of this, a new interface is constantly forming and moving downward into the silicon substrate. Silicon oxidation therefore occurs by the inward diffusion of the oxidant, rather than the outward diffusion of silicon. Conceptually, the simplest way to demonstrate this is to grow an SiO_2 layer with one oxygen isotope and then continue the growth with a second isotope (O^{16} and O^{18}, for example). Profiling through the resulting composite oxide with a mass sensitive technique can then determine whether the second oxide grows at the top or bottom surface. This and other related experiments have consistently shown that the new oxide grows at the Si/SiO_2 interface.

Conceptually one can think of this process in the following way. The Si atoms in the substrate are bonded to other Si atoms. These bonds must be broken, oxygen atoms inserted between the silicon atoms, and finally Si-O bonds formed. The process involves a volume expansion because of the room needed for the oxygen atoms. As illustrated in

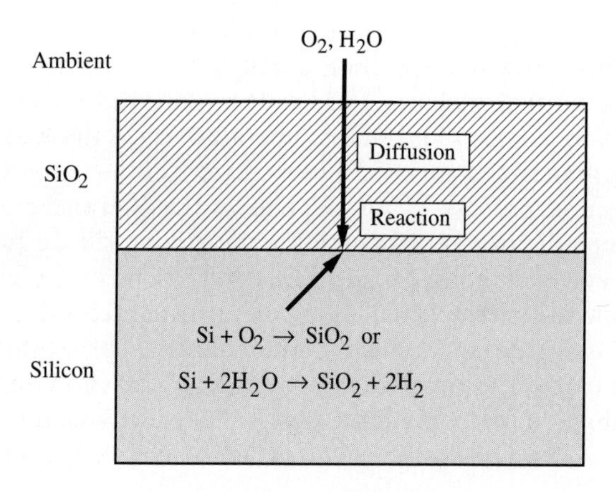

Figure 6–2 Basic process for the oxidation of silicon. The chemical reaction takes place at the Si/SiO_2 interface.

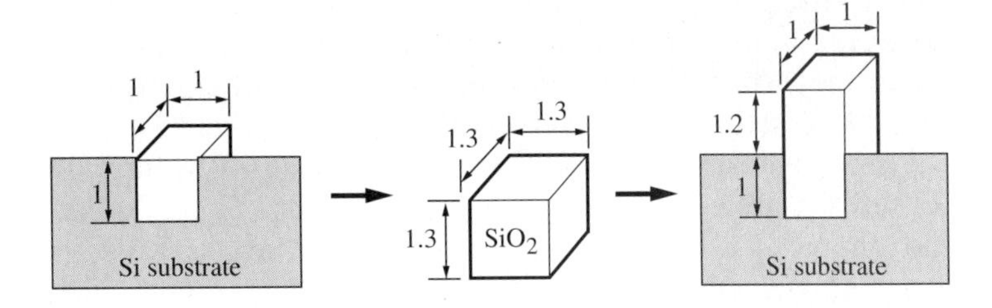

Figure 6–3 Volume expansion that occurs during silicon oxidation. A unit volume of silicon on the left is transformed into SiO_2. In the middle the volume expansion is unconstrained; on the right the substrate restricts the expansion to one dimension.

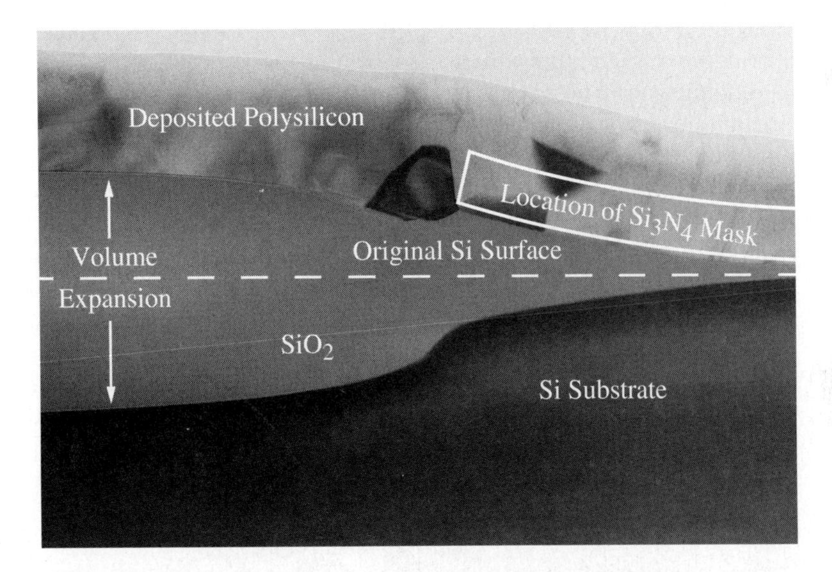

Figure 6–4 Scanning electron micrograph of a simple LOCOS structure. The silicon oxidation was masked on the right side by a Si_3N_4 layer. A polysilicon layer has been deposited on top of the structure, after the Si_3N_4 layer was stripped, to provide contrast in the picture. Note that the grown oxide on the left side occupies approximately twice the volume of the silicon consumed in the oxidation. Courtesy of J. Bravman, Stanford University.

the center of Figure 6–3, the oxide would like to expand by 30% in all three dimensions to accommodate the oxygen atoms. However because the silicon substrate prevents expansion in the two lateral directions, the only option is for the oxide to expand upward as shown on the right of Figure 6–3. The volume is thus accommodated by a 2.2 times upward expansion of the oxide compared to the volume of the silicon oxidized.

Figure 6–4 illustrates this in a real two-dimensional structure. This example is a SEM cross section of a simple LOCOS process like the one we described in Chapter 2. On planar surfaces, most of the volume expansion is accommodated simply by the oxide growing up above the original silicon surface as in Figure 6–3. On shaped surfaces, which are common especially in advanced silicon device structures, the expansion may not be so easily accommodated. LOCOS results in a nonplanar Si/SiO_2 interface between the nitride masked and oxidized regions and an obvious transition region between the two. This transition region takes on a characteristic "bird's beak" shape because of lateral oxidation under the nitride mask.

Oxide layers grown on silicon are amorphous. This might seem surprising initially because we are oxidizing a single-crystal substrate and SiO_2 exists in both crystalline and amorphous phases. However, there are no crystalline forms of SiO_2 whose lattice size closely matches the silicon substrate. Any attempt to grow single-crystal SiO_2 on silicon would therefore result in very large stresses. Such stresses could easily be large enough to generate crystallographic defects in the silicon, which would significantly degrade circuit yield and device performance. Even though the oxide that grows is amorphous, it does have short-range order, which is illustrated in Figure 6–5. SiO_4 tetrahedra are the basic units from which SiO_2 forms. These tetrahedra bond together by sharing oxygen atoms as illustrated on the right of the figure. Such shared atoms are called bridging oxygen atoms. In the amorphous forms of SiO_2 there may also be some nonbridging oxygen atoms present. These phases are often referred to as fused silica. Crystalline forms of SiO_2 such as quartz contain only bridging oxygen bonds. The various crystalline and amorphous forms of SiO_2 arise because of the ability of the bridging oxygen bonds to rotate, allowing the position of one tetrahedron to move with respect to its neighbors. This same rotation is what allows the material to lose long-range order and hence become amorphous. At normal processing temperatures, the thermodynamically stable form of SiO_2 is one of the crystalline forms. These forms are rarely observed in IC structures, however, because the time required for amorphous SiO_2 to rearrange itself into a crystalline form is very long compared to normal diffusion, oxidation, or anneal cycles. Occasionally fused silica furnace tubes that are used in oxidation or diffusion furnaces will crystallize (a process called devitrification) after many months or years at high temperature.

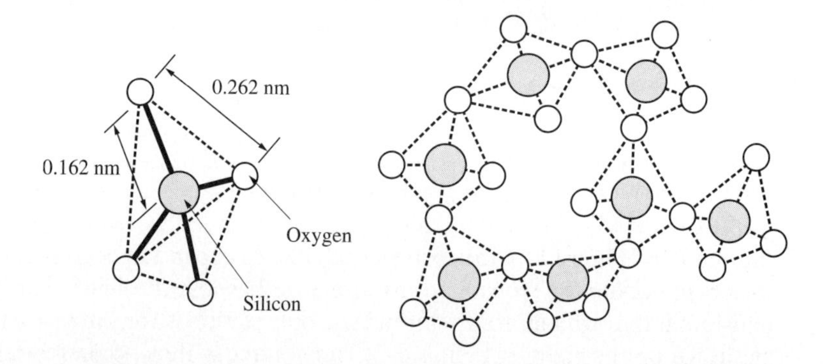

Figure 6–5 Structure of fused silica glass. The silicon atoms are in the center of each of the tetrahedra. The O-O distance is 0.262 nm; and the Si-O distance is 0.162 nm. The Si-Si bond distance depends on the particular form of SiO_2, but is about 0.31 nm. The six-membered ring structure of SiO_2 is shown conceptually on the right.

The oxide layers that grow on Si are normally in compressive stress. At the Si/SiO_2 interface, the growing oxide can expand only upward, not laterally since it must attach to the silicon substrate. This results in compressive stresses that can be as large as 5×10^9 dynes cm^{-2}. At temperatures above about 1000°C, the oxide can relieve some of this stress by viscous flow; at lower temperatures, the oxide viscosity is too high to allow much relief to take place. In addition to these intrinsic stresses which can be present after an oxide is grown, there is also a large difference in the thermal expansion coefficients of Si and SiO_2. As the wafers are cooled down after an oxide is grown, this results in an additional compressive stress in the oxide that can be as high as a few $\times 10^9$ dynes cm^{-2}. These two effects place the silicon substrate in tension; however, the substrate is many times thicker than the oxide layer and as a result, the tensile stresses are scaled down in proportion to the thickness ratio. These effects can easily be observed even on flat silicon wafers. After an oxidation, SiO_2 is normally present on both the top and back surface of the wafer and the stresses from the two oxide films therefore balance. If the oxide is chemically stripped from one surface, however, a distinct bow will be observed in the wafer because of the stresses. In fact measurement of this "wafer curvature" is one way to determine the stress levels in SiO_2 or other thin films on silicon substrates.

Figure 3–15 showed a high-resolution Transmission Electron Micrograph (TEM) of the Si/SiO_2 interface. The atomic resolution in this image clearly shows the silicon crystal structure, the amorphous SiO_2 layer, and the abruptness of the interface. A number of recent studies using TEM and other techniques have shown that the Si/SiO_2 interface is normally characterized by a transition region which is vary narrow (perhaps only one atomic distance). The interface is usually quite flat, although there are steps of one atomic distance which occur occasionally. The abruptness of the interface depends to some extent on the process conditions used to grow the oxide and the interface is a little rougher for oxides which are rapidly grown (H_2O versus O_2 oxidation or high pressure oxidation, for example). The interface is also a little rougher for oxides grown at low temperatures.

The growth kinetics of SiO_2 layers on silicon have been studied for more than three decades and continue to be studied today. Early studies variously reported the growth rate to have a linear, parabolic, logarithmic, inverse logarithmic, or power-law dependence on time. The first widely accepted model of the growth kinetics was due to Deal and Grove in 1965 [6.6]. This work showed that over a wide range of conditions, the growth followed a linear parabolic law which could be explained on a solid theoretical basis. Later work has generally focused on modeling growth conditions for which the Deal-Grove model is inadequate. Examples include very thin oxides, oxides grown in mixed ambients, oxides grown on 2D or 3D silicon surfaces, and oxides grown on heavily doped substrates. We will discuss these and other models later in this chapter.

There has also been for many years a considerable controversy over which oxidant species diffuse through the SiO_2 to grow new layers of oxide. In the gas phase above the wafer, molecular species (O_2 or H_2O) are present. However, these species could dissociate or even ionize to form O, O^-, O_2^-, or many other species once they enter the SiO_2. Some early work [6.2] using an electric field suggested that a charged species was the dominant diffusant. However, later work largely discounted these results and today most workers believe that neutral O_2 and H_2O and/or OH are the dominant species involved in the oxidation process.

The electrical properties of the Si/SiO$_2$ interface have been studied intensively for more than 40 years. A great deal has been learned about these properties, how they depend on process conditions, and how to control them. To first order, the interface is perfect. The densities of defects that are present in modern devices are on the order of 10^9–10^{11} cm^{-2} compared to a silicon surface atom density of about 10^{15} cm^{-2}. Most of the defects that do exist are usually attributed to incompletely oxidized Si atoms or Si atoms with dangling or unsatisfied bonds. However, only about 1 atom in 10^5 has such a defect.

In 1980, in an effort to unify research in this field, Deal [6.7] suggested the nomenclature shown in Figure 6–6 to represent the various types of electrical defects that are found experimentally at the Si/SiO$_2$ interface and in SiO$_2$ layers. There are four basic types of defects or charges that exist. The first, Q_f, is known as the fixed oxide charge. Experimentally we find that a sheet of positive charge (usually 10^9–10^{11} cm^{-2}) exists in the oxide, very close to the interface. It seems to be located within 2 nm of the interface (perhaps closer) and is likely associated with the transition from Si to SiO$_2$. Most physical explanations for Q_f suggest that it is due to incompletely oxidized Si atoms that have a net positive charge. Q_f is called the fixed oxide charge because its charge state does not change during normal device operation. It is positive and invariant under normal conditions.

The second type of charged defect present at the Si/SiO$_2$ interface is Q_{it}, the interface trapped charge. The physical origin of these charges is often suggested to be similar to Q_f. That is, Q_{it} is likely due to some type of incompletely oxidized silicon atom with unsatisfied or dangling bonds located in the oxide, but very close to the interface. However there is a very important difference between Q_{it} and Q_f. The charge associated with Q_f is fixed and positive. The charge associated with Q_{it} may be positive, neutral, or negative and in fact may change during normal device operation because of the capture of holes or electrons. Hence the name trap associated with Q_{it}. These traps behave very much

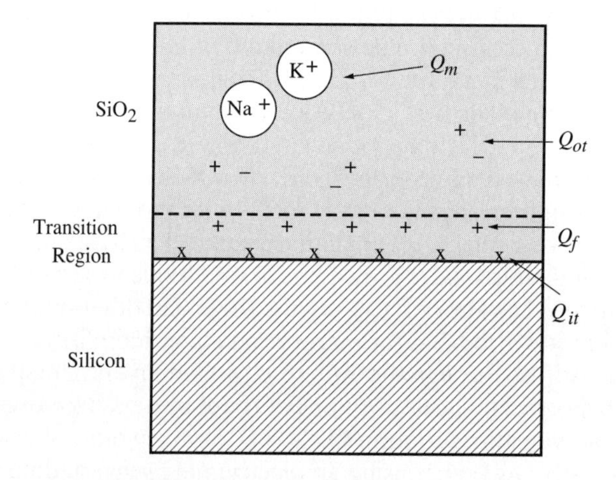

Figure 6–6 Charges associated with the SiO$_2$/Si system. (After Deal [6.7]).

like the bulk deep-level traps we discussed in Chapters 1 and 4 (Figure 1–27). Energy levels associated with Q_{it} exist throughout the forbidden band, although usually there are more traps at energy levels near the conduction and valence band edges than there are in the middle of the bandgap. Oxidizing a silicon surface usually results in a density of Q_{it} on the order of 10^9–10^{11} $cm^{-2}eV^{-1}$, about the same density as is found for Q_f. In fact it is usually the case that a process that results in a high value of Q_f will also result in a high density of Q_{it}. This correlation is one of the experimental results that suggests a common origin for the two charges.

The other two types of charges shown in Figure 6–6 are usually less important today. Q_m is the mobile oxide charge that may be located anywhere in the oxide, and was a serious problem in the 1960s. At that time, it was often the case that MOS structures were unstable after fabrication. We discussed this briefly in Chapter 1 and again in Chapter 4 and observed there that this instability in transistor threshold voltage was traced to the presence of mobile ions like Na^+ and K^+ in the gate oxides—Q_m. With proper attention to cleanliness in wafer fabrication facilities, this problem largely disappeared by the 1970s, although even today it occasionally becomes a problem in manufacturing facilities since ppm concentrations of these mobile ions can cause measurable instabilities. In the example we considered in Chapter 4, we saw that the shift in V_{TH} in MOS devices caused by Na^+ or K^+ is inversely proportional to C_{OX} [Eq. (4.1)]. Thus as gate oxide thickness is scaled down, larger Q_m values can be tolerated.

Q_{ot}, or oxide trapped charge, which also may be located anywhere in the oxide, is the final experimentally observed charge type in the Si/SiO_2 system. These defects are likely broken Si-O bonds in the bulk of the oxide, well away from the Si/SiO_2 interface. Such bonds can be broken by ionizing radiation or by some of the process steps used in manufacturing ICs today. Plasma etching, for example, exposes oxides to energetic ions, electrons and other neutral species. Ion implantation is often done through an oxide layer. These and other processes can damage oxides resulting in traps in the bulk oxide—Q_{ot}. Such traps are normally repaired by a high-temperature anneal before device fabrication is complete which allows the broken bonds to repair themselves. If they exist in the oxide because they are not fully annealed, or because the device is exposed to ionizing radiation, these traps can capture holes or electrons that may be injected into the oxide during device operation, resulting in trapped charge. Hence the name Q_{ot}.

Q_{ot} has taken on increased importance in recent years because of the high electric fields present in scaled devices. These higher fields result in more energetic or "hot" carriers that can achieve energies high enough to be injected into the gate oxides of modern MOS devices. If oxide traps are present, or if they are created by the energetic carriers themselves, charge trapping can occur. This results in device threshold shifts with time [see Eq. (4.1)] and reliability concerns. A common measure of the quality of a gate insulator is Q_{BD} or the amount of charge that can be passed through the oxide before failure (breakdown) occurs. Charge trapping in SiO_2 insulators is also a major issue in programmable devices like EPROMs in which current is purposely passed through the gate oxide as part of the write operation.

All four of the charges in Figure 6–6 can have deleterious effects on device operation. As a result, great care is normally taken during fabrication to choose process sequences that will minimize these charges. Generally this is accomplished by high-temperature inert anneals in Ar or N_2 toward the end of the process flow, and by a final moderate temperature ($\approx 400°C$) anneal in H_2 or forming gas (N_2/H_2) at the end of the process. We will discuss such anneals and charges more carefully in Section 6.5.13 later in this chapter.

A final point with regard to SiO_2 layers on Si is important. One of the earliest and most important uses of SiO_2 layers was for masking against impurity diffusion. Oxides are still widely used for this purpose today and this use depends fundamentally on the fact that most impurities have much lower diffusivities in SiO_2 that they do in Si. It is reasonably simple to calculate the thickness of an oxide layer needed to successfully mask against a diffusion or ion implantation operation. However, we will defer discussion of these points until Chapters 7 and 8 where we discuss diffusion and ion implantation in detail.

The appendix contains a number of useful and important properties of three insulators commonly used in silicon technology. SiO_XN_Y is an insulator usually formed by exposing an SiO_2 layer to an NH_3 or other nitrogen containing ambient to convert the oxide into an oxynitride. The properties of both oxynitrides and Si_3N_4 vary somewhat with deposition and/or nitridation conditions and will be discussed in more detail in Section 6.5.11 and at the end of the chapter when future trends are discussed.

6.3 Manufacturing Methods and Equipment

Oxidation systems are among the simplest types of semiconductor processing equipment. Conceptually all that is needed, as illustrated in Figure 6–7, is an oven capable of temperatures from 600–1200°C and a simple gas distribution system capable of introducing O_2 or H_2O. In practice, such systems are far more complex because of the need for uniformity, reproducibility, and cleanliness in the process. Modern furnaces are capable of handling up to several hundred 8" wafers, with a temperature uniformity of $\pm 0.5°C$.

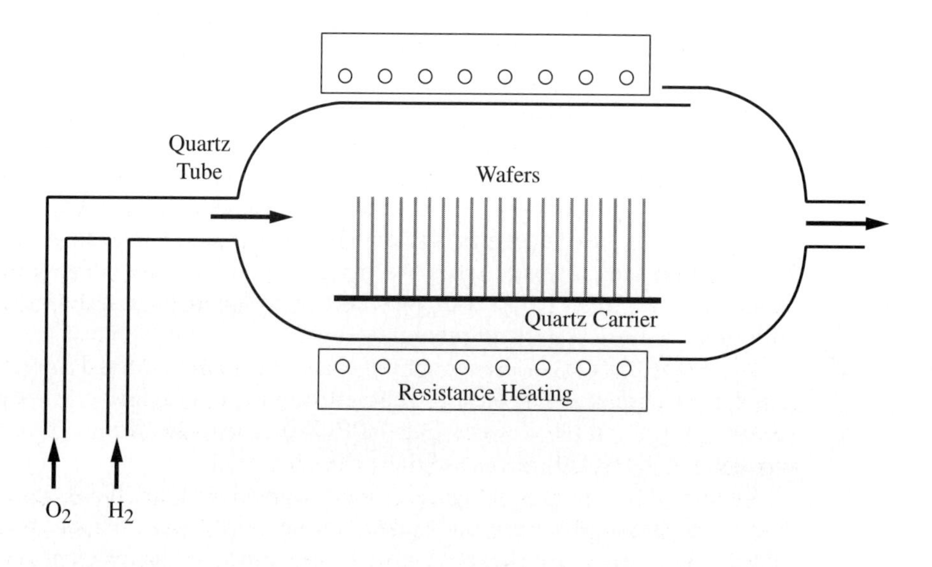

Figure 6–7 Conceptual silicon oxidation system.

Most such systems in use today are horizontally oriented with the oxidant species introduced at the back end and the wafers at the front. Many recently developed furnaces are vertically oriented since these take up less floor space in a manufacturing facility. Liquid sources of O_2 and H_2 are commonly used, with the holding tanks located outside the manufacturing facility. Gases from these liquid sources are carried to the furnaces through high-purity stainless steel lines. For O_2 oxidations, the oxygen is injected directly into the furnace. For H_2O oxidations, O_2 and H_2 are burned in the back end of the furnace to produce H_2O. Additional source lines to the furnace may allow for gaseous HCl or TCA (trichloroethane), both of which provide a Cl source. The Cl may be used to clean the furnace tube prior to oxidation or may actually be used during the oxidation as a small percentage additive. Cl serves the useful purpose of reacting with many unwanted metal ions and producing gas phase byproducts that can be exhausted from the furnace. (Recall our discussion in Chapter 4 of cleaning procedures. HCl is a component of the SC-2 cleaning solution.) If the HCl or TCA are used during the oxidation, some Cl is incorporated in the growing SiO_2 layer. This provides some degree of protection from trace amounts of ionic contaminants such as Na^+ and also changes the growth kinetics. We will discuss these issues more fully later in Section 6.5.6.

The wafers are normally loaded into the furnace on carriers or "boats" which hold 10–50 wafers. These boats are carried into the furnace by automatic loading systems that are usually cantilever arms that move slowly into the furnace hot zone. Early horizontal oxidation systems used sleds, sometimes with quartz wheels that were pushed into the furnace hot zone. However, such systems invariably stir up particles from the furnace system that can deposit on the wafers causing yield loss. Today cantilever systems carry the wafers into the furnace without actually touching the furnace walls. In the case of vertical furnaces, elevators are used to carry the wafers up into the furnace hot zone.

The furnace temperature control system is simple in concept. The furnace is normally divided in three to five zones for temperature control, with the wafers located in the center section during an oxidation. The outer zones are designed to help compensate for heat losses out the ends of the tube, so that a long central section with uniform temperature can be maintained. Thermocouples monitor the temperature in each of the sections and a controller delivers power to the resistive heating elements in each section to maintain a flat temperature profile in the central zone. In order to avoid large thermal gradients across the wafers, which can induce crystallographic defects, the wafers are normally loaded at a moderate temperature (about 800°C) and the furnace is then ramped up to the oxidation temperature after the wafers are in the central hot zone. The furnace controller is usually designed to control the ramp up and ramp down rates so that thermal stress on the wafers is minimized. Ramp rates on the order of $1°C\ sec^{-1}$ are typical.

At 1000°C, oxidation rates in H_2O are on the order of $0.1\ nm\ sec^{-1}$ and approximately double for a 100°C temperature rise. As a result, temperature control on the order of $\pm 0.5°C$ and time control on the order of seconds are required to produce consistent oxide thicknesses from batch to batch.

The vast majority of oxidation furnaces today operate at atmospheric pressure since these are the simplest to operate. However, we will see in Section 6.5.3 that oxide growth rates are proportional to oxidant pressure (to first order), so it is possible to grow a given oxide thickness in less time at high pressure. Such systems exist today and are used in applications in which a thick thermal oxide must be grown with minimum thermal budget (Dt). Pressures lower than atmospheric are simple to obtain by diluting the oxidant gas with an inert gas such as Ar or N_2. In this case, the oxidation rate is slowed down, approximately in proportion to the oxidant partial pressure.

The effort to continue decreasing the size of VLSI devices has in recent years demanded very short high-temperature steps. In addition, gate oxides in modern MOS devices are < 10 nm thick, requiring short, well-controlled growth cycles. These issues have resulted in the investigation of Rapid Thermal Oxidation (RTO) techniques for growing very thin SiO_2 layers. Typically RTO systems use a lamp heated chamber which can heat a wafer up to oxidation temperature at a rate of 100°C sec^{-1}, hold the wafer there while the oxide is grown, and then cool it back down to room temperature, again in a few seconds. Usually such systems are single-wafer machines. When reports of RTO oxide growth kinetics first began to appear in the literature, there were suggestions that the growth kinetics were different from those observed in oxidation furnaces and that new models would be needed to explain the kinetics. This might be the case, for example, if transient effects, which are negligible in a furnace which takes 15 minutes to heat the wafers, become important when the system time constants are measured in seconds. However, it now appears that the conventional models may in fact be satisfactory. One of the very difficult problems in an RTO system is in knowing exactly what the wafer temperature really is. These systems usually support the wafer on a small thermal mass in order to be able to heat the wafer rapidly. This makes it very difficult to use thermocouples for temperature measurement as is done in a furnace. Other techniques such as using a pyrometer are often used, but these methods have their own set of problems. The result is that some of the early RTO experiments which suggested "new" kinetics may have done so because of uncertainties or variations in the wafer temperature. Additional work in the future should clarify whether or not transient effects will require additions to the standard oxidation models.

Some oxidation furnaces today have a "fast ramp" capability (≈ 10°C sec^{-1}) which provides an intermediate capability between conventional furnaces and RTO systems. These new furnaces provide very good temperature control through the use of conventional thermocouples for temperature measurement, along with the fast ramp rates consistent with shorter Dt cycles and better control of thin oxides.

6.4 Measurement Methods

Experimental measurements of the results of an oxidation procedure are an essential part of any manufacturing process. The parameters of interest for an oxide (or other dielectric) layer are usually thickness, dielectric constant, index of refraction, dielectric strength, and defect density. The uniformity of all these parameters across a wafer and from wafer to wafer are also important.

The available measurement techniques can be broadly grouped into three classes. The first of these involves physical measurements that are often destructive. The second involves optical techniques that can measure some, but not all, of the parameters of interest. They are normally nondestructive. The third class of measurements involves electrical measurements. These are also usually nondestructive and are potentially the most powerful because they directly measure the parameters that are of interest in electrical devices.

6.4.1 Physical Measurements

In one of the simplest physical measurements, the dielectric is etched away in some regions using a chemical etchant that attacks the thin film but not the underlying substrate (HF for an SiO_2 layer). A small needle stylus is then moved across the surface step corresponding to the etched edge of the film. Mechanically or electrically amplifying the small signal produces a measurement of the step height. Instruments of this type have been commercially available for many years and have a resolution below 10 nm. The recent development of the scanning tunneling microscope, the Atomic Force Microscope (AFM), and derivative instruments has pushed the resolution of these "stylus" type tools to atomic dimensions. Figure 1–3 showed an example of the capability of these instruments. Other physical techniques for measuring film thickness include cross sectional SEM images similar to Figure 6–4 that can image film thickness, or higher-resolution TEM cross-sectional images such as that shown in Figure 3–15. All of these techniques require sample preparation and as a result are not well suited to in-process measurements on a manufacturing line. They also only provide information on film thickness.

6.4.2 Optical Measurements

Optical techniques are very widely used to measure film thickness and a number of instruments are commercially available. Many depend on the measurement of reflected light from the sample as illustrated in Figure 6–8. If monochromatic light of wavelength λ is incident on the sample surface at an angle ϕ, some light will be directly reflected. If layer x_O is transparent, some light will also reflect from the lower interface. For some values of λ, the two reflected waves will be in phase and will add; for other values of λ,

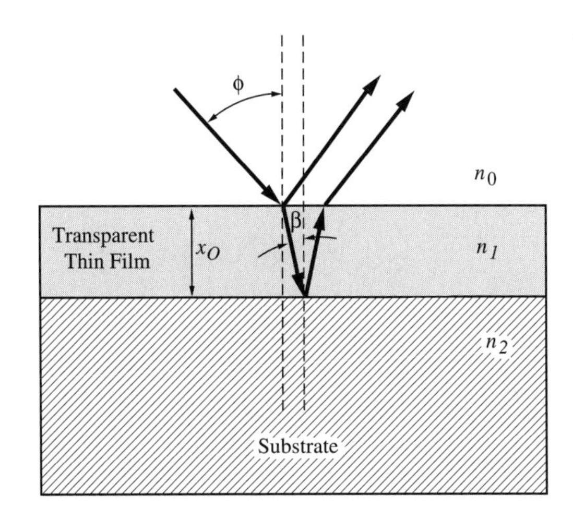

Figure 6–8 Light reflection from a sample with a transparent thin film on its surface. n_O is the index of refraction of air (1.0), n_1 is the index of refraction of the thin film and n_2 is the index of refraction of the substrate. ϕ is the angle of the incident light, β is the angle of the reflecting light at the bottom interface.

destructive interference will occur. The result is that the intensity of the reflected light will go through minima and maxima as λ is varied. These effects are exactly the same as those that cause standing waves during photoresist exposure. (Recall Figures 5–23 and 5–24.) The maxima and minima occur at values of λ given by

$$\lambda_{min,max} = \frac{2n_1 x_O \cos\beta}{m} \qquad (6.1)$$

where

$$\beta = \sin^{-1}\left[\frac{n_0 \sin\phi}{n_1}\right] \qquad (6.2)$$

and $m = 1,2,3,\ldots$ for maxima and $^1/_2, ^3/_2, ^5/_2, \ldots$ for minima. These are simply generalized versions of the simple $\lambda/2n_1$ periodicity we used for the standing waves in photoresist in Chapter 5 for vertically incident light. Commercially available instruments use spectrophotometers to sweep the incident wavelength with ϕ constant. They then measure dielectric film thicknesses by fitting the resulting reflected intensity to Eq. (6.1). This technique works reliably for film thicknesses greater than a few tens of nm. For thinner films, it is difficult to detect the first minimum unless very short wavelength light is used. In using this technique, the index of refraction of the dielectric film must be known since it shows up directly in Eq. (6.1).

There are many cases of interest in silicon technology in which dielectric films thinner than a few tens of nanometers need to be measured, or in which the film dielectric constant is not known precisely. Examples include gate oxides in MOS structures that are now less than 10 nm in thickness and Si_3N_4 or SiO_XN_Y films in which n_1 may vary with processing conditions. For these applications, ellipsometry is a better method to measure film properties. Conceptually, ellipsometry works in a similar fashion to the reflectance technique described above. However, polarized light is used in an ellipsometer and the change in the polarization when the light is reflected from the dielectric/substrate interface is measured. In general the change in polarization depends on the properties of both the film and the substrate. However in the simple case when the optical properties of the substrate are known and the film is transparent at the wavelengths being used, the change in polarization of the reflected light depends only on the film thickness and index of refraction. Commercially available ellipsometers can easily measure films down to 1 nm in thickness and accurately determine the index of refraction. Usually these instruments are computer controlled so that the film properties are calculated automatically.

By far the simplest optical technique to evaluate dielectric film thickness is the use of color charts. These charts were originally described by Pliskin and Conrad [6.8] and are based on the idea that if white light is used to illuminate a thin transparent dielectric film on a reflecting substrate (as in Figure 6–8), destructive interference will occur for some wavelengths in the reflected light, giving the reflected light a characteristic color. This allows a simple observation of the color of the oxide or nitride layer to provide an estimate of the film thickness. Tables in the appendix provide these colors for SiO_2 or Si_3N_4 films on reflecting substrates (usually silicon). The charts assume that the films are being viewed perpendicularly under daylight fluorescent lighting. The colors repeat about every 300 nm for SiO_2 and about every 200 nm for Si_3N_4. For this reason, standards are often used in conjunction with these charts. If the sample under investigation is viewed side by side with a standard of the same color and the observer then views the two at an angle, the colors of both will change as the viewing angle changes. The colors on both will change in the same way, only if the thicknesses are actually the same. This allows one to distinguish where on the color chart a particular sample fits. The eye is remarkably good at distinguishing colors and an estimate of film thickness within about 10–20 nm can be made with these charts, particularly if standards are available as well. The ranges covered by these charts are those normally encountered in silicon technology. Note however, that oxides thinner than about 50 nm do not have any characteristic color so this method is not useful in this thickness range.

6.4.3 Electrical Measurements — The MOS Capacitor

The third category of measurement techniques are those that involve electrical measurements. These are potentially the most powerful methods because they measure parameters that are of direct interest to semiconductor devices—capacitances, electrical charges, and so on. By far the most dominant electrical technique is the Capacitance-Voltage or CV method. This technique is very widely used and provides a large amount of information about dielectric films and the interfaces that such films make with underlying semiconductors. We will describe how this technique works and the information that it provides in the following paragraphs. We will apply the CV technique in this chapter to help understand the properties of the Si/SiO_2 interface. In later chapters (7 and 8 in particular), we will apply it to measurement of doping profiles in semiconductors.

The basic structure used to make CV measurements is the MOS capacitor, consisting of a semiconductor substrate, a dielectric layer and a conducting electrode. We briefly considered this structure in Chapter 4 (Figures 4–15 and 4–19) in connection with measurements of dielectric breakdown and carrier lifetime. Since the primary use of the MOS capacitor is in the characterization and study of insulators and the Si/SiO_2 interface, we will discuss this structure in more detail here.

Generally the MOS system is (polysilicon or Al) SiO_2-Si although any conductor/insulator/semiconductor combination can be used. The basic measurement is illustrated in Figure 6–9 where we consider the specific case of a metal/SiO_2/N silicon structure. This figure shows three regions of operation of the MOS capacitor. Positive voltages on the metal electrode correspond to accumulation [Figure 6–9(a)], negative voltages first cause depletion [Figure 6–9(b)] and then inversion [Figure 6–9(c)] in the substrate. We will define these terms more carefully shortly. The metal part of the structure is often called the gate because that is the role it plays in a MOS transistor that has the same structure. It is important to note that the gate voltage V_G is a DC voltage and it is assumed in the following discussion to be applied for a long enough time for the system to come to a final steady state condition. We will return to this point later when we discuss high-frequency and low-frequency CV curves as well as other applications of the technique.

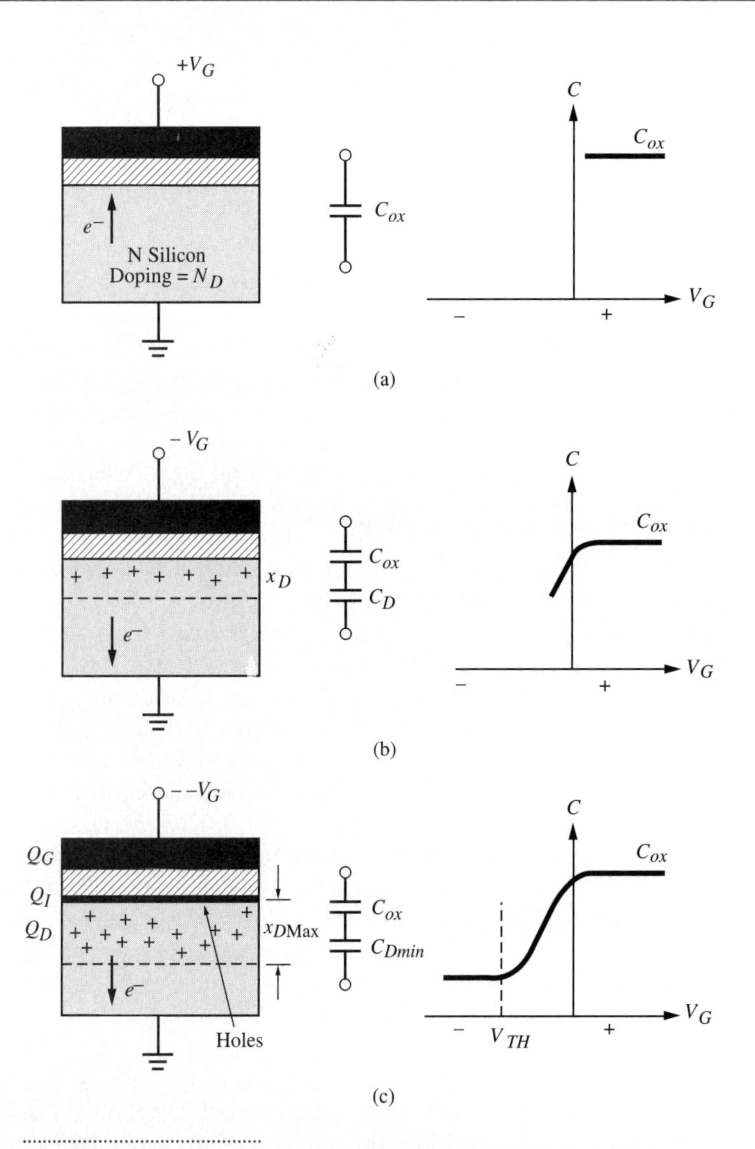

Figure 6–9 MOS capacitor structure and resulting CV plot. (a) corresponds to accumulation, (b) to depletion, and (c) to inversion.

We make the further assumption that the insulator and the insulator/semiconductor interface (SiO_2/Si in this case) have only small numbers of charges or defects. In other words, the four types of charges described in Figure 6–6 are assumed to be relatively small in density. If this is the case, electric field lines that start on charges on the gate will extend through the insulator and into the substrate where there are charges of opposite sign available to terminate the field lines. If there were large numbers of charges or defects in the insulator or at the insulator/semiconductor interface, the electric field lines could terminate on these charges before they reached the underlying semiconductor.

The result would be that applying voltages to the gate would have little effect on the semiconductor. Depletion and inversion could not be controllably achieved and the structure would not be useful in MOS transistors. This is in fact what happens in many insulator/semiconductor systems, but the SiO_2-Si system is close to electrically perfect.

Consider first the case with a DC voltage of $+V_G$ on the gate [Figure 6–9(a)]. Since the substrate is N type, positive gate voltages will attract the majority carrier electrons to the silicon surface. If we now measure the small signal capacitance of the structure by superimposing a small AC signal on V_G, the capacitance measured will be simply the oxide capacitance C_{ox}. The silicon substrate will act simply as a resistor in series with C_{ox} since no depletion region will form for positive gate voltages. The measurement extracts only the capacitive part of the impedance, which will be independent of V_G, as shown in the right-hand part of Figure 6–9(a). Frequencies in the range of 100 kHz to 1 MHz are often used for this measurement.

Consider now the application of negative DC gate voltages in part (b) of the figure. Negative voltages will repel the majority carrier electrons from the surface creating a depleted region. Any negative charge we place on the gate must be balanced by a corresponding positive charge in the substrate to maintain charge neutrality. The positive charge is provided by the substrate donor atoms that have a net positive charge when the mobile electrons are forced away from the surface. Conceptually what happens is that the electrons forced away from the semiconductor surface region flow out the bottom of the substrate, through the power supply connected to the gate and then on to the gate where they provide the negative gate charge. As a result,

$$|Q_G| = |Q_D| = N_D x_D \tag{6.3}$$

where Q_G and Q_D are in units of number of charges cm^{-2}, and N_D is the doping in the substrate which is assumed to be uniform. A depletion region will form to a depth x_D. The concept here is very similar to the PN junction depletion region we discussed in Chapter 1. The depletion region will have a capacitance per unit area associated with it given by

$$C_D = \frac{\varepsilon_S}{x_D} \tag{6.4}$$

where ε_S is the permittivity of silicon. However, x_D is a function of the gate voltage, increasing as V_G increases. The overall capacitance that is measured for the structure is now C_{ox} in series with a varying C_D. The plot on the right of Figure 6–9(b) reflects this, with a capacitance that decreases as V_G becomes more negative because x_D grows as V_G becomes more negative.

For larger values of negative DC gate voltage, the silicon surface will actually "invert" from N type to P type [Figure 6–9(c)]. The negative voltage on the gate will attract the minority carrier holes in the substrate to the surface and if enough of them are present there, they can form an inversion layer of P-type carriers. The gate voltage at which this occurs is called the threshold voltage and is exactly the same voltage that we discussed in earlier chapters in connection with turning on a MOS transistor. Once the inversion layer forms, x_D stops expanding and reaches a maximum value x_{DMax}.

For all regions of operation of the capacitor, the gate charge must be balanced by charge in the substrate. That is

$$Q_G = N_D x_D + Q_I \tag{6.5}$$

where Q_I is the charge density (number of charges per cm^2) in the inversion layer. Q_I is negligible during the depletion condition so that x_D expands during depletion to balance Q_G. Once the inversion layer forms, however, additional gate charge is balanced by Q_I rather than Q_D so that x_D reaches a maximum value. This means that the CV curve will reach a minimum as shown in Figure 6–9(c).

In order to understand why additional Q_G is balanced by Q_I and not by Q_D once inversion occurs, we need to return to the concept of band diagrams that we introduced in Chapter 1. Figure 6–10 shows the band diagram for the MOS capacitor under conditions of accumulation, depletion, and inversion. The oxide prevents any current flow through the structure so the semiconductor is in equilibrium and we can draw the Fermi

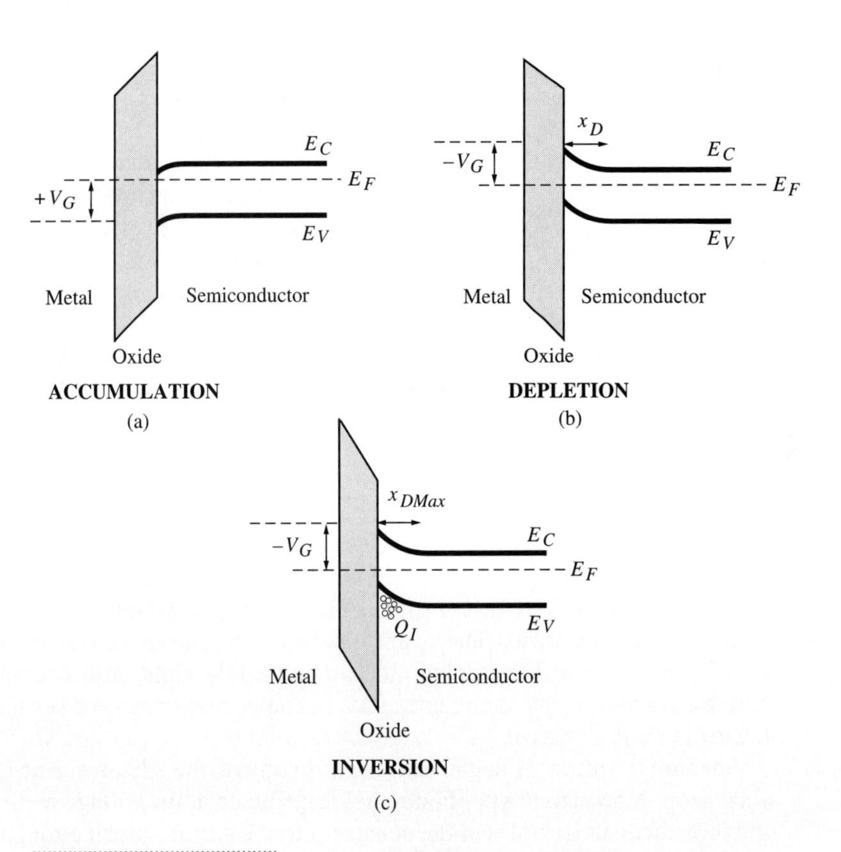

Figure 6–10 Band diagrams for the MOS capacitor in (a) accumulation, (b) depletion, and (c) inversion.

level as flat in the silicon. The Fermi level in the metal is separated from E_F in the silicon by the amount of the applied gate voltage. In Figure 6–10(a), a positive DC gate voltage is applied (recall that positive is downward in these diagrams by convention). This will cause the bands in the semiconductor to bend downward in the near surface region. This places E_F closer to E_C at the surface than is the case in the bulk far away from the surface. As we saw in Chapter 1, this means that the electron population is therefore higher at the surface than it is in the bulk. This accumulates electrons at the surface, the same conclusion we reached when discussing Figure 6–9(a).

In Figure 6–10(b), a negative DC gate voltage has been applied, causing the bands in the semiconductor to bend upward near the surface. This creates the depletion region that we discussed in Figure 6–9(b) since over the distance x_D, E_F is away from both E_C and E_V. This implies that both n and p are small, that is that the mobile carrier concentrations are much less than N_D. In this region, Q_D is given by Eq. (6.3).

Figure 6–10(c) shows the situation in inversion. Here the DC gate voltage is negative enough so that the bands at the surface are bent far enough to place E_F near E_V. This means that the hole population is significant at the surface, that is, that inversion has occurred and the surface is P type. We can now appreciate why additional Q_G is balanced by Q_I rather than by Q_D in inversion. Further increases in the negative voltage on the gate will try to bend the bands further in the semiconductor and move E_F closer to E_V. However, we saw in Chapter 1 that moving E_F nearer to E_V will result in an exponential increase in p. [See Eqs. (1.10) or (1.14) for example.] Because of this, only a very slight movement of E_F with respect to E_V is needed to provide enough Q_I to balance additional Q_G. Referring again to Eq. (6.5), we see that increasing Q_G after inversion is reached, will result in a very small increase in x_D and hence in Q_D, and that most of the Q_G increase will be balanced by an increase in Q_I. We therefore speak of x_D as being "pinned" at x_{DMax} once inversion occurs.

There are a few other basic concepts that we should understand about CV measurements before we discuss how they can be used to evaluate insulators and insulator/semiconductor interfaces. The CV curves we have described to this point are called high-frequency (HF) CV curves. This simply means that the small AC signal used to measure the MOS capacitance is a moderately high-frequency signal (typically 100 kHz to 1 MHz). We need to consider why this frequency is important.

Consider again the inversion condition in Figure 6–9(c) or Figure 6–10(c). Suppose that we have applied the DC gate voltage $-V_G$ for a long enough time for the system to come to equilibrium. (We will define how long this is shortly.) In equilibrium, the inversion layer is present and x_D is "pinned" at x_{DMax}. Suppose we now apply a small HF signal to measure the structure capacitance. The AC signal is superimposed on $-V_G$ and hence modulates Q_G very slightly. This change in Q_G must be balanced by a change in either Q_D or Q_I. In equilibrium, Q_I would change as we saw above. However, high frequency in this context means that Q_G is being modulated faster than Q_I can respond. If this is true, then the only option the system has is to modulate Q_D in order to provide the balancing charge. If this happens, then the charge balancing that occurs is between the gate and the bottom of the depletion region. The bottom edge of the depletion regions moves up and down along with the gate voltage, providing the ΔQ_D needed to balance the ΔQ_G. Hence the capacitance that is measured is between those two plates (C_{ox} in series with C_D). For any $-V_G$ in the inversion region, x_D is at x_{DMax} and so C_D is at C_{DMin}. This is why the HF capacitance measurement produces a minimum capacitance for negative V_G that is independent of V_G.

Now why is it that Q_I cannot change as fast as the high frequency signal on the gate? The answer is simply that there is no source of additional holes available in the substrate to provide the ΔQ_I. There are very few holes present in an N-type semiconductor. The only mechanisms usually available to create or remove holes are thermal generation and recombination, respectively, and these processes are quite slow in materials like silicon which have long carrier lifetimes. As a result Q_I cannot change rapidly and the HF CV curve measures a constant minimum value in inversion.

Now suppose that we slow down the AC signal on the gate. If we reduce the frequency to a low enough value (typically less than 1 Hz for silicon), then generation and recombination processes can keep up with the AC signal and Q_I can follow the changes in Q_G. What do we now measure for the CV curve? The answer, not surprisingly, is that we now measure the Low-Frequency (LF) CV curve. If Q_I follows Q_G, then the capacitance measured in the structure will be just the oxide capacitance because the top and bottom plates of the capacitor where Q is changing are on the two edges of the oxide. Hence we should expect that the CV curve would come back up to C_{ox} in the inversion region. This is in fact what happens and the resulting curve is the LF CV curve. Figure 6–11 illustrates the HF and LF curves. Note that the point at which these ideal HF or LF CV curves reach their minimum corresponds to the onset of inversion and so is the threshold voltage for the MOS structure.

Figure 6–11 also illustrates the deep depletion condition that can be observed in MOS capacitors. We discussed this case qualitatively in Chapter 4 (Section 4.4.3) in connection with measuring the carrier generation lifetime in semiconductors. Deep depletion results if the DC bias voltage on the capacitor is swept too rapidly into the

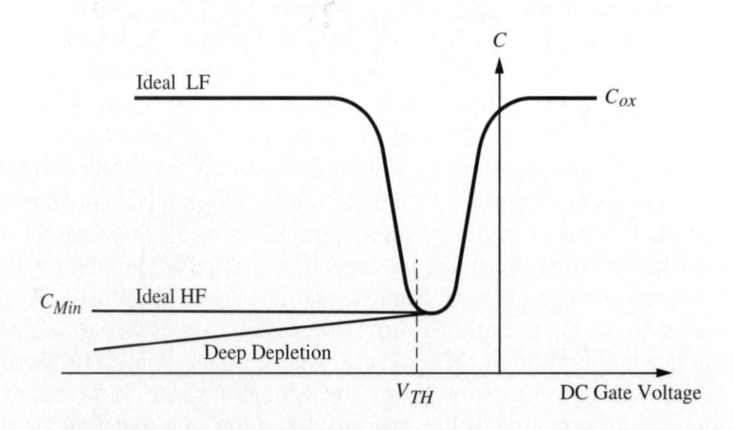

Figure 6–11 Ideal MOS CV curves at high and low frequencies. Also shown is the deep depletion CV curve.

inversion region. If this is done, the holes needed for the inversion layer cannot be generated rapidly enough to follow the applied "DC" bias. If Q_I cannot change rapidly enough, changes in Q_G can only be balanced by Q_D. Thus a deeper depletion region than would be present in equilibrium forms. A smaller capacitance than the equilibrium value is measured, which gradually relaxes back to C_{Min} as hole generation takes place.

Eq. (1.20) gave the net rate of recombination or generation from the Shockley-Read-Hall model. In a depletion region, n and p are negligible and U reduces to

$$U = -\frac{n_i}{\tau_G} \tag{6.6}$$

Assuming that this generation rate holds throughout the volume of the depletion region, then the current density corresponding to U is simply

$$J_{gen} = \frac{qn_iW}{\tau_G} \tag{6.7}$$

This current will flow to the surface, providing the holes for the inversion layer. In order to avoid deep depletion, the rate at which the "DC" bias voltage is swept on the MOS capacitor must be less than

$$\frac{dV}{dt} \le \frac{J_{gen}}{C} \approx \frac{J_{gen}}{C_{OX}} = \frac{qn_iW}{\tau_G C_{OX}} \tag{6.8}$$

In practice, this means that "DC" sweep rates less than about 0.1 V sec^{-1} must be used.

Example In an experimental structure in Figure 6–12, a phosphorus N^+ region is formed by ion implantation using a 50-nm SiO_2 mask. A metal electrode is then

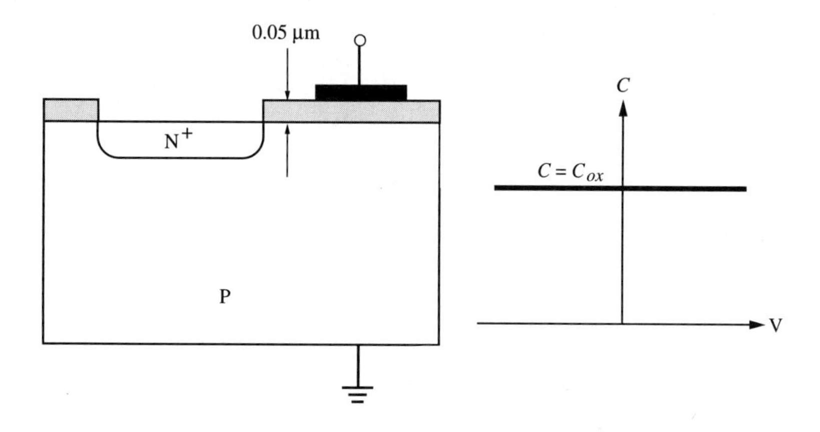

Figure 6–12 MOS capacitor structure with "anomalous" CV measurement.

formed as shown and a CV measurement is made in the region outside the N$^+$ region. The measurement gives $C = C_{ox}$ for all values of applied voltage as shown. Explain what might have gone wrong in this experiment. That is explain why no surface inversion is observed in the CV measurement.

Answer While a number of explanations are possible, the basic observation here is that the gate voltage appears to have essentially no effect on the underlying silicon. This can happen if there are charges at or very close to the Si/SiO$_2$ interface which terminate the field lines before they penetrate into the silicon. This could be caused by a very poor Si/SiO$_2$ interface, but there is nothing in the process flow to suggest that this should have happened (unless there is damage from the implant that was not properly annealed). A more likely explanation is that the 0.05-μm oxide was not thick enough to mask the implant and as a result the N$^+$ implant penetrated everywhere. If this happened, there would be plenty of donor atoms available to terminate the gate field very close to the surface. Thus as $+V_G$ is applied, the material tries to start depleting, but since the doping is so high close to the surface, the depletion region x_d is extremely shallow. Thus the capacitance associated with x_d is very large and the total capacitance (C_O in series with C_D), is essentially just C_O. We will discuss implantation and masking issues more carefully in Chapter 8.

We saw in Section 6.2 that a number of charges are generally associated with insulator/semiconductor interfaces. These charges cause shifts and distortions in CV curves because they require gate charge Q_G to balance them. Figure 6–13 illustrates these effects on the "ideal" HF CV curve. Q_f is a fixed positive charge that is present in the oxide,

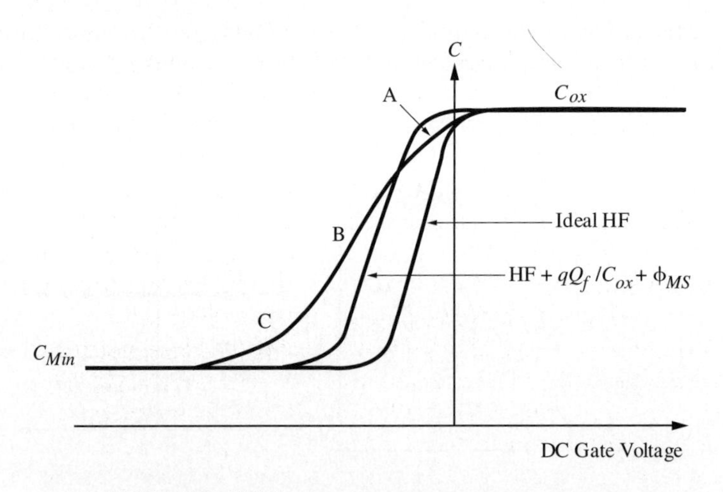

Figure 6–13 HF MOS CV curves illustrating some of the nonidealities that can be present in actual experimental structures. A, B, and C illustrate the effects of interface states with different energy levels in the silicon bandgap.

near the SiO_2/Si interface. Such a positive charge will induce a corresponding negative image charge in the silicon, effectively making the silicon surface more N type and therefore harder to invert to P type. This shows up as a lateral shift in the CV curve, with the magnitude of the shift simply given by qQ_f/C_{ox}. Measurement of this shift thus allows calculation of the magnitude of Q_f. An additional lateral shift occurs in general because of a difference in the work functions of the metal and the semiconductor ϕ_{MS}. The work function is by definition the energy required to remove an electron in the material at energy E_F to a position just outside the material. This is a measurable property of a material and is generally known for any given experiment. The lateral offset in the CV curve due to ϕ_{MS} is thus known. These two terms, ϕ_{MS} and qQ_f/C_{ox}, together account for an increase in the gate voltage required to cause inversion and are often lumped together and called the flat band voltage V_{FB} since if a gate voltage of this magnitude is applied, the bands in the semiconductor will be flat. These terms also show up in the turn-on voltage of a MOS transistor [see Eq. (4.1)].

If mobile charges (Q_m) or oxide trapped charge (Q_{ot}) are present, they produce a similar effect to Q_f. That is, they cause a lateral shift in the CV curve. The only real difference is that these charges are usually not located directly at the SiO_2-Si interface and so the magnitude of the shift they cause is reduced in proportion to their distance away from the interface. (A positive charge located in the central portion of the oxide will induce a balancing negative image charge partially on the gate and partially in the silicon.)

The "distorted" CV curve shown in Figure 6–13 illustrates what happens when interface traps Q_{it} are present. We saw in Section 6.2 that these traps can have energy levels throughout the forbidden band. As applied gate voltage causes the semiconductor surface to move from accumulation to depletion to inversion, sweeping out a CV curve, E_F at the semiconductor surface will move from one band edge to the other (E_C to E_V in the N type example we have been considering). As a result, the Q_{it} traps will fill and empty as E_F moves through their energy levels. As this happens, the CV curve will distort from its ideal shape. The form of the distortion depends on the density and energy levels of the Q_{it} traps. In Figure 6–13 the region labeled A corresponds to interface states near E_C, B corresponds to states near the middle of the bandgap, and C corresponds to states near E_V. The assumption is often made that the interface states cannot follow the HF signal used to measure the capacitance. That is, they do not charge and discharge as the HF signal changes. But these traps will respond to the DC signal applied on the gate since we assume that this signal is applied for a long enough period of time to reach equilibrium. Thus Q_G is partially balanced by Q_{it}. The result is a stretching out of the CV curve along the horizontal (DC voltage) axis.

A number of methods have been developed to experimentally extract the interface state density from CV measurements on MOS capacitors. Many of these are described in detail in references like [6.9, 6.10]. The most commonly used method is the "quasi-static" or LF method that is illustrated in Figure 6–14. In this method HF and LF CV curves are superimposed from measurements on the same MOS capacitor. It is assumed that interface states cannot respond to the HF measurement and that they do respond to the low-frequency measurement. In practice, this means that the HF must be high enough that the traps cannot charge and discharge at the measurement frequency, and

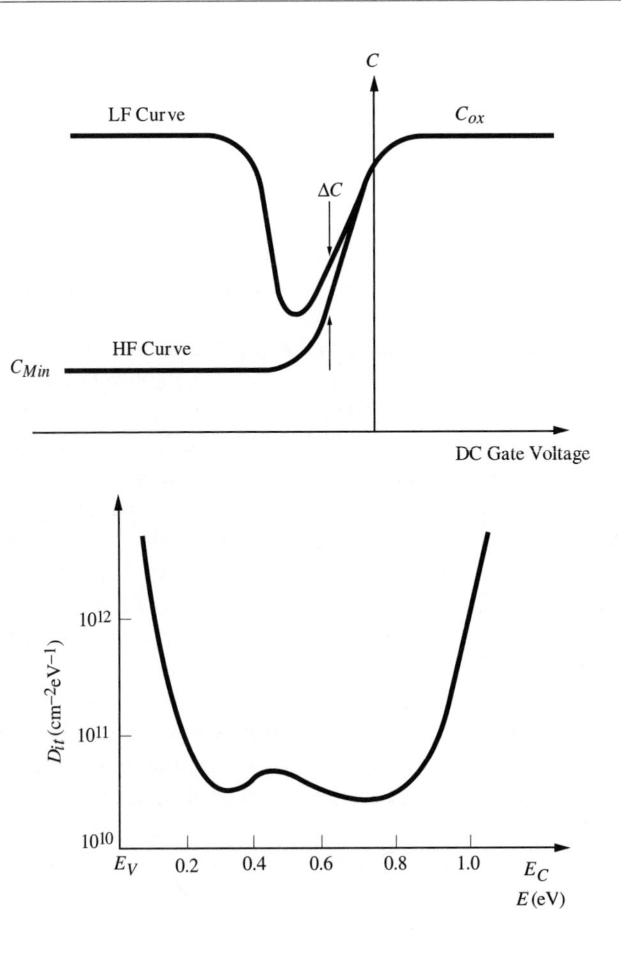

Figure 6–14 Typical experimental HF and LF CV curves used to extract the interface state density D_{it} as a function of energy in the bandgap. The D_{it} plot is typical of extracted data.

the LF must be low enough to allow the traps to charge and discharge as the LF signal varies. If this is the case, then the traps will behave as an additional capacitance for the low frequency measurement and ΔC in Figure 6–14 will be proportional to the trap density at the DC potential corresponding to the measurement point. This information can be used to generate a plot like that shown on the bottom in Figure 6–14. D_{it} is the interface state density at a particular position in the bandgap. Q_{it} has units of coulombs cm^{-2}, while D_{it} has units of traps $cm^{-2}\ eV^{-1}$. The U shape qualitatively shown in the figure is typical of what is generally observed for the Si-SiO_2 interface.

Another CV measurement that is sometimes useful characterizes Q_m, the mobile charge density in the insulator. Typically these ions are Na^+ or K^+, both of which are mobile in SiO_2, especially at slightly elevated temperatures. The measurement method is called Bias Temperature Stressing or simply BTS and involves making an initial HF CV measurement at room temperature. The MOS capacitor is then heated to $\approx 200°C$ with an applied DC bias on the gate. At this temperature Na^+ and K^+ are very mobile and will easily drift upwards or downwards in the SiO_2. The capacitor is then cooled to room temperature (still under bias), and a second HF CV curve is measured. If drifting of Q_m has occurred, a lateral shift in the HF CV curve will be measured, like the lateral shift in Figure 6–13 due to Q_f. The extent of the shift is proportional to Q_m. Sometimes a second BTS procedure with opposite polarity bias is used to drift the Q_m to the other SiO_2 interface so that the lateral difference between the two CV curves corresponds to the total Q_m present regardless of where it was originally located in the insulator.

Another simple measurement of insulator properties that is possible with the MOS capacitor is the I-V characteristic of the insulator. For thin oxides (< 10 nm), this measurement can directly measure tunneling currents which are used in some types of memory devices. For thicker oxides, these currents are too small to measure easily, but a destructive measurement of the dielectric breakdown strength of the oxide is sometimes made simply by ramping the voltage across the oxide until breakdown occurs. (See Figure 4–15.) For high-quality SiO_2 layers, this normally occurs at about 10–15 MV cm^{-1}. If a large number of capacitors are measured on a wafer, a histogram plot of the measured breakdown fields can provide information on defect densities in the oxides.

We briefly mentioned earlier Q_{BD} or the charge to breakdown that can be passed through a thin SiO_2 layer before breakdown occurs. The process of oxide degradation as charge passes through it is the trapping of charge at defect sites in the oxide. This process can also be monitored using a MOS capacitor. If a DC current is forced through a MOS capacitor for a period of time and CV measurements were made before and after this process, then trapped charge will show up as Q_{ot}. Thus the CV curves before and after will show a horizontal shift whose magnitude is proportional to Q_{ot} as illustrated in Figure 6–13. A series of such experiments produce a plot of Q_{ot} versus the time the current is forced through the oxide. Forcing current through an insulator can also create damage at the Si/SiO_2 interface. If this happens, such damage is also evident in CV curves through the distortion of the curve Q_{it} creates (also shown in Figure 6–13).

Finally, in most modern MOS structures, the doping is not constant with depth as we have assumed in our discussion to this point. In fact this provides another powerful opportunity for CV measurements. Since the depletion depth x_D depends on doping, a CV measurement can also be used to extract N_D or N_A versus depth. This is a powerful doping profiling capability, which we will discuss in Chapter 7.

The MOS capacitor can thus provide a tremendous amount of information about insulators and the Si/SiO_2 interface. This simple structure has had such a profound influence on the semiconductor industry that entire books have been written on it [6.10].

In summary then, we see that a variety of measurement techniques are available to determine insulator properties. The thickness of a deposited or grown insulating layer is obtainable through physical, optical, or electrical measurements. The interface properties between the insulator and underlying semiconductor are directly measurable through CV methods. And defect densities are available through destructive breakdown tests on large numbers of capacitors. All of these techniques have been widely applied to both thermally grown oxide/Si interfaces, and to more general insulator/semiconductor structures. We will find many examples of such measurements throughout this text. A final point, although it may be obvious, is that although all the examples we have shown in this section have been for N-type substrates. P-type substrates produce similar CV plots except that the horizontal axis is flipped (mirror imaged).

6.5 Models and Simulation

A substantial amount of effort over more than 25 years has been devoted to understanding and modeling silicon oxidation kinetics. We will focus in this section on a hierarchy of models that have been developed to explain and predict oxidation kinetics and the properties of the Si/SiO_2 interface. The first general models date back to the work of Deal and Grove in the early 1960s [6.6]. This work resulted in the linear parabolic model that is still used today to model the planar oxidation of silicon. This model cannot fully explain the oxidation of shaped surfaces, which are often encountered in modern VLSI devices, and it also cannot fully explain the oxidation kinetics in mixed ambients or for very thin oxides. Finally, it cannot explain why oxidation affects other process phenomena like dopant diffusion, often at great distances away from the oxidizing surface. However, it provides a useful starting point for our discussion and much of the more recent work on modeling builds on Deal and Grove's pioneering work.

Many of the models we will describe in this chapter have been implemented in process simulation programs. We will illustrate the use of these simulation tools as we describe the models. The simulator we will use is the Stanford University program SUPREM IV that has been implemented in commercially available versions like TSUPREM IV [6.11] and ATHENA [6.12]. These programs implement many (but not all) of the models we will discuss. SUPREM IV is a 2D simulator, which is generally available and used fairly widely in the semiconductor industry. The simulation examples in this chapter were run on commercially available versions of this program.

It is important to note that many of the oxidation models we will describe were developed specifically to deal with one aspect of the problem—for example, the oxidation of heavily doped substrates. The fabrication of real device structures involves many processes acting simultaneously. The only real way to model such technologies is to use a computer program that integrates all the individual models and allows them to operate simultaneously during a high-temperature step. This is the real power of simulation programs. However, the very fact that such programs integrate individual models, perhaps even models that were developed independently of each other, means that the interactions between the models may not have been fully tested experimentally. In fact, the simulators really become a means of testing the generality of the individual models. At the end of the chapter we will show some examples of more complete oxidation process simulation—examples that integrate many models simultaneously.

6.5.1 First-Order Planar Growth Kinetics—The Linear Parabolic Model

The central ideas behind the Deal-Grove or linear parabolic model are illustrated in Figure 6–15. (Note the similarity of this model to the photoresist development model we discussed in connection with Figure 5–48.) We assume that an oxide of some thickness x_i is already present on the silicon surface. We also assume that the structure is one dimensional so that this model will only apply to oxide films grown on flat substrates. The oxide grows by indiffusion of the oxidizing species to the oxide/silicon interface, where a simple chemical reaction such as

$$\mathrm{Si} + \mathrm{O_2} \rightarrow \mathrm{SiO_2} \tag{6.9}$$

or

$$\mathrm{Si} + 2\mathrm{H_2O} \rightarrow \mathrm{SiO_2} + 2\mathrm{H_2} \tag{6.10}$$

takes place. We initially assume that three sequential steps are necessary for this to happen, although it will turn out that only two of them are important. Figure 6–15 illustrates three fluxes associated with the process. The first represents the transport of the oxidant in the gas phase to the oxide surface. We can describe this flux as

$$F_1 = h_G(C_G - C_S) \tag{6.11}$$

where F_1 is the flux in molecules cm^{-2} sec^{-1}, $(C_G - C_S)$ is the concentration difference between the main gas flow and the oxide surface, and h_G is the mass transfer coefficient in cm sec^{-1}. The process represented by F_1 is the gas phase diffusion of the oxidant species through the boundary or stagnant layer that always forms adjacent to a solid object placed in a gas which is flowing over its surface. In the case of oxidation, this diffusion process is very fast compared to the other steps that must occur and hence F_1 will turn out to be unimportant in determining the overall growth kinetics. Other processing techniques such as epitaxy and CVD that also involve reactant transport from the

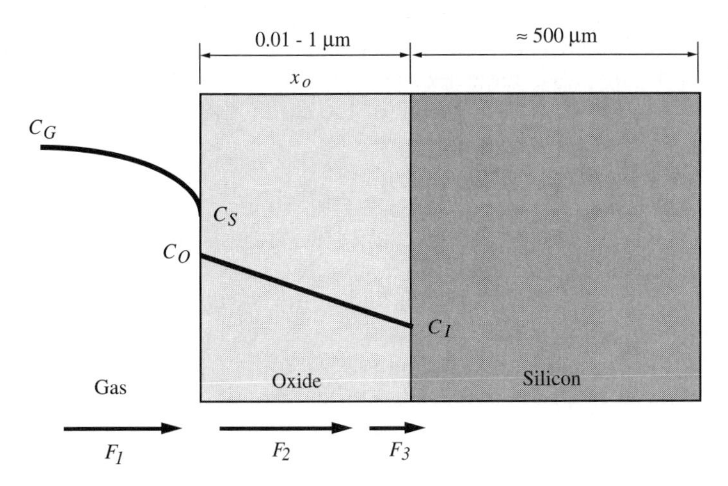

Figure 6–15 Oxidant flux from the gas phase to the silicon surface during thermal oxidation. The bold line represents the O_2 or H_2O concentration.

gas phase to the wafer surface, may be limited by this transport process. We will discuss these technologies in Chapter 9.

We can relate the concentration of the oxidant just inside the oxide surface C_O to the pressure in the gas phase adjacent to the surface, through Henry's law:

$$C_O = HP_S \tag{6.12}$$

This law states that the equilibrium concentration of a gas species dissolved in a solid is proportional to the partial pressure of that species at the solid surface. It holds for molecular species, so we are assuming that O_2 or H_2O are absorbed into the oxide. P_S is not usually a known experimental parameter, so it is convenient to write the oxidant concentration in the oxide in terms of P_G the bulk gas pressure, which is known.

$$C^* = HP_G \tag{6.13}$$

We define C^* to be the oxidant concentration in the oxide that would be in equilibrium with P_G. Since it will turn out that F_1 is not the rate limiting step in the oxidation process, this implies that $C^* \approx C_O$, and $P_G \approx P_S$. C^* therefore really represents the solubility of the oxidant in the SiO_2 .

From the ideal gas law, we have that

$$C_G = \frac{P_G}{kT} \quad \text{and} \quad C_S = \frac{P_S}{kT} \tag{6.14}$$

Substitution of Eqs. (6.12)–(6.14) into (6.11), now leads directly to the result that

$$F_1 = h(C^* - C_O) \tag{6.15}$$

where $h = h_G/HkT$. Experimentally we find that wide changes in gas flow rates in oxidation furnaces, changes in the spacings between wafers on the boat or carrier in the furnace and changes in wafer orientation (standing up or lying down in the furnace) make little difference in oxidation rates. These results imply that h is very large, or that only a small difference between C^* and C_O is required to provide the necessary oxidant flux.

Flux F_2 in Figure 6–15 represents the diffusion of the oxidant through the oxide to the Si/SiO$_2$ interface. Using Fick's law, we can express this as

$$F_2 = D\frac{\partial C}{\partial x} = D\left(\frac{C_O - C_I}{x_O}\right) \tag{6.16}$$

where D is the oxidant diffusivity in the oxide, C_O and C_I are the concentrations at the two interfaces, and x_O is the oxide thickness. In writing this expression, we have assumed that the process is in steady state (not changing rapidly with time), and that there is no loss of oxidant as it diffuses through the oxide. Under these conditions, F_2 must be constant through the oxide and hence the derivative can be replaced simply by a constant gradient. The oxidant concentration falls off linearly through the oxide as shown in Figure 6–15. The experimental evidence seems to suggest that O_2 diffuses in molecular form through the SiO_2, likely interstitially between the atoms in the oxide. H_2O on the other hand, seems to diffuse in a more complex manner, interacting with the SiO_2 matrix. The effective diffusivities of both O_2 and H_2O are on the same order (about 5×10^3 $\mu m^2\ hr^{-1}$ at 1100°C).

The third part of the oxidation process is the reaction at the Si/SiO_2 interface. We represent this with a third flux given by

$$F_3 = k_S C_I \tag{6.17}$$

The rate at which this reaction takes place should be proportional to the oxidant concentration at the interface C_I. There are also many other factors that are likely involved in the reaction such as Si-Si bond breaking, Si-O bond formation, and possibly O_2 or H_2O dissociation. All of these effects and others are lumped into k_S which is termed the interface reaction rate constant (cm sec^{-1}). We will return to a more detailed discussion of this interface reaction later in this chapter.

Under steady-state conditions, the three fluxes representing the oxidation process must be equal since they occur in series with each other and the overall process will proceed at the rate of the slowest process. Thus $F_1 = F_2 = F_3$. Combining Eqs. (6.15)–(6.17) then leads to

$$C_I = \frac{C^*}{1 + \frac{k_S}{h} + \frac{k_S x_O}{D}} \cong \frac{C^*}{1 + \frac{k_S x_O}{D}} \tag{6.18}$$

$$C_O = \frac{C^*\left(1 + \frac{k_S x_O}{D}\right)}{1 + \frac{k_S}{h} + \frac{k_S x_O}{D}} \cong C^* \tag{6.19}$$

In writing the right-hand expressions in these equations, we have made use of the experimental observation that h is very large. Physically, we can think of the overall process as involving two interface reactions (h and k_S) and a diffusion process. Of the two interface reactions, the process at the oxide surface (gas absorption) occurs very rapidly compared to the chemistry occurring at the Si/SiO_2 and hence h can be neglected compared to k_S.

There are two limiting cases that are of interest in Eqs. (6.18) and (6.19). These are illustrated in Figure 6–16. These cases occur when $k_S x_O/D$ is much less than 1 or much greater than 1. The left-hand side of Figure 6–16 illustrates the case when $k_S x_O/D << 1$. In this case $C_I \approx C^*$ and the oxidant profile is essentially flat through the oxide. Physically this means that the diffusion process is not rate limiting or in other words that oxidant is being supplied to the Si/SiO_2 interface at a rate which is fast compared to that required to sustain the chemical reaction occurring there. This condition is often referred to as reaction rate controlled since the interface is determining the rate at which

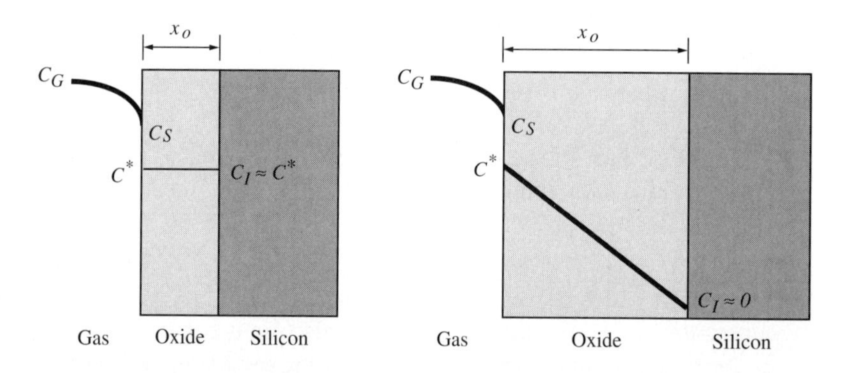

Figure 6–16 Limiting cases in silicon oxidation. The interface reaction is the rate limiting step on the left; the oxidant transport through the SiO_2 rate limits on the right.

the oxide grows. Generally this is the case for thin oxides since $k_S x_O/D << 1$ when x_O is small. The oxide thickness at which $k_S x_O/D \approx 1$ varies with temperature since k_S and D change with temperature, but is usually in the range of 50–200 nm.

For oxide thicknesses above this value, the growth tends more and more toward the limiting case shown on the right of Figure 6–16. In this case, $k_S x_O/D >> 1$ and the oxidant profile in the oxide becomes linear, with $C_I \approx 0$. In this case, the oxidant is reacting at the interface as fast as it arrives and the overall growth rate is limited by the diffusion process. This is often referred to as the diffusion controlled regime.

Combining Eqs. (6.17) and (6.18), we have that

$$\frac{dx_O}{dt} = \frac{F}{N_1} = \frac{k_S C^*}{N_1\left[1 + \frac{k_S}{h} + \frac{k_S x_O}{D}\right]} \tag{6.20}$$

where N_1 is the number of oxidant molecules incorporated per unit volume of oxide grown. $N_1 = 2.2 \times 10^{22}\ \text{cm}^{-3}$ for O_2 oxidation and twice this value for H_2O oxidation. Integrating this equation from an initial oxide thickness x_i to a final thickness x_O leads us to our final result describing the oxide growth kinetics:

$$N_1\int_{x_i}^{x_o} 3 1 + \frac{k_S}{h} + \frac{k_S x_O}{D} 4 dx_0 = k_S C^* \int_0^t dt \tag{6.21}$$

$$\therefore \frac{x_O^2 - x_i^2}{B} + \frac{x_O - x_i}{B/A} = t \tag{6.22}$$

where

$$B = \frac{2DC^*}{N_1} \tag{6.23}$$

and
$$\frac{B}{A} = \frac{C^*}{N_1\left(\frac{1}{k_S} + \frac{1}{h}\right)} \cong \frac{C^* k_S}{N_1} \tag{6.24}$$

B and B/A are often termed the parabolic and linear rate constants respectively because of the x^2 and x terms in which they appear. Physically, they represent the contributions of fluxes F_2 (oxidant diffusion) and F_3 (interface reaction), respectively.

It is sometimes convenient to rewrite the linear parabolic growth law in the following form:

$$\frac{x_O^2}{B} + \frac{x_O}{B/A} = t + \tau \tag{6.25}$$

where
$$\tau = \frac{x_i^2 + Ax_i}{B} \tag{6.26}$$

In these expressions, x_i or τ account for any oxide present at the start of the oxidation. They can also be used to provide a better fit to data in the "anomalous" thin oxide regime in dry O_2 as we will see later. Solving the parabolic equation leads to the following explicit expression for oxide thickness in terms of growth time:

$$x_O = \frac{A}{2}\left\{\sqrt{1 + \frac{t + \tau}{A^2/4B}} - 1\right\} \tag{6.27}$$

There are two limiting forms of the linear parabolic growth law that may be seen directly from Eq. (6.25). These occur when one of the two terms dominates, leading to

$$x_O \cong \frac{B}{A}(t + \tau) \quad \text{or} \quad x_O^2 \cong B(t + \tau) \tag{6.28}$$

The reasons for referring to B/A and B as the linear and parabolic rate constants are clear when the growth law is expressed in these forms. The linear term will dominate for small x values, the parabolic term for larger x values. SiO_2 growth on a bare silicon wafer therefore usually starts out with a linear x versus t characteristic, which becomes parabolic as the oxide thickens.

Eqs. (6.23) and (6.24) suggest that we should be able to calculate values for B and B/A and therefore test the predictions of the linear parabolic model against experiment. In fact, B and B/A are normally determined experimentally by extracting them from growth data. The reason for taking this approach is simply that we usually do not know all the parameters in Eqs. (6.23) and (6.24). k_S in particular contains a lot of "hidden" physics associated with the interface reaction. What we can do, however, is compare experimental values of B and B/A with the form of Eqs. (6.23) and (6.24) to test the reasonableness of the linear parabolic model.

Figure 6–17 suggests how the oxidation rate constants can be extracted from experimental data. By replotting oxide thickness versus time data in the form shown on the

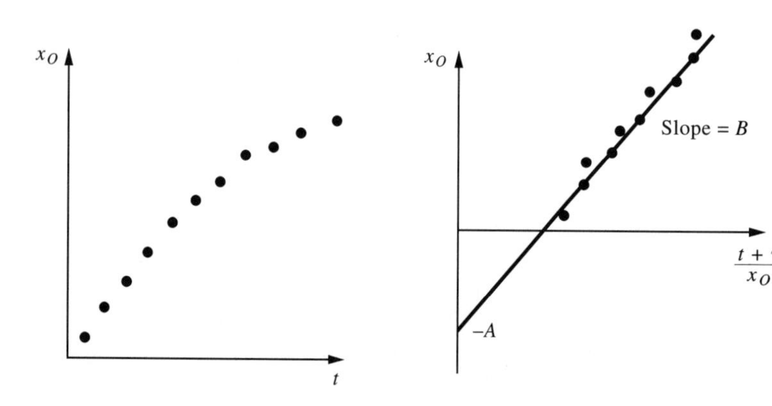

Figure 6–17 Extraction of rate constants from oxide thickness versus time experimental data.

right in the figure, B is directly extracted from the slope of the line and A and hence B/A, is extracted from the intercept. This approach has been widely used to determine values for B and B/A for a wide range of experimental conditions. If the experimental data do fall on a straight line when plotted in the form of Figure 6–17, then the data are well described by a linear parabolic growth law. In fact, there are many growth conditions that do not result in data that lie on a straight line, some of which we will discuss in later sections of this chapter. In these cases, we can conclude that the data are not well modeled by the simple linear parabolic model we have described thus far.

When oxidations are performed on flat unpatterned surfaces, on lightly doped substrates, in simple O_2 or H_2O ambients and when the oxide thickness is larger than about 20 nm, the growth kinetics are usually well described by the linear parabolic law. Under such conditions, values for B and B/A can be readily extracted. Experimentally, we find that both B and B/A are well described by Arrhenius expressions of the form

$$B = C_1 \exp(-E_1/kT) \tag{6.29}$$

$$\frac{B}{A} = C_2 \exp(-E_2/kT) \tag{6.30}$$

In these expressions, E_1 and E_2 are the activation energies associated with the physical processes that B and B/A represent; C_1 and C_2 are the preexponential constants.

It is often the case that considerable physical significance can be attached to activation energies that are measured experimentally when Arrhenius relationships are followed. Table 6–2 below lists the experimental values for the parameters in Eqs. (6.29) and (6.30). The corresponding values for B and B/A are also plotted in Figure 6–18. In Table 6–2, the middle oxidation ambient ("wet O_2") corresponds to an oxidation system in which O_2 is bubbled through H_2O at 95°C. The result is an oxidation ambient which is mostly H_2O, but also contains some O_2. These kinds of systems were common some years ago, although most H_2O oxidation systems today directly react H_2 and O_2 to produce H_2O in the back of the furnace.

Consider first the parabolic rate constant B. We find experimentally, that the activation energy E_1 is quite different for O_2 and H_2O ambients. Eq. (6.23) suggests that the

Table 6–2 Rate constants describing (111) silicon oxidation kinetics at 1 Atm total pressure. For the corresponding values for (100) silicon, all C_2 values should be divided by 1.68.

Ambient	*B*	*B/A*
Dry O_2	$C_1 = 7.72 \times 10^2$ µm² hr⁻¹ → $C_1 = 7.72 \times 10^2\ \mu m^2\ hr^{-1}$	$C_2 = 6.23 \times 10^6\ \mu m\ hr^{-1}$
	$E_1 = 1.23$ eV	$E_2 = 2.0$ eV
Wet O_2	$C_1 = 2.14 \times 10^2\ \mu m^2\ hr^{-1}$	$C_2 = 8.95 \times 10^7\ \mu m\ hr^{-1}$
	$E_1 = 0.71$ eV	$E_2 = 2.05$ eV
H_2O	$C_1 = 3.86 \times 10^2\ \mu m^2\ hr^{-1}$	$C_2 = 1.63 \times 10^8\ \mu m\ hr^{-1}$
	$E_1 = 0.78$ eV	$E_2 = 2.05$ eV

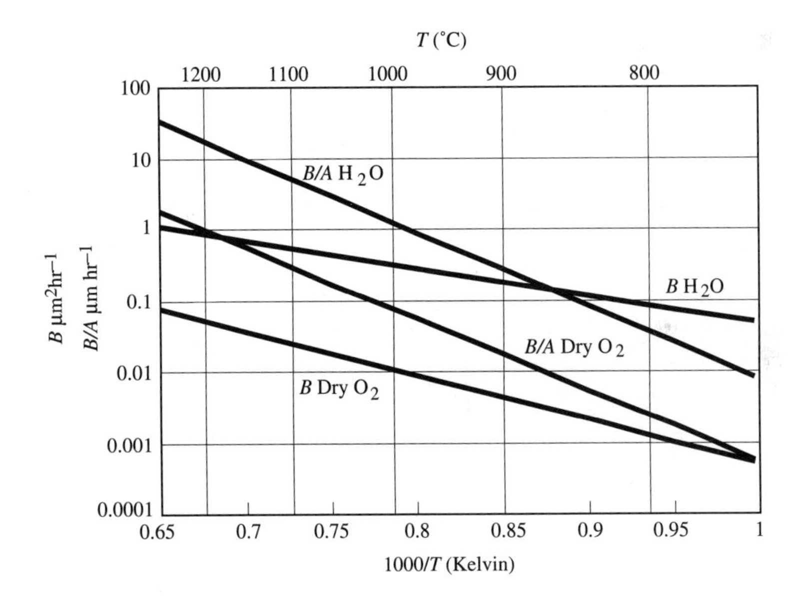

Figure 6–18 *B* and *B/A* for O_2 and H_2O oxidation of <111> silicon. Values taken from the parameters in Table 6–2.

physical mechanism responsible for E_1 might be the oxidant diffusion through the SiO_2. (N_1 is a constant and C^* is not expected to increase exponentially with temperature.) In fact, independent measurements of the diffusion coefficients of O_2 and H_2O in SiO_2 show that these parameters vary with temperature in the same way as Eq. (6.29) and with E_1 values close to those shown in Table 6–2. The clear implication is that *B* in the linear parabolic model really does represent the oxidant diffusion process.

The E_2 values for *B/A* in the table are all quite close to 2 eV. Eq. (6.24) suggests that the physical origin of E_2 is likely connected with the interface reaction rate constant k_S. k_S really represents a number of processes occurring at the Si/SiO_2 interface. These may

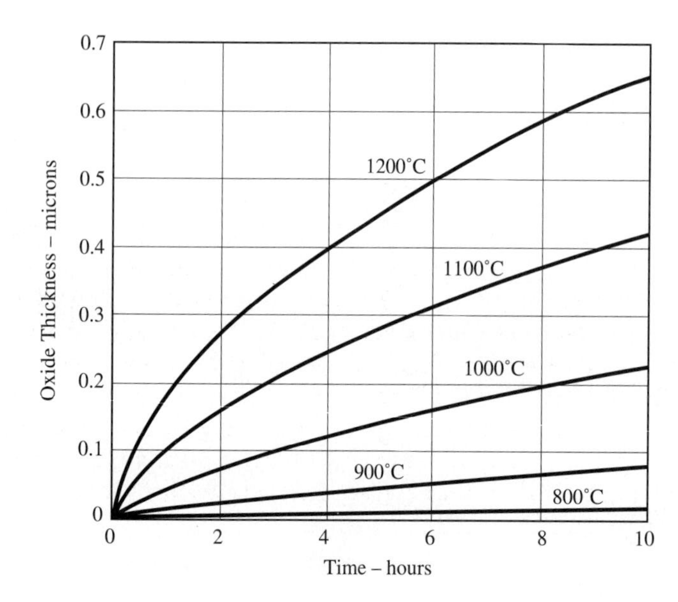

Figure 6–19 Calculated oxidation rates for (100) silicon in dry O_2 based on the Deal-Grove model. Parameter values taken from Table 6–2. The initial fast oxidation for the first ≈ 20 nm is not included ($\tau = 0$).

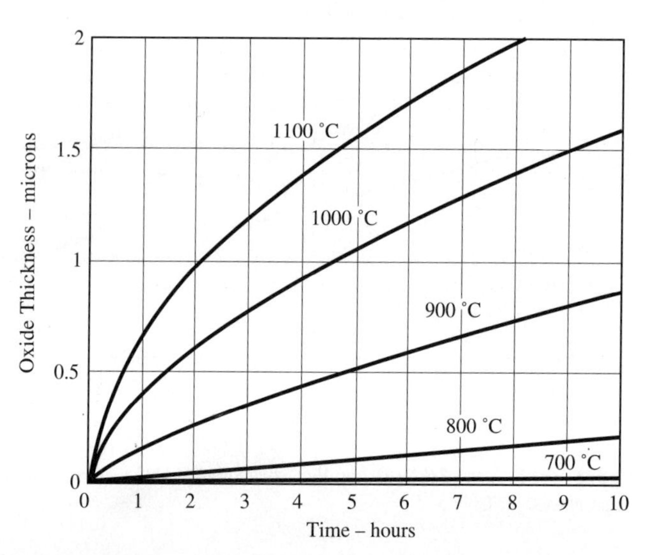

Figure 6–20 Calculated oxidation rates for (100) silicon in H_2O based on the Deal-Grove model. Parameter values taken from Table 6–2.

include oxidant dissociation ($O_2 \rightarrow 2O$), Si-Si bond breaking, and/or Si-O bond formation. Traditionally, the 2-eV activation energy has been associated with the Si-Si bond breaking process because of measurements by Pauling that suggested that the Si-Si bond energy was in the correct range to explain the B/A values. However, the interface reaction is very complex and it is likely that other effects also affect the experimental

B/A values. An additional observation that supports the idea that it is something associated with the Si substrate that determines E_2, is that E_2 is essentially independent of oxidation ambient. It is also essentially independent of substrate crystal orientation, which suggests that E_2 represents a fundamental part of the oxidation process, not something only associated with the substrate.

Using the values for B and B/A in Table 6–2, Figures 6–19 and 6–20 show the calculated oxide thickness versus time curves predicted by the Deal-Grove model. The general behavior of an initially linear growth rate that becomes parabolic as the oxide grows is apparent in these calculated curves. It is also apparent from the figures that SiO_2 grows much faster in an H_2O ambient than it does in dry O_2. The principal reason for this is that the oxidant solubility in SiO_2 [C^* in Eqs. (6.23) and (6.24)], is much higher for H_2O than for O_2. At 1100°C, typical values for C^* are $\approx 5 \times 10^{16}$ cm^{-3} for dry O_2 and $\approx 3 \times 10^{19}$ cm^{-3} for H_2O. As a result, both rate constants, B and B/A are much larger for H_2O than for O_2. Dry O_2 oxidations are thus generally useful for producing oxide films up to 100–200 nm. Films thicker than this would normally be grown using H_2O ambients.

Example Local oxidation is a process that is widely used to provide lateral isolation between devices in IC chips. In some cases, it is desirable to end up with a more planar surface than standard LOCOS provides, and so a silicon etch is used prior to the oxidation step as illustrated in Figure 6–21. For the structure shown on the left, with 0.5 μm of silicon etched prior to the oxidation, how long must the wafer be oxidized at 1000°C in H_2O to produce the planar oxide shown on the right?

Answer There is a 2.2X volume expansion during thermal oxidation, so growing 1 μm of SiO_2 consumes 0.45 μm of silicon. Thus the growing oxide will consume an additional thickness of silicon (y in Figure 6–22) in filling up the etched trench. Thus we need to grow a total thickness of SiO_2 given by

$$\frac{y}{0.45} = y + 0.5 \Rightarrow y = 0.41\,\mu\text{m}$$

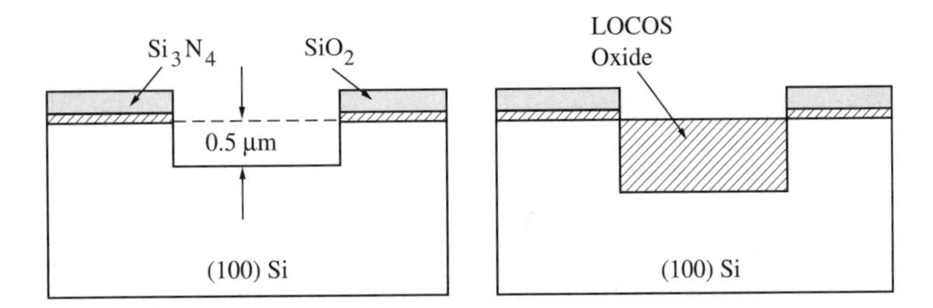

Figure 6–21 Recessed LOCOS process in which the silicon is etched prior to LOCOS to produce a final planar surface. The "bird's beak" produced at the boundaries of such structures is not illustrated here (see Figure 6–41 later in the chapter).

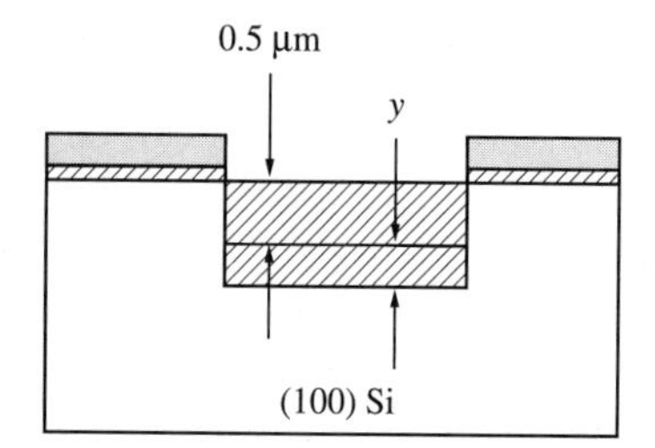

Figure 6–22 Recessed LOCOS geometry showing additional silicon consumed during the oxidation.

Thus we need to grow a total of 0.91 μm of SiO_2. At 1000°C in H_2O we have

$$B = 3.86 \times 10^2 \exp\left(-\frac{0.78\text{ eV}}{kT}\right) = 0.316\ \mu\text{m}^2\text{hr}^{-1}$$

$$\frac{B}{A} = \frac{1.63 \times 10^8}{1.68} \exp\left(-\frac{2.05\text{ eV}}{kT}\right) = 0.75\ \mu\text{m hr}^{-1}$$

$$\therefore t = \frac{x_0^2}{B} + \frac{x_0}{B/A} = \frac{(0.91)^2}{0.316} + \frac{0.91}{0.75} = 3.83\text{ hrs}$$

6.5.2 Other Models for Planar Oxidation Kinetics

The linear parabolic model described above is the most widely accepted oxidation model. However, it does not explain a number of experimental observations, many of which we will discuss in subsequent sections of this chapter. One fact of particular importance is that experimental measurements of oxide growth rates in dry O_2 are not accurately predicted by the Deal-Grove model for thin oxides less than about 20 nm. Because of this and other problems, many other models have been proposed, each claiming to be an improvement over the linear parabolic approach. However, none of these models has gained widespread acceptance. We will briefly discuss here a few of these alternative models, in order to provide a broader picture of oxidation kinetics.

In 1987, Reisman and colleagues [6.13] suggested that a very simple power law of the form

$$x_O = a(t + t_i)^b \quad \text{or} \quad x_O = a\left(t + \left(\frac{x_i}{a}\right)^{\frac{1}{b}}\right)^b \tag{6.31}$$

where a and b are constants for a given set of process conditions and t_i is the time corresponding to the growth of any existing oxide (x_i) at the start of the process, could fit all published dry O_2 oxidation data. In fitting this equation to experimental data, they extracted b values between 0.25 and 1.0, depending on temperature and oxidant partial pressure. This equation has two fitting parameters (a and b), just as the Deal-Grove model has two (B and B/A). There are key differences between the models, however. First, Reisman and colleagues claim that Eq. (6.31) can fit data down to an oxide thickness of essentially 0. There is no anomalous thin regime as there is with the Deal-Grove model. Second, the physical bases for the models are quite different. The Deal-Grove model as we have seen is based on the idea of oxidant diffusion and an interface reaction, with each process dominating the growth under different conditions. In a follow-up paper to [6.13], Nicollian and Reisman suggested that the interface reaction actually controlled the oxidation process at all times and that the volume expansion necessary at that interface to accommodate the growing oxide was provided by viscous flow (relaxation) of the oxide layer [6.14]. The time-dependent viscous flow of the oxide, in their model, is used to explain the extracted pressure and temperature dependence of the parameters in their model (b and a).

The model expressed in Eq. (6.31) has not yet been widely implemented in process simulation programs. These programs generally still rely on the Deal-Grove linear parabolic model. However, the physical approach used in [6.13, 6.14] is interesting because the concepts of volume expansion and oxide viscous flow are also the basic ideas used to explain oxidation on nonplanar silicon surfaces as we will see in Section 6.5.7.

Another approach to modeling oxidation kinetics was recently suggested by Han and Helms [6.15]. They showed that a wide body of oxidation data, including the dry O_2 thin regime, could be modeled by an expression of the form

$$\frac{dx_O}{dt} = \frac{B_1}{2x_O + A_1} + \frac{B_2}{2x_O + A_2} \tag{6.32}$$

The two terms represent parallel oxidation processes, perhaps O_2 and O diffusing through the SiO_2 in parallel, or perhaps O_2 and oxygen vacancies. This type of parallel diffusion and reaction was first proposed by Hirabayashi and Iwamura [6.16], to model O_2/HCl oxidations, a topic we will return to later in Section 6.5.6. All of the rate constants in Eq. (6.32) were found to fit Arrhenius expressions of the form

$$B_1 = C\exp(-E_A/kT) \tag{6.33}$$

with the values given in the Table 6–3 below for dry O_2 oxidation.

Except for the B_2/A_2 values, all numbers in Table 6–3 apply to either (111) or (100) silicon orientations. Note that no values are given for B_1/A_1 since Han and Helms found that setting this term to ∞ ($A_1 = 0$), produced reasonable agreement with experiment.

Table 6–3 Experimental rate constants for the parallel oxidation model of Han and Helms [6.15]

	B_1	B_1/A_1	B_2	B_2/A_2
C	3.9×10^5 μm² hr⁻¹	∞	1.56×10^4 μm² hr⁻¹	4.98×10^6 μm hr⁻¹ (111) 1.56×10^6 μm hr⁻¹ (100)
E_A	2.2 eV		1.6 eV	1.9 eV

Presumably this implies that whatever process the first term in Eq. (6.32) represents, the interface reaction associated with that process is very fast. Integrating (6.32) produces a closed form expression for oxide thickness versus time :

$$(x_O^2 - x_i^2) + C(x_O - x_i) - G\ln\left(\frac{2Ex_O + F}{2Ex_i + F}\right) = Et \qquad (6.34)$$

where $C = \dfrac{A_1B_1 + A_2B_2}{B_1 + B_2}$, $E = B_1 + B_2$, $F = A_1B_2 + A_2B_1$, $G = \dfrac{B_1B_2(A_1 - A_2)^2}{2(B_1 + B_2)^2}$

As mentioned above, Han and Helms found that they could fit experimental data satisfactorily with $A_1 = 0$ which simplifies these expressions somewhat. This model has not been applied to H_2O oxidations. However, the simple linear parabolic model works quite well for H_2O, and it is really just a special case of Eq. (6.32) in which only one of the two terms is used.

Another model that has been proposed is due to Ghez and van der Meulen [6.17]. The model was motivated by a series of oxidation experiments done by van der Meulen with various partial pressures of O_2 in the oxidizing ambient. The linear parabolic model predicts that both B and B/A should be linearly proportional to pressure. (This is a consequence of assuming that Henry's law holds during the oxidant adsorption into the SiO_2 and that only a molecular species is involved in the transport through the oxide and reaction at the Si/SiO_2 interface.) van der Meulen's measurements showed that

$$\frac{B}{A} \propto P^n \qquad (6.35)$$

where n approached 0.5 at low oxidation temperatures and 1 at high temperatures. (In contrast, n is experimentally equal to 1 for H_2O oxidations, suggesting that the assumptions made in the Deal-Grove model are more accurate in that case.)

To explain their results, Ghez and van der Meulen proposed a model in which molecular O_2 is absorbed from the gas phase and diffuses through the SiO_2 to the silicon surface. At the oxidizing interface, two parallel reactions were proposed, one involving molecular O_2 and the other atomic O. This results in a complicated growth law with no simple analytic formulation. However the atomic O reaction does lead to an n value of 0.5 for the interface reaction; the molecular O_2 reaction leads to an n value of 1. van der Meulen's data can therefore be explained by assuming that the atomic reaction dominates at low temperature and the molecular reaction at high temperatures. We will discuss these results more carefully in Section 6.5.4.

Figures 6–23 and 6–24 compare the predictions of several of these alternative models with the Deal-Grove model. The model parameters for these plots were taken from Tables 6–2 and 6–3 for the Deal-Grove and Han and Helms models, respectively. For the Reisman and colleagues model at 800°C, a = 0.302 nm, b = 0.704 and t_O = 13.1 min. At 1000°C, a = 3.02 nm, b = 0.701 and t_O = 1.26 min [6.13].

At 800°C (Figure 6–23), the differences in these models for very thin oxides are apparent. The Han and Helms and Reisman and colleagues models agree fairly well with each other and both match experimental data in the thin regime well. The Deal-Grove

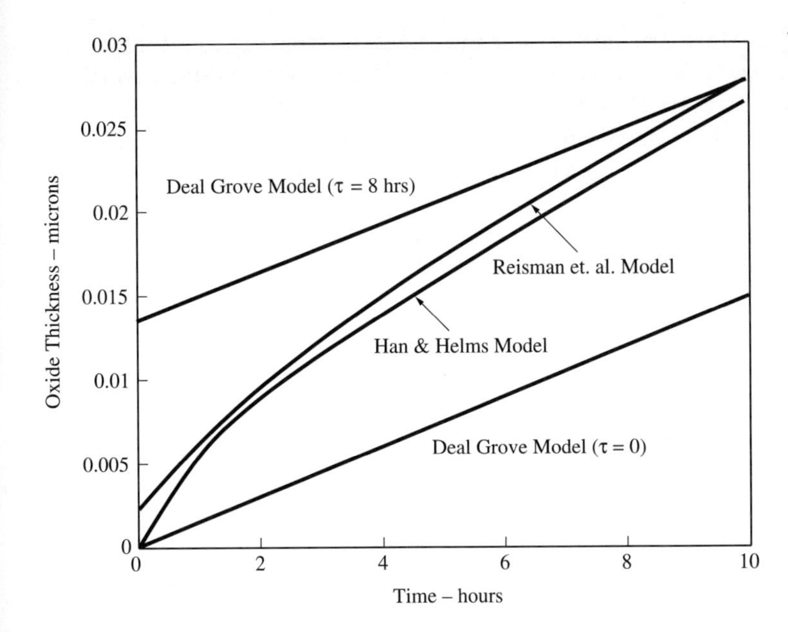

Figure 6–23 Comparison of three oxidation models for 1 atmosphere dry O_2 oxidation at 800°C.

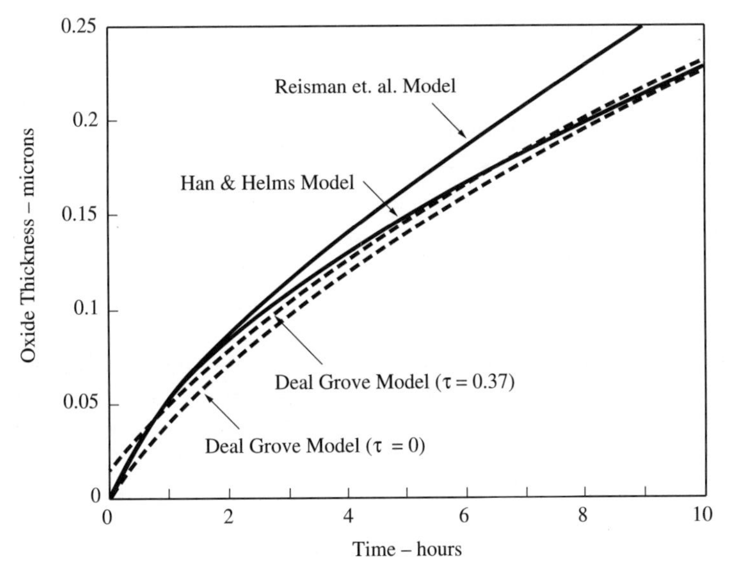

Figure 6–24 Comparison of three oxidation models for 1 atmosphere dry O_2 oxidation at 1000°C. The dashed lines are the Deal-Grove model.

model does not do a very good job for thin oxides even with τ set at 8 hours (the value Deal and Grove extracted in their original work [6.6]). We will see in Section 6.5.3, that the Deal-Grove model can be "fixed" to do a better job in the dry O_2 thin regime. Note that for oxides thicker than about 20 nm all three models converge to approximately the same result, as long as we use $\tau = 8$ hours in the Deal-Grove model.

At 1000°C (Figure 6–24), the differences in the models in the very thin regime are less apparent since much thicker oxides grow at the higher temperature on the same time scale. Including or not including τ in the Deal-Grove model also makes less difference, for the same reason. For the particular parameters chosen for this plot, the Reisman and colleagues model diverges from the predictions of the other models for thicker oxides.

In summary, many other models for oxidation kinetics have been proposed, all of them motivated by shortcomings in the linear parabolic model. However, none of these models has found the widespread acceptance of the linear parabolic model. Most modeling efforts today use the Deal-Grove model as a starting point and then add to it or modify it as necessary to include effects that the basic model itself either does not include or does not model well. We will consider many of these effects in the sections below.

6.5.3 Thin Oxide SiO$_2$ Growth Kinetics

The very earliest oxidation studies suggested that there was something unusual about the initial growth of oxides in dry O_2 on bare silicon wafers. Deal and Grove in their original paper describing the linear parabolic model observed that the model did not fit the first 20 nm of growth in dry O_2 and we saw an example of this in Figure 6–23. They attributed the fast growth rate they experimentally observed in this regime to the effect of a space charge region in the oxide, set up by the indiffusing oxygen ions (presumably O_2^-). If the principal diffusing species really were ionic, then positive charge carriers would also be present to maintain charge neutrality. The two species O_2^- and holes (h^+) would diffuse as a coupled pair. The holes, however, diffuse much faster than the O_2^- and would tend to move on ahead. This sets up an electric field due to the charge separation, which acts to keep the two together. The effect of this field is to slow the holes down and to speed up the O_2^- ions. This coupled diffusion is observed anytime a charged species diffuses. The distance over which the electric field exists is on the order of the extrinsic Debye length, given by

$$L_D = \sqrt{\frac{kT\varepsilon_S}{2q^2C^*}} \tag{6.36}$$

Substituting in numbers for O_2 oxidations gives a Debye length of about 15 nm which agrees with the thickness over which fast growth occurs. For H_2O oxidations, C^* is about 10^3 times higher, resulting in a Debye length of less than 1 nm even if a charged species were involved in water oxidations. Deal and Grove used this observation to suggest why an anomalous fast initial growth is not observed in H_2O oxidations. The difficulty with this explanation, however, is that the original assumption that O_2^- was the species involved in oxidant transport was based on experiments done by Jorgenson in the early 1960s [6.2]. These results have been subsequently largely discounted.

If neutral O_2 and H_2O are the dominant diffusing species, space charge effects cannot be responsible for the anomalous high initial growth rate observed in O_2. This has led to a large number of new proposals over the past 20 years, all attempting to explain thin oxide kinetics. There is still great debate about the physical mechanism(s) responsible; no consensus has emerged. The problem has taken on new importance recently, because MOS gate oxides are now routinely grown with thicknesses in this "anomalous" range. This is an example of industrial application outpacing basic scientific understanding. From an industrial perspective, it is more important to be able to grow these thin oxide layers reproducibly and uniformly, and with good electrical properties than it is to understand the governing physical principles. However this is sometimes a dangerous approach because lack of physical understanding may mean that manufacturing problems which arise may not be understood and may have to be solved by trial and error experiments. This is the reason why so much effort has been invested in understanding thin oxide growth kinetics.

One of the factors which confuses model development and data interpretation in the thin regime is that chemical cleaning procedures prior to oxidation have been shown to significantly affect the oxide growth kinetics. We discussed wafer cleaning and some of these effects in detail in Chapter 4 (Figure 4–3). Most experimental studies of thin growth kinetics have not carefully controlled this parameter with the result that data on oxide thickness versus time vary from experiment to experiment even when the same temperatures and other parameters have been used. This makes model development very difficult.

Perhaps the most extensive experimental study yet reported was that by Massoud and colleagues [6.18]. They reported that growth in the thin regime could be fitted by an addition to the Deal-Grove model given by

$$\frac{dx_O}{dt} = \frac{B}{2x_O + A} + C\exp\left(-\frac{x_O}{L}\right) \tag{6.37}$$

where

$$C = C^0\exp\left(-\frac{E_A}{kT}\right)$$

and $C^0 \approx 3.6 \times 10^8$ μm hr^{-1}, $E_A \approx 2.35$ eV, and $L \approx 7$ nm. All these numbers apply to either (111) or (100) oriented silicon substrates. The first term in Eq. (6.37) is, of course, the Deal-Grove model. The second term represents an additional oxidation mechanism that is important for the first few tens of nm but which decreases exponentially with a decay length of about 7 nm. With this addition to the Deal-Grove model, the predictions of this model also match the data well over the whole thickness range. In Figure 6–24, for example, Eq. (6.37) provides an x_O versus t curve that matches the Han and Helms and Reisman and colleagues models. There are thus several ways of modeling the dry O_2 thin regime. Process simulation programs like SUPREM IV have generally implemented Eq. (6.37) rather than the alternatives given by Eqs. (6.31) and (6.32) because models for many other oxidation effects have also been tied to the basic Deal-Grove formulation as we will see later.

Many physical mechanisms have been suggested for the thin regime. Deal and Grove proposed O_2^- coupled diffusion with holes as was discussed above. Other suggestions have included considering the role of thermionic emission of electrons from the silicon into the SiO_2 [6.19], micropores or channels in the oxide which allow parallel oxidant transport when the oxide is thin [6.20], parallel O_2 and O reactions at the Si/SiO_2 interface [6.15], blocking layers near the Si/SiO_2 interface which form as the oxide grows and slow down the rate for thicker layers [6.21], and a silicon surface layer which provides additional sites for the oxidation reaction in its initial phases [6.18]. None of these mechanisms has been shown to be clearly correct and none of them has gained widespread acceptance. We are left with several empirical expressions that can be used to model the thin regime kinetics, but with no completely satisfactory physical explanation. Additional work in the future may help to clarify some of these issues.

6.5.4 Dependence of Growth Kinetics on Pressure

The linear parabolic model predicts that the oxide growth rate should be directly proportional to oxidant pressure. Eq. (6.13) shows this. If Henry's law holds and the concentration of oxidant just inside the oxide at the gas/SiO_2 interface C^* is proportional to P_G, then both B and B/A are proportional to P_G from Eqs. (6.23) and (6.24). The oxide growth rate should therefore be proportional to P_G.

Experimental measurements have shown that in H_2O oxidations this prediction is correct. Pressures below atmospheric [6.6] and well above atmospheric [6.22] have been investigated. These results suggest that the assumptions made in the linear parabolic model are correct for H_2O oxidation. However, the situation is a little less clear for dry O_2 oxidation. A considerable body of data has consistently shown that in order to model dry O_2 results with a linear parabolic equation, $B \propto P$ and $B/A \propto P^n$ where $0.5 < n < 1$. This pressure dependence is inconsistent with the linear parabolic model. One can only conclude that the linear parabolic model must be incomplete. Within the context of that model, we can infer that since $B \propto P$, then $C^* \propto P$ from Eq. (6.20). If B/A is not linearly proportional to P, then from Eq. (6.21), k_S must depend on P in a nonlinear fashion.

There have been a number of attempts to modify the Deal-Grove model to account for these experimental results. Ghez and van der Meulen (Section 6.5.2) attempted to extend the linear parabolic model to include both O and O_2 reacting at the Si/SiO_2 interface. This model can explain the observed pressure dependence because an O-based reaction would vary as $P^{0.5}$ and an O_2 reaction would vary as $P^{1.0}$. A mixed reaction could give any value between these two limits. However, this model contains many parameters and it has not been fit to a wide range of oxidation data. As a result, it cannot easily be used today to model the complete range of O_2 growth kinetics. More recently, Hu [6.23] attempted to treat the parallel O/O_2 interface reaction in terms of a chemisorption model. Other attempts to account for the pressure dependence of B/A have departed more radically from the Deal-Grove model. These attempts have almost all been based on a modified Si/SiO_2 interface reaction. None of these models has found widespread acceptance.

Lacking a widely accepted first principles model to explain the pressure dependence of O_2 growth kinetics, the best we can do today to model these effects is to simply use the Deal-Grove model with the following corrections:

$$\frac{B}{A} = \left(\frac{B}{A}\right)^i P \quad B = (B)^i P \quad \text{for } H_2O \tag{6.38}$$

$$\frac{B}{A} = \left(\frac{B}{A}\right)^i P^n \quad B = (B)^i P \quad \text{for } O_2 \tag{6.39}$$

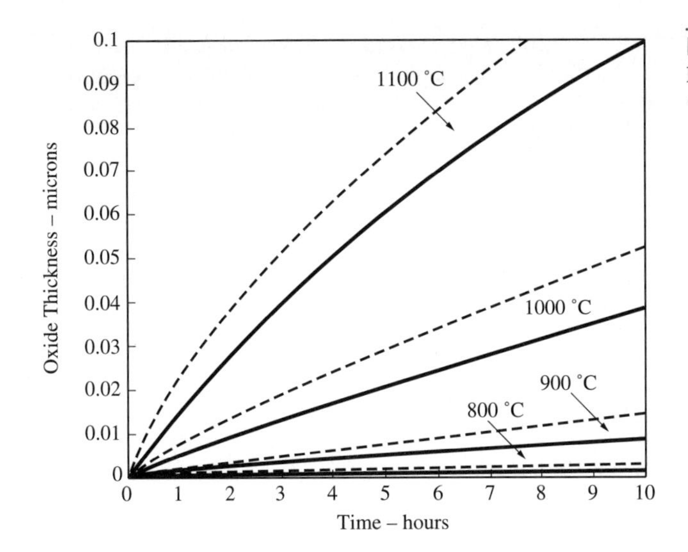

Figure 6–25 Oxidation at 0.1 atmosphere in dry O_2 using the Deal-Grove model. The solid lines correspond to $B \propto P$ and $B/A \propto P$. The dashed lines correspond to $B \propto P$ and $B/A \propto P^{0.8}$.

where $n \approx 0.7$–0.8. The i superscripts refer to the respective values at 1 Atm. A similar $P^{0.8}$ pressure dependence has been noted in the thin regime (< 20 nm). This may be included in Eq. (6.34) by making $C \propto P^{0.8}$. The decay length L in that equation does not seem to have any significant pressure dependence.

Figures 6–25 and 6–26 illustrate the effects of these pressure models on oxidation kinetics, using the Deal-Grove model and Eqs. (6.38) and (6.39), without the added thin oxide model. Note that for pressures below 1 atmosphere, the actual oxide thickness is increased by the sublinear pressure dependence of B/A, while the reverse is true for pressures above 1 atmosphere. Process simulators like SUPREM IV generally implement equations like (6.38) and (6.39) to model these effects.

6.5.5 Dependence of Growth Kinetics on Crystal Orientation

As we saw in Chapter 3, historically two principal crystal orientations have been used in manufacturing ICs. (111) crystals were used in the 1960s almost exclusively. However, as it became clear that the electrical properties of the Si/SiO_2 interface were superior on the (100) crystal surface, a gradual shift to that orientation began, with the result that (100) wafers are almost exclusively used today. Oxidation studies which have investigated orientation effects have usually concentrated on these two types of crystals and it has been shown many times that oxidation growth rates are faster on (111) surfaces than they are on (100) surfaces. In recent years, it has become important to understand orientation effects on oxidation more generally because many structures now use etched trenches and other shaped silicon regions as part of their structure.

Even before the development of the linear parabolic model, it had been observed that crystal orientation affected oxidation rate. Ligenza in 1961 [6.24] suggested that the

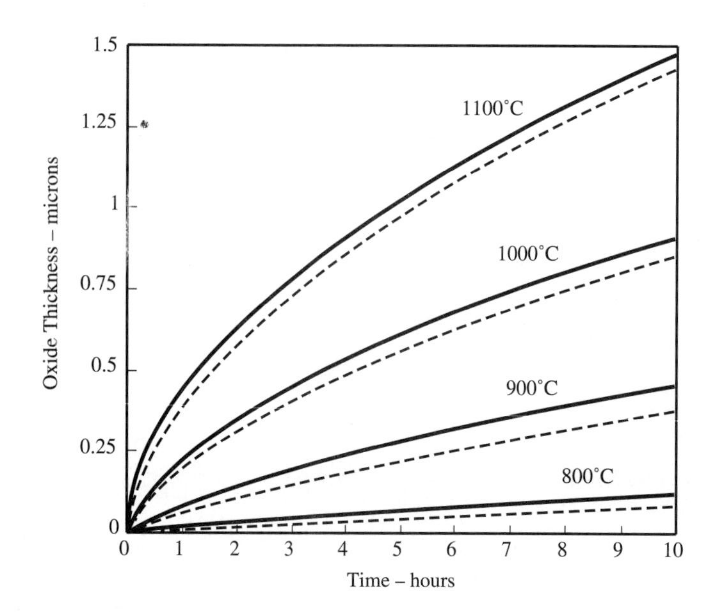

Figure 6–26 Oxidation at 10 atmospheres in dry O_2 using the Deal-Grove model. The solid lines correspond to $B \propto P$ and $B/A \propto P$. The dashed lines correspond to $B \propto P$ and $B/A \propto P^{0.8}$.

effect might be caused by differences in the surface density of silicon atoms on the various crystal faces. He argued that since silicon atoms are required for the oxidation process, crystal planes that have higher densities of atoms should oxidize faster. He further argued that it was not simply the number of silicon atoms cm^{-2} that was important, but also the number of bonds since it is necessary for Si-Si bonds to be broken for the oxidation to proceed.

Ligenza calculated the number of "available" bonds cm^{-2} on the various silicon surfaces and concluded that oxidation rates in H_2O should be in the order (111) > (100). This is in fact what is observed experimentally in both H_2O and dry O_2. For most oxidation conditions of interest in silicon technology, these two orientations represent the upper and lower bounds for oxidation rates. For very thin oxides grown at very low pressures in dry O_2, there is some evidence that the (110) rate becomes fastest [6.25]. This also appears to be the case at very high pressures and low temperatures in H_2O [6.24].

We can incorporate these effects in the linear parabolic model in the following way. Except perhaps in the region very near the Si/SiO$_2$ interface, the oxide that grows on silicon is amorphous; that is, it does not incorporate any information about the underlying silicon crystal structure. Because of this, the parabolic rate constant B should not be orientation dependent since B represents oxidant diffusion through the SiO_2. If the oxide structure is unrelated to the underlying substrate, there should be no crystal orientation effect on B. This is in fact what is found experimentally when kinetic data are analyzed in the context of the linear parabolic model and the rate constants B and B/A are extracted. B/A, on the other hand, should be orientation dependent because it involves the reaction at the Si/SiO$_2$ interface. This reaction surely involves Si atoms and so should be affected by the number of available reaction sites. We can thus incorporate orientation effects as follows:

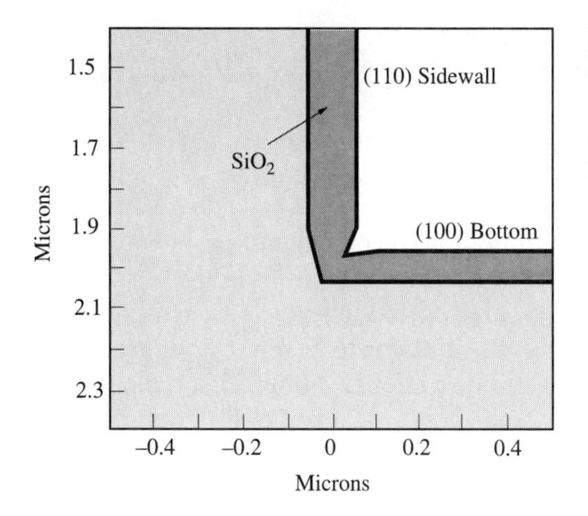

Figure 6–27 Example of an oxidation simulation involving orientation effects using the ATHENA simulator [6.12]. The top and bottom surfaces of the etched trench are (100) surfaces. The trench sidewall is a (110) surface. The oxidation was 30 min at 900°C in H_2O.

$$\left(\frac{B}{A}\right)_{111} = 1.68\left(\frac{B}{A}\right)_{100} \tag{6.40}$$

All other orientations are normally in between these two extremes and B values are the same for all orientations. The (110) B/A value is often taken as 1.45 times the (100) rate although the amount of data available is not sufficient to be certain of this value.

An example of a simulation showing orientation effects is shown in Figure 6–27. A silicon trench is first etched 2 μm deep and then oxidized. Note the thicker oxide along the (110) sidewall surface compared to the (100) wafer surface and trench bottom. Actually the most interesting part of this simulation is at the trench corner, shown on the right, where 2D effects dominate. We will discuss these issues in Section 6.5.7.

Finally, it may be interesting to speculate about why the orientation effect apparently changes for very thin oxides grown at low O_2 partial pressures and also for high pressure steam oxides grown at low temperatures. These two conditions represent the two extremes of oxide growth rates, one extremely slow and the other very fast. In the former case, we have already seen that the growth kinetics are different for thin oxides grown in dry O_2. Since the mechanism is apparently different in this regime, it is perhaps not too surprising that other effects such as the orientation dependence also change. In the case of high-pressure steam oxides, Ligenza observed the (100) surface to oxidize faster than the (111) surface at 800°C and below. These experiments were done at pressures up to 150 atm so the growth rates were extremely high. We will see in Section 6.5.7 on 2D growth kinetics that relaxation of grown-in stresses in SiO_2 layers takes place through viscoelastic flow of the oxide layer. In essence the glass flows as it is grown to relieve the stresses due to volume differences between the oxide and the silicon from which it is grown. At low temperatures this relaxation is more difficult because the oxide cannot flow as easily. It is also more difficult if the oxide is growing very rapidly because there is less time for the oxide to relax before new layers grow. It may be the case in Ligenza's experiments, then, that very high stresses built up in the growing oxides. This may be the origin of the unusual orientation effects that Ligenza observed. The stresses that build up and the oxide flow to relieve those stresses might well be dependent on the substrate crystal orientation. Perhaps future work will resolve these issues.

6.5.6 Mixed Ambient Growth Kinetics

Situations are sometimes encountered in silicon technology in which mixed ambients are used during an oxidation process. The most common example is a mixture of H_2O and O_2. This occurs when H_2 and O_2 are reacted to form H_2O in modern pyrogenic systems. An excess of O_2 is always present in order to ensure that there is no excess H_2 at the furnace exhaust. The result is a mixture of H_2O (about 95% typically) and O_2 (about 5%) in the furnace. In other cases, small concentrations of HCl are sometimes added to O_2 oxidants because this has been found to help reduce oxide defect densities and to reduce contamination levels. The HCl likely helps because it reacts in the furnace to produce Cl_2 and H_2O according to the reaction

$$4HCl + O_2 \leftrightarrow 2H_2O + 2Cl_2 \tag{6.41}$$

and the Cl_2 readily reacts with trace metals and other contaminants in the furnace to produce volatile chlorides as byproducts. In some cases, other Cl sources are used such as trichloroethane that is a liquid, but the reaction that takes place is similar.

Modeling of mixed ambients can be approached in a straightforward manner, if it is assumed each of the oxidants acts independently. The Han and Helms model we discussed for oxidation kinetics allows for independent parallel processes [6.15, 6.16].

$$\frac{dx_O}{dt} = \frac{B_1}{2x_O + A_1} + \frac{B_2}{2x_O + A_2} \tag{6.32}$$

Choosing B_1 and A_1 to correspond to one of the oxidants (H_2O for example) and B_2 and A_2 to correspond to the other oxidant (O_2 for example) allows calculation of the resulting oxide thickness. Note that each B and B/A value must be corrected for the appropriate partial pressure of the corresponding oxidant, using the relationships described in Section 6.5.4.

This simple approach works well in some cases and poorly in others, presumably because the assumption of independence is better in some cases than in others. H_2O/O_2 mixtures can be described by Eq. (6.32) to first order [6.26] although there is some evidence that the H_2O and O_2 reactions at the oxidizing interface are not completely independent (the B/A values seem to be somewhat different than those suggested by the above approach). H_2O/HCl mixtures can be described by Eq. (6.32) because the HCl in this case seems to only dilute the H_2O and plays no role in the oxidation process. This is likely because the H_2O and HCl do not react significantly in the furnace. As a result, only one term in Eq. (6.32) is needed, with rate constants corresponding to H_2O at the appropriate partial pressure [6.27]. O_2/HCl mixtures are not well described by Eq. (6.32). Clear interactions between the oxidant species occur in this case. The Cl generated by Eq. (6.41) is known to be incorporated into the growing SiO_2 film (mostly near the Si/SiO_2 interface). B and B/A values extracted from growth kinetic data monotonically increase with HCl percentage, but not in a well understood manner. Process modeling programs like SUPREM IV generally resort to empirical look-up tables to model these processes. The rate constants are simply expressed as

$$\frac{B}{A} = \left(\frac{B}{A}\right)^{i} \delta \quad \text{and} \quad B = (B)^{i} \chi \tag{6.42}$$

where δ and χ are functions of the HCl concentration in the furnace ambient and are determined empirically. Other mixed ambient reactions could be dealt with in a similar empirical manner, although the principal ones that have been investigated experimentally are those described above.

6.5.7 2D SiO_2 Growth Kinetics

It has been known for many years that shaped silicon structures oxidize differently than simple flat surfaces. This was not of much technological importance until about 1980 when structures became small enough that 2D and even 3D effects began to be noticeable. We saw a simple example of this in Figure 6–4, which illustrated LOCOS processing, and the 2D growth of oxide layers under the edges of Si_3N_4 layers. Even when they were first observed, the origin of these effects was correctly believed to be the volume expansion that SiO_2 undergoes when it grows. We saw previously that SiO_2 grows upward above the silicon surface as it forms, and that the volume expansion involved is more than 2:1. It is perhaps easy to visualize that oxidation occurring in a confined corner in which the volume expansion is more difficult might be different from oxidation on a flat surface.

A quantitative understanding of the physical mechanisms responsible for these effects came only recently from an elegant set of experiments done by Kao and colleagues [6.28, 6.29]. In those experiments, a number of shaped silicon structures were prepared by anisotropic dry etching of silicon wafers. The structures were then oxidized under a variety of conditions and the resulting oxide thicknesses measured using SEM techniques. The data produced oxide thickness as a function of the radius of curvature of the structure being oxidized. Figures 6–28 to 6–30 illustrate the experimental structure and some of the results.

Several interesting observations can be made from the results of Kao et al. The first is that the retardation is a very significant effect in sharp corners—a factor of two in oxide thickness for nominally 500-nm oxides. Second, the retardation is much more pronounced for low-temperature oxidations than it is for high temperatures. In fact there is virtually no corner effect for oxidations done at 1200°C. Finally, interior (concave) corners show a more pronounced effect than do exterior (convex) corners although both are significantly retarded compared to flat surfaces.

Several physical mechanisms are important in understanding these results.

1. Crystal orientation: Shaped surfaces involve many surface orientations. As we saw in Section 6.5.5, orientation affects oxidation rate in the thin oxide or linear regime.

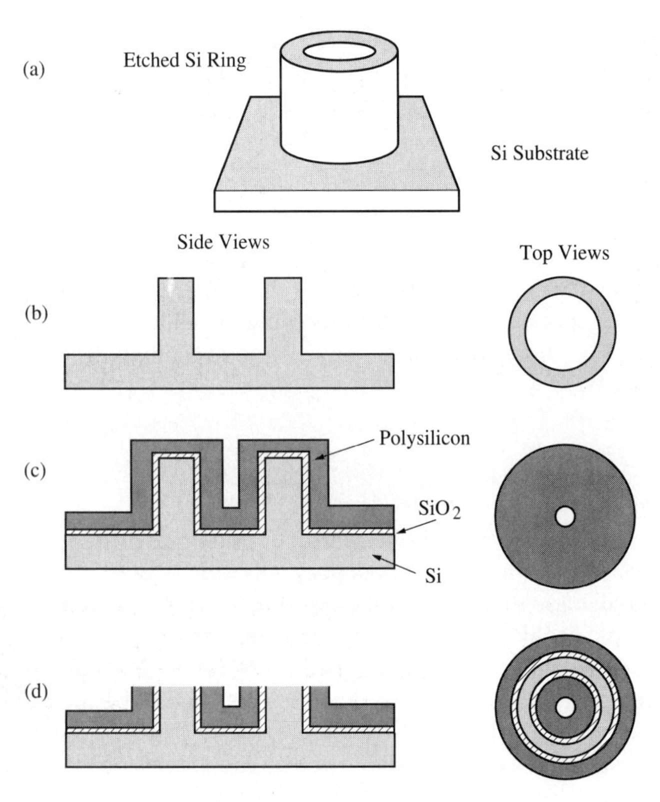

Figure 6–28 Experimental procedure used in the 2D oxidation experiments of Kao [6.28, 6.29]. Silicon wafers were plasma etched to produce a variety of shaped structures including the cylinder illustrated in (a). (b) shows a cross section and top view of the cylinder. In (c) the structure has been oxidized and then coated with a CVD layer of polysilicon. In (d), the structure has been lapped down so that a top view shows the oxide thickness on the sides of the cylinder.

This effect can be modeled in a straightforward manner through Eq. (6.40), although values for the multiplicative constant on B/A for all orientations are needed.

2. 2D Oxidant Diffusion: In corner regions and other shaped structures, oxidant transport to the Si/SiO_2 interface is a 2D or perhaps even 3D transport problem. Since the oxide is amorphous, the diffusion coefficients of O_2 or H_2O should not be direction dependent, but numerical techniques are generally required to solve the diffusion equation in multiple dimensions.
3. Stress due to volume expansion: Oxide layers formed on silicon are under significant compressive stress. This stress is due to the volume expansion that takes place during oxidation and to the difference in thermal expansion coefficients of Si and SiO_2 which causes additional stress when the wafers are cooled from the oxidation temperature

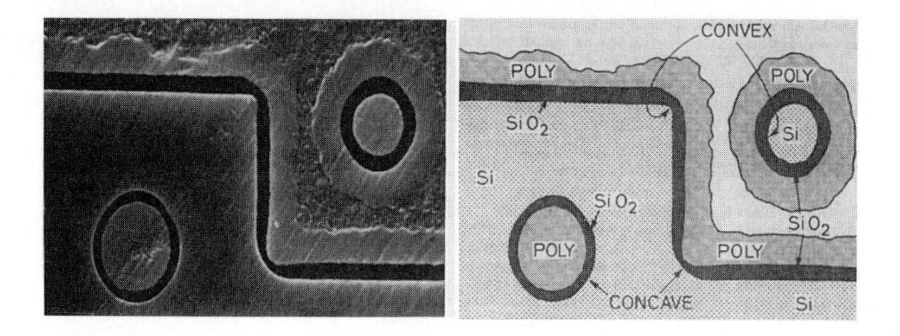

Figure 6–29 Typical experimental result from Kao [6.28, 6.29]. The drawing on the bottom labels the structure shown experimentally on the top. The oxide is thinner on both concave and convex corners than it is on flat regions. Reprinted with permission from IEEE.

back to room temperature. On shaped silicon surfaces, these stresses can be much larger than they would be on a flat surface simply because the volume expansion is dimensionally confined on shaped structures. Such stresses could in principle affect both oxidant transport through the SiO_2 and the interface reaction at the Si/SiO_2 interface.

To model these stress effects, Kao et al. suggested the following modifications to the parameters usually used in the linear parabolic model.

$$k_S(\text{stress}) = k_S \exp\left(-\frac{\sigma_n V_R}{kT}\right)\exp\left(-\frac{\sigma_t V_T}{kT}\right) \tag{6.43}$$

$$D(\text{stress}) = D\exp\left(-\frac{(P)(V_D)}{kT}\right) \tag{6.44}$$

$$C^*(\text{stress}) = C^*\exp\left(-\frac{(P)(V_S)}{kT}\right) \tag{6.45}$$

where k_S is the normal interface reaction rate, σ_n is the stress normal to the growing interface, σ_t is the stress tangential to the growing interface, D is the normal oxidant diffusivity (at 1 Atm), C^* is the normal oxidant solubility used in Eqs. (6.23) and (6.24) and P is the hydrostatic pressure in the growing oxide. V_R, V_T, V_D, and V_S are considered to

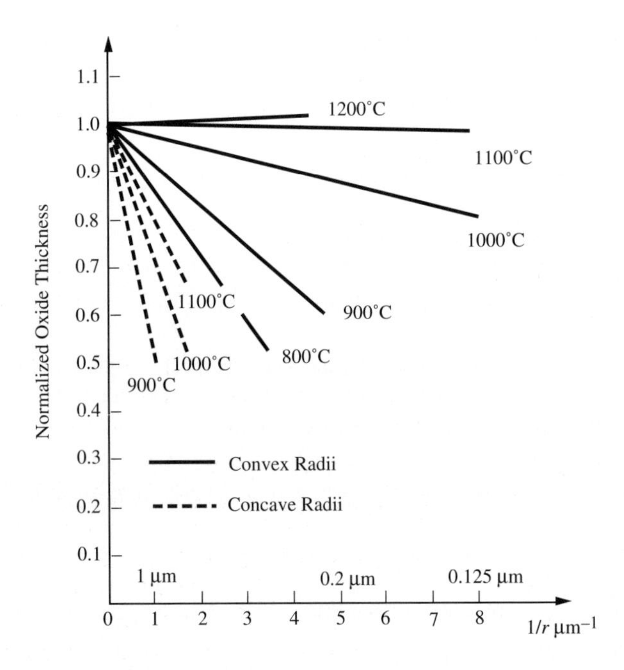

Figure 6–30 Typical experimental data after Kao [6.28, 6.29]. The oxide thickness is plotted versus the radius of curvature of the structure being oxidized. For each temperature, about 500 nm of oxide was grown on a flat surface ($1/r = 0$). These results are for H_2O oxidations. Similar results were found for O_2. Note the retardation of the oxidation for sharp corners (more than a factor of 2 in some cases).

be stress-dependent activation volumes and should be regarded as fitting parameters. They are used in the SUPREM IV implementation of this model.

The final oxide parameter that is needed to calculate growth on shaped surfaces is the oxide viscosity. SiO_2 is a glass and can relax some of the stresses that build up during oxidation by viscoelastic flow. In fact, the stresses that can build up during oxidation are so large, that the oxide viscosity itself needs to be modeled as a function of stress. A relationship of the following form has been found to produce good agreement with experiment [6.30, 6.31]

$$\eta(\text{stress}) = \eta(T)\frac{\sigma_S V_C/2kT}{\sinh(\sigma_S V_C/2kT)} \tag{6.46}$$

where $\eta(T)$ is the stress-free, temperature-dependent oxide viscosity, σ_s is the shear stress in the oxide, and V_C is again a fitting parameter.

Much of the interest in recent years in extending oxidation models has been driven by the need to accurately model advanced isolation processes. LOCOS, poly-buffered LOCOS, shallow trench structures, and the like all involve thermal oxidation of shaped structures. As a result, volume expansion during oxidation, stress-dependent oxidation parameters and oxide viscosity have all taken on first-order importance. Beyond the properties of SiO_2 itself, however, many of the modern isolation structures involve other materials like polysilicon and Si_3N_4. Thus the viscoelastic properties of these materials have also become important.

The nonlinear viscous nature of oxide films at high temperatures has been parameterized by Rafferty [6.31] as described in Eq. (6.46). Subsequent work determined that thin nitride films are viscous at high temperatures, with the viscosity being dependent on the film stoichiometry [6.32]. Similar work with polysilicon thin films has shown that more complex viscosity behavior can be assigned to polysilicon, possibly dependent on the grain size in the film.

Since the shape of the growing oxide changes with time, k_S(stress), D(stress), and η(stress) all change with time during an oxidation. As a result, numerical simulation is required to implement these models. This has been done in SUPREM IV which can successfully predict time-dependent oxide shapes and the stress levels present in both the oxide and the underlying silicon [6.31]. Typical parameters for the SUPREM IV stress-dependent oxidation model are shown in Table 6–4 for wet oxidations [6.30—6.32]. A number of these parameters are fitting parameters (V_R, V_D, V_S, and V_C in particular) and the values should not be regarded as having significant physical meaning. The fact that $V_S \approx 0$ implies that C^* is not highly stress dependent.

An example of the impact of including stress dependent parameters during an oxidation simulation is shown in Figure 6–31. The simulation on the left did not include any stress dependence whereas on the right the types of models for viscosity and stress dependence discussed above were included. Notice that the bird's beak extends much further under the Si_3N_4 mask on the left. Without stress effects, the oxidation rate is not retarded under the masking nitride.

There is a very important implication of the results described in this section. It is quite common in silicon processes to use multiple oxidations during device fabrication. Suppose, for example, that we grow an oxide at 900°C in one step and then further oxidize the silicon in a later step at 1000°C. At the end of the 900°C oxidation, certain stress levels will exist in the SiO_2. If we then heat the wafer to 1000°C, the stress levels cannot immediately take on the values that would be observed in steady state for a 1000°C oxidation. These stresses would in general be lower because the oxide can flow more easily at high temperatures to relieve them. However, this will take some time,

Table 6–4 Typical parameter values in SUPREM IV stress dependent oxidation model

Parameter	Value (Wet Oxidation)
V_R	0.0125 nm^3
V_D	0.0065 nm^3
V_S	0
V_C	0.3 nm^3 @ 850°C
	0.72 nm^3 @ 1050°C
V_T	0
$\eta(T)$—SiO_2	3.13×10^{10} exp(2.19 eV/kT) poise
$\eta(T)$—Si_3N_4	4.77×10^{10} exp(1.12 eV/kT) poise

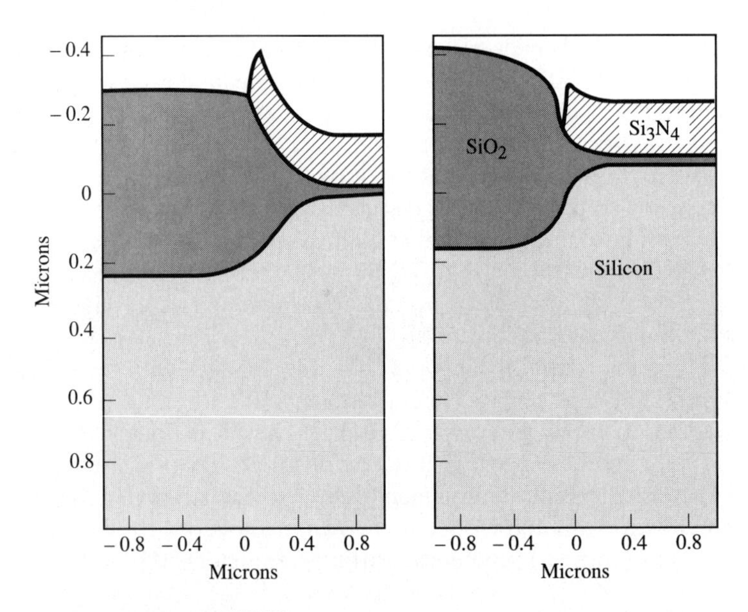

Figure 6–31 Example of an oxidation simulation showing the effects of including stress effects in oxidation using the ATHENA simulator [6.12]. A 20-nm SiO_2 pad oxide is first grown and a 150-nm Si_3N_4 layer is then deposited. The nitride is then etched on the left side of each structure. A 90-minute 1000°C H_2O oxidation was then performed. In the simulation on the left, no stress-dependent parameters were included in the simulation. Stress-dependent parameters were included in the simulation on the right.

and so we should expect a transient at the beginning of the 1000°C oxidation when the oxidation rate constants will not have the values we normally expect for that temperature. These kinds of transients have in fact been observed experimentally and the dominant effect appears to be on B [6.33]. That is, the grown-in stress levels in the oxide change the density of the oxide from that normally expected at the second oxidation temperature; the diffusivity of the oxidant is therefore affected until the oxide relaxes to its "normal" state for the second oxidation. If the first oxidation is at a high temperature and the second at a lower temperature, the second oxide will initially grow faster than expected because the stress levels will be lower than expected at the lower temperature. If the first oxidation is at a lower temperature and the second at a higher temperature, the rate in the second oxidation will be initially slower than expected. These kinds of effects are only beginning to be modeled today in process simulation programs. In essence they imply that wafer history has an effect on the process parameters observed in a given process step.

One of the current trends in the semiconductor industry is toward the use of single-wafer rapid thermal processing type equipment. These systems rapidly ramp wafers from room temperature to process temperatures, typically in a few seconds, using lamp heating. Memory effects like those described in the last paragraph will be exacerbated by such systems because there will be essentially no time during the temperature ramp for the oxide properties to reach the values characteristic of the processing temperature. If rapid thermal processing is combined with oxidation, the effective oxidation rates may be quite different than expected and will certainly depend on wafer history. This is a largely unstudied area that may be increasingly important in the future.

Finally, two interesting recent results have shown that it is possible to oxidize shaped silicon structures and grow uniform oxide layers on them. This can be done if a means is found to relieve the stresses that build up during the oxidation and hence to eliminate the stress effects on oxidation rate coefficients. It is, of course, possible to do this by oxidizing at very high temperatures since around 1200°C, the oxide can flow easily enough to relieve the stresses. However, such high temperatures are generally not compatible with small geometry devices. Two other ways to achieve essentially the same result involve doing the oxidation in an O_2/NF_3 mixture [6.34], or utilizing a corona discharge above the wafer during the oxidation [6.35]. The physical reasons why these processes apparently relieve the stresses in the growing oxide are not understood at present.

6.5.8 Advanced Point Defect Based Models for Oxidation

The models that we have described to this point have been primarily aimed at explaining the growth kinetics of oxide layers. If that were all that we were required to explain, then the set of models we have considered to this point would be fairly complete. However, there are other experimental results that these models cannot explain, most of which have to do with interactions between oxidation and other process steps like diffusion. One of the earliest indications that more was actually going on during oxidation than the effects we have considered to this point were observations more than 20 years ago that surface oxidations changed the rate of diffusion of dopants in the underlying silicon substrate. This phenomenon is now known as Oxidation Enhanced Diffusion (OED) in cases in which dopant diffusion rates are increased by surface oxidation, or Oxidation Retarded Diffusion (ORD) in cases in which diffusion is slowed down by surface oxidation. We will consider these cases in more detail in Chapter 7. However, we will introduce here some additional ideas about oxidation that will be needed to explain OED, ORD, and other related effects.

All of the oxidation mechanisms we have considered to this point are purely local phenomena. That is, they help to explain why oxides grow at the rates they do, but they offer no suggestions as to why surface oxidation should, for example, perturb dopant diffusion rates tens of microns away from the surface. Clearly some nonlocal phenomenon must be involved. Current thinking regarding such effects centers on the interface reaction itself (B/A or k_S in the Deal-Grove model). We have seen that there is a very large volume expansion that occurs during oxidation. This volume expansion results in very large compressive stresses in the oxide layer and tensile stresses in the silicon in the near surface region. Dobson was among the first to suggest that there might be mechanisms at the atomic level available to the oxidizing interface to help relieve these stresses [6.36]. These mechanisms in essence provide some of the "volume" that is needed for the oxide to grow. Figure 6–32 illustrates these ideas. At a microscopic level, Si-Si bonds are broken at the Si/SiO_2 interface, O atoms are inserted between the Si

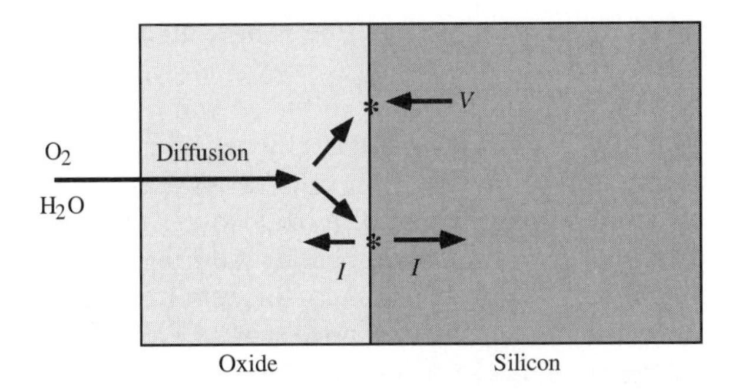

Figure 6–32 Point-defect reactions taking place at the Si/SiO_2 interface during oxidation. Oxidation reactions (*) can consume V or generate I in order to provide the volume needed for the reaction to take place.

atoms, and Si-O bonds are formed. The volume expansion requirement comes from the room needed for the O atoms.

There are two major types of point defects present in crystalline materials like Si—Vacancies (V) or missing Si atoms and Interstitials (I) or excess silicon atoms. We introduced a number of basic ideas about these defects in Chapter 3 where we saw that they can exist in both neutral and charged states and that their concentrations generally increase exponentially with temperature. Volume for the oxidation reaction can be provided at the Si/SiO_2 interface either by consuming vacancies or by generating interstitials. These are the two reactions illustrated in Figure 6–32. We can represent these reactions in the same way we modeled the formation of SiO_2 precipitates in Chapter 3 (Figure 3–25):

$$(1 + 2\gamma)\mathrm{Si} + 2\mathrm{O}_\mathrm{I} + 2\beta V \leftrightarrow \mathrm{SiO}_2 + 2\gamma I + \mathrm{stress} \tag{6.47}$$

The reaction forming SiO_2 consumes vacancies and generates interstitials because the vacancies provide some of the volume needed for the oxidation to proceed, as can removing Si atoms as I. γ is the number of I that contribute to the process per O atom joining the SiO_2, and β is a similar fraction for V. A stress term is also included on the right-hand side because experimentally we know that the point defects do not provide all the necessary volume.

The generation of I is thought to explain the interactions between oxidation and other processes like diffusion (i.e., OED and ORD) because the I which are generated can diffuse far away from the Si/SiO_2 interface and change the diffusivity of dopants which interact with I. We will discuss this further in Chapter 7. The consumption of V as a path to provide the volume required for the oxidation should be favored whenever there are large numbers of V present. This is believed to be the case in heavily doped silicon regions (as we saw in Chapter 3) and this reaction has been used to explain why oxidation proceeds at a much higher rate on heavily doped substrates than it does on lightly doped substrates. We will discuss this more fully in Section 6.5.9.

It is quite clear that the mechanisms proposed in Eq. (6.47) do not provide all the volume required at the oxidizing interface. The fact that grown oxides are under very high compressive stresses is clear evidence for this. In fact, estimates of the number of I which diffuse into the substrate during oxidation, suggest that less than 1 in 10^3 Si atoms does this. The rest are consumed by the oxidation process and end up in the SiO_2 layer. In fact, the number of I actually generated by the oxidation process may be much larger than 1 in 10^3 of the silicon atoms oxidized. Most of them may end up diffusing into the SiO_2 layer where they are oxidized. Nonetheless, the effects that the few point defects that do diffuse into the substrate have on process phenomena in the underlying silicon are quite remarkable.

The coupling between oxidation kinetics and other process phenomena is usually modeled today using reaction diffusion equations and a conceptual framework like that shown in Figure 6–33 [6.37]. An oxidizing interface is characterized by generation and recombination rates for point defects. The balance between G and R determines whether there is a net flux of point defects into or away from the surface. In the case of oxidation, the net result is a flux of interstitials away from the surface and into the bulk. These interstitials interact in the silicon bulk with dopant atoms, producing dopant diffusivities that are proportional to the local concentration of point defects (Chapter 7). This modeling approach has been quite successful in recent years, but it depends on experimentally determined values for G, R, point-defect diffusivities, bulk recombination rates, and many other parameters. The connection to oxidation kinetics is through G and R. For example, in SUPREM IV, G and R for an oxidizing Si/SiO_2 interface are modeled as

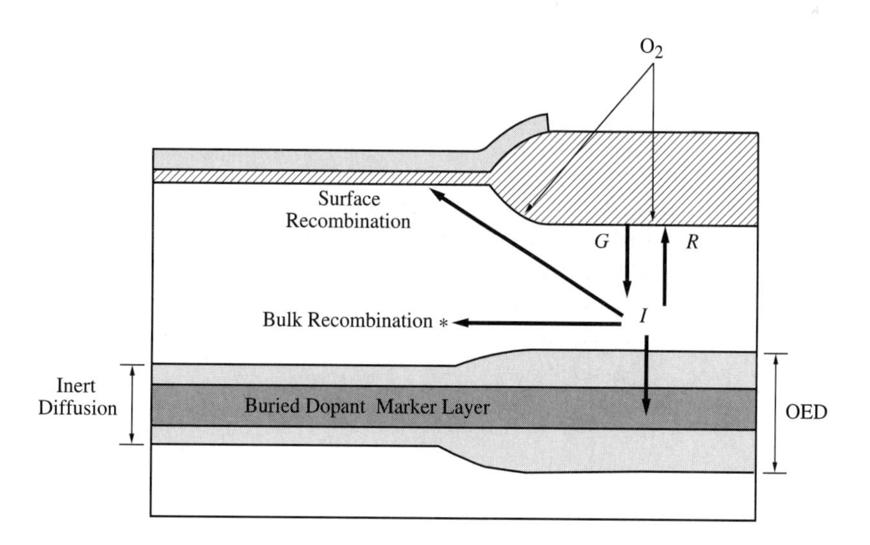

Figure 6–33 Generalized representation of point-defect generation (G), recombination (R, K_B, and K_S) and diffusion processes in silicon. In this example, local oxidation (right side) generates interstitials that diffuse away from the Si/SiO_2 interface, locally enhancing the downward diffusion of the epilayer (OED).

$$G = \Theta \frac{dx_O}{dt} N \tag{6.48}$$

$$R = K_{inert} K_{rat} \left(\frac{dx_O/dt}{B/A} \right)^{K_{pow}} + K_{inert} \tag{6.49}$$

where Θ is the fraction of oxidized silicon atoms that are injected into the substrate as interstitials, dx/dt is the oxidation velocity, N is the number of silicon atoms per unit volume, K_{inert} is the recombination velocity at an inert Si/SiO_2 interface, and K_{rat} accounts for the increased recombination rate at an oxidizing interface. Note that Θ is not the same as γ in Eq. (6.47), since Θ represents only the I which are injected into the silicon. All of the K values and Θ are experimentally determined. Other surfaces, such as Si/Si_3N_4 interfaces are modeled with similar expressions but with different parameter values. This modeling approach should be regarded as phenomenological at present because there is no generally accepted underlying physical model.

Models have been proposed to try to explain G and R on a more fundamental level. Hu suggested a regrowth model in which kink sites at the interface act as sites for interstitial recombination [6.38]. Dunham suggested a three-flux model including generation, surface regrowth and segregation of interstitials into the SiO_2 [6.39]. However all of these models must be regarded as speculative at the present time.

Figure 6–34 shows an example of the simulation of these OED effects. The structure is similar to the conceptual drawing in Figure 6–33. After a uniform boron implant, the

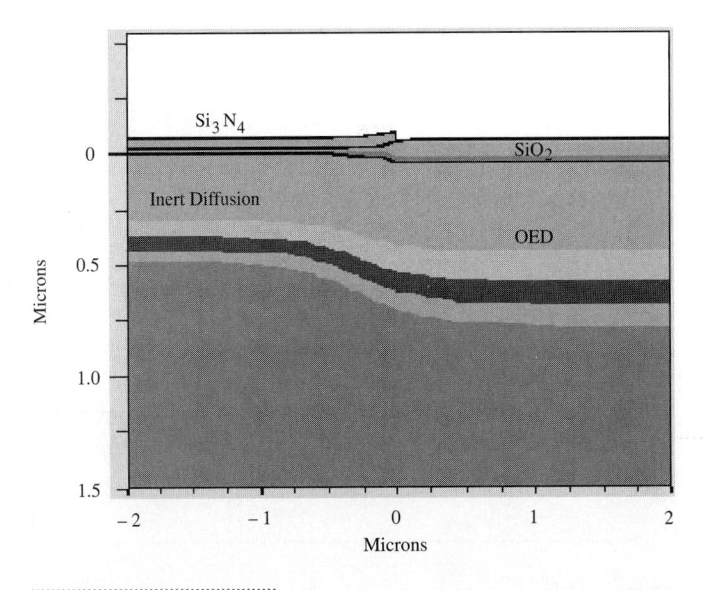

Figure 6–34 Example of the simulation of the OED effect using the ATHENA simulator [6.12]. A uniform 3×10^{14} cm^{-2}, 15-keV implant was performed through a pad oxide, followed by deposition of a nitride masking layer on the left half of the structure. A 60-min H_2O oxidation at 850°C produced the deeper diffusion on the right side.

right half of the structure is oxidized. The I injected by the oxidizing interface enhance the boron diffusivity, producing a deeper junction on the right side. Note the two-dimensional effects associated with the I diffusion away from the surface. The OED effect extends almost a micron under the nitride mask.

6.5.9 Substrate Doping Effects

It has been known for many years that highly doped substrates oxidize more rapidly than do lightly doped wafers. The effect is particularly important at lower temperatures and for thinner oxides. Under these conditions, the difference in oxidation rates between heavily doped and lightly doped regions can be three to four times [6.40]. The difference is more pronounced for N^+ regions than for P^+ regions and is more pronounced for low-temperature compared to high-temperature oxidations. Analysis has indicated that the mechanism associated with the faster oxidation is occurring at the Si/SiO_2 interface. In other words, B/A and not B is affected in the Deal-Grove model. This is perhaps not too surprising because N-type dopants tend to segregate into the silicon during oxidation. As a result, the dopant concentrations in the growing SiO_2 layer are usually fairly small, even if the substrate is heavily doped. As a result, the properties of the grown SiO_2 layer are to first order independent of the substrate doping. Therefore, B, which is primarily determined by the diffusion process of the oxidant through the SiO_2, should not be greatly affected.

While a number of possible physical mechanisms might explain the effect of high doping on B/A, the most widely accepted model relies on the V mechanism illustrated in the top portion of Figure 6–32. The basic idea is as follows. Oxidation requires volume expansion. This volume can be provided by consuming V at the growing Si/SiO_2 interface. We saw in Chapter 3 that the total number of V is much higher in extrinsic, highly doped regions than in intrinsic, lightly doped material. Physically, this is because vacancies can exist in a number of charge states (V^0, V^+, V^- and $V^=$) and the charged vacancies have discrete energy levels in the silicon bandgap. As the Fermi level E_F moves away from the middle of the bandgap in extrinsic material, it crosses over the V^- or $V^=$ levels in N^+ material or the V^+ level in P^+ material, causing large increases in the charged vacancy populations. In Chapter 3 we expressed these ideas mathematically and found that we could calculate the numbers of vacancies present in the crystal at any given temperature and doping level.

If these vacancies are now able to provide sites for the oxidation reaction, then it should be the case that [6.40]

$$\frac{B}{A} = R_1 + KC_{V^T} \tag{6.50}$$

where R_1 represents all mechanisms other than the vacancy driven process and C_{V^T} is the total vacancy population in all charge states present in the material at the oxidation temperature. Given a temperature and a doping level (i.e., E_F), we can calculate C_{V^T} using the equations developed in Chapter 3.

Eq. (6.50) is usually rewritten in the following form for convenience:

$$\frac{B}{A} = \left(\frac{B}{A}\right)^i \left(1 + 2.62 \times 10^3 \exp\left(-\frac{1.1\ \text{eV}}{kT}\right)\left(\frac{C_{V^T}}{C_{V_i^T}} - 1\right)\right) \tag{6.51}$$

$C_{V_i^T}$ is the total vacancy concentration in intrinsic material at the oxidation temperature. The $2.62 \times 10^3 \exp\left(-\frac{1.1\ \text{eV}}{kT}\right)$ factor is an empirically determined parameter that presumably physically represents something to do with the effectiveness of the vacancy reaction compared to other components in B/A. This expression has been quite successful in modeling the oxidation of highly doped regions and is implemented in SUPREM IV.

Several points should be made with regard to this model. The first is that since it is based on V populations and these depend only on T and E_F, it makes no difference if the N^+ regions are formed with arsenic or phosphorus. The same electrically active surface concentration should produce the same E_F and hence the same B/A. Second, the relevant concentration that should be used in calculating E_F and hence C_{V^T} is the surface concentration since that is where the oxidation reaction is taking place.

Segregation and pileup effects may increase this concentration above bulk values. We introduced the idea of segregation in Chapter 3 in connection with crystal growth. In that case we were concerned with the distribution of an impurity across the solid/liquid interface of the growing crystal. In the oxidation process, we have a Si/SiO_2 interface where dopant segregation also occurs. N-type dopants tend to segregate into the silicon whereas boron prefers to be in the SiO_2. As a result, the surface concentration for N-type dopants will tend to build up as the oxidation proceeds, and it will tend to decrease during oxidation for P type. Because of this, the B/A values calculated from Eq. (6.51) will change with time during the oxidation. The oxidation rate will therefore change with time. Recent experiments that carefully measured the dopant profiles near the surface clearly showed the time dependence of the oxidation rate and its correlation with the dopant pileup process [6.41]. A significant fraction of the dopant in the piled up layer at the surface may not be electrically active and hence, according to the C_{V^T} model, would not affect the oxidation rate.

The model also predicts that P^+ substrates should not show nearly as large an increase in oxidation rate as do N^+ regions, because as we saw in Chapter 3, there are fewer total vacancies present in P^+ regions for a given doping level. This agrees with experiments. Finally, because P-type dopants like boron tend to segregate into the growing oxide layer, rather than staying in the silicon substrate, high boron concentrations in the growing SiO_2 can result. There are indications that this may change the structure of the oxide layer sufficiently to observe changes in oxidant diffusivity through these films. As a result, the parabolic rate constant B may be slightly different (larger usually) than it would be at the same temperature if the oxide were being grown on a lightly doped or N^+ region. This effect has not been characterized well enough to model.

Other models have been proposed to explain the doping dependence of oxidation. Some are based on the idea that high dopant concentrations at the Si/SiO_2 interface could change the Si-Si bond energy and hence affect *B/A*. Others are based on the idea that the structure of the Si/SiO_2 interface region is changed by the high dopant concentration, again resulting in a change in *B/A* in the Deal-Grove model [6.42, 6.43]. At this point in time, none of these models has been sufficiently quantified to use them in oxidation simulators so Eq. (6.48) is the model normally used.

An example of a simulation involving heavily doped oxidation is shown in Figure 6–35. On the left side, a low temperature oxidation (800°C) was simulated whereas a higher temperature (1000°C) was simulated in the right side. In each case, the right side of the structure is heavily doped and the left side is lightly doped. The heavily doped region grows about five times as much oxide as the lightly doped control at 800°C, compared to only about twice as much at 1000°C. The transition region between the lightly doped and heavily doped areas in each simulation can only be properly modeled using 2D diffusion and 2D oxidation models and requires a numerical simulator such as SUPREM IV used in this example.

6.5.10 Polysilicon Oxidation

It is not uncommon in silicon technology for there to be thin films of other materials locally on the wafer surface when an oxidation takes place. The most common examples are thin films of polysilicon, Si_3N_4, and various silicides. We saw several examples of these kinds of processes in Chapter 2. In the next three sections, we briefly consider the effect of oxidation on these thin film materials.

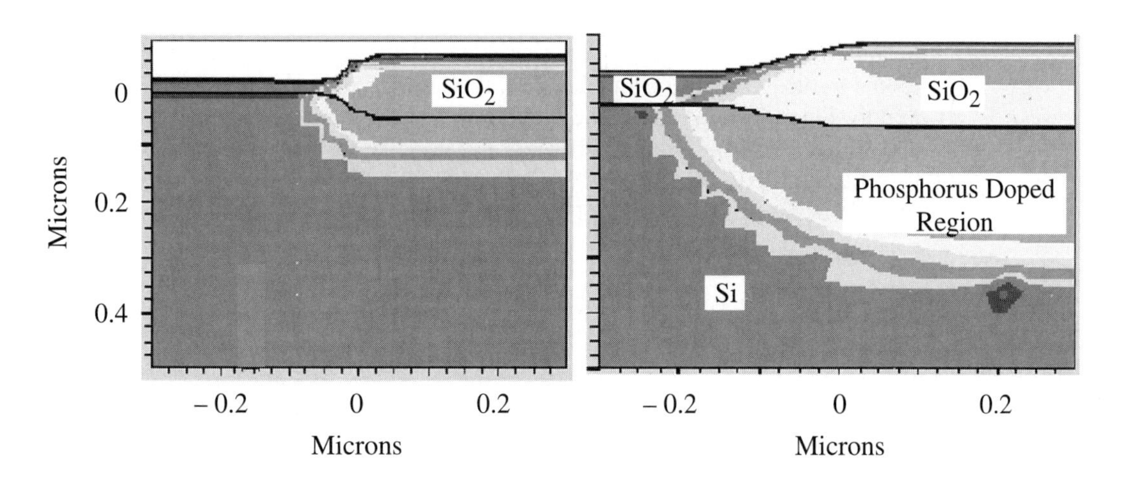

Figure 6–35 Oxidation of heavily doped regions using the ATHENA simulator [6.12]. A 5×10^{15} cm^{-2} 20-keV phosphorus implant was performed on the right half of the structure. An oxidation was then performed for 30 min in H_2O at 800°C (left) and for 5 min in H_2O at 1000°C (right). The contours correspond to the diffused doping profiles. The solid lines at the top of the structure define the grown SiO_2 layers.

To first order, the same set of models described above for single-crystal silicon can also be used for polysilicon. This is, in fact, the strategy used in most process modeling programs. However, this approach is not always completely satisfactory for two fundamental reasons. First, polysilicon is a polycrystalline material. Second, polysilicon films are thin- or finite-volume structures.

The fact that polysilicon materials are polycrystalline means that a variety of crystal orientations may be present in various grains. The grain structure associated with the polysilicon layers is a strong function of deposition conditions and subsequent heat treatments. In general, deposition at lower temperatures results in smaller grain sizes. In fact depositions below about 600°C tend to produce amorphous rather than polycrystalline films. Annealing at high temperatures generally causes the grains to grow and the number of grains to be reduced. The dominant crystal orientation is often (110). An excellent reference on polysilicon, its properties and applications is [6.44].

There are several implications of the polycrystalline nature of these films for oxidation kinetics. The most obvious is simply that B/A will vary from grain to grain and perhaps with time if the poly grain structure changes during the oxidation. We discussed orientation effects in Section 6.5.5 and saw there that B/A can change by up to 70% depending on the orientation. (110) surfaces oxidize at a rate intermediate between (111) and (100) (the two extremes) and often what is done to model polysilicon oxidation is to simply use an average B/A value characteristic of the (110) orientation. For relatively thin oxides, where B/A is important, we should expect to see variations in oxide thickness across a polysilicon surface because of the varying grain orientations. For thicker oxides, these differences tend to disappear because as we saw in Section 6.5.5, the parabolic rate constant B is not a function of the underlying crystal structure.

Most polysilicon thin films used in silicon technology are heavily doped because they are usually used as local interconnects, gate electrodes in MOS devices, or for bipolar emitter regions. In these situations, modeling any oxidation that takes place will have to include doping effects. This becomes a complicated problem because of the polycrystalline nature of the film, and because of its finite volume. Dopants diffuse very rapidly in polysilicon films, because they tend to migrate along grain boundaries and then into the grains. Grain boundary diffusion is a very rapid process (at least 10^2 times faster than bulk diffusion). As a result, dopant profiles tend to be uniform in polysilicon thin films after a very short time at high temperatures. To first order the dopant chemical concentration is simply given by

$$[\text{Dopant}]_{\text{chem}} = \frac{\text{ImplantDose}}{\text{PolyThickness}} \tag{6.52}$$

when the poly is doped by ion implantation. However, the electrically active concentration may be much lower than this because some of the doping atoms segregate to grain boundaries where they are not electrically active and because some of the free carriers are also trapped at grain boundaries. The net result is that n or p and hence E_F may be quite different from the values one would normally find in single-crystal silicon for the same doping concentration. The result of these effects is that applying models like Eq. (6.51) is often not straightforward in polysilicon. It is often possible to do so, but the correct n or p value must be used to find E_F and hence C_{V^T}.

The finite volume of polysilicon thin films also has some interesting implications. Many of these issues also apply to silicon on insulator (SOI) structures such as that illustrated in Figure 3–26. Most often, the polysilicon layer is deposited on an underlying SiO_2 layer. During an oxidation, the polysilicon is consumed and the layer will therefore get thinner. Most N-type dopants prefer to stay in silicon or polysilicon rather than segregating into growing SiO_2 layers. This implies that the chemical and probably electrically active dopant concentrations will increase during the oxidation. In fact, very high doping levels may be reached since poly layers are usually quite heavily doped to improve their conductivity. The electrically active dopant concentrations may easily reach maximum solubility levels and in extreme cases, new phases like SiP may be formed. Such phases may result in unusual process problems. For example, SiP is soluble in HF which may be used later as an oxide etch. If the SiP dissolves, "holes" may be left in the polysilicon layer resulting in yield problems. Finally, there are some processes in which the polysilicon layer is fully oxidized. Usually this is done locally as part of a LOCOS type process. Modeling of such process steps is challenging because extreme conditions of dopant concentrations and other effects may be encountered as the poly gets very thin toward the end of the oxidation process. If the polysilicon layer is deposited on an underlying silicon layer (as in a bipolar emitter region, for example), the process physics will be quite different because there is no blocking oxide layer below the poly in that case.

A number of studies of polysilicon oxidation have been done as a function of temperature, poly doping level, and so forth. To first order, these experiments can be explained by the single-crystal models we described earlier and this is the approach normally taken in simulators like SUPREM IV. However, the effects of grain boundaries and the poly finite volume can result in greatly different oxide growth kinetics than those found on single crystal substrates under some conditions. At this point in time, no general-purpose models have been developed, beyond those we have described, to account for these effects.

Figure 6–36 shows an example of a simulation involving polysilicon oxidation using ATHENA. The silicon substrate is (100) orientation and hence has a slower oxidation rate than the poly (both are undoped in this example). The poly is mostly consumed by the oxidation. Notice also the encroachment of the growing oxide under the poly because of 2D oxidation.

6.5.11 Si_3N_4 Growth and Oxidation Kinetics

We have seen several examples in earlier chapters of the use of thin deposited Si_3N_4 films in silicon technology. By far the most common use is as a mask against oxidation in LOCOS type processes. In this application, we are interested in the ability of CVD Si_3N_4 to withstand oxidizing environments for reasonably long times at high temperatures. The use of Si_3N_4 in this way is illustrated in Figure 6–37. The process forms a surface layer of SiO_2 on the nitride.

Conceptually, the following reactions may take place

$$Si_3N_4 + 3O_2 \rightarrow 3SiO_2 + 2N_2 \quad (6.53)$$

$$Si_3N_4 + 6H_2O \rightarrow 3SiO_2 + 6H_2 + 2N_2 \quad (6.54)$$

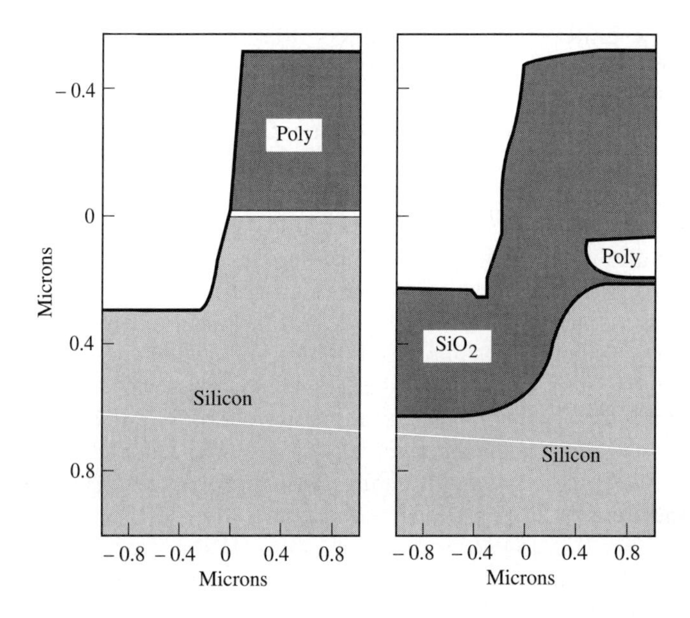

Figure 6–36 Example of an oxidation simulation involving polysilicon using the ATHENA simulator [6.12]. The initial structure (left) has a polysilicon layer on SiO_2 on silicon. The left half of the structure is etched to expose the Si substrate. A 60-min H_2O oxidation at 1000°C is simulated on the right.

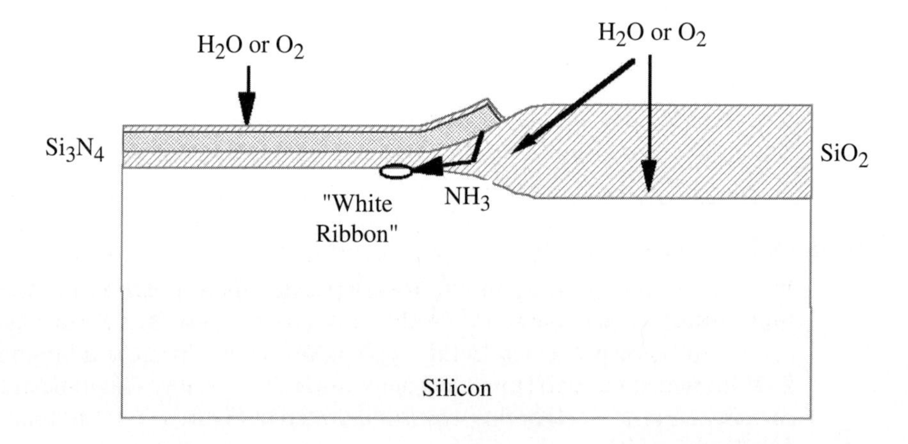

Figure 6–37 LOCOS process illustrating local oxidation of silicon, oxide formation on the Si_3N_4 surface, and "white ribbon" formation due to oxidation of the Si_3N_4.

$$Si_3N_4 + 6H_2O \rightarrow 3SiO_2 + 4NH_3 \tag{6.55}$$

From a practical point of view, we are usually most interested in the latter two reactions because LOCOS type processes attempt to grow fairly thick field oxides and this usually implies an H_2O oxidation. Physically, the oxidation process should be somewhat similar to silicon oxidation. The H_2O must diffuse through the growing SiO_2 layer and then react at the SiO_2/Si_3N_4 interface to form new oxide layers. If this is how the oxide grows, then we might expect a linear parabolic growth law similar to the Deal-Grove model for silicon oxidation. However, the process is apparently not that simple because more complex growth kinetics have been reported [6.45, 6.46]. It has been suggested that the reaction byproducts (N_2 or NH_3) have an effect on the oxidation, either by modifying the interface reaction, or by changing the diffusion process of the indiffusing oxidant as they diffuse out through the oxide.

Lacking a clear physical model, empirical relationships have been developed to allow prediction of Si_3N_4 oxidation kinetics. One such relationship suitable for H_2O oxidations is as follows [6.46]:

$$\Delta x_N = 1.1 \times 10^7 \exp\left(-\frac{1.9\text{ eV}}{kT}\right) t^{0.7} P \tag{6.56}$$

where Δx_N is the thickness of the nitride consumed in nm, t is the oxidation time in min, and P is the H_2O oxidant pressure in Atm. The oxidation process involves a volume expansion just as silicon oxidation does; the resulting oxide thickness is about 1.6 Δx_N. A typical Si_3N_4 film of 80 nm would therefore be completely consumed by a 1050°C oxidation in about 16.6 hours.

In dry O_2 oxidations, it has been suggested that the reaction that takes place is actually more complicated than Eq. (6.53) would suggest [6.47]. The oxidation may actually take place in two steps with a layer of Si_2N_2O forming on the Si_3N_4 surface and then a layer of SiO_2 forming on top of the Si_2N_2O. In any case, the oxidation rate is much slower than in an H_2O ambient and the SiO_2 grown on Si_3N_4 during O_2 oxidations can normally be neglected.

One of the subtleties of LOCOS type processes is also illustrated in Figure 6–37. H_2O diffusing through the growing SiO_2 layer can also react with the underside of the Si_3N_4 layer, generating NH_3 as a byproduct of the oxidation process. [See Eq. (6.55).] It is found experimentally that the NH_3 can then diffuse to the Si/SiO_2 interface and react there to form a thermally grown Si_3N_4 layer. This is sometimes called the "white ribbon" effect or the Kooi effect after the person who first explained the process. The "white ribbon" name came about because of the characteristic appearance in a microscope of the Si_3N_4 layer as a ribbon around the edge of device active regions (just under the edge of the top deposited Si_3N_4 layer). This grown Si_3N_4 layer can sometimes cause problems if it is not removed in later processing because it can slow down or stop later oxidations locally where it is present. Fortunately it is easily removed by chemical etching in hot H_3PO_4 or by oxidizing it after the top Si_sN_4 layer is removed.

The white ribbon effect is a specific example of the fact that it is possible to thermally grow thin Si_3N_4 layers directly on silicon by exposing the silicon to N_2 or NH_3 at high temperature. This process step is rarely used in VLSI structures because the thickness of Si_3N_4 that can be grown is limited. However the process does have potential for future thin dielectrics in MOS structures and it is of interest as a technique in studying dopant diffusion as we will see in Chapter 7, so we will briefly consider it here.

Most attempts to thermally grow Si_3N_4 layers directly on silicon have used NH_3 rather than N_2 because the growth rates are substantially faster. This may be a result of the hydrogen byproduct of the NH_3 reaction which may react with trace amounts of O_2 in the ambient to prevent competing oxidation processes from taking place although this is speculation at this point. At temperatures below about 900°C, oxidation is thermodynamically favored. Films of Si_3N_4 grown in NH_3 are usually between 2.5 and 7.5 nm thick. The chemical reaction is believed to be

$$3Si + 4NH_3 \rightarrow Si_3N_4 + 6H_2 \tag{6.57}$$

The films appear to grow very rapidly to about half their final thickness and then grow slowly to a final thickness that depends primarily on temperature. The growth kinetics are not fully understood but are generally thought to occur via a surface reaction limited process at the Si/Si_3N_4 interface at first (the fast part of the growth), followed by a slower diffusion limited growth phase. This sounds very much like the Deal-Grove model for oxidation. However, kinetic data for the nitridation process has generally been fit with either a logarithmic or a power law expression. One example is the following empirical growth law [6.48]:

$$x_N = at^b \tag{6.58}$$

where

$$a = 92\exp\left(-\frac{0.38\text{ eV}}{kT}\right) \quad \text{and} \quad b = 0.018\exp\left(\frac{0.24\text{ eV}}{kT}\right) \tag{6.59}$$

a is in nm and t is in min. The thermally grown Si_3N_4 layers reach thicknesses of 2.5–6 nm in several hours of growth at temperatures of 950–1200°C. A number of recent studies have shown that these growth rates and final thicknesses can be substantially enhanced by growing the Si_3N_4 layers in an N_2 or NH_3 plasma. Such plasmas create highly reactive species, both neutral and ionized, and may also create electric fields to help drive transport processes. It has been possible to grow Si_3N_4 layers 10–30 nm thick with these processes. The growth kinetics have not been modeled as yet.

Commercially available process simulators generally have not yet implemented models for Si_3N_4 oxidation or for the nitridation of silicon. In many applications it is not a bad approximation to assume that Si_3N_4 is not oxidized at all in an O_2 or H_2O ambient and this is by default what simulators like SUPREM IV currently do.

6.5.12 Silicide Oxidation

Beginning in the late 1970s, it became apparent that the resistivity of polysilicon would soon become a limitation on the speed of ICs. In virtually all modern MOS technologies, polysilicon is used both for the gate electrodes and for short-distance interconnects. When it is used as an interconnect, the RC delays associated with charging and discharging the interconnect lines can become appreciable if the line resistance is too high. Polysilicon resistivities cannot be made much lower than about 400 $\mu\Omega$cm (or about 10Ω/sq. for a 0.4 μm thick film). This is unacceptable in many applications. As a result, silicides like $TiSi_2$ and WSi_2 began to be investigated by 1980. We will discuss the principal properties of these films in Chapter 11 when we deal specifically with contacts and interconnects. However, in many cases, silicides are deposited on top of polysilicon to reduce the resistance of poly lines and the composite structure is sometimes thermally oxidized. We did not use thermal oxidation of silicides in the process flow in Chapter 2 (a deposited oxide layer was used on the $TiSi_2$ instead—see Figure 2–38).

The structure most commonly encountered when silicides are oxidized is shown in Figure 6–38. The silicide/poly part of the structure forms the gate electrode; the lower SiO_2 layer is the gate dielectric and the upper oxide is grown or deposited to insulate the silicide from other metal layers that may be deposited above it. Silicides are generally not used directly on gate oxides because there may be adhesion problems, oxidation problems, gate oxide reliability problems, or simply undesired work functions in the MOS structure.

When such composite structures are thermally oxidized in O_2 or H_2O, a layer of SiO_2 is normally found to grow on the upper surface of the silicide. In principle, either SiO_2 or the metal oxide MO_x could grow. Thermodynamic calculations [6.49] suggest that the MO_x is actually favored on Hf, Zr, and perhaps Ti silicides and the difference between the heats of formation of MO_x and SiO_2 are small on many of the other silicides. Some uncertainty exists in these calculations, but they do suggest that kinetics must play an important role in the system choosing to form SiO_2 rather than MO_x in most cases. MO_x is found to be the preferred oxide on $HfSi_2$ and on $TiSi_2$ at temperatures below 900°C. With these few exceptions, SiO_2 appears to grow in all other cases. By kinetics playing an important role, we mean that Si atoms must react more rapidly with the oxidant than do the metal atoms, even though both reactions may be possible thermodynamically.

The oxidation process appears to proceed in a manner very similar to silicon oxidation. O_2 or H_2O diffuse through the SiO_2 layer to the SiO_2/silicide interface where a reaction similar to that which occurs in silicon oxidation takes place. The silicon atoms needed to form the SiO_2 can be provided either by diffusion upward from the poly, or by M-Si bonds being broken. In the later case, the metal atoms would then diffuse downward to form a new layer of silicide at the silicide/poly interface. In both cases, the silicide layer is conserved. Both possibilities are observed in practice. $CrSi_2$, $CoSi_2$, $NiSi_2$,

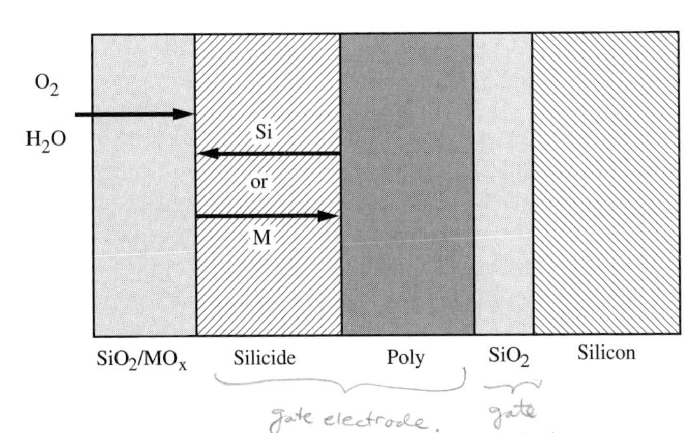

Figure 6–38 Oxidation of a polycide (silicide on poly) structure. M is the metal used to form the silicide.

PdSi, and PtSi all appear to grow oxides primarily by dissociation of the silicide and diffusion of the metal to the silicide/poly interface where new silicide is formed. $TiSi_2$, WSi_2, $TaSi_2$, and perhaps others form oxides by the diffusion of Si atoms from the poly layer. In all cases, the growth kinetics are well described by the familiar linear parabolic model

$$\frac{x_O^2 - x_i^2}{B} + \frac{x_O - x_i}{B/A} = t \tag{6.22}$$

B is found to be exactly the same for silicide oxidations as it is for silicon oxidation. This should not be too surprising because the process is the same in the two cases—oxidant diffusion through SiO_2. B/A values extracted from silicide oxidation data are all significantly larger than the values found for silicon oxidation (typically 10–20 times larger) [6.50]. Apparently the processes contributing to B/A in the silicide structure, metal or silicon diffusion, M-Si or Si -Si bond breaking, and so on, are much faster than the corresponding processes in silicon oxidation. In practice, this means that the oxide growth is often simply parabolic ($B/A \rightarrow \infty$).

Difficulties can be encountered in oxidizing silicide structures like that shown in Figure 6–38. For example, if a barrier layer such as a thin native oxide exists between the poly and silicide layers (due to improper cleaning between poly and silicide depositions for example), the reaction at that interface may be slowed down significantly. This can result in voids forming at the poly/silicide interface, apparently because the Si needed to form the growing SiO_2 can be obtained only from localized regions where pinholes exist in the blocking layer. In $TiSi_2$ in which the metal oxide forms at low temperatures, it is important to ensure that the oxidizing ambient is not turned on until the wafers have reached high temperature in the furnace. There have also been reports of oxidation difficulties in O_2 ambients although these are not uniformly observed. Most data in the literature are for H_2O oxidations. Finally, there are also many reports of problems with gate oxide integrity if the polysilicon layer under the silicide shrinks to below about 200 nm during the oxidation. The poly is consumed during the process, so this constraint may limit the maximum thickness of oxide that can be reliably grown. Commercially available simulation tools have generally implemented models for silicide deposition and for reactions between refractory metals and silicon to form silicides (see Chapter 11), but have not yet implemented oxidation models for silicides, probably because deposited oxides are commonly used in silicide processes.

6.5.13 Si/SiO_2 Interface Charges

Toward the beginning of this chapter, we discussed the four basic kinds of charges that are typically found at semiconductor/insulator interfaces. Figure 6–6 summarizes these charges. Of the four charges illustrated, only two (Q_f and Q_{it}) will be discussed in detail here. Mobile charges in dielectric layers (Q_m), have been largely eliminated from silicon technology because of careful attention to cleanliness during manufacturing. They occasionally are still a problem, but such situations are rare and usually quickly eliminated by discovering the source of the contamination (chemicals, handling etc.) and eliminating it. Oxide trapped charge (Q_{ot}) is of concern in applications in which the device structure is exposed to ionizing radiation either during manufacturing or during later use of the IC (in space applications, for example). It is also of concern in devices which pass current through oxides as part of normal device operation (EPROMs, for example), and more generally in very small MOS devices because of hot carrier effects which can inject carriers into the gate dielectric. However little quantitative modeling of Q_{ot} has been done to this point. Experiments have determined ways of growing oxides in order to minimize susceptibility to Q_{ot}, largely through proper anneals and choice of growth temperature and ambient. Q_{BD} measurements have also become common for characterizing thin gate insulators. Much of this work on Q_{ot} is, however, empirical at present. Much more work has been aimed at understanding and predicting Q_f and Q_{it} and we will focus on that work here.

Virtually all of the experimental techniques that are available to investigate interface charges are electrical in nature. The problem is easily visualized in connection with the TEM photo in Figure 3–15. Normal densities of Q_f and Q_{it} are around 10^9–10^{12} cm^{-2} or about 1 charge for every 10^3–10^6 silicon atoms at the interface. Physical techniques such as TEM are simply not sensitive enough to "find" such charges. It is quite literally like "looking for a needle in a haystack." Electrical methods, such as the CV technique described earlier, do have the required sensitivity and are commonly used to measure Q_f and Q_{it}. Such electrical measurements are also the quantities directly of interest from the point of view of devices. However, it is usually not straightforward to relate the electrical results to a physical, atomic-level model.

Many attempts have been made to relate the Si/SiO_2 interface charges to specific atomic level structures. Figure 6–39 illustrates some of these ideas, although the ideas represented by this figure should be regarded as speculative. Most workers today agree that the interface is almost atomically abrupt. If there is a transition region between the two materials, it is not more than one or two atomic distances thick. The bulk of the oxide consists mainly of rings of SiO_4 tetrahedra (see Figure 6–5), each with six silicon atoms in the ring. In the near interface region rings with smaller numbers of tetrahedra may be present. Many of the models for interface charges associate them with incompletely oxidized silicon atoms, often designated as ≡Si· for trivalently bonded silicon atoms. The · is meant to represent a dangling or unsatisfied bond. Both Q_f and Q_{it} have been modeled in this way, although there are clear experimental differences between the two and so there must be some structural difference between the two charges.

The principal electrical difference between Q_f and Q_{it} is that Q_f is a fixed positive charge which does not change during normal device operation, while Q_{it} is in communication with the silicon surface and can trap holes or electrons to become positively or negatively charged depending on where the Fermi level is at the surface. One explanation for this that has been suggested is that the ≡Si· corresponding to Q_f are located physically further away from the interface and thus are unable to trap carriers. Another explanation is that the energy levels corresponding to Q_f are located outside the silicon bandgap whereas those associated with Q_{it} are inside the bandgap. Thus Q_{it} states can be charged and discharged as E_F moves around in the bandgap. Other explanations

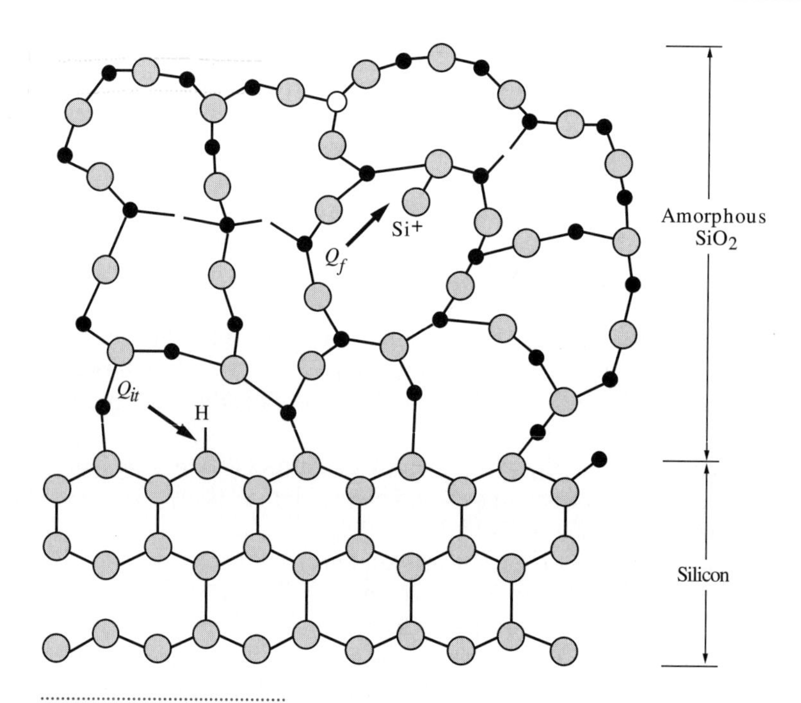

Figure 6–39 Conceptual atomic level picture of the Si/SiO$_2$ interface showing possible structural origins of Q_f and Q_{it}. Q_f corresponds to the excess Si$^+$ atom; Q_{if} is shown as an incompletely bonded Si atom near the interface, passivated in this example with an H bond. The larger circles correspond to Si atoms; the smaller circles to O atoms.

have suggested that the charges are due to stretched or distorted bonds at the interface, that is stress at the interface caused by the size mismatch between Si and SiO$_2$, and that different bonding arrangements account for the different charge types and the different energy levels in the bandgap found for Q_{it} states. There does appear to be a correlation between the roughness of the Si/SiO$_2$ interface and the resulting charge densities (the rougher the interface, the higher Q_f and Q_{it}). In addition, there is nearly always a strong correlation between the values of Q_f and Q_{it} that result from a given process, again suggesting a common origin [6.51]. Many other models have also been suggested, but none has been shown to be conclusively correct.

Whatever the physical origins of Q_f and Q_{it}, much is known about how they vary with process conditions. One of the earliest sets of such experimental data was presented by Deal in the form of the "Q_f triangle" shown in Figure 6–40 [6.52]. The experiments behind this data were done by oxidizing a wafer in a furnace (or annealing it in Ar) at the indicated temperature, and then pulling the wafer from the furnace fairly rapidly (few seconds) to "freeze in" the Q_f corresponding to that condition. Each curve appears to represent equilibrium values for that ambient and that temperature. That is, as the arrows on the figure illustrate, any point on any curve can be reached simply by changing the ambient and temperature in the furnace [6.53].

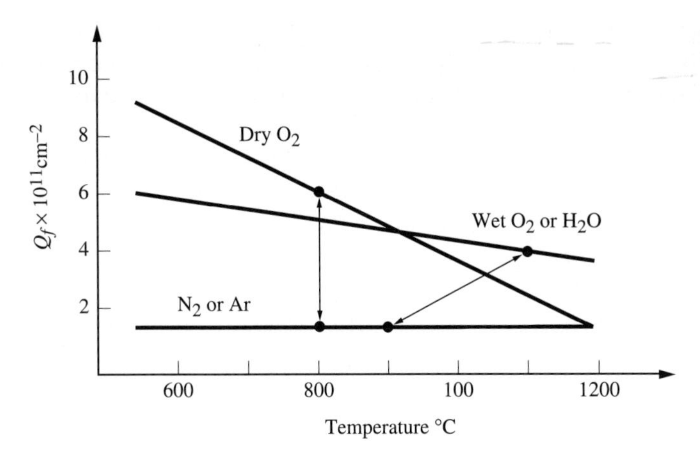

Figure 6–40 Variation of fixed oxide charge Q_f with oxidation temperature and ambient [6.52]. The arrows indicate that changes in temperature or ambient result in equilibrium values of Q_f after a transient time that depends on the temperature. Values shown are for (111) silicon; (100) values are about a factor of 3 lower.

In general, if such a change is made, a transient time will be required to reach the new Q_f value. This time is longer at lower temperatures. These transients and the final value of Q_f achieved after a high temperature Ar anneal can be empirically described by [6.53]

$$Q_f(t) = (Q_f(0) - Q_{fe})\exp\left(-\frac{t}{\tau}\right) + Q_{fe} \tag{6.60}$$

where

$$\tau = 5.41 \times 10^{-10}\exp\left(\frac{2.42\text{ eV}}{kT}\right)\text{ min}$$

$$Q_{fe} = 5.24 \times 10^{9}\exp\left(\frac{0.36\text{ eV}}{kT}\right)\text{cm}^{-2}\quad\text{for (111)}$$

$$Q_{fe} = 5.22 \times 10^{7}\exp\left(\frac{0.69\text{ eV}}{kT}\right)\text{cm}^{-2}\quad\text{for (100)}$$

Q_f is the fixed oxide charge density per cm^2 and Q_{fe} is the final or equilibrium value in Ar for any process temperature (the bottom curve in Figure 6–40). In almost all cases of practical interest, it is desired to minimize Q_f and so a final high temperature Ar anneal is used toward the end of a device fabrication sequence. The time required to reach Q_{fe} is only a few minutes at 1000°C, but many hours at 700°C. N_2 was the most common anneal ambient until recently because it is less expensive than Ar. However, as control of Q_f has become more important in modern device structures, it has been found that Ar is a better choice. The reason is that Q_f has been found to increase with time in N_2 after the transient described by the above equations is complete. That is, Q_f reduces to Q_{fe} and then begins to increase again in N_2. The reason likely is that Si/N_2 reactions can take place at the Si/SiO_2 interface whereas such reactions do not take place in Ar. The anneal conditions are thus less critical in terms of time and temperature if Ar is used.

Finally, it should be pointed out that Figure 6–40 indicates that Q_{fe} is essentially independent of temperature. This is historically how the "Q_f triangle" has been presented [6.51]. More recent data on which Eq. (6.60) is based, indicate that Q_{fe} is actually smaller at higher temperatures [6.53].

We mentioned above that the interface states or traps (Q_{it}) can interact with carriers during normal device operation, by capturing or releasing holes and electrons. This distinguishes Q_{it} from Q_f. Another very important distinction between the two is that the Q_{it} states can be passivated through hydrogen annealing at fairly low temperatures (300–500°C) whereas Q_f is unaffected by such an anneal. By passivated we mean that once the Q_{it} traps are bonded with H atoms, they are no longer electrically active and no longer trap carriers. The interface state conceptually illustrated in Figure 6–39 is shown passivated with a bonded H atom. The mechanism of passivation is believed to simply be hydrogen diffusion through the SiO_2 layer to the Si/SiO_2 interface and reaction there to form Si-H bonds. Since the process takes place readily at temperatures metal layers can tolerate, this step is normally done at the very end of the chip fabrication process. If it is done earlier, the Si-H bonds may break at the higher temperatures used for diffusions, implant anneals, and so on, and the hydrogen may then outdiffuse.

Because of the importance of this passivation process, it has been carefully studied over many years in order to understand not only the origins of the interface states themselves, but also how the passivation works. Most of the atomic level models for interface states are based on excess silicon or incompletely bonded silicon atoms with the trivalent silicon defect $\equiv Si\cdot$ we discussed above being a leading candidate. The annealing or passivation process is usually modeled with molecular hydrogen diffusion to the Si/SiO_2 interface followed by hydrogen dissociation to form atomic hydrogen and then chemical bonding between the $\equiv Si\cdot$ defect and H. This is often expressed simply as

$$H_2 \leftrightarrow 2H \quad \text{followed by} \quad \equiv Si\cdot + H \leftrightarrow \; \equiv SiH \tag{6.61}$$

Both reactions are reversible. The annealing process itself has been shown to follow a power law dependence on time, of the following form [6.54].

$$Q_{it} = \frac{Q_{it}(0)}{(1 + Kt)^{\eta}} \tag{6.62}$$

where $K = 8.4 \times 10^{11} \exp\left(-\frac{1.21\ \text{eV}}{kT}\right)\ \text{sec}^{-1}$ and $\eta \approx 0.55$ for (100) substrates.

The final annealed value is below $10^{10}\ \text{cm}^{-2}$ at all normal anneal temperatures (350–500°C). Times on the order of 30 minutes are required to reach this minimum at 350°C; shorter times are adequate at higher temperatures. The kinetics appear to be a little different for (111) surfaces [6.54]. A number of detailed physical models have been proposed to account for these kinetics [6.54–6.56].

Several additional points should be made regarding Q_{it}. Usually the diffusion process of H_2 getting from the ambient to the Si/SiO_2 interface is neglected in the annealing kinetics. This is nearly always a reasonable thing to do because

$$D_H \cong 7.2 \times 10^{-5} \exp\left(-\frac{0.58 \text{ eV}}{kT}\right) \text{cm}^2 \text{ sec}^{-1} \tag{6.63}$$

which implies quite short time delays for diffusion through normal oxide layers. The fact that Q_{it} annealing kinetics are generally independent of oxide thickness further substantiates this argument. However, many modern IC technologies use polysilicon gates and H_2 may have to go under the edges of such films and then diffuse laterally under them. In large area structures such as MOS capacitors, this can involve significant diffusion times [6.56]. Polysilicon gates have the advantage, however, of preventing outdiffusion of H_2, so that the annealing process is more tolerant of high-temperature exposure than are bare oxide surfaces or Al covered structures.

Al covered oxides actually do not need an external source of H_2 because of the reaction

$$\text{Al} + \text{OH} \rightarrow \text{"AlO"} + \text{H} \tag{6.64}$$

which occurs at the Al/SiO_2 interface. It is believed that cleaning steps prior to Al deposition leave trace amounts of water on the oxide surface, which accounts for the presence of the OH in the above reaction. This process is sometimes called the "Alneal" reaction. The oxide is denoted "AlO" rather than Al_2O_3 because the composition is not known and likely changes during the annealing process. Finally, it is also possible to implant H ions through the oxide to the vicinity of the Si/SiO_2 interface. This process can provide the H needed for the Q_{it} annealing, although the process is not very common since other techniques using annealing furnaces are simpler.

In summary, modern silicon technologies use a combination of a high temperature Ar (or N_2) anneal at a temperature on the order of 900–1000°C as the last high-temperature step to reduce Q_f to a minimum value. In addition, a lower temperature 400–500°C anneal, usually in "Forming Gas" (10% H_2 in N_2), is used to minimize Q_{it}. The combination of these two process steps reduces both types of charges to about 10^{10} cm^{-2} (or lower) on (100) surfaces with slightly larger values on (111) surfaces. These values are low enough that they do not have a significant effect on most devices.

Commercially available process simulation programs generally do not contain models to predict Si/SiO_2 interface charges. Since these charges can have significant effects on device electrical performance, device simulators often allow the user to input Q_f and Q_{it} values that are then used in calculating I-V characteristics.

6.5.14 Complete Oxidation Module Simulation

Many modern device structures involve complex geometries and many process steps. The only real way to simulate such processes is with a computer simulation code like SUPREM IV. It is important to note, however, that many of the models we have discussed in the previous sections were developed largely in isolation of each other. For example, a researcher studying thin oxide growth kinetics might propose a new growth law based on experimental measurements. But such models are very often developed based on simple experimental structures, perhaps planar oxidations in this example. When such a new model is implemented in a program like SUPREM, it may well be applied to nonplanar structures or at temperatures outside the range of the original experiments that led to the model development. New models are also often applied in situations in which many physical effects are occurring simultaneously. For example, the new thin oxide model in this example might be applied to a very heavily doped substrate and as a result, dopants might segregate into the oxide during growth, perhaps changing the growth kinetics in ways that were unanticipated by the researcher doing the model development. Because of all these issues, complete process simulators often provide the most comprehensive test of new models. Figures 6–41 and 6–42 show two examples.

Figure 6–41 shows a simple example of the simulation of a typical isolation process. In this case, the silicon is etched prior to the field oxide growth, so that the final oxide surface is at roughly the same level as the original silicon surface. This produces the well-known "bird's head" shape in the simulation because of lateral oxidation under the masking nitride. Figure 6–41 illustrates one of the powerful features of modern simulators—the ability to "observe" things that are not easily observable experimentally. In this case the time evolution of the structure is shown.

Figure 6–42 shows an example of a more complex isolation process. In this case two nitride depositions (of different thickness) are needed to form the initial structure, along with a silicon etch to form a recessed field oxide. The second (thinner) nitride masks the sidewall of the etched silicon, minimizing oxidation in the active device region under the thicker nitride. In the final structure on the top right of the figure, this thin nitride "flap" has lifted up to control the stresses developed during the oxidation. This simulation invoked many of the stress-dependent models that we described earlier

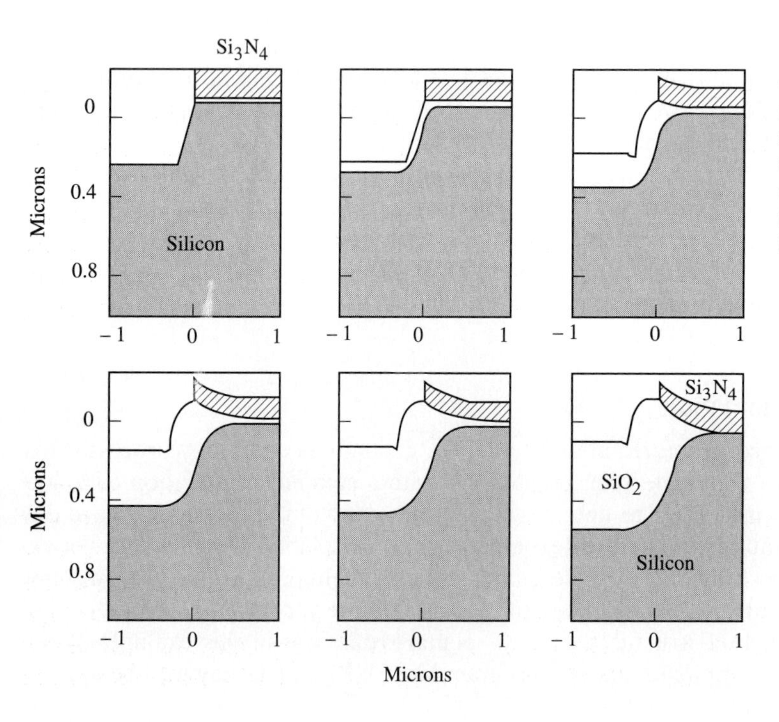

Figure 6–41 Simulation of a recessed LOCOS isolation structure using the ATHENA simulator [6.12]. The initial structure (top left) is formed by depositing a SiO_2/Si_3N_4 structure followed by etching of this stack on the left side. The silicon is then etched to form a recessed oxide and the structure is oxidized for 90 min at 1000°C in H_2O. The time evolution of the bird's head shape during the oxidation is shown in the simulations.

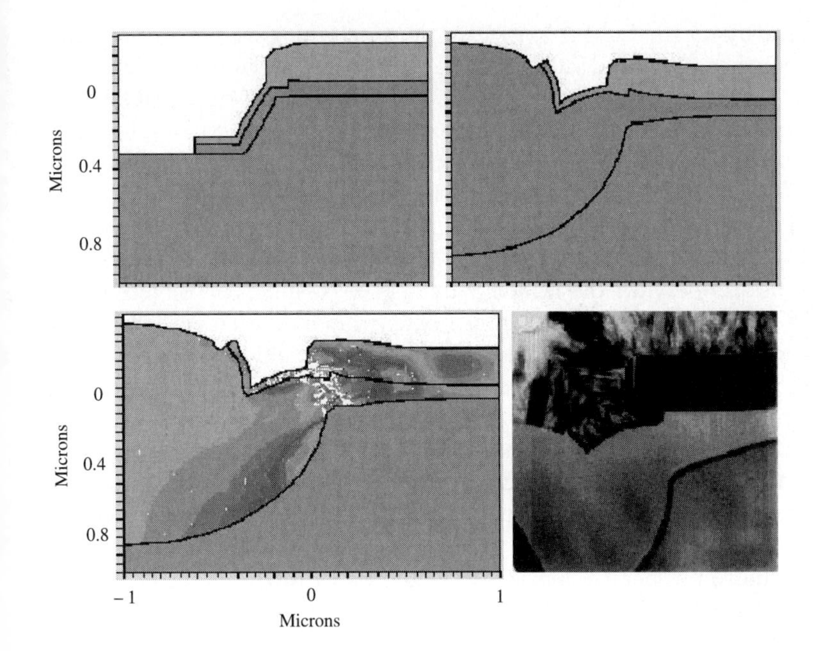

Figure 6–42 Simulation of an advanced isolation structure (the SWAMI process originally developed by Hewlett-Packard), using the ATHENA simulator [6.12]. The structure prior to oxidation is on the top left. This structure is formed by depositing an oxide followed by a thick Si_3N_4 layer, both of which are etched away on the left side. A silicon etch on the left side is then followed by a second oxide and nitride deposition. These layers are then etched away on the far-left side, leaving the thin SiO_2/Si_3N_4 stack covering the sidewall of the silicon. A 450-min H_2O oxidation at 1000°C is then performed which results in the structure on the top right. An experimental structure fabricated with a similar process flow is shown on the bottom right. The stress levels in the SiO_2 are shown at the end of the oxidation on the bottom left.

in this chapter. Note that there is reasonable agreement with the experimental structure also shown in the figure. This example again also illustrates one of the unique capabilities of simulators. The calculated stress levels in the SiO_2 are shown in the lower-left portion of the figure. Information like this is often useful in understanding whether a particular process will create defects in the underlying substrate. The stress contours themselves are usually not observable experimentally at all. About all that can be done experimentally is to observe at the end of the process whether or not defects were created in the substrate. Simulation thus provides a powerful design tool in understanding processes and their effects.

6.6 Limits and Future Trends in Technologies and Models

Oxidation is certain to remain an integral part of silicon technology. However, as device structures shrink in size, some changes may occur in how the process is used. There will certainly be more use made of lower-temperature processes in order to control impurity diffusion. Oxides grow more slowly at low temperatures. There are two basic approaches to obtaining relatively thick SiO_2 layers at lower temperatures. The first is to use high pressures during the oxidation, a strategy that is already finding some use in manufacturing. Systems that operate at 10–25 atmospheres are commercially available and are sometimes used, particularly for LOCOS processes in which thick oxides are required. The second option is to use deposited SiO_2 films. We will discuss deposition in Chapter 9 but relatively simple CVD or LPCVD processes can be used to deposit thick SiO_2 layers. Such processes are increasingly being used. The ideal properties of the Si/SiO_2 interface can be preserved with deposited oxides either by first growing a thin thermal oxide and then depositing SiO_2 on top of it, or by annealing the deposited oxide after deposition. (Such anneals often consist of a short thermal oxidation step which grows a thin thermal oxide underneath the deposited oxide, again producing a virtually ideal interface.)

A second trend that is likely for the future, is the use of "composite" dielectric layers. The SIA NTRS (Table 6–1) calls for extraordinarily thin gate dielectrics in future technology generations. It is unlikely that pure SiO_2 films will be able to meet all the requirements of this roadmap. Very thin layers of SiO_2 conduct excessive currents (due to tunneling) and they are not adequate masks against dopant penetration from polysilicon gates. Boron diffusion through these thin SiO_2 layers is a particular problem. It would also be desirable to have a gate dielectric with a higher dielectric constant than SiO_2 in order to improve the electrical characteristics of MOS transistors or to increase charge storage in DRAM cells.

For these reasons, there has been a considerable amount of work in recent years on composite oxynitride dielectrics. These films were first commonly prepared by exposing thermally grown SiO_2 films to an NH_3 ambient. This results in a dielectric film which is generically called an oxynitride, often labeled as SiO_xN_y, but which usually varies in composition throughout the film. For relatively short NH_3 exposures, chemical profiling through the resulting composite dielectrics has shown that nitrogen rich regions are formed both at the Si/SiO_2 interface and at the top SiO_2/ambient interface. These two "nitride" layers seal the intervening SiO_2 layer and can trap hydrogen in the SiO_2. Because this trapped hydrogen can cause instability problems in the devices, more recent work has focused on using N_2O or NO ambients to create the oxynitride. These ambients do not contain hydrogen. Alternatively, processes that strip off the top "nitride" region and allow the trapped hydrogen to escape, have also been explored. Finally, nitrogen implants into the substrate and subsequent oxidation have also been investigated.

The benefits of the oxynitride dielectric arise because of the stronger Si-N bonds that are formed near the Si/SiO_2 interface. This oxynitride interface can result in more rugged gate dielectrics because the stronger Si-N bonds are more resistant to breaking during hot carrier stressing. Oxynitrides are also more resistant to dopant penetration through the dielectric. Finally, the relative dielectric constant of Si_3N_4 is significantly higher than SiO_2 ($\approx$ 7.5 versus 3.9). While oxynitrides do not achieve values as high as 7.5 because they are composite materials, they usually do improve upon SiO_2. For all these reasons, oxynitirides are likely to find increased use in the future as gate dielectrics.

2D and even 3D effects will become increasingly important in small structures. These include not only predicting the shapes of oxides grown on nonplanar structures, but also accurate prediction of the stresses generated in the oxide and in the silicon substrate. Control of oxide thicknesses at the atomic level will be required for thin dielectrics. The Si-Si bond distances in SiO_2 are a fraction of a nm; this is a significant percentage of the total thickness of films that will be grown in the future for gate dielectrics and other applications. Finally, statistical issues may also become important. For example, an oxide charge density of 10^{10} cm^{-2} corresponds to one charge in an area of about $0.1 \times 0.1\mu$m. As device sizes approach these dimensions, we may find variations from one device to another in the number of such charges that are contained in the device active area.

6.7 Summary of Key Ideas

Thermal oxidation has been a cornerstone of silicon technology since its inception. In fact it is really the ability to easily grow SiO_2 layers that distinguishes silicon technology from all other semiconductors. SiO_2 layers adhere well to silicon, are relatively chemically inert, mask dopant diffusion, block ion implantations, and are easily patterned. However the real strength of SiO_2 lies in the almost perfect electrical interface it makes with silicon. Electrical charges are reproducible and small and the interface is almost atomically abrupt. These features allow junctions to be almost ideally passivated at silicon surfaces and they allow a variety of device structures that critically depend on surface properties to be easily built in silicon (MOS structures in particular). Even devices which are not primarily surface controlled such as bipolar transistors, do not have their electrical characteristics degraded by parasitic surface effects. No other semiconductor/insulator interface has all these desirable properties.

Since SiO_2 is such an important part of silicon technology, the growth kinetics of these layers on silicon have been carefully studied over many years. The basic growth mechanism is oxidant transport through the SiO_2 layer to the Si/SiO_2 interface where a simple chemical reaction produces the new layers of oxide. The growth generally follows a simple linear parabolic law. This basic model of oxidation has been extended in recent years to handle many situations for which the original formulation falls short. These include heavily doped substrates, mixed ambients, 2D effects and thin oxides. The same basic ideas have been applied to other materials like polysilicon and silicides which are common in silicon technology and which are often oxidized. We have not dealt in this chapter in detail with the interaction of oxidation with other process steps such as diffusion. Oxidation enhanced or retarded diffusion and impurity redistribution and segregation during oxidation are important effects. We will discuss them in more detail in Chapter 7 after we describe the basic ideas of dopant diffusion. Finally, many of the models and physical mechanisms described in this chapter have been implemented in process simulators. These simulators today are capable of accurately predicting the oxidation processes in modern VLSI structures. As new understanding develops, particularly with respect to very small structures, new models are incorporated in these simulators so that their capability is constantly improving.

6.8 References

[6.1]. "National Technology Roadmap for Semiconductors," SIA, 1997

[6.2]. P. J. Jorgensen, "Effect of an Electric Field on Silicon Oxidation," *J. Chem. Phys.*, vol. 37, p. 874, 1962.

[6.3]. J. R. Ligenza and W. G. Spitzer, *Phys. and Chem. Solids*, vol. 14, p. 131, 1960.

[6.4]. E. Rosencher, A. Straboni, S. Rigo, and G. Amsel, "An ^{18}O Study of the Thermal Oxidation of Silicon in Oxygen," *Appl. Phys. Lett.*, vol. 34, p. 254, 1979.

[6.5]. R. Pretorius, *J. Electrochem. Soc.*, vol 128, p. 107, 1981.

[6.6]. B. E. Deal and A. S. Grove, "General Relationship for the Thermal Oxidation of Silicon," *J. Appl. Phys.*, vol. 36, p. 3770, 1965.

[6.7]. B. E. Deal, "Standardized Terminology for Oxide Charges Associated with Thermally Oxidized Silicon," *IEEE Trans. Elec. Dev.*, vol. ED-27, p. 606, 1980.

[6.8]. W. A. Pliskin and E. E. Conrad, "Nondestructive Determination of Thickness and Refractive Index of Transparent Films," *IBM J. Res. and Dev.*, vol. 8, p. 43, 1964.

[6.9]. D. K. Schroder, *Semiconductor Material and Device Characterization*, John Wiley & Sons, 1990.

[6.10]. E. H. Nicollian and J. R. Brews, *MOS (Metal Oxide Semiconductor) Physics and Technology*, John Wiley & Sons, 1982.

[6.11]. TSUPREM IV is the version of SUPREM IV by Avanti! Inc. SUPREM IV was originally written at Stanford University by M. E. Law, C. S. Rafferty, and R. W. Dutton.

[6.12]. ATHENA is the version of SUPREM IV by Silvaco Inc.

[6.13]. A. Reisman, E. H. Nicollian, K. C. Williams, and C. J. Merz, "The Modeling of Silicon Oxidation from 1×10^{-5} to 20 Atmospheres," *J. Elect. Mat.*, vol. 16, p. 45, 1987.

[6.14]. E. Nicollian and A. Reisman, "A New Model for the Thermal Oxidation Kinetics of Silicon," *J. Electronic Mat.*, vol. 17, p. 263, 1988.

[6.15]. C. J. Han and C. R. Helms, "Parallel Oxidation Mechanism for Si Oxidation in Dry O_2," *J. Electrochem. Soc.*, vol.134, p. 1297, 1987.

[6.16]. K. Hirabayashi and J. Iwamura, "Kinetics of Thermal Growth of HCl-O_2 Oxides on Silicon," *J. Electrochem. Soc.*, vol. 120, p. 1595, 1973.

[6.17]. R. Ghez and Y. J. van der Meulen, "Kinetics of Thermal Growth of Ultra-Thin layers of SiO_2 on Silicon, Part I: Experiment and Part II: Theory," *J. Electrochem. Soc.*, vol. 119, pp. 530 and 1100, 1972.

[6.18]. H. Z. Massoud, J. D. Plummer, and E. A. Irene, "Thermal Oxidation of Silicon in Dry Oxygen: Growth-Rate Enhancement in the Thin Regime I. Experimental Results, II. Physical Mechanisms," *J. Electrochem. Soc.*, vol. 132, pp. 2685 and 2693, 1985.

[6.19]. E. A. Irene and E. A. Lewis, "Thermionic Emission Model for the Initial Regime of Silicon Oxidation," *Appl. Phys. Lett.*, vol. 51, p. 767, 1987.

[6.20]. A. G. Revesz, *Phys. Stat. Sol.*, vol. 58, p. 107, 1980.

[6.21]. W. A. Tiller, *J. Electrochem. Soc.*, vol. 130, p. 501, 1983.

[6.22]. R. R. Razouk, L. N. Lie, and B. E. Deal, "Kinetics of High Pressure Oxidation of Silicon in Pyrogenic Steam," *J. Electrochem. Soc.*, vol. 128, p. 2214, 1981.

[6.23]. S. M. Hu, "A New Oxide Growth Law, and the Thermal Oxidation of Silicon," *Appl. Phys. Lett.*, May 1983.

[6.24]. J. R. Ligenza, "Effect of Crystal Orientation on Oxidation Rates of Silicon in High Pressure Steam," *J. Phys. Chem.*, vol. 65, p. 2011, 1961.

[6.25]. E. A. Irene, H. Z. Massoud, and E. Tierney, "Silicon Oxidation Studies: Silicon Orientation Effects on Thermal Oxidation," *J. Electrochem. Soc.*, vol. 133, p. 1253, 1986.

[6.26]. B. E. Deal, D. W. Hess, J. D. Plummer, and C. P. Ho. "Kinetics of the Thermal Oxidation of Silicon in O_2/H_2O and O_2/Cl_2 Mixtures," *J. Electrochem. Soc.*, vol. 125, p. 339, 1978.

[6.27]. B. E. Deal, "Thermal Oxidation Kinetics of Silicon in Pyrogenic H_2O and 5% HCl/H_2O Mixtures," *J. Electrochem. Soc.*, vol. 125, p. 576,1978.

[6.28]. D. B. Kao, J. P. McVittie, W. D. Nix, and K. C. Saraswat, "Two-Dimensional Thermal Oxidation of Silicon—I. Experiments," *IEEE Trans. Elec. Dev.*, vol. ED-34, p. 1008, 1987.

[6.29]. D. B. Kao, J. P. McVittie, W. D. Nix and K. C. Saraswat, "Two-Dimensional Thermal Oxidation of Silicon—II. Modeling Stress Effects in Wet Oxides," *IEEE Trans. Elec. Dev.*, vol. ED-35, p. 25, 1988.

[6.30]. P. Sutardja and W. G. Oldham, "Modeling of Stress Effects in Silicon Oxidation," *IEEE Trans. Elec. Dev.*, vol. 36, p. 2415, 1989.

[6.31]. C. S. Rafferty, "Stress Effects in Silicon Oxidation—Simulation and Experiments," Ph.D. Thesis, Stanford University, 1989.

[6.32]. P. B. Griffin and C. S. Rafferty, "A Viscous Nitride Model for Nitride/Oxide Isolation Structures," *IEDM Technical Digest*, p. 741, 1990.

[6.33]. L. M. Landsberger and W. A. Tiller, "Two-Step Oxidation Experiments to Determine Structural and Thermal History Effects in Thermally-Grown SiO_2 Films on Si," *J. Electrochem. Soc.*, vol. 137, p. 2825, 1990.

[6.34]. K. Imai and K. Yamabe, "Nonplanar Silicon Oxidation in Dry O_2 + NF_3," *Appl. Phys. Lett.*, vol. 56, p. 280, 1990.

[6.35]. L. M. Landsberger, D. B. Kao, and W. A. Tiller, "Conformal Two-Dimensional SiO_2 Layers on Silicon Grown by Low Temperature Corona Discharge," *J. Electrochem. Soc.*, vol. 135, p. 1766, 1988.

[6.36]. P. S. Dobson, "The Effect of Oxidation on Anomalous Diffusion in Silicon," *Philosophical Mag.*, vol. 24, p. 567, 1971.

[6.37]. P. M. Fahey, P. B. Griffin, and J. D. Plummer, "Point Defects and Dopant Diffusion in Silicon," *Reviews of Modern Physics*, vol. 61, p. 289, 1989.

[6.38]. S. M. Hu, *J. Appl. Physics*, "Formation of Stacking Faults and Enhanced Diffusion in the Oxidation of Silicon," vol. 45, p. 1567, 1974.

[6.39]. S. Dunham, *J. Appl. Physics*, "Interaction of Silicon Point Defects with Silicon Oxide Films," vol. 71, p. 685, 1992.

[6.40]. C. P. Ho and J. D. Plummer, "Si/SiO_2 Interface Oxidation Kinetics: a Physical Model for the Influence of High Substrate Doping Levels. I. Theory and II. Comparison with Experiment," *J. Electrochem. Soc.*, vol. 126, pp. 1516 and 1523, 1979.

[6.41]. E. Biermann, H. H. Berger, P. Linke and B. Muller, "Oxide Growth Enhancement on Highly N-Type Doped Silicon Under Steam oxidation," *J. Electrochem. Soc.*, vol. 143, p. 1434 , 1996.

[6.42]. S. S. Choi, M. Z. Numan, W. K. Chu, and E. A. Irene, "Anomalous Oxidation rate of Silicon Implanted with Very High Doses of Arsenic," *Appl. Phys. Lett.*, vol. 51, p. 1001, 1987.

[6.43]. F. Lau, L. Mader, C. Mazure, C. Warner, and M. Orlowski, "A Model for Phosphorus Segregation at the Silicon-Silicon Dioxide Interface," *Appl. Phys. A*, vol. 49, p. 671, 1989.

[6.44]. T. Kamins, *Polycrystalline Silicon for Integrated Circuit Applications*, 2d ed., Kluwer Academic Publishers, 1998.

[6.45]. T. Enomoto, R. Ando, H. Morita, and H. Nakayama, "Thermal Oxidation Rate of a Si_3N_4 Film and Its Masking Effect Against Oxidation of Silicon," *Jpn. J. Appl. Phys.*, vol. 17, p. 1049, 1978.

[6.46]. T. I. Kamins, private communication.

[6.47]. H. Du, R. E Tressler and K. E. Spear, "Thermodynamics of the Si-N-O System and Kinetic Modeling of Oxidation of Si_3N_4," *J. Electrochem. Soc.*, vol. 136, p. 3210, 1989.

[6.48]. M. M. Moslehi and K. C. Saraswat, "Thermal Nitridation of Si and SiO_2 for VLSI," *IEEE Trans. Elec. Dev.*, vol. ED-32, p. 106, 1985.

[6.49]. M. Bartur and M-A. Nicolet, "Thermal Oxidation of Transition Metal Silicides on Si: Summary," *J. Electrochem. Soc.*, vol. 131, p. 371, 1984.

[6.50]. J. E. E. Baglin, F. M. d'Heurle, and C. S. Petersson, "Interface Effects in the Formation of Silicon Oxide on Metal Silicide Layers Over Silicon Substrates," *J. Appl. Phys.*, vol. 54, p. 1849, 1983.

[6.51]. R. R. Razouk and B. E. Deal. "Dependence of Interface State Density on Silicon Thermal Oxidation Process Variables," *J. Electrochem. Soc.*, vol. 126, p. 1573, 1979.

[6.52]. B. E. Deal, "The Current Understanding of Charges in the Thermally Oxidized Silicon Structure," *J. Electrochem. Soc.*, vol. 121, p. 198C, 1974.

[6.53]. A. I. Akinwande and J. D. Plummer, "Quantitative Modeling of Si/SiO_2 Interface Fixed Charge I. Experimental Results and II. Physical Modeling," *J. Electrochem. Soc.*, vol. 134, pp. 2565 and 2573, 1987.

[6.54]. M. L. Reed and J. D. Plummer, "Chemistry of Si-SiO_2 Interface Trap Annealing," *J. Appl. Phys.*, vol. 63, p. 5776, 1988.

[6.55]. K. L. Brower and S. M. Meyers, "Chemical Kinetics of Hydrogen and (111) Si-SiO2 Interface Defects," *Appl. Phys. Lett.*, vol. 57, p. 162, 1990.

[6.56]. G. J. Gerardi, E. H. Poindexter, and P. J. Caplan, "Interface Traps and Pb Centers in Oxidized (100) Silicon Wafers," *Appl. Phys. Lett.*, vol. 49, p. 348, 1986.

6.9 Problems

6.1. A spherically shaped piece of silicon is cut and polished from a Czochralski single-crystal ingot and oxidized in a thermal oxidation furnace. Upon pulling the silicon sphere from the furnace, the color is observed to vary significantly over the surface. Why?

6.2. Using Eqs. (6.1) and (6.2), explain why oxides thinner than about 50 nm do not have any characteristic color associated with them. You do not need to do any calculations. Simply explain the physical reason for the lack of color in thin oxides.

6.3. An experimental Metal Insulator Semiconductor (MIS) (I = insulator) structure is fabricated by depositing Si_3N_4 (silicon nitride) on a silicon substrate. The nitride is deposited by directing a jet of silane and ammonia at the surface:

$$3SiH_4 + 4NH_3 \rightarrow Si_3N_4 + 12H_2$$

A metal electrode is deposited and a CV plot is made as shown below. A representative CV plot is also shown for an identical structure except with thermally grown SiO_2 as the insulator.

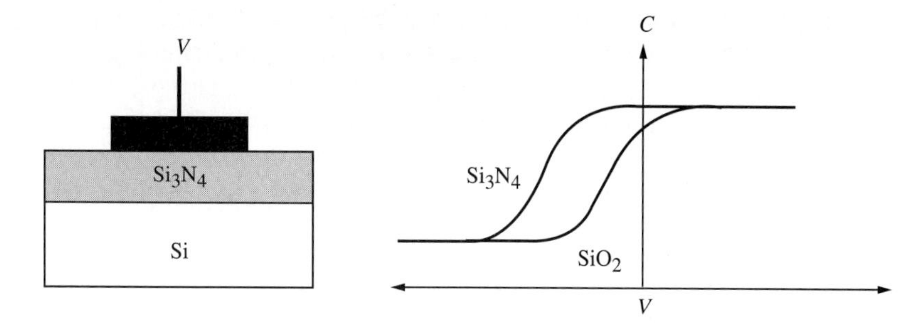

Explain the lateral shift in the CV curve of the Si_3N_4.

6.4. Construct a HF CV plot for a P-type silicon sample, analogous to Figure 6–9. Explain your plot based on the behavior of holes and electrons in the semiconductor in a similar manner to the discussion in the text for Figure 6–9.

6.5. A MOS structure is fabricated to make CV measurements as shown below. The CV plot shows the result if the P^+ diffusion is *not* present. Sketch the expected shape of the CV plot with the P^+ diffusion. Explain.

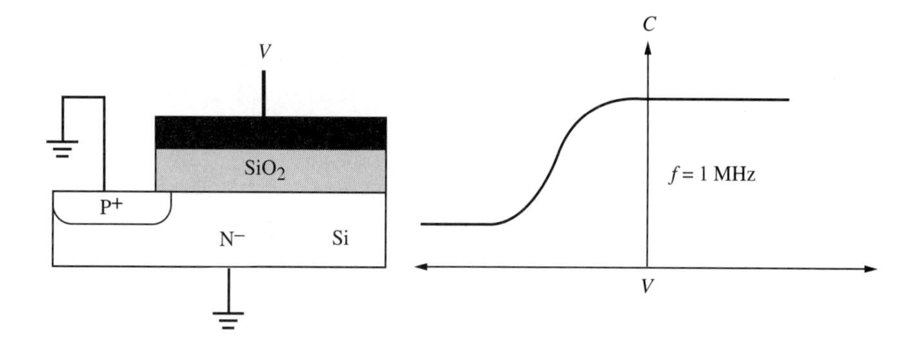

6.6. In a small MOS device, there may be a statistical variation in V_T due to differences in Q_F from one device to another. In a 0.13-μm technology minimum device (gate oxide area = 0.1 μm × 0.1 μm) with a 2.5-nm gate oxide, what would the difference in threshold voltage be for devices with 0 or 1 fixed charge in the gate oxide?

6.7. Why is steam oxidation more rapid than dry O_2 oxidation?

6.8. Under what conditions is the thermal growth rate of SiO_2 linearly proportional to time?

6.9. According to the Deal-Grove model, oxidation kinetics start out linear and become parabolic as the oxidation proceeds. Calculate the oxide thickness at which this transition takes place and plot this versus oxidation temperature.

6.10. Does the oxide thickness at which there is a transition from linear to parabolic rates change if we perform an oxidation at a pressure of 20 Atm rather than at 1 Atm.

6.11. A MOS device requires a gate oxide of 10 nm ± 0.5 nm. Assume the growth is done at 900°C in dry O_2. Neglect any effect of the anomalous initial growth. Derive a simple expression which gives the sensitivity of the oxide thickness to growth temperature (dx/dt). Evaluate this expression to see how well controlled the furnace T must be in order to obtain 10 nm ± 0.5 nm at 900°C.

6.12. A silicon wafer is covered by an SiO_2 film 0.3 μm thick.
   a. What is the time required to increase the thickness by 0.5 μm by oxidation in H_2O at 1200°C?
   b. Repeat for oxidation in dry O_2 at 1200°C.

6.13. Suppose an oxidation process is used in which (100) wafers are oxidized in O_2 for three hours at 1100°C, followed by two hours in H_2O at 900°C, followed by two hours in O_2 at 1200°C. Use Figures 6–19 and 6–20 in the text to estimate the resulting final oxide thickness. Explain how you use these figures to calculate the results of a multi-step oxidation like this.

6.14. What is the approximate oxide thickness (use charts) after a 100-minute dry O_2 oxidation followed by a 35-minute H_2O oxidation at 900°C?

6.15. The structure shown below is formed by oxidizing a silicon wafer (x_O = 200 nm) and then using standard masking and etching techniques to remove the SiO_2 in the center region. An N^+ doping step is then used to produce the structure shown. The structure is next placed in an oxidation furnace and oxidized at 900°C in H_2O. The oxide will grow faster over the N^+ region than it will over the lightly doped substrate. Assume that B/A is enhanced by 4X over the N^+ region. Will the growing oxide over the N^+ region ever catch up in thickness to the other oxide? If so, when and at what thickness? Use the Deal-Grove model for the oxidation kinetics.

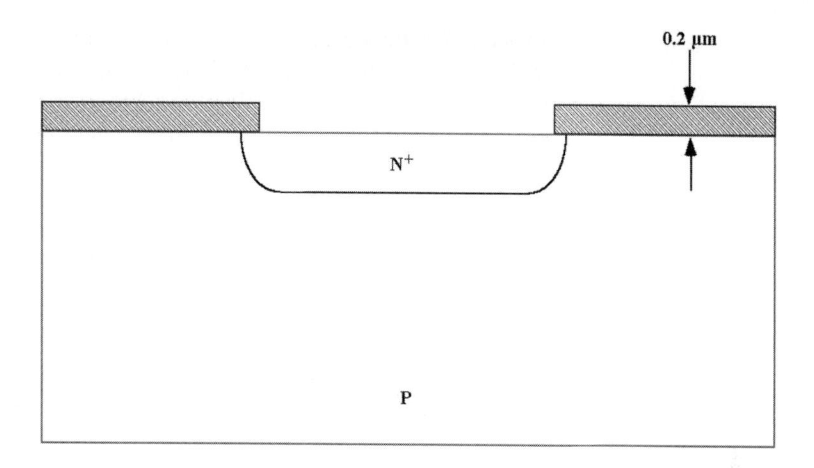

6.16. A 1-μm wide trench is etched in a <100> silicon wafer, so that the sides of the trench are <110> planes. An angled implant is performed, doping the sidewall N^+ and thereby enhancing the linear rate constant by a factor of 4. The structure is then oxidized in steam at 1100°C. At what time during the oxidation will the groove be filled with SiO_2? Assume the appropriate oxidation coefficient scale as [(111 : 110 : 100) = (1.68 : 1.2 : 1.0)].

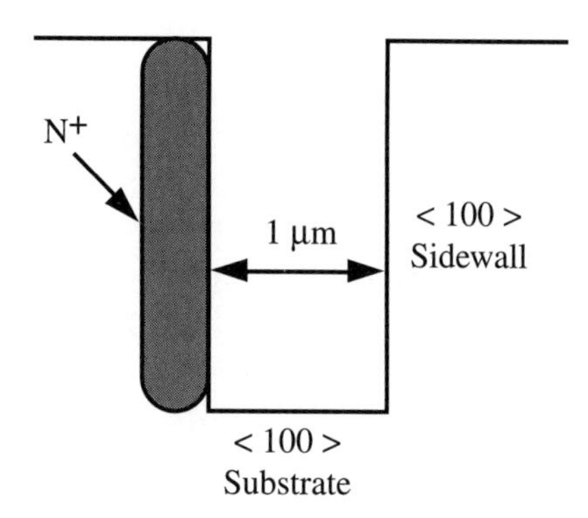

6.17. A uniform oxide layer of 0.4-μm thickness is selectively etched to expose the silicon surface in some locations on a wafer surface. A second oxidation at 1000°C in H_2O grows 0.2 μm on the bare silicon.

a. Sketch a cross section of the SiO_2 in all locations on the wafer and the position of the Si/SiO_2 interface.

b. Would your picture be the same if the second oxidation grew the 0.2 μm at a different temperature? Explain.

6.18. Silicon On Insulator or SOI is a new substrate material that is being considered for future integrated circuits. The structure, shown below, consists of a thin single-crystal silicon layer on an insulating (SiO_2) substrate. The silicon below the SiO_2 provides mechanical support for the structure. One of the reasons this type of material is being considered is because junctions can be diffused completely through the thin silicon layer to the underlying SiO_2. This reduces junction capacitances and produces faster circuits. Isolation is also easy to achieve in this material, because the thin Si layer can be completely oxidized, resulting in devices completely surrounded by SiO_2. A LOCOS process is used to locally oxidize through the silicon as shown on the right below. Assuming the LOCOS oxidation is done in H_2O at 1000°C, how long will it take to oxidize through the 0.3-μm silicon layer? Calculate a numerical answer using the Deal-Grove model.

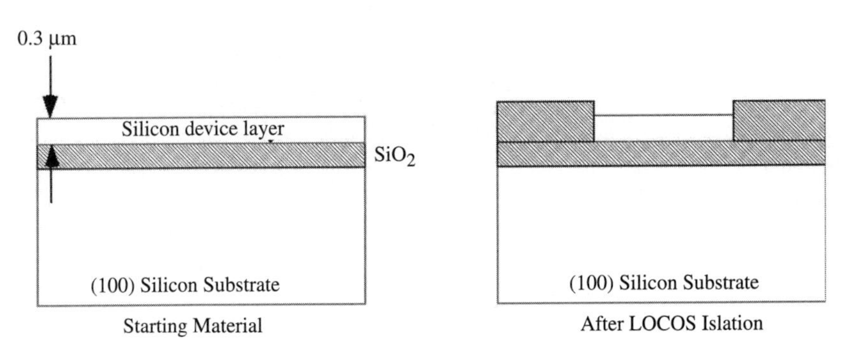

6.19. As MOS devices are scaled to smaller dimensions, gate oxides must be reduced in thickness.

a. As the gate oxide thickness decreases, do MOS devices become more or less sensitive to sodium contamination? Explain.

b. As the gate oxide thickness decreases, what must be done to the substrate doping (or alternatively the channel V_{TH} implant, to maintain the same V_{TH}?

6.20. A SiO_2 layer is thermally grown at 1000°C using a 10–20–30 min dry-wet-dry oxidation cycle. Upon pulling the (100) wafer from the furnace, the oxide color is observed to be tan. Is this right? If not, suggest what might have gone wrong in the experiment.

6.21. In the simulation example in Fig. 6.35, the difference in oxidation rate between the heavily doped and lightly doped regions is much more pronounced at low temperatures (the 800°C example) than at high temperatures (the 1000°C example). Explain physically why this is the case using the mechanisms in the Deal-Grove model and the behavior of point defect (V) concentrations versus temperature.

6.22. The structure shown below is implanted with oxygen using a 1×10^{18} cm^{-2} implant at 200 keV. This places the implanted oxygen in a profile centered at 0.35 μm ($R_P = 0.35$ μm) below the surface. The left-hand side is masked from the implant. Following the implant, a high-temperature anneal is performed which forms stoichiometric SiO_2 in a buried layer on the right side. Calculate the structural dimensions on the right side following this anneal (oxide thickness, distance from the surface, and all other important dimensions). You can assume the silicon atomic density is 5×10^{22} atoms cm^{-3}, and the Si lattice planes are 0.25 nm apart. State any other assumptions you make.

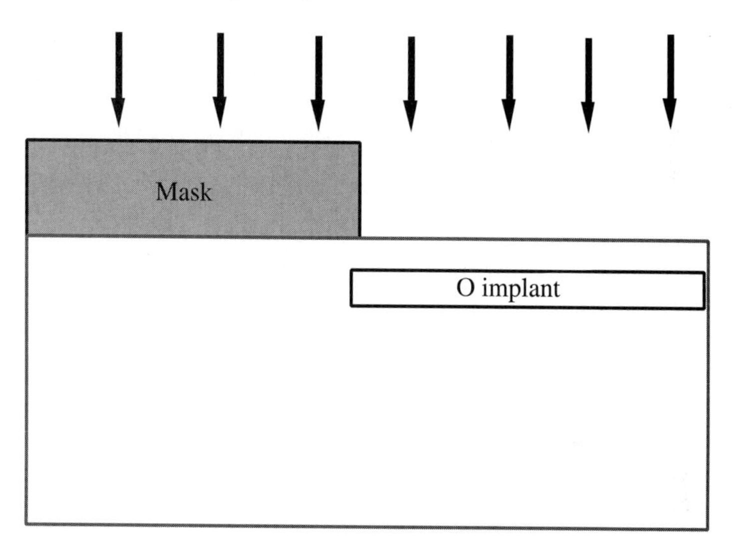

6.23. As part of an IC process flow, a CVD SiO_2 layer 1.0-μm thick is deposited on a <100> silicon substrate. This structure is then oxidized at 900°C for 60 minutes in an H_2O ambient. What is the final SiO_2 thickness after this oxidation? Calculate an answer. Do not use the oxidation charts in the text.

Dopant Diffusion

7

7.1 Introduction

One of the main challenges in designing a front-end process for building a device is accurate control of the placement of the active doping regions. Understanding and controlling diffusion and annealing behavior are essential to obtaining the desired electrical characteristics. If the gate length in a MOS device is scaled down by $1/K$, where K is a scaling factor > 1, ideally the dimensions of all doped regions should also scale down by the same factor to maintain the same $\mathcal{E}$-field patterns (assuming the operating voltage also scales proportionally) [7.1]. With the same $\mathcal{E}$-field patterns, the device operates in the same manner as before, except the shorter channel length allows for faster switching speed. Thus there is a continuous drive to decrease junction depth with each new technology generation. The diffusion cycles required to electrically activate the implanted dopant atoms are often the limiting factor on the junction depth that can be obtained. High activation levels are required so the parasitic resistances of the source/drain and extension regions do not limit the drive current of the device as illustrated in Figure 7–1. There may be requirements that the polysilicon gate is doped at the same time that the source and drain regions are formed, imposing further constraints on the doping levels and thermal cycles that can be used.

We introduced the concept of sheet resistance in Chapters 2 and 3 (see Section 3.4.1.2). Since this concept is central to doped regions, we revisit it here. Consider a region that is uniformly doped. We want to obtain the resistance between contacts at either end of the region as shown in Figure 7–2. The ability of the region to carry current will depend on the doping and the velocity of carriers, so that the current density J is

$$J = nqv = nq\mu\mathcal{E} \tag{7.1}$$

where n is the doping, q is the electron charge, and v is the velocity. The velocity is in turn written as the product of the mobility μ and the electric field $\mathcal{E}$. The conductivity of the doped region σ is then defined as the relationship between the current density and the electric field, with the resistivity being simply $1/\sigma$.

$$J = nq\mu\mathcal{E} = \sigma\mathcal{E} = \frac{1}{\rho}\mathcal{E} \tag{7.2}$$

The resistivity defines the relationship between the electric field and the current density (similar to $R = V/I$)

$$\rho = \frac{\mathcal{E}}{J}\ \Omega\text{cm} \tag{7.3}$$

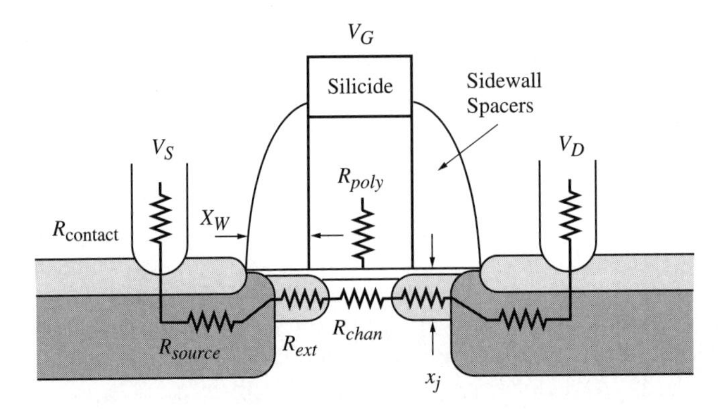

Figure 7–1 Schematic of a MOS device cross section, showing the parasitic resistances compared with the intrinsic channel resistance, the shallow extension (or tip) region to control short channel effects, and the deeper source/drain region (contact junction) to allow good silicide contacts. x_W is the spacer width and x_j is the extension junction depth at the channel as listed in Table 7–1.

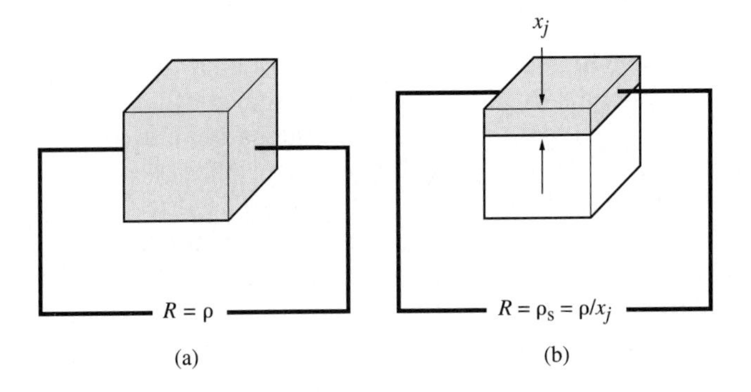

Figure 7–2 The relationship between resistivity and sheet resistance is schematically illustrated. In (a), the resistivity is the resistance that would be measured between the sides of a cube of any dimension, while in (b) the sheet resistance is the resistance that would be measured between the sides of a square of any dimension with junction depth x_j.

and can be thought of as the resistance that would be measured between the sides of a cube. Note that a larger cube would have more area for a given current to flow through, but also more distance for the current to flow, and so would have the same measured resistance between the edges. In other words, the resistivity of a material would not depend on the size of the cube on which the measurement was made. If instead of a cube, the resistance were measured between the shallow edges of a square with depth x_j [Figure 7–2(b)], the resistance would be higher and would measure

$$R = \frac{\rho}{x_j}\ \Omega/\text{square} \equiv \rho_S \tag{7.4}$$

Dimensionally, the sheet resistance is expressed in ohms but has the geometrical significance that the sheet resistance is the same for any square. A smaller square has less area for the current to flow through and thus higher current density, but proportionally a higher field, giving the same measured resistance. It is extremely useful to be able to specify the resistance of a doped region, without having to specify the dimensions of the region or the depth of the junction, once it is known that the resistance applies to any surface square. This concept is so useful in device design that this particular resistance is known as the sheet resistance ρ_S of a junction and is given the units of ohms/square. The sheet resistance of a junction can be measured by using the four-point probe technique or the Van der Pauw method, as described in Section 3.4 of Chapter 3.

The above derivation applies only when the doping is constant throughout the junction. If the doping varies in the conducting region, an integral of the doping and mobility (which varies with doping) must be performed from the surface to the junction depth x_j. An accurate value for the sheet resistance of a diffused layer can be calculated from the integral

$$\rho_s = \frac{1}{\bar{\sigma} x_j} = \frac{1}{q\int_0^{x_j} [n(x) - N_B]\mu[n(x)]dx} \tag{7.5}$$

The junction depth is where the impurity profile meets the background doping concentration N_B. We will see examples of such calculations later in the chapter.

The general guideline when designing modern VLSI transistors is that the resistance of the source or drain region ($R_{\text{contact}} + R_{\text{source}} + R_{\text{ext}}$) should not amount to more than 10% of the channel resistance (R_{chan}). It seems obvious from the definition of sheet resistance that a simple way to reduce the sheet resistance of a layer is to simply increase the junction depth to allow more room for the current to flow. However, this causes an immediate problem in MOS devices—the deeper junctions make it easier for the voltages on the drain to affect the current flow from the source. Ideally, only the gate voltage causes current to flow from the source to drain by inverting the surface of the channel if $V_G > V_{TH}$. But in a submicron MOSFET, the two-dimensional spreading of the electric field from the drain can attract carriers from the source even when the device is supposed to be off with $V_G < V_{TH}$. This off-current in the device is a key design parameter and can be minimized by keeping the junctions shallow. The change in off-current with drain voltage is called DIBL (Drain-Induced Barrier Lowering) and is a key design parameter for a MOS device.

The challenge in designing VLSI MOS devices is thus to keep the junctions shallow, so DIBL is reduced and at the same time keep the resistance of the source and drain regions small so that the drive current is maximized. These are conflicting requirements. The requirements for shallow junctions in future technology generations can be seen in Table 7–1 taken from the SIA NTRS [7.2].

The trends in the NTRS are apparent. Very shallow junctions with very high doping concentrations are required to simultaneously meet DIBL and ρ_S requirements. Of course, VLSI devices also use deeper, less critical doped regions for wells and shallow, more lightly doped regions in the channel region as described in the process flow in

Table 7–1 Channel doping requirements from the NTRS roadmap, showing the continuing drive to obtain shallow junctions (From [7.2])

Year of First DRAM Shipment	1997	1999	2003	2006	2009	2012
Min Feature Size	0.25 μ	0.18 μ	0.13 μ	0.10 μ	0.07 μ	0.05 μ
DRAM Bits/Chip	256M	1G	4G	16G	64G	256G
Minimum Supply Voltage (volts)	1.8–2.5	1.5–1.8	1.2–1.5	0.9–1.2	0.6–0.9	0.5–0.6
Gate Oxide T_{ox} Equivalent (nm)	4–5	3–4	2–3	1.5–2	<1.5	<1.0
Sidewall Spacer Thickness x_W (nm)	100–200	72–144	52–104	20–40	7.5–15	5–10
Contact x_j (nm)	100–200	70–140	50–100	40–80	15–30	10–20
x_j at Channel (nm)	50–100	36–72	26–52	20–40	15–30	10–20
Drain Ext Conc (cm^{-3})	1×10^{18}	1×10^{19}	1×10^{19}	1×10^{20}	1×10^{20}	1×10^{20}

Chapter 2. These regions are generally easier to produce than the shallow, highly doped source and drain regions. We will see examples of all these types of doping applications later. In this chapter we will explore the basic process of dopant diffusion which is one of the fundamental processes used to form junctions in modern silicon ICs. We will be concerned with the fundamental mechanisms that cause diffusion and methods to accurately predict dopant profiles. The NTRS requirements in the future will require knowledge of dopant positions with almost atomic-scale accuracy.

7.2 Historical Development and Basic Concepts

In Chapter 1 we described some of the historical techniques that have been used to produce doped regions in silicon devices. Formation methods like alloy junctions, mesa junctions, and the like were used only until the invention of the planar process because of the far superior manufacturing capability and the improved electrical characteristics of planar junctions. Thus by 1960, the basic junction formation method shown in Figure 7–3 was in widespread use and these techniques continue to dominate today.

The only fundamental change that has occurred in this process in the past 40 years is the preferred method for "predeposition." This step is designed to controllably introduce a desired dose of dopant atoms into the silicon crystal. Throughout the 1960s the dominant predeposition methods were solid-phase diffusion from glass layers deposited on the wafer surface, or high-temperature gas-phase depositions in which the wafers were placed in a furnace with a gas containing the desired doping species. Typical examples included B_2H_6, PH_3, and AsH_3, all of which are gases. Aside from the safety issues associated with using these gases (many of them are toxic), both of these deposition methods have significant limitations in practice. In order to form reproducible junctions in a manufacturing environment they are limited to introducing dopants at the solid solubility level. There are many situations in IC fabrication in which relatively small doses of dopant are required (the threshold adjust steps in the CMOS process we described in Chapter 2 in Figures 2–22 and 2–23 are one example). These kinds of processes are almost impossible to perform with solid-phase or gas-phase predeposition.

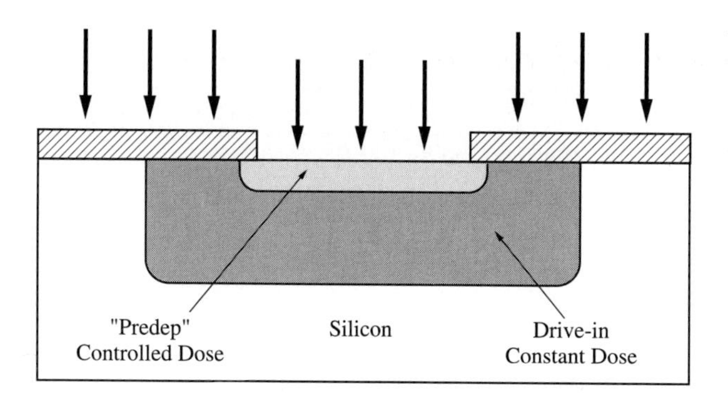

Figure 7–3 Two-step process for producing a junction at the desired depth. The predeposition step introduces a controlled number of impurity atoms, while the drive-in step thermally diffuses the dopant to the desired junction depth.

Ion implantation was studied extensively in the 1960s as an alternative predeposition method. Because it provides much better control of the predeposition dose, it became the dominant doping method by the mid 1970s and continues to be so today. We will discuss this process in detail in Chapter 8. Ion implantation has proven to be a highly flexible, highly manufacturable process with really only one significant drawback. The process causes damage to the silicon crystal which must be annealed at high temperatures and during this step diffusion and redistribution of dopant atoms occur. For relatively deep junctions, this is of little consequence because the drive-in step illustrated in Figure 7–3 diffuses the junctions deeper than any transient effects due to implantation damage. However for today's very small structures and very shallow junctions, the anomalously high diffusion rate observed during damage annealing is a real issue. This Transient Enhanced Diffusion or TED is beginning to limit how shallow junctions can be made and is a subject of intense study today. We will discuss this topic in detail later in Chapter 8.

In fabricating shallow junctions, the challenge is thus to minimize the redistribution of dopants during any subsequent drive-in or anneal following implantation. Because of TED effects, there is a resurgence of interest in solid- or gas-phase diffusion techniques today, driven by the need to form shallow junctions without any damage. However it is likely that ion implantation will remain the dominant predeposition method in the future because of its large installed base in current manufacturing. Table 7–2 summarizes the advantages and disadvantages of these doping techniques.

7.2.1 Dopant Solid Solubility

The maximum concentration of a dopant that can be dissolved in silicon under equilibrium conditions, without forming a separate phase, is termed the solid solubility. Many of the elements used as dopants exhibit a retrograde solid solubility, where the maximum concentration that can be dissolved occurs below the melting point as shown in Figure 7–4. Above the solid solubility, a separate phase forms. Techniques like SIMS measure the total chemical concentration of dopants, which includes the dopants in precipitates. However, it is the electrically active concentration that is most important to device designers. Though the solid solubility is the thermodynamic maximum concentration that

Table 7–2 Comparison of ion implantation versus solid- or gas-phase doping methods

Advantages	
Ion Implantation and Annealing	**Solid-/Gas-Phase Diffusion**
Room temperature mask	No damage created by doping
Precise dose control	Batch fabrication
$10^{11} - 10^{16}$ atoms cm^{-2} doses	
Accurate depth control	
Disadvantages	
Ion Implantation and Annealing	**Solid-/Gas-Phase Diffusion**
Implant damage enhances diffusion	Usually limited to solid solubility
Dislocations caused by damage may cause junction leakage	Low surface concentration hard to achieve without a long drive-in
Implant channeling may affect profile	Low dose predeps very difficult

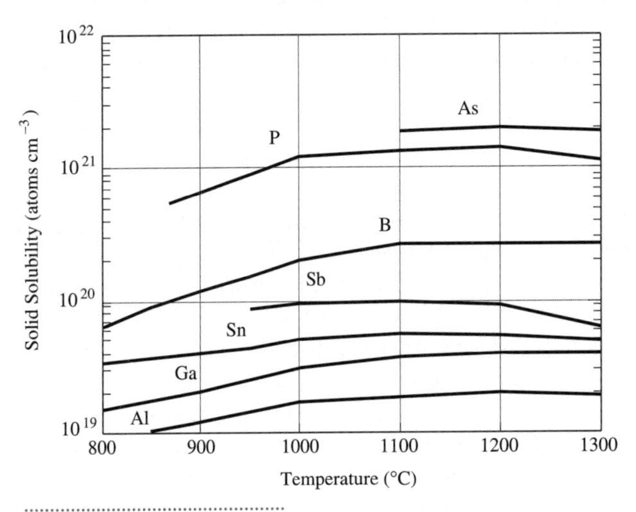

Figure 7–4 Solid solubility curves for various dopants in silicon. These values are the equilibrium solubilities at each temperature and may not be achieved in device doped regions. (After [7.3].)

can be accommodated in a solid without a separate phase forming, kinetic effects may limit the electrically active dopant concentration that can be achieved under typical processing conditions. By this we mean that if the wafer temperature is changed, some time is required for the dopant solubility to reach the value characteristic of the new temperature. In addition, the electrical solubility limit may be considerably lower than the maximum solid solubility, shown in Figure 7–4, because of neutral cluster formation with point defects in the silicon lattice. Typically dopants above the electrical solubility limit form an inactive complex which is electrically neutral and do not contribute free carriers to the doped region. An example is discussed below.

Solid solubility data, like those in Figure 7–4, suggest that arsenic might be active up to concentrations of 2×10^{21} cm^{-3}, but in practice it is difficult to actually achieve electrically active arsenic concentrations above 2×10^{20} cm^{-3}. The origin of this discrepancy is of enormous practical interest. It is true that techniques such as laser melting of the silicon can introduce arsenic into silicon in metastable electrically active concentrations near the solubility limit. However, there is an enormous driving force which tends to inactivate the arsenic during any subsequent thermal cycling. Upon annealing, some of the arsenic, while not strictly forming a separate precipitate phase, forms an electrically inactive structure. One such proposed structure, shown in Figure 7–5, which is consistent with the experimental evidence, is that of several arsenic atoms surrounding a vacancy. The arsenic atoms remain on substitutional sites but adjoin a vacancy which leaves the arsenic threefold coordinated with the silicon lattice while retaining two electrons in a dangling bond for a full shell of eight electrons. Thus the As atoms are not electrically active in this form and do not contribute free electrons to the crystal.

7.2.2 Diffusion from a Macroscopic Viewpoint

Diffusion can be discussed from either a macroscopic or a microscopic viewpoint. The macroscopic viewpoint considers the overall motion of a dopant profile and predicts the amount of motion by solving a diffusion equation subject to some boundary conditions. This is a very useful approach for the practical problem of designing dopant profiles in devices. Diffusion can also be examined by considering the motion of the dopant on an atomic scale, where an attempt is made to relate the overall motion of the whole profile to the individual motions of unseen atoms based on interactions of atoms and point defects in the lattice. This second approach is needed to explain the complex behavior exhibited by dopants diffusing in modern devices and forms the physical basis for the models used in today's simulation tools. From a historical perspective, there is a lot to be gained by looking at the overall macroscopic diffusion process first, because analytical solutions are available for some simple cases.

The assumptions made in this section were first used by Fick to describe the diffusion process. It is a tribute to the power of the approach that even today the most sophisticated diffusion models can trace their origins to an intelligent application of Fick's laws. Fick's first law relates the diffusion of dopant atoms to the concentration gradient. If we consider a block of material in which the concentration varies in different places, as

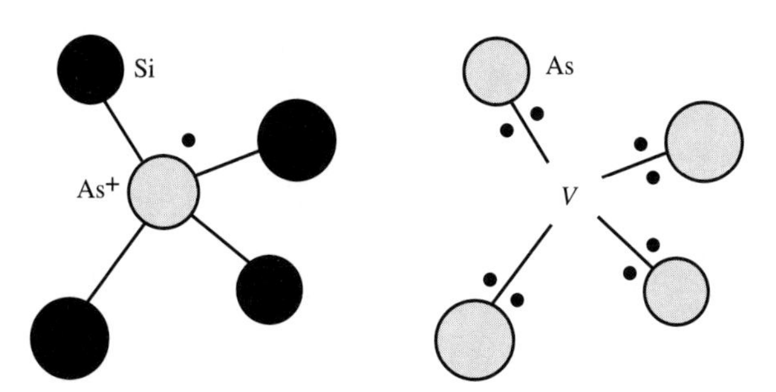

Figure 7–5 Three-dimensional representation of arsenic in a substitutional position versus four arsenic atoms around a vacancy in an inactive configuration.

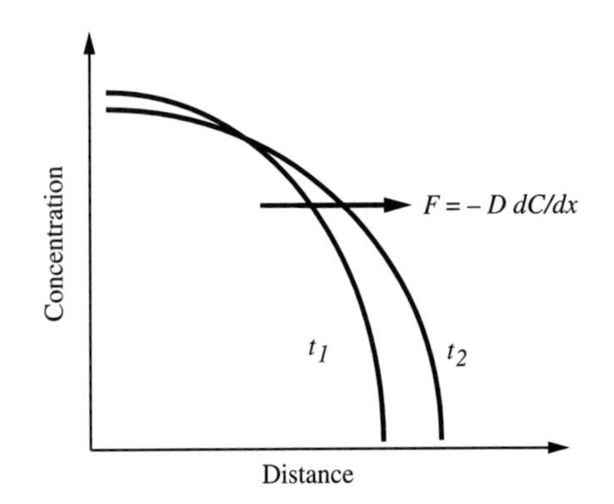

Figure 7–6 Fick's first law states that diffusion is driven by the concentration gradient.

shown in Figure 7–6, this law says there will be a flow of material because of these concentration variations, and postulates that the flow is proportional to the concentration gradient. The proportionality constant is the diffusivity. In essence, this law says that the amount of flow is proportional to the effect causing the flow. Intuitively, this seems to make sense. When the concentration gradient goes to zero and everything is homogeneously distributed, the flow goes to zero. Fick's first law is mathematically described by the equation

$$F = -D\frac{\partial C}{\partial x} \tag{7.6}$$

where F is the flux (atoms cm^{-2} sec^{-1}), D is the diffusivity (cm^2 sec^{-1}) and $\partial C/\partial x$ is the concentration gradient.

In a diamond lattice (Si, GaAs) which has cubic symmetry, D has the same value in all directions. The first law is similar to Fourier's law of heat flow which we used in Chapter 3, which states that the flow of heat is proportional to the temperature gradient, or to Ohm's law, which relates the current to the potential gradient. The negative sign indicates that the flow is down the concentration gradient.

A more useful practical description of the concentration profile is given by Fick's second law, which relates the concentration to both time and space variables. It is obtained by examining the flux in and out of a volume element, as shown in Figure 7–7. Fick's second law is a fundamental conservation law for matter, which says that the increase in concentration in a cross section of unit area with time is simply the difference between the flux into the volume and the flux out of the volume.

$$\frac{\Delta C}{\Delta t} = \frac{\Delta F}{\Delta x} = \frac{F_{in} - F_{out}}{\Delta x} \tag{7.7}$$

In other words, "what goes in and does not go out, stays there" [7.4]. Fick's first law is valid at any instant, even if the concentration and concentration gradient are changing with time. Therefore, substituting from Eq. (7.6) and taking the limit gives

$$\frac{\partial C}{\partial t} = \frac{\partial}{\partial x}\left(D\frac{\partial C}{\partial x}\right) \tag{7.8}$$

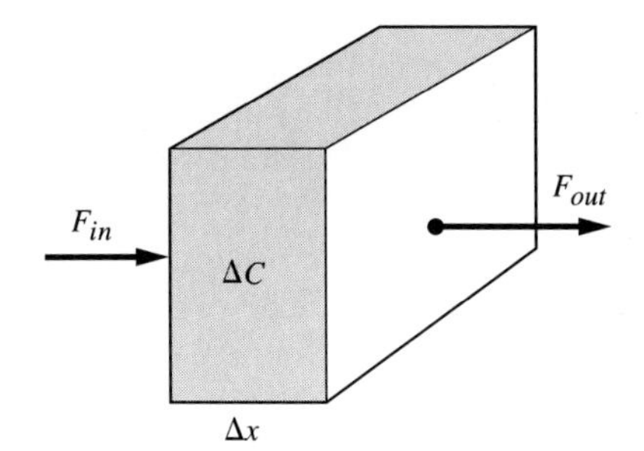

Figure 7–7 Flux in and out of a volume element, used to derive Fick's second law.

If D is a constant (at a particular temperature, perhaps), then the diffusivity can be taken outside the differential to give

$$\frac{\partial C}{\partial t} = D\frac{\partial^2 C}{\partial x^2} \tag{7.9}$$

The three-dimensional generalization of this equation is

$$\frac{\partial C}{\partial t} = -\nabla \cdot F = \nabla \cdot (D\nabla C) \tag{7.10}$$

This is often referred to as Fick's second law of diffusion. It states that the divergence of the flux F gives the rate at which the concentration in a unit volume is being depleted. The flux of material in turn is proportional to the gradient of the concentration, where the proportionality constant is the diffusivity D.

7.2.3 Analytic Solutions of the Diffusion Equation

The simplest solution of the diffusion equation occurs when a steady-state condition applies and there is no variation in the concentration with time. Then,

$$D\frac{\partial^2 C}{\partial x^2} = 0 \tag{7.11}$$

Integrating twice gives,

$$C = a + bx \tag{7.12}$$

This steady-state solution gives a linear concentration profile over distance. This solution was of particular interest when we solved the diffusion equation for the oxidant in the oxide during the oxidation of silicon. (Note the linear oxidant profiles in Figure 6–16.)

There are two other particular analytic solutions of Fick's second law that are of interest to diffusion problems in silicon technology. These arise from differences in boundary conditions.

7.2.4 Gaussian Solution in an Infinite Medium

Consider first the case where we introduce a spike or delta function of dopant in the middle of a lightly doped region as illustrated in Fig 7.8. To build such a structure, we could perhaps use a low-temperature epitaxial growth of single-crystal silicon on a silicon wafer and introduce dopant gas into the growth ambient for a very short time. Or, we might implant a very narrow peak of dopant at a particular depth, which approximates a delta function. Taking the origin to be at the delta function, the boundary conditions are

$$\begin{aligned} C \to 0 \quad \text{as} \quad t \to 0 \quad \text{for} \quad x > 0 \\ C \to \infty \quad \text{as} \quad t \to 0 \quad \text{for} \quad x = 0 \end{aligned} \tag{7.13}$$

and

$$\int_{-\infty}^{\infty} C(x,t)dx = Q \tag{7.14}$$

where Q is the total quantity or dose of dopant which is contained in the spike. The key here is that the initial profile can be approximated as a delta function and that a fixed, constant dose is introduced and remains at all times. The solution of Fick's second law that satisfies these boundary conditions is

$$C(x,t) = \frac{Q}{2\sqrt{\pi Dt}}\exp\left(-\frac{x^2}{4Dt}\right) = C(0,t)\exp\left(-\frac{x^2}{4Dt}\right) \tag{7.15}$$

which is provable by differentiation to be a solution which also satisfies the boundary conditions. This equation describes a Gaussian profile, which evolves with time and retains the same Gaussian form. It is clearly symmetrical about the origin, so that the profile is mirrored about a plane at $x = 0$.

There are several immediate consequences of the solution. The peak concentration decreases as $1/\sqrt{t}$ and is given by $C(0,t)$. When the distance from the origin $x = 2\sqrt{Dt}$ the surface concentration has fallen by $1/e$, which is easily seen by substituting $x = 2\sqrt{Dt}$ in Eq. (7.15). An approximate measure of how far the dopant has diffused is thus

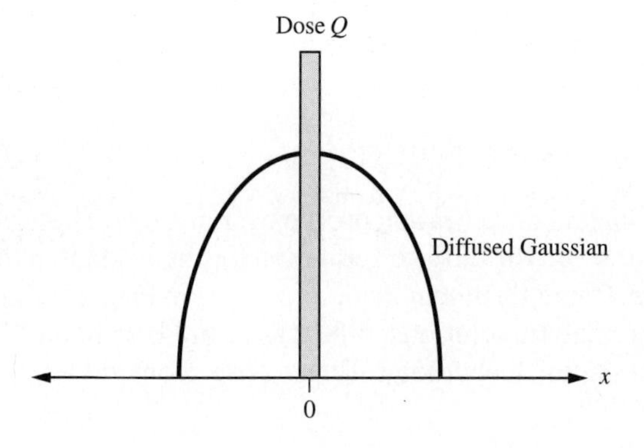

Figure 7–8 A delta function of dopant containing a dose Q is introduced into an infinite medium and subsequently diffused.

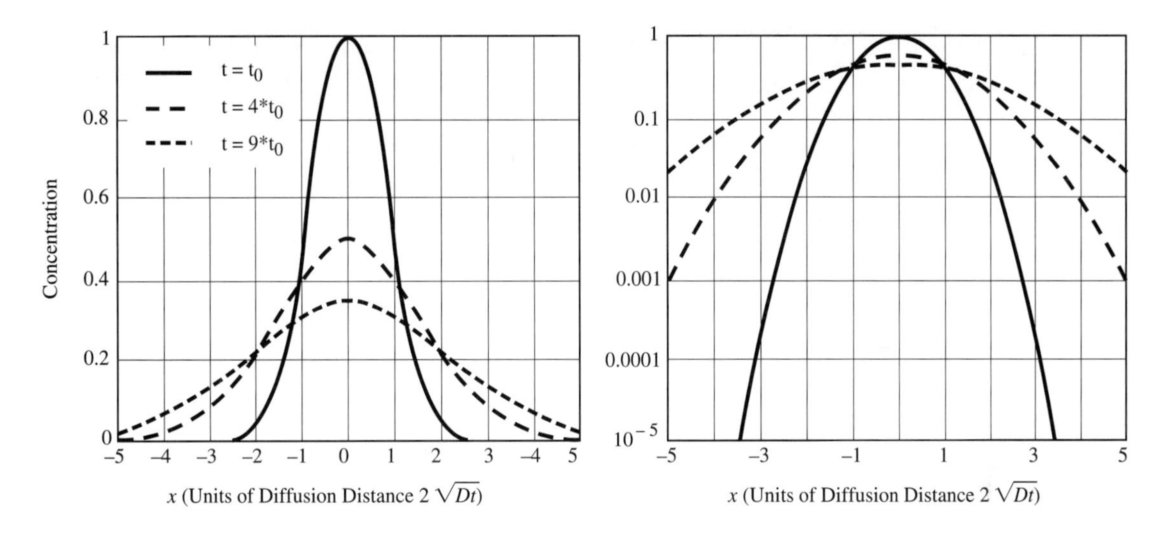

Figure 7–9 Time evolution of a Gaussian diffusion profile.

given by $x = 2\sqrt{Dt}$. This factor is such a convenient measure of the extent of the profile motion that it is often termed the diffusion length. The time evolution of a Gaussian profile is plotted in Figure 7–9 on both linear and logarithmic scales. Note that a Gaussian solution remains Gaussian when more diffusion time is added. Thus, the effect of successive Dt cycles on a Gaussian profile can be easily calculated. Since ion implanted profiles are, to first order, Gaussian profiles, Eq. (7.15) can often be used to make approximate predictions of the evolution of these profiles during subsequent heat cycles.

7.2.5 Gaussian Solution near a Surface

The symmetry represented by Figure 7–8 and Eq. (7.15) allows another very useful solution of Fick's diffusion equation to be easily derived when one considers a dopant dose Q that is introduced near a surface as shown in Figure 7–10. In practice this might be done by low-energy ion implantation. One assumption is that no dopant is lost through evaporation or segregation during the anneal, so the dopant dose is again fixed and constant.

As Figure 7–10 makes clear, a surface at $x = 0$ can be treated as a reflecting or mirror boundary condition, so that effectively a dose of $2Q$ is introduced into a (virtual) infinite medium, giving the following solution for diffusion of a dopant near a surface:

$$C(x,t) = \frac{Q}{\sqrt{\pi Dt}}\exp\left(-\frac{x^2}{4Dt}\right) = C(0,t)\exp\left(-\frac{x^2}{4Dt}\right) \tag{7.16}$$

The surface concentration is given by

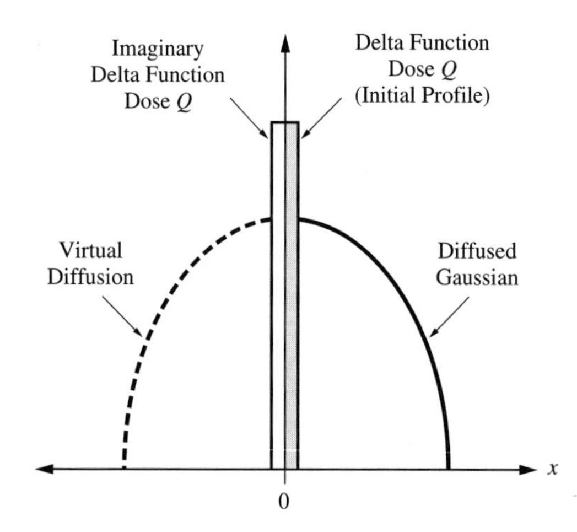

Figure 7–10 A surface Gaussian diffusion can be treated as a Gaussian diffusion with dose $2Q$ in an infinite bulk medium.

$$C(0,t) = \frac{Q}{\sqrt{\pi D t}} \tag{7.17}$$

and falls with time. These surface boundary conditions may be unrealistic in practice because there is generally segregation into a deposited or growing oxide layer or evaporation into the ambient, requiring the use of numerical simulation to accurately characterize the profile. However, Eq. (7.16) represents a useful analytical solution when a dose Q is introduced "near" the surface (generally by ion implantation) and annealed for long enough that the initial distribution is reasonably approximated by a delta function, that is, the spatial extent of the initial profile is much less than $x = 2\sqrt{Dt}$.

7.2.6 Error-Function Solution in an Infinite Medium

The other solution that is useful in silicon processing is the case where we consider the diffusion from an infinite source of dopant. This might correspond to putting a heavily doped epitaxial layer on a lightly doped wafer as in Figure 7–11. The question is: How far does the dopant from the heavily doped region diffuse into the lightly doped region? In this case, the boundary conditions are

$$\begin{aligned} C &= 0 \quad \text{at} \quad t = 0 \quad \text{for} \quad x > 0 \\ C &= C \quad \text{at} \quad t = 0 \quad \text{for} \quad x < 0 \end{aligned} \tag{7.18}$$

It is instructive to consider that the problem is made up by a sum of the previous Gaussian solutions. Consider a series of slices, each of width Δx and of unit cross section, as shown in Figure 7–11.

Each slice initially contains a dose of $C\Delta x$ dopant atoms, which in the absence of the rest of the structure is exactly analogous to the previous condition and would diffuse according to Eq. (7.15). To obtain the solution for the present case, we can make use of a simple linear superposition of solutions for each of the thin slices to give

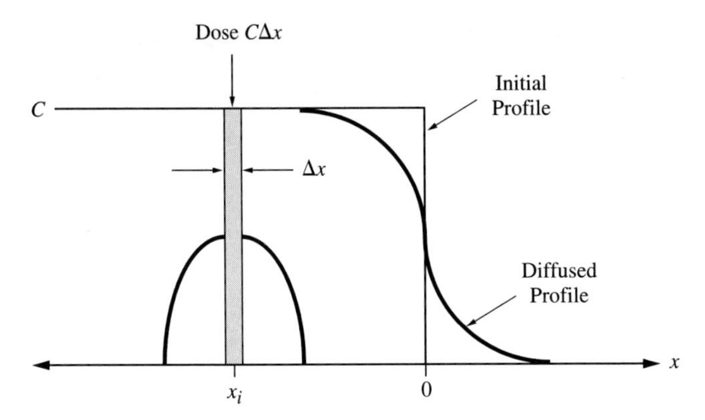

Figure 7–11 An infinite source of material in the half-plane can be considered to be made up of a sum of Gaussians. The diffused solution is also given by a sum of Gaussians, known as the error-function solution.

$$C(x,t) = \frac{C}{2\sqrt{\pi Dt}} \sum_{i=1}^{n} \Delta x_i \exp - \frac{(x - x_i)^2}{4Dt} \tag{7.19}$$

In the limit of thin slices, the sum becomes an integral and the solution is

$$C(x,t) = \frac{C}{2\sqrt{\pi Dt}} \int_{-\infty}^{0} \exp - \frac{(x - d)^2}{4Dt} d \tag{7.20}$$

Letting

$$\frac{(x - \alpha)}{2\sqrt{Dt}} = \eta \tag{7.21}$$

and substituting gives

$$C(x,t) = \frac{C}{\sqrt{\pi}} \int_{x/2\sqrt{Dt}}^{\infty} \exp(-\eta^2) d\eta \tag{7.22}$$

A related integral is tabulated because it is common in the solution of diffusion equations and is not easy to calculate otherwise. This function is called the error function and is defined by

$$\text{erf}(z) = \frac{2}{\sqrt{\pi}} \int_{0}^{z} \exp(-\eta^2) d\eta \tag{7.23}$$

This function is plotted and tabulated in the appendix where some additional properties of the erf are also given. Thus the solution of the diffusion equation from an infinite source becomes

$$C(x,t) = \frac{C}{2} \left[1 - \text{erf}\left(\frac{x}{2\sqrt{Dt}} \right) \right] \tag{7.24}$$

To simplify the notation, the complementary error function can be defined,

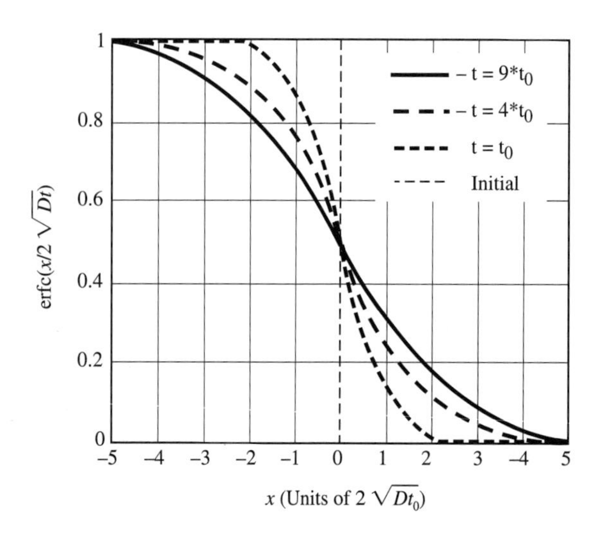

Figure 7–12 Time evolution of erfc diffused profiles. The horizontal axis units are in terms of the diffused distance $2\sqrt{Dt_0}$, a crude measure of how far the profile has diffused.

$$\mathrm{erfc}(x) = 1 - \mathrm{erf}(x) \tag{7.25}$$

so that

$$C(x,t) = \frac{C}{2}\left[\mathrm{erfc}\left(\frac{x}{2\sqrt{Dt}}\right)\right] \tag{7.26}$$

The time evolution of the error-function profile is shown in Figure 7–12.

7.2.7 Error-Function Solution near a Surface

The error function also describes the diffusion kinetics when the profile is characterized by a constant surface concentration at all times. Such a diffusion profile might occur if the diffusion occurred from a gas ambient with a concentration above the solid solubility of the dopant in the solid.

That the error-function type solution is valid for diffusion from a constant surface concentration can easily be seen by a symmetry argument. Because of symmetry, it is clear that the midpoint in Figure 7–12, ($C = C/2$ at $x = 0$) must remain stationary in the solution of the diffusion equation. The solution on either side of $x = 0$ is also equivalent by symmetry. Using this property, if a source concentration is held constant at a value of C_S, we can write

$$C(x,t) = C_S\left[\mathrm{erfc}\,\frac{x}{2\sqrt{Dt}}\right] \tag{7.27}$$

The time evolution of the profile thus looks exactly the same as the $x > 0$ portion of Figure 7–12.

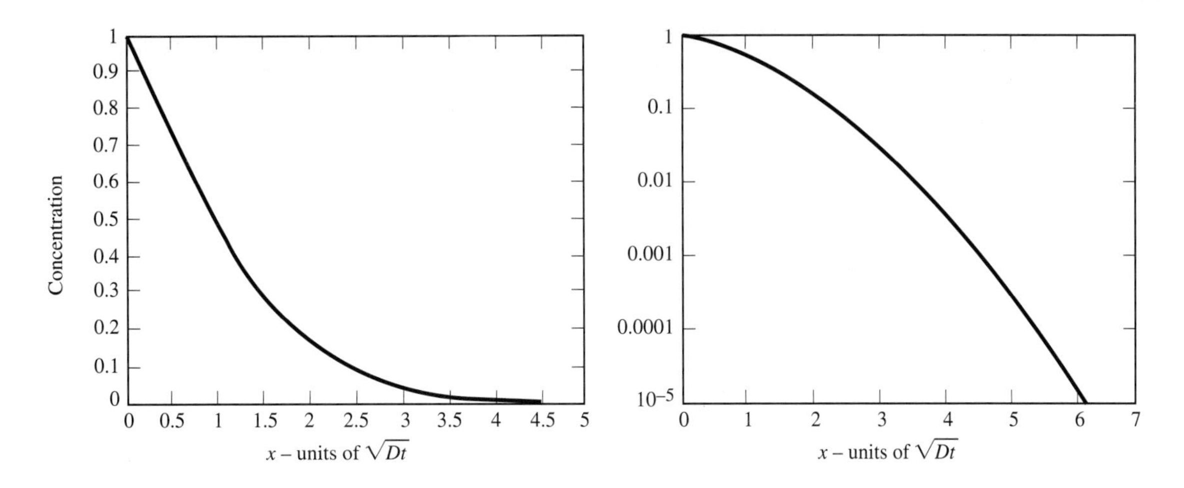

Figure 7–13 Plot of the complementary error-function solution on linear and logarithmic scales.

As seen in Figure 7–13, the error-function solution is (very approximately) triangular on a linear scale, so the dose introduced can be approximated by the area of a triangle of height C_S and a base equal to the diffusion distance $2\sqrt{Dt}$, giving $Q = C_S\sqrt{Dt}$. More accurately,

$$Q = \int_0^{\infty} C_S\left[1 - \operatorname{erf}\left(\frac{x}{2\sqrt{Dt}}\right)\right]dx = \frac{2C_S}{\sqrt{\pi}}\sqrt{Dt} \tag{7.28}$$

The spatial forms of the error-function and the Gaussian solutions are similar when normalized by the same surface concentration, as shown in Figure 7–14. The major difference between these solutions is that the error-function solution applies when there is an infinite supply of dopant, which implies that an increasing dose of dopant is introduced into the substrate during the diffusion process to maintain a constant surface concentration. The Gaussian solution applies when the initial dose of dopant is fixed and, consequently, the surface concentration must drop as the dopant diffuses deeper into the bulk. Thus, while a snapshot at a particular time may show similar profiles, the time evolution of the Gaussian and error-function profiles is vastly different. (Compare Figures 7–9 and 7–12.)

With the exception of the Gaussian and erfc analytical solutions to the diffusion equations, most practical problems in silicon technology today require numerical solutions because the simple boundary conditions required for an analytical solution are not usually satisfied. Modern VLSI structures employ doped regions in which concentration-dependent diffusion, electric field effects, dopant segregation, and complicated point-defect driven diffusion processes take place. All of these effects generally require numerical methods to calculate the resulting dopant profiles. We will return to these issues in Section 7.5 later in the chapter.

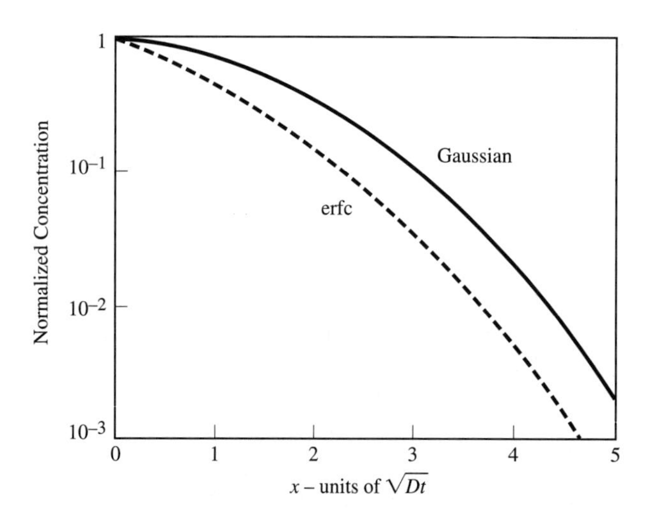

Figure 7–14 The spatial form of the Gaussian and erfc solutions are similar for a particular normalized value of Dt.

7.2.8 Intrinsic Diffusion Coefficients of Dopants in Silicon

The diffusion coefficients of common impurities in silicon are found to depend exponentially on temperature, so they have the form

$$D = D^0 \exp\left(\frac{-E_A}{kT}\right) \tag{7.29}$$

where k is the Boltzmann constant and T is the temperature in degrees Kelvin. The activation energy E_A has units of eV, and is typically 3.5–4.5 eV for impurity diffusion in silicon. We will discuss the physical reasons responsible for this behavior in detail in later sections of this chapter. Plots of the intrinsic diffusion coefficient of common dopants in silicon are shown in Figures 7–15 and 7–16, corresponding to the prefactors and activation energies in Table 7–3. This table represents an Arrhenius fit to the diffusivity under intrinsic conditions. We will update this table later to account for high- concentration diffusion effects in extrinsic regions.

It is important to recall that the intrinsic carrier concentration in silicon is quite high at normal diffusion temperatures (recall Figure 1–16). Thus there are many practical conditions in which dopant diffusion in silicon is described by the data in Figures 7–15 and 7–16. For example, at 1000°C, $n_i = 7.14 \times 10^{18}\ \text{cm}^{-3}$ so that for all N_D and $N_A < n_i$, the material behaves as an intrinsic material. This also means that the analytical solutions given above can be valid if the doping is not extrinsic at the diffusion temperatures. (The analytic solutions, of course, also require specific boundary conditions in order to be valid.)

It is interesting that the dopant diffusivities cluster into groups of "slow" diffusers (As and Sb) and "fast" diffusers (P, B, and In). As junctions have become shallower in recent years, the need for "slow" diffusers has become more important. For N-type regions, this has led to the dominance of As as a dopant because it has both a small D and a high solid solubility. For P-type regions, B is unfortunately the only dopant with a high solid solubility and its higher diffusivity means that fabricating shallow P-type regions is usually

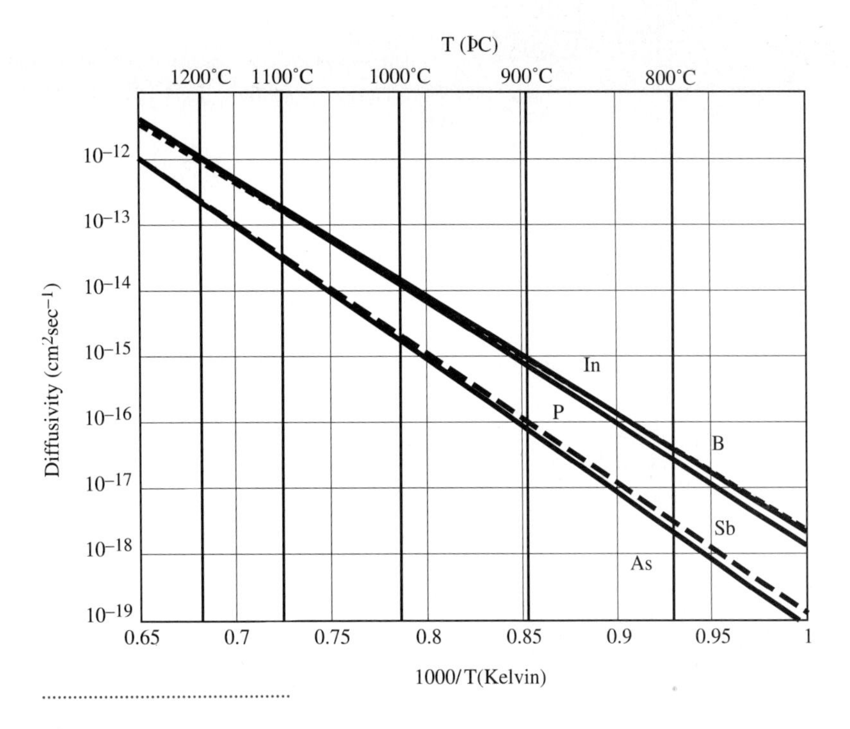

Figure 7–15 Arrhenius plot of the intrinsic diffusivity of the common dopants in silicon.

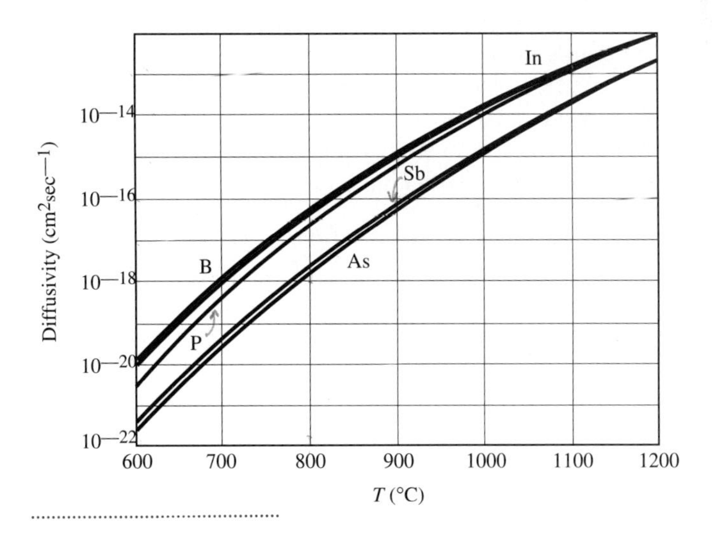

Figure 7–16 Temperature dependence of the intrinsic diffusion coefficient of common dopants in silicon.

Table 7–3 Intrinsic diffusivity in $cm^2 sec^{-1}$ for silicon self-diffusion and of common dopants in single-crystal silicon, fitted to an Arrhenius expression

	Si	B	In	As	Sb	P	Units
D^0	560	1.0	1.2	9.17	4.58	4.70	$cm^2 sec^{-1}$
E_A	4.76	3.5	3.5	3.99	3.88	3.68	eV

more difficult than forming shallow N-type regions. In addition, as we saw earlier in this chapter, modern devices often require both shallow and heavily doped junctions. When dopant concentrations are very large, diffusivities are not well described by the intrinsic values given in this section. Under extrinsic conditions, all dopants show much higher D values than those given here. We will discuss these issues later in the chapter.

7.2.9 Effect of Successive Diffusion Steps

Since there are often multiple diffusion steps in a full IC process, they must be added in some way before the final profile can be predicted. It is clear that if all the diffusion steps occurred at a constant temperature where the diffusivity is the same, then the effective Dt product is given by

$$(Dt)_{\mathrm{eff}} = D_1(t_1 + t_2 + \ldots) = D_1t_1 + D_1t_2 + \ldots \tag{7.30}$$

In other words, doing a single step in a furnace for a total time of $t_1 + t_2$ is the same as doing two separate steps, one for time t_1 and one for time t_2. We often consider the effective Dt product to be a measure of the thermal budget that is used in a process. It is this time-temperature product that occurs in the diffusion equations.

Mathematically, we could increase the time t_2 by a numerical factor (D_2/D_1) and write

$$(Dt)_{eff} = D_1t_1 + D_1t_2\left(\frac{D_2}{D_1}\right) = D_1t_1 + D_2t_2 \tag{7.31}$$

and thus derive a formula for the total effective Dt for a dopant that is diffused at a temperature T_1 with diffusivity D_1 for time t_1 and then diffused at temperature T_2 with diffusivity D_2 for time t_2. Thus, the total effective Dt is given by the sum of all the individual Dt products.

Because the diffusion coefficient is exponentially activated, the highest temperature steps in the process generally dominate the thermal budget (or the effective Dt product). Some of the steps in the process may thus be negligible in determining the overall amount of diffusion.

These concepts also allow us to calculate the equivalent time needed at temperature T_2 to diffuse a profile as far as a time t_1 at a temperature T_1—the time needed is related to the ratio of the diffusivities at each temperature.

$$t_2^{\text{equiv}} = t_1 \times \frac{D_1}{D_2} \tag{7.32}$$

In many cases in real device structures, dopant diffusivities are not constant during a particular process step even if the temperature is constant. In fact, in many cases, D is a function of both time and position. This can result from effects like Transient Enhanced Diffusion (TED) following an ion implantation, from concentration-dependent diffusivities, and from many other effects. In these cases, numerical simulation is the only viable way to calculate accurately the final impurity profile. Equations like (7.31) are only really useful if D is constant over time and position during each process step.

7.2.10 Design and Evaluation of Diffused Layers

The key parameters that are important in designing a diffused layer are the sheet resistance, the surface concentration, and the junction depth. The metallurgical junction is where the chemical concentration in the diffused region equals the chemical concentration of the background doping. This may differ slightly from the electrical junction because of carrier spilling effects, but we will ignore these here. These three parameters are interdependent and any two of them fully define a simple erfc or Gaussian profile. There are useful design curves known as Irvin's curves which have numerically integrated Eq. (7.5) for the sheet resistance of simple Gaussian and erfc profiles and plotted the average conductivity of these layers versus the surface concentration. An example of these curves is shown in Figure 7–17 for p-type Gaussian diffusions. Additional curves are in the appendix.

When designing a process, a key step is to use any available information to decide which (if any) analytic solution to Fick's laws applies. For example, a surface concentration at the solid solubility limit might imply that the profile is likely to be described

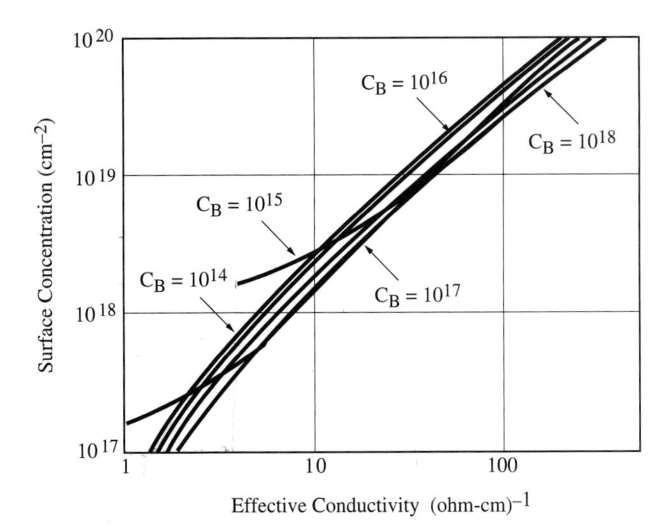

Figure 7–17 Example of Irvin's curves, in this case for P-type Gaussian profiles in an N-type background of concentration C_B. (After [7.5].)

by an error-function-type solution. A low surface concentration might mean that the profile was driven in with a long heat cycle, indicating a Gaussian type solution. It is always important to check these initial assumptions later to verify that the boundary conditions implicit in the solutions of the equations are valid.

Example Design a boron diffusion process (say for the well or tub of a CMOS process), such that $\rho_s = 900\ \Omega$/square, $x_j = 3\ \mu$m, and $C_B = 1 \times 10^{15}\ \text{cm}^{-3}$ (substrate concentration). These specifications might correspond to the P well in Figure 2–10 in the CMOS process we considered in Chapter 2.

Answer The average conductivity of the layer is given by

$$\bar{\sigma} = \frac{1}{\rho_s x_j} = \frac{1}{(900\Omega/\square)(3 \times 10^{-4}\ \text{cm})} = 3.7\ (\Omega \cdot \text{cm})^{-1}$$

We know that $\sigma = nq\mu$, but we cannot calculate n or μ directly because both are functions of depth. Since CMOS N and P wells are moderate concentration profiles, we can initially assume that the P profile is Gaussian. Thus we can use Irvin's curve in Figure 7–17, from which we obtain

$$C_S \approx 4 \times 10^{17}\ \text{cm}^{-3}$$

This surface concentration is well below the solid solubility, so we can surmise that the likely profile is approximately Gaussian and was driven in to a deep junction depth from an initial dose that was introduced into the silicon probably by ion implantation (as in Figure 2–10). Given that the profile is a Gaussian, we can calculate the extent of the thermal anneal (the Dt product) used to diffuse it to the required junction depth, from Eq. (7.16):

$$C_B = \frac{Q}{\sqrt{\pi Dt}} \exp\left(-\frac{x_j^2}{4Dt}\right) = C_S \exp\left(-\frac{x_j^2}{4Dt}\right)$$

so that

$$Dt = \frac{x_j^2}{4\ln\frac{C_S}{C_B}} = \frac{(3 \times 10^{-4})^2}{4\ln\left(\frac{4 \times 10^{17}}{10^{15}}\right)} = 3.7 \times 10^{-9}\text{cm}^2$$

Now that we have the thermal budget for the anneal, we can choose a diffusion temperature (which fixes the diffusivity) and see if the time required at that temperature makes sense, given the constraints of typical manufacturing equipment. If the drive-in is done at 1100°C, then the boron diffusivity from Figure 7–16 is $D = 1.5 \times 10^{-13}\,\text{cm}^2\,\text{sec}^{-1}$.

The drive-in time is therefore

$$t_{\text{drive-in}} = \frac{3.7 \times 10^{-9}\,\text{cm}^2}{1.5 \times 10^{-13}\,\text{cm}^2/\text{sec}} = 6.8 \text{ hours}$$

Thus, to form the deep, low-concentration-boron well requires 6.8 hours at 1100°C. Such long high-temperature steps need to occur early in the process to avoid the effects of this high-thermal budget step on other more sensitive and shallower junction profiles. The well process was in fact performed near the beginning of the CMOS process described in Chapter 2. (See Figure 2–12 and the associated text.)

Given both the surface concentration and the Dt product, the initial dose can be calculated for this Gaussian profile:

$$Q = C(0,t)\sqrt{\pi Dt} = (4 \times 10^{17})(\sqrt{\pi})(\sqrt{3.7 \times 10^{-9}}) = 4.3 \times 10^{13}\,\text{cm}^{-2}$$

This dose could easily be implanted in a narrow layer close to the surface, justifying the implicit assumption in the Gaussian profile that the initial distribution approximates a delta function.

Alternatively, a gas or solid-phase predeposition step might be used to deposit the required dose at the surface. The assumption is made that the dopant is introduced at the solid solubility limit because of manufacturing control issues, and the surface concentration is maintained constant at the solid solubility. We can assume a reasonable temperature like 950°C for the predeposition. We choose a relatively low temperature because of the small dose involved. For boron, the solid solubility at 950°C is $2.5 \times 10^{20}\,\text{cm}^{-3}$ from Figure 7–4 and the diffusivity is $4.2 \times 10^{-15}\,\text{cm}^2\,\text{sec}^{-1}$ from Figure 7–16. The dose for an erfc profile from Eq. (7.28) is

$$Q = \frac{2C_s}{\sqrt{\pi}}\sqrt{Dt}$$

so that the time required for the predeposition is

$$t_{\text{pre-dep}} = \left(\frac{4.3 \times 10^{13}}{2.5 \times 10^{20}}\right)^2 \left(\frac{\sqrt{\pi}}{2}\right)^2 \frac{1}{4.2 \times 10^{-15}} = 5.5 \text{ sec}$$

(Note that the use of this boron diffusivity is really not valid in this example because Figure 7–16 gives intrinsic diffusivities and the boron is certainly not intrinsic if a solid solubility predeposition is being performed.)

We must now check that the delta function approximation is valid for this combination of predeposition step and drive-in, so that our assumption of a final Gaussian profile is reasonable:

$$Dt_{\text{predep}} = 2.3 \times 10^{-14} << Dt_{\text{drive-in}} = 3.7 \times 10^{-9}$$

which is completely adequate in this particular case. In other words, the erfc predeposition profile sufficiently approximates a delta function when compared with the Gaussian drive-in profile.

However, in this particular case, the predeposition time is too short to be "reasonable" in a manufacturing environment. A lower predeposition temperature could be used which would increase t_{predep}. However, an alternative would be to simply use ion implantation to introduce the low dose of dopant required in this process. This is, in fact, what was done in the process flow in Chapter 2 (Figure 2–8). This simple example shows how the analytic solutions of the diffusion equation can be used to design a simple process, provided the underlying assumptions are valid.

7.2.11 Summary of Basic Diffusion Concepts

Fick's first and second laws have formed the basis for understanding and predicting diffusion profiles for many years. However, there are only a few simple analytic solutions to these equations because such solutions require a time- and position-independent dopant diffusivity. These constraints are rarely met in modern VLSI structures. Thus while first-order designs of profiles can be accomplished analytically, accurate design today requires numerical solutions to Fick's equations. We will return to this topic in Section 7.5.

7.3 Manufacturing Methods and Equipment

Diffusion equipment is conceptually very simple—a high-temperature system capable of heating wafers up to temperatures of 800–1100°C is all that is needed. Indeed, the same type of furnace is used for thermal annealing and oxidation processes. These modern furnace systems were described in Chapter 6 (see Figure 6–7). It is clear that simply maintaining the gas flows in an inert ambient such as nitrogen or argon allows an inert anneal to be performed. It is usually important to have some oxide or other capping layer on the wafers to prevent evaporation of the dopant to the atmosphere. If the capping oxide layer is not present or is so thin that pinholes are present, trace amounts of oxygen in the furnace ambient can form SiO, which is volatile at high temperatures, leaving pits on the wafer surface where silicon is removed. Because of these subtle problems, anneals are often performed in a low partial pressure of oxygen sufficient to grow a thin oxide layer on the surface or are performed with a reasonable thickness of oxide present.

Large diffusion furnaces typically idle at a temperature between 750–800°C, at which temperature a batch of wafers are loaded in a cantilevered boat. The wafers stabilize at the loading temperature to ensure repeatable thermal cycles, and then the furnace ramps slowly (5–10°C min^{-1}) to the final anneal temperature which may be as high as 1000–1100°C. There is no inherent problem with using higher anneal temperatures other than potential wafer warpage and accelerated sagging of the furnace tubes. After a diffusion step for a specified time, the wafers are ramped down to the idling temperature and slowly removed from the furnace. These careful ramps and loading steps are designed to ensure that the wafers do not experience any severe thermal shocks, leading to wafer warpage and slip (see the discussion of dislocations in Section 3.2.2). These furnace steps frequently couple oxidation and diffusion steps. During oxide growth, the thermal cycles for growing a certain thickness of oxide also causes dopants to diffuse. Indeed, oxidation can alter the diffusion coefficient of dopants through OED which was discussed in Section 6.5.8.

It is simple to calculate the dopant diffusion at the lower loading and ramp temperatures and show that it is insignificant compared to the highest temperature because of the exponential dependence of the dopant diffusivity on temperature. However, this often turns out to be an overly simplistic analysis because anomalous TED caused by the implantation of dopants can dominate how far the dopant moves. Surprisingly, if the dopants are introduced by ion implantation, they can end up diffusing more (!) at the lower temperatures because the ion-implantation-induced defects last longer at low temperature and continue to enhance the dopant diffusivity. Chapter 8 discusses the ion implantation technique and the anomalous TED that it causes in more detail. Suffice it to say that the effort to reduce the time-temperature (Dt) budget to minimize dopant diffusion in an attempt to get shallower junctions in scaled devices has run into a severe problem. The effort to reduce the anneal temperature in furnaces may simply not work for future generations of devices.

A new generation of fast-ramp, vertical furnaces has been designed to minimize loading and ramp times, using ramp rates of 100°C min^{-1}. However, these have primarily been designed to minimize floor space and particulates in the fabrication facility and to improve the cycle time of the overall furnace operation. It is unlikely that they will be able to reduce the anomalous diffusion effects that are beginning to dominate in shallow junction processing.

As junction depths have decreased in VLSI devices, the thermal cycles required to achieve specified junction depths have also decreased. In fact modern devices often use a thermal cycle simply to electrically activate implanted dopant atoms and process designers would often be very happy if no diffusion took place during this step. For these reasons, Rapid Thermal Annealing (RTA) is becoming a key process in diffusion annealing. RTA has become synonymous with machines which use a bank of lamps that rapidly heat a single wafer resting on sharp pins or on a low-thermal mass holder. Figure 7–18 conceptually illustrates this type of machine. Ramp rates of 100°C sec^{-1} are typical. The heating occurs by optical energy transfer between the radiating lamps and the silicon wafer, so that the transparent walls of the reaction chamber may remain relatively cool during short time processing. This is a very different thermal environment to a furnace, which depends on conductive, convective, and radiative heat transfer from hot resistively heated walls in thermal equilibrium with the wafer. This explains why RTA machines can perform short anneals (seconds) compared with the long stabilization and anneal times required for a typical batch furnace.

Very few RTA machines were used in manufacturing until relatively recently. The major obstacles to acceptance have been concerns about the temperature uniformity and the fact that these are single-wafer machines in contrast to batch furnaces. However, an interesting economic argument may be made in favor of single-wafer RTA—if there is any step in a process that is serial, such a lithography, then throughput will not

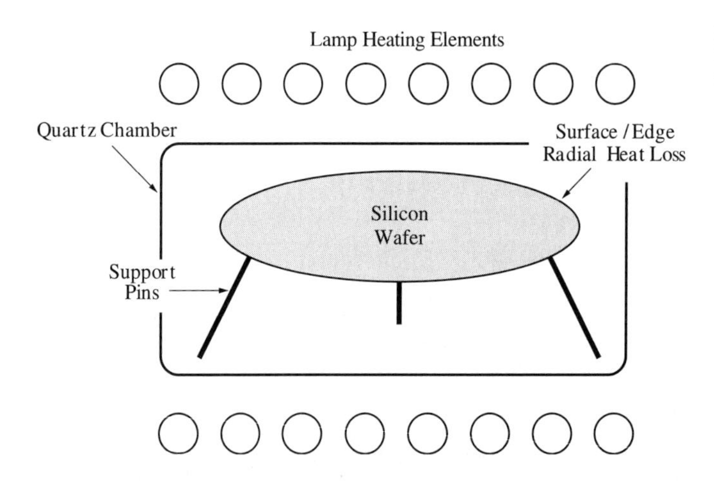

Figure 7–18 Conceptual schematic of an RTA machine.

Table 7–4 Summary of furnace and RTA diffusion and annealing system characteristics

Furnace	RTA
Batch	Single wafer
Long time	Short time
Slow ramp	Fast ramp
Long stabilization	Short steady state
Excellent temperature control	Accurate temperature control difficult

necessarily be further compromised by additional serial steps. Also, 300-mm (12-inch) diameter wafers may simply be too valuable to risk having a complete lot ruined by a single faulty batch operation. Annealing steps that remove damage from implants and require that transient-enhanced diffusion is minimized will likely use RTA to meet the narrow process window available for future device generations. Table 7–4 summarizes the features of furnace and RTA systems for annealing and diffusion processes.

A simple calculation based on the thermal conductivity of silicon shows that a silicon wafer subject to incident radiation will achieve a uniform temperature across and through the wafer in a time of a few milliseconds (see problem 7.18). Thus, heating times in the range of 1–100 seconds can easily be used to anneal implant damage and activate dopants as well as to diffuse these dopants.

It is interesting to consider how the optical energy is absorbed at the surface of a wafer in an RTA system, because that will determine its temperature. Even if there is a perfectly uniform incident radiation flux, the wafer edges will be cooler than the center of the wafer because of radiant heat loss at the edge of the wafer. This radial temperature nonuniformity could be severe enough to cause slip in the wafer. It can be suppressed by surrounding the wafer with a polysilicon slip ring, in effect making the environment around the wafer edge look like silicon. Heat loss at the wafer edges can also be suppressed by using multiple circular zones of lamps with independent power control to each zone, or by designing the chamber reflections so that more of the radiation emitted from the hot wafer is reflected from the chamber walls and back onto the edges of the wafer. The thermal design of a modern RTA machine attempts to balance the primary heat flux and the emitted radiation from the wafer to achieve a steady-state uniform temperature profile.

A number of techniques can be used to monitor the temperature in an RTA environment. Embedded thermocouples in a test wafer can give temperature readings, but the effect of the thermocouple wires acting as cooling fins can introduce large errors in the absolute measurement of the temperature. Thermocouples are generally difficult to use in RTA systems in a manufacturing environment because of maintenance, reliability, and contamination issues.

Many RTA machines use optical pyrometry to measure the wafer temperature. The major problem here is that the emissivity of the wafer can vary depending on the thickness of films on the wafer and can be different for bare and patterned wafers. Once again, the absolute measurement of temperature is difficult.

The problems in patterned wafers are even more severe, because of local differences in the absorption of radiation by different material stacks. The principles are the same here as in optical lithography in which standing waves, reflections, and absorption of the optical energy all play a role. We discussed many of these issues in Chapter 5. There is not much of a problem from local temperature nonuniformity because of the high thermal conductivity of silicon. The more severe effect is on the emissivity variations and the subsequent problems with pyrometer calibration.

In summary, rapid thermal annealing was originally developed for implant annealing because of its potential for simultaneously reducing thermal budgets (short times) while allowing high temperatures for damage removal and dopant activation. One of the critical concerns for manufacturing is temperature uniformity and hence stress control. Partly for this reason, one of the first applications of RTA machines in manufacturing was in silicide annealing, which occurs at the relatively low temperatures of 700–800°C. Here, the issue of slip-induced dislocations due to nonuniform temperature profiles during ramping and steady-state heating is not nearly as severe as for higher-temperature annealing. However, the demand for small thermal budgets and simultaneous activation of dopants will make RTA machines the equipment of choice for manufacturing future generations of devices.

7.4 Measurement Methods

If we consider the cross section of a modern CMOS device, like those considered in Chapter 2, we see that there are several profiles of interest for understanding how the device operates. These might include the channel doping profile, the source drain profile, the well profiles, and the field region profiles. These diffusion profiles can be characterized by measuring the concentration versus depth. These one-dimensional diffusion measurements are useful for calibrating process simulators and form an essential first step in characterizing the process. A number of methods are available to measure dopant profiles, several of which we will consider in this section.

7.4.1 SIMS

The primary doping measurement technique is Secondary Ion Mass Spectrometry (SIMS), as illustrated in Figure 7–19. The basics of this method were outlined in Chapter 4 (see Figure 4–16 and the associated text). SIMS is used to measure the chemical concentration of dopants. It would be useful to be able to directly probe a particular location in a submicron device and obtain a dopant profile. However, this is difficult to do, because SIMS needs to count atoms to obtain a dopant profile and the sensitivity of the technique depends on the statistics obtained. For this reason, special SIMS test areas, which are large squares (200 × 200 μm), are often incorporated in the layout, particularly during process development. This large area is then physically sputtered by an incident ion beam, and the sputtered ions are typically collected from a smaller, central probe area to minimize edge effects on the count statistics. The sputtered atoms which happen to be ionized can be accelerated in an electric field, mass analyzed, and counted. By sputtering away the surface of the sample at a constant rate, a depth profile of the chemical species can be obtained.

Since only a small, random fraction of the sputtered atoms are ionized, the incident ion beam is chosen to produce a high ion yield and a small mass interference due to unintentional ion complexing for the species being examined. In general, the n-type dopants (As, P, Sb) produce a high ion yield when a cesium primary beam is used, while the p-type dopants (B, In) produce a high ion yield when an oxygen primary beam is used. The ion yield at a given sputter rate determines the sensitivity of the technique. Modern SIMS machines are capable of sensitivities in the ppm range, enabling dopant profiling down to concentrations of $10^{16} - 10^{17}$ cm^{-3}.

Cesium is a heavy atom and tends to "knock on" atoms of the species being analyzed, thus degrading the depth resolution for the species. By "knock on" we mean the Cs atoms physically strike and recoil atoms deeper into the substrate. An oxygen primary beam is lighter and minimizes this problem and thus can be used to obtain better depth resolution for a sharp arsenic profile, but at the expense of not being able to profile the full concentration range, that is, a higher background or noise floor.

SIMS is an excellent technique for profiling dopants in a bare silicon area. However as junctions depths have decreased in recent years, the near-surface profile has become of more interest. In ultrashallow depth profiling, a steady-state sputter rate may not be

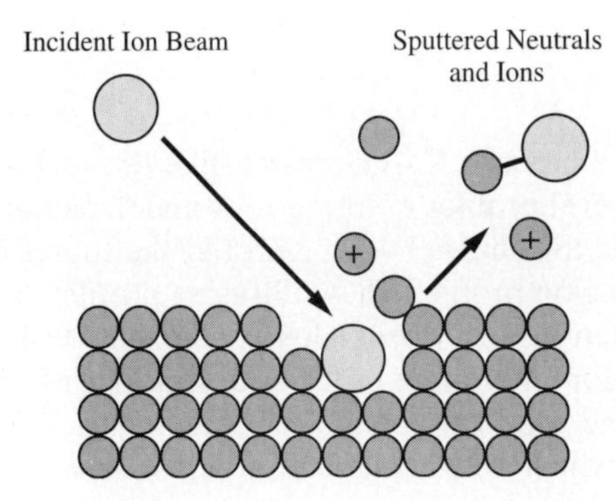

Figure 7–19 Schematic of SIMS process, where an incident ion beam, typically at 1–15 keV, sputters atoms from the surface of a sample. Some of the sputtered atoms are ionized and can be collected and mass analyzed.

reached close to the surface and the SIMS profile may be unreliable in this region. In addition, if an oxygen beam is used, the initial sputter rate may be higher than when the layer being sputtered has become partially oxidized by subsequent incorporation of the oxygen atoms. The use of low-energy primary ion beams with energies from 200 eV to 5 keV can reduce the sputter rates and help to mitigate these problems.

Profiling through multilayer structures still poses many problems for SIMS. Consider the basic MOS structure, consisting of a highly doped polysilicon gate on a thin (< 10 nm) gate oxide above a complex channel profile. Profiling through this structure is difficult because the different materials have inherently different ion yields for the dopant, leading to a "matrix effect." The matrix effect occurs because each different layer in the matrix has its own unique ion yield. In addition, if a cesium primary beam is used, it can lead to "mixing" of layers when trying to sputter through ultrathin layers. The mixing effects can be minimized by using a low sputter ion energy and a shallow angle of incidence.

Ultrashallow or surface SIMS profiles, useful for determining contaminant concentrations of sample surfaces or profiles over the first 50 nm, can be obtained by lowering the primary beam current and energy and optimizing the angle of incidence. Samples can also be measured in the presence of a low-pressure oxygen bleed which gives time for the surface to become saturated with oxygen and thus maintains the ionization yield constant for more accurate quantification in the near-surface region.

Techniques to improve the resolution and sensitivity of SIMS continue to be made. For example, sputtered neutrals make up about 99% of the sputtered atoms. Improved SIMS techniques use a laser tuned to the atom species of interest to deliberately ionize a large fraction of the sputtered neutrals by resonance absorption, generating a large concentration of ionized species which improves the count statistics and the sensitivity. This technique is called sputter neutral mass spectrometry.

7.4.2 Spreading Resistance

Spreading resistance measurements provide an electrical measurement of the active concentration using a pair of fine metal probes to step down the beveled surface of a sample. By measuring the resistivity and comparing it against resistivity standards, the doping concentration can be obtained. The first step in analyzing a sample is to bevel the sample at a shallow angle as illustrated in Figure 7–20. This provides a substantial magnification of the depth scale. The beveling is done by gluing a small sample to a precision-machined holder with typical bevel angles between $8'$ and $34'$. The sample is then polished using a diamond slurry and a rotating wheel. The metal probes are then stepped down the beveled surface in increments of a 2–10 μm and a resistance measurement is made between the probes at each step. The probe spacing is typically 25 μm and the name spreading resistance derives from the spreading pattern of the current flow between the point contacts on the silicon surface. The raw spreading resistance data are converted to active dopant concentration by comparison with resistivity standards. The bevel angle can easily be measured using a stylus profiler or by optical methods and the corrected depth scale calculated.

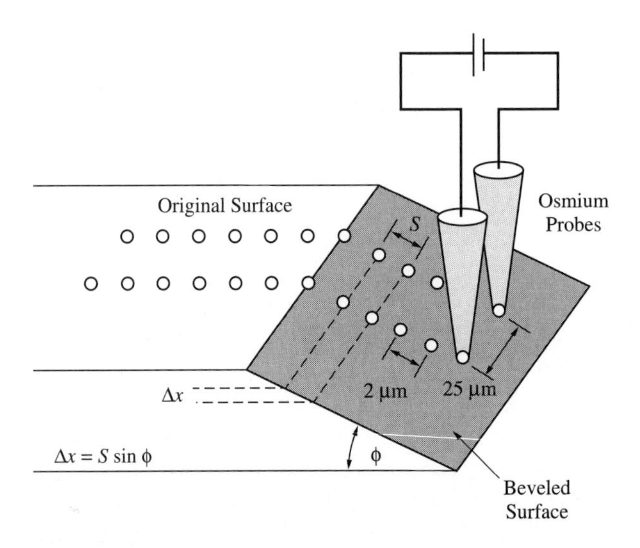

Figure 7–20 Schematic of a spreading resistance measurement, where metal probes step down the surface of a beveled sample and measure the resistance between the probes at each step.

Clearly, it is important that the probes make good electrical contact with the silicon surface yet not penetrate too deeply into the bulk. This imposes conflicting requirements on the condition of the probe tips. The tips of the probes are generally roughened by stepping them on a diamond abrasive paste. If the tip is too smooth, then the microasperities on the tip will not be able to fracture any native oxide layer on the sample and this will provide a poor contact resistance. If the tip is too rough, it penetrates too deeply into the sample and measures the resistance in regions other than directly under the probes. Probe pressure, probe conditioning (an art form), and sample polishing all play a role in obtaining the carrier profile data.

Since SIMS provides a chemical concentration profile, and spreading resistance provides an electrical concentration profile, any difference between these two profiles corresponds to dopants which are not electrically active. Such dopant atoms may be off lattice sites (due to incomplete annealing after ion implantation), or they may be clustered or precipitated, especially at high doping concentrations.

7.4.3 Sheet Resistance

Simple sheet resistance measurements are similar in principle to spreading resistance profiling but provide an integrated electrical conductivity over the whole profile. Typically, four probes contact the surface, the outer two of which force a current with the inner probes measuring a voltage to obtain a resistivity reading. The probes may be stepped over the surface to produce a map of the average conductivity at each location on the wafer. For shallow junctions, the mechanical probes penetrate too deeply into the silicon and other methods of measuring the sheet resistance must be used. A Van der Pauw measurement structure can be patterned lithographically on the wafer and accurate measurements made, even for very shallow junctions. These methods were described in Section 3.4 in Chapter 3. (See Figure 3–12 and the associated text.)

7.4.4 Capacitance Voltage

Capacitance-voltage profiling is particularly useful for lightly doped regions, such as the channel of a MOS device. The MOS structure itself can be used as a capacitor, typically in a large area (100 μm × 100 μm) configuration. By varying the gate and substrate voltages, a family of CV curves is obtained which is characteristic of the doping profile. These one-dimensional MOS CV measurements are remarkably sensitive to the doping concentration profile in the channel region of a device.

The basic CV method was discussed in detail in Chapter 6. From that discussion, recall that a DC voltage is placed on the MOS gate, producing a depletion region in the underlying silicon. A small AC signal is superimposed on the DC voltage to measure the capacitance, essentially by measuring how deep the depletion region is. Since the depletion region depth, x_D, depends on the substrate doping, a measurement of capacitance versus DC voltage can be used to extract the doping profile in the substrate. Commercially available machines and software can perform this kind of measurement automatically.

7.4.5 TEM Cross Section

Several 2D measurement methods have been proposed and are beginning to be used to obtain doping profiles in the cross section of a device. These include TEM, electrical inverse methods, and direct CV or Kelvin probe measurements.

The TEM method was described in Chapter 3 (see Figure 3–15 and the related text). This method can be extended to reveal doping information although the information obtained is largely qualitative today. TEM specimens suitable for imaging dopant profiles can be made by examining a cross-sectional sample where an etch has been used to delineate the doping contours as illustrated in Figure 7–21 [7.6]. Cross-sectional sample preparation for TEM imaging is a time-consuming art form. Specialists in TEM imaging claim that a cross-sectional sample can be produced in a few hours. However, these are not routine procedures. Focused Ion Beam (FIB) milling machines have simplified the preparation of cross-sectional samples at specific locations. A new idea which may simplify the procurement of specimens thin enough for atomic resolution TEM imaging uses a layer of resist to define a thin stripe by e-beam lithography. Anisotropically etching everything surrounding the stripe then leaves a sample standing up above the surface, ready to be imaged [7.7].

Etching mixtures of HF:HNO_3:CH_3COOH (1:40:20) have been used to selectively etch cross-sectional TEM samples to reveal doping information. This is a standard silicon etch, where the nitric acid (HNO_3) oxidizes the silicon and the hydrofluoric acid (HF) dissolves the oxide as it is formed. The acetic acid (CH_3COOH) acts as a dilutant. The etch rate and chemistries for intrinsically doped silicon are well known [7.8]. Etch

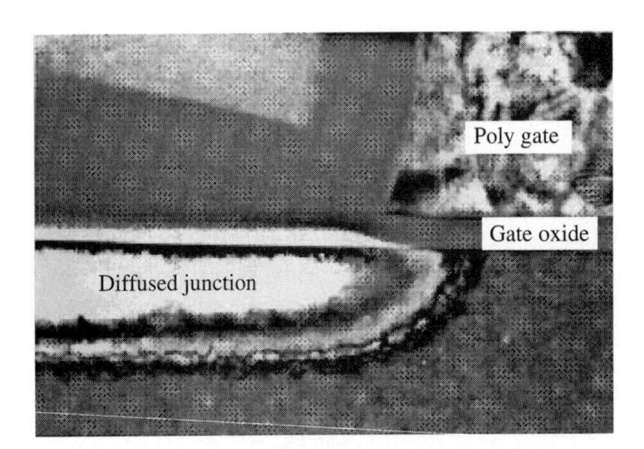

Figure 7–21 TEM image of an etched cross section of the source/drain region of a MOS device at the poly gate edge [7.6]. Reprinted with permission of *J. Vac. Science and Technology*.

rates depend on the doping concentration and appear to be similar for n-type and p-type silicon [7.9]. The TEM images of the sample cross sections show contours corresponding to the thickness of the sample, which are indicative of the doping concentrations. This technique can provide useful qualitative information on the two-dimensional extent of doping profiles. Because it is time consuming and difficult to prepare the samples and the image quality relies on thickness variations, it is not a routine technique.

7.4.6 2D Electrical Measurements Using Scanning Probe Microscopy

All electrical measurements measure carrier concentrations and not the positions of dopant atoms. Dopant atoms are sparsely distributed if a random 3D distribution is assumed. The average distance between randomly distributed dopant atoms depends on the doping concentration and is 1.3 nm at 10^{20} cm^{-3}, 6.2 nm at 10^{18} cm^{-3}, and 28.8 nm at 10^{16} cm^{-3}. However, it is the carrier profiles that determine the device characteristics and due to carrier spilling, these tend to smooth out the discrete, random nature of the underlying donor or acceptor atoms. Because of this, 2D electrical measurements are of enormous interest to device and process engineers.

Scanning probe methods are techniques based on derivatives of the Scanning Tunneling Microscope (STM). Scanning tunneling microscopes have been used to image single-dopant atoms in gallium arsenide cross sections and an example of their patterning capability was shown in Figure 1–3. However, cleaved silicon cross sections are not atomically smooth and reconstruct into low-energy surface configurations where the surface potential is pinned. Scanning tunneling microscopy has not provided useful information on doping profiles in silicon.

However, derivatives of this scanning probe technology show considerable promise for routine imaging of silicon cross sections. In particular, scanning capacitance and scanning resistance probes which are based on atomic force microscopy offer a great deal of potential. The SCM illustrated in Figure 7–22 operates by using laser deflection

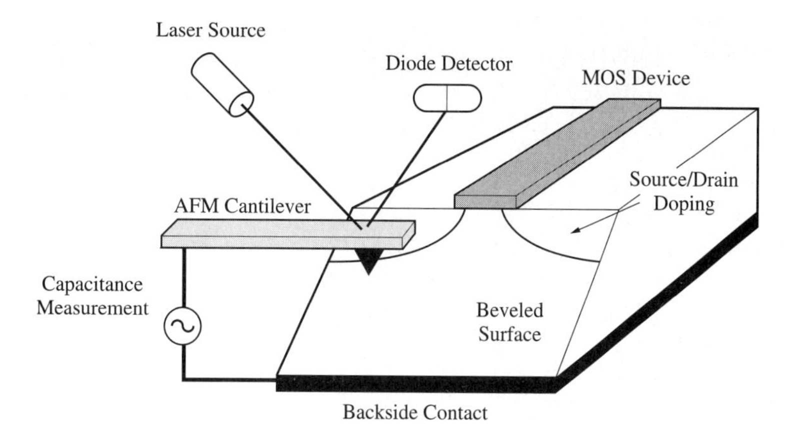

Figure 7–22 Schematic of the scanning capacitance microscope measurement technique. An AFM cantilever is positioned in close proximity to the surface and a capacitance measurement is made.

from a cantilever arm which bends and thus senses when a metal probe is in soft contact with the sample surface. Either a deposited or grown oxide on the beveled surface produces a structure on which MOS CV measurements can be made. The probe tip serves as the "gate electrode" in this case. Once the probe is positioned in contact, a high frequency bias is applied between the tip and the sample and the capacitance is measured, just as in the macroscopic CV method we discussed in Chapter 6. In the SCM, the technique is extended to much smaller areas. The probe is then scanned to adjacent pixels in x and y using a piezoelectric scanner capable of translating the probe with atomic-scale accuracy. The change in capacitance that is measured is a function of the doping level in the pixel. Thus, the SCM image is composed of pixels of varying brightness, where the brightness is related to the doping concentration. The spatial resolution is limited by the probe tip size, fringing fields, and the electrical depletion width at the probe-sample contact.

The problems with the technique are that cross-sectional samples must be prepared at the desired location. The surface of the silicon cross section or the metal probe must then be coated with an oxide layer to form a stable surface and allow for reproducible measurements. Finally, image interpretation is difficult since it involves a deconvolution of doping from capacitance data, and the one-dimensional deconvolution method commonly used for macroscopic MOS capacitors is not valid for many 2D profiles. An example of the current capability of the SCM method is shown in Figure 7–23.

An alternative scanning probe technique is to measure resistance rather than capacitance. The limitations of conventional two-probe SRP can be overcome by using a much smaller probe mounted on an atomic-force microscope cantilever. The use of a hard, conductive tip on an AFM cantilever allows a small point contact to be made on a thin sample cross section. By measuring the resistance between the point contact and a large backside contact, information on the doping concentration can be obtained. This

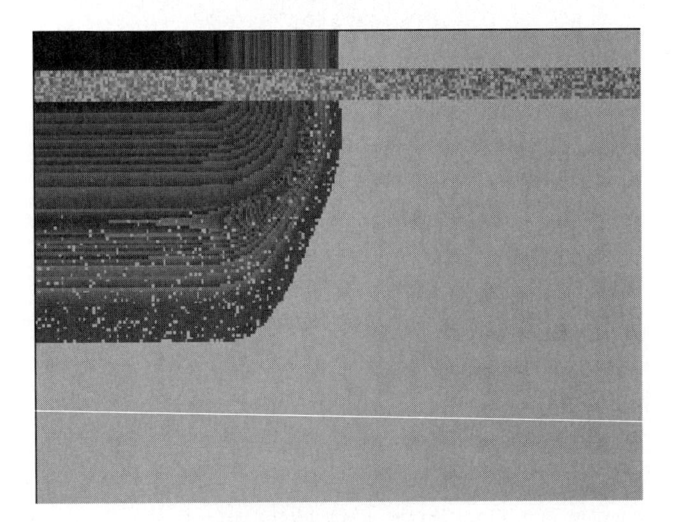

Figure 7–23 Raw scanning capacitance image of a 50keV, 10^{13} cm^{-2} phosphorus implant annealed for 30 seconds at 1050°C. The image is taken near an abrupt mask edge. (Courtesy of Guanyuan Yu, Stanford University).

requires a comparison with a calibration curve from standard samples at similar applied probe pressures. However, if we consider the case of the tip in contact with a low concentration region, it is quite possible that much of the current will flow through an adjacent more highly doped part of the sample that has a lower resistivity path. The deconvolution of the doping profile from the resistivity measurements is thus a three-dimensional problem, very similar to the problem mentioned previously with capacitance measurements.

It is also possible to operate such probes in a mode where the work function is measured. Measuring the potential difference which minimizes the electrostatic force between a probe and the surface of a sample gives an estimate of the work function difference between the sample and the probe. Since the work function difference depends on the doping concentration near the sample surface, this can be used to infer the doping concentration.

7.4.7 Inverse Electrical Measurements

Another broad class of techniques involve trying to infer the doping profiles from electrical measurements. Device IV or CV experimental measurements are made and these are then compared with simulation results based on coupled process and device simulations. Essentially, the assumption is made that the device physics is well understood, and that if there is a problem matching the measured device electrical data, it is the doping profiles in the simulation that are incorrect. This is a reasonable assumption, since the device equations for electrons and holes are well known, whereas the process models for dopant and point-defect interactions are less well understood. If the simulated and measured electrical characteristics do not agree, the doping profiles are varied until they do. However, there are often too many variables to modify in order to get a physically reasonable fit to measured data. Thus, it is important to have a strategy for calibrating the physical models to the electrical measurements in a way that will have some predictive value. A number of recent studies have suggested methods to do this [7.10 – 7.12].

7.5 Models and Simulation

We saw earlier in the chapter that there are only a few useful analytic solutions to the diffusion equation, principally the Gaussian and erfc profiles. Real VLSI device structures require numerical methods in order to describe their dopant profiles accurately. Modern process simulators use such numerical methods, along with sophisticated physical models of the diffusion process. In this section we will focus on such models and use simulation tools to illustrate the effects of various physical models.

Many of the models we will describe in this chapter have been implemented in process simulation programs. We will illustrate the use of these simulation tools as we describe the models. The simulators we will use are based on derivatives of the Stanford University program SUPREM IV [7.13] which has been implemented in commercially available versions like TSUPREM IV [7.14] and ATHENA [7.15]. These programs implement many (but not all) of the models we will discuss. The SUPREM class of programs are 2D simulators which are generally available and fairly widely used in the semiconductor industry. The simulation examples in this chapter were run on commercially available versions of this program.

After briefly discussing some issues associated with the numerical implementation of diffusion models, we will consider a number of modifications to Fick's first and second laws which account for additional physical effects beyond those which can be included in analytic solutions. Recall from our discussion earlier in the chapter that analytic solutions generally require that the dopant diffusivity be constant over space and time during a particular process step. Neither of these is generally true in real VLSI fabrication sequences. We will thus consider modifications to Fick's laws which broaden their applicability and are capable of incorporating better physics.

7.5.1 Numerical Solutions of the Diffusion Equation

It is interesting to think about how to solve the diffusion equation numerically, because the numerical approach will not be restricted to the simple initial and boundary conditions we have examined. For example, the diffusion of an arbitrary initial profile that is non-Gaussian could easily be examined numerically but would have no tractable analytic solution.

Following Crank [7.16], let us consider the physical situation where we have atoms hopping from one plane to another in the crystal as shown in Figure 7–24. If we divide up the crystal into planes Δx apart, labeled 0,1,2 . . . and we have a number of atoms at each plane $N_0, N_1, N_2, \ldots$, that is, the planar density is N_i atoms cm^{-2}. The average volume concentration at any point is then $C_i = N_i \, \Delta x$ cm^{-3}. The atoms remain relatively fixed in the lattice but vibrate about their equilibrium position at the Debye frequency, which is about 10^{13} sec^{-1} in silicon. Sometimes, an atom will be able to surmount the energy barrier keeping it in place and will hop to an adjacent plane if a

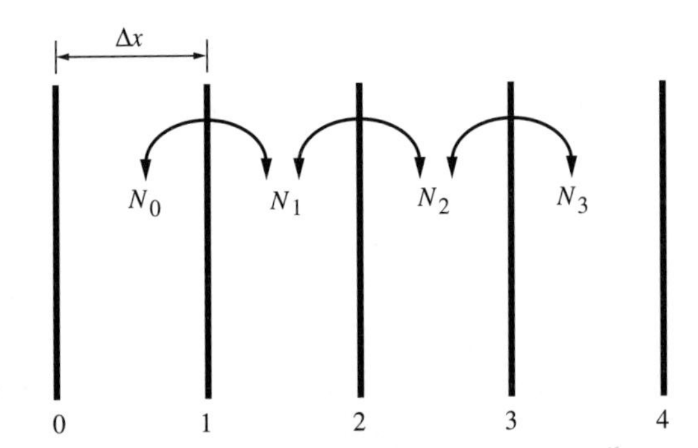

Figure 7–24 Atomic planes Δx apart, with N_i atoms at each plane. Atoms at a plane have an equal probability of jumping left or right.

free site exists (a vacancy) or exchange directly with an adjacent atom. The frequency of hopping is given by

$$\upsilon_b = \upsilon_d \exp\left(-\frac{E_b}{kT}\right) \tag{7.33}$$

where υ_d is the Debye frequency and E_b is the energy barrier. The jump frequency is υ_b. Any given atom will have an equal probability of jumping to the left or to the right so there will be $(\upsilon_b/2)$ atoms jumping right and $(\upsilon_b/2)N$ atoms jumping left per unit time.

The number of atoms crossing the plane with N_2 atoms on one side and N_1 atoms on the other is simply

$$F = -\frac{\upsilon_b}{2}(N_2 - N_1) = -\frac{\upsilon_b}{2}\Delta x(C_2 - C_1) = -\frac{\upsilon_b}{2}\Delta x^2\frac{\Delta C}{\Delta x} = -D\frac{\Delta C}{\Delta x} \tag{7.34}$$

where we have defined

$$D = \frac{\upsilon_b}{2}\Delta x^2 \tag{7.35}$$

This provides some atomic-scale insight into the origins of Fick's first law. It is our first indication that diffusion processes have an origin in atomic-scale jumps of atoms, which we will return to in a later section. It is, at first sight, surprising that independent hops with equal probability of going left or right for each individual atom in a dilute mixture leads to a flow of atoms down the concentration gradient.

Consider for a moment all the atoms hopping to or from plane i only. Atoms at plane $i-1$ can jump to plane i, atoms at plane i can jump to $i-1$ or $i+1$, and atoms at plane $i+1$ can jump back to plane i. Summing all the atom hops at plane i, we have at the end of an interval of time Δt,

$$N_i^+ = N_i + \frac{\upsilon_b}{2}\Delta t(N_{i-1} - 2N_i + N_{i+1}) \tag{7.36}$$

In terms of concentrations, we have

$$C_i^+ = C_i + \frac{\upsilon_b}{2}\Delta t(C_{i-1} - 2C_i + C_{i+1}) \tag{7.37}$$

Making the substitution for diffusivity defined above, we get

$$C_i^+ = C_i + \frac{D\Delta t}{\Delta x^2}(C_{i-1} - 2C_i + C_{i+1}) \tag{7.38}$$

This forms the core of our numerical solution. Given initial concentrations at different places, we can calculate the subsequent concentrations after a small interval of time Δt. We have considerable flexibility in choosing the magnitude of Δt and Δx. These parameters should be chosen such that they are relevant to the problem we are attempting to solve. For example, Δx should be such that the profile is uniformly divided up into a sufficient number of distance intervals that the profile can be fitted in a reasonable manner by these piecewise linear approximations. Similarly, Δt should be chosen so that the time interval is divided into a sufficient number of time steps to resolve the diffusion process. Each iteration of the numerical solution for C_i^+ advances the solution of the diffusion equation at each of the distance intervals Δx by an amount of time Δt.

What are the limits on the values of Δt and Δx that we choose? We can investigate this in a little more detail by considering a simplification of this equation that is mathematically clever if we take

$$\frac{D\Delta t}{\Delta x^2} = \frac{1}{2} \tag{7.39}$$

Then, our numerical solution becomes

$$C_i^+ = \frac{1}{2}(C_{i-1} + C_{i+1}) \tag{7.40}$$

which simply relates the new value at a node to the average of the values at the adjacent nodes. This may be considered a mathematical trick to simplify the equation, but it contains some interesting physics and numerics. For example, if we were to take the increment in the numerical solution in $D\Delta t/\Delta x^2 > 0.5$ in Eq. (7.38), we would find that the solution becomes unstable—oscillations in the values of the concentration increase for each succeeding numeric interval. Thus, $D\Delta t/\Delta x^2 = 0.5$ represents the maximum value of the numeric interval that can be used before the numerical solution becomes unstable. Physically, we can interpret this as meaning that we are asking more than the available number of atoms at a plane to jump within a time Δt.

This very simple derivation allows us to solve the diffusion equations for any arbitrary initial dopant profile. It provides an introduction to the numerical solution of diffusion equations, which takes on a heightened importance when the diffusivity is no longer constant and when the diffusion of one species affects the motion of another. It also provides an introduction to the numerical issues that must be tackled in a process simulator such as SUPREM.

7.5.2 Modifications to Fick's Laws to Account for Electric Field Effects

When the doping concentrations exceed the intrinsic carrier concentration at the diffusion temperature, electric fields set up by the doping atoms can affect the diffusion process. This is an example of an extrinsic effect which is not observed below the intrinsic carrier concentration.

If there is an external force acting on the diffusing species in addition to normal diffusion, then there is an additional flux or flow of species $F' = Cv$, where v is the velocity of the particles in the external force field. The overall flux is then

$$F_{total} = F + F' = -D\frac{\partial C}{\partial x} + Cv \tag{7.41}$$

where the first term on the right is the normal diffusion flux term from Eq. (7.6). If F' and consequently v are independent of x, the application of Fick's second law to the fluxes is straightforward and the change in doping concentration with time is given by

$$\frac{\partial C}{\partial t} = \frac{\partial}{\partial x}\left(D\frac{\partial C}{\partial x}\right) - v\frac{\partial C}{\partial x} \tag{7.42}$$

The most common case that we find in silicon is where the force on the diffusing particles is generated by an internal electric field. The electric field can be generated by the diffusing species itself if the dopant concentrations are high enough. The origin of the field comes from the higher mobility of electrons and holes compared to dopant atoms. Consider the case of an abrupt arsenic profile. Electrons from the donor atoms will tend to diffuse ahead of the profile because they have a very high mobility. This leaves behind positively charged donor arsenic atoms. Thus, an electric field is set up which tends to prevent the electrons from diffusing further and a steady-state condition exists when the electron diffusion flux is balanced by the electron drift flux as shown in Figure 7–25.

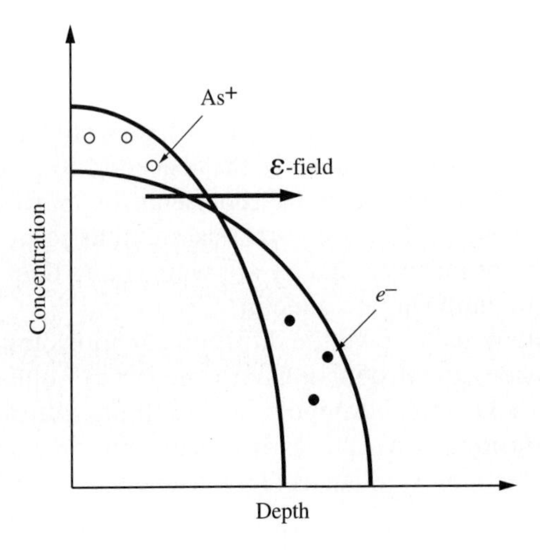

Figure 7–25 Schematic of the electric field. This develops because the electron or hole mobility exceeds the dopant mobility, so that electrons or holes diffuse ahead until they reach a steady-state condition where the drift flux from the internal electric field balances the diffusion flux.

This field continues to act on the charged donor atoms, tending to drag them into the bulk. Thus, the internal electric field tends to enhance the dopant diffusivity through a drift term. The velocity of particles in an electric field is given by

$$v = \mu \mathcal{E} \tag{7.43}$$

where μ is the mobility. The electric field itself is given by the gradient of the potential,

$$\mathcal{E} = \frac{\partial \psi}{\partial x} \tag{7.44}$$

and the potential is given by

$$\psi = -\frac{kT}{q}\ln\frac{n}{n_i} \tag{7.45}$$

Now, there is a relationship between diffusivity and mobility developed by Einstein when he investigated Brownian motion:

$$\mu = \frac{q}{kT}D \tag{7.46}$$

which, together with the above equations, allows us to write an equation for the flux when there is an electric field:

$$F = -D\frac{\partial C}{\partial x} - DC\frac{\partial}{\partial x}\ln\frac{n}{n_i} \tag{7.47}$$

There are two ways to proceed and simplify the form of this equation. One, which is commonly used in process simulation programs, uses the fact that

$$\frac{\partial}{\partial x}\ln x = \frac{1}{x} \tag{7.48}$$

and writes Eq. (7.47) as

$$F = -DC\frac{\partial}{\partial x}\ln\left(C\frac{n}{n_i}\right) \tag{7.49}$$

This is the equation that is solved in process simulators like SUPREM under equilibrium conditions and is useful when multiple dopants contribute to the field term.

A simple analytic estimate of how the electric field increases the apparent dopant diffusivity can be obtained as follows. The flux can be expressed in terms of the dopant concentration only, if charge neutrality and Boltzmann statistics apply. From Chapter 1,

$$N_D^+ + p = N_A^- + n \tag{1.15}$$

$$np = n_i^2 \tag{1.5}$$

If all of the dopant is ionized ($N_D^+ \cong N_D$ and $N_A^- \cong N_A$) the flux can be written as

$$F = -hD\frac{\partial C}{\partial x} \tag{7.50}$$

where C is the net doping concentration at position x ($C = |N_D - N_A|$) and the electric field enhancement factor h, which increases the apparent diffusivity, is given by

$$h \equiv 1 + \frac{C}{\sqrt{C^2 + 4n_i^2}} \tag{7.51}$$

h has an upper bound of 2 which means that this electric field enhancement term can enhance the diffusivity of the dopant causing the field by a maximum factor of two, when the doping concentration term is much greater than the intrinsic electron concentration.

However, in a case where there are species at different concentrations, the field term can cause even bigger changes in the diffusivity of a low-concentration dopant in the vicinity of the field as illustrated in Figure 7–26. While the field can only double the flux of the high-concentration species, the magnitude of this term can completely dominate the diffusion flux of a lower-concentration dopant. This is basically because in the example in Figure 7–26, the high-concentration As profile determines the $\mathcal{E}$ field. But the same field acts on the boron profile which is flat to begin with and hence would not diffuse at all if it were driven only by its own gradient and a constant D. Note in the figure that the direction of the field pulls the B^- atoms into the N^+ region and depletes the boron in the region past the junction.

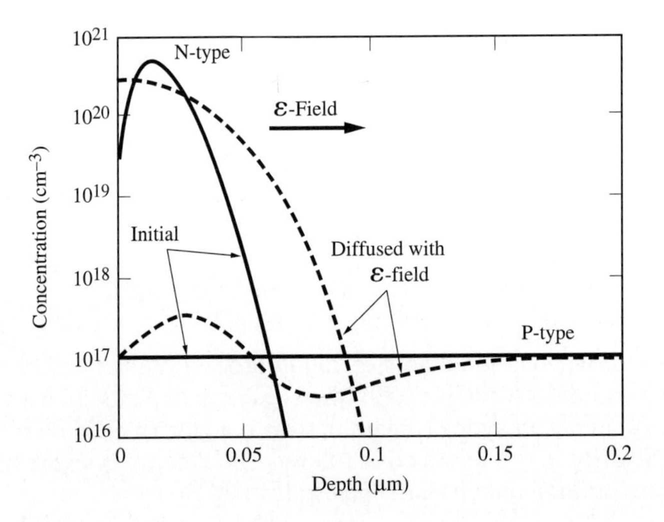

Figure 7–26 Simulation of the $\mathcal{E}$-field effect using TSUPREM IV [7.14] at 1000°C. The electric field causes the diffusion of the low-concentration boron to be drastically affected in the vicinity of the junction.

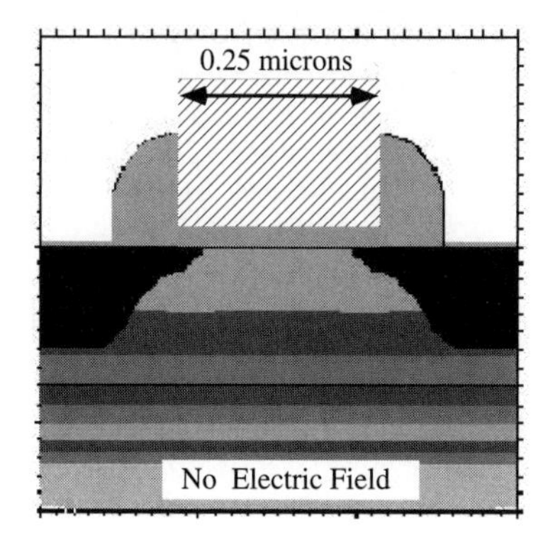

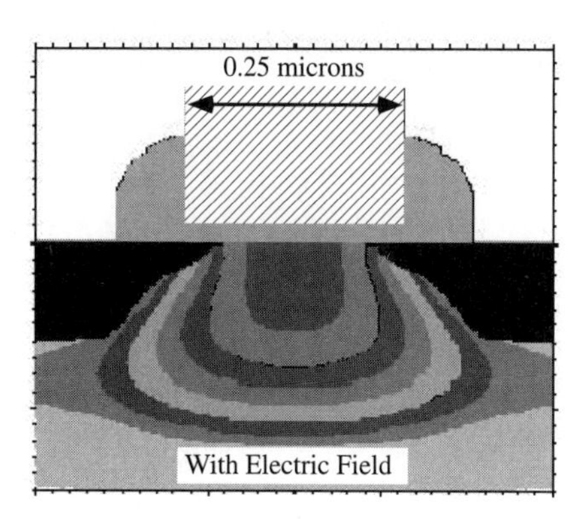

Figure 7–27 NMOS process simulation using TSUPREM IV [7.14]. The boron channel doping profiles are diffused without any electric field on the left. Including the electric-field effect from the highly doped arsenic source/drain and extension on the right gives rise to a field-aided flux which dramatically alters the boron profile in the channel. This effect is particularly severe in a short channel device.

Figure 7–27 illustrates a SUPREM simulation of $\mathcal{E}$-field effects in a real device. The structure here is an NMOS transistor, similar to that considered in the CMOS process in Chapter 2. In the left simulation, the implanted boron channel region is diffused without field effects being considered. Laterally uniform boron profiles result. On the right side, the As N^+ source and drain regions' $\mathcal{E}$-field effects are added. A high-temperature diffusion now results in significant changes in the boron profile, similar to those illustrated in one dimension in Figure 7–26. Note in the simulation the dramatic loss of boron from the channel region into the device N^+ regions. Obviously this effect could have a significant impact on the device electrical characteristics.

7.5.3 Modifications to Fick's Laws to Account for Concentration-Dependent Diffusion

When the doping concentration exceeds the intrinsic electron concentration at the diffusion temperature, another extrinsic diffusion effect in addition to electric field effects is seen. Fick's first law is really based on the premise that the flux or flow is directly proportional to the concentration gradient. However, if we examine the actual concentration profile of many diffused dopants, we find that the diffusion profile is boxlike—that is, the diffusion appears to be faster in the higher-concentration regions. An example is shown in Figure 7–28. Here an experimental constant surface concentration, low-concentration ($C_S = 10^{18}\ \text{cm}^{-3}$) diffusion is fit quite well with a simple erfc profile (constant D). The higher concentration constant surface concentration profile ($C_S = 10^{20}\ \text{cm}^{-3}$) is often not well modeled by a simple erfc profile with constant D. The reason for this discrepancy is that the diffusivity varies with concentration, with the higher-concentration regions diffusing faster and smoothing the concentration gradient. This observation represents a major revision of the original intent of Fick's laws, where the flux depended only on the concentration gradient, not the absolute

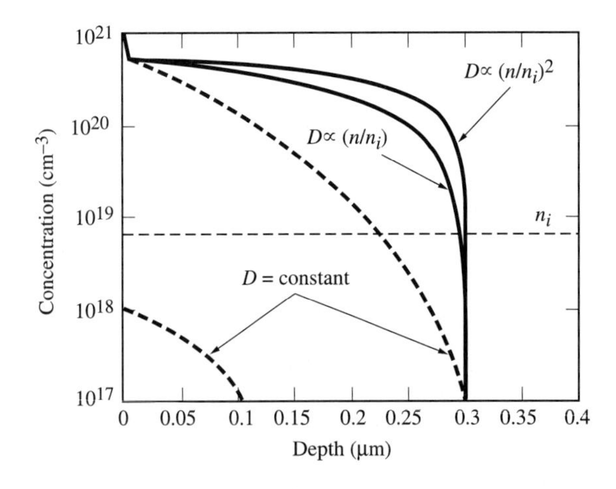

Figure 7–28 Simple erfc profiles (symbols) of constant surface concentration boron diffusions with C_S values of 10^{18} and 5×10^{20} cm^{-3}. The dashed lines show the erfc profiles. The solid lines are numerical simulations of the 5×10^{20} cm^{-3} example using TSUPREM IV [7.14] which agree with experimental results.

value of the concentration. All of the common dopants in silicon exhibit this behavior and tend to have more box-shaped profiles than would be expected from simple error-function or Gaussian solutions.

If we define the diffusivity as being a function of concentration, then Fick's formulation with nonconstant D still represents a very useful way of describing dopant diffusion in silicon. The modified form of Fick's law where the diffusivity is a function of concentration cannot usually be integrated directly, so that the solution of the equation

$$\frac{\partial C}{\partial t} = \frac{\partial}{\partial x}\left(D_A^{\text{eff}} \frac{\partial C}{\partial x}\right) \tag{7.52}$$

must be computed numerically. Experimentally, it often appears that the profile can be well modeled by assuming that the diffusivity is directly proportional to the free carrier profile as illustrated in Figure 7–28 where $D \propto (n/n_i)$ or $D \propto (n/n_i)^2$. The box-shaped profiles characteristic of concentration dependent diffusion are evident.

Information on the concentration dependence of the diffusivity can be obtained from isoconcentration experiments, which we now describe. Boron is a particularly interesting element on which to perform isoconcentration experiments, because there are two common isotopes B^{10} and B^{11}. If a high-concentration background doping is set by one isotope, and a profile of the other isotope is introduced into the background, the diffusivity of the tracer can be measured as a function of the background concentration. This is a particularly nice experiment, because it is all boron diffusion, albeit different isotopes. Any complications that might occur due to dopant-dopant interactions are removed. SIMS is a particularly convenient analysis tool because its mass sensitivity allows a B^{10} profile to be measured inside a uniform B^{11} background, for example. This kind of experiment gives the diffusivity of boron as a function of concentration.

Based on many results like these, the diffusivity of the common dopants in silicon has been characterized and found to depend linearly or sometimes quadratically on the carrier concentration as shown in Figure 7–28. The effective diffusivity to be used in Eq. (7.52) can be written as

$$D_A^{\text{eff}} = D^O + D^-\left(\frac{n}{n_i}\right) + D^=\left(\frac{n}{n_i}\right)^2 \quad \text{for Ntype dopants} \tag{7.53}$$

$$D_A^{\text{eff}} = D^O + D^+\left(\frac{p}{n_i}\right) + D^{++}\left(\frac{p}{n_i}\right)^2 \quad \text{for Ptype dopants} \tag{7.54}$$

The superscripts D^O, D^+, and so forth, are chosen, because on an atomic level, these different terms are thought to occur because of interactions with neutral and charged point defects.

The diffusivity under intrinsic conditions for an n-type dopant (when $p = n = n_i$) is

$$D_A^* = D^O + D^- + D^= \tag{7.55}$$

Each of these individual diffusivities can be written in Arrhenius form

$$D = D.0 \exp\left(-\frac{D.E}{kT}\right) \tag{7.56}$$

with a preexponential factor and an activation energy.

By rewriting the above equations, the diffusion coefficient measured under extrinsic conditions can be elegantly described as

$$D_A^{\text{eff}} = D_A^*\left(\frac{1 + \beta\frac{n}{n_i} + \gamma\left(\frac{n}{n_i}\right)^2}{1 + \beta + \gamma}\right) \tag{7.57}$$

where $\beta = D^-/D^O$ and $\gamma = D^=/D^O$. Expressed in this manner, the β factor represents the linear variation in the diffusion coefficient in highly doped material and the γ factor represents a square law variation in the diffusion coefficient in highly doped material. For P-type dopants, n would be replaced by p in this equation. A set of reasonable values for these parameters as defined in Eqs. (7.53), (7.54) and (7.56) is shown in Table 7–5.

Table 7–5 Concentration-dependent diffusivities of common dopants in single-crystal silicon. D.0 values in cm^2 sec^{-1}, D.E values in eV.

	Si	B	In	As	Sb	P
$D^0.0$	560	0.05	0.6	0.011	0.214	3.85
$D^0.E$	4.76	3.5	3.5	3.44	3.65	3.66
$D^+.0$		0.95	0.6			
$D^+.E$		3.5	3.5			
$D^-.0$				31.0	15.0	4.44
$D^-.E$				4.15	4.08	4.0
$D^=.0$						44.2
$D^=.E$						4.37

Example Calculate the effective diffusion coefficient at 1000°C for two different box-shaped arsenic profiles grown by silicon epitaxy, one doped at 1×10^{18} cm^{-3} and the other doped at 1×10^{20} cm^{-3}.

Answer At 1000°C, the intrinsic electron and hole concentrations are 7.14×10^{18} cm^{-3}, so for dopant concentrations less than this the profile appears intrinsic.

For the 1×10^{18} cm^{-3} profile:

$$D_{As} = 0.011 \exp\left(-\frac{3.44}{k(1000+273)}\right) + 31.0 \exp\left(-\frac{4.15}{k(1000+273)}\right)$$

$$= 2.67 \times 10^{-16} + 1.17 \times 10^{-15}$$

$$= 1.43 \times 10^{-15} \text{ cm}^2 \text{ sec}^{-1}$$

The value calculated from the Arrhenius fit in Table 7–3, which was obtained by fitting a single activation energy to the two activation energies above under intrinsic conditions, is

$$D_{As} = 9.17 \exp\left(-\frac{3.99}{k(1000+273)}\right)$$

$$= 1.48 \times 10^{-15} \text{ cm}^2 \text{ sec}^{-1}$$

For the 1×10^{20} cm^{-3} profile:

$$D_{As} = 0.011 \exp\left(-\frac{3.44}{k(1000+273)}\right) + 31.0 \exp\left(-\frac{4.15}{k(1000+273)}\right)\left(\frac{1 \times 10^{20}}{7.14 \times 10^{18}}\right)$$

$$= 2.67 \times 10^{-16} + 1.63 \times 10^{-14}$$

$$= 1.66 \times 10^{-14} \text{ cm}^2 \text{ sec}^{-1}$$

Note that the highly doped layer has a ten-fold higher diffusion coefficient in the extrinsic material.

Simulators like SUPREM implement Eqs. (7.49) and (7.52) in a straightforward manner and are thus capable of modeling complex profiles. An example is shown in Figure 7–29. In this example, a bipolar transistor structure is simulated. A boron dose Q approximating a delta function of doping is introduced into the wafer to form the initial

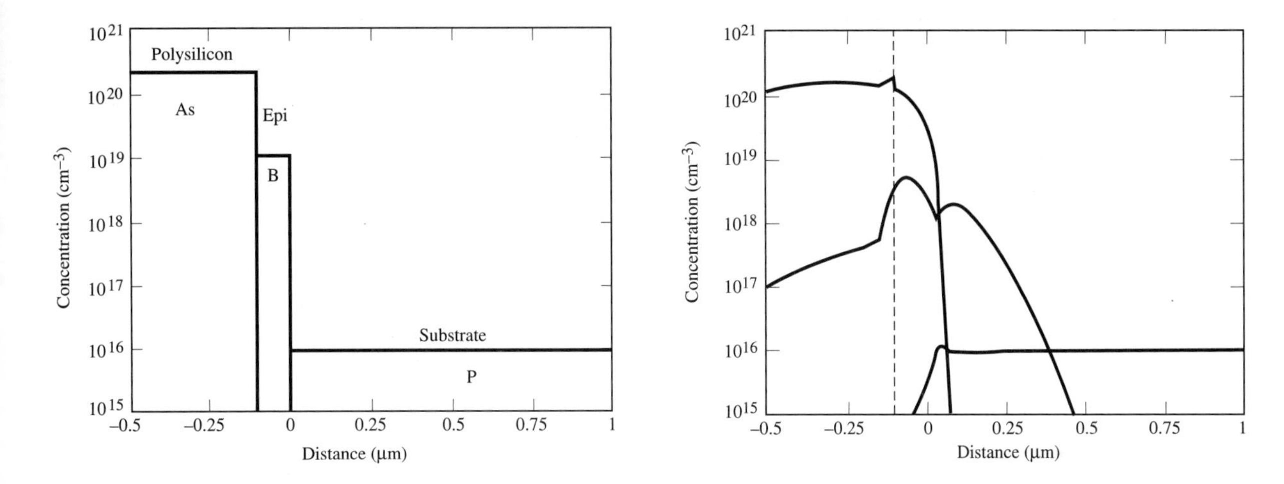

Figure 7–29 Example of bipolar transistor designed with TSUPREM-IV [7.14] simulations using concentration and $\mathcal{E}$-field-dependent diffusion coefficients (solid lines). The initial boron concentration (left) is a box-shaped layer doped at 10^{19} grown on the silicon surface with 0.1 microns of epitaxial silicon. After a 60-min 1000°C anneal, an arsenic-doped polysilicon layer is deposited and annealed for 30 mins at 1000°C (right).

base profile. This is then annealed at high temperature to fully activate the dopant and form a narrow diffused base region. Subsequently, a highly As-doped polysilicon layer is deposited on the surface of the wafer and an emitter region is outdiffused from the poly. The final result is shown at the right of Figure 7–29. There are several interesting things to observe about this simulation. First note that the simple analytic formulas (a Gaussian profile for the base and an erfc profile for the emitter) would not do a very good job of matching the full numerical simulations. In the case of the boron profile, $\mathcal{E}$-field effects significantly affect the profile near the junction. In the As emitter profile, concentration-dependent diffusivity effects are apparent because the simulated profile is much more abrupt and "boxlike" than the erfc approximation. Even the background (substrate) phosphorus profile is not a simple profile. The phosphorus diffuses upward during the heat cycle, but the shape is affected by $\mathcal{E}$-field effects. This example clearly illustrates the need for numerical simulators to accurately model modern device structures.

7.5.4 Segregation

Interfaces between different materials occur frequently in silicon processing. Dopants have different solubilities in different materials and so redistribute at an interface until the chemical potential is the same on both sides of the interface. The ratio of the equilibrium doping concentration on each side of the interface is defined as the segregation coefficient. We used this same concept in Chapter 3 in connection with dopant behavior during CZ crystal growth. (See Section 3.5.2.) This difference in a dopant's solubility in each phase drives a diffusion flux until the chemical potential equalizes and for this reason is an important boundary condition.

For example, consider two separate phases A and B (which might be oxide and silicon); we want to derive the transfer of a component X between A and B having concentrations C_A in A and C_B in B. The basic first order assumption is that the species interchange at the interface according to the chemical reaction:

$$X_A \underset{k_2}{\overset{k_1}{\Leftrightarrow}} X_B \tag{7.58}$$

so that the flux or flow of material from A to B is

$$F_{AB} = k_1 C_A - k_2 C_B \tag{7.59}$$

In steady state,

$$F_{AB} = 0 \Rightarrow \frac{C_B}{C_A} = \frac{k_1}{k_2} = k_O \tag{7.60}$$

$$\therefore F = k_1\left(C_A - \frac{C_B}{k_O}\right) = h\left(C_A - \frac{C_B}{k_O}\right) \tag{7.61}$$

where h is the interface transfer coefficient (cm sec^{-1}) across the interface and k_O is the segregation coefficient at the interface. Both h and k_O may be exponentially activated. In equilibrium F goes to zero.

It might seem to be easy to determine the segregation coefficients between different materials. However, if we consider the simple problem of profiling a doping concentration across an Si/SiO_2 interface using SIMS, matrix effects on the yield and mixing effects at the interface complicate the measurements. Similarly, stripping the cap layers and measuring the concentration profiles in the underlying substrate do not unambiguously define the segregation coefficient because the profile in the substrate can depend not only on the segregation parameters, but also on the diffusivity in the capping layers. Especially for boron at the oxide/silicon interface, the apparent segregation coefficient is strongly influenced by the amount of moisture in the oxidizing ambient.

For thick oxides, the segregation coefficient can be determined from careful SIMS profiles. For thin oxides, SIMS does not have adequate resolution and the electrical effects of segregation provide a better monitor of the dopant segregation. Measurements such as threshold voltage or capacitance measurements are sensitive indications of the segregation of dopants at interfaces. Process simulators like SUPREM contain experimentally determined values for k_O for the common dopants in silicon across the Si/SiO_2 interface. These parameters are often temperature activated but are in the range of the values given below [7.17, 7.18]. There is a real need for additional data of this type, especially for interfaces other than the Si/SiO_2 interface.

$$k_O = \frac{C_{Si}}{C_{SiO_2}} \approx \left\{ \begin{array}{l} 0.3 \text{ for boron} \\ 10 \text{ for arsenic} \\ 10 \text{ for antimony} \\ 10 \text{ for phosphorus} \end{array} \right\} \tag{7.62}$$

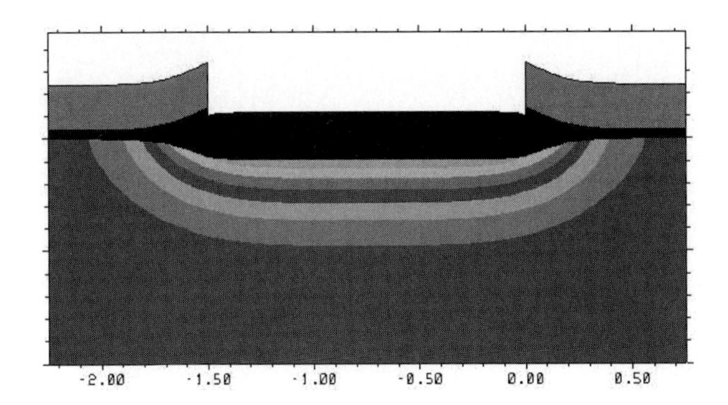

Figure 7–30 TSUPREM IV [7.14] plot of boron contours after an oxidation of an initially uniform boron-doped substrate. The boron depletes from the bulk into the oxide layer due to segregation.

Boron segregates into oxide layers, tending to deplete the boron concentration in the silicon near the oxide silicon interface. Figure 7–30 shows a two-dimensional simulation of the depletion of boron by a local oxidation at the silicon surface. Phosphorus on the other hand, tends to "pileup" on the silicon side of the interface. This leads to a "snowplow" effect when a phosphorus-doped substrate is oxidized and there is a moving interface which attempts to reject the phosphorus from the growing oxide into the silicon. Figure 7–31 illustrates these effects for As, P, and B in silicon. The As profile is steeper than the P profile in the silicon because of arsenic's smaller diffusivity compared to phosphorus.

7.5.5 Interfacial Dopant Pileup

As junctions become more shallow, it has been observed that dopants may pileup in a very narrow interfacial layer between SiO_2 and Si, as illustrated in Figure 7–32. This pileup is separate from any segregation that may occur. The interfacial layer may be as thin as a monolayer and can act as a sink for dopant atoms and is able to trap on the order of an atomic layer of dopant at the oxide/silicon interface. The dopants are inactive in the interfacial layer and can be removed if the oxide layer is stripped in dilute hydrofluoric acid. An actual SIMS profile of the dose loss from an implanted Arsenic layer is shown in Figure 7–33, before and after an anneal. The "lost" dose in this example has been incorporated into a thin layer just at the interface, which is not resolved in the SIMS data.

Because the amount of interfacial dose loss may be a significant fraction of the dose of dopants that are used in the tip or extension regions of small MOS devices, this effect can take on a dominant role in determining the electrical characteristics of these devices. Transient-enhanced diffusion of the implanted dopant atoms (see Chapter 8) can allow many of the dopant atoms to reach the interface where they can be trapped. Some of the dopant can return to the silicon upon subsequent annealing.

This dose loss is important because it occurs on the same time scale as the rapid thermal cycles that are used to anneal implants. Understanding this process is important for designing the source/drain profiles in MOS devices. At present, trapping models in

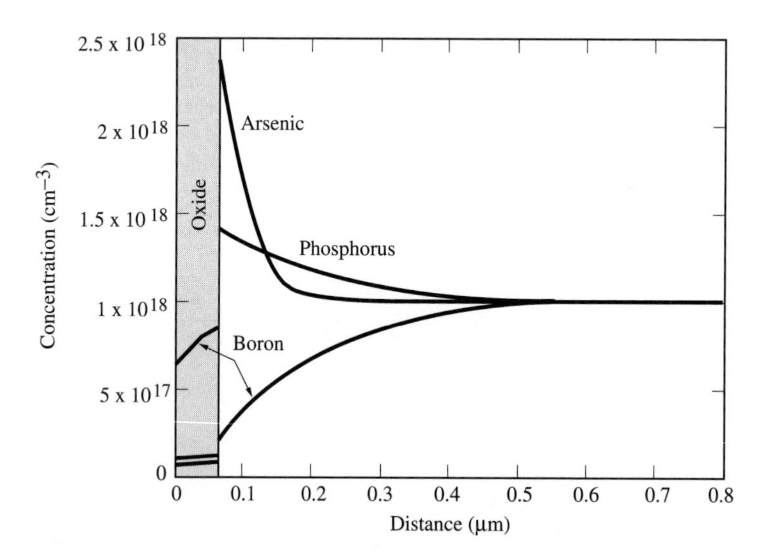

Figure 7–31 TSUPREM IV [7.14] plot of initially uniform arsenic, phosphorus, and boron profiles after an oxidation of the silicon surface. Arsenic and phosphorus pileup in front of the moving interface, while boron is depleted.

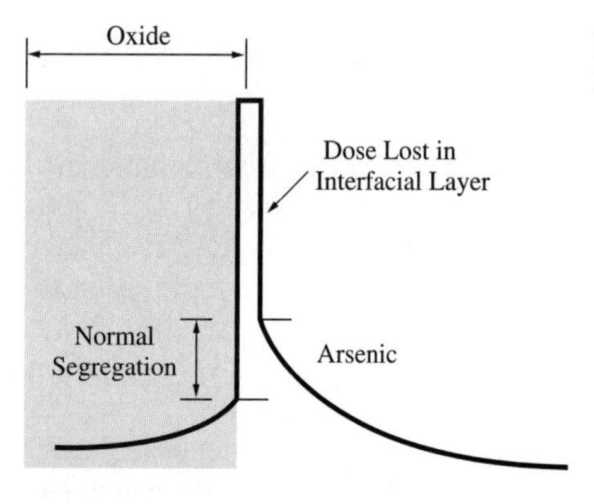

Figure 7–32 Schematic diagram of interfacial dopant dose loss.

TSUPREM IV account for a flux of dopant to unfilled traps at the interface and consider a trapping flux:

$$F = h\left(C\left(f + r\frac{\sigma}{\sigma_{max}}\right) - k\sigma\right) \tag{7.63}$$

where h is a transport coefficient, C is the dopant concentration near the interface, f is the fraction of unfilled interface traps, σ and σ_{max} are the available and maximum trap

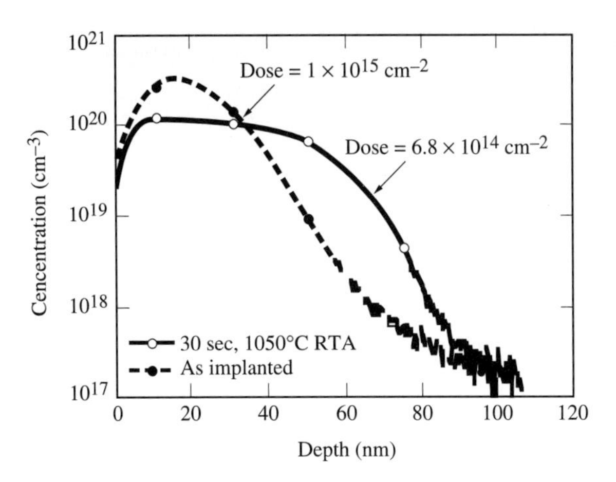

Figure 7–33 SIMS data showing 32 percent arsenic dose loss after a 30-sec 1050°C RTA [7.19]. The dose loss results in the areas under the two curves being different by 32 percent.

density, respectively, and r and k are rate constants for trapping and detrapping. In general this dose loss effect is poorly understood and only preliminary models are available in process simulators.

7.5.6 Summary of the Macroscopic Diffusion Approach

We have discussed many of the issues related to macroscopic dopant diffusion in silicon. Darken and Gurry [7.4] make the point that Fick's first law is a fundamental physical law in the sense that it appears to properly describe diffusion behavior in the limit of sufficiently low concentrations or for small concentration differences. We have modified the original intent of Fick's first law because experimental data suggested that it was not adequate to describe the evolution of doping profiles by adding electric-field effects and concentration-dependent diffusivities. It is at this stage that we run out of steam in dealing with a macroscopic description of the diffusion process. The complexities from these ad hoc descriptions begin to outweigh their usefulness. In order to progress further, we need to understand a little more about how dopants diffuse on an atomic scale. Understanding at the atomic scale forms the physical basis for the models used in most process simulation programs used today.

We will see later that Fick's laws, intelligently applied to the mobile diffusing species on an atomic level, will provide a useful description of the full range of anomalous dopant diffusion in silicon.

7.5.7 The Physical Basis for Diffusion at an Atomic Scale

Point defects (vacancies and interstitials) and dopant diffusion are intimately linked on the atomic scale. Understanding the behavior of point defects can help to provide a unified explanation of the atomic mechanisms underlying dopant diffusion. This provides

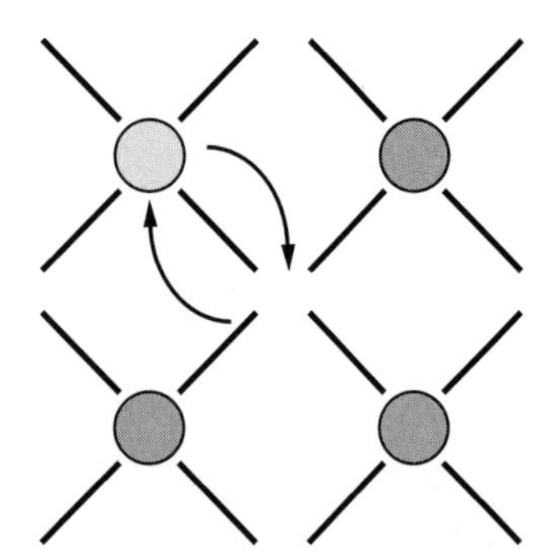

Figure 7–34 Schematic of vacancy-assisted diffusion mechanism.

a clear picture of many effects that previously seemed anomalous. The basic concepts relating to point defects were introduced in Chapter 3 (Section 3.5.4).

Intuitively, it seems clear that a vacancy adjacent to a dopant atom provides a mechanism for the dopant atom to hop to the adjacent site, thus effecting a single migration jump for the dopant atom as shown in Figure 7–34. This is precisely the mechanism of diffusion that occurs in metals. In fact, the vacancy concentrations in metals are so high that changes in the lattice constant can be observed directly by X-Ray Diffraction (XRD). If the metal temperature is changed and the lattice constant measured as a function of temperature, the change in lattice constant can be used to extract the vacancy concentration versus temperature. A similar experiment in silicon does not reveal a measurable change in the number of lattice sites, which implies that the vacancy concentrations are below the detection limit of this technique. The change in the length of a specimen is related to the change in volume by $\Delta L/L = \Delta V/3V$, so that the length of a silicon specimen changes by only 0.7×10^{-7} for a vacancy concentration of $1 \times 10^{16}/\text{cm}^{-3}$ [7.20]. This is below the detection limit of the XRD technique.

The success of the "vacancy-only" theory of impurity diffusion in metals was initially applied with great enthusiasm to diffusion in silicon. It had some early dramatic successes, in that it allowed many of the observations of high-concentration dopant diffusion to be explained in a consistent manner using a single set of vacancy concentrations which depended only on the Fermi level [7.21]. Much of the current success in modeling dopant diffusion in simulators such as SUPREM IV stems directly from this idea that an atomic-level understanding of the process is both possible and powerful.

It is also easy to imagine how a silicon interstitial might "kick out" a substitutional dopant atom from its lattice site and enable it to quickly diffuse down the relatively open channels in the silicon lattice as illustrated on the left in Figure 7–35. Eventually, the mobile dopant interstitial will regain its place on a substitutional site by displacing a silicon atom or perhaps by finding a vacant site. The interstitial-assisted diffusion of the dopant then takes place by a series of these hops or episodes of mobility. Each hop of the diffusing dopant is actually a random walk through the channels of the silicon lattice, interspersed with long periods in a stable, substitutional site.

It is perhaps less easy to imagine that a dopant and a silicon interstitial could diffuse as a bound pair as also illustrated on the right in Figure 7–35, but this could correspond

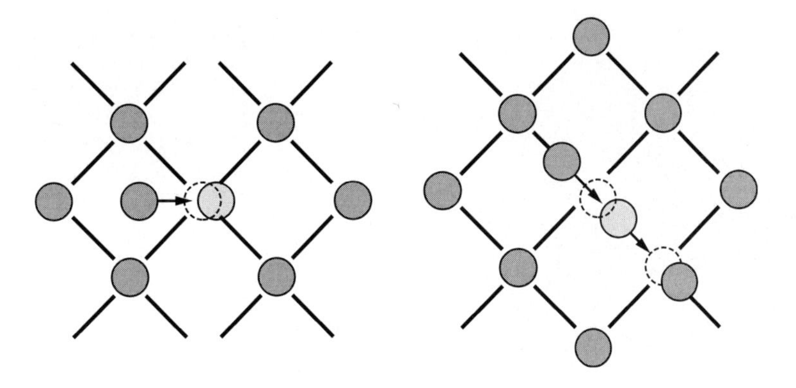

Figure 7–35 Schematic of interstitial assisted kick-out diffusion (left) and interstitialcy-assisted diffusion (right) mechanisms.

to diffusion along the bond directions rather than through the open channels in the lattice. A dopant and a silicon atom could share a lattice site and by moving in the bond directions could effectively migrate as a bound pair through the lattice. Once again, a free silicon interstitial is temporarily bound with a dopant atom while the pair migrates as a mobile species, before the pair breaks up leaving the dopant atom on a substitutional site and releasing the silicon interstitial. To distinguish this process from the kick-out process, the mechanism on the right in Figure 7–35 is known as the interstitialcy mechanism. Mathematically it is identical to the kick-out process and in the literature, both the kick-out and interstitialcy processes are often simply referred to as "interstitial-" assisted diffusion. We will adopt this terminology in this text.

7.5.8 Oxidation-Enhanced or -Retarded Diffusion

It is known that some dopants(e.g., P, B) appear to have their diffusion coefficients enhanced when the surface of the silicon is oxidized, while antimony appears to have its diffusion coefficient reduced, as shown in Figure 7–36. We introduced these ideas in Chapter 6 (Section 6.5.8). These experimental observations were important in elucidating the microscopic mechanisms of diffusion, because the variations in the diffusion coefficients were postulated to be due to perturbed point-defect concentrations caused by the surface oxidation. The fact that the diffusion of one dopant was enhanced while that of another was retarded is evidence that two different diffusion mechanisms are operating on an atomic scale.

The original insights that led to postulating dual roles for interstitials and vacancies in mediating dopant diffusion arose from recognizing that the growth of oxidation stacking faults and the oxidation-enhanced diffusion of dopants were different manifestations of the same underlying phenomena [7.22]. Oxidation-induced stacking faults are nonequilibrium defect structures which have been shown by TEM image contrast to be composed of an extra partial plane of interstitials (see Figure 3–4 in Chapter 3).

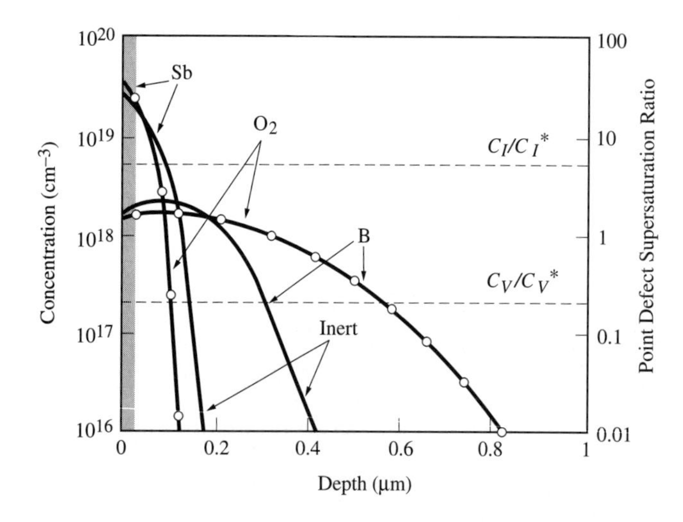

Figure 7–36 TSUPREM IV [7.14] simulations of Oxidation-Enhanced Diffusion (OED) of boron and Oxidation-Retarded Diffusion (ORD) of antimony during the growth of a thermal oxide on the surface of silicon. The two shallow profiles are antimony, the two deeper profiles are boron. Oxidation increases C_I and decreases C_V from their equilibrium values.

These stacking faults grow during oxidation of the silicon surface, indicating that oxidation is injecting interstitials as illustrated in Figure 7–37. This makes intuitive sense, because when a cube of silicon is oxidized there is an expansion of 30% to form the SiO_2 structure. (Recall Figure 6–3 in Chapter 6.) Some of the resulting compressive stress can be relieved by injection of a silicon interstitial to make space at the silicon surface where oxidation is occurring. We discussed these mechanisms in some detail in Chapter 6 and Figure 7–39 extends the ideas from Section 6.5.8 by including the experimental stacking fault growth observations.

Oxidation-enhanced diffusion of boron or phosphorus is seen under the same conditions that cause stacking faults to grow. Antimony, on the other hand, undergoes oxidation-retarded diffusion, that is, the diffusion of antimony is slower than normal during an oxidation process. This implies that boron and phosphorus prefer to diffuse with interstitials and Sb prefers to diffuse with vacancies. The oxidation injected interstitials recombine with vacancies in the bulk, depressing the vacancy concentration and therefore retarding Sb diffusion. (Note the I and V supersaturation and undersaturation, respectively, in Figure 7–36.) Physically, the preference of antimony for a vacancy mechanism may be related to its large size in the silicon lattice. The elastic interaction between a point defect and a dopant atom depends on the mismatch in size, so that a large dopant atom may prefer to migrate with a vacancy, while a small dopant atom may prefer to migrate with an interstitial. Figure 7–38 shows the simulated interstitial supersaturation that occurs during oxidation of the silicon surface.

Models for the interstitial supersaturation generated by oxidizing the surface of the silicon are available in process simulators like SUPREM IV. The interstitial level depends on the balance between the generation rate G of interstitials (indicated schematically in Figure 7–37) and the recombination rate R at an oxidizing interface and is found to depend on the oxidation rate as follows:

$$C_I \propto \sqrt{\frac{dx}{dt}} \tag{7.64}$$

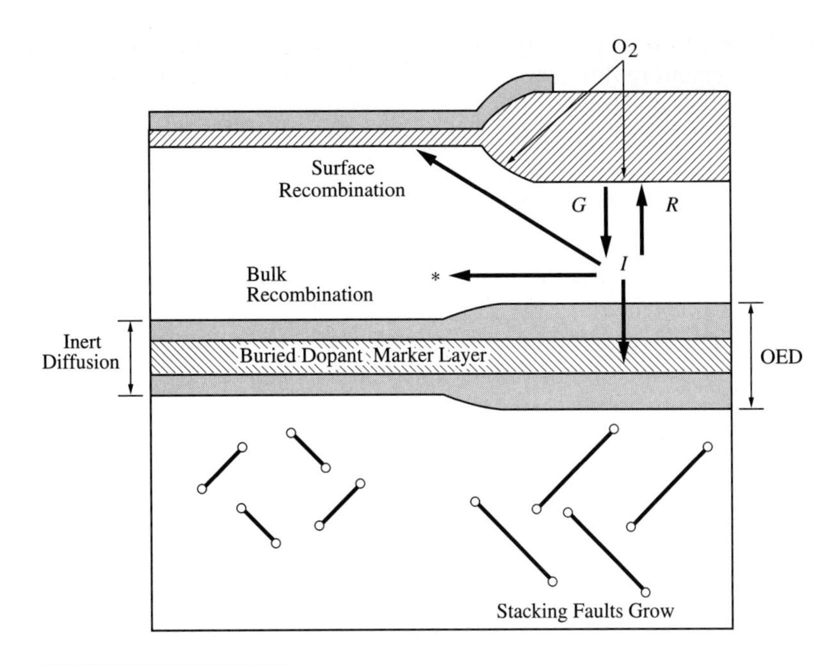

Figure 7–37 Generalized representation of point-defect generation (G), recombination (R), and diffusion processes in silicon. In this example, local oxidation (right side) generates interstitials which diffuse away from the Si/SiO_2 interface, locally enhancing the diffusion of dopants like B or P, while causing interstitial type stacking faults to grow.

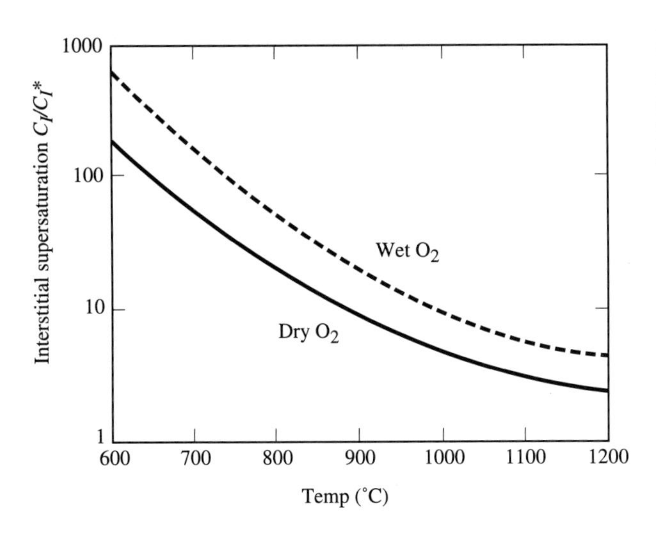

Figure 7–38 TSUPREM IV [7.14] simulations of the interstitial supersaturation generated by oxidation in wet and dry O_2 at various temperatures. The oxidation time is chosen to be at the transition between the linear and parabolic regimes.

This equation is a specific version of the more general forms given in Eqs. (6.48) and (6.49). The interstitial supersaturation results from the balance between the generation rate and the recombination rate of interstitials at the oxidizing interface. The interstitial excess above the equilibrium value (or supersaturation) depends primarily on temperature and is larger at lower oxidation temperatures, as shown in Figure 7–38. The enhancement in diffusion coefficient is small at high temperatures but can be very large at low temperatures.

7.5.9 Dopant Diffusion Occurs by Both I and V

The idea that both I and V contribute to dopant diffusion in silicon is now generally accepted based on both experimental observations and theoretical calculations. The theoretical calculations have only recently become possible based on a direct quantum mechanical description of solid-state systems on powerful computers. The experimental results that dramatically capture the existence of a dual diffusion mechanism are based on the observation that under certain identical conditions such as oxidation of the silicon surface, one dopant has its diffusion enhanced while another dopant has its diffusion retarded.

For example Figure 7–39 shows the diffusion of arsenic and antimony (both n-type dopants) during oxidation of the silicon surface. The diffusion of the arsenic is enhanced while, simultaneously, the diffusion of the antimony is retarded below the normal values that would be observed if the anneal were carried out in an inert ambient such as argon. In this particular experiment, the retarded diffusion of the antimony is observed even inside the arsenic layer which is undergoing enhanced diffusion. Thus, by perturbing the point-defect populations by oxidation, the existence of two different fundamental mechanisms of diffusion is demonstrated.

It is important to note that this information could not be obtained by observing the diffusion of the dopants in an inert (argon or nitrogen) atmosphere. In that case, the only observation that could be made is that one dopant diffused faster or slower than another one. Instead, it is because the point-defect levels are perturbed from their equilibrium values by oxidation that some inference can be made about dopant diffusion mechanisms.

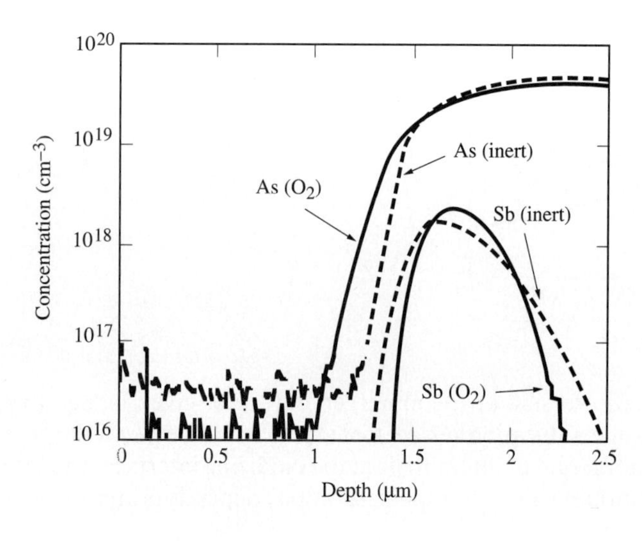

Figure 7–39 SIMS plot showing arsenic diffusion enhanced during oxidation at the same time that antimony diffusion is retarded below normal values. This is a strong indication that two different diffusion mechanisms are taking place. (After [7.23].)

It has also been found that nitridation of the silicon surface in an ammonia ambient has exactly the opposite effects to oxidation. In other words, B and P exhibit retarded diffusion, while the diffusion of Sb is enhanced. Preexisting stacking faults also shrink in a nitriding ambient. Thus the conclusion is that nitridation injects vacancies. This complementary set of observations "weaves a seamless logic" for the dual roles of interstitials and vacancies in assisting dopant diffusion in silicon [7.24, 7.25].

These observations can be formalized by saying that dopants diffuse with a fraction f_I interstitial-type diffusion mechanism and with a fraction $f_V = 1 - f_I$ vacancy-type mechanism. Under perturbed conditions, when the interstitial (C_I) or vacancy (C_V) concentrations are different from their equilibrium concentrations (C_I^*, C_V^*), the diffusivity of a dopant can be written

$$D_A^{\text{eff}} = D_A^*\left(f_I\frac{C_I}{C_I^*} + f_V\frac{C_V}{C_V^*}\right) \tag{7.65}$$

where D_A^{eff} is the effective diffusivity of the dopant measured under conditions where the point-defect populations are perturbed and D_A^* is the normal, equilibrium diffusivity measured under inert conditions and by definition $f_I + f_V = 1$.

It is interesting to note that if two different diffusion mechanisms are operative (i.e., interstitial- and vacancy-assisted mechanisms) and if they have very different activation energies (Q_A), then a plot of D_A versus $1/T$ would show distinct regions with different slopes. For dopants in silicon, there has never been such an observation in the intrinsic Q_A versus $1/T$ plot (Figure 7–15). We might expect that this slope change or curvature would be most obvious for arsenic, which has approximately equal I and V components of diffusion. This indicates that the activation energies of diffusion via both I and V mechanisms are comparable at processing temperatures.

It is the observation of retarded diffusion that allows the extent of diffusion by an I or V mechanism to be quantified. What is measured experimentally is how much the dopant is retarded compared with its normal diffusion in an inert ambient, that is, the extent of retardation for a dopant whose diffusion is retarded (superscript R) is given by

$$\left(\frac{D}{D^*}\right)^R = f_I^R\frac{C_I}{C_I^*} + f_V^R\frac{C_V}{C_V^*} = (1 - f_V^R)\frac{C_I}{C_I^*} + f_V^R\frac{C_V}{C_V^*} \tag{7.66}$$

A very conservative assumption under conditions of interstitial excess and a resulting vacancy deficit is that the vacancy component of diffusion is reduced to zero ($C_V/C_V^* = 0$) so that

$$\left(\frac{D}{D^*}\right)^R \geq (1 - f_V^R)\frac{C_I}{C_I^*} \tag{7.67}$$

An even more conservative assumption under conditions of interstitial excess is that $C_I/C_I^* = 1$ so that

$$f_V^R > 1 - \left(\frac{D}{D^*}\right)^R \tag{7.68}$$

This provides a mathematical justification for the statement that a dopant whose diffusivity is reduced to 1/10 of normal when there is an interstitial excess present must diffuse at least 9/10 by a vacancy mechanism. This is an absolute lower bound on the extent of diffusion by a V-type mechanism.

If another dopant is enhanced by some factor under the same conditions of an interstitial excess, then for the dopant that is enhanced (superscript E)

$$\left(\frac{D^{\text{eff}}}{D^*}\right)^E = f_I^E \frac{C_I}{C_I^*} + f_V^E \frac{C_V}{C_V^*} \tag{7.69}$$

Since the interstitial fraction of the dopant diffusion $f_I^E \leq 1$ and vacancy-assisted component of diffusion $f_V^E\,(C_V/C_V^*) \geq 0$, a conservative estimate is that

$$\left(\frac{D}{D^*}\right)^E \leq \frac{C_I}{C_I^*} \tag{7.70}$$

Simply stated, the measured enhancement in the diffusivity of a dopant won't exceed the interstitial supersaturation value. By substituting for C_I/C_I^*, Eq. (7.67) can now be used to show that the vacancy component of the dopant whose diffusivity is retarded can be better approximated by

$$f_V^R \geq 1 - \frac{\left(\dfrac{D}{D^*}\right)^R}{\left(\dfrac{D}{D^*}\right)^E} \tag{7.71}$$

An even stricter bound on the preference for a particular microscopic diffusion mechanism is possible if the interstitials and vacancies recombine to reach a steady-state condition given by

$$C_I C_V = C_I^* C_V^* \tag{7.72}$$

In this case, a strict lower bound on f_V can be derived as (see problem 7.19)

$$f_V^R \geq 0.5 + 0.5\sqrt{1 - \left[\left(\frac{D}{D^*}\right)^R\right]^2} \tag{7.73}$$

Thus by observing how much a dopant is enhanced or retarded under different conditions where the point defects are perturbed, an estimate of their propensity to diffuse via a vacancy- or interstitial-assisted mechanism can be made.

If an independent measure of the vacancy or interstitial supersaturation can be made, the fraction of diffusion by a vacancy or interstitial mechanism can be directly computed from Eq. (7.66). Such an estimate of the supersaturation might be made by observing the growth rate of stacking faults, for example. However, these methods tend to be less reliable than the self-consistent approach which relies on observing enhanced and retarded dopant diffusion in the same experiment as described above. Remember that this problem of inferring the mechanism of dopant diffusion occurs because there is no reliable way to directly observe the interstitial or vacancy populations themselves at processing temperatures because of their low concentrations. In spite of this limitation, a self-consistent picture of the atomic-scale mechanisms of dopant diffusion in silicon can be deduced by following the trail of physical evidence. These kinds of experiments have been widely done, resulting in the f_I and f_V values for the common dopants in silicon shown in Table 7–6.

We have now "split" the overall dopant diffusivity into components dominated by interstitial- and vacancy-assisted mechanisms. Though this contains a lot more insight than a purely macroscopic description of the diffusion process, it is still a crude description of the atomic-level mechanisms. Consider that the dopant may diffuse much faster with the interstitial component than the vacancy component. Or that the activation energy for diffusion with interstitials might be different from the activation energy for diffusion with vacancies. How are these physical effects captured in our description of the diffusion process?

As described previously, the effective diffusivity of a dopant at low concentration in silicon is given by

$$D_A^{\text{eff}} = D_A^0 \exp\left(\frac{-E_A}{kT}\right) \tag{7.74}$$

where E_A is the activation energy of diffusion and D_A^0 is the preexponential factor. The description above showed that this effective, intrinsic diffusivity is given by the sum of the diffusivities by each mechanism:

$$D_A^{\text{eff}} = D_{AI} + D_{AV} \tag{7.75}$$

where D_{AI} and D_{AV} are the contributions due to the I and V components of diffusion, respectively. Each of these terms depends on both the diffusivity of the mobile species and the fraction of the dopant atoms that are mobile, so that

$$D_A^{\text{eff}} = d_{AI}\left[\frac{C_{AI}}{C_A}\right] + d_{AV}\left[\frac{C_{AV}}{C_A}\right] \tag{7.76}$$

Table 7–6 Approximate values for f_I and f_V for silicon self-diffusion and for the common dopants in silicon

	f_I	f_V
Silicon	0.6	0.4
Boron	1.0	0
Phosphorus	1.0	0
Arsenic	0.4	0.6
Antimony	0.02	0.98

where d_{AI} or d_{AV} is the diffusivity of the actual mobile species causing the migration and C_{AI}/C_A and C_{AV}/C_A are the fractions of the dopant in the particular migrating state.

This is a much more rigorous description of the diffusion process, as it breaks the overall diffusion down into the diffusivity of each individual migrating species and the microscopic concentration of those migrating species. In the following sections, we will consider how these mobile species form on an atomic level and how Fick's laws can be applied to these mobile diffusing species to give a detailed description of the diffusion process on an atomic scale.

7.5.10 Activation Energy for Self-Diffusion and Dopant Diffusion

It is found experimentally that the activation energy [E_A in Eq. (7.74)] is about 1 eV lower for dopant diffusion in silicon than it is for self-diffusion (3 – 4 eV versus 4 – 5 eV). This raises a fundamental question regarding this difference. Because dopants have a lower activation energy for either I or V or mixed mechanisms of diffusion, there must be a lowering of the activation barrier specifically related to group III and V elements that is not present for group IV elements (Si or Ge). Coulombic effects can contribute to some but not all of this barrier lowering. (The dopant atoms are charged on substitutional lattice sites and the Si atoms are not.) If Coulombic effects alone dominated dopant-defect interactions, then all n-type or p-type dopants would have the same activation energy. Since this not the case, there must be additional dopant-defect interactions to be considered. One such possibility is the relaxation of the silicon lattice around a dopant, related to the size of the dopant atom. For example, theoretical calculations indicate that a substitutional boron atom causes the lattice to relax inwards by about 12% [7.26]. It is easy to imagine that lattice distortions when both dopants and defects are in close proximity could significantly alter the activation energy for diffusion. Another possibility relates to the electronic interactions due to charge transfer between the dopant and the defect. These effects lead to a higher probability of a point-defect binding to a dopant atom or interacting with a dopant atom to kick it out of its normal, substitutional lattice site. It is this interaction between dopant atoms and point defects that is the key to understanding dopant diffusion on an atomic scale. The difference in activation energies between self-diffusion and dopant diffusion plays a key role in how native point defects and mobile dopants interact as the temperature is changed, generating complex diffused profiles, as described in the following sections.

7.5.11 Dopant-Defect Interactions

We have seen that the macroscopic diffusivity of dopants is dominated by terms of the form $d_{AI}C_{AI}$ (or $d_{AV}C_{AV}$) on a microscopic scale. These terms describe the diffusivity of the mobile species and the concentration of the mobile species in the lattice. The mobile species come about via interactions of individual dopant atoms and individual point defects. We can consider a dopant atom A interacting with an interstitial I as follows:

$$A + I \leftrightarrow AI \tag{7.77}$$

where AI is the actual interstitial-assisted mobile species on an atomic scale. The substitutional dopant is immobile by itself, unless it interacts with a point defect. (For a vacancy mechanism, I is replaced by V in this equation and the subsequent discussion.) This equation might represent either a migrating bound pair or a substitutional dopant "kicked out" of a lattice site by an interstitial to become a mobile dopant in an interstitial site. The justification for considering that the bound pair might migrate as a single entity comes from the difference in activation energy between self-diffusion and impurity diffusion. This activation energy difference indicates that there is a binding energy between an impurity and an intrinsic point defect. Our later mathematical treatment of Eq. (7.77) shows that there is no difference between a bound pair migrating and a pure dopant interstitial migrating. The overall picture in either case is that a silicon interstitial is temporarily consumed to generate the mobile species, which then migrates into the interior of the silicon sample, where the mobile dopant settles down on a lattice site to become a substitutional dopant once again, releasing a silicon interstitial in the process.

Eq. (7.77), although simple, contains a surprising amount of physics. It is clear that an interstitial supersaturation will drive more dopant atoms into a mobile state by shifting the equation to the right, thus enhancing the dopant diffusivity. This explains the phenomena of oxidation-enhanced diffusion, where the interstitial supersaturation during oxidation enhances the dopant diffusivity. A suppression of I, by nitridation of the silicon surface which introduces vacancies, can occur through the reaction

$$I + V \leftrightarrow Si_S \tag{7.78}$$

where Si_S represents a silicon atom on a lattice site. This will lead to retarded diffusion for dopant species that diffuse with interstitials.

Even under inert conditions where we consider the diffusion of a dopant from the surface (say, a shallow phosphorus implant), the atomic-level description says that the interior of the sample soon contains a lot of AI species, which drives Eq. (7.77) to the left, releasing interstitials in the interior when the mobile dopant regains a substitutional lattice position. In this way, silicon interstitials are "pumped" from the surface region into the interior region by the dopant diffusion. If there is a strong source of interstitials at surface kinks and ledges which maintains near-equilibrium levels of interstitials in the surface region, this leads to a supersaturation of interstitials in the interior of the sample. But a supersaturation of interstitials causes enhanced dopant diffusion. Thus, the tail of the phosphorus profile can diffuse much faster than expected, which is exactly what is observed experimentally. This demonstrates that diffusion pumping of point defects leads to point-defect supersaturations, which in turn feed back and enhance the diffusion process itself, as illustrated in Figure 7–40.

This description of "chemical pumping" of point defects also explains an anomalous interaction between emitter and base diffusions in some bipolar processes. The "emitter-push" or "emitter-dip" effect refers to the enhanced diffusion of the base profile below a phosphorus emitter as shown in Figure 7–41. This manifests itself in a much wider base width than expected. It is now understood to be caused by the pumping of interstitials by the diffusion of phosphorus which builds up a high supersaturation of

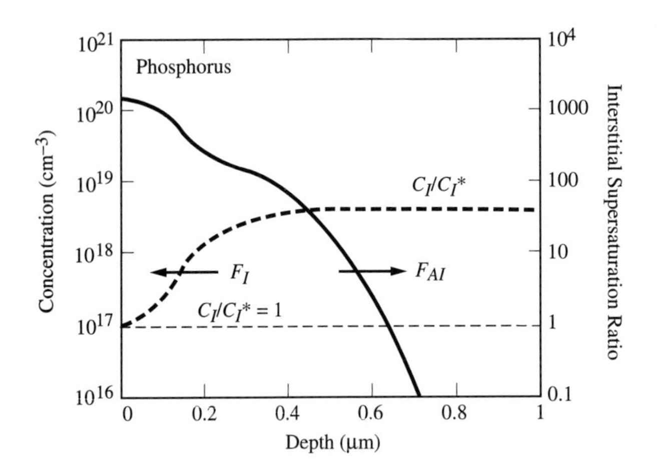

Figure 7–40 TSUPREM IV [7.14] simulation of the chemical or diffusion pumping of native point defects from the surface region into the bulk region by dopant-defect coupling. A quasi-steady state situation exists when the flux of free interstitials balances the flux of mobile dopant-interstitial pairs (or equivalently, mobile dopant interstitials). See text for a discussion of the C_I/C_I^* plots (right axis).

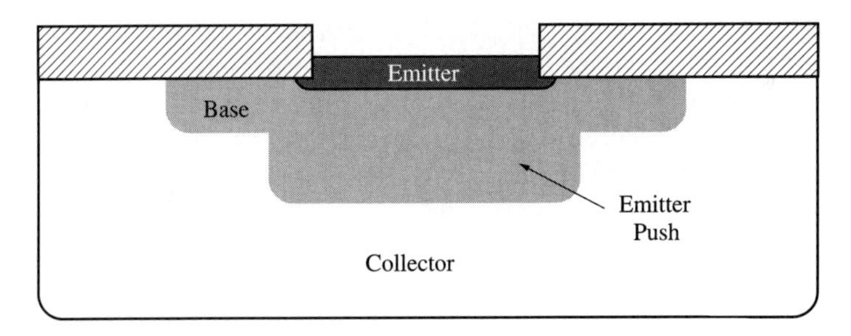

Figure 7–41 Schematic of the emitter-push effect in a bipolar transistor. The diffusion of the emitter junction affects the base region underneath the emitter and causes the base to "push out" further than expected [7.28]. This interaction is now known to be due to the chemical pumping of native point defects from the emitter region to the deeper bulk regions.

these point defects in the interior of the sample, well beyond the phosphorus diffusion front. The interstitial supersaturation then enhances the base (typically boron) diffusion in accordance with Eq. (7.76). We will return to this example later and show some SUPREM IV simulations that elucidate this coupling between dopant and self-interstitial fluxes.

In beginning this section we indicated qualitatively how a diffusing dopant atom transported interstitials into the bulk of the silicon, where it could enhance the tail diffusion of the diffusing dopant. We can now understand the origin of this effect if we properly account for the full coupling between the defects and the dopants when we consider the diffusion equation for the defects.

As seen in Figure 7–42, it is often important to include the full coupling between dopant and defects in simulations. Using only the concentration-dependent diffusivity for boron gives rise to a box-shaped simulated profile that does not match the experimental data. The β coefficient for boron [Eq. (7.57)] is the experimentally determined

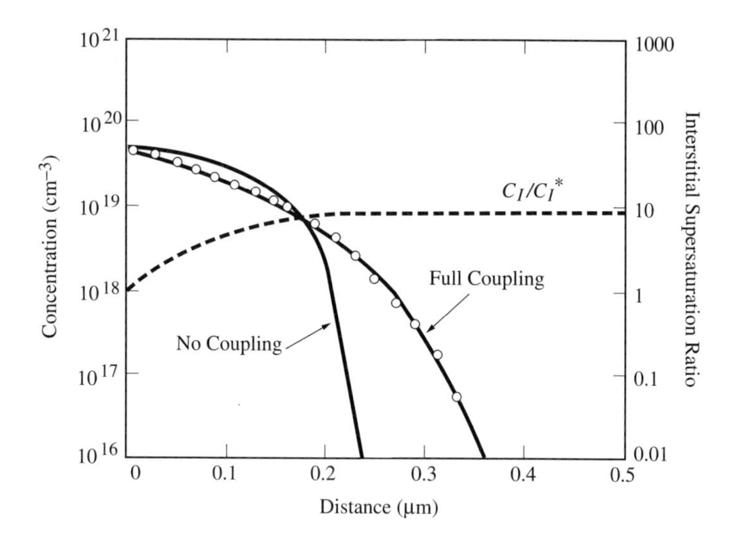

Figure 7–42 TSUPREM IV [7.14] simulations of boron diffused from a polysilicon source for eight hours at 850°C, with experimental data (circles) from [7.29]. The simulations use identical coefficients, but with and without full coupling between dopants and defects. The C_I/C_I^* curve (right axis) is for the fully coupled case. Without full coupling, $C_I/C_I^* = 1$.

value of 19 from highly doped extrinsic experiments (Table 7–5). One might be able to "fit" the experimental profile by adjusting the coefficients for neutral and positively charged boron diffusivity to make the profile less boxlike. However, by simply accounting for the coupling between boron and interstitials and therefore the enhanced diffusion in the tail region, the simulated profile agrees with the experimentally measured profile.

We want to be able to calculate how the supersaturation of point defects in the bulk is affected by the dopant transport in from the surface. The simplest interstitial diffusion equation is given by applying Fick's continuity equations to the native interstitial species:

$$\frac{\partial C_I}{\partial t} = -\frac{\partial}{\partial x}(F_I) \tag{7.79}$$

but this does not account for the fact that an interstitial is temporarily consumed and transported along when a mobile dopant atom diffuses through the lattice (this is most easily envisioned for the interstitialcy mechanism of dopant diffusion). The full coupling between the native interstitials and mobile dopant atoms is accounted for by including the flux of mobile dopant in the total interstitial continuity equation as follows:

$$\frac{\partial}{\partial t}(C_I + C_{AI}) = -\frac{\partial}{\partial x}(F_I + F_{AI}) \tag{7.80}$$

We can make some simplifying assumptions to estimate how this modification affects the interstitial supersaturation in the bulk. If we consider a quasi-steady state when the time derivative terms are small, then

$$\frac{\partial}{\partial x}(F_I + F_{AI}) = 0 \tag{7.81}$$

Integrating gives

$$F_I + F_{AI} = 0 \tag{7.82}$$

where we have taken the constant of integration to be zero. This is reasonable for many boundary conditions of interest. For example, the dopant flux (F_{AI}) deep in the crystal is certainly negligible and in quasi-steady state the interstitial flux deep in the crystal is also negligible, justifying our choice for the integration constant [7.29].
Thus,

$$F_I = -F_{AI} \tag{7.83}$$

which indicates that in steady state, the flux of dopant is balanced by a reverse flux of silicon interstitials, as shown in Figure 7–40. This balance between the dopant and defect fluxes is the key effect that results from a full coupling between the dopant and point-defect fluxes.

We can use this flux balance to investigate the magnitude of the interstitial supersaturation in the bulk, which is what causes the enhanced tail diffusion of dopants like phosphorus, the emitter-push effect, and boron profiles as in Figure 7–42. Since the flux of free interstitials is

$$F_I = -d_I\frac{\partial C_I}{\partial x} \tag{7.84}$$

we can use the flux balance equation [Eq. (7.82)] to write

$$\frac{\partial C_I}{\partial x} = \frac{F_{AI}}{d_I} \tag{7.85}$$

and we can obtain the depth dependence of the interstitial supersaturation by introducing the equilibrium interstitial concentration on both sides of the equation to give

$$\frac{\partial(C_I/C_I^*)}{\partial x} = \frac{F_{AI}}{d_I C_I^*} \tag{7.86}$$

We can relate the overall, observable macroscopic diffusion of the dopant to the microscopic diffusivity of the mobile species by realizing that the flux of the dopant is equivalent to the flux of the mobile species, giving

$$D_A^{\text{eff}}\frac{\partial C_A}{\partial x} = d_{AI}\frac{\partial C_{AI}}{\partial x} \tag{7.87}$$

Thus,

$$D_A^{\text{eff}} C_A = d_{AI} C_{AI} \tag{7.88}$$

which holds if the concentration of the mobile species bears some constant relationship to the substitutional dopant. This formulation for the effective dopant diffusivity brings out the importance of the (Diffusivity Concentration) or "DC" product of the mobile species in determining the overall motion of the dopant species. A more mathematical derivation of Eq. (7.88) is given in Section 7.5.12.

Since the flux of the mobile dopant species $F_{AI} = d_{AI}\nabla C_{AI}$ is equivalent to the overall flux of dopant $F_A = D_A^{\text{eff}}\nabla C_A$, we can write

$$\frac{\partial\left(C_I/C_I^*\right)}{\partial x} = \frac{D_A^{eff} C_A}{d_I C_I^*} \tag{7.89}$$

For an interstitial-type diffusion process, this equation indicates that the depth dependence of the interstitial supersaturation depends on the ratio of the dopant flux to the interstitial component of the self-diffusion flux. The severity of the chemical pump effect for different dopants relates to how the DC product for the dopant ($D_A^{\text{eff}} C_A$ or equivalently $d_{AI}C_{AI}$) compares with the DC product for the interstitial component of native silicon self-diffusion ($d_I C_I^*$).

Because of the difference in activation energies between self-diffusion (4.8 eV) and dopant diffusion (3–4 eV), Eq. (7.89) indicates that the magnitude of the interstitial supersaturation gets larger at lower temperatures, as shown in Figure 7–43. This is also the reason that the emitter-push effect is more pronounced for a fast diffusing dopant with a high solubility like phosphorus (high D_A^{eff}, high C_A) compared with a slow diffuser with a low solubility like arsenic, as shown in Figure 7–44. Thus, it explains why the emitter-push effect is more severe at lower temperatures and for fast diffusing emitter dopant species. Once again, this detailed understanding of the full coupling between mobile dopant atoms and native point defects on an atomic scale provides answers to questions that would otherwise remain a puzzle.

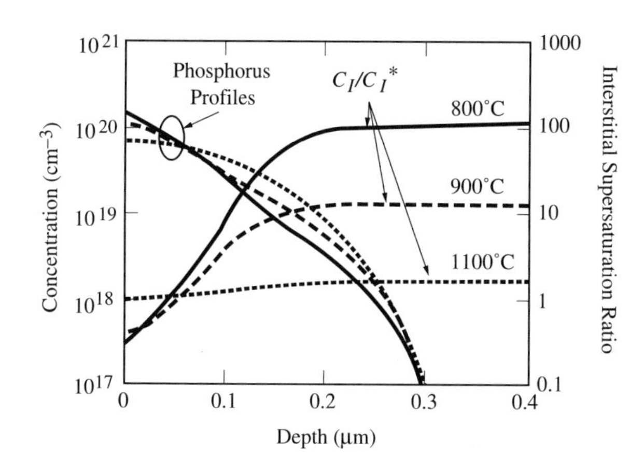

Figure 7–43 TSUPREM IV [7.14] simulations of the interstitial supersaturation generated by considering the fully coupled diffusion of phosphorus at different temperatures. The interstitial excess (right axis) generated by the diffusing dopant (left axis) can exceed a hundred-fold at lower temperatures, making the fully coupled effect an important contribution to high-concentration diffusion modeling. The diffusion times at each temperature were chosen to give the same junction depth.

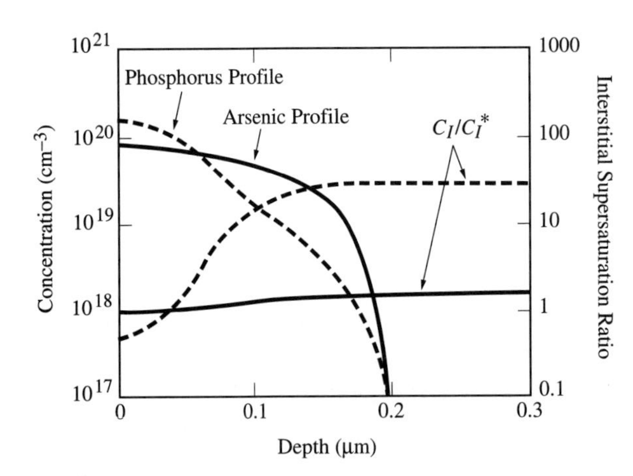

Figure 7–44 TSUPREM IV [7.14] simulations of the interstitial supersaturations generated by a phosphorus versus an arsenic diffusion to the same depth. The fast-diffusing phosphorus profile has a larger effect on C_I/C_I^* than the slow-diffusing arsenic profile.

7.5.12 Chemical Equilibrium Formulation for Dopant-Defect Interactions

In the previous section, we have seen how important a simple point-defect mediated reaction can be for determining how high-concentration dopants diffuse. The implications of such a reaction are now considered in more detail. Without loss of generality, if we consider an interstitial mediated reaction

$$A + I \leftrightarrow AI \tag{7.90}$$

to be in chemical equilibrium, then we can apply the law of mass action to the solid-state system and relate the concentrations by

$$C_{AI} = kC_A C_I \tag{7.91}$$

This particular description of the diffusion process is in "chemical equilibrium" in the sense that the mobile pairs are directly related to the reacting species by the equilibrium reaction constant. Experimentally this is justified because large enhancements in the diffusivity when excess interstitials are present can be seen for short diffusion times and remain the same for longer anneals. This indicates that the mobile species forms quickly and that the equilibrium assumption is valid.

Applying Fick's law to the mobile species C_{AI} gives

$$F_{AI} = -d_{AI}\frac{\partial C_{AI}}{\partial x} \tag{7.92}$$

At this point, our description of the diffusion flux is in terms of the unseen mobile species parameters ($d_{AI}C_{AI}$), the diffusivity and concentration of the mobile species in the lattice. These mobile species are not readily observable. Thus, the description as it stands is not very helpful. If we had numbers for the diffusivity of the mobile species itself and the concentration of the mobile species, we would have a useful description of the evolution of the profile shape. To make this description useful, we must relate these parameters to what can be observed, namely the overall dopant concentration (measured say, by SIMS) and the apparent or effective diffusion coefficient of the total dopant concentration. A primary goal of this section will be to relate the microscopic diffusivity and concentration to parameters that can be measured at the macroscopic scale.

Differentiating Eq. (7.91) with respect to x and using the chain rule for differentiation gives

$$F_{AI} = -d_{AI}\left(kC_I\frac{\partial C_A}{\partial x} + kC_A\frac{\partial C_I}{\partial x}\right) \tag{7.93}$$

Now, we are interested in the overall observable diffusion of the dopant. But the substitutional dopant is immobile on an atomic scale, so F_A itself is zero. The only way for the substitutional concentration C_A to change in a small-volume element is if there is a difference in the flux of mobile species into and out of the volume element (similar to the argument used in Figure 7–7), giving

$$\frac{\partial C_A}{\partial t} = -\frac{\partial F_{AI}}{\partial x} = \frac{\partial}{\partial x}d_{AI}\left(kC_I\frac{\partial C_A}{\partial x} + kC_A\frac{\partial C_I}{\partial x}\right) \tag{7.94}$$

Note that the concentration of mobile species $C_{AI} << C_A$. We can infer that $C_{AI} << C_A$ experimentally. Silicon and phosphorus have similar mass and create similar interstitial and vacancy damage profiles in the lattice when they are implanted. Experimentally, the point defects from this damage enhance the diffusion of nearby buried dopant layers by the same amount (for low-implant doses, where there is no chemical pumping of the point defects). If a significant fraction of the damage-induced point defects were tied up with migrating phosphorus atoms (large C_{PI} or C_{PV} population), there would be a difference in the amount of enhanced diffusion seen at the buried layer for silicon and phosphorus implants at short diffusion times. There is not, so the dopant-defect complexes must be dilute.

The overall profile motion that is measured for a substitutional dopant C_A with an apparent measured diffusion coefficient D_A is in fact generated by a very small number of species on the atomic scale that become mobile intermittently (C_{AI}) and that migrate with a high diffusivity d_{AI} in the silicon lattice [illustrating the importance of the (DC) product again].

From Eq. (7.91), the equilibrium balance between the chemical species gives

$$C_{AI} = kC_AC_I \Rightarrow kC_I = \frac{C_{AI}}{C_A};\ kC_A = \frac{C_{AI}}{C_I} \tag{7.95}$$

so we can write the flux expression in the form

$$\frac{\partial C_A}{\partial t} = \frac{\partial}{\partial x}d_{AI}\left[\frac{C_{AI}}{C_A}\frac{\partial C_A}{\partial x} + \frac{C_{AI}}{C_I}\frac{\partial C_I}{\partial x}\right] \tag{7.96}$$

When we compare this to our original diffusion equation which claimed to describe the dopant diffusivity [Eq. (7.52)]

$$\frac{\partial C_A}{\partial t} = \frac{\partial}{\partial x}D_A^{\text{eff}}\left(\frac{\partial C_A}{\partial x}\right) \tag{7.97}$$

we see that there are both similarities and differences. Eqs. (7.96) and (7.97) are similar if the second term in Eq. (7.96) (the defect gradient term) is negligible, and then we can define the effective dopant diffusivity to be

$$D_A^{\text{eff}} = d_{AI}\frac{C_{AI}}{C_A} \tag{7.98}$$

which indicates that the macroscopic dopant diffusivity actually depends on the diffusivity of the mobile species and the fraction of the dopant that is actually mobile. This "effective diffusivity" is loosely considered to be the dopant diffusivity. It can easily be measured when the extra point-defect gradient term is negligible, which is most of the time for dopant diffusion in silicon. The effective diffusivity of a dopant should not be measured when there are large point-defect sources and sinks present, such as near a surface sink when large amounts of damage are present. Since we are considering an interstitial-assisted diffusion mechanism in this section, the effective diffusivity that can be measured is given by Eq. (7.65) for an interstitial type diffuser ($f_I = 1$)

$$D_A^{\text{eff}} = D_A^*\frac{C_I}{C_I^*} \tag{7.99}$$

Under equilibrium conditions where the interstitials are at their equilibrium level C_I^*, the measured diffusivity is the equilibrium, intrinsic, inert value D_A^*. The effective diffusivity that is enhanced by an interstitial supersaturation can also be measured by SIMS, providing there are no steep gradients in the interstitial profile in the region where the dopant is diffusing that could interfere with the measurement of the dopant diffusivity.

Combining the last two equations gives

$$d_{AI}C_{AI} = D_A^*C_A\frac{C_I}{C_I^*} \tag{7.100}$$

The microscopic parameters are now expressed in terms of the measured, macroscopic dopant diffusivity measured under equilibrium, inert conditions, the overall dopant concentration, and the supersaturation in the point-defect concentration which is easily estimated by observing how much the diffusion of an interstitial-type diffuser (P or B) is enhanced over its diffusion under normal, inert conditions (see problem 7.17). We have thus obtained a useful expression for the microscopic parameters of the mobile species that determine the diffusion flux.

7.5.13 Simplified Expression for Modeling

Because the derivative of the natural logarithm of x is $1/x$, we can further simplify the expression in Eq. (7.96) for the flux to

$$F_{AI} = -D_A^*C_A\frac{C_I}{C_I^*}\left[\frac{\partial}{\partial x}\ln(C_AC_I)\right] \tag{7.101}$$

Since C_I^* is a constant, we can include it in the gradient and in doing so we express the flux in terms of the gradient of the supersaturation rather than the absolute number of interstitials, giving

$$F_{AI} = -D_A^* C_A \frac{C_I}{C_I^*}\left[\frac{\partial}{\partial x}\ln\left(C_A \frac{C_I}{C_I^*}\right)\right] \tag{7.102}$$

This is really a nice accomplishment, because we have related the diffusion on an atomic scale to measurable parameters like the overall dopant diffusivity under inert equilibrium conditions, the overall dopant concentration, and the supersaturation of point defects which can be gauged by how much the dopant diffusivity is enhanced over its inert diffusivity. Thus, all the parameters in the equation are susceptible to measurement, even though the equation itself describes the atomic-scale motion of a short-lived intermittently migrating species which is responsible at the atomic scale for the overall motion of the dopant profile.

This expression is almost precisely the equation that is solved in most process simulators, with one omission. We left out the effect of an electric field on the diffusion of the mobile species. This modifies the flux equation for the mobile species to

$$F_{AI} = -d_{AI}\left[\frac{\partial C_{AI}}{\partial x} + \frac{q}{kT}C_{AI}\frac{\partial \psi}{\partial x}\right] \tag{7.103}$$

The potential ψ is given by

$$\psi = -\frac{kT}{q}\ln\frac{n}{n_i} \tag{7.104}$$

Thus, this simply adds another term in $\ln(n/n_i)$ to the overall flux equation, so with the inclusion of the electric field effects it becomes

$$F_{AI} = -D_A^* C_A \frac{C_I}{C_I^*}\left[\frac{\partial}{\partial x}\ln\left(C_A \frac{C_I}{C_I^*}\frac{n}{n_i}\right)\right] \tag{7.105}$$

The overall continuity equation for the dopant that is solved in a process simulator like SUPREM IV (with a similar term for the vacancy fraction of the diffusion flux) is

$$\frac{\partial C_A}{\partial t} = \frac{\partial}{\partial x}D_A^* C_A \frac{C_I}{C_I^*}\left[\frac{\partial}{\partial x}\ln\left(C_A \frac{C_I}{C_I^*}\frac{n}{n_i}\right)\right] \tag{7.106}$$

According to Eq. (7.106), there are three distinct effects that drive the diffusion flux—the gradient in dopant concentration, the gradient in the interstitial supersaturation, and the $\mathcal{E}$ field. The contribution from the point-defect gradient term is often overlooked [the interstitial gradient term in Eq. (7.106)]. The mathematical origin came from the application of the chain rule to the gradient in the mobile species, while the physical interpretation is that areas with high point-defect populations have faster diffusion, so a gradient in point defects can drive a diffusion flux. This cross term is of paramount importance in the neighborhood of point-defect sources and sinks, where point-defect gradients are large. In these cases, it can dominate the overall diffusion of the dopant.

The full implications of this equation were realized only recently [7.30], when the impact of the gradient in point defects on the dopant profiles was shown to be responsible for altered threshold voltages in submicron MOS devices. The damage from implants in the source/drain regions (discussed in Chapter 8) combined with the local sink for point defects under the gate of the MOS device creates large gradients in the point-defect profiles in the channel region. An interesting practical example of this is the reverse short-channel effect in MOS devices, where point defects generated by implant damage in the source/drain regions flow toward the surface sink at the gate oxide interface, thereby creating large point-defect gradients which drive the overall dopant diffusion "uphill" toward the surface. These gradients in point defects drive dopant diffusion in a manner that is unexpected based on a simple application of Fick's law to the gradient in the doping profile itself. But Eq. (7.106) provides a complete description of the microscopic diffusion mechanisms and their otherwise unexpected impact on device operation. A simulation of how gradients in point-defect profiles affect the doping profile in a small MOS device is shown in Figure 7–45. The pileup of dopant under the gate oxide leads to an increase in the threshold voltage which we will discuss in Chapter 8. This effect is captured by the physically based diffusion model we have derived.

7.5.14 Charge State Effects

So far, we have ignored how the charge states of the defects or dopants affect the diffusion process, with the exception of mentioning that the overall concentration dependent dopant diffusivity can be written in the form

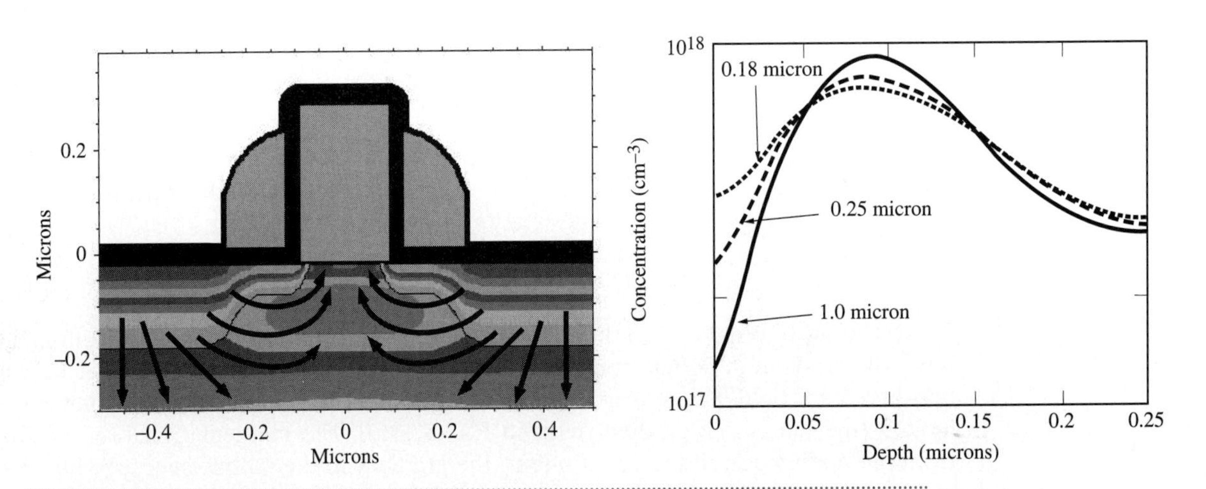

Figure 7–45 TSUPREM IV [7.14] simulation of short-channel MOS devices. The doping profiles are shown on the left with arrows that indicate the interstitial fluxes emanating from the diffusing heavily doped source drain regions. The doping profiles on the right are vertical plots through the center of the channel showing that as the device becomes smaller, more of the channel dopant piles up at the surface.

$$D_A^{\text{eff}} = D^O + D^-\left(\frac{n}{n_i}\right) + D^=\left(\frac{n}{n_i}\right)^2 \quad \text{N type} \tag{7.53}$$

$$D_A^{\text{eff}} = D^O + D^+\left(\frac{p}{n_i}\right) + D^{++}\left(\frac{p}{n_i}\right)^2 \quad \text{P type} \tag{7.54}$$

where each term is thought to originate from atomic-scale interactions with charged point defects.

However, because the dopant concentrations of interest in building devices are usually above the intrinsic concentration, high-concentration effects are often the dominant effect that should be taken into account in describing the diffusion profiles. This rather simplistic observation is the reason that effective diffusivities of the form shown in Eqs. (7.53) and (7.54) had such early success in process modeling programs—they capture the important first-order effects related to concentration-dependent diffusion that determine the shape of the diffused profiles. The concentration of charged point defects depends on the Fermi level. Thus, a deeper understanding of the interactions of dopants and charged defects to form mobile dopant species is required to understand the changes in the diffusion profiles that occur at high doping concentrations in real devices.

Fortunately, the process is very simple to sketch out in our description of the atomic-level transport process. We can take a concrete example of a boron dopant which interacts with an interstitial to form a mobile boron-interstitial species, with no loss of generality. Consider a substitutional boron acceptor (which donates a mobile hole to the electronic structure) that remains negatively charged on its lattice site, where it may interact with either neutral or positive interstitials. If no additional electrons or holes are involved in the reaction, this leads to the following two equations which describe the process:

$$B^- + I^0 \overset{K_A}{\leftrightarrow} BI^- \tag{7.107}$$

$$B^- + I^+ \overset{K_B}{\leftrightarrow} BI^0 \tag{7.108}$$

These two reactions give rise to fluxes of mobile species that we can sum to obtain the overall flux of mobile dopant:

$$F_{BI}^{\text{total}} = F_{BI^-} + F_{BI^0} \tag{7.109}$$

where each flux component can be specified using Fick's laws applied to the mobile species. In this case, we will take into account the effect of the electric field generated by the dopant profile only in the case where the mobile diffusing species is charged.

$$F_{BI^-} = -d_{BI^-}\left(\frac{\partial C_{BI^-}}{\partial x} + C_{BI^-}\frac{\partial}{\partial x}\ln\frac{p}{n_i}\right) \tag{7.110}$$

$$F_{BI^0} = -d_{BI^0}\left(\frac{\partial C_{BI^0}}{\partial x}\right) \tag{7.111}$$

Given the importance of understanding how charge-state information affects the diffusion process, it is desirable to try to connect the atomic-level description to the observed shape of the overall dopant diffusion profile. The assumption that the reaction of point defects and dopants are in chemical equilibrium is useful and is certainly valid for most of the processes of interest in silicon technology. This allows the concentration of the mobile species to be written in terms of the dopant and free point defects as follows:

$$C_{BI^-} = k_A C_{I^0} C_{B^-} \tag{7.112}$$

$$C_{BI^0} = k_B C_{I^+} C_{B^-} \tag{7.113}$$

Another major simplification occurs because electronic processes occur much faster than the atomic jumps that mediate diffusion steps, which occur on a time scale of the Debye frequency for lattice vibrations. Thus, the electronic charging process is fast compared to any of the diffusion processes that occur in silicon. This allows the concentration of defects in the charged state to be directly related to the concentration of neutral defects in the silicon, according to Shockley-Last statistics [7.31]. (See Chapter 3, Section 3.5.4.)

$$C_{I^+} = C_{I^0} \exp\left(\frac{E_F - E_{I^+}}{kT}\right) \tag{7.114}$$

By a similar analysis to the previous charge neutral case, we can show that

$$D_{BI}^{\text{eff}} = D_{BI}^{*} \cdot \frac{\left(1 + \beta \frac{p}{n_i}\right)}{1 + \beta} \cdot \frac{C_{I^0}}{C_{I^0}^{*}} \tag{7.115}$$

where β represents the enhancement in the boron diffusivity due to the Fermi level and is dependent on the diffusivity of the pairs, the concentrations of the pairs, and the energy level of the charged point defect in the bandgap.

Quite a bit of the microscopic physics is lumped into the β constant—it contains information on the diffusivities of the individual charged pairs, the charged concentrations of the native point defects that form the pairs, and the relative concentrations of the pairs in each charge state (through the ratio of the reaction constants). However, it has a very physical interpretation at the macroscopic scale—it simply represents how much the overall diffusivity is enhanced in highly doped regions and was already considered in an empirical model for high concentration diffusivity in Eq. (7.57). Its microscopic origins are now more clearly elucidated.

The overall diffusivity of the mobile boron pairs is thus given by a product of three easily interpreted terms—the intrinsic, inert equilibrium diffusion coefficient that can be measured for low concentration boron profiles, the extent to which this intrinsic diffusion coefficient is enhanced in highly doped material by the Fermi-level, and the supersaturation of interstitials.

The final equation representing the flux which includes all the Fermi-level effects can be written as

$$F_{BI}^{tot} = D_{BI}^{*} \cdot \left(\frac{1 + \beta \frac{p}{n_i}}{1 + \beta} \right) \cdot \frac{C_{I^0}}{C_{I^0}^{*}} \cdot C_{B^-} \frac{\partial}{\partial x} \ln\left(C_{B^-} \frac{C_{I^0}}{C_{I^0}^{*}} \frac{p}{n_i} \right) \tag{7.116}$$

This equation represents a remarkable step in our understanding of dopant diffusion in silicon. What is most interesting is that we started with a detailed atomic-level description of the diffusion by point defects and mobile dopant species in different charge states and ended up with an equation containing only macroscopic terms that can easily be measured experimentally. Each one of the terms represents a distinct physical effect that can easily be investigated experimentally by doing measurements on the total concentration of the dopant, using techniques such as SIMS. This gives us numbers to plug into the equation for parameters like D_{BI}^{*} and β.

But there is a downside to our successful development of Eq. (7.116)—it means that it is very difficult to say anything definite about the underlying atomic-level processes by making macroscopic measurements on the overall dopant motion. Instead, we can try to infer what is happening on an atomic scale by using clever test structures and by comparing and contrasting how different dopants diffuse under various conditions. But in the end, we must build an atomic-scale model for how the dopant moves and see if the equations based on that atomic-scale model are a useful description of the physical world where we make measurements.

7.6 Limits and Future Trends in Technologies and Models

A tremendous amount has been learned in the past 20 years about dopant diffusion and doping profiles in silicon. The simulation tools used today are very powerful and are widely used to develop new generations of technology. While we have focused our discussion on the issues associated with CMOS technology, these tools are also used in many other types of silicon device structures. In many cases they are crucial in reducing the number of experiments required to develop new processes. They are also very useful in understanding process sensitivities and manufacturing tolerances.

The SIA NTRS for mainstream CMOS technology makes it very clear that the main challenges for the future lie in making very shallow junctions to minimize short-channel effects, with low sheet resistances to maximize drive currents. An obvious limit to device scaling occurs when the junctions are so shallow that the doping concentrations are at the solubility limit—making the junctions even shallower only increases the sheet resistance and degrades drive current. Other doped regions (deeper junctions like wells, for example), will continue to be used, but these are easily fabricated with today's technology. There will thus be continued emphasis on understanding dopant diffusion and activation at the atomic level because the shallow doping profiles required in future devices may have metastable activation levels and will have to be controlled almost to the point of knowing where individual doping atoms are located. The physical understanding and the simulation tools described in previous sections will likely not be adequate for these kinds of applications. Thus the sophistication and the complexity of models will likely continue to increase. We describe in this section a few extensions to the technologies and the models described above which indicate some of the directions current research is taking to address these issues.

7.6.1 Doping Methods

Most workers believe that the dominant doping method used today—ion implantation—will continue to dominate in the future. Ion implantation affords tremendous flexibility in terms of the doping species, the physical location of the dopants, and in manufacturing throughput. Deeper doped regions in device structures are straightforward to form by moderate- or high-energy implants. The very shallow junctions required in future devices can be formed by very low energy implants. The only real drawback to this technology is the damage produced by the implantation process and the transient diffusion and extended defects that result when implants are annealed. In order to minimize these effects, rapid thermal processing is likely to dominate annealing and diffusion processing in the future. We will discuss ion implantation and some of the issues associated with extending it to future device fabrication in Chapter 8.

A number of alternative doping methods are currently being investigated and may find some use in the future. These methods range from very old methods like outdiffusion from deposited thin films, to very new processes like laser-assisted annealing or doping. In the latter category, processes such as Gas Immersion Laser Doping (GILD) have been suggested, in which the wafers are placed in a controlled environment containing the dopant in a gas phase. A laser is used to heat the wafer either by scanning the laser beam or selectively using a mask. The dopant is incorporated into a thin surface layer where the silicon is melted by the laser [7.32]. This process can produce ultrashallow junctions, sometimes with very high, metastable active doping concentrations.

7.6.2 Advanced Dopant Profile Modeling—Fully Kinetic Description of Dopant-Defect Interactions

Even more sophisticated models than those described previously may be required for very shallow junctions produced by ion implantation and very short anneals. This is because in our previous modeling, we considered the reaction

$$A + I \leftrightarrow AI \tag{7.117}$$

to be in equilibrium. However, there are experimental hints that the chemical reaction between the dopants and the intrinsic point defects to form the intermediate mobile diffusing species may not be in chemical equilibrium for very short diffusion times at very low temperatures (e.g., 15 minutes at 450°C). The experimental observations show exponential tails on the diffusion profiles, rather than the expected Gaussian profiles, indicating a single hop or migration event for the mobile species [7.33]. A more general description of the diffusion process is to consider that the reaction terms are not yet in chemical equilibrium and are described atomistically by their forward and backward reaction rates, so that the fully kinetic reaction rate is given by

$$R = k_f C_A C_I - k_r C_{AI} \tag{7.118}$$

where k_f and k_r are the forward and reverse reaction rates. The diffusion of the dopant is then atomistically described by a series of reaction-diffusion equations. These are standard rate equations for chemical kinetics.

For example, the substitutional dopant A, which is immobile on an atomic scale, can only decrease its local concentration by reacting with an interstitial in a reaction which is proportional to both the local concentration of A and the local concentration of I,

$$\left.\frac{\partial C_A}{\partial t}\right|_{\text{forward}} = -k_f C_A C_I \tag{7.119}$$

Similarly, it can increase its local concentration by dissociation of the mobile species, that is, if the reaction goes to the left so that

$$\left.\frac{\partial C_A}{\partial t}\right|_{\text{reverse}} = +k_r C_{AI} \tag{7.120}$$

Similar terms govern the time evolution of the mobile species C_{AI} and C_I, with the exception that their time rate of change is also governed by their ability to diffuse. We know how to describe that process by Fick's laws, so that the overall system of reaction-diffusion equations that describes the diffusion process is given by

$$\frac{\partial C_A}{\partial t} = -k_f C_A C_I + k_r C_{AI} \tag{7.121}$$

$$\frac{\partial C_{AI}}{\partial t} = d_{AI}\frac{\partial^2 C_{AI}}{\partial x^2} + k_f C_A C_I - k_r C_{AI} \tag{7.122}$$

$$\frac{\partial C_I}{\partial t} = d_I \frac{\partial^2 C_I}{\partial x^2} - k_f C_A C_I + k_r C_{AI} \tag{7.123}$$

Here, we have assumed that d_{AI} and d_I are both constants. This is a fully kinetic formulation of the diffusion process.

The above example actually considered only a reduced set of the possible reactions that could occur when a particular dopant diffuses. Generalizing these ideas produces a complex set of equations with many parameters which at first glance seems almost intractable. However this approach has been taken successfully in a number of cases in recent years and may be required for more cases in the future. For example, the reactions which are thought to be involved in modeling high-concentration phosphorus diffusion have been solved based on the work of Dunham [7.27] and of Mulvaney and Richardson [7.34]. What is impressive is that a large number of these highly coupled, nonlinear differential equations can be solved numerically and can generate a lot of physical insight into the diffusion process.

One characteristic of the fully kinetic approach is that it contains a large number of parameters. Some method for estimating these parameters must be used, as there is no easy means to directly measure these quantities. Fortunately, chemists have a fundamental interest in reaction rate kinetics and have well developed theories to describe the rate constants of simple reactions.

So, what is really known about the coefficients that are needed to solve these reactions and where does that information come from? About the only thing that is known with certainty is what can be directly measured, that is, the overall diffusion coefficient of a dopant species or of a silicon isotope in the silicon lattice. The goal of the fully kinetic approach to modeling is to estimate the microscopic diffusion parameters (such as the concentration of mobile species and their diffusivities), based on what is known.

Recently, due to breakthrough developments in theoretical methods and the availability of powerful computers, direct quantum mechanical calculations of some of the microscopic parameters have been made. These *ab initio* (from first principles) calculations currently give reliable information for the ground state properties of the system and calculations for the charged states are under development. More approximate quantum mechanical methods (tight-binding methods) allow the silicon lattice defects to be directly simulated at high temperatures, where their migration in the lattice can be observed and values for the diffusivity can be calculated. Such computational approaches will play a more important role in understanding the atomic-level details of the process kinetics in the future. However, the full set of parameters needed for solution of a system of reaction-diffusion equations has been attempted to date only in a few special cases.

7.7 Summary of Key Ideas

Doping of semiconductors is the fundamental process by which devices are fabricated. To make dopants electrically active and therefore useful in devices, they must generally sit on substitutional lattice sites. Both the concentration and the spatial variation (profile) of these dopants are critical to device performance. Diffusion is thus the basic process by which we produce these doping profiles.

Ion implantation is the dominant method used today to introduce dopants into silicon. This process allows precise control of the numbers of doping atoms and their physical position. Annealing and sometimes additional diffusion are required following implantation in order to allow the dopants to diffuse to their final, substitutional lattice sites. For short times, this process is dominated by transients associated with the implantation damage. During this period, the dopant diffusivity is much larger than its equilibrium value because of the high concentration of point defects present. Following this transient, the dopant diffusivity drops to a more reproducible value.

Dopants diffuse in silicon by interacting with point defects through a number of possible atomic-scale mechanisms. The dopant diffusivity is basically proportional to the number of such defects present in a crystal. Point-defect concentrations depend exponentially on temperature and as a result, dopant diffusivities do also. However point-defect concentrations are also changed by Fermi-level effects, by ion implantation damage, and by surface processes like oxidation. The result is that dopant diffusivities may vary spatially and with time during the diffusion of a particular doped region. This greatly complicates the modeling of dopant profiles and generally requires that numerical simulation tools be used to calculate such profiles. Only in the simplest cases in which D is constant can simple analytical solutions be used to calculate impurity profiles.

Much progress has been made in recent years in developing physically based models for dopant diffusion and in implementing these models in simulators. These simulators today allow full coupling of the point defects and the dopants and can accurately predict very complex experimental dopant profiles in silicon. Many complex insights such as point-defect gradient-driven up-hill diffusion and chemical pumping of point defects appear as a trivial consequence of these physically based atomistic models of dopant diffusion. In the future, even deeper understanding of these atomistic mechanisms and more complete models may be required. The reaction-diffusion approach described above is suitable for treating nonlinear processes far from equilibrium (such as transient-enhanced diffusion after ion implantation) and is conceptually simple. It also offers the possibility that theoretical models of reaction pathways (i.e., binding energies and cross sections for reactions) can integrate seamlessly into the overall picture of diffusion in silicon. For these reasons, this description of transport processes is now favored for the silicon system.

7.8 References

[7.1]. R. H. Dennard, F. H. Gaensslen, H. N. Yu, V. L. Rideout, E. Bassous, and A. R. LeBlanc, "Design of Ion-implanted MOSFET's with Very Small Physical Dimensions," *IEEE Journal of Solid State Circuits*, vol. 9, no. 5. p. 256, 1974.

[7.2]. "National Technology Roadmap for Semiconductors," SIA, 1997.

[7.3]. F. A. Trumbore, "Solid Solubilities of Impurity Elements in Germanium and Silicon," *Bell System Technical Journal*, vol. 39, p. 205, 1960.

[7.4]. L. S. Darken and R. W. Gurry, *Physical Chemistry of Metals*, McGraw-Hill, 1953.

[7.5]. J. C. Irving, "Resistivity of Bulk Silicon and Diffused Layers in Silicon," *Bell System Technical Journal*, vol. 41, p. 387, 1962.

[7.6]. R. Alvis, S. Luning, L. Thompson, R. Sinclair, and P. Griffin, "Physical Characterization of Two-dimensional Doping Profiles for Process Modeling," *J. Vac. Sci. Technology B*, vol. 14., no. 1, p. 231.

[7.7]. H. J. Cho, P. B. Griffin, and J. D. Plummer, "Cross sectional TEM Sample Preparation Using e-beam Lithography and Reactive Ion Etching," Paper Z2.18, 1997 MRS Spring Meeting, San Francisco, April 1997.

[7.8]. B. Schwartz and H. Robbins, "Chemical Etching of Silicon. IV. Etching Technology," *Journal of the Electrochemical Society*, vol. 123, no.12, p.1903, 1976.

[7.9]. D. P. Gold, J. H. Wills. G. R. Booker, M. C. Willson, and D. J. Godfrey, *Microscopy of Semiconductor Materials*, edited by A. G. Cullis and J. L. Hutchinson, Institute of Physics Conference Series, vol. 100, p. 537, 1989.

[7.10]. N. Khalil, J. Faricelli, D. Bell, and S. Selberherr, "The Extraction of Two-dimensional MOS Transistor Doping via Inverse Modeling," *IEEE Electron Device Letters*, vol. 16. no. 1. p.17, 1995.

[7.11]. Z. K. Lee, M. B. McIlrath, and D. A. Antoniadis, "Inverse Modeling of MOSFETs Using I-V Characteristics in the Subthreshold Region," *IEDM Technical Digest*, p. 683, 1997.

[7.12]. G. J. L. Ouwerling, "A Problem-specific Inverse Method for Two-dimensional Doping Profile Determination from Capacitance-voltage Measurements," *Solid State Electronics*, vol. 34, no. 2, p. 197, 1991.

[7.13]. SUPREM IV is a computer program written by Mark Law, Conor Rafferty, and Robert Dutton at Stanford University.

[7.14]. TSUPREM IV is the version of SUPREM IV by Avant! Inc.

[7.15]. ATHENA is the version of SUPREM IV by Silvaco Inc.

[7.16]. J. Crank, *The Mathematics of Diffusion*, Oxford University Press, 1979.

[7.17]. R. B. Fair and J. C. C. Tsai, "Theory and Direct Measurement of Boron Segregation in SiO_2 in Dry, Near Dry, and Wet O_2 Oxidation," *J. Electrochem. Soc.*, vol. 125, pp. 2050, 1978.

[7.18]. A. S. Grove, *Physics and Technology of Semiconductor Devices*, John Wiley & Sons, 1967.

[7.19]. R. Kasnavi, P. Pianetta, Y. Sun, R. Mo, P. Griffin, and J. D. Plummer, "Characterization of Arsenic Dose Loss at the Si/SiO2 Interface Using High Resolution X-ray Photoelectron Spectrometry," *IEDM Technical Digest*, p. 721, 1998.

[7.20]. S. M. Hu, private communication.

[7.21]. R. B. Fair, in *Impurity Doping Processes in Silicon*, edited by F. F. Y. Wang, North-Holland, 1981, p. 315.

[7.22]. S. M. Hu, "Formation of Stacking Faults and Enhanced Diffusion in the Oxidation of Silicon," *Journal of Applied Physics*, vol. 45, p. 1567, 1974.

[7.23]. E. A. Perozziello, P. B. Griffin, and J. D. Plummer, "Retarded Diffusion of Sb in a High Concentration as Background During Silicon Oxidation," *Applied Physics Letters*, vol. 61, no. 3. p.303, 1992.

[7.24]. P. M. Fahey, P. B. Griffin, and J. D. Plummer, "Point Defects and Dopant Diffusion in Silicon," *Reviews of Modern Physics*, vol. 61, p. 289, 1989.

[7.25]. S. M. Hu, "Nonequilibrium Point Defects and Diffusion in Silicon," *Materials Science and Engineering*, vol. R13, no. 3–4, pp. 105–192, 1994.

[7.26]. J. Zhu, T. Diaz de la Rubia, L.H. Yang, C. Mailhiot, and G. H. Gilmer, "Ab Initio Pesudopotential Calculations of B Diffusion and Pairing in Si," *Physical Review B*, vol. 54, no. 7, p. 4741, 1996.

[7.27]. S. T. Dunham, "A Quantitative Model for the Coupled Diffusion of Phosphorus and Point Defects in Silicon," *Journal of the Electrochemical Society*, vol. 139, no. 9, p. 2628, 1992.

[7.28]. R. B. Fair, "Explanation of Anomalous Base Regions in Transistors," *Applied Physics Letters*, vol. 22. no. 4. p. 186, 1973.

[7.29]. W. A. Orr Arienzo, R. Glang, R. F. Lever, R. K. Lewis, and F. F. Morehead, "Boron Diffusion in Silicon at High Concentrations," *J. Appl. Phys.*, vol. 63, no. 1, p. 116, 1988.

[7.30]. C. S. Rafferty, H. H. Vuong, S. A. Eshraghi, M. D. Giles, M. R. Pinto, and S. J. Hillenius, "Explanation of Reverse Short Channel Effect by Defect Gradients," *IEDM Technical Digest*, p. 311, 1993.

[7.31]. W. Shockley and J. Last, "Statistics of the Charge Distribution for a Localized Flaw in a Semiconductor," *Phys. Rev.*, vol. 107, p. 392, 1957.

[7.32]. K. H. Weiner, P. G. Carey, A. M. McCarthy, and T. W. Sigmon, "Low-temperature Fabrication of p-n Diodes with 300Å Junction Depth," *IEEE Electron Device Letters*, vol. 13, no. 7, p. 369, 1992.

[7.33]. N.E.B. Cowern, G.F.A. van de Walle, P.C. Zalm, and J.J. Oostra, "Reactions of Point Defects and Dopant Atoms in Silicon," *Physical Review Letters*, vol. 69, no.1, p. 116, 1992.

[7.34]. B. J. Mulvaney and W. B. Richardson, "The Effect of Concentration-dependent Defect Recombination Reactions on Phosphorus Diffusion in Silicon," *Journal of Applied Physics*, vol. 67, no. 6, p. 3197, 1990.

7.9 Problems

7.1. A resistor for an analog integrated circuit is made using a layer of deposited polysilicon 0.5 μm thick, as shown below.

Polysilicon

SiO_2

Si

a. The doping of the polysilicon is 1×10^{16} cm^{-3}. The carrier mobility $\mu = 100$ cm^2 V^{-1} sec^{-1} is low because of scattering at grain boundaries. If the resistor has $L = 100$ μm, $W = 10$ μm, what is its resistance in ohms?

b. A thermal oxidation is performed on the polysilicon for two hours at 900°C in H_2O. Assuming B/A for polysilicon is $^2/_3$ that of <111> silicon, what is the polysilicon thickness that remains?

c. Assuming that all of the dopant remains in the polysilicon (i.e., does not segregate to oxide), what is the new value of the resistor in (a). Assume the mobility does not change.

7.2. A resistor is made as part of a high-frequency analog integrated circuit as shown below. The N$^-$ epi layer forms the body of the resistor. If the width of the resistor in the direction into the paper is 2.5 μm, what should the length X be to give a resistor of approximately 50 kΩ?. The epilayer is doped with phosphorus at a concentration of 1×10^{15} cm^{-3} and is 3 μm thick.

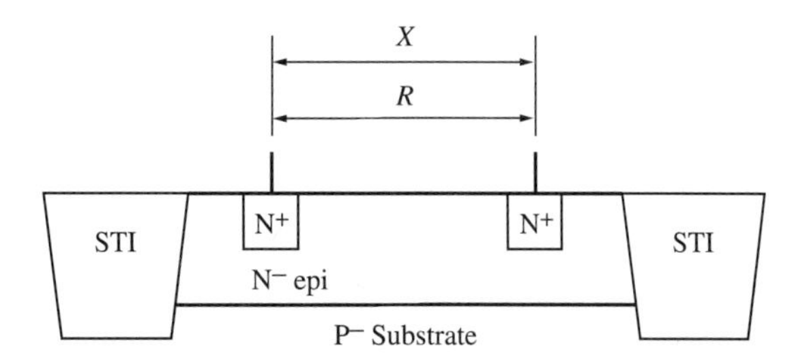

7.3. A p-type (boron) diffusion is performed as follows:
Predep: 30 minutes, 900°C, solid solubility
Drive in: 60 minutes, 1000°C
a. What is the deposited Q?
b. If the substrate is doped 1×10^{15} cm^{-3} phosphorus, what is x_j?
c. What is the sheet resistance of the diffused layer?

7.4. Suppose we perform a solid solubility limited predeposition from a doped glass source which introduces a total of Q impurities / cm^2.
a. If this predeposition were performed for a total of t minutes, how long would it take (total time) to predeposit a total of $3Q$ impurities / cm^2 into a wafer if the predeposition temperature remained constant?
b. Derive a simple expression for the $(Dt)_{\text{drive in}}$ which would be required to drive the initial predeposition of Q impurities / cm^2 sufficiently deep so that the final surface concentration is equal to 1% of the solid solubility concentration. This can be expressed in terms of $(Dt)_{\text{predep}}$ and the solid solubility concentration C_S.

7.5. A diffused region is formed by an ultrashallow implant followed by a drive in. The final profile is Gaussian. Derive a simple expression for the sensitivity of x_j to the implant dose Q. Is x_j more sensitive to Q at high or low doses?

7.6. From a process control point of view, predeposition times > 10 min are required. From an economic point of view, times < 10 hours are required. Equipment limitations restrict $700°C < T < 1200°C$. You need only consider simple Gaussian- and erfc-type profiles in this problem.
a. Is it possible to dope a MOS channel region by predeposition to shift threshold voltages? The required dose is 5×10^{11} cm^{-2}, boron.
b. What would be a reasonable schedule (T, t) for a MOS source drain predep? The required dose is 5×10^{15} cm^{-2}, arsenic. The junction depth cannot be deeper than 0.2 μm for device reasons. Assume the channel doping is 1×10^{18} cm^{-3}.
c. What sheet resistance would your profile in (b) have if the channel doping is 1×10^{18} cm^{-3} P type?

7.7. A boron diffusion is performed in silicon such that the maximum boron concentration is 1×10^{18} cm^{-3}. For what range of diffusion temperatures will electric field effects and concentration-dependent diffusion coefficients be important?

7.8. An N$^+$ region is formed in a P$^-$ substrate with a junction depth is x_j as shown below. For the device being fabricated it is important to minimize the sheet resistance of the N$^+$ region.

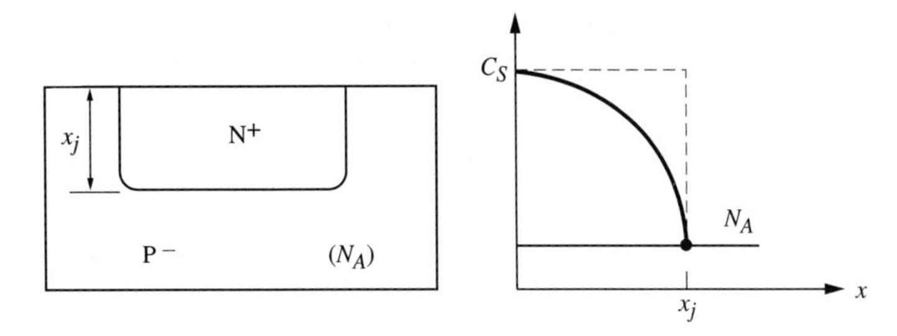

a. If the ideal "box" profile shown could be obtained, it would provide an absolute minimum limit on ρ_s. Derive an approximate expression for this lower bound on ρ_s.

b. If As had been used as the dopant and a metastable doping at the solid solubility of 2×10^{21} cm^{-3} had been obtained in a box-shaped profile by laser melting, estimate the absolute minimum ρ_s for an x_j of 0.1 μm if the limiting carrier mobility in N$^+$ silicon is 85 cm^2 volt^{-1} sec^{-1}.

c. If a normal error function profile were used with the surface at the metastable solid solubility, what value of ρ_s would be realized with an x_j of 0.1 μm?

d. Repeat the calculation in (c) if the arsenic had deactivated to its normal "electrical solubility" in silicon.

7.9. A bipolar transistor is fabricated by implanting the boron base with a dose of $Q_B = 2 \times 10^{13}$ cm^{-2}. Then an in situ arsenic-doped polysilicon emitter region doped at 10^{20} cm^{-3} is deposited on the surface. A drivein is performed for 60 min at 1100°C. Assume that the implant can be treated as a delta function. The substrate is 10^{15} cm^{-3} N type. Calculate the base width of the final NPN bipolar transistor. You can neglect all second-order effects like concentration-dependent diffusion, $\mathcal{E}$-field effects, segregation, rapid diffusion in polysilicon, and so forth.

7.10. A special twin-well (twin-tub) CMOS technology requires that the wells have precisely the same depth at the substrate concentration of 1×10^{15} cm^{-3}, with arsenic used for the n tub and boron used for the p tub. A shallow implant dose of 1×10^{14} cm^2 is used for both and the slow diffusing arsenic is introduced first and partially driven in. Then the boron is introduced and the rest of the anneal is performed until both junctions reach 2.5 microns. Calculate all of the drivein times and temperatures used.

7.11. A process engineer on the day shift started a boron isolation diffusion for a structure in which the boron diffusion needs to penetrate completely through a 6-μm-thick N-type epitaxial layer that is lightly doped with phosphorus ($N_D = 1 \times 10^{15}$ cm^{-3}) on a P-type substrate ($N_A = 1 \times 10^{14}$ cm^{-3}). The purpose of the diffusion is to provide isolation between different N-type regions. The day shift engineer left no information on what he or she did. On a monitor wafer, you make measurements and find that probing between adjacent N-type regions shows they are not isolated from each other and that the sheet resistance between the probes is 20 kΩ. The sheet resistance of the p-type diffusion measured using a four-point probe is 25 Ω/square. What time and temperature are needed to complete the isolation diffusion?

7.12. A bipolar transistor is fabricated by implanting the base and emitter regions and then driving them in together. Boron is used for the base and arsenic for the emitter. The implants are $Q_B = 2 \times 10^{13}$ cm^{-2} and $Q_E = 2 \times 10^{15}$ cm^{-2}. The drive in is 60 min at 1100°C. Assume that the implants can be treated as delta functions at the surface. The substrate is 10^{15} cm^{-3} N type.

a. Calculate and plot the resulting impurity profiles. Assume that the B and As diffusivities are the values from Table 7–5. You can neglect all second order effects like concentration dependent diffusion, $\mathcal{E}$-field effects, and so forth.

b. A parameter of interest in bipolar transistors is the base Gummel number which is the total dose (atoms cm^{-2}) in the base region under the emitter. Estimate this parameter for the device in part (a).

7.13. All semiconductor devices are really "unstable" at device operating temperatures because dopants will continue to diffuse and hence, given long enough, profiles will change and devices will stop functioning correctly. How long would it take at a 150°C operating temperature for the base width in the device in problem 7.12 to double? Assume the As does not move, just the boron moves.

7.14. An epitaxial layer is grown with uniform concentrations of B and P impurities ($B = 2 \times 10^{15}$ cm^{-3}, $P = 1 \times 10^{15}$ cm^{-3}) so that the net doping is p type. The wafer is oxidized at 1000°C for 60 minutes. Approximately (use $2\sqrt{Dt}$ as a measure of the profile motion) sketch the resulting impurity profiles for both boron and phosphorus under the oxide which result from the redistribution that occurs.

7.15. A silicon wafer is uniformly doped with boron (2×10^{15} cm^{-3}) and phosphorus (1×10^{15} cm^{-3}) so that it is net P type. This wafer is then thermally oxidized to grow about 1 μm of SiO_2. The oxide is then stripped and a measurement is made to determine the doping type of the wafer surface. Surprisingly it is found to be N type. Explain why the surface was converted from P to N type. *Hint*: Consider the segregation behavior of dopants when silicon is oxidized.

7.16. An engineer wants to use analytical solutions to diffusion equations in a programmable calculator to make rapid estimates for process changes on junction depths. Consider the following possible diffusion regimes: (a) high temperatures, (b) low temperatures, (c) long times, (d) short times. Which of them are most appropriate for analytical solutions (i.e., which would minimize $\mathcal{E}$-field or concentration-dependent effects). Explain.

7.17. A shallow phosphorus implant with a dose of 1×10^{14} cm^{-2} is covered in some regions with a deposited layer of inert nitride. An anneal is performed at 1000°C in dry O_2 and a junction depth below the original surface is measured in the inert region of 0.5 μm and of 1.2 μm under the oxidizing region. What is that diffusivity enhancement that the phosphorus in the oxidizing region experiences? If f_I for phosphorus is 0.9 and I-V recombination is efficient at 1000°C, what is the interstitial supersaturation that is generated by the oxidation?

7.18. Rapid Thermal Annealing (RTA) systems are becoming common for activating dopants. Silicon has quite a high thermal diffusivity of 0.88 cm^2 sec^{-1}, which describes how fast heat flows through silicon. Calculate the time required for a silicon wafer of thickness 500 μm to reach a constant temperature if a thin surface layer absorbs all the incident light and quickly reaches a reaches a steady-state temperature of T_S, that is, when does the center reach $T/T_S = 0.5$, since the wafer is heated from both sides?

7.19. By using Eq. (7.72) ($C_I C_V = C_I^* C_V^*$) and letting $C_V/C_V^* = x$, solve for x and use the fact that the solution must be real and positive to derive Eq. (7.73). Using the fact that $f_I = 1 - f_V$ and completing the square simplifies the solution. Alternatively, use Eq. (7.72) to substitute for C_V/C_V^* in Eq. (7.66) and take the derivative with respect to C_I/C_I^* and find an extreme (maximum or minimum).

7.20. Figure 7–38 shows that a wet oxidation produces a significantly higher C_I/C_I^* than does a dry O_2 oxidation. Explain quantitatively why this should be the case.

Ion Implantation

8

8.1 Introduction

Ion implantation has been the dominant doping technique for silicon ICs for the past 20 years. It is expected to retain this position of dominance for the foreseeable future. In this process, dopant ions are accelerated to hundreds or thousands of volts of energy and smashed into a perfect silicon lattice, creating a cascade of damage that may displace a thousand silicon atoms for each implanted ion. It is the purpose of this chapter to understand how such an energetic and violent technique has become the dominant and preferred method of doping silicon wafers in manufacturing. At first glance, it seems that the technique would not be of much use in the precise art of fabricating integrated circuits. Indeed, although the original patent for ion implantation was issued to William Shockley in 1954, it was not until the late seventies that ion implantation was used in manufacturing. To appreciate the power of the technique, we will investigate its ability to control precisely the distribution and dose of various dopants in the silicon and examine how the implant damage is annealed and how the dopant is introduced to active sites in the silicon lattice.

8.2 Historical Development and Basic Concepts

Ion implantation provides a very precise means to introduce a specific dose or number of dopant atoms into the silicon. The reason this is possible is because the electrical charge on the ion allows them to be counted by collection in a Faraday cup. Electrical measurements are very precise, so numbers of dopant atoms ranging from 1×10^{12} cm^{-2} to 1×10^{16} cm^{-2} are routinely introduced during the fabrication of a MOS device, and even lower and higher doses are possible. To increase the dose simply requires a longer implant time or a higher beam current. This allows subtle tailoring of implant doses for such critical steps as the threshold adjusting implant in a MOS device or the base dose in a bipolar device. This and other applications were illustrated in the CMOS process flow in Chapter 2. For example, Figures 2–22 and 2–23 illustrated threshold adjusting implants.

In spite of the precision with which the dose can be controlled, at its heart ion implantation is a random process, because each ion follows a random trajectory, scattering off the lattice silicon atoms before losing its energy and coming to rest at some location as illustrated in Figure 8–1. The reason the technique can be used successfully is because large numbers of ions are implanted so an average depth for the implanted dopants can be calculated.

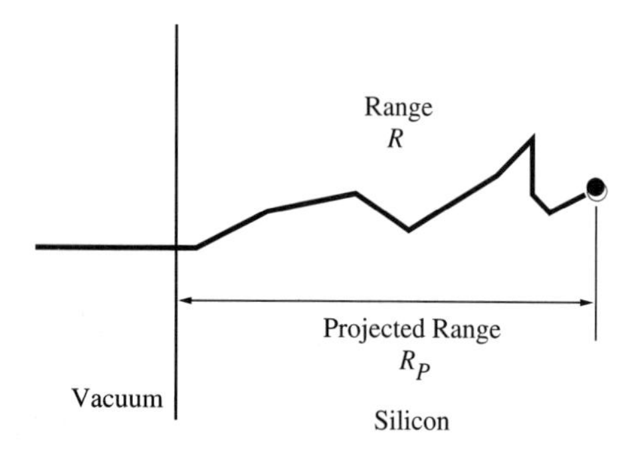

Figure 8–1 Schematic of the actual range of an implanted ion and the projected range normal to the surface. The projected range describes the peak of the implanted profile.

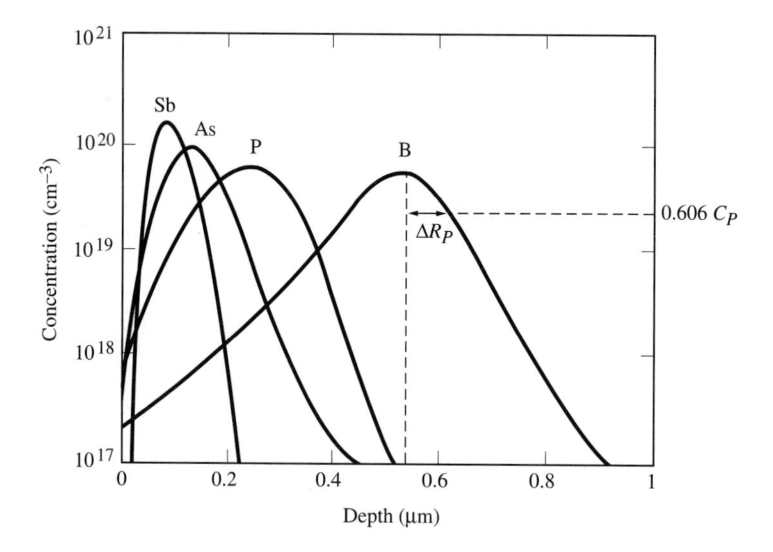

Figure 8–2 Distribution of ions implanted into crystalline silicon at an energy of 200 keV. The light ions travel further and have a broader distribution than the heavy ions.

The first step is to investigate the distribution of ions implanted at a given energy. Heavy ions like antimony do not travel as far in the crystal as light ions like boron. If different ions are implanted with the same energy, the heavy ions stop at a shallower depth, as shown in Figure 8–2. The projected range R_P depends on the energy that is used for the implant, with higher energies giving a deeper range. While each implanted ion itself follows a random trajectory with a range R, on average the distribution of a large group of ions will peak at a projected depth R_P below the surface of the wafer. Because of the random nature of the process, some ions will stop sooner because of more collisions, while some will travel further. The spread of the ions depends on the range traveled with deeper ranges allowing for more random stopping events. This gives rise to a distribution of ions where most of the ions are within a standard deviation $\pm\Delta R_P$ of the projected range. The heavy ions with the smaller range have a more narrow distribution than the light ions.

Since the number of ions implanted is usually greater than 10^{12} cm^{-2}, the distribution can be described statistically and is often modeled to first order by a symmetric Gaussian distribution given by

$$C(x) = C_p \exp\left(- \frac{(x - R_P)^2}{2\Delta R_P^2} \right) \tag{8.1}$$

where R_P is the average projected range normal to the surface, ΔR_P is the standard deviation or straggle about that range, and C_p is the peak concentration where the Gaussian is centered. Figure 8–3 plots the range and standard deviation for common dopants in silicon. Note that the profiles in Figure 8–2 are not perfectly symmetrical. We will return to these details later.

The total number of ions implanted is defined as the dose and is simply

$$Q = \int_{-\infty}^{\infty} C(x)dx \tag{8.2}$$

Making use of the fact that the sum (or integral) of Gaussian functions is an error function (Chapter 7), and using the formula which defines the error function gives

$$\int_{-\infty}^{\infty} \exp^{-u^2} du = \frac{\sqrt{\pi}}{2}[\text{erf}(\infty) - \text{erf}(-\infty)] \tag{8.3}$$

so that

$$Q = \sqrt{2\pi}\Delta R_P C_P \tag{8.4}$$

This provides a useful relationship between the dose and the peak concentration of the implant. The range and standard deviation for typical dopants in silicon have been measured and tabulated.

So far, we have considered a blanket implant over the whole silicon surface. It is interesting to think about what the implant profile would look like if we left the beam centered on a particular spot ($x,y,z = 0,0,0$). The distribution of 1000 ions implanted at a random position in a silicon unit cell centered at (0,0,0) is shown in Figure 8–4.

The side view shows the depth distribution of the ions which is approximated by Eq. (8.1), with a projected range of 50 nm and a straggle about the projected range of 20 nm. The beam direction view shows that the ions scatter laterally around the impact point centered at ($y,z = 0,0$). This lateral distribution around the peak can also be described statistically by a Gaussian distribution with a lateral straggle $\Delta R_\perp$ replacing the vertical straggle. Most of the time we are not concerned with implanting at one spot on a wafer, but we are very interested in implanting in a window with the surrounding areas masked from the implant. The two-dimensional projection near the window edge is of interest, because it indicates how many of the ions scatter under the window because of the lateral straggle. Because it is very difficult to experimentally measure lateral dopant profiles, the two-dimensional distribution is often assumed to be composed of just the product of the vertical and lateral distributions, so that

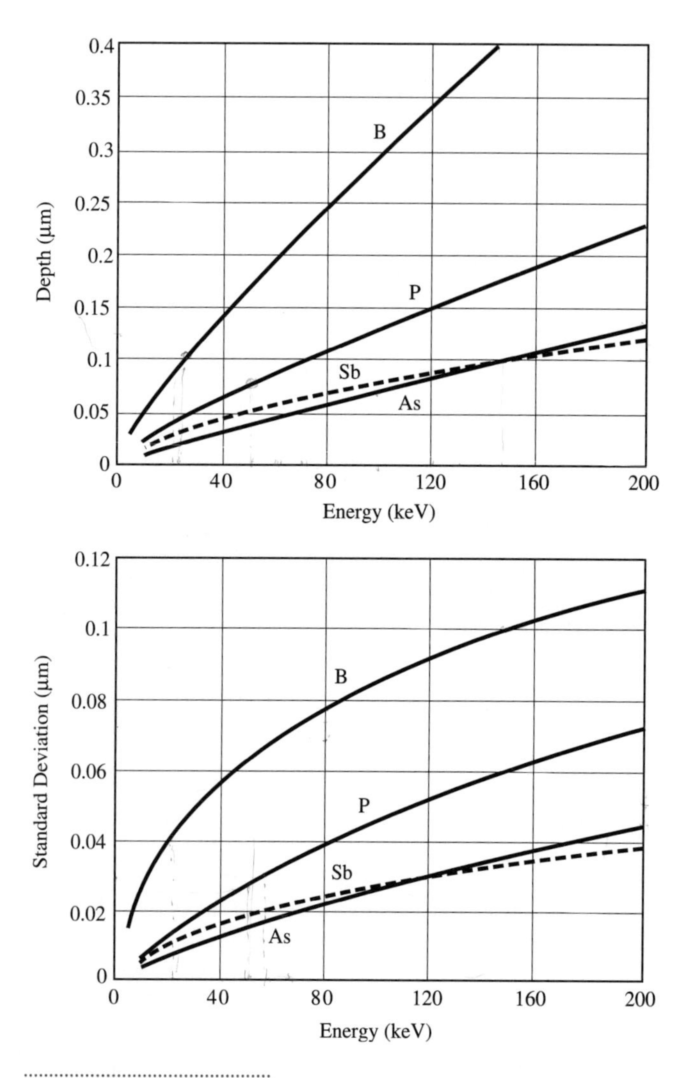

Figure 8–3 Plot of the range R_P (top) and standard deviation ΔR_P (bottom) of common dopants in crystalline silicon tilted and rotated to simulate a random direction. (After [8.1].)

$$C(x,y) = C_{\text{vert}}(x) \exp\left(-\frac{y^2}{2\Delta R_\perp^2}\right) \tag{8.5}$$

Any layer thick enough to capture the implanted ions can be used as a masking layer. For example, photoresist is often used as a convenient mask, because implants are performed at room temperature. Near a mask edge, the profile is dominated by the lateral straggle and is given by a sum of point response functions with the Gaussian form of Eq. (8.5). This means that the profile under a mask edge, such as under the gate

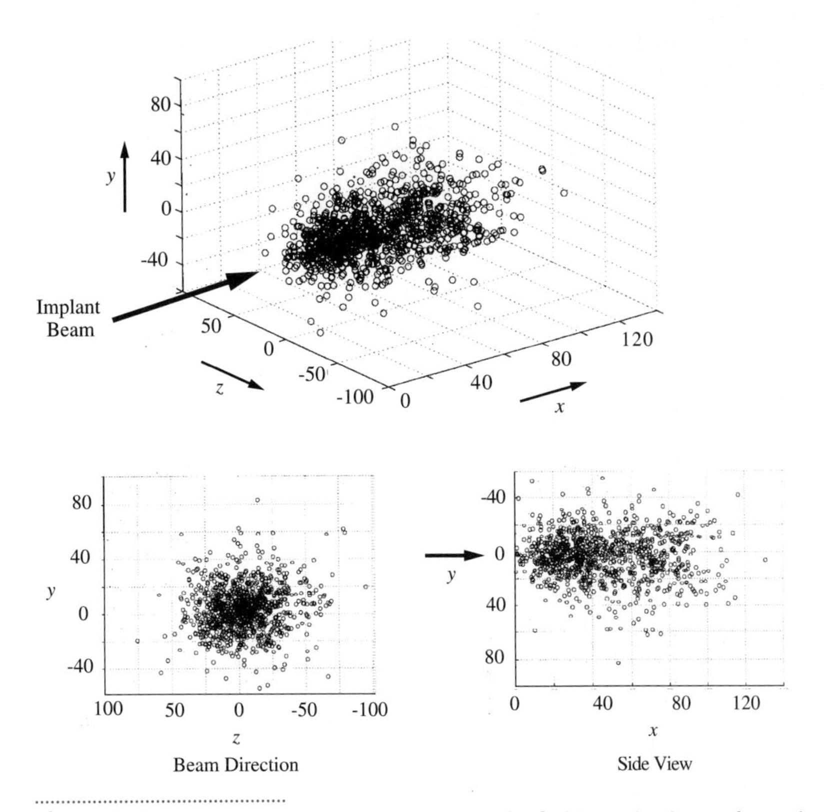

Figure 8–4 Monte Carlo simulations using UT-Marlowe [8.2] of the 3D distribution of 1000 phosphorus ions implanted at 35 keV. The 2D projection (side view) and top view are also shown. The implant beam is centered at (y,z = 0,0) and the axes are in units of nm.

of a MOS transistor, can be dominated by the lateral straggle of the implant and by how far this moves during subsequent annealing. With decreasing device geometries, the implant straggle under the mask edge is becoming a more important feature in modern MOS devices.

How thick does a masking layer have to be to block the transmission of ions through the mask? The range can be measured in different materials and denser materials have better masking properties. The range and standard deviation are very similar in silicon and silicon dioxide, while a thin layer of metal or a thick photoresist layer could efficiently mask an implant. In order to act as an efficient mask, the thickness of the mask should be large enough that the tail of the implant profile in the silicon is at some specified background concentration as illustrated in Figure 8–5. We will use a superscript * to identify the ranges and standard deviations in the masking material, since they will in general be different from those in the silicon. Then, the criterion for efficient masking is that

$$C^*(x_m) = C_P^*\left(\exp - \frac{(x_m - R_P^*)^2}{2\Delta R_P^{*2}}\right) \leq C_B \tag{8.6}$$

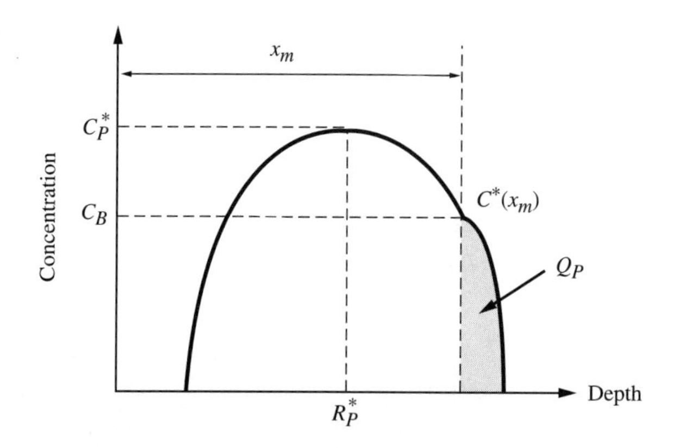

Figure 8–5 Schematic of a masking process, where a dose Q_P penetrates the mask of thickness x_m.

where $C^*(x_m)$ is the concentration at the far side of a mask of thickness x_m and C_B is the background concentration in the substrate. Setting $C^*(x_m) = C_B$ and solving for the mask thickness gives

$$x_m = R_P^* + \Delta R_P^* \sqrt{2\ln\left(\frac{C_P^*}{C_B}\right)} = R_P^* + \mathrm{m}\Delta R_P^* \tag{8.7}$$

where the parameter m indicates that the mask thickness should be equal to the range plus some multiple m times the standard deviation in the masking material. Values of m for different levels of masking efficiency can easily be calculated from this equation.

If Q_P is the dose that penetrates the mask (the dashed area in Figure 8–5), then

$$Q_P = \frac{Q}{\sqrt{2\pi}\Delta R_P^*} \int_{x_m}^{\infty} \exp - \left[\frac{x - R_P^*}{\sqrt{2}\,\Delta R_P^*}\right]^2 dx \tag{8.8}$$

Since the integral or
sum of Gaussian functions can be described as an error function, where

$$\int_d^{\infty} \exp(-u^2)du = \frac{\sqrt{\pi}}{2}\mathrm{erfc}(u) \tag{8.9}$$

the dose that penetrates is

$$Q_P = \frac{Q}{2}\mathrm{erfc}\left(\frac{x_m - R_P^*}{\sqrt{2}\,\Delta R_P^*}\right) \tag{8.10}$$

One case of practical interest which involves both of the previous calculations is the case where the mask edge is tapered or the implant is performed at a tilted angle. In these cases, the mask is not perfectly efficient and the distribution near the mask edge is more complex. An experimental result of etch delineated dopant contours under the gate of a MOS device was shown in Figure 7–21. Note in that figure that the dopant profile extends under the edge of the polysilicon gate.

Example A process engineer building an NMOS device wants to dope the polysilicon at the same time as doing the arsenic source/drain diffusion. The source drain implant dose is 2×10^{15} cm^{-2} at an energy of 50 keV. (a) For the above implant conditions, what is the minimum polysilicon thickness that can be used if the implant is not to affect the channel doping which is 1×10^{16} cm^{-3} near the surface? (Assume the gate oxide is negligibly thick compared to the polysilicon.) (b) Assuming that this polysilicon thickness is actually used, how much of the implant dose will penetrate the polysilicon mask if the process engineer decides to change the implant energy to 80 keV?

Answer (a) From Figure 8–3, 50-keV arsenic has a range of 35 nm and a standard deviation of 15 nm, so the implant profile in the polysilicon is equal to the channel profile when

$$C(x_m) = 1 \times 10^{16} = \frac{Q}{\sqrt{2\pi}\Delta R_P} \exp\left[-\frac{(x_m - R_P)^2}{2\Delta R_P^2}\right]$$

$$C(x_m) = 1 \times 10^{16} = \frac{2 \times 10^{15}}{\sqrt{2\pi}(150 \times 10^{-8})} \exp\left[-\frac{(x_m - (350 \times 10^{-8}))^2}{2(150 \times 10^{-8})^2}\right]$$

$$\therefore x_m = 10.5 \times 10^{-6} \text{ cm} = 0.105 \mu\text{m}$$

(b) If the implant energy is raised to 80 keV, the range from Figure 8–3 is 55 nm and the standard deviation on the implant is 22.5 nm. The dose that penetrates the mask of thickness $x_m = 0.105$ μm is

$$Q_P = \frac{Q}{2} \text{erfc}\left[\frac{x_m - R_P^*}{\sqrt{2}\Delta R_P^*}\right]$$

$$Q_P = \frac{2 \times 10^{15}}{2} \text{erfc}\left[\frac{0.105 \times 10^{-4} - 550 \times 10^{-8}}{\sqrt{2} \times (225 \times 10^{-8})}\right]$$

$$= 1 \times 10^{15}(1 - \text{erf}(1.571)) = 2.7 \times 10^{13} \text{ cm}^{-2}$$

In the general case in which the mask edge is not vertical or an angled implant is performed, numerical methods must be used to calculate the 2D doping profile. There may be reasons to use a high-angle implant to try to introduce dopants underneath the gate in a MOS device. For example, in order to minimize short-channel effects in small

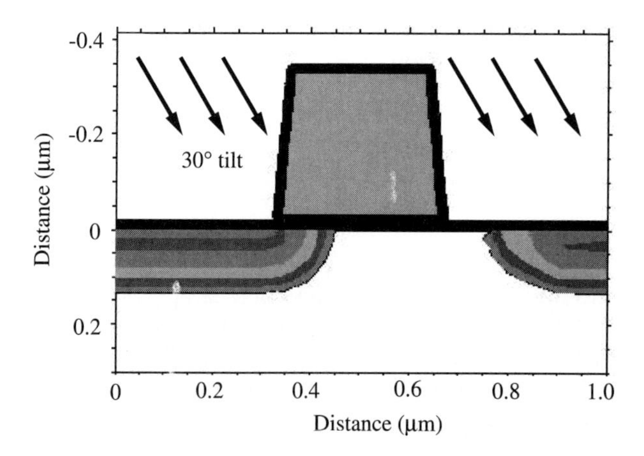

Figure 8–6 TSUPREM IV [8.1] simulation of a 50-keV phosphorus implant at a high-tilt angle of 30°, showing the asymmetrical implant distribution and the shadowing cause by the gate polysilicon.

devices, some doping may be introduced below the tip extension region under the gate. This "halo" of doping is formed by a high-tilt implant under the edge of the gate. Tilted implants can cause shadowing effects due to the topography already on the wafer. A numerical simulation of a tilted implant near a mask edge is shown in Figure 8–6, which clearly shows the asymmetric distribution and the shadowing caused by the gate polysilicon thickness. To get a symmetrical distribution on all devices, the wafer is often rotated during the implant or is implanted at four separate rotations. To completely avoid shadowing effects requires that the implant be performed at a zero-tilt angle.

To understand how these implanted profiles evolve in time during subsequent annealing, we can compare the Gaussian formulation from the implant distribution with that from a delta-function distribution that has diffused. The solutions for both Gaussian distributions in a semi-infinite medium are

$$C(x) = C_p \exp\left(-\frac{(x-R_p)^2}{2\Delta R_p^2}\right) \quad \Leftrightarrow \quad C(x) = C(0)\exp\left(-\frac{x^2}{4Dt}\right) \tag{8.11}$$

Implanted Diffused

By comparing these solutions, we can see that an implanted Gaussian profile with a standard deviation ΔR_p has the same form as an initial delta-function distribution that has diffused for an effective time-temperature cycle of $\Delta R_p = \sqrt{2Dt}$. Because we simply add successive Dt cycles to predict how a diffused profile continues to evolve with time (Section 7.2.9 in Chapter 7), we can easily consider the effect of additional time-temperature cycles on the implanted Gaussian distribution by using the formula

$$C(x,t) = \frac{Q}{\sqrt{2\pi(\Delta R_p^2 + 2Dt)}} \exp\left(-\frac{(x-R_p)^2}{2(\Delta R_p^2 + 2Dt)}\right) \tag{8.12}$$

From this, it is clear that a Gaussian remains a Gaussian and that it preserves its shape upon further annealing in an infinite medium although its standard deviation or straggle about the peak concentration increases with the diffusion distance as shown in Figure 8–7.

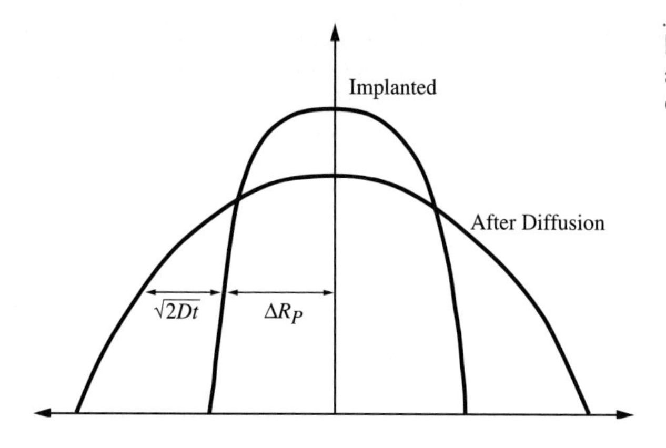

Figure 8–7 Evolution of a Gaussian profile after annealing. The Gaussian preserves its shape as it diffuses in an infinite medium.

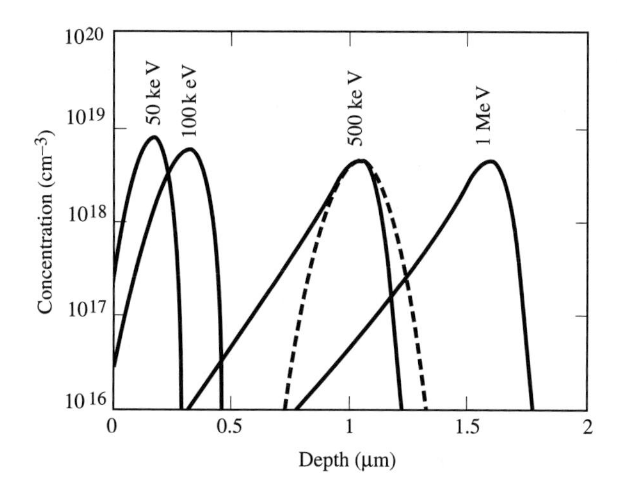

Figure 8–8 TSUPREM IV [8.1] simulated profiles of boron implanted into amorphous or polycrystalline silicon at a range of energies. The profiles show a noticeable skew toward the surface because of backscattering of the light boron ions. These skewed profiles are described by a four-moment Pearson distribution. A Gaussian fit to the profile at 500 keV is shown as a dashed line and only matches the peak of the profile. (After [8.3].)

While these Gaussian distributions are very simple mathematically, we find experimentally that they often only match the central (peak) region of the implanted profiles, while there are significant deviations in the tails of the distributions. For example, in Figure 8–8, the boron distribution is skewed toward the surface and a Gaussian profile provides a good fit only near the peak of the distribution.

We can understand this physically by considering how light ions like boron scatter off silicon atoms compared with how heavy atoms like arsenic scatter off silicon atoms. There is a greater tendency for light ions to backscatter and fill in the front side of the distribution and vice versa for heavy ions. Figure 8–9 shows how dramatic this effect can be for light and heavy ions implanted into amorphous silicon. Clearly, to accurately describe implanted profiles, higher-order moments other than the range and standard deviation are needed.

An arbitrary distribution can be described by a series of moments. The normalized first moment is the projected range and is given by

$$R_p = \frac{1}{Q}\int_{-\infty}^{\infty} xC(x)dx \tag{8.13}$$

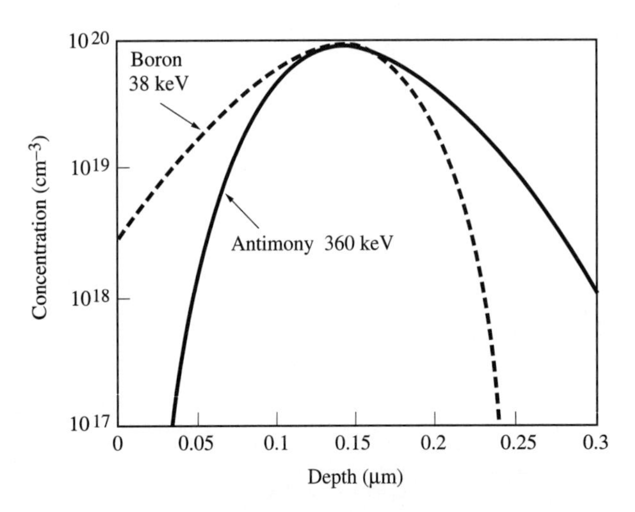

Figure 8–9 TSUPREM IV simulation [8.1] of ion-implanted boron and antimony profiles with the implant energy adjusted to give the same range. The light boron ion skews toward the surface while the heavy antimony ion skews toward the bulk.

The second moment is the straggle or standard deviation

$$\Delta R_p = \sqrt{\frac{1}{Q}\int_{-\infty}^{\infty} (x - R_P)^2\, C(x)dx} \tag{8.14}$$

The third moment describes the skewness and is given by

$$\gamma = \frac{\int_{-\infty}^{\infty} (x - R_p)^3 C(x)dx}{Q\Delta R_p^3} \tag{8.15}$$

and the fourth moment is the kurtosis

$$\beta = \frac{\int_{-\infty}^{\infty} (x - R_p)^4 C(x)dx}{Q\Delta R_p^4} \tag{8.16}$$

These four moments can be used to get a more accurate description of a wide range of implanted species in silicon. The integral representation of the moments is not particularly convenient, so in practice the equivalent moments are described by coefficients in a functional form known as Pearson's equation. Tabulated values of the moments can then be used to generate a profile. A plot of the first two moments for the common dopants was shown in Figure 8–3.

At this stage, we have an accurate description of implanted profiles in an amorphous or random silicon matrix, perhaps capped with an amorphous masking material like oxide or nitride. This provides a useful description for implants in amorphous silicon and fine-grain polycrystalline silicon. The description can also be applied to crystalline silicon if care is taken to make the substrate appear amorphous by tilting and rotating the wafer. However, the level of sophistication needed in describing implant profiles in most devices requires that we consider the atomic-scale structure of the silicon lattice to accurately describe profiles.

8.2.1 Implants in Real Silicon—The Role of the Crystal Structure

One crucial property of real silicon wafers that we have ignored is the crystalline symmetry of the lattice which leads to planar and axial channels that can have quite dramatic effects on the implant profile. Images from a silicon crystal viewed in different directions are shown in Figure 8–10, showing some of the different channels that exist and including a "random" orientation where the crystal appears amorphous. Even a wafer tilted and rotated to appear amorphous, as in Figure 8–10, can allow a scattered ion to enter the channels which, of course, continue to exist no matter how we rotate the crystal in space.

Most of the scattering events that do occur are through relatively small angles, so that a tilt and rotation can minimize the number of ions that immediately find the relatively open channels in the silicon lattice. However, once an ion does enter a channel, the small-angle scattering events from the atoms that line the walls of the channel mean that the ion can be steered quite a long distance along the channel before coming to rest from the electronic drag forces or from a sharp collision that causes the ion to exit the channel. The effect of channeling on the implant profile is to cause a tail that continues

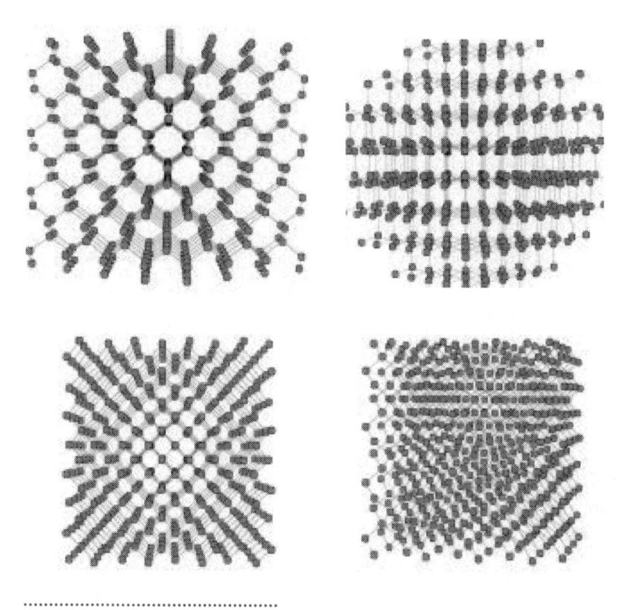

Figure 8–10 Image of a silicon crystal looking down the 110 axial channels (top left), the 111 planar channels (top right), the 100 axial channels (lower left), and with a tilt and rotation to simulate a "random" direction (lower right).

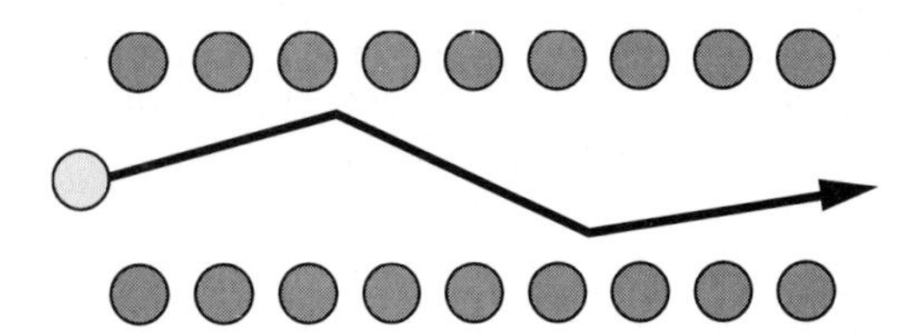

Figure 8–11 Schematic of a channeling direction in silicon where an ion undergoes many small-angle deflections.

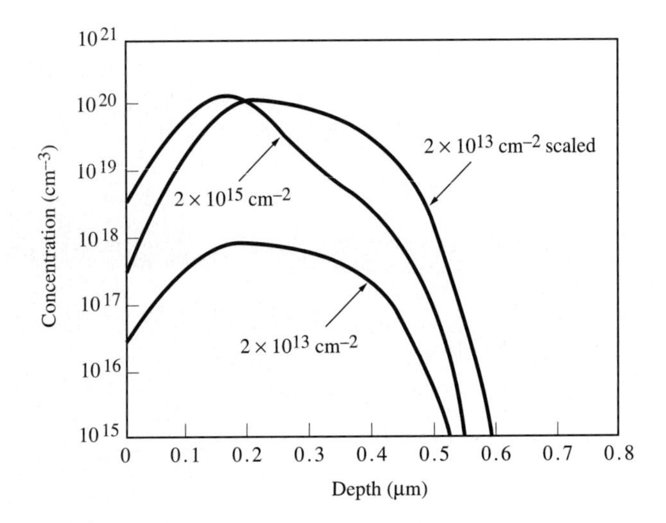

Figure 8–12 TSUPREM IV simulations [8.1] of boron profiles implanted into <100> crystalline silicon wafers with zero tilt and rotation. The implant energy is 35 keV. Note the deep channeling tails in crystalline silicon, which depend on the implant dose, in marked contrast with Figure 8–8 (After [8.4] and C.S. Rafferty [private communication].)

much further than expected. Small-angle scattering from silicon channels is depicted in Figure 8–11.

If we examine the channeled profiles in Figure 8–12, they appear to be composed of two portions, one corresponding to the main peak and the other corresponding to the channeled part. Note that the origin of this skewed tail is different from the skewness caused by heavy ions being implanted in amorphous silicon. In the case of crystalline silicon, it is due to some fraction of the ions entering channels in the silicon lattice and traveling further because of fewer collisions with lattice atoms. However, it has a similar effect in that it modifies the profile so that it requires higher-order moments to fit it. The effects of channeling in Figure 8–12 are so severe that two distributions are required to fit the profiles—one distribution to describe the main part of the profile and another to describe the channeled part of the profile. This leads to a dual-Pearson approach to modeling implant profiles in crystalline silicon, with an additional parameter to specify the ratio of the dose in the main and channeled profiles. A further parameter is needed to describe the dose dependence that is present in the profiles. As shown in

Figure 8–12, simply scaling up a low-dose implant does not give the same profile as a high-dose implant. As the crystal gets damaged by the implanted ions, the channels are less evident to subsequent incoming ions. Relatively speaking, higher implanted doses are less prone to channeling effects.

To attempt to minimize channeling, a thin screen oxide which is amorphous is often used, causing some randomization of the incident beam before it enters the lattice. For example, this was done in the implants used in the CMOS process in Chapter 2. A complete description of the implanted profile requires that the effect of the thickness of the screen oxide on the Pearson parameters be included. Finally, this functional form should be tabulated for each tilt and rotation angle that is likely to be used, because the distributions in the channels clearly vary depending on the orientation of the wafer.

Though tabulating all possible parameters that affect implant profiles is a tedious task, it does provide simulation programs with the ability to use a look-up table of coefficients and to estimate the shape of a profile for various implant conditions. Because of extensive characterization using SIMS, the implanted profiles can be well modeled in crystalline silicon for blanket implants.

Often however, the two-dimensional distribution of the ions near a mask edge is critical for device performance. To illustrate the complexity of this task, several different implant models are compared in Figure 8–13. The profile is shown close to a polysilicon gate edge coated with a thin liner oxide (similar to the structure in Figure 7–21). Three of the models use look-up tables of varying complexity, while the fourth model takes a more atomistic view of the implant process. The disagreement between the phenomenological models is perhaps expected, as they are usually calibrated to one-dimensional SIMS data and the lateral straggle is arbitrarily taken to be some fraction of the vertical straggle. Implanting near a mask edge may cause an ion to travel through multiple different layers (thin spacer, polysilicon, gate oxide) before ever entering the silicon and all of these affect the ion's trajectory, particularly in the lateral direction. The biggest problem in verifying which model is correct is that two-dimensional measurements of doping profiles are very difficult, although one-dimensional measurements in large areas using SIMS are easy. Recent developments in 2D dopant profiling such as scanning capacitance microscopy (Figure 7–23) will help to resolve these issues however.

It is at this stage that the phenomenological description of the implanted profiles becomes insufficient to describe many of the effects that are crucial for VLSI processes. Of particular importance is how well the lateral profile under a mask edge is modeled by these ad hoc descriptions. In order to achieve an adequate description, an atomic-scale view of the implant process will be discussed in the modeling section.

8.3 Manufacturing Methods and Equipment

Conventional ion implanters have much in common with linear accelerators. Indeed, the early history of ion implantation made much progress when research in nuclear physics shifted to such high energies that laboratory machines were no longer useful and were instead used to investigate the relatively low energies of ion-solid interactions that are useful for ion implantation. A schematic of an ion implanter is shown in Figure 8–14.

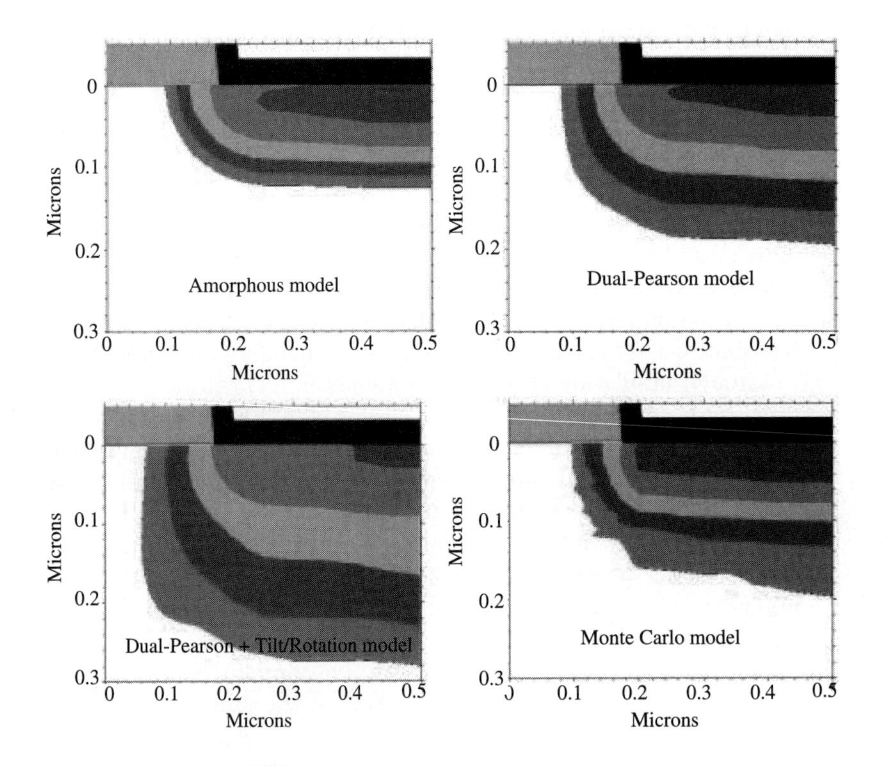

Figure 8–13 TSUPREM IV [8.1] implant simulations using four different implant models of varying complexity. The implant contours are shown near a polysilicon gate edge (thick enough to block the implant) coated with a thin oxide layer. Only the Monte Carlo model considers the atomic structure of the silicon lattice in detail, a factor which is lacking in the other models which use tabulated coefficients for Gaussian, dual Pearson, or dual Pearson with a tilt/rotation dependence.

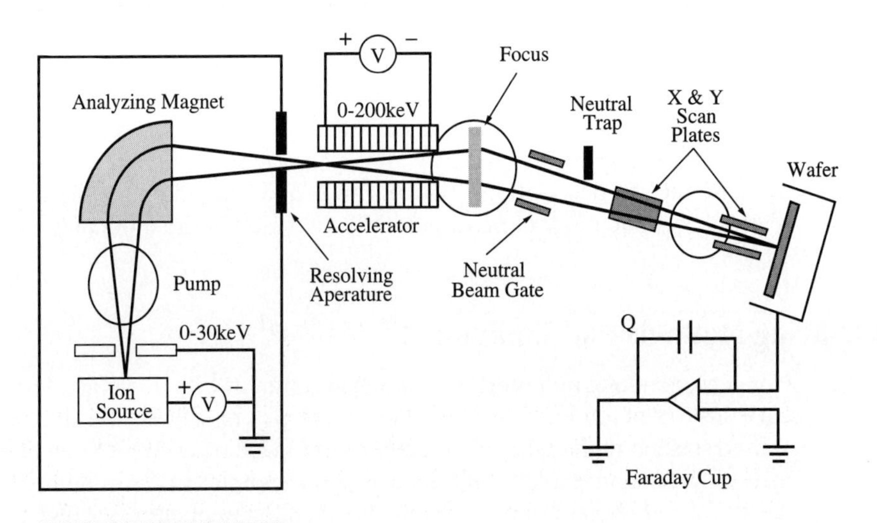

Figure 8–14 Schematic of an ion implanter.

The basic requirement is a source of ions of sufficiently high density to be useful. Either a solid source that is vaporized or a gas source is conventionally used to deliver the material to the ion implanter. Arsine, phosphine, and BF_2 gas sources are extremely toxic and have historically been used in dilute mixtures (15% in H_2) in high-pressure (> 400 psi) cylinders. Because of safety concerns, solid sources of elemental arsenic or phosphorus are sometimes preferred. The advantage of a solid feed source is that any element can be vaporized and implanted. New gas source systems use a zeolite matrix which acts as a molecular sieve to adsorb and store the gas in cylinders below atmospheric pressure, neatly avoiding the possibility of high-pressure rupture and release. Even a catastrophic failure releases gas at a rate driven only by molecular diffusion. These gaseous systems allow rapid beam tuning, which is important if multiple implants are to be performed through a single mask.

The gas from the feed source is ionized by energetic electrons boiled off a hot filament or by a plasma discharge. The ions are extracted by a voltage bias on a grid and mass analyzed to select only one ion species and perhaps even a single isotope of an ion species. This mass analysis is necessary because a gas like BF_2, for example, will dissociate into many ions such as B^{++}, B^+, F^+, BF^+, and BF_2^+ for both the boron mass-10 and mass-11 isotopes. The mass analysis relies on balancing the force exerted on the charged ions in a magnetic field with their centrifugal force, so that the path of the ion is given by the solution of the equation

$$\frac{mv^2}{R} = q \cdot \vec{v} \times \vec{B} \tag{8.17}$$

where m is the mass of the ion, q is the charge on the ion, v is the ion velocity, R is the radius of curvature, and B is the magnetic field intensity. The magnetic field intensity depends directly on the current in the electromagnet coils, so that $B = \alpha I$ where α depends on the magnet design. Because the magnetic field is designed to be perpendicular to the ion velocity, $|\vec{v} \times \vec{B}| = vB$. The ion velocity is related to the extraction voltage by

$$v = \sqrt{\frac{2E}{m}} = \sqrt{\frac{2qV_{ext}}{m}} \tag{8.18}$$

The field can be tuned to allow an ion of particular mass m to exactly follow an arc of radius r and exit the analyzer through a narrow slit. Using the above equations, we can show that

$$\sqrt{m} = \frac{q}{\sqrt{2E}}(\alpha r)I \tag{8.19}$$

For a fixed magnet design and fixed position of the resolving aperture in a machine, this indicates that tuning the analyzer magnet current will cause different mass ions to be selected depending on the square root of their mass. This is the reason that very heavy isotopes are difficult to separate using electromagnetic methods, though it is not a severe problem for most of the species used in semiconductor fabrication. In ultralow energy machines no further acceleration of the selected ions takes place and they continue toward the sample at the extraction energy.

For most situations, the selected ions are further accelerated in a small linear accelerator to the final energy of implantation. Some beam neutralization may occur during this acceleration phase and this is a problem because neutral atoms cannot be electrostatically scanned or counted as ion current. They implant an uncontrolled dose in the center of the wafer. For this reason, the ion path typically undergoes an electrostatic deviation from the linear path just before final implantation, which acts to trap the neutrals which continue undeflected. This bend in the column is often noticeable near the end station. The ion beam may then undergo an x-y electrostatic deflection which scans the beam onto the wafer, perhaps combined with a mechanical translation and scan of the wafer holder.

The implant dose is measured by locating the sample at the end of a deep Faraday cup, which collects the current and integrates it over time. The normalized dose is given by

$$D = \frac{1}{A}\int \frac{I}{q}dt \tag{8.20}$$

where I is the collected beam current, A is the implant area, t is the integration time, and q is the charge on the ion.

8.3.1 High-Energy Implants

While most implanters cover a range of 30 keV to 200 keV for singly ionized species, this imposes practical limits on the depth that dopant atoms can be introduced into the silicon. The upper energy limit is determined by breakdown in systems with air insulation. The effective ion energy can be extended by using doubly charged species, but the beam current is lower since fewer doubly charged species are generated in the source. However, there are particular applications where implant energies in the MeV range are useful, such as for the deep wells in a CMOS technology. Implanting the well allows cost savings because multiple sequential implants can be performed through the same mask, allowing an optimized profile for the deep well, a shallower punchthrough implant, and a threshold voltage adjust implant to be performed in the same load step and pump-down. Because of the nature of ion implantation, it is also possible to produce a retrograde well profile with higher doping deep in the substrate and low doping at the surface, something that is impossible to do using diffused wells. For example in the P and N wells produced in the CMOS process in Chapter 2, a high-temperature diffusion was used after the implants (Figure 2–12). This would result in wells in which the highest dopant concentrations are near the surface.

We can examine the impact of introducing high-energy implantation technology in a standard CMOS process. One of the major problems with CMOS devices is the susceptibility to latchup, whereby a parasitic n-p-n-p thyristor latches in the on state, destroying the circuit operation. Figure 8–15 illustrates this problem. The CMOS structure inherently contains parasitic NPN and PNP bipolar transistors. Under normal CMOS

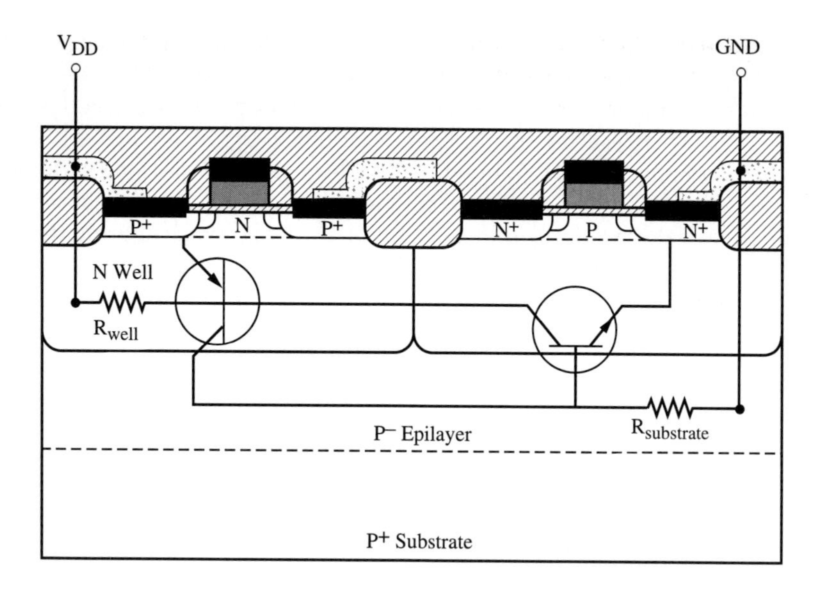

Figure 8–15 Schematic of latchup structure which occurs in a CMOS technology. The parasitic bipolar transistors are overlaid on the technology discussed in Chapter 2. The resistors are normally connected as shown in the schematic.

circuit operation, these devices are not active since $V_{BE} = 0$ volts. However under transient conditions, *IR* drops in the parasitic resistors shown in Figure 8–15 can become large enough (≈ 0.7 volts) to turn on one or both bipolar devices since voltage drops across these resistors also appear across the bipolar base emitter diodes. If this happens, the bipolar devices can behave like a thyristor because they are inherently wired in a cross-coupled configuration. Once triggered, the thyristor structure can carry large currents, shorting the supply voltage to ground and causing catastrophic failure of the chip.

This problem can be solved for all practical purposes by building CMOS devices in an epitaxial layer above a highly doped substrate, using the high conductivity of the substrate to reduce the parasitic resistances in the critical parasitic path. But epitaxial wafers are expensive and there is a possibility of using high-energy MeV implants to introduce a similar buried layer shunt path in a bulk wafer. This requires a relatively high dose (above 10^{14} cm^{-2}) but could be used to replace epitaxial wafers.

The more immediate use of high-energy implants is to simplify the well-formation process in CMOS while simultaneously decoupling the isolation design from the transistor design. A typical sequence of implants includes all of the implants for the n well such as a deep well, a punchthrough implant, and a threshold adjust implant, using thick (2-micron) photoresist as the implant mask. Note that the high-energy implants can be performed after the isolation regions have been formed. This can provide some advantages in terms of reduced thermal cycles when the implants are performed after the field oxide formation or the shallow trench isolation step. The p-well regions can subsequently be defined and a similar series of implants performed to optimize the various dopant profiles. The thick photoresist provides an adequate mask but is often not hard-baked (Chapter 5) to avoid photoresist flow and degradation of the sidewall angle. The masking qualities of the resist can be measured by doing implants in the resists and subsequently measuring the implanted profiles using SIMS analysis.

It is likely that MeV implant technology will be increasingly used to reduce the number of process steps associated with forming the wells and for the ability to optimize each sequential implant, thereby decoupling the isolation design and the transistor design.

8.3.2 Ultralow Energy Implants

As seen from the technology roadmap (Table 7–1 in Chapter 7), the ability to form junctions shallower than 100 nm is needed to continue CMOS scaling. Forming such shallow junctions is not an inherently difficult problem—for example, energies below 100 eV have been used for doping shallow layers grown by Molecular Beam Epitaxy (MBE). At this low energy, the ions are not implanted into the material but land softly onto the growing surface where they are buried by the incoming molecules from the MBE evaporation source. The real question for this chapter is whether it is possible to form shallow junctions by ion implantation in an economically viable manner, allowing an extension of current technology to future technology generations.

The reason most current ion implanters cover an energy range above 30 keV is because the low-energy limit is set by the extraction voltage for the ions from the source plasma. In order to get sufficient beam current, a reasonably large extraction voltage has traditionally been used. The beam current determines the throughput and hence the economic viability of using ion implantation in large-scale production and needs to be in the range of several milliamps.

The source current available from a typical plasma source is not a limiting factor on the ion flux that is available. Instead, it is the space charge in the beam that limits the beam current at low energies. At some current level, the amount of charge in transit shields the source from the applied field, limiting the current in the beam. The space charge limited ion current density is given by Child's Law:

$$J \propto V_{\text{ext}}^{1.5} d^{-2} \tag{8.21}$$

where V_{ext} is the extraction voltage and d is the distance over which the voltage is applied. Thus, the available beam current scales as the extraction voltage $V^{1.5}$, so the beam current at 2 keV is only one-quarter of that available at 5 keV. Careful attention to the ion optics and the design of the extraction electrodes has enabled useful currents to be obtained at low energies, within this scaling limitation.

Since the extracted ions are often accelerated to higher energies, why is it not possible to simply decelerate the beam? Deceleration can produce higher currents at low energies. This particular mode of operation is sometimes used (decel mode) but may cause subtle problems in manufacturing. Because charge exchange between neutrals and ions in the beam may occur continuously, some of the neutrals will not be decelerated and there can be a variable energy spectrum leading to a deeper than expected profile which directly affects the junction depth. This means that extraordinary care has to be taken with the machine design. However, the latest generations of optimized low-energy machines have beam currents that are comparable with those achieved in decel mode, without the problems of beam instabilities. These machines operate in a drift mode, where ions are extracted from the source at the final energy required, mass analyzed, after which the ions drift toward the sample. Implants at energies less than 250 eV can be performed, suggesting that there is no lower limit on the economical throughput for ion implantation in shallow junction formation. The absolute lower energy is determined by the energy needed to penetrate the lattice and is approximately 50 eV for boron. High doses cannot be introduced at extremely low energies, because the incoming ions sputter off some surface atoms, leading to a self-limiting dose. For very low energies, the profiles appear to be still affected by Transient Enhanced Diffusion (TED), discussed in Section 8.5.9. The final junction may need careful annealing to minimize TED, but junctions a few tens of nanometers deep are still within reach. Similar {311} defects (described later) are seen, as in higher-energy implants, though with a preferred orientation parallel to the surface, suggesting that the TED kinetics will continue to be controlled by evaporation of interstitials from clustered defects. It appears that there is no unusual behavior for ultralow energy implants, other than enhanced interactions with the surface. We will return to many of these issues later in the chapter.

8.3.3 Ion Beam Heating

The temperature rise in the silicon caused by ion implantation is determined by the dose, acceleration voltage, and thickness of the silicon wafer. The energy deposited is

$$E_{\text{dep}} = V \int I dt = VQ \tag{8.22}$$

One important limiting temperature regime is at about 120°C, where photoresists which are used for masking begin to flow, crack, and deteriorate. For many normal dose-energy combinations even an uncooled wafer will not reach this temperature.

8.4 Measurement Methods

Since ion implantation is used to provide doped regions in silicon, the measurement methods associated with this process are generally designed to measure dopant profiles. Thus the same methods as those described in Chapter 7 are used. Total chemical concentration profiles are generally measured with SIMS. Electrically active profiles are measured with spreading resistance, sheet resistance, or CV methods. The more advanced methods described in Chapter 7 (cross sectional TEM, scanning capacitance microscopy, and inverse electrical measurements) can also be used to characterize implanted profiles in 2D.

Because the ion implantation process creates damage, most dopants are not electrically active at the end of the implantation. Thus profile measurement at this point must carefully distinguish between total chemical concentrations and the portion of the dopant that is electrically active. Following an appropriate activation anneal, most of the dopant is electrically active, unless the concentrations are so high that precipitation, clustering, or other processes occur.

8.5 Models and Simulations

While the phenomenological description of ion distributions in silicon in terms of distribution functions is useful, a complete description of the detailed atomic-scale events that take place along an ion trajectory has proven to be the only viable method for accurately modeling the final ion distribution in crystalline silicon. Much of the theoretical description of the stopping of charged ions by matter came from original work on the structure of the nucleus. Following Ziegler [8.5], we provide a brief review of some of the interesting historical highlights.

Rutherford, in 1911, observed that about 0.01% of alpha particles were backscattered from thin aluminum foils and proceeded to show that these came from a single collision with a positively charged nucleus, thereby altering the prevailing view of the nature of matter. In the terminology of ion implantation, the alpha particle is just a double ionized helium atom, though the source of Rutherford's particles came from radioactive decay. Soon after, Bohr attempted one of the first unified theories of ion stopping by matter and made the hypothesis that the energy loss of ions could be divided into two components: the nuclear energy loss to the positive atomic cores of the target and the electronic energy loss to the free electrons in the target. The major unknown in calculating the energy loss was the effective charge state of a moving ion in the target. Bohr assumed that the ion's electrons with an orbital velocity less than the ion velocity would be stripped off, leaving a highly charged particle interacting with the orbiting target electrons which could be treated as harmonic oscillators. Bethe and Bloch later introduced a quantum mechanical treatment of the electronic energy loss of a charged particle to a free electron gas, while Fermi considered how the charged particle would polarize the electron gas and alter the interaction. Fermi and Teller extended this work and found that the electronic energy loss would be directly proportional to the particle's velocity. The nuclear energy loss was treated as an elastic collision of the charged particle with the Coulomb field of a positively charged nucleus, partially screened by the outer valence electrons.

The culmination of this work by Lindhard, Scharff, and Schiott in 1963 in what has become known as LSS range theory brought all the pieces together and allowed the stopping powers to be calculated for any arbitrary atomic species and elemental targets within a factor of two. The improvements in range calculations since the LLS theory have come about from considering the shell structure of the atoms using quantum mechanical atomic structure calculations, by numerically calculating the path of the ion trajectory during interactions with a target atom rather than making asymptotic collision approximations, by improved effective charge approximations [8.6], and by considering the lattice structure of crystalline materials.

Computers are now powerful enough to literally follow the atomic-scale trajectory of a representative sample of a few thousand ions through the lattice, accurately accounting for an arbitrary screen oxide thickness together with any tilt and rotation used during implantation. By combining the information on the final resting positions of the ions, a picture of the final distribution can be obtained. Because of the random nature of the starting condition, this approach is often called a Monte Carlo simulation. In amorphous silicon, the position of the silicon atoms is also randomly chosen so the overall density is correct. Given the atomic density for the target, the average distance between atoms in an amorphous target is $(1/N)^{1/3}$, which gives the average path length between nuclear interactions in amorphous material.

In crystalline silicon, the trajectory is completely determined by the structure of the lattice after the ion is set in motion. The ion scatters deterministically from target atoms through angles determined from classical two-body collision theory, slowing down by an additional drag force from electronic interactions. The rate at which an ion loses energy depends on both the nuclear and electronic stopping power of the target, giving

$$\frac{dE}{dx} = -N[S_n(E) + S_e(E)] \tag{8.23}$$

where N is the target atom density (5×10^{22} cm^{-3} for silicon) and $S_n(E)$ and $S_e(E)$ are the nuclear and electronic stopping powers in eV cm^2. Both are in general functions of energy.

If $S_n(E)$ and $S_e(E)$ are known, then the range of the ion can be calculated using

$$R = \int_0^R dx = \frac{1}{N}\int_0^{E_0} \frac{dE}{S_n(E) + S_e(E)} \tag{8.24}$$

8.5.1 Nuclear Stopping

When an ion with mass m_1, atomic number Z_1 and kinetic energy E_0 collides with a stationary target atom with mass m_2 and atomic number Z_2, it loses energy by interacting with the electric field of the nucleus of the target. Not all collisions are head-on collisions, so the nuclear energy loss depends on the distance of closest approach, often called the impact parameter. As the ion interacts with the electric field of the nucleus, it exchanges its kinetic energy for potential energy, reaching a maximum transfer at the distance of closest approach. This potential energy is partitioned between the ion and target atom in accordance with their masses, and the ion continues on a deflected path while the lattice atom recoils. The velocities and trajectories can be found from the conservation of momentum and energy in a classical treatment of two colliding particles. Thus, the nuclear energy loss is elastic in that the energy lost by the ion is transferred to the lattice atom, providing the atomic-scale basis for the damage created by the incoming ions. These nuclear interactions give rise to scattering and deflected trajectories, with the deflection angle depending on the impact parameter. The energy transferred by the incoming ion and its subsequent scattering angle depends on the distance of closest approach to the target atom. If the ion and target atoms were bare nuclei, the scattering potential would be given by the simple Coulomb potential

$$V(r) = \frac{q^2 Z_1 Z_2}{4\pi\varepsilon r} \tag{8.25}$$

Because of the electrons which surround the target nucleus, the full effect of the positive core potential is screened from the incoming ion. Modifying the potential by an exponential screening function gives the Thomas-Fermi model of the atom

$$V(r) = \frac{q^2 Z_1 Z_2}{4\pi\varepsilon r} \exp\left(-\frac{r}{a}\right) \tag{8.26}$$

where a is some screening distance. To predict the scattering angle, the interaction of the ion with the screened Coulomb potential is integrated over the path length where the nuclear force is important, as shown in Figure 8–16. Since the scattering is deterministic in the binary collision approximation, tables of precalculated scattering angles for each impact parameter and energy speed up the calculations in practice, trading memory for speed in the simulations.

For a head-on collision, the maximum energy transferred in the nuclear encounter is given from classical two-body collision theory

$$E_{\text{Trans}} = \frac{4m_1 m_2}{(m_1 + m_2)^2} E \tag{8.27}$$

where E is the impact energy. This allows an estimate of the maximum recoil energy given to an atom in the substrate.

The nuclear stopping power $S_n(E)$ depends on the ion energy. The nuclear energy loss is small at very high energies, because fast particles have less interaction time with

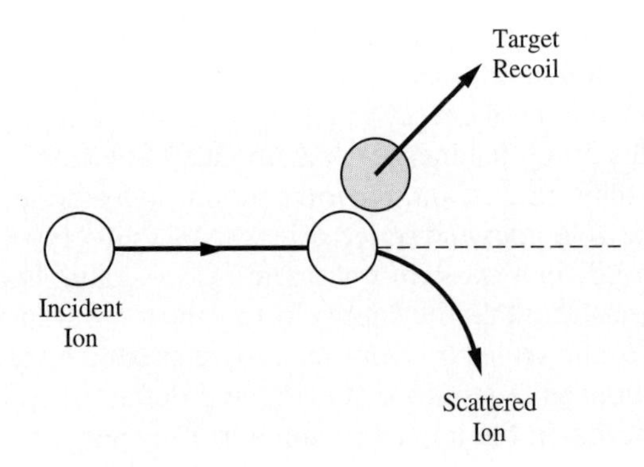

Figure 8–16 Schematic of a nuclear collision or scattering encounter between an ion and a stationary target atom.

the scattering nucleus (reduced cross section). Thus, the nuclear energy loss tends to dominate toward the end of the range when the ion has lost much of its energy and where the nuclear collisions produce most of the damage. While more sophisticated models are used in modern computer simulation tools, $S_n(E)$ can sometimes be usefully approximated as a constant value at energies below where electronic stopping is important by [8.7]

$$S_n(E) = 2.8 \times 10^{-15} \frac{Z_1 Z_2}{(Z_1^{2/3} + Z_2^{2/3})^{1/2}} \frac{m_1}{m_1 + m_2} \text{ eV cm}^2 \tag{8.28}$$

where m_1 and Z_1 refer to the ion and m_2 and Z_2 are the substrate atom mass and atomic number. Note that this simple expression does not include any energy dependence in $S_n(E)$. We will look at more accurate ways of modeling $S_n(E)$ later (Figure 8–20).

8.5.2 Nonlocal Electronic Stopping

The other important components of energy loss are due to electronic effects. The major component of electronic stopping is due to the drag that a moving ion experiences in a dielectric medium. Consider first a stationary ion in a dielectric medium. A polarization of the dielectric medium occurs around the ion to minimize the overall electric field. As the ion is set in motion, the polarization field must adjust by realignment of the electrons in the valance bonds, which at sufficient ion velocities causes the polarization field to lag behind the charged ion, leading to a drag force on the moving ion as illustrated in Figure 8–17.

An analogy is sometimes made with particle transport in a viscous medium, where the viscosity is caused by the sea of electrons from the target lattice. This drag force is directly proportional to the ion velocity at all energies of interest for ion implantation. It depends strongly on the effective ionization state of the ion in the medium (the Brandt-Kitagawa effective charge [8.6]). Because this electronic stopping mechanism is an overall characteristic of the target medium, it is referred to as nonlocal electronic stopping. It acts as a dissipative energy loss which does not alter the direction of the ion's trajectory.

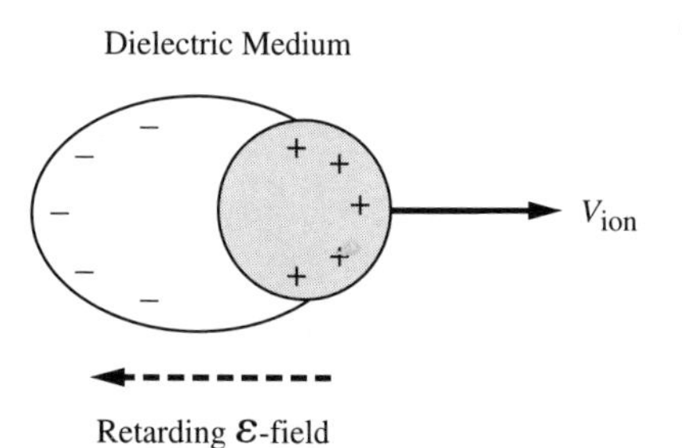

Figure 8–17 Schematic of drag force exerted on a moving ion in a dielectric medium. (After [8.2].)

Much of the progress in modeling implanted profiles has come from better models for the electronic stopping. One effect we have not considered is that the shell structure of the ion varies with the atomic mass of the ion and there are thus oscillations in the electronic stopping powers as the ion mass increases. These subtle but important effects are not shown in Figure 8–19 (discussed later), where an average electronic stopping power versus energy is plotted.

Recent work [8.8] has used a single adjustable parameter which provides an effective ionization radius to describe electronic stopping for different species in silicon. It remains to be seen if this is a sufficiently good description of the electronic stopping, or if an additional local component for electronic stopping is also needed.

8.5.3 Local Electronic Stopping

An argument can be made that the local electronic environment around the lattice atoms also contributes to electronic stopping, through collisions with electrons and consequent momentum transfer. If an ion passes close enough to a lattice atom so that their electron wavefunctions overlap, there can be charge exchange and momentum exchange, as shown in Figure 8–18. This reduces the ion energy and gives rise to a force on the ion which slows it down. The ion-target electronic collisions give rise to a momentum transfer $m_e v_{\text{ion}}$, where m_e is the electron mass and v_{ion} is the velocity of the ion. Because of the momentum transfer, it can subtly alter the ion trajectory, though this effect is minor compared to the scattering from the nuclear core. To compute the total momentum transfer, the momentum transfer from a single electron is multiplied by the electron current transferred between the ion and target during the course of an electronic interaction. The momentum transfer is proportional to the local electron concentration in the vicinity of the target atom multiplied by the orbital velocity of the electrons. Both the local electron concentration and the orbital velocity of the electrons depend strongly on the distance from the atoms. This gives rise to a long-range (compared with nuclear stopping) local electronic stopping which depends directly on the ion velocity and decreases as the fifth power of the impact parameter.

Since both forms of electronic stopping depend directly on the ion velocity, we can write

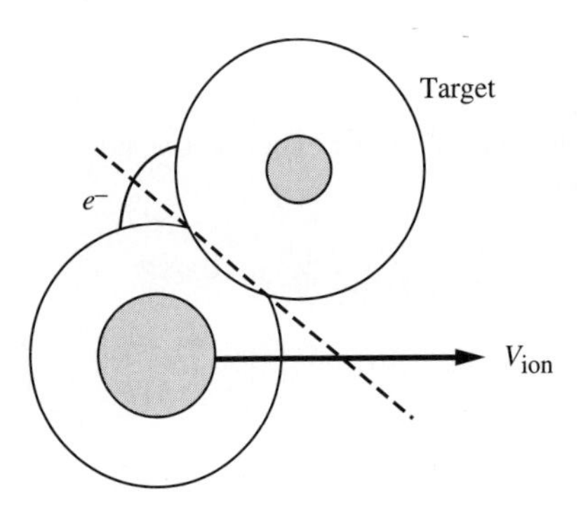

Figure 8–18 Schematic of charge and momentum exchange due to local electronic interactions. (After [8.2].)

$$S_e(E) = cv_{\text{ion}} = kE^{1/2} \tag{8.29}$$

where c and k are parameters that depend on the ion, the substrate, and the particular electronic stopping process being modeled. In the simplest case, in which the substrate is assumed to be amorphous, k is roughly independent of the ion being implanted and is given by [8.7]

$$k \cong 0.2 \times 10^{15}\ \text{eV}^{1/2}\ \text{cm}^2 \tag{8.30}$$

In summary, electronic stopping is inelastic and is responsible for dissipating the energy of the incoming ions. Both the overall dielectric response of the target medium and the local electronic structure of the target atoms contribute to the electronic stopping.

8.5.4 Total Stopping Powers

Both the nuclear and electronic stopping powers depend on energy and contribute to the total stopping, as seen in Figure 8–19. For some range of ion energies, the total stopping power is approximately constant, which explains why the ion ranges in Figure 8–3 are approximately linear with energy.

Clearly, the local environment (such as whether the ion is in a channel or amorphous region) will have a dramatic effect on the nuclear encounters that will be faced by the ion. To adequately model implanted profiles, especially in channeling directions, accurate models for the electronic stopping must also be available. Many modern processes have implants at zero tilt to avoid shadowing effects (Figure 8–6). In addition, some channeling component always exists because of the inherent structure of the lattice. For these reasons, accurate modeling of both the nuclear and electronic stopping in a Monte Carlo simulator is the only feasible way to obtain accurate implanted profiles.

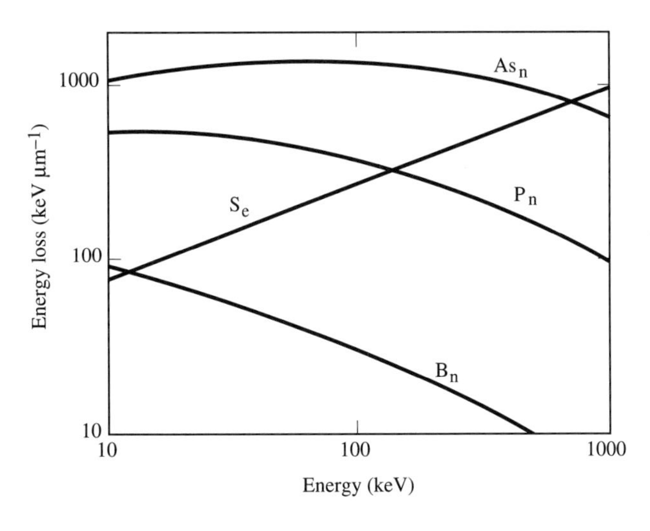

Figure 8–19 The total stopping power is composed of the sum of the nuclear and electronic stopping. An average electronic stopping power is plotted, though the details depend on the shell structure of the incident ion. The nuclear stopping dominates at low energies while the electronic stopping dominates at higher energies. (After [8.2].)

8.5.5 Damage Production

The major disadvantage of ion implantation is that the nuclear stopping creates a lot of damage in the lattice that must be repaired by annealing at high temperatures. The energy required to displace a silicon atom just far enough from its lattice site to create a stable separated interstitial and vacancy (a Frenkel pair) is the displacement energy E_d and is approximately 15 eV in silicon. Because the implant energy is often in the range of kilovolts, a large number of displacements will be caused.

Example How many displaced lattice atoms are created by a single incident 30-keV arsenic atom?

Answer For a heavy ion like arsenic, this energy is mainly dissipated due to nuclear collisions [8.9]. From Figure 8–3, a 30-keV arsenic implant has a range of 25 nm, which means it transverses 100 planes of atoms (0.25 nm average interplanar spacing), so that on average it loses 300 eV in a nuclear collision at each plane, as illustrated in Figure 8–20. This is much more than the displacement energy, so the lattice atom that is displaced by the incident ion (the primary knock-on) can continue and itself lose energy and displace other secondary lattice atoms. This is essentially equivalent to a silicon implant with 300 eV of energy at each point where a nuclear collision occurred. When the energy of the incident ion or the secondary knocked-on atoms reach E_d, they can be considered stopped, because if they do manage to transfer all their energy to a lattice atom, they can cause a single displacement but remain at rest in the lattice position themselves. Thus, an energetic particle can only increase the number of moving particles if it has energy greater than $2E_d$. This allows an estimate of the number of displaced atoms created by an energetic particle to be made (the Kinchin-Pease formula):

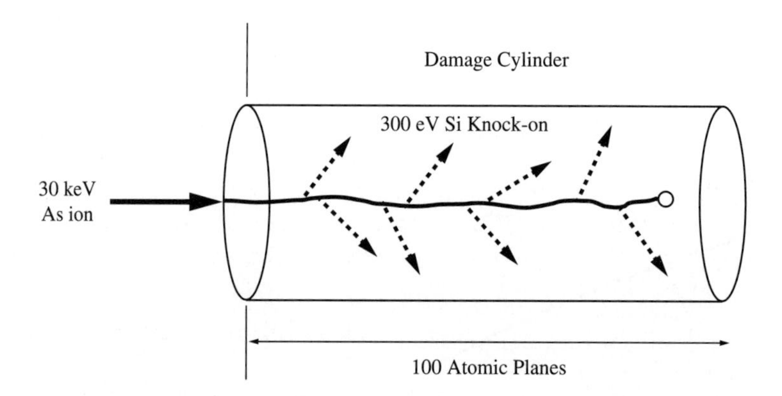

Figure 8–20 Schematic of the damage caused by a 30-keV arsenic implant into silicon, with a range of 25 nm. The ion crosses approximately 100 atomic planes. (After [8.9].)

$$n = \frac{E_n}{2E_d} \tag{8.31}$$

where E_n is the energy lost in nuclear collisions. For a 30-keV arsenic ion,

$$n = \frac{30{,}000}{2 \times 15} = 1000 \text{ displaced atoms}$$

$$\text{Equivalently, n} = 100 \text{ planes} \times \frac{300}{2 \times 15} \text{ atoms/plane} = 1000 \text{ atoms}$$

Thus, each incident arsenic ion creates a trail or cascade of 1000 displaced lattice atoms.

What is the time scale on which this damage production occurs? We can estimate that the time it takes the ion to come to rest is given by the range divided by its velocity:

$$t = \frac{R_p}{\sqrt{E/2m}} \approx 10^{-13} \text{ sec} \tag{8.32}$$

while the thermal vibrations decay on the order of the Debye frequency (10^{-12} sec). Some recombination occurs within the cascade due to elementary diffusion hops on the time scale of 10^{-9} sec after which the primary damage generated by the incident ion can be considered stable. This damage is primarily small defect clusters and dopant-defect complexes and some isolated interstitials and vacancies. Such a detailed picture of the damage evolution has been obtained from molecular dynamics calculations of ions impacting a crystalline silicon lattice. Since the damage evolution is primarily determined by the silicon atoms that are knocked on, the well-characterized silicon interatomic potentials should provide a physically accurate description of the damage evolution. An example of these calculations is shown in Figure 8–21.

The question now is how this primary damage accumulates when other ions are implanted. Some of the defects generated can recombine with defects from other cascades, so the damage accumulation depends on the existing local defect density. Thus the amount of damage that accumulates [8.11] depends on the number n generated in an isolated cascade, on the fraction f_{rec} that recombine within a cascade and from overlapping cascades, along with a factor for the existing local defect density. The increment in the primary damage in a volume element for an additional implanted ion is given by

$$\Delta n(x) = n f_{rec}\left(1 - \frac{N}{N_\alpha}\right) \tag{8.33}$$

where N is the local defect density and N_α is a threshold defect density where the crystal is considered amorphous. Clearly, if the crystal is amorphous $N = N_\alpha$ and $\Delta n = 0$,

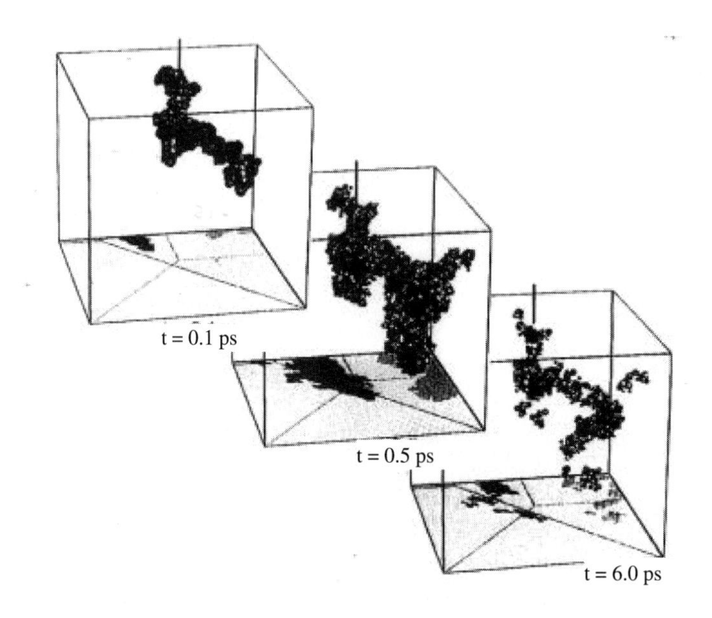

Figure 8–21 Molecular dynamics simulations of a 5-keV boron implant into silicon, showing the damage evolution and stabilization. The simulation temperature was 40K and the atoms plotted have a potential energy greater than 0.2 eV. Reprinted with permission of *Nucl. Instrum. Methods Phys.* [8.10].

so that there is no incremental disorder introduced by additional cascades. In UT-Marlowe [8.2], the values of f_{rec} are chosen to be 0.1, 0.4, 0.6, 0.6 for boron, phosphorus, arsenic, and BF_2 implants. Physically, the dense damage cascades from heavy species like arsenic and BF_2 allow for more efficient recombination than the more dispersed damage distribution from a light ion like boron. The threshold damage density for amorphization, N_α, is often taken to be 10% of the silicon lattice density. It is clear that the primary damage builds up until eventually an amorphous state is reached, after which no channeling occurs and the damage accumulation saturates.

Since the number of displacements n produced by an ion depends on the amount of energy deposited into nuclear collisions, the damage production is a maximum where the nuclear energy losses are highest. For heavy ions like arsenic, whose stopping may be dominated by nuclear collisions, this means that the damage profile is relatively flat over the whole range up to R_P. For lighter ions like boron, which have an appreciable component of electronic stopping at higher energies, the damage accumulation is concentrated near R_P where the ion energy is lower. For light ions then, the amorphous region will form first at the peak of the damage density profile near R_P and expand on both sides of this depth as the implant dose is increased. Experimental measurements of the amorphization layer thickness as a function of implant dose support this picture and indicate a U-shaped distribution for the amorphous layer thickness depending on implant dose, as shown in Figure 8–22. A buried amorphous layer first forms, and it may

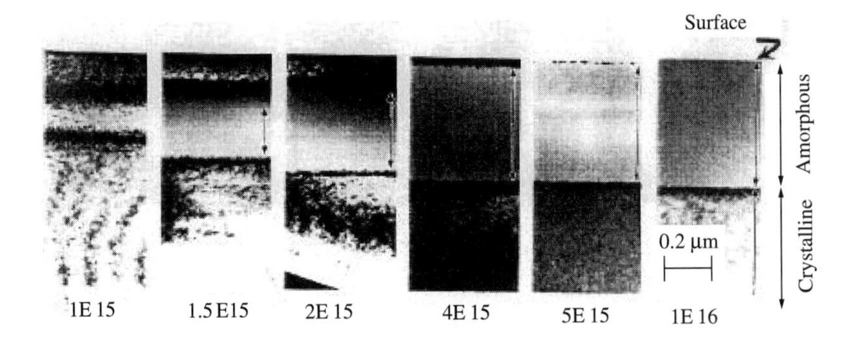

Figure 8–22 Cross-sectional TEM images of the formation of an amorphous layer for increasing Si implant doses. The layer begins to form where the nuclear damage is highest, spreading wider with higher doses. Reprinted with permission of J. Appl. Phys. [8.12].

take a considerably higher implant dose before a continuous amorphous layer extending down from the surface forms [8.12]. The experimental results also indicate that it is easier to form an amorphous layer at low temperatures (liquid nitrogen) rather than at room temperature or higher. This observation is easily explained by the larger fraction of ions that recombine within a cascade at higher implant temperatures.

These ideas suggest the possibility of preamorphizing the silicon substrate to eliminate ion channeling, perhaps by preimplanting the substrate with silicon or germanium ions. If an amorphous layer is created, then a subsequent implant of a dopant will not channel and a shallow implant profile can be formed.

8.5.6 Damage Annealing

The goal of damage annealing is to remove the primary damage created by the implant and restore the silicon lattice to its perfect crystalline state, leaving the dopants on active substitutional sites. This damage removal can be divided into two distinct regimes: one below and the other above the amorphous threshold.

The primary damage begins to anneal at relatively low temperatures of about 400°C. First, the vacancy complexes (di-vacancies and vacancy-type clusters) begin to break up and the released vacancies annihilate with interstitials. The final result of the initial stages of annealing is to remove most of the Frenkel pairs, leaving only interstitial-type defects whose origin stems from the extra atom introduced into the lattice. This gives rise to the "+1" model for residual damage due to implants, that is, to a good approximation, all of the original damage recombines, leaving only one interstitial created when the implanted ion finally occupies a lattice site. Figure 8–23 illustrates some of these effects. Note the very short time scale on which the Frenkel pairs recombine in this simulation through bulk I-V recombination [8.13]. Some vacancies recombine independently at the surface. After 10^{-2} seconds, only interstitials remain in small clusters, and these slowly dissolve by recombining interstitials at the surface. Though this

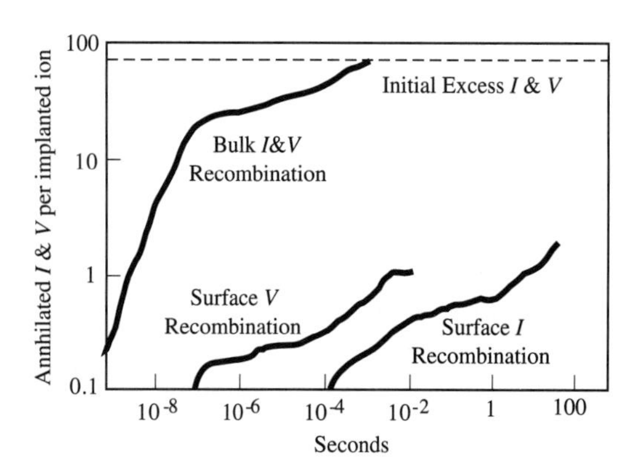

Figure 8–23 Monte Carlo simulation of the recombination of I and V damage generated by an implant. After a short time, only excess interstitials remain and these form clusters in a fraction of a second at 800°C. (After [8.13].)

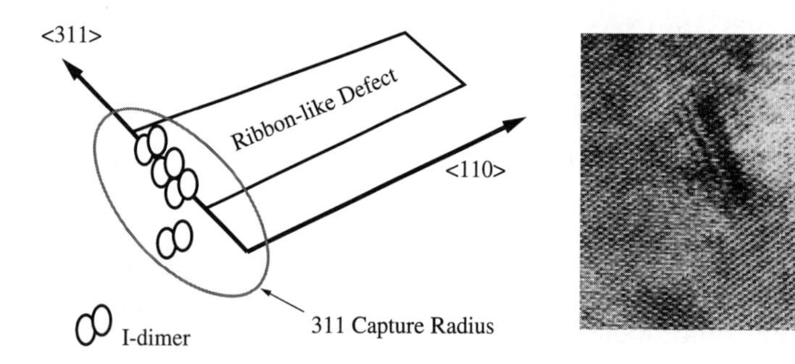

Figure 8–24 Schematic (left) and cross section TEM (right) of {311} clusters that form by capturing a row of interstitial dimers that lie on the {311} plane and grow by extending in the 110 directions. Photo courtesy of H. Chao, Stanford University.

picture is simple, it captures much of the essential physics that occurs during implant damage annealing.

The silicon interstitials generated by this "+1" amount of damage very quickly condense into characteristic rod-shaped defect clusters upon further annealing at temperatures above 400°C. These rod-shaped defects are composed of ribbons of silicon atoms that lie on {311} planes as illustrated in Figure 8–24. An actual TEM image of such a defect is also shown in Figure 8–24.

The {311} defects are typically composed of rows of a few silicon dimers that precipitate on {311} planes and extend in the <110> directions to form a planar defect. After a 5-second anneal at 900°C, there may be a very high concentration ($\approx 10^{11}$ cm^{-2}) of these {311} defects, which are only about 10 nm long. The {311} defects start to dissolve upon further annealing by the evaporation of silicon interstitials from the ends of the defects.

If the amount of primary damage is below a critical value, these {311} defects dissolve completely and the crystal is restored to its perfect state. Above this critical damage level, some of the {311} defects grow at the expense of others which shrink. The larger

{311} defects can turn into stable dislocation loops which are much more difficult to remove. These stable dislocation loops are called secondary defects and remain when the primary damage is completely annealed. The dislocation loops can be approximated by an extra circular atomic layer of silicon atoms precipitated on a {111} plane of silicon. They can be shown from TEM images to be extrinsic loops, that is, they are composed of an extra plane of silicon interstitials.

Stable dislocation loops are a much more dominant feature of higher-dose implants, which drive the silicon amorphous. The largest concentration of these loops is seen at the interface between amorphous and crystalline silicon after an anneal which regrows the amorphous region by solid phase epitaxy. These defects at the original amorphous/crystalline (a/c) interface are referred to as End-Of-Range (EOR) defects as illustrated in Figure 8–25. They occur because there is a large amount of damage which is just below the threshold of amorphization beyond the a/c interface. By definition, just beyond the a/c interface is the maximum possible amount of damage that can exist in the crystal at the implant temperature without its being amorphous. This damage is sufficiently high to be able to nucleate a mixture of {311} defects and a band of dislocation loops in a very narrow region just beneath the a/c interface on the crystalline side of the interface.

The loops have a mean radius of approximately 10 nm and ripen to a mean radius of approximately 20 nm during subsequent annealing at a typical RTA anneal temperature of 1000°C, as shown in Figure 8–26 [8.14]. This ripening of the loops happens because a few big loops are energetically more favorable than many small loops since this minimizes the total circumference and the total energy of the system. The ripening process appears to conserve the total number of interstitials trapped in the loops, which

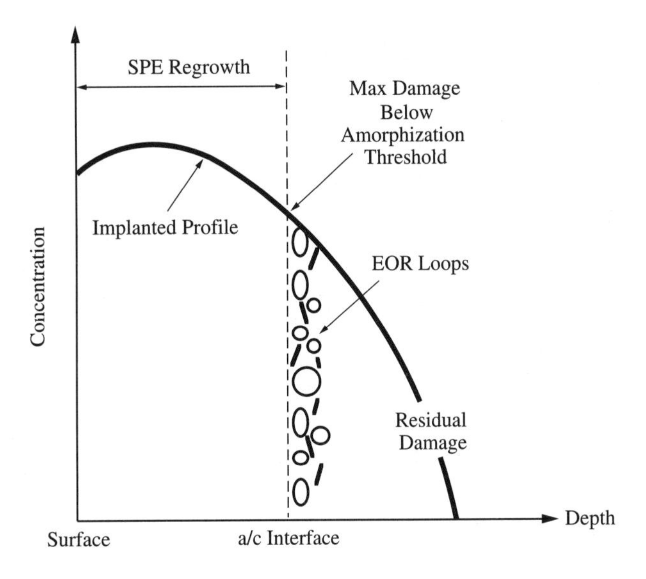

Figure 8–25 Schematic of the stable End-Of-Range (EOR) dislocation loops that form at the amorphous/crystalline (a/c) interface after solid-phase epitaxial regrowth.

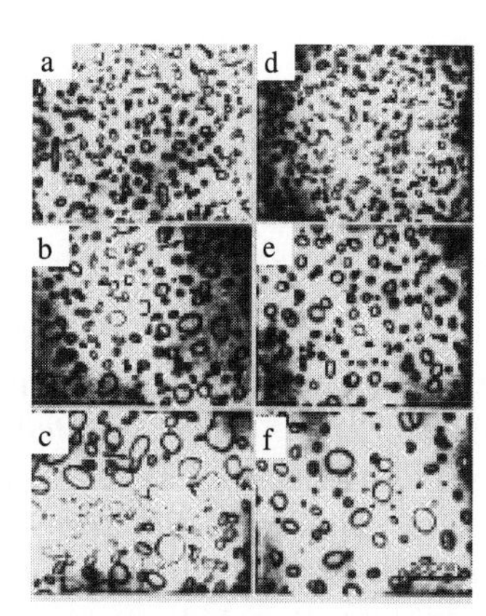

Figure 8–26 Plan view TEM images of the EOR dislocation loops for annealing times of 5, 60, and 960 min at 850°C (a–c) and for 1, 60, and 400 sec at 1000°C (d–f). The loops show some ripening (large circumference loops grow at the expense of smaller loops to minimize the total energy) but remain very stable for typical anneal temperatures. Reprinted with permission of *J. Appl. Phys.* [8.14].

indicates just how stable this secondary damage is at 1000°C. The dislocation loops will disappear at high enough temperatures, and times of 60 sec at 1100°C have been reported to remove loops in some instances.

If the dislocation loops are in the depletion region of a PN junction during device operation, they can give rise to large leakage currents, in particular if they become decorated with metal impurities. Thus, they are often detrimental to device performance. Annealing cycles are chosen to cause just enough dopant diffusion so that the loops are contained in the highly doped regions and are shielded from any depletion regions during device operation. This is a critical optimization problem, since there are often conflicting requirements to minimize the amount of dopant diffusion and maintain shallow junction depths.

The implant process can also be optimized to minimize the nucleation of the loops. In particular, if the implant is performed at liquid nitrogen temperatures rather than room temperature, a lower implant dose can be used to form the same amorphous layer depth. Because of this, the amount or dose of damage in the tail of the damage distribution beyond the a/c interface is much less for the liquid nitrogen temperature implant and may be small enough to preclude stable dislocation loop formation. For example, 75-keV Germanium with a dose of 5×10^{14} cm^{-2} gives rise to an amorphous layer 100 nm deep for a room temperature implant, while only 4×10^{14} cm^{-2} is needed to form the same amorphous layer thickness at liquid nitrogen temperatures and the a/c interface is also sharper. A band of EOR loops at a depth of 100 nm is seen for the room temperature implant, where the loop diameter is 25 nm and their concentration is about 10^{10} cm^{-2} after an anneal at 900°C for 15 min. No loops are seen at all for the LN_2 sample after the same anneal [8.15].

8.5.7 Solid-Phase Epitaxy

If the substrate is amorphous, then it can regrow by layer-by-layer epitaxial realignment beginning from the amorphous/crystalline interface. This process is similar to the crystallization process that occurs from the melt onto a single-crystal seed or from a gas

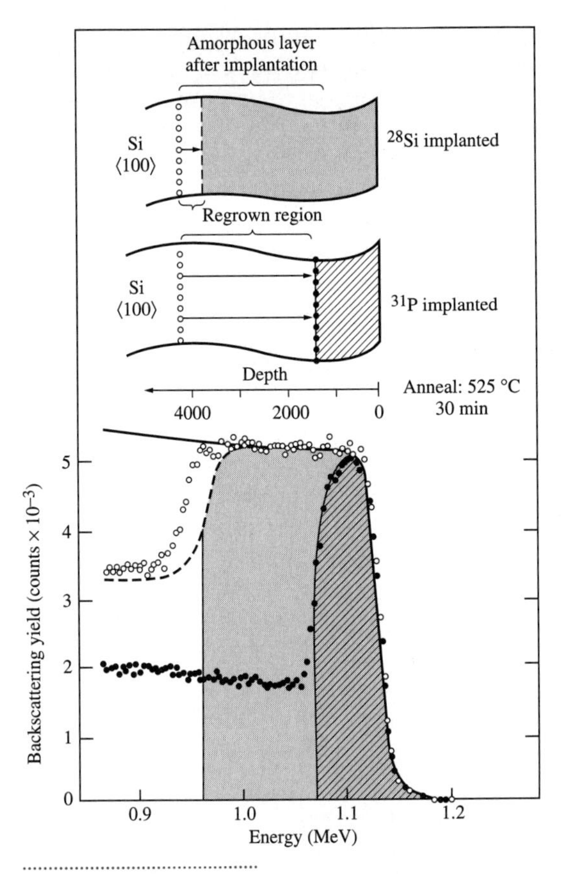

Figure 8–27 Channeling RBS images of the regrowth of an amorphous layer during annealing. The layer regrows from the substrate and undoped silicon regrows more slowly than doped silicon. Reprinted with permission of *J. Appl. Phys.* [8.16].

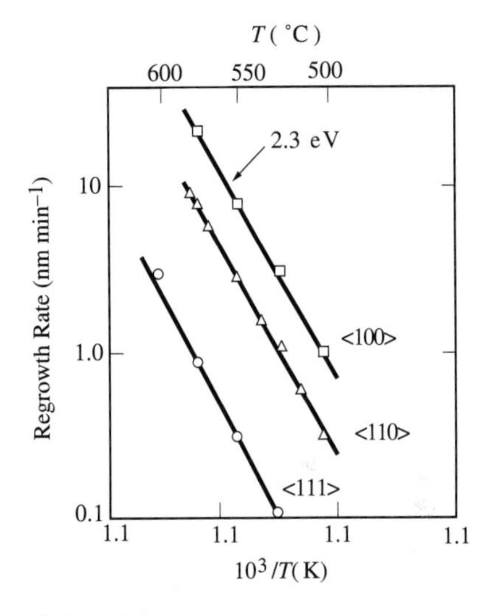

Figure 8–28 Plot of the regrowth velocity during solid phase epitaxy as a function of temperature. (After [8.17].)

phase onto a crystalline substrate, except that it is now occurring from a solid phase rather than a liquid or gas phase. Figure 8–27 shows a time lapse series of channeling Rutherford Backscattering Spectrometry (RBS) images of this regrowth process. It occurs quite quickly, with regrowth rates in undoped silicon at 600°C of 50 nm min^{-1} for <100> orientations, 20 nm min^{-1} for <110> orientations, and 2 nm min^{-1} for <111> orientations, as illustrated in Figure 8–28. The activation energy for the regrowth process on any orientation is 2.3 eV, which is indicative of a silicon-silicon bond breaking and formation process. The regrowth rate is given by

$$v = A \exp\left(-\frac{2.3}{kT}\right) \tag{8.34}$$

where v is the regrowth rate and A is an experimentally determined parameter. The regrowth rate can be enhanced by a factor of 10 for doping levels characteristic of the source and drain in MOS devices. The regrowth at these low temperatures quickly eliminates all the primary damage in the amorphous region, so that no anomalous dopant diffusion occurs there. Most of the dopant atoms in the amorphous regions are incorporated onto substitutional lattice sites during regrowth, so that high levels of activation are possible even at these low temperatures. Indeed, were it not for the residual band of EOR defects just below the a/c interface, solid-phase epitaxy would provide an ideal method for simultaneously removing all the implant damage and obtaining high levels of dopant activation without any noticeable dopant diffusion.

If the implant energy is high enough, a buried amorphous layer can be created. Solid-phase regrowth occurs from both the top and bottom interfaces and leaves a band of dislocations in the center when the two moving interfaces collide.

8.5.8 Dopant Activation

In order to contribute to the electrical activity, the implanted dopant atoms must occupy substitutional sites in the lattice. In addition, the broken bonds in the lattice must be repaired so that the carrier mobility is returned to a reasonable value. At a sufficiently low level of primary damage, all the damage anneals out and high activation levels are obtained. As indicated above, for very high levels of damage where amorphization takes place, solid-phase epitaxial regrowth provides a nearly ideal method to remove damage and obtain high levels of dopant activation. It is much more difficult to anneal a sample that has only been partially damaged at levels below the amorphization threshold. This difficult regime is where secondary damage forms—then the annealing behavior is more complex. For example, Figure 8–29 shows both regimes clearly. Above the amorphization threshold ($\approx 1 \times 10^{15}$ cm^{-2} dose), an anneal temperature of 600°C is sufficient to get high activation. For very low doses ($\approx 10^{12}$ cm^{-2}), the damage also anneals out at 600°C, giving high levels of activation. However, for increasing doses where secondary defects form, up to the amorphous threshold, the damage becomes increasingly difficult to anneal. Typically, temperatures of 950°C to 1050°C are required to obtain useful levels of activation when secondary damage has formed.

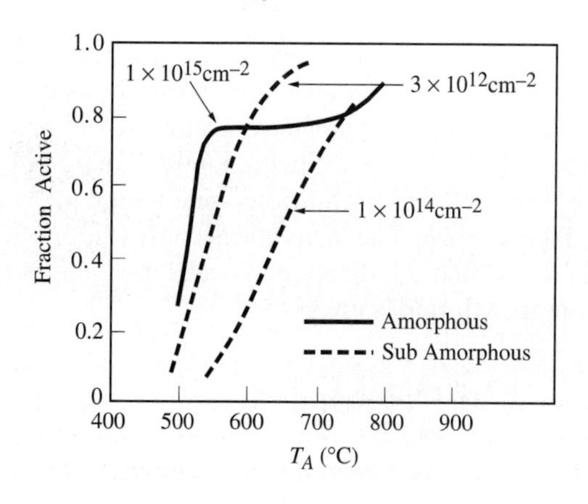

Figure 8–29 Plot of the fraction of an implant activated as a function of anneal temperature for various doses. Note the distinct difference between doses below and above the amorphization threshold (After [8.18].)

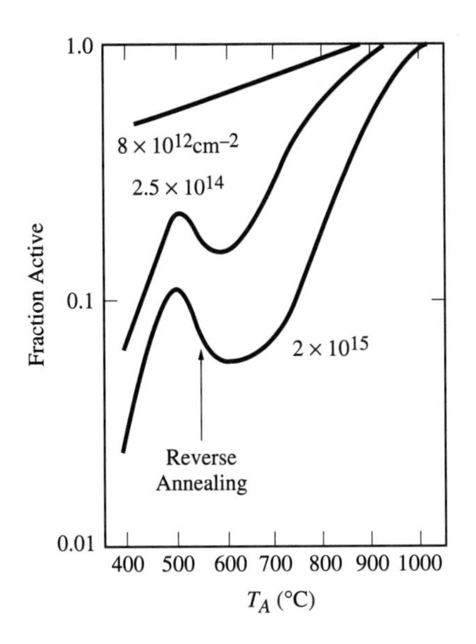

Figure 8–30 Plot of the fractional activation of a boron implant as a function of anneal temperature, showing a region where there is reverse activation. This reverse annealing behavior is thought to be due to competition between boron atoms and native silicon point defects for substitutional lattice sites. Isochronal anneals (30 min at each temperature) were used in these experiments. (After [8.19].)

The behavior of the activation process as a function of temperature provides some indication of the complex interactions that occur between the dopants and the defects. Figure 8–30 shows anneals for different implanted boron doses below the amorphization threshold as a function of temperature. For very low doses, much of the boron is active even after very low temperature anneals and it quickly gains full activity as the anneal temperature is increased. For higher doses, the initial activation level is very low. The damage created by the implant creates deep-level traps which increase the resistivity in either n- or p-type silicon. Some of these traps begin to anneal out at temperatures below 400°C, causing a reduction in the resistivity and an increase in the carrier concentration. However, between approximately 450°C and 550°C, the interstitial damage that remains is responsible for a "reverse annealing" effect, where the carrier concentration abruptly drops. This is caused by silicon interstitials competing with boron atoms for substitutional sites or by interstitials pairing with boron to form inactive complexes. Above 550°C, the activation level slowly rises, approaching full activation at the highest anneal temperatures. Similar annealing behavior is seen for phosphorus below the amorphization threshold.

The problem with using these higher anneal temperatures to activate the dopant is that diffusion also occurs, making it difficult to form shallow junctions. The problem of minimizing the amount of dopant diffusion after implantation is exacerbated by the presence of the excess interstitials which give rise to a transient enhancement in the dopant diffusion (TED). This transient-enhanced diffusion is anomalous because there are conditions where the dopant can diffuse more at lower temperatures than at higher temperatures. It might seem that only the $\sqrt{Dt}$ product should determine the extent of profile motion, that is, a longer time at low temperature could be chosen to be equivalent to a short time at high temperature. A longer time at lower temperature would allow a controllable anneal to be performed in a furnace environment. However, when

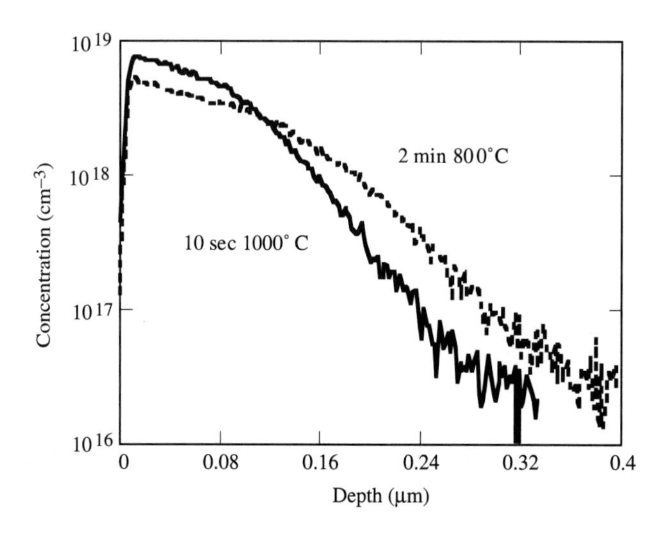

Figure 8–31 Temperature dependence of transient-enhanced diffusion, showing more diffusion for lower temperatures. (After [8.20].)

implant damage is present, the result is very surprising and is shown in Figure 8–31 [8.20]. Here, the profile annealed at the lower temperature diffused further than the one annealed at high temperature.

The reason is that at lower temperatures the damage can stay around longer and enhance the dopant diffusion, while at higher temperatures the damage annihilates faster. Historically, long anneals at high temperatures masked this effect, because eventually normal thermal diffusion will occur and is exponentially faster at higher temperatures. However, for the small thermal budget anneals used in present day devices, this anomalous TED has become the dominant effect that determines how far an implanted dopant moves during an anneal.

The magnitude of this anomalous TED can be quantified by examining how large the enhancement in dopant diffusivity is at each temperature. The results are astonishing, with enhancements ranging from 20,000 at 700°C to 400 at 1000°C. In the following section, we will examine the phenomena of TED and show how its impact on devices can be mitigated.

8.5.9 Transient-Enhanced Diffusion

There now exists a much deeper understanding of how Transient-Enhanced Diffusion (TED) due to implant damage affects dopant motion and consequently device performance. This is a direct result of understanding at an atomic level the physical processes that control TED. Transient-enhanced diffusion occurs when an attempt is made to anneal implant damage and restore the lattice to its crystalline perfection. It consists of a burst of diffusion many thousands of time faster than what is normally observed for similar anneals when no implant damage is present.

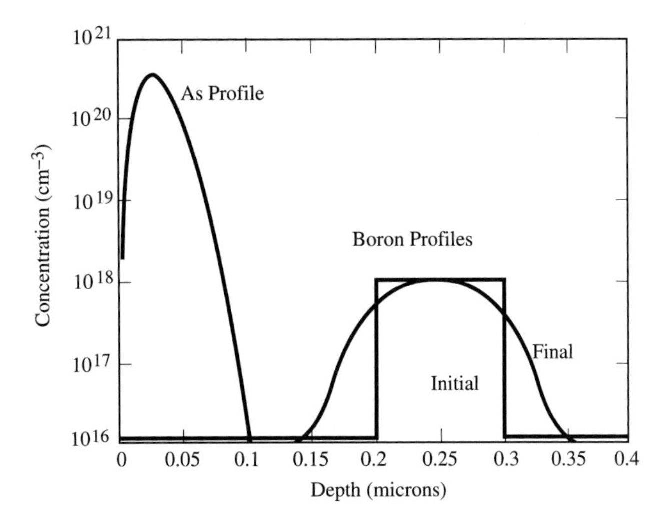

Figure 8–32 Simulation of an arsenic layer implanted above a buried boron layer that gives rise to damage beyond the amorphization/crystalline interface that is able to cause substantial diffusion in the nearby boron layer during a 1-sec, 900°C anneal. (After [8.21].)

Where is TED important and how are its effects measured? Consider for example the arsenic implant in Figure 8–32, which is performed above a buried, lightly doped boron layer. The boron layer might be grown using epitaxial silicon growth, followed by a lightly doped intrinsic silicon layer. The arsenic implant amorphizes the surface region of the substrate, and solid-phase epitaxial regrowth removes much of the implant damage. But there is still a sufficient amount of damage below the a/c interface to cause an enormous enhancement in the diffusion of the nearby boron buried layer, which would not normally show any appreciable motion for the short anneal at 900°C. The arsenic profile itself also shows some slight but significant diffusion, but it is less for arsenic than for boron because of the lower component of arsenic diffusion that takes place by an interstitial mechanism and also because of the lower intrinsic diffusivity of arsenic.

Figure 8–32 illustrates the effect that TED can have in determining how the damage introduced by one dopant affects its own diffusion and also that of a nearby dopants. The structure in Figure 8–32 represents a unique experimental structure that also provides a means to quantify the amount of enhancement seen by a "marker layer" when damage is introduced into the crystal. It is a particularly useful structure because the amount of profile motion can easily be measured using SIMS. Its most important feature is that it decouples the damage itself from the effects of the damage on a nearby region. This test structure is a one-dimensional analog of the source/drain to channel coupling in a MOS device. Thus, experiments on this test structure allow models to be developed which are directly relevant to how TED affects MOS device characteristics. This kind of test structure has allowed many crucial experiments about the nature of TED to be performed.

8.5.10 Atomic-Level Understanding of TED

Atomic-level understanding of TED has come from key experimental [8.22] and theoretical studies. An important experimental finding was that the point defects responsible for TED are interstitial-type extended defects in the form of {311} clusters, whose evaporation rate matches the kinetics of TED [8.23]. Figure 8–33 shows the experimentally measured dissolution rate of the {311} defects. The same time dependence is seen experimentally in TED. These {311} defects appear in transmission electron microscope images as ribbonlike structures that lie on {311} planes and grow and extend in the <110> direction. They form during the very early stages of the anneal, being visible after 1 second at 600°C. The key theoretical results come from molecular dynamics simulations of the collision cascade process in silicon [8.10] and from Monte Carlo simulations of the point-defect evolution and clustering [8.13]. The molecular dynamics simulations show that although a large cascade of damage is generated immediately after an ion strikes the silicon lattice, there is much local recombination and only a small amount of damage remains after a nanosecond. (Recall Figure 8–21.) The Monte Carlo simulations of the subsequent anneal indicate that the small vacancy clusters first decay and the free vacancies start to annihilate interstitial-type defects. After a hundredth of a second at 815°C, only interstitial-type defects remain that are caused by the imbalance introduced in the lattice by the extra implanted ion, as shown in Figure 8–23. Recent experimental work using Deep-Level Transient Spectroscopy (DLTS) confirms this picture [8.24], where interstitial-type defects are found after annealing ion implanted samples but are not found after annealing comparable damage produced by electron beam impact where extra atoms are not introduced.

The microscopic explanation of the energy dependence of TED is even more interesting for the insights it provides into the nature of the residual implant damage. In a clever experiment, Giles and colleagues [8.25] implanted a dopant at the same depth below the surface using both a normal angle of incidence for the ion beam and using a higher energy at a tilted angle of incidence. One expects that the higher energy creates more damage, but the amount of TED in both profiles is identical. This indicates that though more primary damage is created, the bulk recombination process is efficient

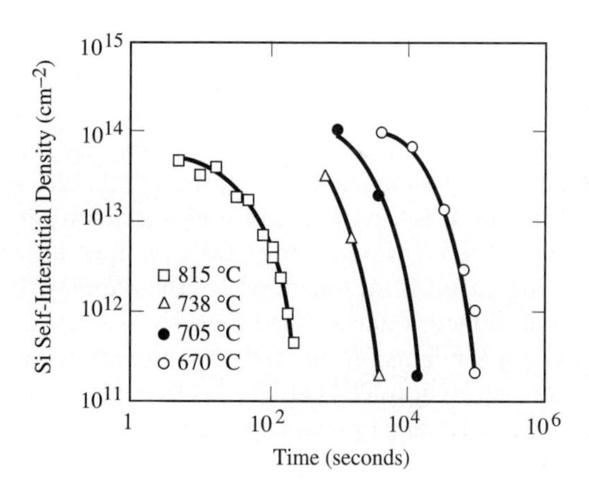

Figure 8–33 Plot of the number of interstitials contained in {311} defect clusters as a function of anneal time at various temperatures. The {311} defects dissolve and provide the interstitial supersaturation that controls TED. (After [8.23].)

enough that essentially all the interstitials and vacancies produced by the implant annihilate in the early stages of the anneal, leaving only a dose of interstitials due to the extra ions introduced into the lattice. This provides a remarkable confirmation of the "+1" approach to implant damage modeling [8.26], where the assumption is made that the net effect of an implant is to introduce one extra interstitial when a dopant atom is introduced into the lattice. This "+1" dose of interstitials then proceeds to cluster and control the kinetics of the TED.

A simulation of how this "+1" interstitial profile from a boron implant evolves in time is shown in Figure 8–34. Rapid clustering of interstitials into {311} defects reduces the enormous supersaturation of interstitials immediately after implant in a time scale of 10^{-2} seconds, and subsequently the supersaturation level is maintained approximately constant while the clusters are dissolving, until the clusters eventually disappear. Most of the TED occurs during this period when the supersaturation of interstitials is at a high, constant level allowing the maximum doping motion to occur.

While the +1 model is more physically correct than considering the thousandfold damage excess introduced by an incoming ion, it should perhaps be better termed a "+n" model where n is of order unity. Clearly, the details of the cascade evolution and in particular the effects of atoms lost to sputtering near the surface along with any of the net vacancies captured in the screen oxide all modify the effective dose of interstitials introduced by the implant. In most simulation programs, this number is taken as a fitting parameter, though detailed Monte Carlo calculations of the implant cascades and

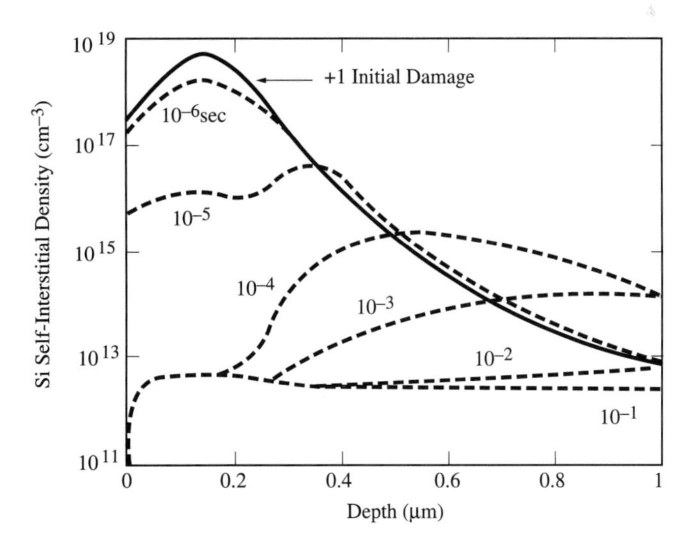

Figure 8–34 TSUPREM IV simulation [8.1] of the time evolution of the "+1" damage from a 40-keV, 10^{14} cm^{-2} boron implant, for anneals from 10^{-6} sec to 10^{-1} sec at 750°C. The equilibrium interstitial concentration is approximately 10^8 cm^{-3}, so the flat concentration profile at 10^{-1} sec represents an interstitial supersaturation of more than 10,000 fold, and TED occurs until surface recombination reduces this to equilibrium levels.

their subsequent evolution allow trends in the "$+n$" value to be obtained as a function of implant species, dose, and energy.

Given these atomic-level insights, we can now quantitatively model the impact of TED on dopant diffusion [8.27] and hence device characteristics. The fact that the {311} defects form remarkably quickly, as shown in Figure 8–34, implies that the TED transient is controlled by the evaporation of interstitials from these aggregated defects. The process of cluster growth and evaporation can be atomistically described by

$$I + Cl_n \Leftrightarrow Cl_{n+1} \tag{8.35}$$

where the subscript n indicates a cluster with n interstitials. If we assume that the properties of the cluster remain the same with size, we can write an equation [8.27] for the time rate of change of the cluster growth as

$$\begin{aligned} -\frac{\partial C_I}{\partial t} = \frac{\partial Cl}{\partial t} &= k_f C_I Cl - k_r Cl \\ &= \text{growth} - \text{shrinkage} \end{aligned} \tag{8.36}$$

where the forward reaction rate for {311} cluster growth is given by k_f and the reverse reaction rate for cluster shrinkage is given by k_r. We can assume that the growth of the clusters is diffusion limited so that the forward reaction rate is given by

$$k_f = 4\pi a d_I \tag{8.37}$$

where a is an encounter distance equal to the nearest neighbor distance in silicon and d_I is the interstitial diffusivity. The reverse reaction constant which describes the rate of evaporation will be given by the attempted hop frequency of the bound interstitial d_I/a^2, times a Boltzmann factor to account for the binding energy to the cluster, so that

$$k_r = \frac{d_I}{a^2} \exp\left(-\frac{E_b}{kT}\right) \tag{8.38}$$

For longer anneal times, the growth of the clusters is not important, leaving only the second term

$$\frac{\partial Cl}{\partial t} = -k_r Cl \tag{8.39}$$

which is the origin of the exponential decay kinetics of the clusters and the consequent change in the dopant diffusivity for longer time anneals. This accounts for some attempts to model the effective diffusivity during TED with terms of the form

$$D_{eff} = D_0 + D_{\text{II}} \exp\left(-\frac{t}{\tau}\right) \tag{8.40}$$

However, this formulation ignores the initial stages of the anneal, where a steady state exists between the cluster growth and evaporation. The steady-state period turns out to be the dominant source of the amount of TED observed. This balance between growth and evaporation when $\partial Cl/\partial t = 0$ gives rise to a constant interstitial concentration during the steady state period of

$$C_I^{\max} = \frac{k_r}{k_f} = \frac{1}{4\pi a^3} \exp\left(-\frac{E_b}{kT}\right) \tag{8.41}$$

It is more useful to write this as a constant interstitial supersaturation during the steady-state period, since this will determine the enhancement in the dopant diffusivity, giving

$$\frac{C_I^{\max}}{C_I^*} = \frac{1}{4\pi a^3 C_I^0} \exp\left(-\frac{E_b - E_F}{kT}\right) \tag{8.42}$$

where we used the formula for the equilibrium interstitial concentration from Chapter 3,

$$C_I^* = C_{\text{Si}} \exp\left(-\frac{(E_F - TS_F)}{kT}\right) = C^0{}_I \exp\left(-\frac{E_F}{kT}\right) \tag{8.43}$$

Example Calculate the interstitial supersaturation versus temperature using the above equations. Assume the binding energy of an interstitial to a {311} cluster is 1.77 eV.

Answer From Table 7–5, we have the self-diffusion coefficient for silicon

$$D_{\text{Self}} = 560 \exp\left(-\frac{4.76}{\text{kT}}\right) \text{cm}^2 \text{ sec}^{-1}$$

This is the overall measured diffusion coefficient for silicon atoms, so the self-diffusion flux is given by

$$D_{\text{Self}} C_{\text{Si}} = 560 \exp\left(-\frac{4.76}{\text{kT}}\right) [\text{cm}^2 \text{ sec}^{-1}](5 \times 10^{22})[\text{cm}^{-3}]$$

$$= 2800 \times 10^{22} \exp\left(-\frac{4.76}{\text{kT}}\right) [\text{cm}^{-1} \text{ sec}^{-1}]$$

The interstitial fraction of the self-diffusion (using Table 7–6) is

$$d_I C_I^* = (0.6) 2800 \times 10^{22} \exp\left(-\frac{4.76}{kT}\right) = 1680 \times 10^{22} \exp\left(-\frac{4.76}{kT}\right) [\text{cm}^{-1} \text{s}^{-1}]$$

This equation describes the magnitude and temperature dependence of the interstitial flux. Note that the activation energy is large compared to the activation energy for dopant diffusion. This will become important in the later discussion.

A reasonable value for the diffusion coefficient of interstitials is given by

$$d_I = 51 \exp\left(-\frac{1.8}{kT}\right) [\text{cm}^2 \text{s}^{-1}]$$

allowing C_I^* to be calculated

$$C_I^* = 33 \times 10^{22} \exp\left(-\frac{2.96}{kT}\right) [\mathrm{cm}^{-3}]$$

The jump distance can be taken as half the lattice constant, so that

$$a = \frac{5.41 \times 10^{-8}}{2} = 2.7 \times 10^{-8} \text{ cm}$$

The binding energy of interstitials to {311} clusters is 1.77 eV, which was obtained by fitting the decay kinetics of the 311 defects in Figure 8–33 [8.27]. It is a pure coincidence that this is so similar to the activation energy for interstitial diffusion. Using these values gives

$$\frac{C_I^{max}}{C_I^*} = \frac{1}{4\pi a^3 C_I^0} \exp\left(-\frac{E_b - E_F}{kT}\right)$$
$$= \frac{1}{4\pi(2.7 \times 10^{-8})^3 (33 \times 10^{22})} \exp\left(-\frac{1.77 - 2.96}{kT}\right)$$
$$= 1.22 \times 10^{-2} \exp\left(\frac{1.19}{kT}\right)$$

which is plotted in Figure 8–35.

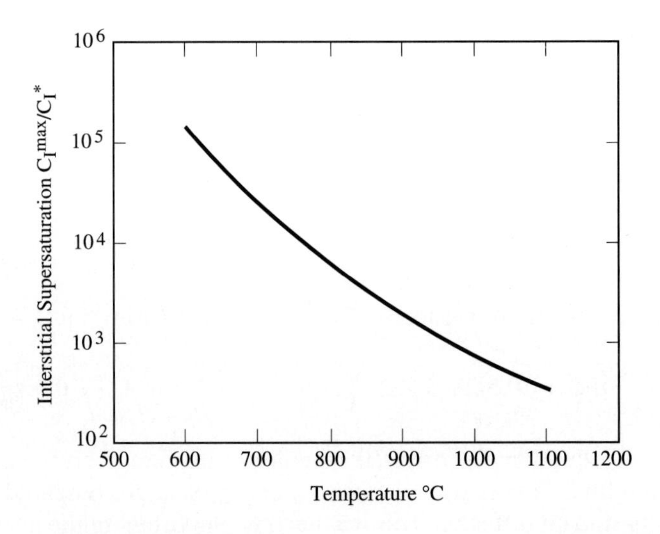

Figure 8–35 The maximum interstitial supersaturation as a function of anneal temperature.

The enhancement in diffusivity observed during TED is determined by the balance between cluster growth and evaporation. As long as there are a sufficient number of clusters around, some will shrink and others will grow, maintaining a steady-state interstitial supersaturation. It is during this steady-state condition that most of the profile motion occurs because the interstitial supersaturation is large and constant. This supersaturation has been measured experimentally and is as large as 10,000 at 750°C [8.21]. It reduces to a factor of 800 at a typical RTA temperature of 1000°C.

An example is shown in Figure 8–36, where the effects of TED on boron profile motion are dramatic for times as short as 1 minute at 750°C. The reason is that the normal, inert diffusivity of the boron is enhanced by a factor of 10,000 during the steady-state period when the clusters exist. The clusters continually supply interstitials to maintain this supersaturation by dissolving slowly, and the excess interstitials diffuse into the bulk producing the flat supersaturation profile and also recombine at the surface. After approximately 10 minutes at 750°C, the interstitial supersaturation decays rapidly and the boron profile will have experienced the maximum profile motion. Further annealing at 750°C will move the profile only with the inert diffusivity.

A second critical parameter is how long this steady-state condition lasts. If we assume the "+1" model for damage, then an implanted dose Q introduces an equivalent dose Q of excess interstitials which rapidly form clusters, and we wish to determine how long these excess interstitials survive. The interstitials in the clusters will eventually diffuse into the bulk or recombine at the surface. Since the damage is in general near the surface, the surface is the dominant sink for the excess interstitials and the flux of interstitials toward the surface can be estimated from Figure 8–37 to be $d_I C_I^{\max}/R_p$, where R_p is the range of the implant.

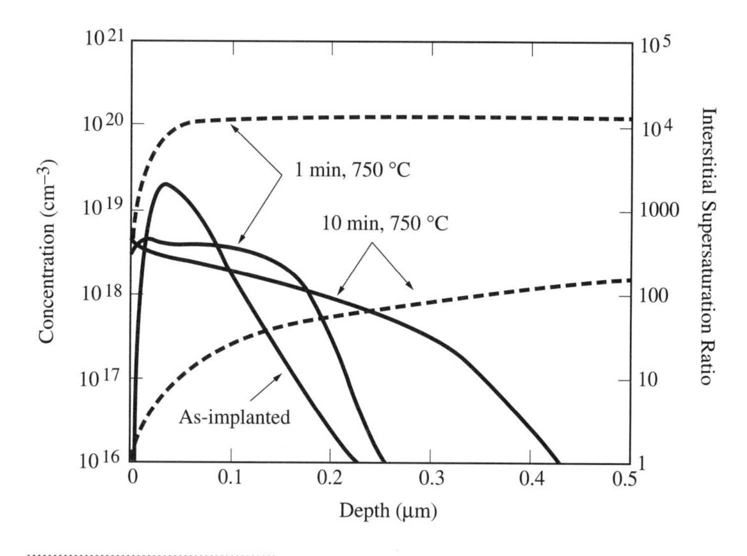

Figure 8–36 TSUPREM IV simulations [8.1] of boron TED (solid lines) at 750°C. A 10-keV, 10^{14} cm^{-2} boron implant experiences a steady-state enhancement of 10^4 while TED lasts at 750°C. The TED effect is beginning to decay rapidly after 10 min at 750°C. The dashed lines are the interstitial supersaturations.

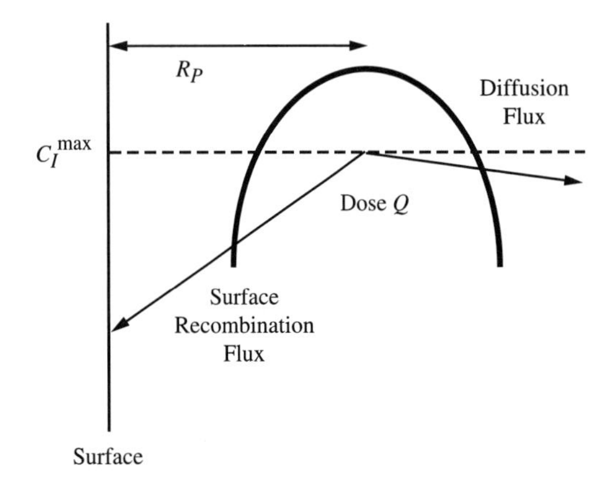

Figure 8–37 A schematic of the recombination flux at the surface which removes the +1 damage introduced by an implant at a range R_p [8.27].

The time to dissolve the clusters is given by the dose divided by the flux,

$$\tau_{\text{enh}} = \frac{4\pi a^3 R_P Q}{d_I} \exp\left(\frac{E_b}{kT}\right) \tag{8.44}$$

To clearly see the activation energy for the steady-state period, we can substitute for the self-interstitial diffusivity

$$d_I = d_I^0 \exp\left(-\frac{E_m}{kT}\right) \tag{8.45}$$

giving

$$\tau_{\text{enh}} = \frac{4\pi a^3 R_P Q}{d_I^0} \exp\left(\frac{E_b + E_m}{kT}\right) \tag{8.46}$$

Example Calculate and plot how the duration of TED depends on temperature for a 40-keV, $1 \times 10^{14}\ \text{cm}^{-2}$ phosphorus implant into silicon.

Answer From Figure 8–3, a 40-keV phosphorus implant has a range of 60 nm:

$$\therefore \tau_{\text{enh}} = \frac{4\pi a^3 R_P Q}{d_I^0} \exp\left(\frac{E_b + E_m}{kT}\right)$$

$$= \frac{4\pi(2.7 \times 10^{-8}\ \text{cm})^3(60 \times 10^{-7}\ \text{cm})(1 \times 10^{14}\ \text{cm}^{-2})}{51[\text{cm}^2\ \text{sec}^{-1}]} \exp\left(\frac{1.77 + 1.8}{kT}\right)$$

$$= 2.9 \times 10^{-15} \exp\left(\frac{3.57}{kT}\right)\ \text{sec}$$

which is plotted in Figure 8–38.

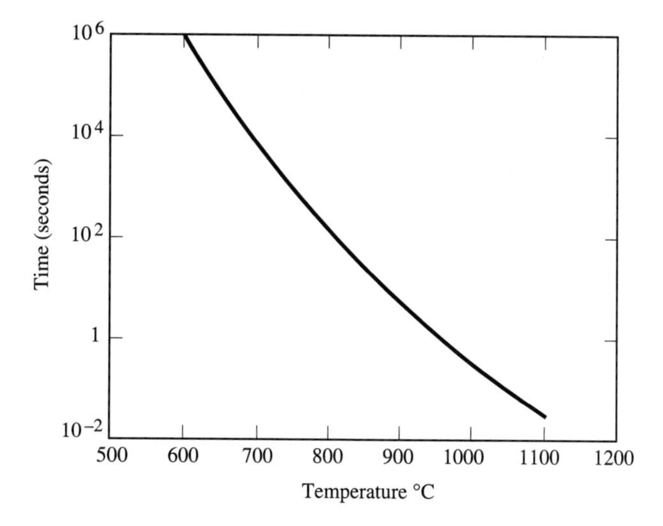

Figure 8–38 Duration of TED plotted versus temperature.

We can estimate the overall amount of profile motion after TED by combining the above information and taking the product of the dopant diffusivity, the steady-state interstitial supersaturation, and the steady-state time to give

$$D_A^{\text{eff}} t_{\text{eff}} = \left(D_A \frac{C_I^{\max}}{C_I^*} \right) \tau_{\text{enh}} = D_A \times \frac{QR_P}{d_I C_I^*} = \frac{D_A}{f_I^{\text{self}} D^{\text{self}} C_{\text{Si}}} \times QR_P \tag{8.47}$$

which immediately makes clear the anomalous temperature dependence of TED. Though the dopant diffusivity has an activation energy of approximately 3.5 eV, it is overwhelmed by the activation energy of self-diffusion D^{self} (i.e., $E_F + E_m$) $\approx$ 4.8 eV, which causes more profile motion at lower temperatures. Thus, this equation neatly explains the single most anomalous observation about TED—the fact that profiles diffuse more at lower temperatures than at higher temperatures, even for similar Dt as shown in the experimental SIMS plots in Figure 8–31. Though puzzling, this observation can be rationalized by considering that a fixed amount of damage is introduced by the implant, while the background point-defect concentration and interstitial self-diffusion coefficient fall sharply with temperature. Thus, the supersaturation in the point-defect levels rises sharply with falling temperature and the excess defects remain around longer due to the lower interstitial diffusion coefficient, leading to greater overall motion in the dopant profile. A simulation of how this comes about is shown in Figure 8–39, where the higher interstitial supersaturation which also lasts longer at low temperatures causes more profile motion at the lower temperatures.

The general form of the TED dependence in Eq. (8.47) also indicates that the amount of profile motion measured by $\sqrt{Dt}$ has a square root dependence on the dose of damage and also on the range at which the damage is introduced. For implants close to the surface, this also contains information on how the energy of the implant will

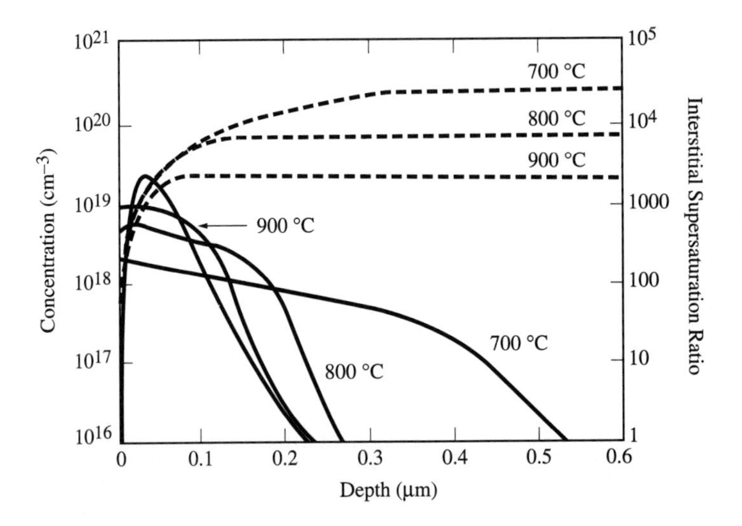

Figure 8–39 TSUPREM IV simulations [8.1] of boron profile motion after TED at various temperatures. The steady-state enhancement in the interstitial supersaturation is shown on the right axis and is higher at low temperatures and also lasts longer at low temperatures, leading to more profile motion at low temperatures.

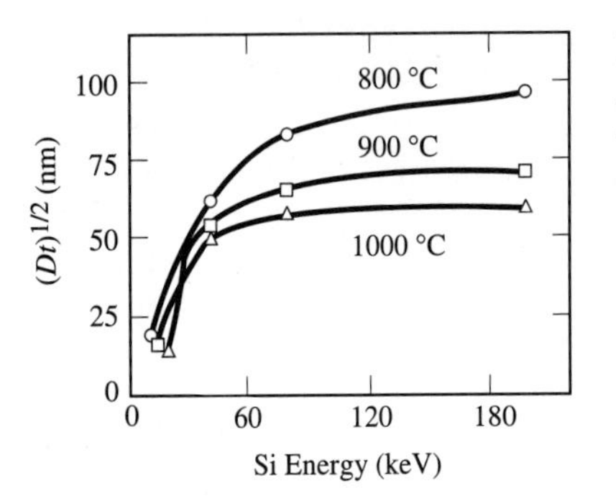

Figure 8–40 Energy dependence of TED. In these experiments, an experimental structure similar to that shown in Figure 8–32 was used, with different Si implant energies used to create the surface damaged region and the impact of TED on a buried marker layer was observed. (After [8.22].)

affect the overall profile motion. Since the range is roughly linearly proportional to the energy, it indicates that higher energies will give rise to higher overall profile motion. For large enough energies, the surface is no longer the dominant sink and diffusion to the bulk limits the flux away from the clusters. At this point, the amount of profile motion will be independent of the implant energy. Higher implant energies do give rise to more TED, as shown in Figure 8–40. The explanation appears to be obvious, in that higher implant energies create more damage. Though eminently reasonable, this is not the whole story for the energy dependence of TED and the physics contained in Eq. (8.48) provides a more complete explanation of the shape of the curves versus energy.

Another puzzling experimental observation relates to the dose dependence of TED—how do different damage doses give rise to the same amount of TED for short anneal times, but more damage produces more TED for longer anneal times? An example of

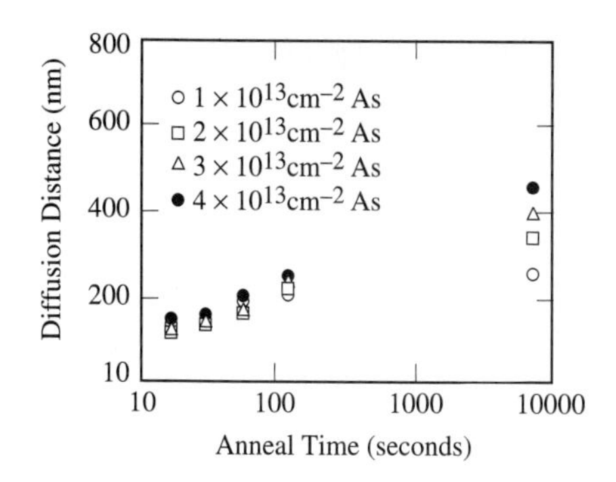

Figure 8–41 Dose dependence of TED. In these experiments, an experimental structure similar to that shown in Figure 8–32 was used, with different As implant energies used to create the surface damaged region and the impact of TED on a buried marker layer was observed. (After [8.22].)

the amount of profile motion after different As implant damage doses is shown in Figure 8–41. These data suggest that there is a maximum cap in the amount of enhancement that a dopant can experience, but a detailed understanding of the dose dependence requires an atomic-level model for the damage evolution. The microscopic cluster mechanism solves the dilemma of the unusual dose dependence of TED. Supersaturations higher than C_I^{max}/C_I^* do not exist because of the balance between cluster growth and dissolution. This provides a maximum cap on the diffusion enhancement regardless of the implant dose. Larger implant doses simply mean that the steady-state interstitial supersaturation is maintained for a longer time period before the clusters eventually decay. This provides the atomic-level explanation for why the enhancement is the same for different doses at short times but is greater for higher doses at longer times.

Thus, two parameters control the duration of TED for practical purposes—the critical supersaturation level and the time that the steady-state condition lasts, as shown schematically in Figure 8–42. This has been validated experimentally for As, P, and Si implant damage [8.21]. Boron TED appears to be more complex, perhaps because of the enormous strain that boron atoms introduce in the lattice, leading to the preferential formation of Boron Interstitial Complexes or BICs [8.28]. There are fewer {311} defects seen in high-concentration boron layers, but there is still substantial TED. Small dots that appear on TEM images may be related to Boron Interstitial Clusters or BICs. There appears to be competition between BICs and {311} defects for the excess interstitials. The BICs appear to have a higher binding energy for interstitials, so retain them longer during an anneal, giving rise to a longer time transient for boron TED than for the other dopants. However, the general picture holds, in that the magnitude and duration of TED are controlled by the evaporation of interstitials from microscopic defect aggregates.

8.5.11 Effects on Devices

MOSTEK in the early seventies was the first company to make major use of ion implantation to adjust the threshold voltage in MOS transistors. This application is ideally suited to the strengths of ion implantation and is still one of its key uses today. Because ion implantation can control even very low implant doses accurately, this allows the threshold voltage of MOS devices to be made uniform, without regard to the initial

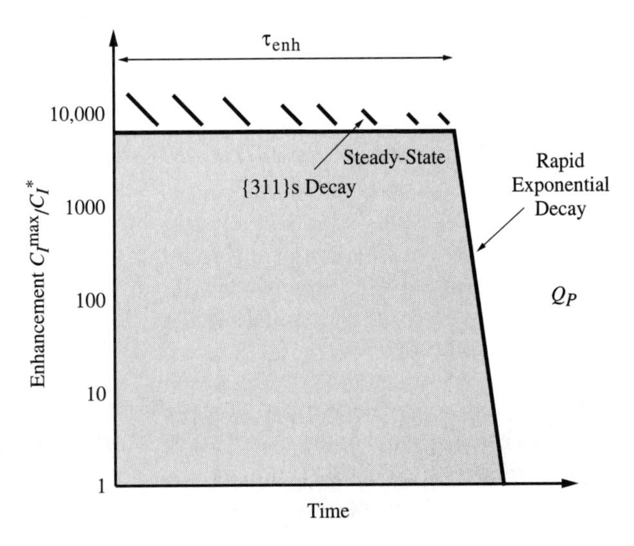

Figure 8–42 Schematic of the magnitude and duration of TED, determined from Eqs. (8.45) and (8.48). The shaded area is primarily responsible for the profile motion observed during TED.

variations in the substrate. When an ion implant dose Q is introduced into the channel of a MOS device such that all of the dose is contained in the depletion region during normal operation, this introduces a threshold voltage shift of

$$\Delta V_T = \frac{qQ}{C_{OX}} \tag{8.48}$$

where C_{OX} is the oxide capacitance per unit area, given by

$$C_{OX} = \frac{\varepsilon_0}{x_o} \tag{8.49}$$

In this way, MOS transistors can be fabricated on a lightly doped substrate or in a lightly doped well without much regard to the precise surface doping level. Later in the process, a threshold adjust implant can tailor the surface concentration in the channel region to the precise value needed for correct device operation. The ability of ion implantation to control the dose of ions introduced means that uniform thresholds can be obtained. This approach is universally used today and was illustrated in the CMOS process in Chapter 2.

Ion implantation has also made a major contribution to MOS scaling by allowing a deeper implant under the channel to be introduced, thereby avoiding punchthrough between the source and the drain through the bulk of the silicon. Once predicted to be a limiting factor on the scaling of MOS devices, this bulk punchthrough can now easily be avoided by using a punchthrough implant below the channel of the MOSFET. Typically, this is a higher dose than used for the threshold adjust implant, but the ability of ion implantation to introduce a retrograde profile below the surface was a key factor to its success.

Today, the focus of much effort is on even deeper implants to replace the deep well diffusions in a CMOS device. The ability to introduce a retrograde well profile, a punchthrough implant, and a threshold adjust implant through the same mask allows for considerable process simplification and mask savings. The reader may note that the implants in Figures 2–10 and 2–22 in Chapter 2 use exactly the same mask, for example.

Quite apart from the possibility that dislocations may be introduced by implants, there are more subtle effects on devices that are caused by ion-implant-induced TED. One example is the so-called Reverse Short-Channel Effect (RSCE), where a gradient in the interstitial profile toward the gate oxide causes the channel dopant to pile up under the gate giving rise to a higher threshold voltage for shorter gate lengths [8.29]. (Recall Figure 7–45 and the associated text.) Understanding TED allows suggestions to be made for avoiding the RSCE. For example, the dopant can be piled up in both long- and short-channel devices by using a silicon damage implant at the same time as the threshold adjust implant. The existing gradient of dopant atoms will inhibit further pileup, thus reducing the RSCE effects from later thermal anneals and source/drain implants. Alternatively, indium can be used as the channel dopant instead of boron. Even though indium exhibits diffusion characteristics very similar to boron, including identical susceptibility to TED, it segregates very strongly to an oxide interface. Thus, while some of the channel dose is lost to the oxide interface, further indium does not pile up at the interface during TED. It thus maintains its retrograde profile, which gives rise to less severe RSCE.

In summary, recent advances in understanding the physically based origins of TED on an atomic scale have led to breakthrough abilities to model its impact on devices. Key device effects such as DIBL, short-channel rolloff behavior, and RSCE can now be quantitatively modeled.

8.6 Limits and Future Trends in Technologies and Models

Ion implantation seems destined to retain a key role in doping semiconductors into the foreseeable future. The limits of the technology range from energies low enough to "soft-land" dopant atoms on the silicon surface at one extreme, to energies in the MeV range which may provide a replacement for buried layer epitaxial wafers. Energies at either extreme can be realized in a conventional implanter, consisting of ion separation, ion acceleration, and ion counting in a Faraday cage.

Alternative technologies have been suggested in the ultralow-energy regime, where conventional ion sources may have difficulty producing the required beam current. When the implant energies are in the hundreds of electron volts, they are comparable to the ion energy that is available across the sheath in an ion plasma (see Chapters 9 and 10). A plasma source can provide a large ion current and thus allow high doses to be implanted at low energies. The one drawback is that there is no ion separation possible, so multiple ion complexes are implanted into the wafer. In spite of this drawback, plasma source ion implantation is being investigated as a high-dose, low-energy doping method.

Diffusion from doped layers still remains attractive for obtaining the shallowest possible junctions, without the complication of transient-enhanced diffusion caused by implant damage. The possibility that the ultrashallow tip or extension region in a MOS device can be formed by out-diffusion from a doped spacer layer remains attractive. Dopant is introduced at the solid solubility limit without accompanying damage, providing the minimum possible junction depth.

The future trends in ion implantation are dominated by the need for the equipment manufacturer to supply a process module that will provide a shallow junction meeting the NTRS requirements. Many of the auxiliary steps not directly related to the ion implant equipment play a key role, such as how to anneal the implant damage to provide a shallow junction with high activation. The equipment maker must also be familiar with the associated technology to provide the complete solution required by the semiconductor manufacturer. The trend is for the equipment makers to combine several steps, such as ion implant and RTA, and provide detailed process recipes that produce an optimized process step. In the future, it is likely that a detailed physical understanding of the underlying atomic-scale mechanisms that affect implantation and diffusion will be required by the equipment process developer. Models for the process steps, not just raw machinery, will likely be provided to the semiconductor customer.

8.7 Summary of Key Ideas

Ion implantation is a technique which combines ion separation, acceleration, and dose measurement to introduce a precise number of dopant atoms into the silicon substrate. The ions that impact the silicon wafer slow down by a combination of nuclear and electronic interactions with the lattice atoms. Ion implant energies range from hundreds of eV to millions of eV, with higher energy producing a deeper doping profile. This energy is much larger than the 15 eV needed to displace a silicon atom from the lattice and create a stable interstitial and vacancy pair. Large numbers of displaced atoms are created by a single implanted ion. The damage can accumulate and eventually produce a completely disordered or amorphous layer where the implant has occurred. Damage produced by an implant causes a large enhancement in the diffusion coefficient of dopants, until such time as the damage is completely repaired. This effect is known as transient-enhanced diffusion of ion-implanted layers and often limits how shallow a junction can be made.

Simple models for the ion implanted profile rely on a Gaussian distribution, though higher-order moments are needed to characterize profiles even in amorphous material. The relatively open structure of the silicon lattice leads to channeled profiles at low doses, where ions that enter a planar or axial channel travel further. Accurate models for ion implanted profiles in silicon require that the nuclear and electronic collisions be considered for a number of ions so that the implanted profile can be constructed. Provided that means can be found to minimize TED and provide highly active layers, ion implantation is likely to remain the technology of choice for doping silicon.

8.8 References

[8.1]. TSUPREM4 is a version of SUPREM-IV from Avant! Inc. SUPREM IV was originally written at Stanford University by M. E. Law, C. S. Rafferty, and R. W. Dutton.

[8.2]. Simulation performed with computer code UT-MARLOWE, distributed by the University of Texas, Austin.

[8.3]. W. K. Hofker, D. P. Oosthoek, N. J. Koeman, and A.M. De Grefte, "Concentration Profiles of Boron Implantations in Amorphous and Polycrystalline Silicon," *Radiation Effects*, vol. 24, no. 4, p. 223, 1975.

[8.4]. S. J. Morris, B. Obradovic, S. H. Yang, and A. F. Tasch, "Modeling of Boron Phosphorus and Arsenic Implants into Single-crystal Silicon over a Wide Energy Range (Few keV to Several MeV)," *IEDM Technical Digest*, p. 721, 1996.

[8.5]. J. F. Ziegler, "The Stopping and Range of Ions in Solids," in *Ion Implantation Science and Technology*, edited by J. F. Ziegler, Academic Press, 1984.

[8.6]. W. Brandt and M. Kitagawa, "Effective Stopping-power Charges of Swift Ions in Condensed Matter," *Physical Review B (Condensed Matter),* vol. 25, no. 9, p. 5631, 1982.

[8.7]. J. F. Gibbons, "Ion Implantation in Semiconductors, Part 1, Range Distribution Theory and Experiments," *Proc. IEEE*, March 1968, vol. 56, no. 3, p. 295.

[8.8]. D. Cai, C. M. Snell, K. M. Beardmore, and N. Gronbech-Jensen, "Simulation of Phosphorus Implantation into Silicon with a Single parameter Electronic Stopping Power Model," *International Journal of Modern Physics C*, vol. 9, no. 3, p. 459, 1998.

[8.9]. I. Brodie and J. J. Muray, *The Physics of Microfabrication*, Plenum Press, 1982.

[8.10]. M. J. Caturla, T. Dias de la Rubia, and G. H. Gilmer, "Disordering and Defect Production in Silicon by keV Ion Irradiation Studied by Molecular Dynamics," *Nucl. Instrum. Methods Phys. Res. B* (*Beam Interactions with Materials and Atoms*), vol. B106, no. 1–4, p. 1, 1995.

[8.11]. S. Tian, M. F. Morris, S. J. Morris, B. Obradovic, G. Wang, A. F. Tasch, and C. M. Snell, "A Detailed Physical Model for Ion Implant Induced Damage in Silicon," *IEEE Transactions on Electron Devices*, vol. 45, no. 6, p. 1226, 1998.

[8.12]. W. P. Maszara and G. A. Rozgonyi, "Kinetics of Damage Production in Silicon During Self-implantation," *Journal of Applied Physics*, vol. 60, no. 7, p. 2310, 1986.

[8.13]. M. Jariz, G. H. Gilmer, J. M. Poate, and T. D. de la Rubia, "Atomistic Calculations of Ion Implantation in Si, Point Defect and Transient Enhanced Diffusion Phenomena," *Applied Physics Letters*, vol. 68, no. 3, p. 409, 1996.

[8.14]. G. Z. Pan, K. N. Tu, and A. Prussin, "Size-distribution and Annealing Behavior of End-of-range Dislocation Loops in Silicon-implanted Silicon," *Journal of Applied Physics,* vol. 81, no. 1, p. 78, 1997.

[8.15]. J. R. Liefting, J. S. Custer, R. J. Schreutelkamp, and F. W. Saris, "Dislocation Formation in Silicon Implanted at Different Temperatures," *Materials Science and Engineering B (Solid-State Materials for Advanced Technology),* vol. B15, no. 2, p. 173, 1992.

[8.16]. L. Csepregi, E. F. Kennedy, T. J. Gallagher, J. W. Mayer, and T. W. Sigmon, "Reordering of Amorphous Layers of Si Implanted with P, As and B Ions," *J. Appl. Physics*, vol. 48, p. 4234, 1977.

[8.17]. J. Fletcher, J. Narayan, and O. W. Holland, "Studies of Defects and Solubility Limits in SPE grown In and Sb Implanted Silicon," *Microscopy of Semiconducting Materials*, 1981, Proceedings of the Second Oxford Conference, p. 295, editors, A. G. Cullis and D. C. Joy, 1981.

[8.18]. B. L. Crowder and F. F. Morehead, "Annealing Characteristics of N-type Dopants in Ion Implanted Silicon," *Appl. Phys. Lett.,* vol. 14, p. 313, 1969.

[8.19]. T. E. Seidel and A. U. MacRae, "The Isothermal Annealing of Boron Implanted Silicon," in *First International Conference on Ion Implantation*, editors, F. Eisen and L. Chadderton, Gordon and Breach, 1971.

[8.20]. S. W. Crowder, "Processing Physics in Silicon-on-Insulator Material," Ph.D. thesis, Stanford University, 1995.

[8.21]. H. S. Chao, S. W. Crowder, P. B. Griffin, and J. D. Plummer, "Species and Dose Dependence of Ion Implantation Damage Induced Transient Enhanced Diffusion," *Journal of Applied Physics*, vol. 79, no. 5, p. 2352, 1996.

[8.22]. P. A. Packan and J. D. Plummer, "Transient Diffusion of Low-concentration B in Si Due to Si Implantation Damage," *Applied Physics Letters*, vol. 56, no.18, p. 1787, 1990.

[8.23]. D. J. Eaglesham, P.A. Stolk, H.-J. Gossmann, and J. M. Poate, "Implantation and Transient B Diffusion in Si: The Source of the Interstitials," *Applied Physics Letters*, vol. 56, no.18, p. 2305, 1994.

[8.24]. J. L. Benton, S. Libertino, P. Kringhoj, D. J. Eaglesham, J. M. Poate, and S. Coffa, "Evolution from Point to Extended Defects in Ion Implanted Silicon," *Journal of Applied Physics*, vol. 82, no. 1, p. 120, 1997.

[8.25]. M. D. Giles, S. Yu, H.W. Kennel, and P.A. Packan, "Modeling Silicon Implantation Damage and Transient Enhanced Diffusion Effects for Silicon Technology Development," in *Defects and Diffusion in Silicon Processing Symposium*, San Francisco, 1997, edited by T. Diaz de la Rubia, S. Coffa, P.A. Stolk, and C. S. Rafferty, Materials Research Society, 1997.

[8.26]. M. D. Giles, "Transient Phosphorus Diffusion from Silicon and Argon Implantation Damage," *Applied Physics Letters*, vol. 62, no. 16, p. 1940, 1993.

[8.27]. C. S. Rafferty, G. H. Gilmer, M. Jaraiz, D. Eaglesham, and H.-J. Gossmann, "Simulation of Cluster Evaporation and Transient Enhanced Diffusion in Silicon," *Applied Physics Letters*, vol. 68, no. 17, p. 2395, 1996.

[8.28]. K. S. Jones, J. Liu, and L. Zhang, "Evidence of Two Sources of Interstitials for TED in Boron Implanted Silicon," in *Proceedings of the Fourth International Symposium on Process Physics and Modeling in Semiconductor Technology*, p. 116, edited by G. R. Srinivasan, C. S. Murthy, and S. T. Dunham, Pennington, NJ, Electrochemical Society, 1996.

[8.29]. C. S. Rafferty, H.-H. Vuong, S. A. Eshraghi , M. D. Giles, M. R. Pinto, and S. J. Hillenius, "Explanation of Reverse Short Channel Effect by Defect Gradients," *IEDM Technical Digest*, p. 311, 1993.

8.9 Problems

8.1. Arsenic is implanted into a lightly doped p-type Si substrate at an energy of 75 keV. The dose is 1×10^{14} cm^{-2}. The Si substrate is tilted 7° with respect to the ion beam to make it appear amorphous. The implanted region is assumed to be rapidly annealed so that complete electrical activation is achieved. What is the peak electron concentration produced?

8.2. An engineer worried about avoiding punchthrough in an NMOS device decides to perform a deep punchthrough implant while keeping the surface concentration at a maximum value of 1×10^{17} cm^{-3}. What is the maximum implant dose that would be suitable if the peak of the profile is aligned at twice the depth of the deep source/drain contact junction in a 180 nm technology? (See NTRS Table 7–1 for parameter values.)

8.3. We want to design an implant step which will implant phosphorus ions through 50 nm of SiO_2 into an underlying silicon substrate such that the peak concentration in the substrate is 1×10^{17} cm^{-3} and the concentration at the SiO_2/Si interface is

1×10^{15} cm^{-3}. What energy and dose would you use to achieve these conditions? Assume that the stopping power of SiO_2 is the same as that of silicon. Neglect channeling effects.

8.4. How thick does a mask have to be to reduce the peak doping of an implant by a factor of 10,000 at the mask/substrate boundary? Provide an equation in terms of the range and the standard deviation of the implant profile.

8.5. In a particular application, it is important to produce a fairly flat profile over an extended distance by ion implantation, as indicated below. One way to do this is to superimpose several implants at different energies. If phosphorus implants with energies of 0.5 R_P, R_P, $2R_P$ are used with a dose of 1×10^{14} cm^{-2} in the middle peak, approximately what doses should be used in the adjacent peaks if the initial peak concentrations are to be the same?

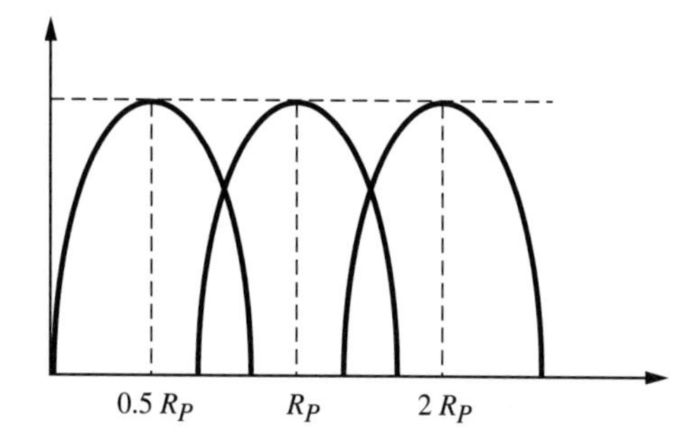

8.6. The equations below provide a reasonable analytical description for some of the diffusion processes indicated schematically in the diagrams on the following page. Put the equation number [(a)–(f)] on each figure that is the best match. Equations may be reused, or multiple equations may describe the same figure. A brief explanation is required for each figure.

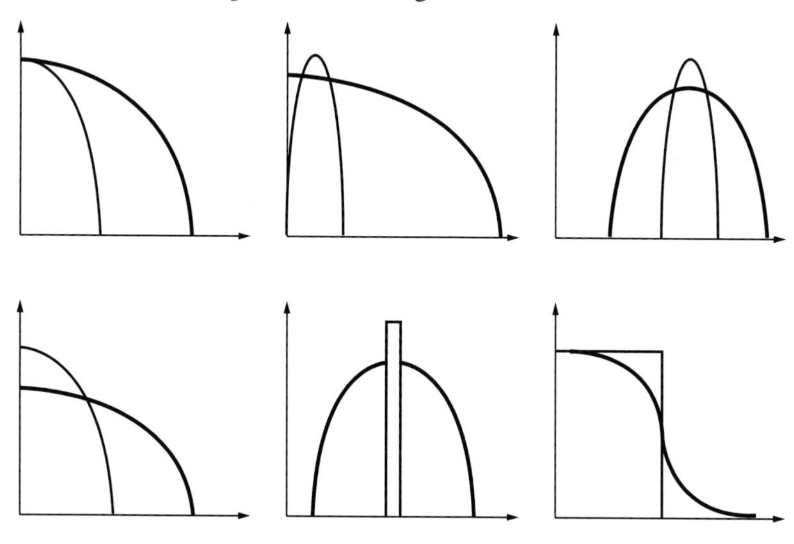

a. $C(x,t) = \frac{C}{2} \operatorname{erfc}\left(\frac{x}{2\sqrt{Dt}}\right)$

b. $C(x,t) = \frac{Q}{\sqrt{\pi(D_1t_1 + D_2t_2)}} \exp\left(-\frac{x^2}{4(D_1t_1 + D_1t_1)}\right)$

c. $C(x,t) = \frac{Q}{2\sqrt{\pi Dt}} \exp\left[-\left(\frac{x}{2\sqrt{Dt}}\right)^2\right]$

d. $C(x,t) = C\operatorname{erfc}\left(\frac{x}{2\sqrt{Dt}}\right)$

e. $C(x,t) = \frac{Q}{\sqrt{\pi Dt}} \exp\left(-\frac{x^2}{4Dt}\right)$

f. $C(x,t) = \frac{Q}{\sqrt{2\pi(\Delta R_P^2 + 2Dt)}} \exp\left(-\frac{(x - R_P)^2}{2(\Delta R_P^2 + 2Dt)}\right)$

8.7. An 80-keV, 5×10^{13} cm^{-2} boron implant is performed into bare silicon. A subsequent anneal at 950°C is performed for 60 min.

a. Can the annealed profile evolution be described by the following formula?

$$C(x,t) = \frac{Q}{\sqrt{\pi D_B t}} \exp\left(-\frac{x^2}{4D_B t}\right)$$

b. Assume that all the dopant remains in the silicon and that none evaporates to the ambient. By considering a virtual or imaginary image profile on the ambient side of the interface (a reflecting boundary), calculate the surface concentration after a 60-min 950°C anneal.

8.8. A 1×10^{14} cm^{-2} phosphorus implant through a 200-nm SiO_2 mask layer is performed so the peak concentration is at the silicon/SiO_2 interface. An anneal is then performed for 30 min at 1000°C. Calculate the location of the junction with the substrate doped at 1×10^{15} cm^{-3}. Assume no diffusion in the masking layer and ignore any segregation effects. Assume the same range statistics for SiO_2 and Si.

8.9. Phosphorus is implanted at 50 keV with a dose of 1×10^{14} cm^{-2}. Calculate the junction depth where the phosphorus meets the substrate (p type, 1×10^{15} cm^{-3}) after (a) a 900°C, three-hour anneal and (b) a 1200°C, three-hour anneal.

8.10. An implant machine for 300-mm wafers is required to have a throughput of 60 wafers per hour. What beam current is required in order to implant a source/drain region in a CMOS device with a dose of 1×10^{15} cm^{-2}?

8.11. In the ion implantation process, positively charged ions impact on the semiconductor surface. Normally these ions are neutralized by capturing an electron from the conducting substrate. However, when the mask is an insulator like SiO_2, the charge on the ions may not be neutralized as easily. Consider the case where a dose Q is implanted into the surface of an SiO_2 layer (assume all the charge resides at the oxide surface). Further assume that the oxide can withstand an electric field of 10^7 Vcm^{-1} before it breaks down. What implant dose Q is required to cause electrical failure of the mask? That is, what dose will cause a field of 10^7 Vcm^{-1} across the oxide?

8.12. An engineer investigating solid-phase epitaxial regrowth after amorphizing ion implants of various species (P, B, Si, Ge, As, Sb) makes the following observations:

1. N-type dopants of very different size or atomic radius (e.g., antimony versus phosphorus) show identical regrowth rates, approximately an order of magnitude faster than the regrowth of silicon implanted and amorphized with silicon ions.
2. P-type and N-type ion implanted regions have much faster regrowth rates than Si or Ge implanted regions, although they are not identical.
3. B-doped regions compensated with an equal dose of an arsenic implant show identical regrowth rates to Ge implanted and amorphized regions.

Construct a unified physical explanation of all three phenomena, considering possibilities such as size or stress effects, dopant charge or electric field effects, or point-defect-based effects (no calculation required).

8.13. In two separate experiments, As and then B are implanted through a thin SiO_2 layer into the underlying substrate. As a result of the implantation, some of the oxygen atoms in the SiO_2 layer are knocked into the silicon substrate. Would you expect the As or the B to produce more oxygen knock-ons? Why?

8.14. A boron implant is performed into silicon at 100 keV. The boron beam is aligned with the silicon crystal so that channeling is present. Estimate the range of the channeled boron profile by considering that electronic stopping is the only mechanism for slowing the boron ions.

8.15. An amorphizing implant is performed using a high dose of arsenic (5×10^5 cm^{-2}, 200 keV) and TEM cross-section images indicate complete amorphization to a depth of 50 nm. If Solid-Phase Epitaxial (SPE) regrowth instantly removes all of the damage in the amorphous region, calculate the fraction of the "+1" implanted dose that is available for TED.

8.16. Calculate the change in junction depth for a 40-keV boron threshold adjust implant of 5×10^{13} cm^{-2} annealed at 750°C in a furnace or at 1000°C in an RTA for a time just long enough to remove all the damage that causes TED. Assume a uniform well doping of 5×10^{16} cm^{-3}.

8.17. The diffusion of a buried antimony layer is only 20% of its normal diffusion in an inert ambient after a phosphorus implant is performed at the surface of a silicon wafer. The phosphorus diffusion coefficient is itself enhanced by a factor of 4 (400%).

a. Suggest a qualitative reason for this observation.

b. Assuming that the phosphorus diffuses completely by an interstitial mechanism, calculate how much of the antimony diffusion is mediated by interstitials and how much by vacancies.

8.18. A phosphorus implant is performed into a bare p-type silicon wafer with a background doping of 1×10^{15} cm^{-3}, at an energy of 50 keV, and a dose of 1×10^{14} cm^{-2}. After an anneal at 900°C for 10 min, the junction depth is measured to be 0.25 μm. Calculate the enhancement in the phosphorus diffusion coefficient that was caused by the implantation damage.

8.19. An engineer wants to form a shallow boron-doped source/drain junction for an advanced technology. The manager wants to know whether the company should buy an inexpensive batch furnace and achieve the required junction depth using a low-thermal budget anneal (one hour at 800°C) or an expensive single-wafer RTA (Rapid Thermal Annealer) using a high-temperature anneal.

a. Calculate the time required to achieve the target junction depth if the annealing temperature is 1050°C in the RTA.

b. Make a crude estimate ($\sqrt{Dt}$ approximation) of how far the dopants move during these anneals

c. Now, consider that the boron is introduced using an implant and that Transient Enhanced Diffusion (TED) due to the implant will be important. Using the charts for the expected enhancement in diffusivity and the time TED lasts, calculate how far the dopants move at each temperature.

d. Which anneal would you recommend?

8.20. An NMOS transistor is being built and an ion implantation is done after the gate oxide is grown and before the gate polysilicon deposition, in order to adjust the threshold voltage by +1volt.

a. Which dopant should be used?

b. Calculate the dose of the dopant if the oxide thickness is 10 nm.

8.21. A phosphorus implant is performed into a bare p-type silicon wafer with a background doping in $1 \times 10^{15}\text{cm}^{-3}$, at an energy of 50 keV and a dose of $1 \times 10^{14}\text{cm}^{-2}$. After an anneal at 900°C for 10 min, the junction depth is measured to be 0.25 μm. Calculate the time averaged enhancement in the phosphorus diffusion coefficient that was caused by implantation damage.

Thin Film Deposition

9

9.1 Introduction

The CMOS process flow in Chapter 2 contained many layers above the silicon substrate. These layers include dielectrics, semiconductors, and metals. In most cases these layers must be deposited which implies that there are typically many deposition steps in an IC process. In this chapter we describe the different techniques used to deposit these thin films. In Chapter 10 the techniques used to etch thin films are discussed.

We begin with several issues related to thin films and their deposition. These issues are important when evaluating deposited films and choosing deposition methods. The first issue is the "quality" of the deposited film. By quality we mean composition, contamination levels, defect density, and mechanical and electrical properties. The composition of films may vary depending on the deposition conditions and it is usually important to achieve a specific composition. This is especially important when a range of compositions is possible, such as with TiN films which can be Ti or N rich, or with alloys of metals like Al/Cu. Generally there needs to be a low level of contaminants, such as unwanted metals, water, oxygen, or halogens. There should also be a minimum of pin holes or other structural defects. These often result from particle contamination on the surface and are a common problem in thin film deposition (recall Figure 4–1). There should also be a minimum of stress in the films, and the films should be mechanically stable during subsequent processing. Finally, good adhesion to underlying films is important.

A second issue is that of uniform thickness across a wafer, from wafer to wafer, and as the film crosses nonplanar topography. Figure 9–1 shows a metal layer deposited over nonplanar topography in which there is a step in the underlying oxide. In Figure 9–1(b) the film thickness decreases as it crosses a step, which can lead to high electrical resistance in metal lines and a greater chance of mechanical cracking and failure. Coverage on the side of a step in topography is called step coverage. It is often defined quantitatively as the minimum thickness deposited on the side of a step divided by the thickness deposited on the top horizontal surface. Conformal step coverage, or conformal coverage, refers to uniform film thickness on both horizontal and vertical surfaces, or a step coverage of one.

A related issue is that of filling spaces between or within topographical structures. This includes filling a via or contact hole with metal, as illustrated in Figure 9–2(a), and filling spaces or gaps in shallow trench isolation structures or between metal lines with an oxide (often called gap filling), as illustrated in Figure 9–2(b). In this figure incomplete filling is shown, leading to a void in the dielectric between the lines. A void in a metal layer can lead to high-contact or -sheet resistance, and in a dielectric layer can

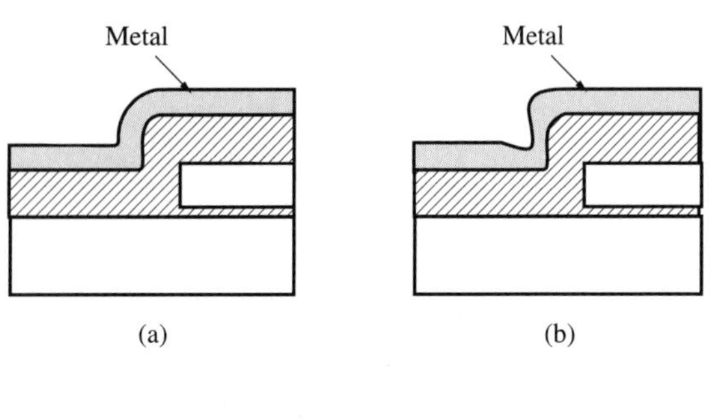

Figure 9–1 Step coverage of metal over nonplanar topography. (a) shows conformal step coverage, with constant thickness on horizontal and vertical surfaces. (b) shows poor step coverage.

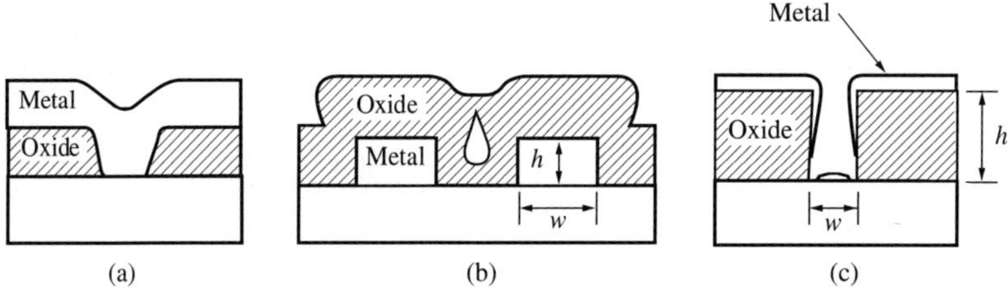

Figure 9–2 Thin film filling issues. (a) shows good metal filling of a via or contact hole in a dielectric layer. (b) shows silicon dioxide dielectric filling the space between metal lines, with poor filling leading to void formation. (c) shows poor filling of the bottom of a via hole with a barrier or contact metal.

result in cracking problems. In addition, a void may trap processing chemicals or moisture, leading to reliability problems. Even if complete filling of a space is not needed, good coverage or filling at the bottom of a space is often required. An example of this is the case of depositing contact and barrier layers, in which good filling of the bottom of contact or via holes is important. Figure 9–2(c) shows poor bottom coverage of a deep contact hole. The sides may also need adequate coverage of an adhesion layer.

An important parameter that can affect filling and bottom coverage is the Aspect Ratio (AR) of a feature, defined as the ratio of the height of a feature to its width:

$$AR = \frac{\text{height of feature}}{\text{width of feature}} = \frac{h}{w} \tag{9.1}$$

The feature could be a metal line, for example, or a space, such as a gap between two metal lines or a contact hole, as illustrated in Figure 9–2(b) and (c). A deep, narrow contact hole would have a large aspect ratio and would be harder to fill.

Two examples of poor filling and coverage are shown in Figure 9–3. Figure 9–3(a) shows poor step coverage of a TiW/Al/TiW metal stack layer over an oxide step. Figure 9–3(b) shows voids in an oxide layer for narrow spaces between metal lines. We will see that in filling or depositing in very deep contacts or vias, conditions that would lead to good step coverage may actually hinder adequate filling of the bottom of the contacts or vias.

We saw in the CMOS process flow in Chapter 2 that as more interconnect levels are used, another property that is desired for thin films is a smooth and flat top surface, as op-

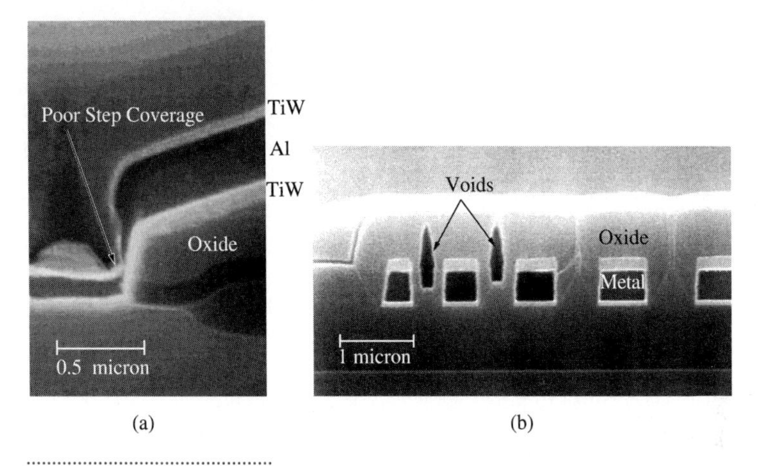

Figure 9–3 SEM images of coverage and filling problems. (a) shows poor step coverage of a TiW/Al/TiW metal stack layer, deposited by sputter deposition, over an oxide step. (b) shows voids in a Chemical Vapor Deposition (CVD) oxide layer for narrow spaces between metal lines. Photos courtesy of VLSI Technology, Inc.

posed to one that just follows the underlying topography. Figure 9–3(b) shows a relatively flat, planarized top surface of the oxide over the metal lines. While planarized topography can be achieved by postdeposition processing using etching or polishing techniques, we will also see how certain deposition techniques can also help attain this feature.

9.2 Historical Development and Basic Concepts

Methods of thin film deposition are usually separated into two main categories: Chemical Vapor Deposition (CVD) and Physical Vapor Deposition (PVD). In each case the silicon wafer is placed in a deposition chamber, and the constituents of the film are delivered through the gas phase to the surface of the substrate where they form the film. In the case of CVD, reactant gases are introduced into the deposition chamber, and chemical reactions between the reactant gases on the substrate surface are used to produce the film. In the case of PVD, physical methods are used to produce the constituent atoms which pass through a low-pressure gas phase and then condense on the substrate. The methods used to produce the atom flux in PVD include (1) heating a solid or molten source until it vaporizes, called "evaporation," and (2) bombarding a solid source with energetic ions formed in a plasma, called "sputter deposition." PVD is sometimes called "vacuum deposition" since very low-pressure environments are required for the transport of the gaseous species from the source to the film surface. (As we will see, low-pressure CVD is commonly used, but not at nearly as low pressures as in PVD.) CVD has historically been used in the integrated circuit industry mainly for silicon and dielectric deposition, primarily due to its good quality films and good step coverage. PVD has been used historically for metal deposition, mostly due to its ability to deposit a variety of metals and alloys not easily deposited by CVD.

A third category for thin film deposition is the technique of coating a wafer with a liquid film that forms a solid film when heated. Spin-On-Glasses (SOGs) are examples of this. This method, which is used for topography smoothing or "planarization," will be discussed in Chapter 11. A fourth category includes electrolytic deposition techniques. These have historically been used for printed circuit board fabrication but have recently been extended to the deposition of Cu interconnect layers.

9.2.1 Chemical Vapor Deposition (CVD)

In CVD, gases are introduced into the deposition chamber that react and form the desired film on the surface of the substrate. The silicon substrate will usually have other films deposited and patterned on it which then form a complex topography on which the new film must be deposited. Either a single gas is used that will decompose when heated to supply the necessary component or components for the film, or multiple gases are used which will react to produce the film. In either case, the film-producing reaction should take place on the surface of the substrate as opposed to in the gas stream. Gas stream reactions can create particulates that form above the wafer which can drop down onto the surface and cause the films to have pinholes or low density. Sometimes appropriate reactants are not available in gaseous form, in which case a liquid source may be used. A carrier gas such as hydrogen is bubbled through the liquid source and carries the source vapor to the reaction chamber. Nitrogen or argon may be used as a diluent or carrier gas.

The simplest CVD process uses an atmospheric deposition chamber, and no plasma-enhanced processes are used. This is appropriately called Atmospheric Pressure Chemical Vapor Deposition, or APCVD. The configuration shown in Figure 9–4(a) is a common type that has been used for APCVD, especially for epitaxial silicon deposition, but several other systems in a variety of configurations such as barrel-shaped chambers, have been used. The walls of the chamber in this case are not heated—a so-called "cold-wall" reactor. The wafers are heated by using a graphite susceptor which is heated by RF induction. This minimizes deposition on the reactor walls since only the susceptor and wafers are hot. APCVD has been used for many films, especially epitaxial silicon and silicon dioxide—both undoped and doped with boron and phosphorus. However, the increasing use of Low-Pressure CVD, or LPCVD, and Plasma-Enhanced CVD, or PECVD, for reasons to be discussed in the following sections, has made the use of APCVD reactors much less common today.

Figure 9–4(b) shows the low-pressure CVD configuration. In this case the wafers are stacked upright, and the deposition is performed at a reduced pressure. Heating is accomplished using resistive heating elements wrapped around the tube (a "hot-wall" reactor), which heats up the tube and everything inside. This is very similar to the oxidation system described in Chapter 6. Very uniform temperatures can be obtained in this type of system.

There are other types of CVD configurations and techniques, but all are based on the idea of supplying gaseous chemical sources and energy to the surface of the wafers. The energy is usually thermal energy, but one can greatly reduce the amount of thermal energy needed by using a plasma to provide for energetic ions and very reactive free radicals to stimulate the deposition.

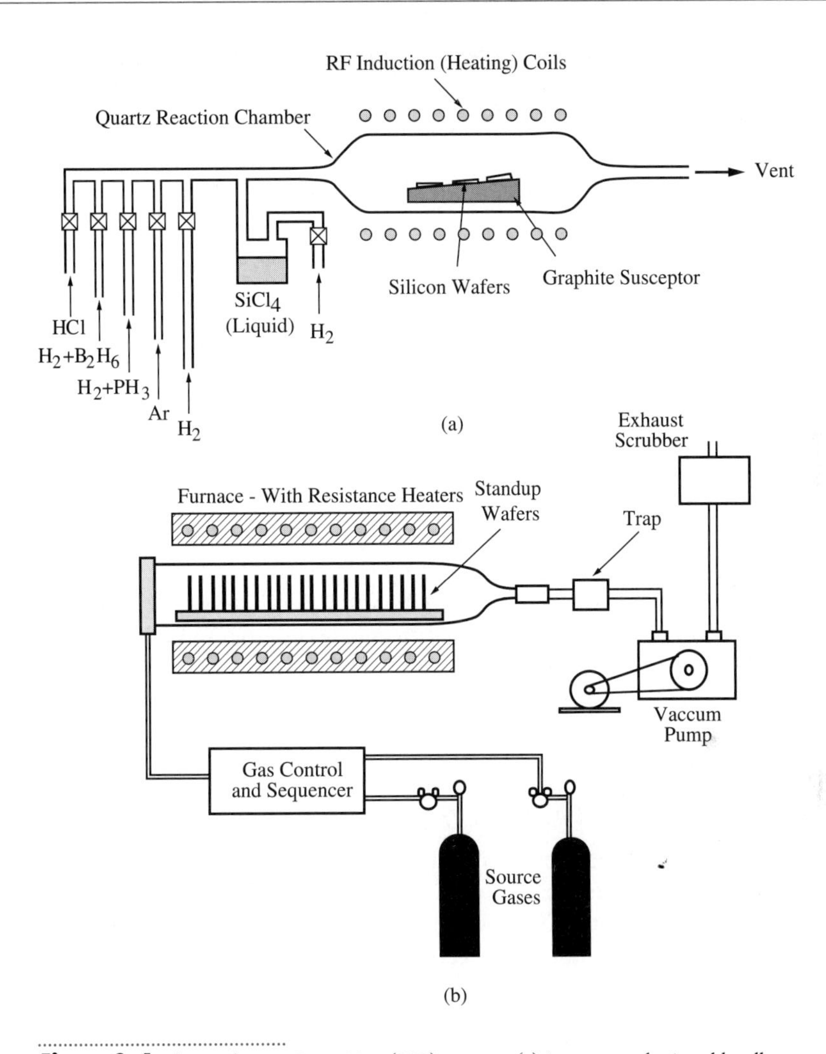

Figure 9–4 Chemical Vapor Deposition (CVD) systems. (a) is an atmospheric cold-wall system used for deposition of epitaxial silicon. (b) is a low-pressure hot-wall system used for deposition of polycrystalline and amorphous films, such as polysilicon and silicon dioxide, respectively.

9.2.1.1 Atmospheric Pressure Chemical Vapor Deposition (APCVD)

Although APCVD systems are not used as commonly today, we will begin with an APCVD system to describe some of the basic concepts of CVD. The steps involved in a CVD process, schematically illustrated in Figure 9–5, are

1. Transport of reactants by forced convection to the deposition region.
2. Transport of reactants by diffusion from the main gas stream through the boundary layer to the wafer surface.

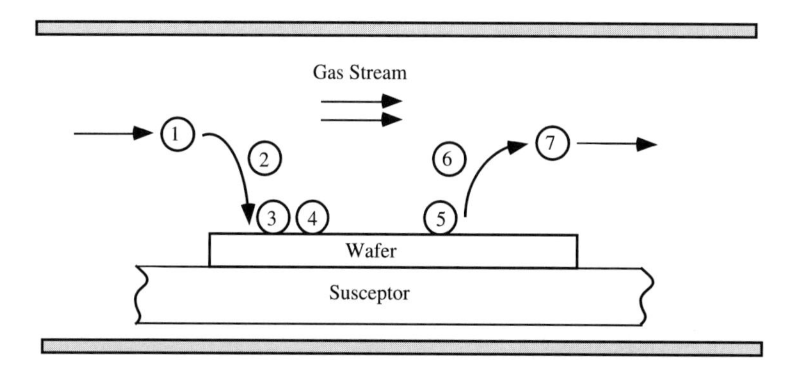

Figure 9–5 Steps involved in a CVD process. Numbered steps are explained in text.

3. Adsorption of reactants on the wafer surface.
4. Surface processes, including chemical decomposition or reaction, surface migration to attachment sites (such as atomic-level ledges and kinks), site incorporation, and other surface reactions.
5. Desorption of byproducts from the surface.
6. Transport of byproducts by diffusion through the boundary layer and back to the main gas stream.
7. Transport of byproducts by forced convection away from the deposition region.

A process not explicitly shown is that of desorption or "reemission," often just called "emission," of the reacting species before any reaction can occur. This is related to the sticking probability or coefficient, which will be discussed in more detail later. This process becomes important in coverage and filling issues, particularly in low pressure systems, since the desorbed species may deposit elsewhere such as on the sidewall of a trench or contact hole. In CVD processes the emission and redeposition process may occur quite readily, corresponding to a low sticking coefficient and can lead to better coverage. Surface migration or diffusion can also occur on a more long-range scale on nonflat topographies, due to surface curvature and surface energy reduction considerations for example. This can affect coverage and filling in a similar manner to reemission and redeposition. In the analysis here we are mainly concerned with deposition kinetics of thin films for relatively large-scale depositions on relatively flat surfaces. Local topography and coverage issues will be examined later focusing on low pressure CVD and PVD systems. We will also not consider gas-phase reactions, which sometimes produce intermediary vapor-phase species.

A full treatment of the kinetics of CVD thin film deposition, or growth, would involve all of the steps in Figure 9–5. However, steps 2–5 are usually the most important as far as determining the overall growth rate and thus we consider only those processes here. Step 2 is the mass transfer of reactants through the boundary layer. To simplify matters, we group steps 3–5 and classify them together as surface reactions. In our simple treatment

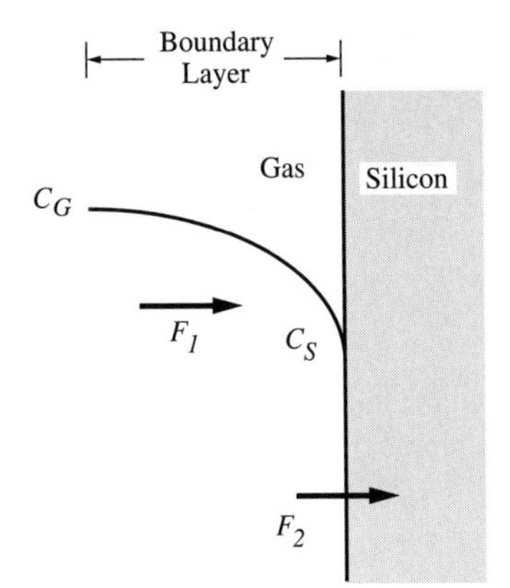

Figure 9–6 Wafer surface region in CVD process showing concentrations and fluxes of reactant species.

we consider the fluxes for the two important processes (mass transfer and surface reactions) and equate them under steady-state conditions. The treatment is very similar to that used for oxidation kinetics in Chapter 6 and for photoresist development in Chapter 5. Figure 9–6 shows the surface region of the depositing films, with the appropriate concentrations and fluxes in the gas-phase boundary layer and at the wafer surface.

The flux of reactant species from the gas phase to the wafer surface through the boundary layer, F_1 (in molecules cm^{-2} sec^{-1}), can be described by

$$F_1 = h_G(C_G - C_S) \tag{9.2}$$

The $(C_G - C_S)$ term is the difference in concentration of the reactant species (in molecules cm^{-3}) between the main gas flow and the wafer surface, and h_G is the mass transfer coefficient (in cm sec^{-1}). This flux represents the gas-phase diffusion through the stagnant boundary layer that forms between a flowing gas and a solid object. F_2 is the flux of reactant consumed by the reaction at the surface. Assuming first-order reaction kinetics, this can be written as

$$F_2 = k_S C_S \tag{9.3}$$

where k_S is the chemical surface reaction rate (in cm sec^{-1}) and C_S is the concentration of the reacting species at the surface (in cm^{-3}). All of the processes involved with the surface chemical reactions and surface diffusion that occur during the actual film formation, steps 3–5 above, are lumped into this one parameter. This is very similar to the strategy used in the Deal-Grove oxidation model. [Recall Eq. (6.17).]

Assuming steady-state deposition conditions, these two processes that act in series must be equal to each other, and the overall process will proceed at the rate of the slower process. Thus

$$F = F_1 = F_2 \tag{9.4}$$

and equating Eqs. (9.2) and (9.3) leads to

$$C_S = C_G\left(1 + \frac{k_S}{h_G}\right)^{-1} \tag{9.5}$$

The growth rate of the film is now given by

$$v = \frac{F}{N} = \frac{k_S h_G}{k_S + h_G}\frac{C_G}{N} \tag{9.6}$$

where v is the deposition rate or velocity in cm sec^{-1}, and N is the number of atoms incorporated per unit volume in the film, or its density, in cm^{-3} (5×10^{22} cm^{-3} for the case of Si deposition).

We now define Y to be the mole fraction of the incorporating species in the gas phase:

$$Y \equiv \frac{C_G}{C_T} \tag{9.7}$$

where C_T is the concentration of all molecules in the gas phase. One example is the case of epitaxial Si deposition by the reaction of $SiCl_4$ and hydrogen:

$$SiCl_{4(g)} + 2H_{2(g)} \Leftrightarrow Si_{(s)} + 4HCl_{(g)} \tag{9.8}$$

Here the incorporating species is Si, C_G is the number of molecules of $SiCl_4$ per cm^3 in the gas phase and C_T would correspond to the total number of $SiCl_4$ and H_2 molecules (plus any other species) per cm^3 in the gas phase. Y is also equal to the partial pressure of the incorporating species, P_G, divided by the total pressure in the system such that

$$Y \equiv \frac{C_G}{C_T} = \frac{P_G}{P_{\text{Total}}} = \frac{P_G}{P_G + P_{G'} + \ldots} \tag{9.9}$$

where P_G is the partial pressure of $SiCl_4$ and $P_{G'}$ corresponds to the partial pressure of H_2. The partial pressures of any other gas species present, such as N_2 or Ar used as carrier or dilutant gases and any byproduct gases, would also have to be added to the total pressure term. The equation for the deposition velocity is now

$$v = \frac{k_S h_G}{k_S + h_G}\frac{C_T}{N}Y \tag{9.10}$$

Example Calculate the deposition rate for a CVD system in which

$h_G = 1.0$ cm sec^{-1}

$k_S = 10$ cm sec^{-1}

Partial pressure of incorporating species $= P_G = 1$ torr

Total pressure $= P_T = 1$ atm $= 760$ torr

Total concentration in gas phase $= C_T = 1 \times 10^{19}\ \text{cm}^{-3}$
Density of depositing film $= N = 5 \times 10^{22}\ \text{cm}^{-3}$

Answer By Eq. (9.10):

$$v = \frac{k_S h_G}{k_S + h_G}\frac{C_T}{N}Y = \frac{1}{\left(\frac{1}{h_G} + \frac{1}{k_S}\right)}\frac{C_T}{N}Y$$

$$v = \frac{1}{\left(\frac{1}{1.0\ \text{cm sec}^{-1}} + \frac{1}{10\ \text{cm sec}^{-1}}\right)}\frac{1 \times 10^{19}\ \text{cm}^{-3}}{5 \times 10^{22}\ \text{cm}^{-3}}\frac{1}{760}$$

$$= 2.4 \times 10^{-7}\ \text{cm sec}^{-1} = 0.14\ \mu\text{m min}^{-1}$$

From Eq. (9.10) one sees that the deposition velocity is determined by the smaller of k_S or h_G, leading to two limiting cases. If $k_S << h_G$, then

$$v \cong \frac{C_T}{N}k_S Y \tag{9.11}$$

This is the surface reaction controlled case. The mass transfer through the gas boundary layer is relatively fast, while the surface reaction is sluggish. From Eq. (9.5) one sees that the surface concentration, C_S, approaches C_G. If $h_G << k_S$, then

$$v \cong \frac{C_T}{N}h_G Y \tag{9.12}$$

This is the mass transfer, or gas-phase diffusion, controlled case. Here the surface reaction is quite fast compared to the mass transfer process. C_S approaches zero because the reactant species are used up at the surface as soon as they arrive. In the above example, $h_G << k_S$ and so that system is operating in the mass transfer controlled regime.

These two limiting cases are analogous to the oxidation cases in Figure 6–15. The analysis in Chapter 6 showed how thermal oxidation leads to two kinetic regimes, one described by a linear rate constant (interface reaction limited or controlled) and the other described by a parabolic rate constant (solid-state diffusion limited). In the case of CVD deposition, there are also two limiting cases: one reaction controlled and one diffusion controlled. But the growth rate in both regimes is linear with time. That is, both regimes have constant growth velocities, and neither is parabolic. This is because the reaction always occurs at the growing surface, and the diffusion-related process is mass transport through a gas region of constant thickness, not a growing solid region as in the oxidation process. The two CVD regimes are therefore not differentiated by different growth laws. However, the two processes dominate in different temperature regimes.

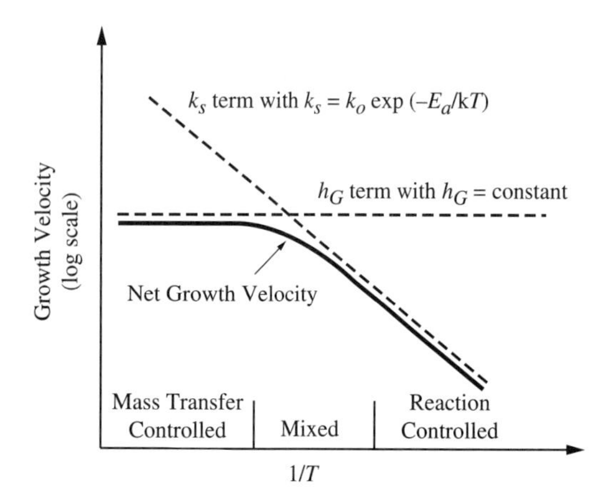

Figure 9–7 Arrhenius plot of growth velocity (or deposition rate) vs. $1/T$ for CVD process. The net growth velocity is the result of the surface reaction and gas-phase mass transfer processes acting in series so that the slower of the two dominates at any temperature.

The temperature dependence of the surface reaction controlled case is Arrhenius just as in the oxidation case. On the other hand, the mass transfer coefficient, h_G, is rather insensitive to temperature. Figure 9–7 plots the growth velocity versus reciprocal temperature. The k_S and h_G components are plotted separately showing their different temperature dependencies. When the two components are combined so that the smaller of the two components dominates (two processes acting in series), as described by Eq. (9.10), the resulting growth velocity behaves as shown in the figure. In practice, the cross-over temperature (where the two processes are equal) and the temperature ranges for the different regimes depend on a variety of factors, such as the specific gases used, the reaction activation energy, wafer configuration, the flow conditions in the reactor, and the pressure.

This basic model for CVD deposition has important implications for deposition conditions and equipment configuration. When the deposition occurs in the mass transfer controlled regime (higher temperatures), the deposition rate is relatively constant with temperature. However because it is limited by mass transfer of species through the gas-phase boundary layer, the flow of the gas over the wafers and transport of the reactants to the wafer surfaces are very important and can place major restrictions on the configuration of the equipment and the placement of the wafers. For example, the wafers must usually be placed face up and edge to edge in the chamber [as in Figure 9–4(a)] to ensure that equal gas flows reach each wafer surface and that equal deposition rates are achieved. By contrast, when the deposition occurs in the surface reaction controlled regime (lower temperatures), the process is very sensitive to temperature. However, the mass transfer through the boundary layer is not as important, leading to fewer restrictions on the gas flow and wafer placement. For example, the wafers may be stacked face-to-face [as in Figure 9–4(b)] without much of a penalty in wafer-to-wafer deposition uniformity.

Figure 9–8 shows typical experimental data for the deposition of silicon at atmospheric pressure. All four silicon sources exhibit similar types of behavior, with surface reaction limited regimes showing Arrhenius behavior, and mass transfer (or diffusion) limited regimes showing little temperature dependence. For all sources, the slopes of the curves in the reaction limited regimes are approximately the same, with an activation

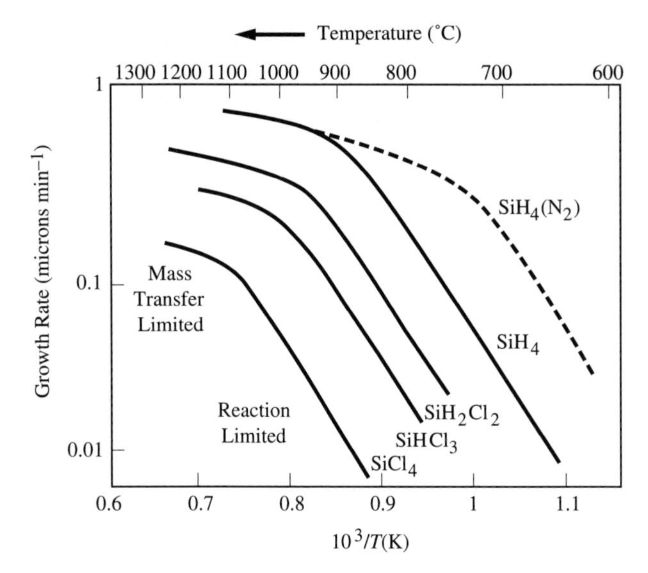

Figure 9–8 Growth or deposition rate versus $1/T$ for silicon deposited by CVD at atmospheric pressure using various silicon source gases. The partial pressure of the reactant gas is 0.8 torr. Hydrogen is used as the carrier or diluent gas for the solid curves. (After [9.1].) Using an inert gas such as N_2 for the diluent shifts the SiH_4 curve to the right, as indicated by the dashed curve and as discussed later in Section 9.3.2.

energy of about 1.6 eV. This suggests that the rate limiting surface reaction process is the same for each of the different sources and may be related to the desorption of hydrogen atoms from the Si surface. The choice of source gas does affect the overall growth velocity. The growth is fastest for a silane (SiH_4) source and slowest for a silicon tetrachloride ($SiCl_4$) source. The growth rate in the mass transfer limited regime is found to be approximately inversely proportional to the square root of the source gas molecular weight. There is also a substrate orientation effect on the growth kinetics. As expected, this is only important at lower temperatures where the surface reaction dominates. The (111) Si surface has a lower growth rate, presumably due to the fewer kink or attachment sites available for atom incorporation.

Epitaxial Si deposition has traditionally been done at higher temperatures to ensure that all the Si atoms being deposited are incorporated into lattice sites in order to obtain a single-crystal thin film. This means that epitaxial Si in these systems is deposited in the mass transfer regime where gas-phase processes are important. On the other hand, polysilicon is usually deposited at lower temperatures and in the surface reaction regime. Here the gas-phase processes are not important (so that stacking of wafers is possible), but the deposition is very temperature sensitive.

Earlier we assumed that the flux of reactant from the main gas flow to the wafer surface could be described simply by

$$F_1 = h_G(C_G - C_S) \tag{9.2}$$

where h_G is a constant. But gas flow in deposition chambers is more complicated than this, and it is worthwhile to take a little deeper look at it. We start with the configuration of Figure 9–4(a) where the wafers lie flat on a susceptor. The simplest model assumes that a completely stagnant boundary layer δ_S exists next to the surface of the wafer. This means that for some distance, away from the surface, the gas is not moving

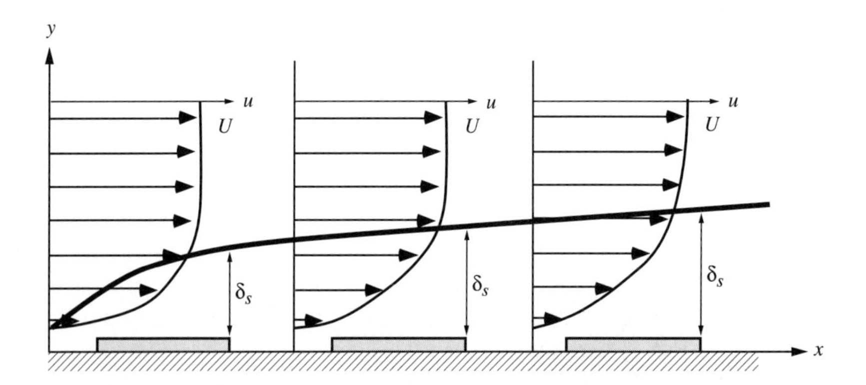

Figure 9–9 Boundary layer velocities along susceptor. δ_S is the thickness of the boundary layer. The boundary layer increases with distance in the direction of the gas flow from Newton's second law. (After [9.2].)

at all. Beyond δ_S, the gas is well mixed and moving at a constant velocity, U, parallel to the substrate surface. Figure 9–9 illustrates this and also the fact that δ_S increases in thickness along the susceptor. The transfer of gas across the boundary layer is assumed to occur via diffusion.

According to Fick's first law, the flux across the boundary layer at steady state is

$$F_1 = -D_G \frac{\partial C}{\partial x} = \frac{D_G}{\delta_S}(C_G - C_S) \tag{9.13}$$

where D_G is the diffusion coefficient of the reacting species across the boundary layer in the gas phase, and C_G and C_S are defined in Figure 9–6. From Eq. (9.2) we see that h_G corresponds to

$$h_G = \frac{D_G}{\delta_S} \tag{9.14}$$

If D_G and δ_S are constant, then h_G is constant. But δ_S is generally not constant with position in the chamber.

Right next to the wafer surface, the gas velocity is zero, and the velocity changes from zero to U within the boundary region. The boundary layer is caused by the frictional force of the gas stream on the stationary susceptor and wafers. If the gas velocity right next to the wafer surface were not zero, an infinitely large frictional force would exist right at the surface which would bring the velocity to zero there. Using Newton's second law ($F = ma$), where F is the friction force, one can determine the position of the boundary layer as a function of x to be [9.2]

$$\delta_S(x) = \left(\frac{\mu x}{\rho U}\right)^{1/2} \tag{9.15}$$

where ρ is the gas density, μ is the gas viscosity, and U is the bulk gas velocity as before. Since δ_S increases along the length of the susceptor, then the effective mass transfer coefficient, h_G, decreases along the length of the susceptor according to Eq. (9.14). Therefore, if the deposition is limited by mass transfer through the boundary layer, then the deposition rate would decrease going from the front of the susceptor to the back.

In addition, source gas depletion occurs down the length of the susceptor. As reacting gases are consumed, their concentrations decrease with distance along the susceptor. Since the growth rate is proportional to the partial pressure of the reacting species, the growth rate will decrease going downstream. While the growth rate decrease due to the increasing boundary layer is important only in the mass transfer regime, this decrease due to reactant depletion occurs in both the mass transfer and surface reaction controlled regimes. This is because Y is important in both regimes [Eqs. (9.11) and (9.12)].

To compensate for both the boundary-layer variation and depletion effects, a change in reactor geometry is needed. The wafer susceptor is tilted, as shown in Figure 9–10. This decreases the cross sectional area of the chamber along the susceptor, which causes the gas velocity to increase. This in turn causes the boundary layer to decrease along the susceptor. This increases the growth rate downstream, compensating for the friction-induced boundary-layer increase as well as the depletion effects. A way to compensate for the depletion effect when operating in the surface reaction limited regime is to impose a 5–25° temperature gradient along the tube or chamber, increasing from front to back. This is often done in LPCVD tubes, which normally operate in the surface reaction limited regime and where depletion is the main problem. For SiO_2 deposition by APCVD, commonly done in the mass transfer limited regime, a different gas flow configuration has been used to help overcome both boundary layer nonuniformities and depletion effects. The wafers still are placed side by side, facing up, but the gas is injected straight down from above. In addition the wafers can be moved horizontally on a conveyor belt. This helps ensure that uniform fluxes of reactant gases are delivered to each wafer.

As we have seen, chemical vapor deposition can be used to deposit compounds, such as SiO_2 and Si_3N_4, as well as elements. However alloys, such as Al(2% Cu), are much

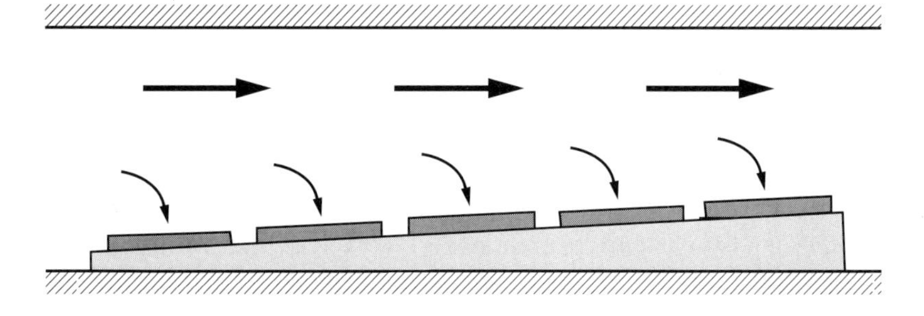

Figure 9–10 The susceptor in a horizontal epitaxial reactor is tilted so that the cross-sectional area of the chamber is decreased, increasing the gas velocity along the susceptor. This compensates for both the boundary layer and depletion effects.

more difficult. The problem is usually that separate reactions are required for each constituent (Al and Cu in our example) and it is often difficult to avoid unwanted reactions between the different reactant species, or precursors. In addition it can be hard to control the exact composition of the alloy, because unlike compounds where limited compositions result (very close to 2:1 oxygen-to-silicon in SiO_2, for example), a wide range of alloy compositions are possible. Physical vapor deposition methods are usually better suited for alloy deposition.

Thin films deposited by CVD may be doped during the deposition process. This is common for oxides, polysilicon, and epitaxial silicon. A gaseous source of the desired dopant is mixed with the other source gases, often along with hydrogen which acts as a carrier gas and a diluent. Common dopant source gases are arsine (AsH_3), phosphine (PH_3), and diborane (B_2H_6). The same steps occur in the incorporation of the dopants as occur in the thin film deposition, including mass transport and surface reactions. The surface reactions include (1) dissociation of the hydride gas, (2) lattice site incorporation, and (3) burying of dopants atoms by the other atoms in the film. It is believed that these are the rate limiting steps for doping of Si during epitaxial growth, and not the mass transport through the boundary layer. Models have been developed to predict the doping concentration in the film as a function of gas partial pressures, temperature, flow rate, and so on. However the models have not been very successful since many factors, especially in regard to the reactor geometry, are not well characterized and not adequately incorporated into the models. In general, for low growth rates the dopant concentration in the growing film C is proportional to the dopant gas-phase concentration (which equals the partial pressure of the dopant species, P_i) at the reactor input. For higher growth rates, C is inversely proportional to v, the deposition velocity.

$$C \propto P_i \text{ for low growth rates} \tag{9.16a}$$

$$C \propto \frac{P_i}{v} \text{ for high growth rates} \tag{9.16b}$$

In practice, the relationship between dopant concentration in a deposited film and the deposition conditions is determined experimentally for each particular reactor.

Unintentional doping of deposited layers can also occur. This is especially common when depositing a lightly doped epitaxial Si film on a highly doped Si substrate—a common occurrence in CMOS technology (Figure 2–20). One way unintentional doping can occur is through normal solid-state diffusion. During the deposition process, dopants from the highly doped substrate can diffuse into the newly deposited, lightly doped region. This is often termed outdiffusion. A large concentration gradient exists and at normal deposition temperatures (800–1100°C), significant diffusion can occur. Another way unintentional doping can occur is when dopant atoms get added to the gas stream and are then subsequently reintroduced into the growing film. This is termed "autodoping." The dopant may be added to the gas during film deposition (or even during an HCl in situ preclean) by evaporation from the wafer frontside, from the wafer backside or edges, other wafers, or from the susceptor.

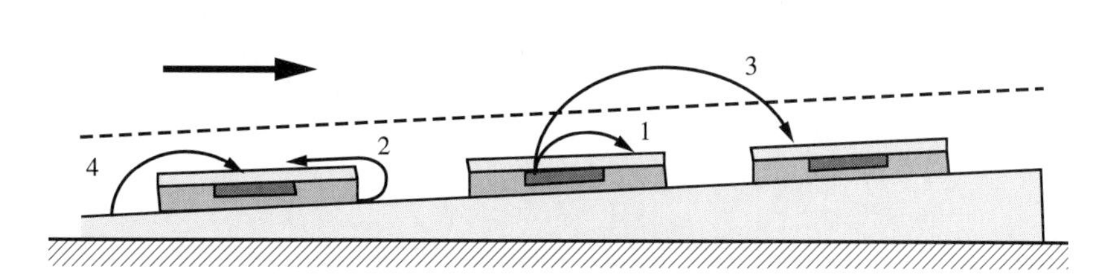

Figure 9–11 Autodoping processes in an epitaxial reactor. Illustrated are evaporation from 1, the wafer frontside; 2, the wafer backside or edges; 3, other wafers; and 4, the susceptor.

Figure 9–11 illustrates these processes. The autodoping effects add to the outdiffusion problem, often making the doping profile in the deposited layer quite complicated. The outdiffusion can be modeled with standard diffusion models. Since the growth of the layer is usually faster than the diffusion from the surface (that is, $vt \gg \sqrt{Dt}$), one can assume this is just diffusion from a doped region into a semi-infinite medium. This is described by a simple error-function profile, as discussed in Chapter 7 and given by Eq. (7.26):

$$C(x,t) = \frac{C}{2}\left[\operatorname{erfc}\frac{x}{2\sqrt{Dt}}\right] \tag{9.17}$$

Here $x = 0$ at the substrate/epitaxial layer interface, and x is positive in the epitaxial layer.

Autodoping from the frontside can usually be modeled with the empirical expression

$$C_{\text{autodoping}} = C_S{}^{*}\exp\left(-\frac{x}{L}\right) \tag{9.18}$$

Here C_S^{*} is the effective substrate surface concentration and L is an experimentally determined parameter, or diffusion length. This decrease in dopant concentration toward the surface arises from the fact that as the film grows in thickness, the dopant must diffuse through more and more film, and less dopant enters the gas phase. Autodoping from the backside, edges, or other sources usually results in a relatively constant level in the deposited film since the source of dopant does not diminish as quickly but is at a much lower level.

Figure 9–12 illustrates these effects in a Si epilayer. The top part of the curve, closest to the substrate, is due to outdiffusion, as described to first order by Eq. (9.17). (In fact, a concentration-dependent diffusivity would model the diffusion profile better than a simple error function.). The next segment, the nearly straight line on the plot, is from frontside autodoping, described by Eq. (9.18). The background portion is due to backside autodoping, and the concentration level is constant. These effects can significantly modify desired doping profiles in epitaxial layers.

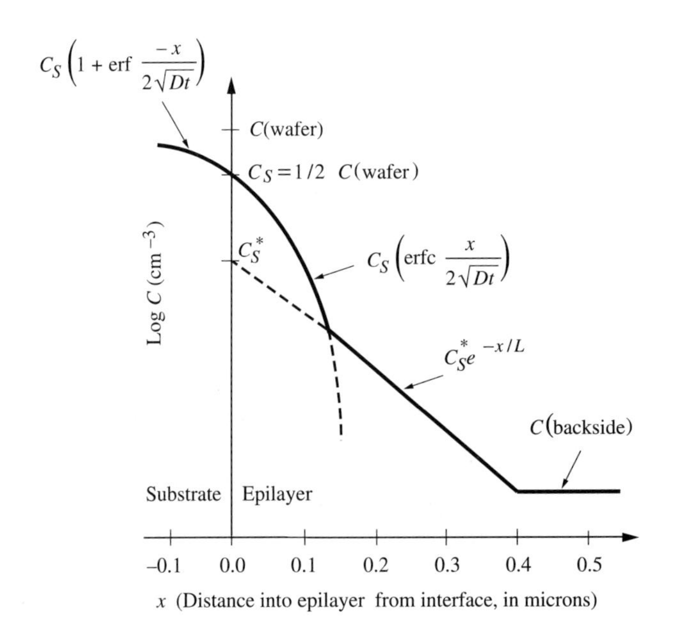

Figure 9–12 Dopant profile in a Si epilayer due to outdiffusion and autodoping. (After [9.3].)

Example Calculate the dopant concentration due to outdiffusion and autodoping in an otherwise undoped epilayer at 0.2 μm from the substrate/epilayer interface (x = 0.2 μm). The deposition time is 1 hour with a deposition rate of 1 μm hour^{-1}. The substrate doping, C(wafer), is 1×10^{19} cm^{-3}, C_S^* is 1×10^{18} cm^{-3}, L is 0.25 μm, D is 6×10^{-15} cm^2 sec^{-1}, and the backside doping concentration, C(backside), is 1×10^{15} cm^{-3}.

Answer The dopant concentration profile looks like Figure 9–12, with the concentration at each depth equal to the sum of the contributions from the outdiffusion, frontside autodoping and backside autodoping. For the outdiffusion term, we first check vt versus $\sqrt{Dt}$:

$$vt = (1 \times 10^{-4}\ \text{cm hr}^{-1})(1\text{hr}) = 1 \times 10^{-4}\ \text{cm}$$

$$\sqrt{Dt} = \sqrt{(6 \times 10^{-15}\ \text{cm}^2\ \text{sec}^{-1})(3600\ \text{sec})} = 4.6 \times 10^{-6}\ \text{cm}$$

Since $vt \gg \sqrt{Dt}$, we can assume the diffusion is occurring into a semi-infinite medium at all times:

$$\therefore\ C(x,t) = \frac{C}{2}\left[\operatorname{erfc}\frac{x}{2\sqrt{Dt}}\right] + C_S^{*}\exp\left(-\frac{x}{L}\right) + C(\text{backside})$$

The outdiffusion and autodoping occur throughout the deposition, so $t = 3600$ sec. We wish to know the doping concentration at $x = 0.2\ \mu\text{m}$, so

$$C(0.2\ \text{micron}, 3600\ \text{sec}) = \frac{1\times10^{19}\ \text{cm}^{-3}}{2}\left[\operatorname{erfc}\frac{0.2\times10^{-4}\ \text{cm}}{2\sqrt{(6\times10^{-15}\ \text{cm}^2\ \text{sec}^{-1})(3600\ \text{sec})}}\right]$$

$$+\ 1\times10^{18}\ \text{cm}^{-3}\exp\left(-\frac{0.20\ \mu\text{m}}{0.25\ \mu\text{m}}\right) + 1\times10^{15}\ \text{cm}^{-3}$$

$$= 0.5\times10^{19}\ \text{cm}^{-3}[\operatorname{erfc}(2.15)] + 1\times10^{18}\ \text{cm}^{-3}\cdot 0.45 + 1\times10^{15}\ \text{cm}^{-3}$$
$$= 1.2\times10^{16} + 4.5\times10^{17} + 1\times10^{15}\ \text{cm}^{-3}$$
$$= 4.6\times10^{17}\ \text{cm}^{-3}$$

The major contribution at this depth is from the frontside autodoping.

9.2.1.2 Low-Pressure Chemical Vapor Deposition (LPCVD)

We saw that when operating CVD reactors in the mass transfer limited regime, one has to ensure that equal fluxes of reactant gases must reach every location in order to achieve uniform depositions across the wafers. This generally implies placing the wafers side by side as in Figure 9–4(a). Otherwise the variability in the boundary layer thickness and transport through that layer would result in nonuniform depositions. Operating in the surface reaction limited regime where transport is not important would avoid these problems and allow stacking the wafers as in Figure 9–4(b). This generally provides higher throughput. This can be achieved by going to a lower deposition temperature (Figure 9–7). However as the temperature is lowered, the deposition rate can decrease significantly. In addition the film quality may suffer.

Lowering the total pressure of the gas stream increases the diffusion and extends the reaction controlled regime to higher temperatures. First recall that the CVD film deposition rate is given by

$$v = \frac{k_S h_G}{k_S + h_G}\frac{C_T}{N}Y \tag{9.10}$$

where k_S is the surface reaction coefficient and h_G is the mass transfer coefficient. The smaller of the two terms dominates and controls the overall deposition process. Diffusion through the boundary layer is given by

$$h_G = \frac{D_G}{\delta_S} \tag{9.14}$$

where D_G is the diffusivity of the reacting species through the boundary layer and δ_S is the boundary layer thickness. The key new point is that D_G is inversely proportional to P_{total},

$$D_G \propto \frac{1}{P_{\text{total}}} \tag{9.19}$$

since the diffusivity is inversely proportional to the number of collisions that the gas species experience. So decreasing the total pressure, which also means decreasing the total concentration of gases in the gas stream but not necessarily decreasing the concentrations or partial pressures of the reactant gases, causes D_G to increase.

Decreasing P_{total} from 1 atm (760 torr) to 1 torr, a typical LPCVD pressure, increases D_G by 760 times. Decreasing P_{total} also increases the boundary layer thickness, δ_S, but not proportionally. Reducing the pressure to 1 torr only increases δ_S by 3 to 10 times. The net effect on h_G is that it increases by about 100 times. In the earlier APCVD numerical example, if h_G were increased by 100 times, with everything kept the same, the deposition rate would increase to 1.4 μm min^{-1} and system operation switches to the surface reaction controlled regime (problem 9.6).

Since h_G is much larger at the lower pressure, mass transport through the boundary layer becomes much less important compared to the surface reactions. Figure 9–13 illustrates this. Now that the deposition velocity is not limited by the mass transfer of reactants through the gas-phase boundary layer, the wafers can be placed much closer together without affecting the deposition uniformity nearly as much. The configuration

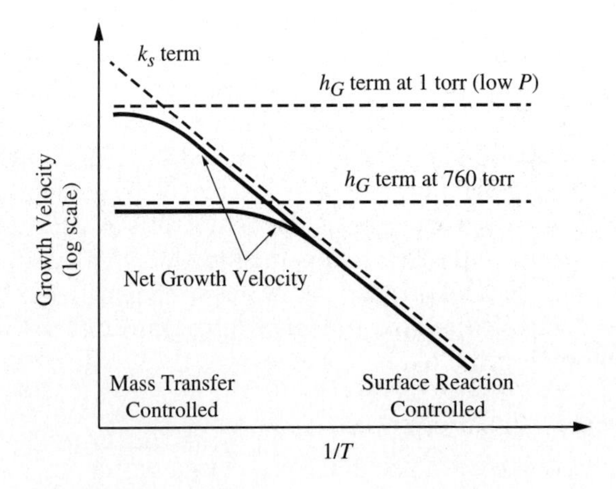

Figure 9–13 Growth velocity vs. $1/T$ for APCVD (760 torr) and LPCVD (1 torr) systems. The lower total pressure (with P_G and C_G remaining fixed) shifts the h_G curve upward, extending the surface reaction regime to higher temperatures.

shown earlier in Figure 9–4(b) is typical for LPCVD reactors. The wafers are stacked vertically. A vacuum pump is needed to reduce and control the pressure, usually in the 0.25–2.0 torr range. Deposition temperatures in LPCVD systems range from 300–900°C. Since these systems are operated in the surface reaction regime, temperature must be controlled typically to ±1°C, but this is easily achieved in hot-walled furnaces. Depletion of reactant gas can still be a problem, as discussed earlier, so a 5–25°C temperature gradient (higher temperature downstream) is often used. This speeds up the reaction rate toward the back of the tube to compensate for the depletion. An alternate method to avoid the depletion problem is to use a distributed feed setup in which the reactant gases are injected at regular intervals down the tube.

There are additional advantages to using a low-pressure system. With the lower pressure and much faster diffusion out through the boundary layer to the main gas stream, less autodoping occurs. In addition, little or no carrier or dilutant gas is needed and gas consumption is much lower. Also, at lower pressures there are usually fewer gas-phase reactions and hence fewer particulates form that can deposit on the wafers. There is of course a limit to how much the pressure can be lowered. At some point the reactant gas concentration, C_G, or pressure, P_G, would have to be lowered to reduce the total gas pressure, which would then decrease the deposition rate.

It should be pointed out that even though we describe operating in the surface reaction limited regime at low pressures to achieve uniform deposition, the transport of the depositing material through the gas phase can still be important, especially on a local level near the surface. It is true that the diffusional flow through a boundary layer is no longer the limiting step. One might assume that under such conditions there would always be enough species available to react and deposit at each position along the surface, resulting in perfectly conformal coverage for local topographical features. However, at these low pressures virtually no gas-phase collisions occur in the near-surface region within the topographical features. Therefore line-of-sight transport occurs over this distance, as opposed to more randomly directed diffusional transport that occurs within the surface features at atmospheric pressure. As a result, shadowing can occur where the flux from the gas phase is impeded locally by surface topography features. This shadowing can directly affect step coverage and filling. Reemission processes may not always occur readily enough (or equivalently, the sticking coefficient low enough) or surface diffusion fast enough to allow for constant flux to reach each point on the surface from the gas phase. Thus nonconformal profiles can still result, as we shall see. These issues will be even more important for PVD systems—not only do they operate at very low pressures, but the deposition processes are usually assumed to occur with very little surface diffusion or reemission.

9.2.1.3 Plasma-Enhanced Chemical Vapor Deposition (PECVD)

Sometimes there are restrictions on the temperature that the substrate can be exposed to when depositing a film. The most obvious example is when depositing a silicon dioxide or silicon nitride film when an aluminum metal level is already in place. The melting point of Al is 660°C, and any subsequent processing temperature must be less than about 450°C. APCVD or LPCVD films can be deposited at these lower temperatures, but the deposition rate is usually quite low because k_S decreases exponentially with temperature. In addition the film quality can be poor, with the films being rather porous and susceptible to moisture absorption. Good film quality is especially important for multilevel metallization schemes where deposited dielectric layers are used to provide electrical and physical barriers between metal interconnect layers. Conformal and void-free films are also important. Therefore a dielectric deposition technique is needed that provides reasonable deposition rates, good film quality, conformality, and low deposition temperatures.

A method developed for these needs is Plasma-Enhanced Chemical Vapor Deposition, or PECVD. In addition to using a thermal source to provide the energy needed for the chemical reactions to occur during the deposition, a plasma source is used. Plasmas are highly ionized gases and will be discussed in more detail later in Section 9.2.2.2. By supplying additional energy from the plasma to the reactant gases, the reactions needed for deposition can occur at temperatures much lower than those needed when only thermal energy is provided. In fact, room temperature depositions are even possible with this method. Usually, though, PECVD depositions of dielectrics are done in the 200–350°C range. In addition to allowing the depositions to occur at lower substrate temperatures, PECVD also allows more easily altering the film's properties (composition, density, stress, etc.) and the tailoring of those properties for particular applications. This is due mainly to the more nonequilibrium nature of the deposition process compared to the nonplasma CVD methods. However, this can also lead to undesirable compositions or properties in the films, such as the incorporation of byproducts or gas molecules into the film.

A typical equipment configuration for PECVD is shown in Figure 9–14. This is similar to the parallel plate plasma etching equipment to be described in Chapter 10. In plasma etching, the energetic species created in the plasma are used to etch materials on

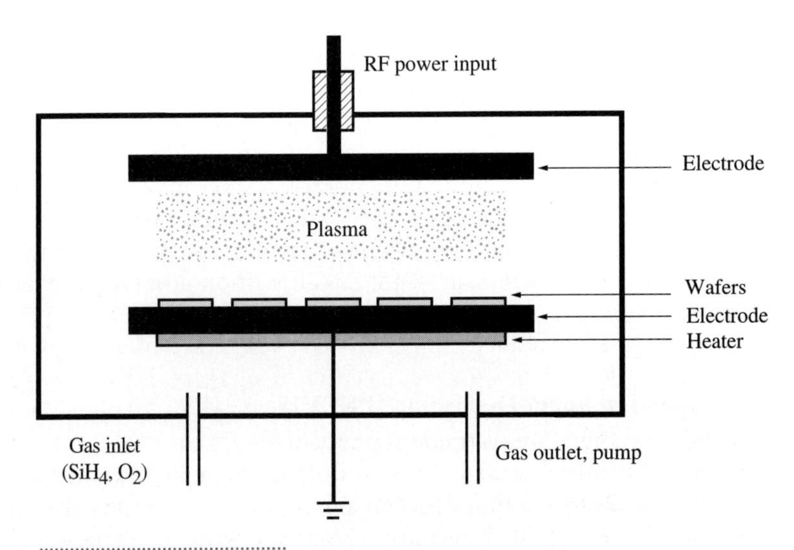

Figure 9–14 Typical PECVD equipment configuration.

the wafer. In plasma-enhanced deposition, the energetic species are used to help form the films on top of wafers. The wafers are placed on the lower plate electrode. Heat can be supplied to the wafers through a heater beneath the electrode. The reactant gases, such as silane and oxygen for the deposition of silicon dioxide, are fed through inlets. A glow discharge, or plasma, is sustained between the lower and upper electrodes. This is formed by applying a high electric field, often at 13.56 MHz, to a low pressure gas (between 50 mtorr and 5 torr), creating ions and free electrons. The plasma is sustained when high-energy electrons strike and ionize atoms and molecules.

In the plasma, interactions with the high-energy electrons cause the reactant gases to dissociate and ionize into a variety of species. These include ionized and excited molecules (or atoms), neutral molecules and neutral and ionized fragments of broken-up molecules, including free radicals. Free radicals are electrically neutral species that have incomplete bonding; that is, they have unpaired electrons. Examples are SiO, SiH_3, and F (the first two are important in plasma deposition and the last one in plasma etching). These species are extremely reactive, and with other species are absorbed onto the wafer surface, migrate, interact, rearrange, and chemically recombine to form the film. In addition, ion and electron bombardment from the plasma onto the wafer surface can occur. As we will see later in the description of RF sputtering systems, a potential difference will exist between the plasma and the wafer surface in RF plasma systems, with the wafer surface electrically negative with respect to the plasma. This will accelerate positive ions to the wafer surface. Even some of the high-energy electrons can escape the plasma to strike the wafers. This bombardment of ions and electrons transfers even more energy to the species on the surface, breaking chemical bonds for example, and further enhances the different surface processes and reactions. The net result from the plasma-induced fragmentation, free radical generation, and ion bombardment is that the surface processes and deposition can occur at much lower temperatures than in nonplasma systems. The byproducts of the deposition reactions are desorbed and exhausted through the outlet ports.

The reactions and processes that occur in a PECVD system are numerous and complicated and not easy to predict or model. The complexity and nonequilibrium nature of the reactions can lead to nonstoichiometric compositions of the films (Si- or O-rich SiO_2, for example), as well as the incorporation of byproducts into the films. Incorporation of H_2, O_2, or N_2 is common and can result in outgassing, peeling, or cracking of the film during subsequent processing. Film density and stress may also vary, depending on the conditions of the deposition.

PECVD depositions can result in fairly good coverage and filling of non-planar topography in some cases (such as TEOS SiO_2 depositions), better than what might be expected at these low temperatures and often similar to higher temperature depositions in non-plasma systems. This has often been attributed in the past to long-range surface diffusion, enhanced by the more energetic species and by ion bombardment. However, as we will discuss later, for oxide deposition this may be instead due to muliple near-surface emission and redeposition events occurring, characterized by a low effective sticking coefficient for the neutral species even at low temperatures, along with the directional ion component of the deposition to help in filling spaces [9.4, 9.5]. While standard PECVD depositions may be adequate for covering and filling larger dimension structures, for smaller dimensions and higher aspect ratio spaces (greater than about 1) other methods are required.

9.2.1.4 High-Density Plasma Chemical Vapor Deposition (HDPCVD)

A newly developed version of PECVD utilizes a very high-density plasma and a separate RF bias applied on the substrate. Called HDP (High-Density Plasma) CVD, this technique combines PECVD deposition with bias sputtering to obtain very good filling of narrow gaps. It is used primarily for silicon dioxide depositions. The high-density plasma can be generated by a variety of sources, including Electron Cyclotron Resonance (ECR) and Inductively Coupled Plasma (ICP). This high-density plasma results in a dense CVD silicon dioxide film at low temperatures, typically 150°C down to room temperature, and with a very low chamber pressure in the 1–10 mtorr range. In fact, there is usually no intentional heating in these CVD systems. The ion bombardment supplies enough energy to raise the substrate temperature and cooling of the wafers is often required to keep the temperature below 400°C.

With a separate RF bias applied on the substrate in HDP systems, the angular dependence of ion sputtering is exploited. Sputtering—the knocking off of atoms from a solid by incident ions when the solid is electrically biased—occurs preferentially on sloped surfaces rather than on vertical or horizontal surfaces. This simultaneous sputtering of the film during its deposition can result in planarized and void-free films. This is the same idea behind the bias sputtering deposition method. Bias-sputter deposition and angle-dependent sputtering will be more fully explained in the next section. The strong directed ion component of the HDP deposition process also helps in the filling of holes, and the ion bombardment helps make the film denser.

9.2.2 Physical Vapor Deposition (PVD)

Rather than relying on chemical reactions to produce the reacting species and to form the film as in chemical vapor deposition, physical vapor deposition methods use mainly physical processes to deposit the films. PVD techniques are generally more versatile than CVD methods, allowing for the deposition of almost any material. The constituent species, individual atoms or molecules, are produced by either evaporation of a solid or molten source, or by using energetic gaseous ions in a plasma to knock off, or sputter, the atoms from a source "target." These atoms or molecules then travel though a vacuum or a very low pressure gas phase, impinge on the wafers, and condense on the surface to form the film. Very few, if any, chemical reactions occur. An exception to this is in reactive sputtering, in which a species is sputtered in the presence of a reactive gas (such as N_2) and a compound is formed and deposited. But in general, physical processes dominate in PVD.

Because of the very low pressures in these systems, very few gas-phase collisions occur. In addition, the surface reactions occur very rapidly and very little rearrangement of atoms usually occurs on the wafer surface. As a result, thickness uniformity, shadowing by surface topography, and step coverage can be very important issues in PVD depositions.

Both PVD techniques, evaporation and sputter deposition, have a long history. Both have been used for over 100 years to coat objects with metal thin films [9.6]. Today sputtering is the dominant PVD technique, but evaporation is still used for some special applications.

9.2.2.1 Evaporation

A schematic of a simple evaporator is shown in Figure 9–15. In this process the source material is heated in a vacuum chamber which has initially been pumped down to less than 10^{-5} torr. Evaporated atoms from the source condense on the surfaces of the wafers. The heater can be of the resistance type, using a tungsten filament which heats up when current passes through it. More popular for microelectronics use is an e-beam heater, in which a high-energy electron beam is focused onto the source material in a crucible using magnetic fields. e-beam heaters can achieve higher temperatures so that a wider range of materials can be evaporated. In addition, the process is cleaner since no metal filaments are used. (Recall our discussion in Chapters 1 and 4 regarding alkali ions as sources of electrical instability in early MOS devices. One source of these contaminants was found to be Al evaporation systems where sodium and potassium were used in the production of the tungsten filaments.) In addition, since only the top of the source in e-beam systems is usually melted, no contamination from the crucible occurs. As a result, purer films are deposited with e-beam evaporation systems. A downside of e-beam systems is that X-rays can be emitted when an e-beam strikes Al. These X-rays can create trapped charges in gate oxides. Annealing of the film is required to remove this damage.

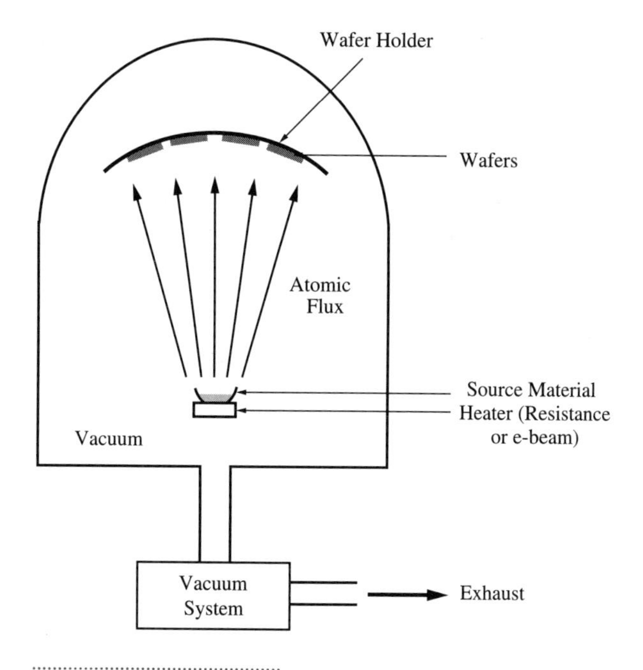

Figure 9–15 Schematic diagram of evaporation equipment.

Since the evaporated atoms are transported through a high-vacuum atmosphere, very little gas-phase scattering occurs. Therefore, unlike CVD systems, the mean free path is very long and the atoms travel in essentially straight lines all the way from the source to the surface of the wafers. This is illustrated in Figure 9–15. Since the source is small, we can first consider it as a point source. For uniform or isotropic emission from a point source, that is, an equal evaporation rate in every direction, the contours of equal flux (atoms per area per time) would be circular in two dimensions or spherical in three dimensions.

For a point source one can derive an expression for the deposition rate or growth velocity, v, of a film deposited on a flat surface as a function of distance along the surface. For this we use the coordinate system of Figure 9–16. We are interested in the amount of material striking a small area on the surface, A_k, per unit time. But first we consider the flux being emitted from the source. If R_{evap} is the evaporation rate from the point source (in either atoms or grams per second), r is the distance from the source to the spot on the surface, and A_k^p is the projected area of A_k facing the source, then the flux F_k^p that strikes A_k^p is simply

$$F_k^p = \frac{R_{evap}}{\Omega r^2} \tag{9.20}$$

Here Ω is the solid angle over which the source emits evaporated material. For a source emitting in all directions (in three dimensions) this would equal 4π. For a source emitting only upward, this would equal 2π.

Eq. (9.20) describes the flux emitting outward from a point source and it is independent of emission angle θ_i for any radius r. Since the deposition rate on A_k depends on the component of the incoming flux that is normal to the surface A_k, we must then mul-

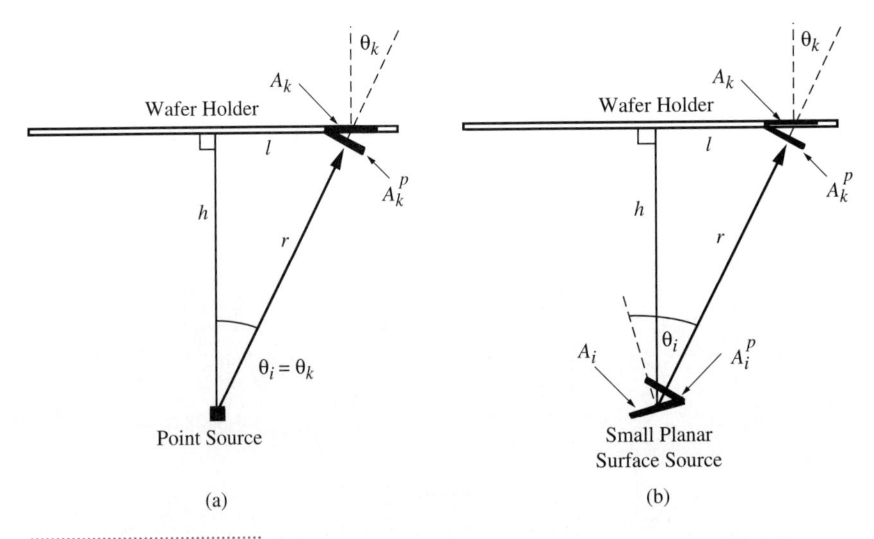

Figure 9–16 Geometries of flux and deposition of small areas on a flat wafer holder for (a), a point source, and (b), a small planar surface source.

tiply this by $\cos\theta_k$. Here θ_k is the angle between the surface normal and the direction of the source to a spot on the surface, as indicated in the figure. We designate the normal component of the incoming flux with respect to A_k to be F_k. This corresponds to the amount of material deposited per time per unit surface area. This leads to

$$F_k = \frac{R_{\text{evap}}}{\Omega r^2} \cos\theta_k \tag{9.21}$$

Another way to look at this is that for a larger angle, the material that is coming through the cone to strike the area A_k^p must be deposited over a larger surface area A_k, and the amount striking A_k per unit area is thereby decreased (by $\cos\theta$). Thus the deposition rate on a surface area will decrease as the area is tilted from an orientation facing the source.

The deposition rate or velocity, v, on area A_k is then just the flux F_k as expressed by Eq. (9.21) divided by the density of the material being deposited, N, so that for a point source:

$$v = \frac{R_{\text{evap}}}{\Omega N r^2} \cos\theta_k \tag{9.22}$$

Eq. (9.22) can be converted to a plot of the relative or normalized deposition rate versus ℓ/h, as is done in Figure 9–17, where ℓ is the distance from the center of the wafer holder and h is the length of the surface normal. Note that $\cos\theta_k = h/r$ and that $r^2 = \ell^2 + h^2$. The thickest deposit is at $\ell = 0$ and leads to v_o (v at $\ell = 0$) being equal to $R_{\text{evap}}/\Omega N h^2$. The nonuniform deposition is obvious. As ℓ increases, not only does r increase, but also the $\cos\theta_k$ term decreases.

Evaporation is usually modeled better as a small surface area source rather than a point source. Evaporation from a small surface area behaves similarly to effusion of gas

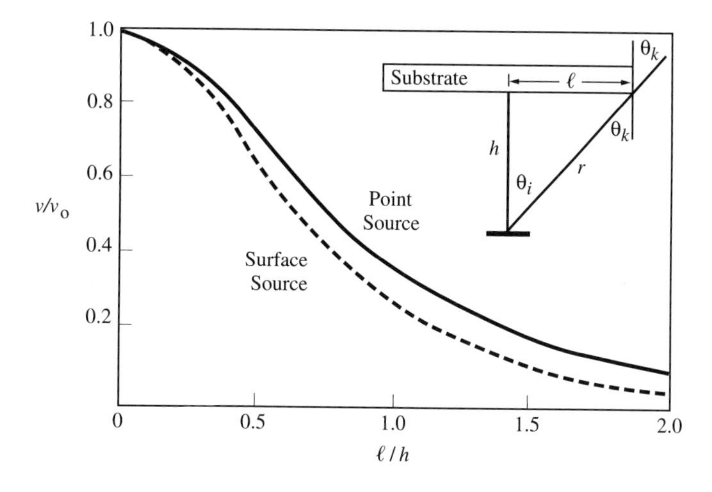

Figure 9–17 Deposition rate of evaporated film as a function of position on substrate for point and surface sources. $\theta_i = \theta_k$ in this configuration for both point and surface sources. (After [9.6].)

out a small opening from a container, as in a Knudsen cell [9.7]. The outward or emitted flux is not uniform in all directions as with an ideal point source but is more directed and dependent on the projected area of the small source area toward the flux direction. Thus the emitted flux is largest in the direction perpendicular to the source surface and less to the sides. The orientation of the 2D surface source to the area being deposited on is defined by the angle θ_i, as shown in Figure 9–16(b), which may be different from θ_K. As θ_i becomes larger, the projected area of the surface source, A_i^P, facing the deposition area, becomes smaller and there is less flux in that direction. Hence the emitted flux for any distance r is greatest in the direction normal to the source, $\theta_i = 0$, falling off as a cosine function toward either side. This is different than the $\cos\theta_K$ factor above used to calculate the deposition rate on a flat surface and instead describes how a certain type of source is seen to emit material differently in different directions, following a cosine relation. This emission behavior from a small planar source is known as the cosine distribution law for evaporation from a planar source, or ideal cosine emission.

An extra $2\cos\theta_i$ factor due to this cosine emission now comes into the expressions for the emitted flux [Eq. (9.20)], the normal component of the incoming flux striking A_K, [Eq. (9.21)], and the deposition rate [Eq. (9.22)]. (The factor of 2 normalizes the total evaporation rate with the $\cos\theta_i$ term.) The deposition rate, v, for a small surface area source becomes

$$v = \frac{R_{\text{evap}}}{\pi N r^2} \cos\theta_i \cdot \cos\theta_k \tag{9.23}$$

Eq. (9.23) is valid for any small area emitting material, with ideal cosine emission behavior, to any other small area in any relative orientation to each other, with r the distance between them and the angles as defined above.

While it may not be intuitively obvious that this Knudsen-cell-like behavior, resulting in cosine emission behavior, should apply to evaporation from a small surface, it has been verified experimentally by Knudsen himself [9.8] and others for many materials. (In radiation theory, this type of emission is called "diffuse" emission or more specifically "perfectly diffuse" emission from a surface, and very similar equations express the radiation behavior from a blackbody [9.9].) Cosine emission behavior not only describes source emission in most evaporation systems, but also describes the reemission of deposited material from a surface area in many cases, as we will discuss later. The contours of equal flux for an evaporation system with a small planar source would not be hemispherical as in the point-source case in Figure 9–15 but would fall off more quickly from the center of the wafer holder to each side.

We can now plot the deposition rate versus ℓ/h curve for a small surface source in Figure 9–17, as we did for a point source. We do this for the special case when the small surface source is parallel to the wafer holder. In this particular situation with the surface source facing the wafer holder, θ_i equals θ_K. The deposition curve for the planar surface source case is similar to the point-source case, except that the deposition is even more directed toward the region directly above it. Not only is r increasing and the $\cos\theta_K$ term decreasing as ℓ gets larger, as with the point source, but due to the $\cos\theta_i$ emission from the planar source, even more deposition occurs upward.

To achieve thickness uniformity over many wafers for either type of source, the wafers obviously cannot be placed on a flat holder. Instead, spherical or hemispherical holders are used, with the wafers all facing inward toward the center. For a point source at the center of the sphere, θ_k and r will be constant giving a uniform deposition rate over the whole wafer holder. (Across each individual wafer, θ_k and r will vary somewhat, giving less than uniform across each wafer, but from wafer to wafer the deposition will be uniform.) It can be shown (problem 9.8) that to obtain uniform deposition around a sphere for a small surface source, the source itself should be placed on the inside surface of the sphere holding the wafers, rather than the sphere's center. Figure 9–18 illustrates these configurations. Since most evaporation sources act more like small surface sources than point sources, it is common practice to place the source at the inside surface of a spherical wafer holder in an evaporation system.

Deviations from ideal point-source or small-area surface source emissions can occur and sometimes even more directed and narrower emission distributions are observed. For small planar surface sources, the flux and deposition rate expressions can be described with a $\cos^n\theta_i$ term rather than a $\cos\theta_i$ term to take this nonideal behavior into account. Values of n greater than 1 correspond to angular distributions of evaporant flux from the source being narrower than from ideal sources. This is conceptually illustrated in Figure 9–19 for a planar source, where a value of $n = 1$ leads to ideal cosine emission

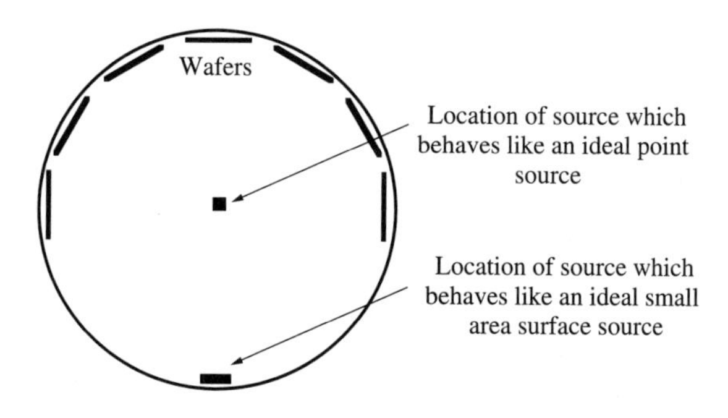

Figure 9–18 Positions of wafers and sources to achieve uniform deposition in evaporation system on all the wafers. Most evaporation sources behave more like a small area surface source and are in that configuration.

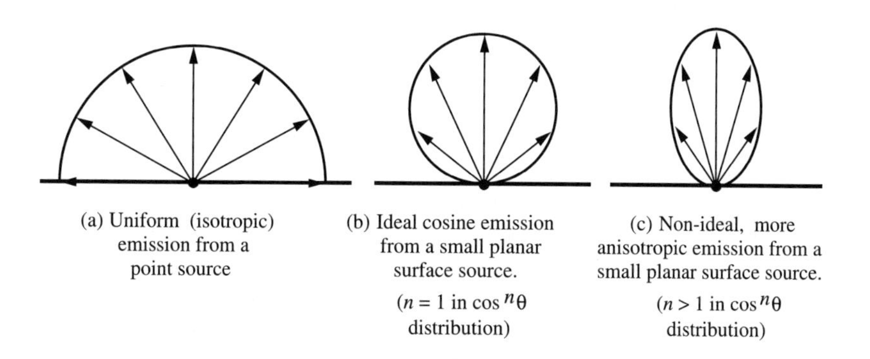

Figure 9–19 Emitted fluxes for point sources and small surface areas sources.

behavior in the emitted angle distribution, and a value of $n > 1$ leads to even more anisotropic behavior.

This nonideal behavior may be due to crucible geometry, the ratio of melt depth to the melt surface area, and other factors. In addition, a large density of evaporated atoms right above the source sometimes causes the gas phase to act more like a viscous medium rather than the preferred near-vacuum condition. (In the latter case, molecular flow, or free molecular flow, is said to occur, with virtually no gas-phase collisions or interactions.) This viscous behavior near the source also causes nonideal, nonuniform behavior. To counter these problems another solution is employed. Not only are hemispherical wafer holders used, but they are rotated. And not only is the entire planetary fixture rotated about the vertical axis, but each group of wafers is also rotated about a second axis. This use of rotating planetaries helps compensate for nonideal deposition behavior and results in more uniform deposition.

The source evaporation rate, R_{evap}, is found to be proportional to the equilibrium vapor pressure (P_e) of the source material at the evaporation temperature. From Langmuir-Knudsen theory, the evaporation rate in g sec^{-1} is estimated to be

$$R_{\text{evap}} = 5.83 \times 10^{-2} A_s \left(\frac{m}{T}\right)^{1/2} P_e \tag{9.24}$$

where A_s is the area of the source in cm^2, m is the gram-molecular mass, T is the temperature in Kelvin, and the vapor pressure, P_e, is in torr. The vapor pressure of the material is a very strong function of temperature, and Figure 9–20 shows the vapor pressure of several metals commonly evaporated. A partial vapor pressure of the element of about 1–10 mtorr or more is required to achieve reasonable deposition rates (on the order of 0.1–1 μm per minute), and one can see that a temperature of about

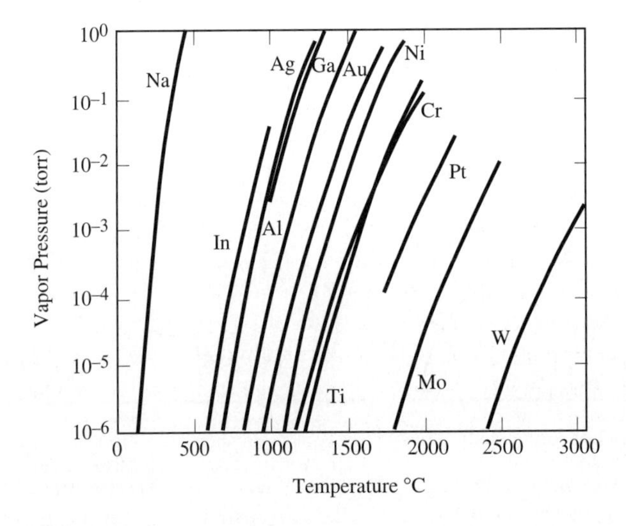

Figure 9–20 Vapor pressure as a function of temperature of commonly evaporated metals. (After [9.10].)

1100°C is needed for the evaporation of aluminum. This means that the aluminum is evaporated from the liquid phase. Tungsten must be heated to a much higher temperature of about 3100°C, where it evaporates or "sublimes" from the solid phase.

Because the vapor pressures of different elements vary so much, evaporating alloys presents a special challenge. Alloying one element with another is common in microelectronics to achieve the desired thin film properties. Alloys of Al with small amounts of Si and Cu for interconnects are examples, as we will see in Chapter 11. But with different vapor pressures at a given temperature (the vapor pressure of Cu is about 5 times lower than that of Al at 1100°C, while that of Si is 10^4 times lower!), the evaporation rates will be different, and the deposited film will have a different composition than the source. When evaporating films from a single, multicomponent source, the differences in evaporation rates of the constituent elements must be taken into account, and the sources must be enriched in the element with the lower evaporation rate. But the source itself will change in composition as one element evaporates faster than the other (called fractionation). This will in turn change the composition of the deposited film, resulting in a deposited film with a composition that varies throughout the thickness of the film. This problem is very similar to the dopant segregation problem during Czochralski crystal growth that we considered in Chapter 3.

The most common solution to this problem is two or more separate e-beams used on separate sources, each containing just one of the elements in the alloy. The e-beam energies, and hence the source temperatures, can be different so that the evaporation rates can be controlled to give the desired deposited film composition. Differences in evaporation rates and changing source compositions are not a problem here. But spatial compositional uniformity when using dual sources is a problem, and it is difficult to obtain constant compositions across the wafer and across the wafer holder.

Compounds, such as SiO_2, are just as hard, if not harder, to evaporate as alloys. The composition of the vapor phase is usually not the same as the source compound, and chemical reactions and molecular changes often occur as the material is evaporated and deposited. Sputter deposition generally does a much better job in depositing compositionally uniform films of both alloys and compounds. This is partly because the sputter rates of elements are usually much closer to each other than their vapor pressures are.

There are advantages in using evaporation to deposit thin films for microelectronics applications. First, there is little damage caused to the wafer, since the wafers are not subjected to energetic particles. Second, the deposited films are usually very pure. Because the deposition is done in a high vacuum, there are no residual gases or particles to get incorporated in the film.

However, there are also disadvantages to this method which have all but eliminated its use from mainstream silicon fabrication. First, metals with low vapor pressures, such as W, and films of alloys or compounds with precisely controlled composition are difficult to evaporate, as discussed above. Second, there is no *in situ* precleaning method available as there is for sputter deposition. The third problem with evaporation has to do with step coverage. Because of the very low chamber pressure which makes the mean free path of the gaseous species very large, the evaporated deposition species travel essentially in straight lines from the source to the wafer surfaces. This and the fact that the source is small means that the atoms arrive at a limited range of angles, leading to poor step coverage. Rotating the planetary and wafers does help to widen the range of arrival angles, but shadowing still occurs.

Step coverage also depends on another property or characteristic of the deposition species, the sticking coefficient. This can be even more important than the line-of-sight issues in regards to step coverage and filling ability. The sticking coefficient is the ratio of the number of species that actually stay or "stick" on the surface relative to the number of incident species. We define the sticking coefficient S_C, or more accurately the effective sticking probability, specifically in terms of incident and reacting fluxes, where a deposition species that has "reacted" on the surface is one that properly deposits and stays there:

$$S_c = \frac{F_{\text{reacted}}}{F_{\text{incident}}} \tag{9.25}$$

The idea of a sticking coefficient is important for step coverage since the deposition species that do not stick or react are desorbed and may deposit elsewhere—on the sidewall of a stop, a trench, or a contact hole, for example. This is illustrated in Figure 9–21. Therefore, deposition processes with a sticking coefficient close to one, in which the species react and stick locally where they first hit without desorbing, will tend to have poorer step coverage and filling ability. Those with a sticking coefficient much less than one, in which the species bounce around before they stick and deposit, such as is generally the case in CVD depositions, will have better step coverage and better filling. In evaporation systems and other PVD methods, the sticking coefficient of the depositing species is usually very close to one, meaning that they deposit where they hit and there is little or no redepositing of desorbed species to other regions. Surface diffusion is also very slow at low temperatures. In addition, there is no resputtering of material in evaporation systems, as can be in the case in plasma CVD or sputter deposition systems where there is significant ion bombardment. As we will see in more detail later, deposition fluxes that have narrow arrival angle distributions and high sticking coefficients with little or no resputtering or diffusion lead to very poor step coverage. Deposition will occur primarily on horizontal surfaces, not on the sides of features. Heating the substrate during the evaporation process increases the surface diffusion and allows for

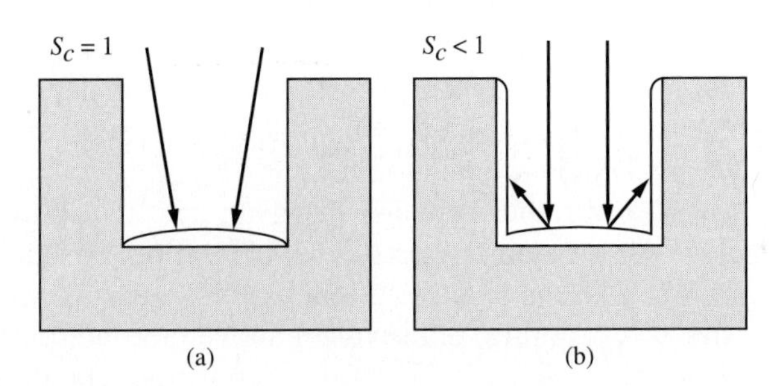

Figure 9–21 In (a) the depositing species have a high sticking coefficient (close to 1) so that they are deposited where they first strike. In (b) the depositing species have a low sticking coefficient ($<<1$) so that many are reemitted and deposited elsewhere on the topography, such as on the sidewalls.

some coverage on sidewalls. But heating can also affect the film composition and microstructure.

For all these reasons—difficulty in depositing alloys, compounds, and high-vapor pressure elements, lack of an in situ preclean, and poor step coverage—evaporation is rarely used today for standard silicon microelectronics technology. CVD and sputter deposition, described next, are now used instead. Nevertheless, we will make extensive use of the basic concepts of emission distribution laws and deposition rates developed in this section.

9.2.2.2 Sputter Deposition

Because the vacuum requirements for sputter deposition are less severe than for evaporation (in the 1–100 mtorr range for sputtering compared to $<10^{-5}$ torr for evaporation), sputter deposition was the preferred method in a variety of technologies prior to the microelectronics age. However, because the higher pressures in sputtering systems allowed significant contamination, evaporation was generally preferred in the early years of silicon microelectronics technology. But with the availability of ultrahigh purity source gases and the use of an initial low-pressure pumpdown, gas incorporation in sputtered films was found to be greatly reduced and contamination became much less of a problem with sputtered films. Because of the problems with evaporation discussed above, as well as the inability to develop manufacturable CVD methods for some materials, sputter deposition is commonly used today in semiconductor technology.

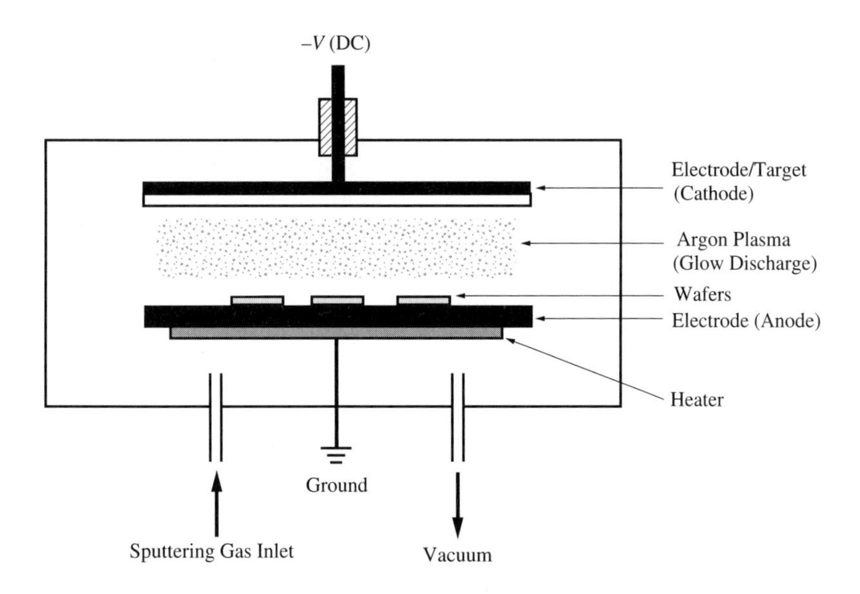

Figure 9–22 Schematic diagram of DC-powered sputter deposition equipment.

DC Sputter Deposition Figure 9–22 illustrates schematically a sputter deposition system. Note the similarity to the PECVD system in Figure 9–14. In the sputter system an inert gas, such as argon, is fed into the sputtering chamber at low pressure. A voltage is applied across the two electrodes and a plasma is created. The plasma contains neutral argon atoms, and roughly equal numbers of positive ions and free electrons, and is a conducting medium. (No free radical species are present here since Ar does not form free radicals in a plasma as O, H, and F species do in plasma deposition and etching systems.) The top electrode, where a negative DC voltage is applied, is actually the source material to be deposited, a plate or "platen" of Al, for example. This electrode becomes the cathode and is called the target. The bottom electrode is a metal platen, which is grounded and becomes the anode. The wafers sit upon the anode electrode. The positive ions in the plasma are accelerated to the negatively biased target, which can be several hundred to several thousand volts negative relative to the plasma. These energetic ions strike the target and dislodge, or sputter, the target atoms. These atoms are then free to travel through the plasma as a vapor and strike the surface of the wafers, where they condense and form the deposited film.

Since the target acts as an electrode in the DC mode of sputter deposition, the target or source material must be conductive. Therefore Al, W, Ti, silicides, and other metals can be sputtered this way. To deposit nonconductors—oxides, nitrides, and lightly doped silicon—another method must be used. We will discuss a technique to do that, the

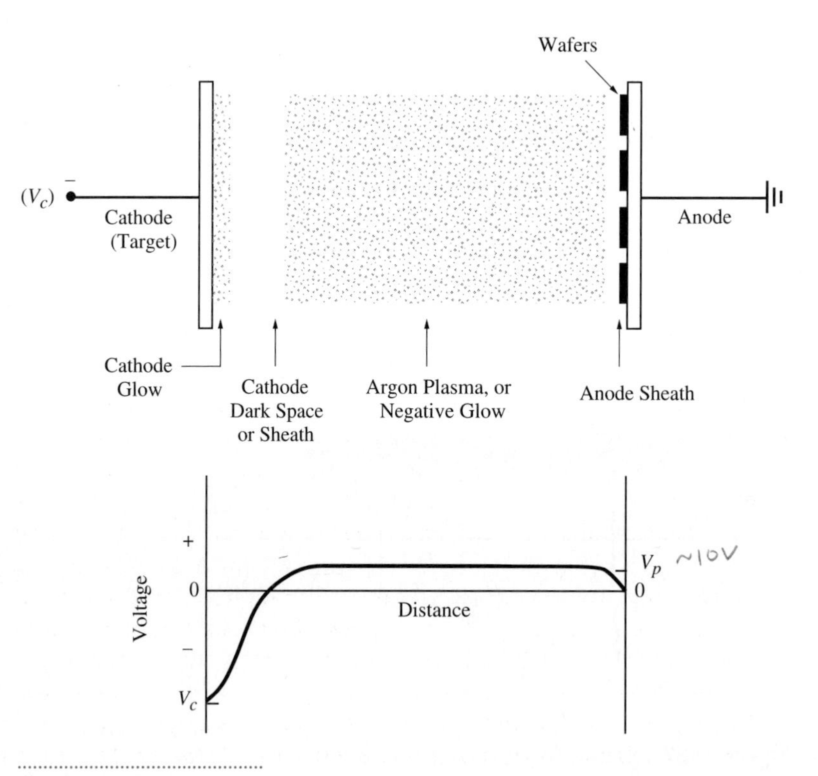

Figure 9–23 Plasma structure and voltage distribution in DC sputter system. (After [9.11].)

RF or AC method, a little later.

The structure and voltage distribution of the plasma in a DC system are shown in Figure 9–23. Most of the space between the electrodes is made up of the argon plasma, called the negative glow due to photon emission from excited Ar atoms. The voltage is fairly constant throughout this region since it has a fairly low resistance. Near the negative electrode, where there is an excess of positive ions and a shortage of electrons, as discussed below, there exists a space charge region that does not glow. This is called either the cathode dark space, the Crookes dark space, or the cathode sheath and is on the order of 0.1 to 10 mm thick. It is across this space charge region that most of the voltage drop in the system occurs. Because of the low density of electrons in the cathode sheath, few collisions between Ar atoms and electrons occur and that region is dark. Right next to the negative electrode is the thin cathode glow region; the light produced in this case is due to the interaction between the incoming ions and the cathode material. In this region incoming argon ions and sputtered target ions are neutralized and secondary electrons created by the ion bombardment are accelerated away from the cathode. These electrons then pass through the cathode sheath and collide with the Ar atoms in the negative glow region, ionizing some of them and sustaining the plasma.

While the electrons are accelerated in one direction across the high electric field in the cathode dark space, the positive argon ions are accelerated in the opposite direction, from the negative glow region to the target. They strike the target surface and sputter off the source atoms, which can then transport to the wafers and form the film.

Additional glow regions and dark spaces can form closer to the anode, such as the Faraday dark space, the positive column region, and the anode sheath [9.11]. But these are not useful in the sputter deposition process, and all but the anode sheath are eliminated or minimized by having the positive electrode close to the negative glow, resulting in the plasma structure and voltage distribution shown in Figure 9–23.

One interesting feature is that the plasma potential, V_p, is positive with respect to the anode (on the order of 10V), as shown in Figure 9–23. In fact, the plasma potential will be positive with respect to any surface within the plasma, with positive space charge regions, or sheaths, formed next to each surface. This is primarily due to the fact that both ions and electrons from the plasma will randomly strike the surface and escape the plasma. But the electrons with their lighter mass and higher mobility will strike the surface more often, causing an imbalance in the ion and electron currents. An electric field develops that opposes this imbalance by opposing the electron flow, raising the voltage (by V_p). Therefore the potential of the plasma will be positive with respect to both the anode and cathode, with a positive space charge region of excess ions and a shortage of electrons forming a sheath at both the anode and the cathode. With the applied negative voltage at the cathode, the voltage distribution shown in Figure 9–23 results, with a net DC current passing through the circuit. In the region near the cathode, this current is predominantly carried by the positive ion flux (which is also responsible for the sputtering). The large voltage drop there accelerates the secondary electrons from the cathode across the sheath and sustains the plasma. In the region near the anode an equal current flows, but is mostly carried by the electrons. Because of the exponential Maxwell-Boltzmann distribution of the electron energy, only a small perturbation of the zero-current plasma potential is needed to supply the net DC current at the anode. Because of the potential drop from the plasma to the anode, some sputtering of the anode

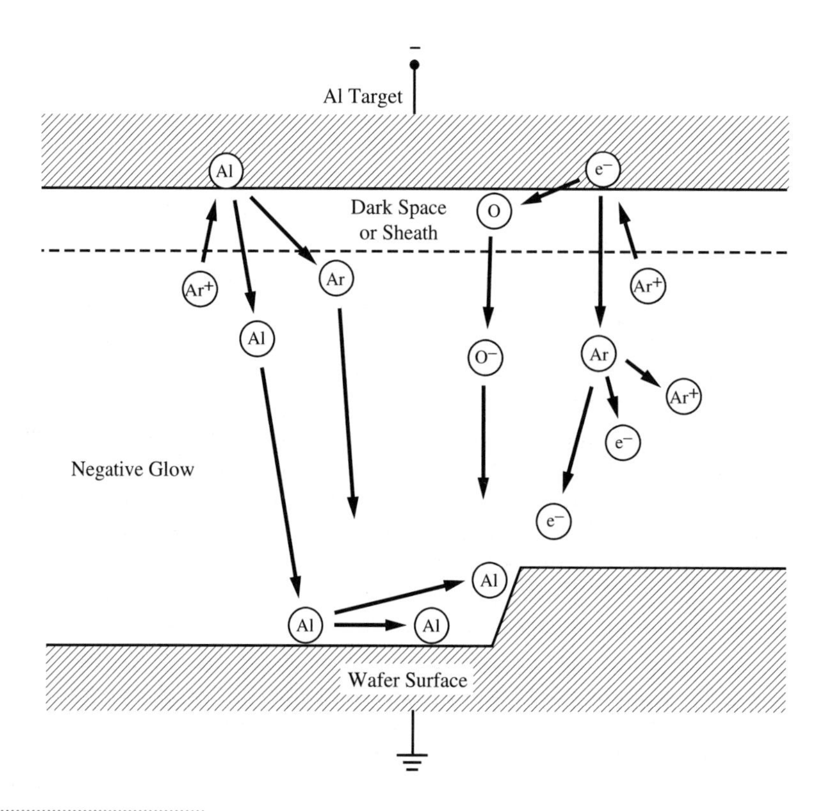

Figure 9–24 Important processes in sputter deposition.

can occur, but very little compared to that at the cathode.

Several of the important processes that occur during sputter deposition are illustrated in Figure 9–24. At the top left, an Ar ion from the negative glow accelerates across the dark space and sputters off an Al atom from the target. (A minimum energy, on the order of 10–20 eV, is needed to sputter an atom, and the sputter yield increases with ion energy.) This Al atom travels through the dark space and negative glow and lands on the wafer surface. If the argon atom is neutralized during gas phase collisions, it can retain enough kinetic energy to also travel to the wafer surface and become incorporated in the growing film. The Al atom now on the wafer surface may stay absorbed and become part of the growing film there. It may also surface migrate or diffuse to another location. Finally, it can leave the surface by either desorbing on its own (though this does not occur very often compared to CVD systems, as we will discuss later), or by being resputtered by another atom hitting the surface. The Al atom could then be redeposited at another location.

In the upper right, an Ar ion strikes the target, and a secondary electron is emitted. The secondary electron can accelerate across the dark space and strike another argon atom, exciting it or ionizing it, and sustaining the plasma. The electron can also ionize an impurity atom, oxygen in this case, which can then be accelerated across the dark space and travel toward the wafer surface. Finally, all the species moving toward the wafer surface can be embedded in the wafer surface. Even a significant number of positively charged ions can be made to strike the wafer surface with high energies by independently biasing the wafer surface relative to the plasma, as will be described later in the sections on bias sputtering and ionized sputtering. Or the atoms or ions can strike the atoms on the wafer surface, imparting energy to them and enhancing their movements and reactions, and even heating the wafer surface. Thus physical reactions and processes, rather then chemical, dominate in PVD.

In evaporation, the deposition rate was seen to depend on the source material vapor pressure. In sputter deposition, it is the source, or target, sputtering rate that is important. The plasma gas ion strikes the target and physically dislodges the target atom. This is a physical, rather than a chemical, process, and is often explained using billiard ball models. Sputtering occurs when the incoming ion transfers enough energy to the target surface to break the bonds holding the target atom in place. This depends on the energy and mass of the ions, and the target material.

The sputter yields for argon sputtering of different target materials do not vary very much for the different target materials compared to the wide range of vapor pressures important in evaporation. Typically this yield, defined as the number of atoms or molecules ejected from the target per incident ion, is in the range of 0.1 to 3. It does depend on the energy of the incoming ion, determined mainly by the voltage across the sheath, and on the direction of incidence of the ions. An ion coming in at a low, glancing angle will not be as successful at dislodging an atom, with the ion itself being reflected off the surface. At the other extreme, ions arriving normal to the surface will push a surface atom further into the target but not necessarily sputter it off. The sputter yield peaks at some angle less than 90°. The angles that the sputtered atoms leave the surface of the targets are usually found to be diffusely distributed, with an ideal cosine-emitted angle distribution, or close to it, from each position on the target. This means that the sputtered atoms are ejected from each location on the target in a broad range of directions.

The targets used in sputter deposition come in a variety of shapes and sizes. Multiple targets may also be used in these systems for cosputtering of alloys and compounds or for multilayer depositions, where Ti and Al layers may be deposited one after the other in the chamber without breaking vacuum. Achieving good thickness uniformity in the different types of systems is accomplished in different ways: having the target larger than the wafer or wafer holder; having the wafers pass by or spin in front of a long rectangular target; or by using the cylindrical wafer holder around an oblong target (similar to having a spherical holder in front of a point source in evaporation.)

Having a large area target also means that the arrival angles of the atoms at the wafer surface are more widely distributed which generally improves step coverage. Having the wafers rotate or pass by a target is somewhat similar to having a large target in this regard and also helps increase the range of arrival angles in the direction of the rotation.

Let us first discuss how we describe or quantify the "arrival angle distribution." Here we are interested in the flux, as a function of arrival angle, arriving at any small area on the wafer surface. In Figure 9–25 on the left we show fluxes arriving at the surface from all angles with equal magnitude; that is, the number of particles or atoms, per time and per area normal to the flux direction, is equal for all incoming directions. We call this isotropic arrival. We could describe this arrival distribution as being constant since the flux relative to the flux direction is constant, similar to the way we characterized the

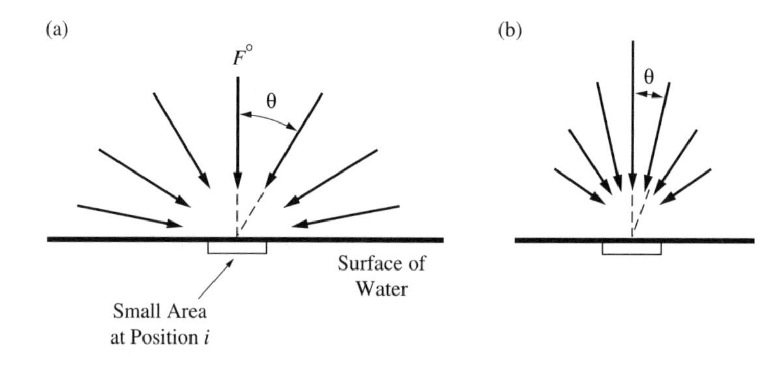

Figure 9–25 Distribution of arrival fluxes for (a) uniform or isotropic arrival distribution; and (b) directed or anisotropic arrival distribution. Arrival angle distribution ($\cos^n\theta$) is defined by arrival flux relative to unit surface area. This flux is equal to the normal component of incoming flux, relative to the vertical direction for a horizontal surface.

emission angle distribution. However, we are going to define the arrival angle distribution a little differently. We are ultimately interested in the deposition on a surface area, so we are concerned with the flux in terms of particles per time per area on the surface, or per unit surface area. This is just the incoming flux, which is constant for isotropic arrival, multiplied by the cosine of the arrival angle θ, where θ is the angle between the incoming flux and the normal direction to the surface. Just as in our treatment of a flux striking and depositing on a flat surface in an evaporation system, the deposition rate depends on the normal component, or the cosine of the angle, of the incoming flux to that surface. Using the cosine function in the arrival angle distribution also allows us to easily describe both isotropic and anisotropic arrival distributions. (This convention may be a little confusing since in our description of the emitted angle distribution for evaporation sources and emission, which uses a different convention, a "cosine distribution" from a small area is not uniform or isotropic as we describe it but is directed toward the surface normal. But to be consistent with normal terminology for emission, as well as with that used to describe arrival angle distributions in our deposition and etch modeling using the SPEEDIE simulator, we will use these two conventions.)

We thus describe the arrival angle distribution in terms of $\cos\theta$, or the normal component of the incoming flux. For isotropic incoming fluxes, the arrival angle distribution by this definition is therefore described as $\cos\theta$, with a maximum at $\theta = 0°$ and decreasing as the angle gets larger, eventually going to 0 at $\theta = 90°$. Another way to look at it is that for isotropic arrival, the atoms that strike the unit surface area from a particular direction, θ, must pass though the projected area of the unit surface area facing the flux direction. As θ increases, the projected area gets smaller. Therefore fewer atoms strike the unit surface area, and the flux relative to the surface area (the atoms per time per unit surface area) decreases. Ultimately, no atoms strike the surface area when $\theta = 90°$, since the flux is parallel to the surface.

For incoming fluxes that are not isotropic, but anisotropic and more directed toward the surface [as shown in part (b) of the figure], a $\cos^n\theta$ distribution can be used. A value of n larger than 1 describes a more directed or anisotropic incoming flux distribution.

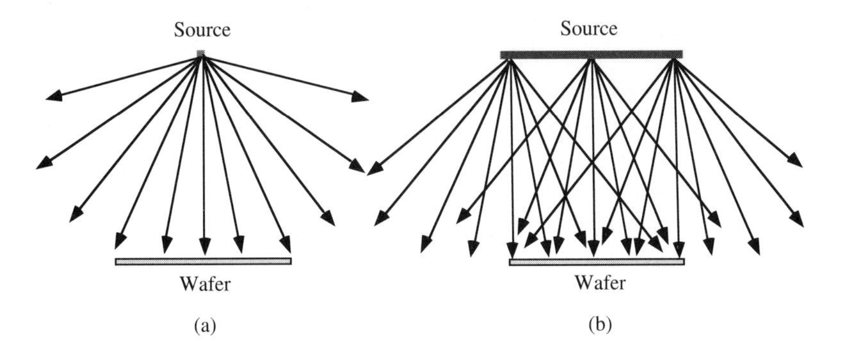

Figure 9–26 Flux lines of atoms from small area and extended sources. In (a) the flux lines from a point or small area source are shown, with a wide emitted angle distribution but a narrow arrival angle distribution. In (b) the flux lines from an extended source are shown. A wider arrival angle distribution is seen with the extended source.

We now return to illustrating the idea that a larger source region, or target area in the case of sputtering, results in a wider arrival angle distribution. In Figure 9–26(a), the flux lines of atoms from either an ideal small area surface source or an ideal point source are shown, in either case emitting in a rather wide angular distribution. While the atoms are emitted from the small source with a wide angular distribution, the distribution of angles arriving at each point or small area on the wafer is very small. This tight or narrow distribution can be described by an arrival distribution of $\cos^n \theta$ with n much greater than 1. Obviously a wide emission or departure distribution of angles does not necessarily mean a wide arrival distribution of angles.

In Figure 9–26(b) an extended source is used, such as a larger target. At each position on the wafer, atoms arrive at a range of angles, as determined by the geometry of the system, and not just from a narrow range of angles. Here n in the $\cos^n\theta$ arrival distribution would be closer to 1, meaning less anisotropic and more isotropic. This can cause more uniform step coverage on steps in the wafer topography, and would also improve thickness uniformity across the substrate.

As we described earlier, the arrival angle distribution for evaporation systems can be made wider by rotating the wafer holder around two axes, effectively making the source wider, and the step coverage can be improved. But there are other reasons that step coverage is usually still better in sputtering systems. Because of the higher pressure in sputtering systems, the atoms experience more gas-phase collisions in sputtering systems. One can estimate the average number of collisions by calculating the mean free path, λ, of a particle in a gas. From kinetic theory, the mean free path of a gas particle is

$$\lambda = \frac{kT}{\sqrt{2}\pi d^2 P} \tag{9.26}$$

where $k = 1.36 \times 10^{-22}$ cm^3 atm K^{-1}, T is the temperature in K, d is the collision diameter of the molecule in cm (approximately 4×10^{-8} cm, or about 0.4 nm, for most molecules of interest), and P is the pressure in atm. In a typical sputtering system with $P =$

5 mtorr, this results in a mean free path on the order of 1 cm, which is a little less than the physical path length the depositing atoms follow.

For evaporation systems, the number of collisions experienced between the source and wafer is virtually zero, while in sputtering systems the average number of collisions experienced is on the order of one to a few. This tends to make the arrival angle distribution somewhat wider. (Increasing the pressure or number of collisions too much to widen the distribution can result in poor film properties, partly due to less energetic species, and contamination problems.) Also, the number of resputtered atoms on the wafer surface is higher for sputtering due to the bombardment of energetic particles. This effectively increases the arrival angle distribution even more. For these reasons, step coverage in sputtering systems is usually better than in evaporation systems. But it is still usually much worse than in CVD depositions, which generally have an isotropic arrival angle distribution and lower sticking coefficients, as we will discuss later. In some cases, though, we actually want to narrow the arrival distribution—for example when filling a deep via with metal in a PVD system. We will see how that can be achieved when we discuss collimated and ionized sputtering systems.

Because the sputtering yields of different elements are much more similar to each other than their vapor pressures are, the deposition of alloys and compounds should be much more controllable using sputtering rather than evaporation. But there is another reason why the compositions of sputter deposited films are more controllable and uniform. Because sputtering occurs just from the top surface of the target and little mixing from the layers below takes place, a steady-state condition soon develops where the atoms are sputtered off at relative rates equal to the target composition, even when the sputtering rate of each type of atom is different. Initially the element with the higher sputtering rate does preferentially sputter off more from the surface. This leaves the top surface enriched, relative to the bulk of the target, with the element with the lower sputtering rate. But now more of the element with the lower sputtering rate is sputtered since the surface region is enriched with that element. A steady state is achieved where the elements leave the surface in a ratio that is the same as the bulk target composition—the difference in sputtering rates is exactly compensated for by the difference in the surface concentration.

The overall target composition thus remains at its original composition, with no depletion or fractionation, since the two elements are being sputtered off in proportion to the overall composition. This does not work for evaporation. Since the evaporation source material is often molten or near molten, the diffusion of atoms is very fast and mixing between the surface and bulk wipes out any concentration gradients. Therefore, the required enriched surface concentration cannot be maintained. But in sputtering, the temperature of the target is much lower—near room temperature—and little diffusion and mixing occur.

Compounds, such as SiO_2 and WSi_2, may be sputtered as well. In some cases, they are sputtered off as individual atoms, and sometimes they are sputtered as molecules. Both alloys and compounds may be sputtered from two different targets, called cosputtering (as opposed to the use of one "composite" target). For example, WSi_2 can be sputtered by simultaneously using a tungsten target and a silicon target. But it is often difficult to control the stoichiometry, and composite targets are more commonly used. Even then the composition may vary.

Reactive Sputter Deposition Another way in which compounds can be sputter deposited is by reactive sputter deposition. Here a reactive gas is introduced into the sputtering chamber in addition to the Ar plasma, and the compound is formed by the elements of that gas combining with the sputtered material. For example, TiN can be deposited by sputtering Ti in the presence of nitrogen. The plasma can furnish energy to the N_2 to allow it to dissociate into atomic nitrogen, which then can easily react with the Ti. The reaction usually occurs either on the wafer surface or on the target itself, and not in the plasma. In the case of TiO_2 reactive sputtering, it is found that the oxygen reacts with the Ti on the surface of the Ti target to form the oxide there, and then it is sputtered onto the wafer surface. Controlling the stoichiometry of reactively sputtered films is sometimes difficult and this method is not used very often—sputtering from compound targets is more common. Sometimes a reactive gas such as O_2 or N_2 is used in conjunction with sputtering from a compound target. This could ensure that the composition of a gaseous constituent is maintained in a sputtered film, or it could be used to improve the properties of a film. Sputtering TiW in the presence of oxygen or nitrogen has been found to improve the barrier properties of these films, as discussed in Chapter 11.

RF Sputter Deposition DC sputter deposition is not suitable for insulator deposition. When applying the necessary DC voltage to the insulating target to sustain a plasma, difficulties arise. With a negative DC voltage applied, positive argon ions from the plasma strike the negatively charged insulator and positive charge would accumulate. The negative surface voltage would become less than that required to sustain the glow discharge, and the plasma would shut down. The time required for this to occur is only about 1–10 μsec.

The solution is to use a high-frequency alternating voltage instead of DC. 13.56 MHz is commonly used. RF voltages can be coupled capacitively through the insulating target to the plasma, so that conducting electrodes are not necessary, and the positive charge buildup is neutralized by electron bombardment over each cycle. The RF frequency is chosen to be high enough so that a continuous plasma discharge is maintained, that is, higher than the effective RC time constant of the system. The difference in mass and hence mobility between the electrons and ions allows for virtually continuous sputtering of the target throughout both half cycles of the RF voltage. The electrons have a high enough mobility to keep up with the changing electric field, but the heavier argon ions do not. During the first few complete cycles more electrons than ions are collected at each electrode, and this negative charge buildup on the electrodes is maintained during subsequent cycles. As a result, both electrodes maintain a self-biasing steady-state (DC) potential that is negative with respect to the plasma voltage, V_p. The value of V_p is set by the requirement that the DC current is zero. A positive V_p aids the transport of the slower positive ions and slows down the negative electrons. The spatial distribution of the voltage that develops is shown in Figure 9–27, with the solid curve for the symmetric RF case (that is, with equal area electrodes). This is similar to

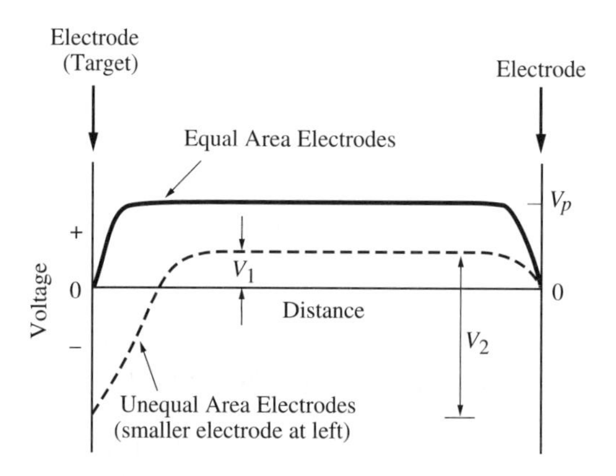

Figure 9–27 Steady-state voltage distribution in RF powered sputtering systems. The wafer sits on the right electrode.

the DC-powered case where electron depletion regions form and the plasma self-biases. However, V_p is generally larger and the net voltage drop at both electrodes would be equal in the symmetric RF powered case. The heavy ions, while they cannot travel across the sheath at the frequency of the RF signal, do respond to the average DC potential that develops across the sheath and strike the negatively biased target.

The induced negative biasing of the target due to the RF powering means that continuous sputtering of the target occurs throughout the RF cycle. But it also means that this occurs at both electrodes. The wafers will be sputtered at the same rate as the target since the voltage drops would be the same at both electrodes for a symmetric system. It would thus be very difficult to deposit any material this way. However, because the RF current must be continuous throughout the system, the voltage drops, V_1 and V_2, across the dark space next to the two electrodes are related to the respective electrode areas, A_1 and A_2, by [9.12]

$$\frac{V_1}{V_2} = \left(\frac{A_2}{A_1}\right)^m \tag{9.27}$$

The smaller electrode requires a higher RF current density to maintain the same total current as the larger electrode. As a result, the fields must be higher at the smaller electrode. Simple theory gives $m = 4$, but experimentally the exponent is found to be between 1 and 2, perhaps due to voltage saturation and sheath collision issues, but the effect is the same. By making the area of the target electrode smaller than the area of the other electrode, the voltage drop at the target electrode will be much greater than at the other electrode. V_p in the asymmetric case would also be smaller. The resulting voltage distribution for unequal electrodes is also shown in Figure 9–27, and closely resembles that for the DC sputter deposition case (Figure 9–23 shown earlier). The volt-

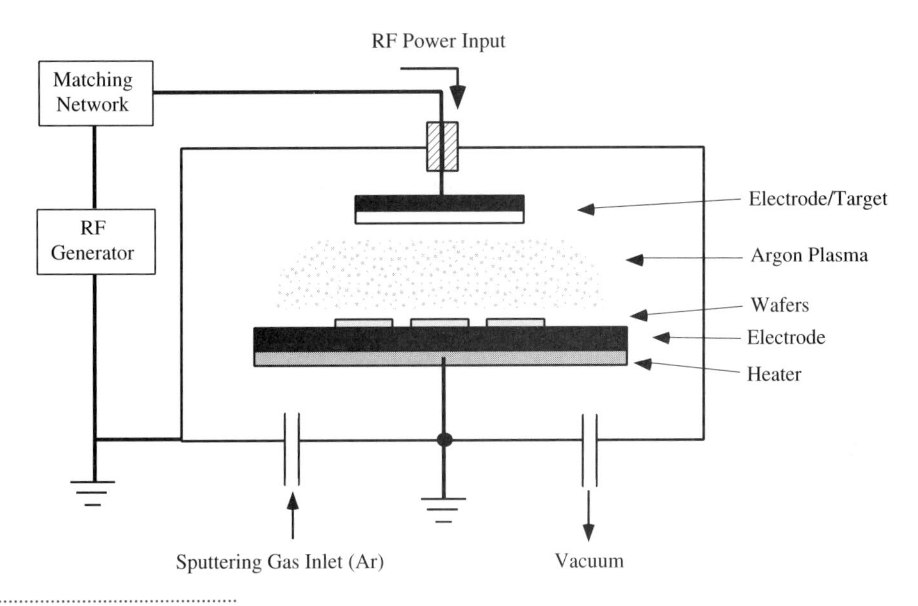

Figure 9–28 Schematic diagram of RF-powered sputter deposition system.

age drop from the plasma to the larger electrode is typically tens of volts while the voltage drop to the smaller electrode is several hundreds or even a thousand volts. Therefore almost all the sputtering will occur at the target electrode, as is desired.

Not only can the target electrode be made relatively small, but the wafer electrode can also be connected to the chamber walls (which would also be grounded), thus making the effective area of that electrode even larger. For typical RF-frequency power supplies (e.g., 13.56 MHz), an impedance matching network is also required. A typical setup for RF sputter deposition is shown in Figure 9–28.

In addition to allowing sputtering of nonconducting material, there are two other advantages of using RF powered systems. In RF plasmas, electrons gain energy directly from the oscillating RF fields because of low-loss elastic collisions with neutral atoms. Thus the plasma can in fact be sustained without the need for secondary electrons from the walls and electrodes. In addition, the efficiency of ionization is increased by these oscillating electrons, allowing for operation at somewhat lower pressures.

Bias Sputtering: Sputter Etching and Bias-Sputter Deposition Sometimes sputtering of the wafer is desirable. One application would be for precleaning the wafer before the actual deposition, or "sputter etching." Another application is in "bias sputtering," where deposition and sputtering of the wafer are done simultaneously. A negative bias relative to the plasma is applied to the wafer electrode, which is now electrically isolated from the chamber walls. Positive Ar ions from the plasma will now be accelerated to the wafers on the substrate carrier and sputter off atoms. The energy of the ions (and hence the sputtering yield) can be controlled by controlling the substrate bias. Usually an RF bias is used since the wafers often have insulating films on them, while the target is given either a DC or RF bias. The target bias is in the range of -700 to -2000 V, while the substrate bias is on the order of -50 to -300 V [9.6].

In sputter etching or cleaning, no deposition is allowed to occur on the wafer by using a shutter to block sputtered material from the target. During this step, a controlled thickness of surface material is sputtered off the wafer, removing any contaminants or native oxides. A film can then be sputter deposited immediately afterward without breaking the vacuum, inhibiting recontamination or reoxidation. Redeposition of contaminants due to sputtering of chamber walls and other parts of the wafer can occur during sputter etching and may be a concern. Charging damage can also be a problem.

In bias-sputter deposition, or sometimes just "bias sputtering," sputter etching of the wafer and deposition on the wafer (by sputtering the target) are allowed to occur concurrently. Conditions are chosen so that more deposition occurs than etching. But by allowing some sputtering of the wafer surface to occur during the deposition, both the topography and the properties of the deposited film can be altered. The most common application is SiO_2, called "bias-sputtered quartz" when deposited this way. By applying bias to the substrate, sharp edges of the SiO_2 due to the underlying structure are reduced during the sputter deposition. This allows for a more planarized film as well as for better filling between metal lines. The common reason given for these results is that the sputtering of the wafer is a function of the geometry of the surface features, with pointed and sloped features being sputtered, and removed, more easily than horizontal or vertical surfaces. Not only does this help planarize the film, but the overhang that can develop when depositing into a trench or hole is preferentially sputtered away, allowing for better filling of the hole, as illustrated in Figure 9–29. Another factor may be that the resputtered atoms allow for some redeposition on sidewalls. We will demonstrate these ideas with simulations of high-density plasma CVD and ionized PVD depositions which make use of these same phenomena later in this chapter. Another technique for filling spaces based on these same ideas is to do the deposition, usually by PECVD, and sputter etching sequentially, as opposed to simultaneously. This can be done in a cluster tool with separate chambers for each process. The wafer is physically moved back and forth between the two.

Because of the energetic ions bombarding the film surface during bias-sputter deposition, the properties of the films being deposited can also be altered by changing the substrate bias. These properties include resistivity, residual stress, density, etch rate, and dielectric constant. SiO_2 that is deposited by regular sputtering (no substrate bias) is very porous and unsuitable for use in microelectronics, while SiO_2 that is deposited using bias sputtering is much denser and has been used for intermetal dielectric applications.

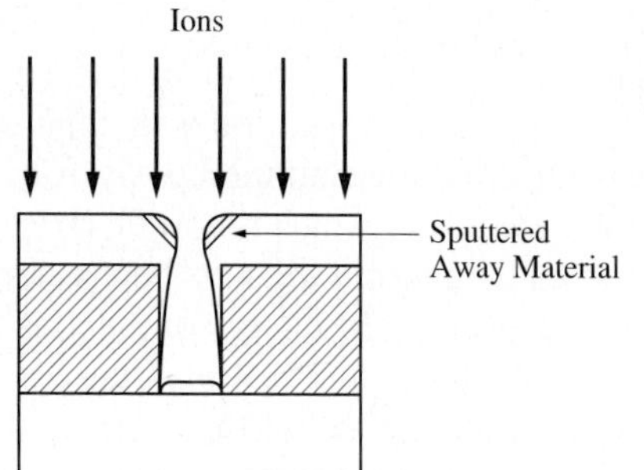

Figure 9–29 Illustration of angle-dependent sputtering which removes nonplanar features in bias-sputter deposition. Here the angled surfaces of the overhang are preferentially sputtered by the directed ions, allowing for better filling of the hole.

However, this method for depositing SiO_2 also has shortcomings. First, because of the combined deposition and etching of the wafer, the net deposition rate is low. Also, the SiO_2 will deposit on the chamber walls and other metal surfaces in the chamber and can flake off and cause contamination and particulate problems. For these reasons bias sputtering is not commonly used today. A method which combines bias sputtering with CVD deposition methods, the High-Density Plasma (HDP) CVD method described earlier, has recently been developed and does not suffer from these problems.

Magnetron Sputter Deposition In both conventional DC and RF sputtering, the efficiency of ionization from energetic collisions between the electrons and gas atoms is rather low. Most electrons lose their energy in non-ionizing collisions or are collected by the anode, and only a small percentage of them take part in ionization processes with the Ar atoms. In RF plasmas electrons gain energy directly from the oscillating RF fields, increasing the ionization efficiency somewhat. But the overall ionization efficiency is still fairly low. As a result, the deposition rates are usually rather low. Few Ar atoms are converted to positive ions and few positive ions strike the target.

In the technique known as magnetron sputtering, magnets are used to increase the percentage of electrons that take part in ionization events, and the ionization efficiency is increased significantly. A magnetic field is applied at right angles to the electric field, usually by placing large rectangular magnets behind the target. This traps the electrons near the target surface, and causes them to move in a spiral motion until they collide with an Ar atom. The ionization and sputtering efficiencies are increased significantly, and deposition rates of up to one μm per minute can be achieved—about 10 to 100 times faster than without the magnetron configuration. Unintentional wafer heating is also significantly reduced, since the dense plasma is confined to near the target and the ion loss to the wafers is less. In addition, a lower Ar pressure can be utilized since the ionization efficiency is so much larger. This can lead to better film quality since less argon will be incorporated in the film. Magnetron sputtering can be done in either DC or RF modes, but the former is more common. At these higher ion currents, cooling of the target can be a problem for RF systems which have insulating targets.

Collimated Sputter Deposition and Ionized Sputter Deposition A small range of arrival angles during deposition can cause nonuniform, or poor, step coverage over a step in topography. However, sometimes a small range of arrival angles is desirable. If material is required to be deposited into of a deep contact or via, as when filling it with Aℓ or depositing Ti/TiN contact and barrier layers, a large arrival angle distribution can cause problems. As illustrated in Figure 9–30(a), a relatively large arrival angle distribution, when little surface diffusion or reemission occurs, can result in little deposition at the bottom of a hole due to shadowing effects. In addition, overhang formation can occur at the top corners of a deep hole, enhancing the shadowing effect. All this leads to poor coverage at the bottom of the hole or incomplete filling.

One way to improve this is by having a narrow range of arrival angles, with most of the depositing atoms arriving at the wafer perpendicular to the surface. Evaporation from a stationary small source would result in a narrow range of arrival angles compared to sputtering due to geometric arguments (Figure 9–26), as well as due to the fewer gas-phase collisions, but sputtering is preferred due to its ability to deposit uniform alloys and compounds and its in situ sputter etch capability. While standard sput-

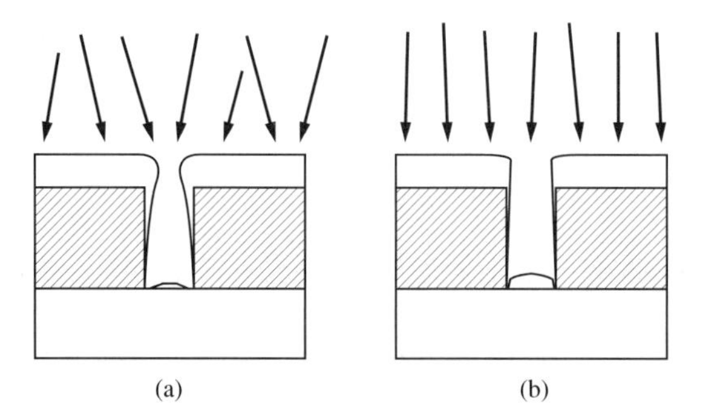

Figure 9–30 Effect of arrival angle distribution of depositing species on filling of trenches or holes in a PVD system. In (a) a relatively wide arrival angle distribution leads to poor bottom filling or coverage, while in (b) a narrower arrival angle distribution leads to better bottom filling. The higher the aspect ratio of the feature, the narrower the arrival angle distribution must be for adequate bottom coverage.

ter deposition equipment may adequately cover the bottoms of holes with low aspect ratios (less than 1 or so), its arrival angle distribution is too large for holes with high aspect ratios. Using a smaller sputtering target would result in a narrower arrival angle distribution at the wafer, with a single angle coming from a point source in the extreme case. But that angle would vary across the wafer. This would result in uneven asymmetric deposition, depositing more on one sidewall of the hole or the other for much of the wafer. (A small evaporation source would have the same problem.) It would be better to somehow filter or focus the incoming atoms in a sputtering system so that a narrow range of angles, all nearly perpendicular to the wafer surface, arrived at the wafer. Better filling of a hole, and more uniform directionality across a wafer, could thus be obtained as illustrated in Figure 9–30(b). Two methods to do this have been developed: collimated sputtering and ionized sputtering.

In collimated sputtering, a plate of circular or hexagonal holes, or cells, is placed between the target and the wafer. The height to width aspect ratio of these cells can range from 1:1 to 3:1. As the sputtered atoms travel through the collimator toward the wafer, only those with a nearly normal incidence trajectory will continue on to strike the wafer. Those at more oblique angles will strike the walls of the collimator, depositing there. The collimator thus acts as a physical filter to low-angle sputtered atoms. A problem with this method is that a significant percentage of the sputtered atoms are filtered out, up to 95 percent, and never make it to the wafers. Thus the deposition rate is significantly reduced and the collimator must be cleaned regularly. As a result, collimated sputtering is rarely used for completely filling contacts or vias where a lot of material needs to be deposited but is more suited for contact and barrier metal deposition where the amounts of material deposited are much less. It does do a fairly good job of covering the bottoms of contacts and vias with contact and barrier metals. Some sidewall coverage, important for via liners, is also obtained from the flux that is slightly off-normal, but the sidewall film is often less dense. In addition, uniformity across a wafer or from wafer to wafer may be affected by shadowing by the collimator.

Another type of sputtering is called "long throw collimation," or "long throw sputtering." No collimation plate is actually used. Instead, a limited size target, about the size of the wafer in a single-wafer system, is used and the distance between the target and wafer is increased (up to about 30 cm compared to about 5 cm in more standard systems), decreasing the distribution of arrival angles at the wafers. In effect the sputtering chamber acts as one collimator cell, with the high-angle atoms not reaching the wafer but striking the chamber wall instead. However, as the spacing is increased, the deposition rate, the target utilization, and the uniformity all decrease; in addition, the chance of gas-phase collision and scattering increases. Low pressures are usually utilized in these systems to minimize gas-phase collisions. Because of the limited target size and target-to-wafer spacing, asymmetric depositions in trenches and vias can occur at the edges of wafers in these systems [9.13].

In ionized sputtering a narrow arrival angle distribution, perpendicular to the surface, is obtained as in collimated sputtering. However, most of the sputtered material reaches the wafers, giving it a significant advantage over collimated sputtering. In this technique, the sputtered atoms—mostly neutral as they leave the target—are ionized as they travel between the target and the wafers. An inductively coupled RF antenna is placed around the plasma region which ionizes the sputtered atoms through collisions with electrons in the plasma, as illustrated in Figure 9–31. Fifty to eighty-five percent of the atoms are ionized. The ionized atoms, Al^+ or Ti^+, for example, will be accelerated and directed across the wafer sheath, striking the wafers in a nearly perpendicular direction. A DC or RF bias is usually applied to the wafer holder, similar to bias sputtering. This will further accelerate these ions to the wafer surface, resulting in a highly directional flux. In addition, the energy of the incoming ions (both Ar and the deposited element) can be tightly controlled, and the deposition behavior and film properties can

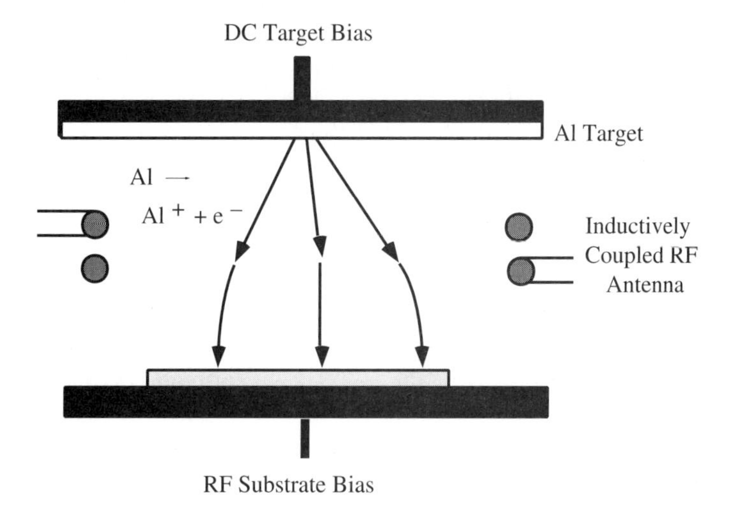

Figure 9–31 Schematic diagram of ionized sputter deposition system (or ionized PVD), showing atomic flux lines. (After [9.15].)

be altered, just as in bias sputtering. The highly directional ionized atoms and angle-dependent sputtering can result in very good coverage at the bottom of deep vias or contacts. However, the sidewall coverage may be poor. By increasing the ion energy, the resputtering and redeposition of the atoms can be increased, resulting in better sidewall coverage [9.14], often still thinner than the bottom, but at least continuous. Bevelling of the top corners due to angle-dependant sputtering may also occur.

Ionized PVD (IPVD) is also referred to as "ionized metal plasma" (IMP) deposition. It is also sometimes called "high density plasma sputtering," analogous to high density plasma CVD, because of the higher density plasma produced which ionizes the metal atoms. With the high density plasma produced, much more efficient deposition occurs compared to bias-sputtering or collimated sputtering, and IPVD is beginning to be more commonly used in chip production. The main problems with ionized PVD have to do with uniformity and manufacturing issues. The ionizing coils are usually located inside the chamber, and not remotely as in HDP CVD and etching systems. (Otherwise metal deposited on the chamber windows would block the signal from a remote RF source.) Having the coils inside the chamber leads to deposition on the coils and other associated problems. Another type of IPVD system utilizes a hollow cathode magnetron source rather than RF coils.

High-Temperature or Hot-Sputter Deposition Another method used to fill spaces during deposition as well as to improve overall coverage is high-temperature, or hot-, sputtering. This will be discussed further in Chapter 11 since it is most often used for Al deposition. The basic idea is to heat the substrate to 450°C or higher during deposition, usually by a wafer backside gas heating system. Surface diffusion is significantly increased so that filling in spaces, smoothing edges, and planarization are accomplished, all driven by surface energy reduction. This can be considered as *in situ* reflow. Usually a thin "cold" deposition is done first with the substrate at room temperature, which serves as a nucleation-wetting layer. CVD deposition of Al may also be used for this. This is then followed by the hot-PVD deposition. High-temperature sputter deposition is still in the development stage. One of the main drawbacks is the relatively high temperature required. Excessive reaction between the hot Al and the liner can occur. The high temperature can also adversely affect other materials and layers already present on the wafer at this stage in the process.

Even more recently developed is high-pressure sputter deposition. In this method, called the aluminum extrusion fill, or the "ForceFill" [9.16] technique, the aluminum is first sputter deposited, which covers and seals the holes. Then the chamber is pressurized with argon to up to 700 atmospheres while the wafer is heated to about 400°C. This forces the aluminum to completely fill any hole and does so quite effectively. Applying the high argon pressure after the deposition minimizes any argon incorporation in the film. The high temperature and specialized equipment are drawbacks to this technique.

9.3 Manufacturing Methods

The different types of equipment used for the deposition of thin films in microelectronics were discussed in the previous section. In this section the techniques used today to deposit specific thin films will be briefly described. Table 9–1 provides a summary.

Table 9–1 Common deposition methods for thin films in integrated circuit fabrication

Thin Film	Equipment	Typical Reactions	Comments
Epitaxial silicon	APCVD, LPCVD	$SiH_4 \rightarrow Si + 2H_2$ $SiCl_4 + 2H_2 \rightarrow Si + 4HCl$ Also $SiHCl_3$, SiH_2Cl_2	1000–1250°C. Reduce pressure for lower-temperature deposition.
Polysilicon	LPCVD	Same as epitaxial Si	575–650°C. Grain structure depends on deposition conditions and doping.
Si_3N_4	LPCVD, PECVD	$3SiH_4 + NH_4 \rightarrow Si_3N_4 + 12H_2$	650–800°C for oxidation mask. 200–400°C (PECVD) for passivation.
SiO_2	LPCVD, PECVD, HDPCVD, APCVD	$SiH_4 + O_2 \rightarrow SiO_2 + 2H_2$ $Si(OC_2H_5)_4\ (+O_3) \rightarrow SiO_2$ + byproducts	200–800°C. 200–500°C (LTO)—may require high T anneal. 25–400°C (TEOS-ozone, PECVD, HDPCVD).
Al	Magnetron sputter deposition		25–300°C (standard deposition). 440–550°C (hot Al for in situ reflow). CVD difficult for alloys (Al-Cu-Si).
Ti and Ti-W	Magnetron sputter deposition (standard, ionized, or collimated)		CVD difficult. Nitrogen can be added to Ti-W to stuff grain boundaries.
W	LPCVD	$2WF_6 + 3SiH_4 \rightarrow 2W + 3SiF_4 + 6H_2$ $WF_6 + 3H_2 \rightarrow W + 6HF$	250–500°C. Blanket deposition with two-step process using both reactions is common.
$TiSi_2$	Sputter and surface reaction Cosputtering or CVD	Ti(sputtered) + Si(exposed) $\rightarrow TiSi_2$	Sputter/reaction gives self-aligned silicide.
TiN	Reactive sputter deposition	Ti + N_2 (in plasma) $\rightarrow$ TiN	Organometallic source possible for MOCVD deposition.
	CVD	$6TiCl_4 + 8NH_3 \rightarrow 6TiN + 24HCl + N_2$	TiN can also be formed in $TiSi_2$ process.
Cu	Electroplating, electroless, sputtering, CVD	$Cu^{2+} + 2e^- \rightarrow Cu$	Electroplating is most common method today.

9.3.1 Epitaxial Silicon Deposition

"Epitaxy" is from the Greek for "arranges upon." Epitaxial silicon is silicon that is deposited on top of single-crystal material (usually the silicon substrate) and "arranges upon" and takes the crystalline form of the substrate. If no underlying single-crystal silicon is present, or if the deposition conditions are not right, then either amorphous or polycrystalline silicon will result. An example of an epitaxial layer is shown in Figure 2–20 in the CMOS process in Chapter 2.

Epitaxial silicon is deposited by CVD by either decomposing silane via the reaction

$$SiH_4 \rightarrow Si + 2H_2 \tag{9.28}$$

or by the reaction of a silicon chloride compound with hydrogen. Silicon tetrachloride, $SiCl_4$, is often used, and the overall reaction is

$$SiCl_4 + 2H_2 \rightarrow Si + 4HCl \tag{9.29}$$

Two other chlorides, $SiHCl_3$ and SiH_2Cl_2, are also sometimes used as the source species, with similar reactions. Eq. (9.29) is the overall, or net, reaction for the tetrachloride source. Actually many intermediate and competing reactions occur, and the process is quite complex. The silicon chloride species are all liquids at room temperature and are delivered to the chamber using hydrogen as a carrier gas. Using silicon chlorides rather than silane as sources of silicon is beneficial in that chlorine removes metal contaminates from the deposited silicon film.

Cold-walled CVD systems have traditionally been used for epitaxial silicon, either in the horizontal tube configuration shown earlier in Figure 9–4(a), or in a "pancake" configuration, with a round vertical wafer holder with source gases coming from above. Systems using quartz halogen radiant heating are also used. In each of these systems the wafers are placed side by side (end-to-end) to ensure uniform depositions.

For conventional epitaxial growth, relatively high deposition temperatures of 1000–1250°C are used, the lower temperature for silane and the higher for $SiCl_4$. These high temperatures are used so that single-crystal layers are readily obtained. High temperatures are required to desorb any native oxide on the surface which would inhibit single-crystal growth. At temperatures over 1000°C at 1 atmosphere, thin silicon dioxide films that may form during the deposition become unstable and vaporize. Also at the higher temperatures the surface reactions for deposition are enhanced, especially the surface migration to kink sites and rearrangement of the atoms, allowing for single-crystal growth. It is important that the atoms on the surface have time to attach at the proper sites before too many more atoms arrive. If the deposition rate is too fast relative to the surface processes, polycrystalline material results. Because of the high temperatures and fast surface reactions, epitaxial growth in these systems usually occurs in the mass transfer limited regime. Therefore thickness uniformity requirements preclude the wafers from being stacked close together. Recently lower temperature systems have been developed, as will be described later in this section.

Conventional Si epitaxial deposition is done either at atmospheric pressure, or at somewhat reduced pressures of 80–200 torr, but still above normal LPCVD pressures which are in the 0.5–2 torr range. Reducing the pressure gives better control over switching on and off dopant source flows and reduces autodoping so that more abrupt doping profiles may be obtained. This works well for arsenic and phosphorus, but not as well for boron. Decreasing the pressure too much may causes the deposition rate to be quite low, by perhaps limiting the reactant species, especially for the chlorine-based sources. In earlier years when most epitaxial deposition was done using these conventional systems, the epitaxial layers were up to 20 μm thick and higher deposition rates were required.

A clean surface is critical to obtaining epitaxial growth. If contaminants or native oxide films are present, single-crystal growth will not occur. Wafers must be carefully cleaned prior to loading into the system. In addition, after the wafers are loaded into the deposition chamber, they may be subjected to an in situ HCl gas clean. This will etch the top surface of the silicon and remove any contaminates or native oxide.

Doping of epitaxial Si films can be done during the deposition by introducing appropriate gas sources of the dopants into the chamber along with the silicon source gases, as discussed earlier in the section on APCVD. Common dopant source gases are arsine (AsH_3), phosphine (PH_3), and diborane (B_2H_6). Unintentional doping due to diffusion and autodoping can be a problem, as discussed earlier. Reducing the pressure and increasing the temperature seem to reduce the problem for arsenic and phosphorus, while increasing the pressure and reducing the temperatures work better for boron. Using antimony instead of arsenic or phosphorus helps due to antimony's low vapor pressure compared to arsenic and low diffusivity compared to phosphorus.

Selective deposition of epitaxial silicon is sometimes desired. Selective deposition means that the silicon deposits on exposed regions of silicon, but not on other films, such as silicon dioxide. Under non-selective conditions, epitaxial silicon would be deposited over the exposed silicon, and amorphous or polycrystalline silicon would be deposited over the other regions. But by using the right conditions, one can actually achieve selective deposition. Conditions are chosen to reduce the nucleation and growth rate on the less-favored nonsilicon regions and to enhance the surface migration of the silicon atoms. Chlorides in the source gas tend to inhibit nucleation on the oxide by Cl etching of Si and by increasing the surface migration of Si atoms. Therefore using $SiCl_4$, $SiHCl_3$, or SiH_2Cl_2 increases the selectivity over using SiH_4. HCl gas is often added to improve selectivity. Reducing the pressure also helps.

Recently the need for low-temperature epitaxial growth of Si has greatly increased. In advanced process technologies, minimizing the thermal processing that the wafer is exposed to is crucial in order to decrease dopant diffusion, control abrupt interfaces and junctions, and reduce damage to device structures. Reducing the growth temperature from 1000°C or higher to temperatures in the 500–900°C range is of great benefit in these regards. Recently techniques have been developed to provide good quality epitaxial silicon films at low temperatures. The key to this is to provide an ultraclean environment so that oxides and other contaminants that would inhibit single-crystal growth are not present on the wafer surface. This can be achieved by using high-vacuum compatible CVD systems, ultrapure gases, and utilizing low pressures. A good predeposition clean is critical, and the wafers can also be initially heated to high-temperatures (above 1000°C) in the chamber prior to the deposition to desorb any native oxide. The low deposition temperatures and pressures usually place the deposition in the surface reaction limited regime. The deposition rates in these systems may be lower than in conventional epitaxial systems, but the layers that are grown today are generally much thinner than in older technologies.

Another technique for low-temperature Si epitaxy is Molecular Beam Epitaxy (MBE). Used for many years to produce III-V epilayers, this method is now being used more frequently for Si and SiGe films. In this technique, the silicon and dopant atoms are evaporated under ultrahigh vacuum conditions onto the Si substrate. Low-temperature epitaxial deposition, in the 500–800°C range, is obtainable, with ultraabrupt interfaces and doping profiles.

9.3.2 Polycrystalline Silicon Deposition

Polycrystalline silicon, unlike epitaxial silicon, can be deposited on arbitrary substrates and does not need exposed silicon underneath. It is used for the gate electrode in CMOS technology and for local interconnects and resistors. Its good thermal stability, good interface to silicon dioxide, good conformality, and ease of deposition and processing have made it a mainstay of silicon microelectronics technology. Polycrystalline silicon, as its name implies, is made up of regions or "grains" of crystalline material, but with each grain oriented differently from the neighboring grain. Separating each grain from the next one is a region called, appropriately, the grain boundary. Polycrystalline structures, grains, and grain boundaries will be discussed in detail in Chapter 11.

Polycrystalline silicon, or polysilicon, can be sputter deposited; however, CVD deposition is the usual method today. This is mainly due to two reasons, one historical and one technological. As we described above, epitaxial silicon must be deposited at relatively high temperatures in order for single-crystal material to be obtained. The low temperatures of sputtering (room temperature up to a maximum of about 400°C) preclude its use in depositing epitaxial film. Once CVD methods were developed for epi, it was a simple matter to use this method for polysilicon, where the conditions are much less restrictive. The other reason that CVD is used for polysilicon rather than sputtering is due to step coverage issues. In actual devices and circuits, polysilicon must often be deposited across steep topography. (See Figure 2–25 for example.) Good step coverage is important, and as we have mentioned many times, CVD usually gives better step coverage than sputtering. The conformality of LPCVD polysilicon is extremely good, with a sticking coefficient of 0.001 or less.

Silane is most often used for polysilicon deposition, following the decomposition reaction in Eq. (9.28). Silane is used rather than the silicon chlorides because better coverage over amorphous materials such as SiO_2 is obtained. This may be related to enhanced surface mobility in the presence of the chlorides or to the chlorine etching of Si over an insulator, leading to better nucleation and growth on the silicon and worse on the oxide. What is better for selective epitaxy is what is worse for depositing polysilicon over oxide layers, and vice versa. In addition, moderately low temperatures are usually used for polysilicon deposition, and silane decomposition occurs at lower temperatures than with the chloride reactions. If a dilutant or carrier gas is used, it is commonly nitrogen or hydrogen. However, using hydrogen increases the reverse reaction of

Eq. (9.28), and can decrease the deposition rate at lower temperatures. This decrease in the surface reaction shifts the deposition rate versus $1/T$ curve to the left compared to when nitrogen or no carrier gas is used, as shown in Figure 9–8 [9.17].

In order to achieve good throughput with uniform films, LPCVD systems with stacked wafers are used for polysilicon. Such a system was shown schematically in Figure 9–4(b). The deposition pressure is generally in the 0.2 to 1 torr range. A dilutant or carrier gas may or may not be used with the silane. By using a low pressure at the relatively low deposition temperatures described below, one ensures that the deposition occurs in the surface reaction limited regime while maintaining adequate deposition rates. The use of low pressure has been seen to greatly improve the uniformity of polysilicon depositions in closely stacked wafer systems at these moderate temperatures. Using lower pressure also results in fewer gas-phase reactions and less gas usage.

The deposition temperature for polysilicon films is moderately low, usually in the 575 to 650°C range. One reason for these low temperatures is to minimize the thermal budget of the wafer, reducing dopant diffusion and material degradation. Also, fewer gas phase reactions occur at the lower temperatures, leading to smoother and better adhering films, and silane depletion is less at lower temperatures. Another reason is that small grains are usually desired for polysilicon films. This is because films with finer grains are easier to mask and etch to give smooth and uniform edges. Deposition of polysilicon at higher temperatures usually results in larger grained films. For temperatures less than 575°C or so, the deposition rate is too low.

The deposition rate depends on the temperature, the silane partial pressure, and the presence of hydrogen or doping gases. At 620°C with a partial pressure of silane (with nitrogen carrier gas) of 0.5 torr, the deposition rate is about 15 nm per minute. According to our simple model for deposition, the deposition rate should be a linear function of the silane partial pressure, as given in Eq. (9.10). But the deposition rate for polysilicon has been found to be a sublinear function of the silane partial pressure, saturating as the silane is increased. This may be due to the desorption of hydrogen from the surface, which could be the limiting step in the deposition mechanism.

The as-deposited grain structure depends on these same factors: the temperature, the silane partial pressure, and the presence of other gases or species [9.17, 9.18]. Usually the polysilicon film is columnar in structure, meaning that most grains span the entire height of the film, with the grains quite tall and narrow in some cases. The average size at the top of the grains is often a little larger than at the bottom. Figure 9–32 shows several TEM cross-section images of deposited polysilicon films with the grain structure evident [9.19]. Polycrystalline films often exhibit a certain crystallographic texture. Crystallographic texture means that while the in-plane orientation of the columnar grains is more or less random, there is a preferred orientation of the grains in the vertical direction or out-of-plane orientation. For example in <110> textured films, which are common for typical polysilicon deposition conditions, most of the grains would have their <110> orientation pointing upward, or close to it. (And a more textured film means that a higher percent of the grains are at, or close to, a single orientation.) These orientations are a function of the deposition conditions, particularly deposition temperature and partial pressure of silane. If the deposition temperature is below 570–600°C, depending on the silane partial pressure, the as-deposited film will not be polycrystalline, but amorphous. Annealing the film at 600–1000°C will convert the struc-

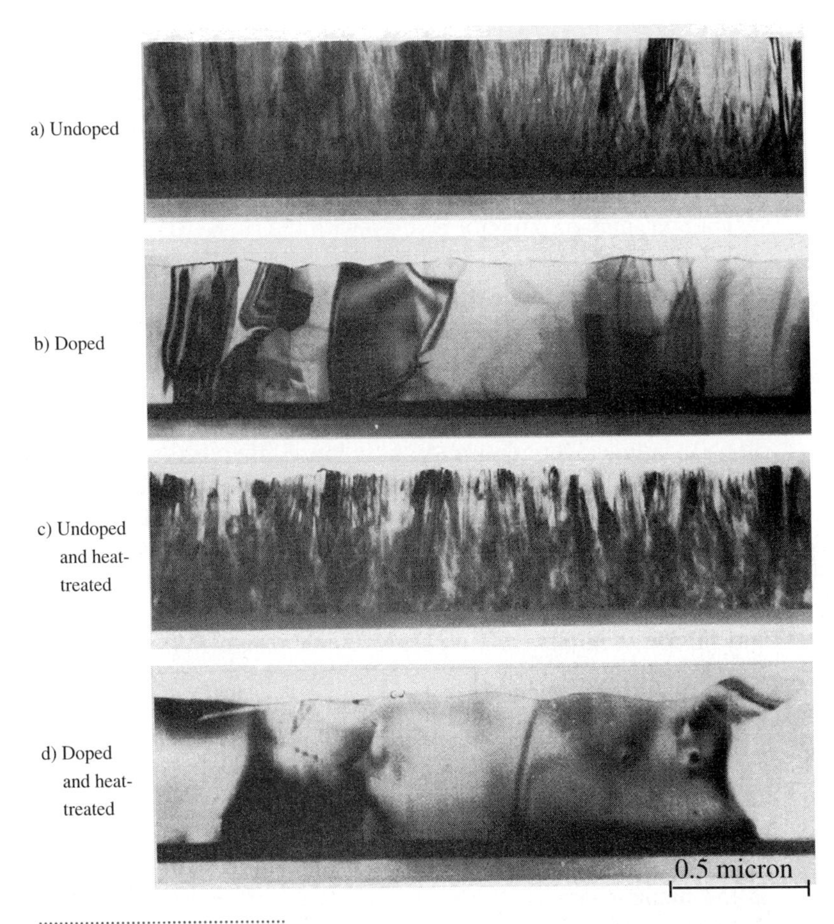

Figure 9–32 TEM cross sections of CVD polycrystalline films deposited at 625°C: (a) as-deposited, undoped film, showing the thin grains in a columnar structure; (b) as-deposited phosphorus-doped film, showing much larger grain size; c) annealed (1000°C), undoped film, showing little grain growth as compared to (a); (d) annealed (1000°C), phosphorus-doped film, showing evidence of grain growth as compared to (b). Reprinted with permission of the Electrochemical Society [9.19].

ture to polycrystalline material.

The average diameter of the columnar grains, the grain size, also depends on the deposition conditions and can range from 0.01 to 0.4 μm, with a typical size of about 0.05–0.1 μm for undoped polysilicon deposited at 625°C. Higher deposition temperatures generally result in larger grain sizes, as do thicker film depositions. High doping with phosphorus or arsenic (greater than about 3×10^{20} cm^{-3} for P and greater than about 1×10^{19} cm^{-3} for As) can greatly increase the grain size of as-deposited films, as shown in Figure 9–32. During any subsequent high-temperature annealing, the average grain size will increase only slightly for as-deposited undoped polycrystalline silicon when annealed at 1000°C (more grain growth occurs at higher temperatures above 1200°C). For as-deposited amorphous silicon, the crystalline grains will nucleate and grow much more, even exceeding the size of the grains of annealed polycrystalline films. They also end up being somewhat less columnar, with some grains nucleating and growing above and below each other. The final size in either case will depend on deposition and anneal temperatures, anneal time, dopants, impurities, and film thickness. For example, phosphorus and arsenic doping will significantly increase the grain growth, while boron does not. This may be related to the increased vacancy concentrations with n-doping [9.20]. Grain growth and the dependence on film thickness will be discussed in more detail in Chapter 11.

Polysilicon can be doped either n type or p type. This can be done either during the deposition or afterward by implantation or diffusion. Doping during deposition is done by adding dopant source gases, such as those used for epitaxial growth, into the chamber along with the silane. However, the addition of arsine (AsH_3) or phosphine (PH_3) greatly decreases the deposition rates, by competing for sites perhaps, as well as creates thickness variations in the films. For these reasons, n-type doping of polysilicon is usually done after the deposition by implantation or diffusion. Diborane (B_2H_6) on the other hand, increases the deposition rate slightly and therefore can be used to dope the film during the deposition. As and P dopant atoms in polysilicon tend to segregate to the grain boundary regions. Here they are electrically inactive, so that only the dopants that remain in the grain interiors contribute to the doping of the film. B does not appear to segregate to grain boundaries. In addition, the grain boundaries can trap carriers regardless of the dopant, also reducing the net doping. The carrier mobility is also decreased by the grain boundaries. As a result, polysilicon must be doped at higher than normal concentrations in order to achieve desired doping and resistivity levels. Figure 9–33 extends the resistivity data we discussed in Chapter 1 (Figure 1–18) to the polysilicon case and shows the resistivity of annealed films as a function of phosphorus doping concentration. One can see that the resistivity for polycrystalline material is higher than single-crystal silicon for the same total doping level. This difference gets smaller at higher doping concentrations, presumably because the finite number of traps at the grain boundaries get saturated above some critical concentration (about 1×10^{17} cm^{-3} here). One sees that for samples deposited at 580°C (indicated by the LP-580 label, for LPCVD deposition at 580°C), the critical doping concentration is less. This is consistent with a larger grain size for annealed amorphous films, as discussed above. Larger grains means less grain boundary area and thus fewer segregated dopant atoms and fewer carrier traps.

9.3.3 Silicon Nitride Deposition

Silicon nitride, Si_3N_4, films are used primarily for two purposes. One is for a mask against oxidation. In earlier chapters we saw how Local Oxidation of Silicon (LOCOS) occurs using silicon nitride as a mask against oxidation (Figure 2–5). The diffusion of oxygen through the film is very slow, preventing the underlying silicon from being oxidized. The other main use of silicon nitride is as a final passivation layer on chips. Silicon nitride is a very good barrier against water and sodium diffusion (unlike silicon dioxide) and it can be deposited conformally, making it an excellent final passivation

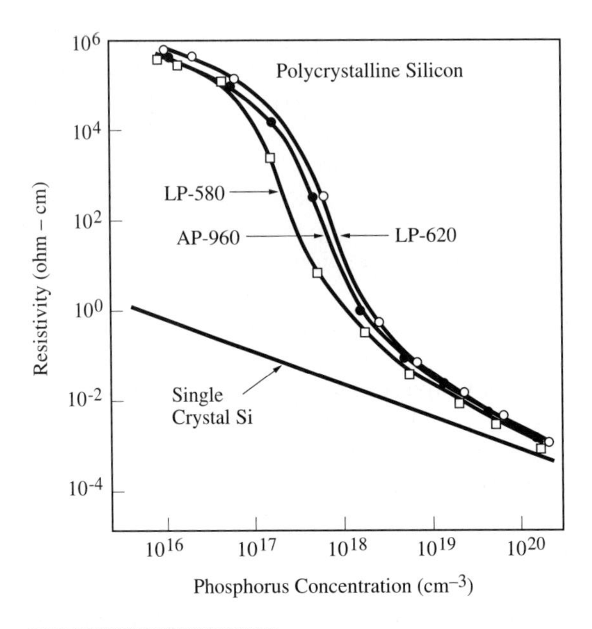

Figure 9–33 Resistivity of annealed phosphorus-implanted silicon films as a function of phosphorus concentration. LP refers to LPCVD deposition, AP refers to APCVD deposition, and the numbers in the labels refer to the deposition temperature. (After [9.21].)

layer for silicon microelectronics. It is generally not used in direct contact with silicon because of its relatively poor interface properties, especially with regard to fixed or interface trapped charges, and its high stress.

The two uses of silicon nitride require different deposition techniques as dictated by the allowable deposition temperatures. The masking nitride film is deposited relatively early in the fabrication process, and the temperature can be high. However, the passivating nitride is deposited after the metallization is in place, and therefore the deposition and processing temperature is limited to 450°C.

Masking silicon nitride films for LOCOS processes are deposited by CVD in the 650–800°C range. Low-pressure CVD is frequently used for good uniformity and high wafer throughput. The source gasses are ammonia and either dichlorosilane or silane, following the reactions

$$3SiH_2Cl_2 + 4NH_4 \rightarrow Si_3N_4 + 6HCl + 6H_2 \tag{9.30}$$

or

$$3SiH_4 + 4NH_4 \rightarrow Si_3N_4 + 12H_2 \tag{9.31}$$

To ensure the proper stoichiometry of the film, an excess of ammonia is used often by as much as 20-to-1 over the chloride or silane. Nitrogen can also be used in place of the ammonia. Significant amounts of hydrogen, up to 8 atomic percent, are incorporated into these films, bonded to both the silicon and nitrogen. This can affect the film properties, such as density and etch rate.

Silicon nitride films used for final passivation films must be deposited at temperatures of 450°C or below, as mentioned above. Because of this, PECVD is the common technique employed here. Silane and ammonia are used, following Eq. (9.31), since silane works better at the lower temperatures than do the chlorides. Typical PECVD nitride deposition temperatures range from 200 to 400°C. The film that is deposited at these low temperatures using PECVD is often not stoichiometric Si_3N_4 and is often referred to as just SiN or Si_XN_Y. In fact, even more hydrogen than in the high-temperature LPCVD films is incorporated, up to 25 atomic percent, and the film is often designated by $Si_XN_YH_Z$. Oxygen can also be present in the film. The deposition rate and the film properties are very dependent on the deposition conditions, including the RF power and frequency, the gas flow, and the chamber pressure. The various film properties, such as composition, stress, dielectric constant, thermal expansion coefficient, and density, can be optimized, or at least traded off between each other, by varying the various deposition conditions.

To reduce the Si/SiO_2 interface trapped charge density in the active devices, an anneal is done in a hydrogen ambient near the end of the fabrication process. Because a nitride film is a barrier to hydrogen diffusion, the hydrogen anneal must be done prior to the deposition of the passivation nitride film.

9.3.4 Silicon Dioxide Deposition

Deposited films of silicon dioxide are utilized throughout silicon microelectronic structures as described in the CMOS process flow in Chapter 2 (see, for example, Figures 2–29 and 2–38). They are used for dielectric layers to electrically separate conducting regions as well as for masks against implantation and diffusion. The requirements for the films will be discussed in more detail in Chapter 11, but obtaining films of good quality in terms of density, purity, and thermal stability, as well as good step coverage and filling properties are of major concern.

Most oxide films today are deposited at relatively low temperatures, from 200°C to 500°C using CVD techniques. Sputtered oxide films have worse coverage and more particulates (mostly due to flaking off of the metal chamber walls) than CVD oxides. Atmospheric systems have been used for many years, but today LPCVD and PECVD systems have become more commonly used.

Silane and oxygen are common source gases for CVD silicon dioxide deposition, following the net reaction

$$SiH_4 + O_2 \rightarrow SiO_2 + 2H_2 \tag{9.32}$$

Oxidants other than O_2 are sometimes used, such as N_2O, NO, and CO_2. When non-plasma, silane-based deposition of SiO_2 is done at temperatures less than 500°C, it is commonly referred to as Low-Temperature Oxide, or "LTO," deposition.

Other sources of silicon are also used. One such source is tetraethooxysilane—$Si(OC_2H_5)_4$—or "TEOS." It can form silicon dioxide by decomposing via the reaction

$$Si(OC_2H_5)_4 \rightarrow SiO_2 + \text{byproducts} \tag{9.33}$$

(O_2 is often added as an extra oxidizer to reduce the carbon content in the film.) This deposition occurs at higher temperatures, in the 650–800°C range, but because of the low sticking coefficient of TEOS compared to silane, more conformal films are produced. The deposition temperature can be lowered to below 400°C by either utilizing plasma enhanced deposition, or by including ozone, O_3, in the chamber:

$$Si(OC_2H_5)_4 + O_3 \rightarrow SiO_2 + \text{byproducts} \tag{9.34}$$

Because at low pressures (<150 torr) the deposition using TEOS and O_3 is limited by O_3 and gives worse film properties, a so-called Sub-Atmospheric CVD (SACVD) system has been developed for doped premetal films and undoped intermetal films [9.22, 9.23]. The deposition pressure in this system is at higher pressures (200–400 torr) and the deposition temperature is 300–550°C. Oxide films with good gap fill and reflow ability can be obtained with this system.

The major drawbacks to using TEOS are that it is a more difficult source to use (it is an organometallic liquid), the relatively high levels of carbon in the deposited film (from the TEOS itself), and the more porous films that are sometimes formed. But TEOS is still commonly used due to the conformality of the films it produces.

Silicon dioxide films deposited using LPCVD or APCVD at low temperatures (less than 500°C) can be nonstoichiometric and are often porous. They can also exhibit inadequate step coverage or filling. The films that are deposited before aluminum is on the wafer are usually annealed at high temperatures after their deposition. This densifies the films, as well as allowing them to flow, or "reflow," in order to achieve better filling and step coverage, as discussed in Chapter 11. This is done at temperatures of 1000–1100°C for undoped films, and as low as 800°C for doped (with B and/or P) films.

For films that are deposited after aluminum is already on the wafer, other measures must be taken. No high temperature densification anneal can be done, so the films must be of adequate quality and have good coverage "as-deposited." TEOS with ozone and plasma enhanced CVD TEOS are commonly used. While PECVD TEOS gives dense films and fairly good coverage and filling at low temperatures, the films usually contain a lot of hydrogen or nitrogen, up to 10 atomic percent, which can affect their properties. TEOS/O_3 films may be more conformal and have better filling ability, but are also much more porous and can absorb moisture.

Another method of silicon dioxide deposition, bias sputtering, has been developed to improve filling and planarizing. But because of its low deposition rate and a high density of particulates, this method is not commonly used today. A relatively new technique called High-Density Plasma (HDP) CVD, which combines PECVD with bias sputtering, is being used for low-temperature deposition (150°C down to room temperature). Figure 9–34 shows examples of SiO_2 deposited by HDPCVD, displaying excellent filling and good planarizing properties. In this method, both silane-and TEOS-based chemistries can be used, giving good quality films in high aspect ratio structures.

Deposited silicon dioxide films are often doped with phosphorus or boron, or both. Phosphorus is used to reduce stress and enhance Na gettering, while the boron allows more reflow at lower temperatures, as will be discussed in Chapter 11. Doping can be done by using hydrides for the silane case and organometallic compounds for the TEOS case in APCVD, LPCVD and PECVD configurations.

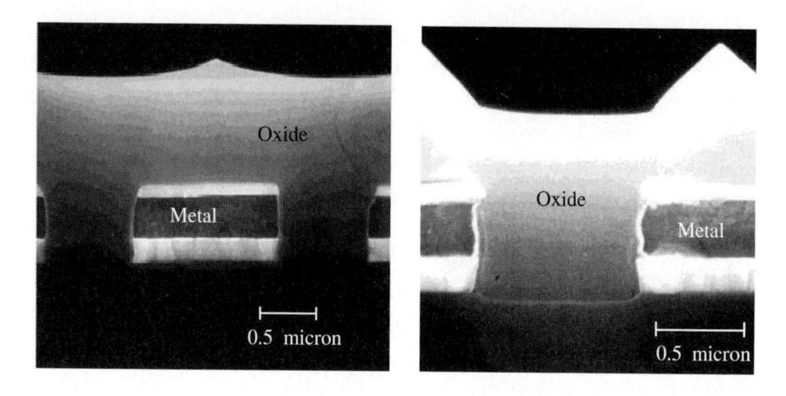

Figure 9–34 SEM images of High-Density Plasma (HDP) CVD deposited SiO_2, showing good planarizing and excellent filling properties. Photos courtesy of VLSI Technology, Inc.

9.3.5 Al Deposition

Aluminum is used as the main interconnect material in silicon microelectronics. As explained in Chapter 11, pure Al is usually not used, but an alloy of Al with 0.5–1 wt. percent Cu (to reduce hillocking, voiding, and electromigration) and sometimes with about 1 wt. percent Si (to prevent spiking and other interactions). The technique almost always used is DC magnetron sputter deposition. CVD techniques are not currently used for Al (but are being investigated) because of the problems with CVD of metal alloys, and Al is almost always used as an alloy. These problems include unwanted reactions between the precursors for the various metals, carbon contamination, rough films, low deposition rate, and inefficient use of the Al precursor which can result in a very costly deposition. Sputter deposition does not have these problems. Magnetron sputtering is used primarily due to its high deposition rate of up to one μm per minute for Al.

The argon pressure and the presence of impurities can affect the deposition and properties of the film. While a higher pressure of argon will increase the number of collisions of the Al atoms in the gas phase, decreasing the mean free path and improving the step coverage, a higher pressure of argon also means that more Ar will be incorporated in the Al film, up to 1 atomic percent. This can have deleterious effects on the film properties, including higher electrical resistivity, more stress, and smaller grain size (the argon acting as nucleation sites for the grains). Therefore lower pressures are usually desired. The presence of other gas species also affects the deposition and film properties. Oxygen, nitrogen, hydrogen, and water vapor may all be present in small amounts in the deposition chamber or on the wafer surface. These can all be incorporated into the film, having the same effects on the film properties: higher electrical resistivity, more stress, and smaller grain size. It is important to minimize the amount of these impurities in the deposition chamber. This is done by pumping down the chamber to very low pressures before the argon is introduced (to less than 1×10^{-10} torr in some cases), by using ultrapure argon, and by heating the wafers and wafer holders before the deposition occurs to desorb any moisture.

It is common to heat the wafers to 150–300°C during Al sputter deposition, mainly to improve step coverage by increasing the surface mobility. Heating the substrates to even higher temperatures, up to 450–550°C, is called high-temperature or hot sputter deposition, or just "hot Al". The surface diffusion (and possibly bulk viscous flow) increases significantly, allowing for filling of deep contact and via holes.

There has been quite an interest recently in CVD Al. This is because of the technique's inherently better step coverage and excellent filling ability. There has been some limited success at depositing an Al-Cu alloy by using different Al and Cu organometallic precursors [9.24]. However, a more common approach involves depositing a film of pure Al by CVD, then doping it with Cu afterward. Al itself can be deposited by CVD using metal-organic sources, such as tri-isobutyl-Al (TIBA), or dimethylaluminumhydride (DMAH). The presence of Al-H bonds in the latter precursor results in less carbon incorporation in the Al film. To alloy or dope the film with Cu, one method is to sputter a layer of Cu, or Al-Cu alloy, on top of or below the CVD Al layer. Then a 250–400°C anneal is done in which the Cu diffuses into the pure Al layer, producing a uniform layer of Al-Cu. However, controlling this process can be difficult.

9.3.6 Ti and Ti-W Deposition

Titanium is often used as an underlayer for contacts, vias, and interconnects because of its good adhesion to other materials, its ability to reduce native oxides, and its good electrical contacting properties (as discussed in Chapter 11). It is usually deposited by sputtering, either using standard magnetron sputtering, or by using collimated or ionized sputtering for good coverage in contact or via bottoms. CVD of Ti is difficult because the precursors are so thermodynamically unstable. Impurities incorporated into the film from the precursors can also be a problem.

Ti-W alloys have been used as barrier metals in contacts and as underlayers and antireflective layers in interconnects, as also discussed in Chapter 11. However, TiN is more commonly used today for these purposes due it its better thin film and barrier properties and will be discussed separately later. Ti-W films are deposited using magnetron sputtering, usually from a single target. The most common target is 10 wt. percent Ti (30 atomic percent) and 90 wt. percent W (70 atomic percent). Nitrogen is commonly added to the chamber and is incorporated into the polycrystalline film, plugging or "stuffing" the grain boundaries. This reduces atomic diffusion along these high diffusion paths and improves the film's barrier performance. Film properties, such as resistivity, stress, composition, and barrier performance, depend mainly on four deposition conditions: sputtering pressure, power, temperature, and Ar/N_2 ratio. [9.25] The films can be rather brittle, leading to cracking on the wafer and to flaking off of deposition chamber walls onto the wafers.

9.3.7 W Deposition

Tungsten is commonly used as a contact or via metal, called "tungsten plugs," or in some cases is used as a first-level metal interconnect. (See, for example, Figure 2–41 in Chapter 2.) It is usually deposited by CVD, due to its very good filling ability and conformal coverage, in a hot-wall, low-pressure system. Temperatures range from 250–500°C, and total pressures are in the 0.1-to 2-torr range.

Tungsten can be deposited either selectively or as a blanket deposition. In selective deposition, W is only deposited where Si is exposed, such as in contact holes, and not on the surrounding SiO_2. In this process, the exposed Si is used to reduce the W source gas, WF_6, depositing W only in those regions.

Much more commonly used is blanket tungsten deposition. Here tungsten is deposited everywhere, both in the contact or via holes, and over the dielectric. (CMP shown in Figure 2–42 or an etchback process described in Chapter 11 can then be used to remove all the tungsten except in the contact or via holes.) Tungsten can be deposited by either the hydrogen reduction reaction

$$WF_6 + 3H_2 \rightarrow W + 6HF \tag{9.35}$$

or the silane reduction reaction

$$2WF_6 + 3SiH_4 \rightarrow 2W + 3SiF_4 + 6H_2 \tag{9.36}$$

A two-step process utilizing both these reactions can also be used, as will be described in Chapter 11.

Tungsten films deposited by CVD have significant amounts of fluorine incorporated in them as a result of the WF_6 source, often 1 atomic percent or more. This increases their resistivity over bulk values by 1.5 to 2 times. The grain size is usually less than 0.2 μm , yet the films are rather rough. This is due to random crystal faceting. This makes the films harder to etch evenly and can also lead to problems in the dielectric overlayers. Overall, good filling of contacts and vias with decent film properties can be achieved, and the use of tungsten plugs in current microelectronics is widespread.

9.3.8 $TiSi_2$ and WSi_2 Deposition

Titanium silicide, $TiSi_2$, and tungsten silicide, WSi_2, are common silicides used today in Si microelectronics. Other common silicides include $CoSi_2$, $TaSi_2$, $MoSi_2$, NiSi, and PtSi. We will focus on $TiSi_2$ and WSi_2 here, but many of the same deposition methods and ideas can apply to the other silicides as well. As we saw in the CMOS example in Chapter 2 and as we will discuss in much more detail in Chapter 11, silicides are used in CMOS technology extensively to reduce sheet resistance of polysilicon lines and n^+ regions. (See Figure 2–36.) They are often part of contact structures, either because they are already on top of the gates, sources, and drains or because they are deposited in contact holes. Silicides can also be used as local interconnects themselves.

The formation of silicides can be done in two general ways: by direct deposition of the silicide; or by deposition of the metal on top of Si followed by the reaction between the metal and Si to form the silicide. The direct deposition method can be accomplished in several ways: (1) sputtering from a composite target, (2) cosputtering from two targets of the metal and Si, (3) co-evaporation of the metal and Si, and (4) CVD.

The reaction method is more common today than the direct deposition method. (See Figures 2–35 to 2–37.) Here the metal, Ti for example, is deposited by sputtering on the exposed gate and/or source drain regions, all of which are silicon. The wafer is annealed and the silicide forming reaction occurs wherever the silicon and metal are in contact, that is, on the gate and source/drain regions. The unreacted metal is then selectively etched away. This method produces self-aligned silicide structures on the gate and/or source drains. This is often called the "salicide" technique, for "self-aligned silicide," and will be discussed more in Chapter 11. Another reaction method deposits the metal and then amorphous Si, both usually by sputtering, then patterns and selectively etches the amorphous Si. The wafer is then annealed so that the metal and amorphous Si react to form the silicide, and the unreacted metal is selectively etched off. This nonself-aligned method produces local interconnects independent of either gate or source/drain regions. For either type of reaction method, it is imperative to have the equipment (both sputtering chamber and annealing chamber) and the wafer surfaces free of oxygen, water, and native oxides. Their presence can result in films that are high resistivity, have uneven thickness and rough surfaces, and have poor adhesion properties.

WSi_2 has historically been used in a "polycide" structure. Here the silicide is blanket deposited over a blanket polysilicon layer, and both polysilicon and silicide are masked and etched at the same time to produce a low-resistivity gate structure. Both sputtered and CVD deposition of the WSi_2 have been used. Sputtering from a composite (WSi_2) target has been used, but CVD has the advantage of better step coverage, lower stress, and better adhesion. (WF_6 and SiH_4 are used in the CVD reaction, but a high SiH_4:WF_6 ratio is used so that WSi_2 is deposited instead of W.) However the trend today is to use the self-aligned silicides (namely $TiSi_2$ or perhaps $CoSi_2$) instead and form the silicide on the gate and source/drain regions all at once.

9.3.9 TiN Deposition

TiN films are used as barrier layers in contacts, and as underlayers and antireflective layers in interconnects, as discussed in Chapter 11. They have mostly replaced Ti-W in these applications due to their better barrier and film qualities. TiN films are often deposited or formed on top of Ti films, which have better contact and adhesion properties to the films underneath.

TiN is commonly sputtered using the reactive sputtering technique. As discussed earlier, reactive sputtering involves sputtering a metal in the presence of a reactive gas, such as nitrogen or oxygen, to form the metal oxide or nitride. In this case, nitrogen gas is mixed with the argon gas while Ti is being sputtered. The plasma breaks up the N_2 molecules into atomic nitrogen, which then react with the Ti to form the compound both on the target and on the wafer surface. The properties vary significantly with the deposition conditions, which include the nitrogen flow or partial pressure, the total pressure, the sputtering power, the substrate temperature, and the substrate bias, if one is applied. While excess nitrogen, or the presence of oxygen, increase the film's resistivity, they also enhance the barrier properties by saturating the grain boundaries. The deposited film is typically fine grained, columnar, and with <111> orientation, although <100> orientation can be achieved under certain deposition conditions [9.25]. The microstructure and orientation also depend on the film underneath. For example, the crystallographic orientation or texture often follows that of the Ti film that is commonly underneath TiN films. TiN is a very hard metal, and the films can be highly stressed and brittle, like Ti-W. TiN is often sputter deposited when the TiN is part of the Al interconnect stack. Step coverage and filling are not usually issues here. Generally it is better to deposit the whole stack by one technique without leaving the deposition chamber to avoid surface oxidation and contamination. Ionized PVD of TiN can be used when TiN is utilized as a liner/barrier in vias.

To improve the step coverage and filling ability of TiN films, CVD methods for deposition of these films have gained a lot of interest recently [9.26]. Titanium tetrachloride, $TiCl_4$, can be reacted with ammonia, NH_3, to form the films at 400–700°C via the reaction

$$6TiCl_4 + 8NH_3 \rightarrow 6TiN + 24HCl + N_2 \tag{9.37}$$

In general, the higher the deposition temperature, the better the film properties. As the temperature increases, the resistivity of the films decreases, the film density increases, and the chlorine content in the films decreases. Chlorine incorporation can be significant, 0.5–5%, which can lead to corrosion problems in Al interconnects. CVD processes using Metal-Organic (MOCVD) precursors instead of ammonia have also been developed. These include tetrakis-dimethyamino titanium (TDMAT) and tetrakis-diethyamino titanium (TDEAT). TiN films can be deposited with these sources at lower temperatures and with no Cl contamination. However, the films typically have carbon and oxygen incorporation, lower density, particulates, and not as good step coverage or filling ability. Methods to improve these properties, including postdeposition annealing treatments, or plasma treatments, are being developed. PECVD methods using ammonia are also being developed.

Another method to deposit TiN films is by first sputtering Ti on the wafers and then annealing them in a nitrogen or ammonia ambient above 600°C [9.25]. This was the process used in the CMOS technology described in Chapter 2. The Ti film reacts with the nitrogen to form the TiN film. The reaction is limited by the diffusion of the nitrogen through the forming TiN film, and the formation rate exhibits a diffusion-limited square root of time dependence, as expected. The reaction is very sensitive to the presence of oxygen, which can actually stop the reaction. The anneal is often done in an RTA system in which the heating time and exposure to oxygen are minimized. This nitridation method is often done in conjunction with silicide formation (Figure 2–36), as discussed in more detail in Chapter 11. Here the anneal done to react the deposited Ti with the underlying Si is performed in a nitrogen ambient. While $TiSi_2$ forms on the bottom of the Ti, TiN forms on top.

9.3.10 Cu Deposition

As we will discuss in Chapter 11, manufacturing processes that use copper instead of Al as a global interconnect metal have recently been developed. Cu has a lower electrical resistivity than Al and has better electromigration resistance. However, there are several processing and process integration issues concerning the use of Cu. One problem with Cu is that it is difficult to plasma etch due to the low volatility of the etch byproducts. Therefore a process that does not require etching, such as selective deposition, would be attractive. However, by using the damascene process, which was described in the CMOS technology in Chapter 2, the deposition and patterning of Cu can be accomplished by doing a blanket deposition in an etched-out dielectric layer, followed by Chemical-Mechanical Polishing (CMP). In this manner, neither etching or selective deposition is required. The damascene process will be described further in Chapter 11.

Copper can be deposited by PVD methods, including both sputter deposition and evaporation. However, the step coverage for these is quite poor and filling small vias is difficult. A high-temperature reflow step can be done, but that raises the thermal budget of the process.

CVD processes for Cu deposition are being developed to give better step coverage and filling properties. Like Al CVD processes, metal-organic sources are commonly used. One such source is 2Cu(hfac)L, where (hfac) is hexafluoroacetylacetoneate and L is a neutral ligand weakly bonded to the Cu. One ligand is vinyltrimethylsilane. Both blanket and selective depositions can be done depending on the ligands and deposition conditions. However, it is difficult to simultaneously achieve low resistivity, good step coverage and via filling, and a high deposition rate with these methods [9.27].

An alternative deposition method that has been developed for Cu is electrolytic plating. This can be done with the use of external electrodes and applied current. Applying an external voltage is generally referred to as electroplating. Deposition without an applied field is called electroless deposition. Both processes are used commonly in printed circuit board manufacturing, and work is being done to apply these processes to on-chip interconnect fabrication. While the electroless method has received a lot of attention in recent years, mostly due to its selective deposition capabilities, the electroplating method has become the current method of choice for Cu deposition in integrated circuits.

In electroplating, the wafers are mounted on a cathode and immersed into a plating solution that contains Cu ions. An inert anode, made of platinum, for example, is also immersed into the solution. A voltage is applied between the two electrodes and the current drives the Cu ions toward the wafer, forming metallic Cu on the surface, according to the electrochemical reaction

$$Cu^{2+} + 2e^{-} \rightarrow Cu \tag{9.38}$$

A thin seed layer, commonly Cu as well, is deposited first over the wafer so that electrical contact can be made to the surface of the wafer and so that Cu is electroplated over the entire wafer surface. This can be done by sputtering or CVD. Excellent filling can be achieved with electroplating of Cu. Filling of gaps is enhanced by using "leveling" agents or additives in the solution. These chemicals inhibit the deposition. They preferentially adsorb on the top surfaces of the topography rather than on the bottom of trenches or vias due to diffusion limitations. The top surfaces and corners then receive less deposition than the bottoms of trenches or vias, resulting in excellent filling ability. Low resistivity and high deposition rate can also be achieved with electroplating, and this method is becoming the most common method to deposit Cu for interconnects.

The electroless deposition technique involves the formation of thin metallic films from electrolytic solution without the use of external electrodes and without applying an external current. Simultaneous oxidation-reduction reactions between two half-reactions occur to deposit the film from solution. By this method, both blanket and selective Cu films of good quality, low resistivity, and good filling properties can be obtained. In a typical process, the solution contains formaldehyde (HCOH) as a reducing agent, and CuEDTA as the oxidizing agent and source of Cu. The two half-reactions with their redox potentials are

$$2HCOH + 4OH^- \rightarrow 2HCOO^- + 2H_2O + H_2 + 2e^- \quad V = 0.32\ (pH = 0.12) \tag{9.39}$$

$$[CuEDTA]^{2-} + 2e^- \rightarrow Cu + EDTA^{4-} \quad V = -0.26 \tag{9.40}$$

The net potential is positive so that the combined reaction is thermodynamically favorable:

$$[CuEDTA]^{2-} + 2HCOH + 4OH^- \rightarrow Cu + 2HCOO^- + 2H_2O + H_2 + EDTA^{4-} \tag{9.41}$$

Therefore by placing the wafer in a very basic solution containing Cu-EDTA and formaldyde, copper will be deposited from the solution. Complexing and surfactant agents are also commonly added to the solution.

In order for the copper to be deposited on the wafer surface, thin seeding layers are required in the electroless process, as in the electroplating process. Here the seed layer is needed to catalyze the electroless process. These are often Pd, Au, or Cu layers, deposited by CVD, sputtering, or evaporation. For selective electroless deposition, the seed layers should only be in the locations where the Cu deposition is desired. This can be done by selectively depositing the seed layer material itself, doing very directional PVD deposition with subsequent etchback or CMP, or using lift-off techniques [9.28]. For nonselective Cu deposition, the seed layer is deposited everywhere followed by the Cu electroless deposition. A problem with the electroless method has to do with contamination. The seed layer materials, Pd, Au, or Cu, can all act as deep-level traps in the underlying Si. Of more concern are the alkali ions needed for the highly basic solution. The hydroxide ion, OH^-, is commonly produced from sodium or potassium hydroxide. Sodium and potassium ions can drift in SiO_2 and alter the electrical properties of the active devices as we saw in Chapter 4. Tetra-methyl-ammonium-hydroxide ($N(C_2H_5)_4OH$), or TMAH, is often used instead of sodium or potassium hydroxide. However, the complex solution and reactions involved with the electroless technique compared to the electroplating method and the slower deposition rate, along with the trend toward blanket deposition of Cu in conjunction with the damascene process, have made the electroless process less attractive than the electroplating method for Cu deposition in IC technology.

9.4 Measurement Methods

The properties of the deposited films can be measured either during the deposition (in situ) or after the deposition is complete. The latter case is much more common. Properties such as thickness, composition, impurity concentration, step coverage, and stress, which often depend on the underlying layers and topography, are usually measured on the films after the deposition is complete, outside the deposition chamber. The measurement of these properties is discussed in the measurement methods section of Chapter 11 for films used in back-end technology. These films include silicon oxide, silicon nitride, silicide, and metal films, but the techniques are also used for other dielectric and interconnect materials, such as polysilicon, as well. In this section we will briefly describe some in situ measurement techniques.

The measurement of properties during the deposition is not very common today during IC fabrication and is mostly limited to film thickness and deposition rate measurements or to research applications. But as the technology progresses and more control is needed over film properties, there is much more interest in having automatic feedback during deposition. This requires in situ measurement of the film properties so that the deposition conditions can be adjusted as the deposition proceeds. The two most common methods of in situ measurement techniques are ellipsometery and the quartz-crystal microbalance.

Ellipsometry was discussed in Chapter 6 and can measure the thicknesses, and hence the deposition rates, of thin films on a reflective substrate. This technique is based on the change of polarization that occurs when a polarized light beam is reflected by a film. When data for multiple wavelengths are acquired, the technique is known as spectroscopic ellipsometry. This provides better measurement when multiple layers are present on the wafer. Ellipsometers are well suited for in situ deposition measurements. This is because the ellipsometer can be placed outside a chamber, using a window to allow the measurement. Even if the window becomes coated with the deposition material or byproducts, the measurement can still be done since the technique relies on relative intensities of light, and not on an absolute intensity which can change with time. The technique is only useful for transparent thin films.

The other common in situ measurement technique, QCM (Quartz-Crystal Microbalance), is based on the fact that the oscillating frequency of a crystal depends on its mass. A quartz crystal, sandwiched between two electrodes, is mounted in the deposition chamber in the same area as the wafers. As the film material is deposited on the wafers and the crystal, the mass of the crystal increases. This changes the oscillating frequency of the crystal in a well-understood manner, which is monitored through an external circuit, and the change in frequency is determined. This is then converted to a change in mass, which is then converted to a change in thickness. This technique is so sensitive that it is often used to calibrate other, less common, techniques, such as atomic emission and atomic absorption methods. This method can be applied to the deposition of any thin film.

9.5 Models and Simulation

While one important goal in thin film deposition is to obtain films with the desirable physical and chemical properties, an equally important goal is to achieve proper coverage and filling of the film over the underlying topography. This becomes even more critical as lateral dimensions decrease and aspect ratios get larger.

In this section we will focus on the modeling of thin film deposition as it relates to film coverage and filling over nonplanar topography. In the first part of the section we will utilize SPEEDIE [9.29], a 2D simulator developed at Stanford University. SPEEDIE uses physically based models for deposition and etching. Many other simulation tools have been developed for deposition and etching in integrated circuit fabrication, such as EVOLVE at Arizona State University, SAMPLE at the University of California, Berkeley, SIMBAD at the University of Alberta, and SHADE at IBM. Many of these are also physically based and contain many of the same basic mechanisms and models as in SPEEDIE. We will use SPEEDIE's simulation capability to predict the thickness and shape, in two dimensions, of deposited thin films as a function of various deposition conditions and configurations. These simulations will be used to illustrate many of the concepts discussed earlier in this chapter. Later in this section we will describe simulations using some commercially available simulation tools.

9.5.1 Models for Deposition Simulations

Figure 9–35 shows a generalized deposition picture of both CVD and PVD techniques. PVD systems use sputtering or heating of a source, whereas CVD systems use gas flow introduction of chemical precursors to provide the reactant species for deposition. The surface processes may also be different. Nevertheless, the steps are in general terms the same and can be modeled with the same components. Only the values used for the specific terms of the model will vary depending on the deposition technique and conditions. This is in fact a good way to analyze and compare the different deposition techniques. By starting with the same basic components and equations, and modeling the different techniques by varying the different parameters, one can more clearly see the similarities and differences between them.

In Figure 9–35 we focus on the wafer surface and the gas phase adjacent to the wafer surface. In the figure we see the direct flux of species, both neutrals and ions, arriving from the gas phase. The deposition species, Al in this case, can be either neutral or ionic. The ions, both Al^+ and Ar^+ in the figure, can also sputter atoms which have been deposited on the surface. In addition the ions, by their surface bombardment, can enhance the deposition rate of the neutral species. We also see in the figure species being desorbed, or "emitted." We see atoms being resputtered by ions. Both emitted and resputtered species can then be redeposited elsewhere, as shown at the bottom of the trench, and are called indirect fluxes. We also see another type of indirect flux: atoms moving due to surface diffusion. The indirect fluxes are all surface, or near-surface, processes.

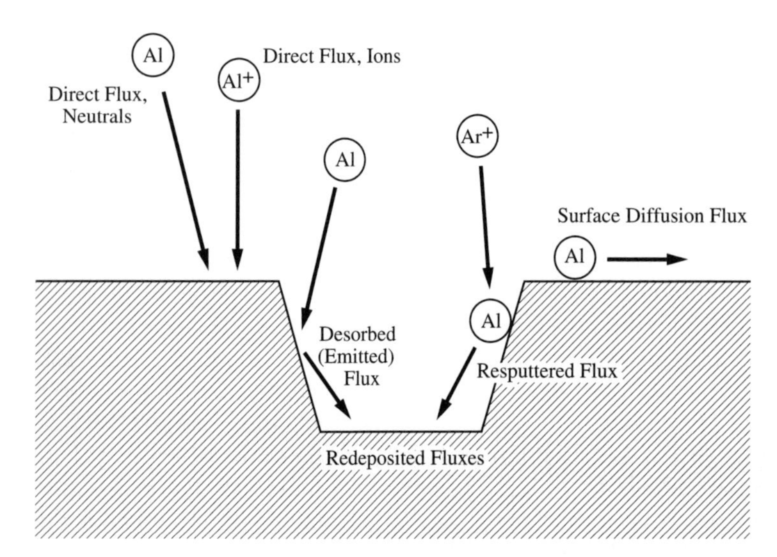

Figure 9–35 Generalized surface region processes in both CVD and PVD deposition systems used in simulation models.

A gas-phase boundary layer is not considered in this formulation since the gas pressure for most deposition systems is low enough so that diffusion through a boundary layer is not important. Because the mean free path in these systems is large compared to the feature sizes of the topography, free molecular flow (i.e., collisionless, nondiffusive flow) is assumed as the transport mechanism near the surface. (Diffusional flow through a boundary layer near the surface is important in APCVD systems, and SPEEDIE has a separate model for that. With many gas-phase collisions occurring within the topographical features in that case, good coverage and filling can result for processes that are reaction limited, such as with TEOS/O_3 SiO_2 [9.5].)

9.5.1.1 Models in Physically Based Simulators Such as SPEEDIE

In physically based topography models such as SPEEDIE all the phenomena depicted in Figure 9–35 should be taken into account. In SPEEDIE the net flux at each position on the surface is calculated based on all the fluxes arriving at and leaving that spot, either from the gas phase—the direct flux—or from other points on the surface—the indirect fluxes. The surface is then moved in the perpendicular direction according to the net flux, normal to the surface, at each point as the film grows. The net flux at each point i, F^i_{net}, can be expressed as the sum of the fluxes that are positive (due to atoms arriving at each point), minus each negative flux (due to atoms leaving each point):

$$F^i_{\text{net}} = F^i_{\text{direct(neutrals)}} + F^i_{\text{direct(ions)}} + F^i_{\text{redep}} + F^i_{\text{diff.in}} - F^i_{\text{emitted}} - F^i_{\text{sputtered}} - F^i_{\text{diff.out}} \tag{9.42}$$

The fluxes are all in units of atoms (or molecules) $\text{cm}^{-2}\,\text{sec}^{-1}$.

The *direct fluxes*, $F_{\text{direct(neutrals)}}$ and $F_{\text{direct(ions)}}$, are the fluxes of the different species at each position (or small area) i on that surface that arrive without any interaction with the wafer surface topography. These arrive directly from the gas phase above the wafer and include both neutral and ionic species. In calculating the direct fluxes, one has to know the distribution of arrival angles of the incoming species relative to the orientation of the surface at that point. Then the distribution can be integrated over all angles to obtain the total direct flux, normal to the surface, at each point.

There are two ways of modeling the direct fluxes. One is to start with the angular distribution of fluxes as the species depart from the target or gas source, or the emitted angle distribution at each source point. Then by taking into account the gas-phase collisions and the geometric configuration of the chamber (distance from target to source, etc.), as well as the surface topography, one can determine the distribution of angles of the precursor arriving at each point on the wafer surface. This is similar in a qualitative way to Figure 9–30 which illustrates deposition from different size sources. But including the gas-phase reactions and the various equipment geometries can get quite complicated. Techniques such as Monte Carlo methods are often used for this and are available in various deposition simulators, but even so, fitting parameters are usually needed.

A simpler way to account for the incoming flux is to just assume some distribution function of fluxes as a function of angle just above the surface of the wafer. This is illustrated in Figure 9–36. If the fluxes were coming in equally at all angles, that is isotropic arrival fluxes, then one would assume a constant flux for all angles in the distribution at each position in that plane. However, as we discussed earlier, we define the arrival distribution in terms of the normal component of the incoming flux relative to a unit area on a surface. In this case the surface is a horizontal plane just above the wafer surface. By simple geometry, the normal component would be proportional to the cosine of the vertical angle. We would therefore express this

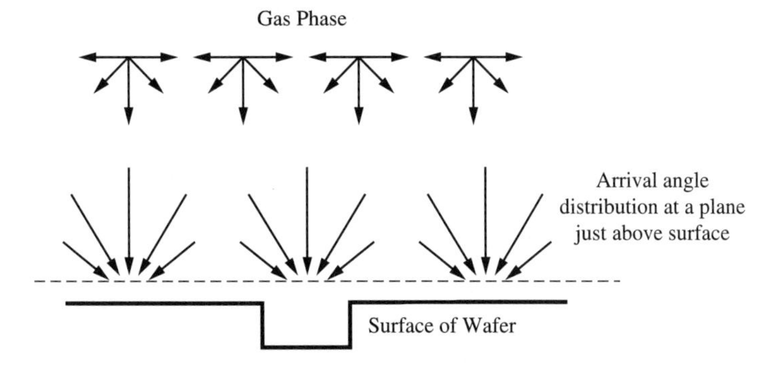

Figure 9–36 Simplified way of considering incoming flux distribution. A distribution of fluxes arriving from the gas phase, with a $\cos^n\theta$ distribution, is assumed in a plane just above the wafer surface. From that plane to the surface features below, no gas-phase collisions occur, just line-of-sight molecular flow.

isotropic arrival as a cosθ distribution, where θ is relative to the vertical direction. To account for nonisotropic distributions as well, this can then be generalized to the form.

$$F_{\text{direct}}(\theta) = F^{\circ} \cos^{n}\theta \tag{9.43}$$

Here F_{direct} is the normal component of the flux coming in at angle θ, F° is the flux at $\theta = 0°$, and θ is the angle from the vertical direction, as was indicated in Figure 9–25. By adjusting n from 1 to large numbers, one can obtain isotropic to very anisotropic distributions of arrival angles, as shown in Figure 9–37. With $n = 1$, the distribution is isotropic, with fluxes coming from above at all directions equally. Higher pressure, more collisions in the gas phase, and shorter mean free path would lead to a more isotropic arrival distribution. A larger source and shorter source-to-wafer distance also give more isotropic arrival. For $n > 1$, a tighter distribution of arrival angles would occur, as shown in the graph in Figure 9–37. This means that the fluxes arriving are more directed in the vertical direction. Lower pressure, fewer collisions in the gas phase, and a longer mean free path would lead to a more anisotropic arrival distribution, as would a smaller source and a longer source-to-wafer distance. For ionic species in biased systems (bias sputtering, ionized sputter deposition, HDPCVD), the n values would be quite high since the ions are accelerated and directed toward the surface by the imposed electric field. In practice, the value of n for the various species is first approximated according to the type of species (ionic or neutral, for example) and type of deposition system, as we will discuss later. The exact value of n for the various species is then often determined by fitting simulations to experimental profiles in calibration structures.

One must also specify the maximum, unobstructed flux of each species to normalize the flux distribution. This is the integrated flux of Eq. (9.43) over all directions above the surface and corresponds to deposition on an unobstructed flat surface.

Knowing the magnitude and distribution of fluxes coming from the gas phase, one must then take into account the local surface topography. This includes the relative orientation of the surface at each position i on the wafer surface, as well as any shadowing

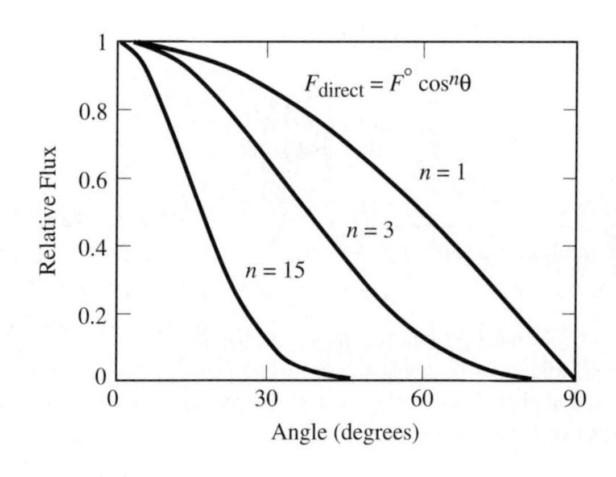

Figure 9–37 Distribution of arrival angles as function of angle to vertical direction, θ, for three values of n. The relative flux is $(F_{\text{direct}}/F^{\circ})$, where F_{direct} is the normal component of flux arriving at point i at angle θ. The $n = 1$ curve corresponds to isotropic arrival, with higher values of n representing more vertically directed arrival.

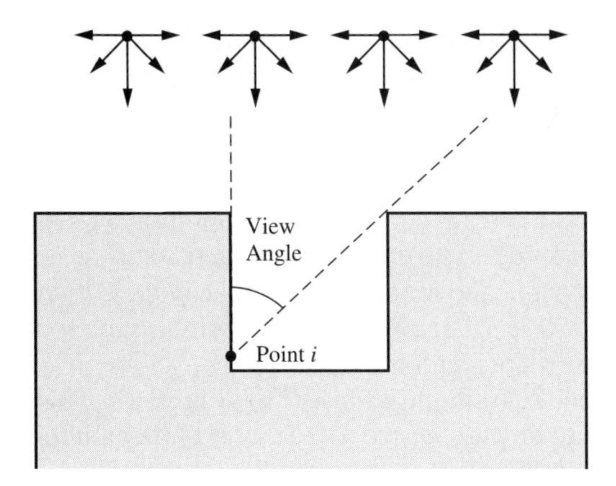

Figure 9–38 Illustration of viewing angle concept. A point, *i*, inside a trench would only see fluxes arriving within a limited range of angles due to geometrical considerations and shadowing.

effects from the topographical features. For example, the position may be on the sidewall of a step or trench and receive little flux from directly above with more coming in at an angle. Or the position may be at the bottom or side of a trench and see a limited amount of direct flux coming in since the fluxes outside the line of sight will be blocked or shadowed. Figure 9–38 illustrates this. One must take into account the line of sight, the "view angle," from the reference plane in the gas phase just above the surface to each position on the surface. (In fact, each small area on the reference plane can be assumed to be an emission source to the topography below, equivalent to a downward pointing Knudsen cell, for these calculations.) Assuming collisionless, line-of-sight transport in this region, all this geometry and shadowing can be taken into account and the total direct flux can be calculated at each position on the wafer surface for each species.

The *indirect fluxes* include the processes that occur on the surface, or near the surface of the wafer during deposition. Surface diffusion, emission, sputtering, and redeposition are all indirect fluxes.

The *surface diffusion fluxes*, $F_{\text{diff.in}}$ and $F_{\text{diff.out}}$, are driven by differences in the curvature in the surface. Here we are not concerned with the short-range diffusion of atoms to attachment sites as part of the surface reaction process, but rather the longer-range diffusion in order to reduce surface energy. The net diffusion flux ($F_{\text{diff.net}} = F_{\text{diff.in}} - F_{\text{diff.out}}$) at each point is calculated by

$$F_{\text{diff.net}} = \frac{D_s}{kT}\gamma_s\Omega\upsilon\frac{\partial^2 K}{\partial s^2} \tag{9.44}$$

D_S is the surface diffusivity of the material, γ_s is the per area surface energy, Ω is the atomic volume of the atom or molecule, υ is the number of atoms per unit area, or the surface density, K is the curvature, and s is the unit length along the surface the atom or molecule travels. In Chapter 11 in the section on reflow modeling we derive the expression for the surface flux and the normal velocity of a surface due to surface diffusion. Here we are interested in the flux relative to the surface normal direction, which is the velocity in that direction times the density. To get this, we multiply the expression for the normal velocity due to surface diffusion of Chapter 11, Eq. (11.37), by the density, which is the same as dividing by Ω, and we end up with Eq. (9.44).

Because of curvature-induced surface diffusion during deposition, filling in of corners is enhanced and smoother and conformal depositions can result, as we will see in the simulations. Because atoms can diffuse along the surfaces to areas in less direct view of the source, better step coverage can be obtained. Surface diffusion also helps with filling vias and trenches and can lead to more planarized depositions as well. Fast surface diffusion is often used to explain, and model, conformal coverage in particular deposition cases. However, as we will see, emission and redeposition can model the same effects and may be more physically correct in some cases.

The *flux due to emission* of species from the surface, F_{emitted}, occurs because not all deposition species or precursors stay, or stick, where they land. A finite number, usually assumed to be a constant fraction of the incident species, will be emitted or desorbed from the surface without properly reacting or depositing there. The emitted flux at each point i is thus

$$F^i_{\text{emitted}} = (1 - S_c)F^i_{\text{incident}} \tag{9.45}$$

where F^i_{incident} includes both direct and indirect deposition fluxes incident at i and S_c is the sticking coefficient.

The sticking coefficient here is defined as the ratio of the flux of species that properly react and stay on the surface to the flux of incident deposition species:

$$S_c = \frac{F_{\text{reacted}}}{F_{\text{incident}}} \tag{9.46}$$

This is really an effective sticking coefficient or probability, since factors such as site availability, reaction competition and completion, and surface recombination are implicitly included in it. It is also sometimes referred to as the reactive sticking coefficient, and is often empirically determined from deposition profiles. The sticking coefficient depends on the type of deposition system, the chemistry, and material being deposited. It can also depend on substrate temperature. The temperature dependence is often difficult to predict because of all the processes that may be involved. A lower value is seen at higher temperatures in some cases, such as in the case of LPCVD SiO_2 [9.30]. In other cases, such as with CVD W deposition, a lower value is sometimes seen at lower deposition temperatures. In more advanced models S_c may not be a constant, as is assumed here.

The fraction that does not stay at a particular position and is emitted is therefore equal to $(1 - S_c)$. The F_{emitted} flux is thus subtracted in the total flux equation [Eq. (9.42)]. It is often assumed that the emitted species are emitted in a range of directions away from the surface in a perfectly diffuse angular distribution, with a cosine emission distribution, independent of the incident angle [9.31, 9.32]. Thus the emission process is modeled as a small planar surface source at each position with $n = 1$ in the $\cos^n\theta$-emitted angle distribution, and the distribution is centered around the surface normal. This implicitly assumes that there is appreciable residence time on the surface so that the species lose their memory of their incident angle. It is also generally assumed that only the neutral species can be emitted from the surface. For ionic species the sticking coefficient is thus taken to be one, except when ion reflection effects are considered.

Those emitted species can then be deposited on other surfaces of the structure, leading to the *redeposited (emitted) flux*, $F_{\text{redep(emitted)}}$, term. So for each point i, there is a flux coming from each of the other points, termed k. It is again assumed that the number of gas-phase collisions near the surface area is negligible, so that the emitted species travel in straight lines to other points on the surface. Knowing the emitted flux distribution from each point k [Eq. (9.45) for k and a cosine distribution] and the geometrical relationship to point i, the flux emitted from each point k to point i can be determined. This is similar to what we did earlier in Section 9.2.2.1 when we calculated the flux and deposition rate onto a surface from a planar evaporation source. Of course, only those points that are in line of sight to point i are included. The redeposited flux at point i due to emission from point k is thus:

$$F^{ik}_{\text{redep(emitted)}} = g^{ik} * F^{k}_{\text{emitted}} = g^{ik} * (1 - S_c) * F^{k}_{\text{incident}} \tag{9.47}$$

Here g^{ik} is the geometrical factor that accounts for the distance and orientation between points i and k, similar to Eq. (9.23) where we derived the expression for deposition on a surface from a planar source. Then all the emitted fluxes from each of the points k to i are summed up and contribute to $F_{\text{redep(emitted)}}$.

We mentioned earlier that fast surface diffusion of deposited species is often used to explain good step coverage. However, the emission and redeposition process can result in the same effect. If the sticking coefficient is less than one, species landing on surfaces can be emitted and deposited elsewhere, including vertical surfaces (recall Figure 9–21). The diffuse emission behavior means that surfaces in all orientations can get material deposited on them. The lower the sticking coefficient, the more conformal step coverage becomes. Whether this redistribution of material and better coverage occur by the emission/redeposition process or the surface diffusion process is sometimes hard to distinguish although this has been done in some studies [9.32, 9.33, 9.34]. Using a clever overhang test structure, these experiments concluded that the emission-redeposition process, and not surface diffusion, was dominant for LPCVD and PECVD deposition of SiO_2. Thus a lower sticking coefficient, and not faster surface diffusion, is the appropriate model, at least in the specific cases studied. For other materials or techniques, surface diffusion may be important. For example, for sputter deposited A1, the sticking coefficient is found to be one [9.33], which implies no emission/redeposition, but surface diffusion at high temperatures is significant. In our simulations later we will show how both the sticking coefficient and surface diffusivity affect the degree of coverage.

The *sputtered flux*, $F_{\text{sputtered}}$, term is from the atoms that are sputtered off the wafer surface. This is a momentum-transfer process in which incoming particles knock and displace surface atoms from the surface of the wafer. This is due mainly to accelerated ions, both argon and ionized deposition atoms, coming directly from the gas phase. These ions can achieve energies of several hundred eV. The flux term at each point i due to sputtering (a negative term since atoms are being taken away from the surface) is therefore

$$F^{i}_{\text{sputtered}} = Y * (F^{i}_{\text{argon}} + F^{i}_{\text{direct(ions)}}) = Y * F^{i}_{\text{ions}} \tag{9.48}$$

Y is the sputtering yield and is defined as the ratio of atoms that are sputtered or knocked off the surface to the number of incident ions or atoms. Y is a function of the target material (the wafer surface material, in this case) and the mass of the incoming ion. However, we assume here for simplicity that it is the same for argon and other ions. It is also a function of ion energy and the incident angle, θ, at point i, with a normal incidence being 0°. Ions coming in at low angles are reflected from the surface and do not transfer significant energy to the surface atoms, while ions coming perpendicular to the surface knock surface atoms further into the film and not off. The maximum sputtering yield occurs usually between 40 and 70°C.

A typical sputtering yield distribution can be seen in Figure 9–39. The specific characteristics of the curve, such as the maximum yield and angle for which it occurs, could vary for different materials and equipment conditions. Also shown is the normalized etch rate due to sputtering, which equals the product of the sputter yield and $\cos\theta$. The latter term is due to the fact that it is the component of the flux normal to the surface that determines the etch or deposition rate on a surface, as we have described. The sputter etch rate also has a maximum at some angle between 40 and 70°C. This angular dependence on sputtering yield and sputter etch rate is often utilized to achieve more planar surfaces during deposition. The sloped surfaces (with incident angles less than 90°) sputter off faster than horizontal or vertical surfaces (with incident angles near 0 or 90°), leading to more planar surfaces.

The emitted angle distribution of the sputtered atoms has been modeled with different types of distributions [9.35]. The sputtered atoms often exhibit an ideal, diffuse angular distribution, being sputtered away at many angles centered around the surface normal, like desorbed or emitted species discussed above. This is illustrated in Figure 9–40(a). The distribution may in fact be more sideways, described by an "under-cosine" distribution (where n is less than 1 in a $\cos^n\theta$ distribution), shown in Figure 9–40(b). In some cases though they can exhibit a specular distribution, being sputtered at just a few angles near an angle opposite that of the incident angle. In this case the angular distribution of the sputtered atoms is described by a $\cos^n\theta$ distribution, with a very large

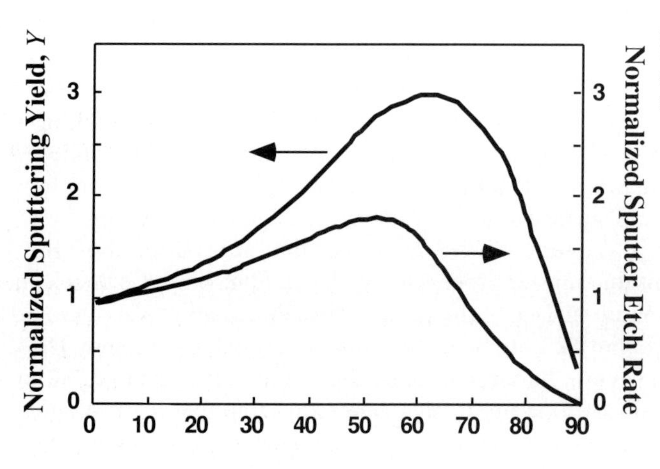

Figure 9–39 Typical example of sputtering yield and sputter etch rate as functions of incident angle, with respect to surface normal.

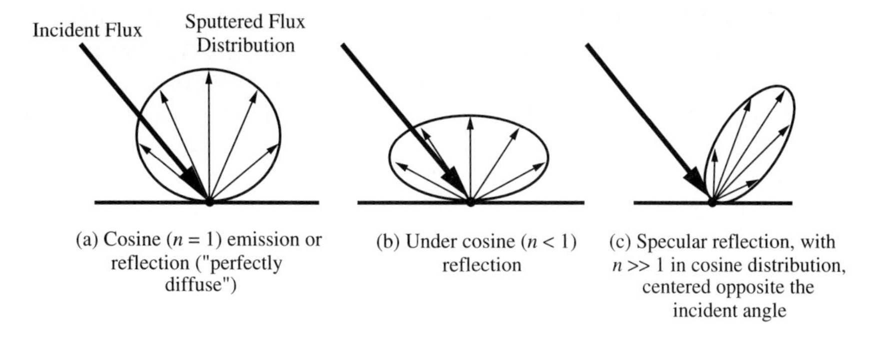

Figure 9–40 Different emitted angle distributions for sputtered atoms.

value of n, and the distribution of sputtered atoms is centered opposite the incident angle. This is illustrated in Figure 9–40(c). Generally distributions like Figure 9–40(a) or (c) are used in simulations. The first type is common when the incident ion energy is high and there are collisions and interactions deeper in the sputtered layer, while the latter type is more common when the incident ion energy is lower and single surface collisions dominate. Also, amorphous materials like SiO_2 tend to sputter off with the first type of distribution.

As was the case with desorbed or emitted species, sputtered atoms can be redeposited elsewhere on the surface. The method to calculate this *redeposited (sputtered) flux* and the equations used are analogous to the redeposition due to emission. At each point i the redeposited flux coming from each other point k is determined:

$$F^{ik}_{\text{redep(sput)}} = g^{ik} * F^{k}_{\text{sputtered}} = g^{ik} * Y * F^{k}_{\text{ions}} \tag{9.49}$$

Again, g^{ik} is a geometrical factor that accounts for the distance and orientation between points i and k, as well as for the angular distribution of sputtered atoms from k. Only those points, k, that are in line of sight of i would contribute.

In addition to sputtering off atoms from the surface, ions striking the surface can also enhance the deposition rate. Ion bombardment can transfer energy to the species on the surface and enhance the different surface processes and reactions. One way to model this is by adding an ion-induced deposition rate enhancement term to the total flux expression (rather than trying to modify the other terms). This term is of the form of

$$F^{i}_{\text{ion-induced}} = K_i * F^{i}_{\text{ions}} \tag{9.50}$$

where K_i is the ion-induced deposition enhancement factor and is usually a fitting factor. Remember that F_{ions} includes all ions, both nonprecursor ions, such as Ar^+, and any ionized precursor species (Al^+ or Ti^+, for example). Non-ionized precursor species are still needed for this ion-enhanced process, but they are not a limiting factor in this process so only the ion flux is included in this term. The competition between ion sputtering and ion-enhanced deposition can be very important in obtaining the final topography.

9.5.1.2 Models for Different Types of Deposition Systems

To simulate deposition, one should include all the terms in Eq. (9.42) and calculate the total net flux at each point *i* on the surface. The deposition rate, or the movement of the surface, at each point is then calculated by dividing the total flux by the film density. For ease of use and computation, one could simplify the net flux equation for the various types of deposition methods (LPCVD, standard PVD, ionized PVD, etc.), including only the important terms for each technique. This is in fact what is done in SPEEDIE. Relative rate constants (K's) are often included in front of some of the flux terms which makes it easier to adjust the parameters when multiple processes are occurring. By examining the expressions that SPEEDIE uses for each type of deposition, one can gain a better understanding of the different deposition techniques.

First we consider *LPCVD deposition*. Figure 9–41 shows an LPCVD system and the relevant fluxes needed to model this type of deposition. In this case we have the direct flux of neutral species, as well as the desorbed or emitted flux and redeposition of these neutral species. There is no flux of ionic species in this system, and no sputtering or redeposition of sputtered species. In addition, long-range surface diffusion is usually not important, as discussed earlier.

Eq. (9.42) becomes

$$F^i_{\text{net}} = F^i_{\text{direct(neutrals)}} + F^i_{\text{redep(emitted)}} - F^i_{\text{emitted}} \tag{9.51}$$

Substituting in Eqs. (9.45) and (9.47) for the emitted and redeposited fluxes leads to

$$\begin{aligned} F^i_{\text{net}} &= F^i_{\text{direct(neutrals)}} + F^i_{\text{redep(emitted)}} - (1 - S_c)(F^i_{\text{direct(neutrals)}} + F^i_{\text{redep(emitted)}}) \\ &= S_c * (F^i_{\text{direct(neutrals)}} + F^i_{\text{redep(emitted)}}) \\ &= S_c * (F^i_{\text{direct(neutrals)}} + g^{ik} * (1 - S_c) * F^k) \end{aligned} \tag{9.52}$$

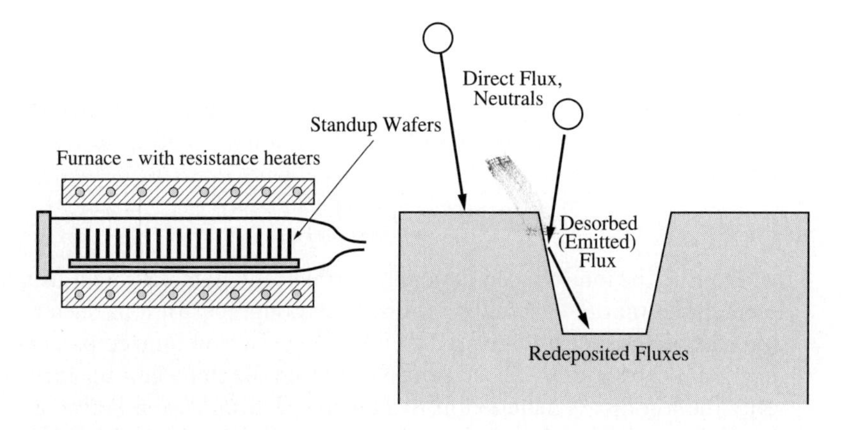

Figure 9–41 LPCVD system and relevant fluxes needed to model this type of deposition.

This must be solved for all points i simultaneously and consistently—emitted flux from one point affects the redeposition flux at another, which in turn affects the flux at the first point, and so on. In the deposition rate equation, the direct neutral and redeposited flux terms ($F^i_{direct(neutrals)} + F^i_{redep(emitted)}$) are combined into one term, and called the local deposition flux, F_d. The net deposition rate at each point is just the net flux, F^i_{net}, divided by the film density, N. So for LPCVD, the deposition rate equation is given as

$$\text{rate} = \frac{S_c F_d}{N} \tag{9.53}$$

The other important parameter would be the value of n in the $\cos^n\theta$ distribution for the incoming (direct) species.

Example Calculate the deposition rate using the expression for LPCVD deposition for SiO_2 on a flat surface with no topography. S_c is equal to 0.3, the maximum, unobstructed flux is equal to 3×10^{15} molecules $cm^{-2}\,sec^{-1}$, and the density of the deposited oxide film is 2.27 gm cm^{-3}.

Answer We are interested in this case in the deposition rate on a flat surface. Therefore there is no shadowing, no redeposited flux, and each surface position is in a horizontal orientation. Thus F_d is just equal everywhere to the maximum, unobstructed flux. The deposition rate for LPCVD in SPEEDIE is given by Eq. (9.53). The density of SiO_2 in terms of molecules cm^{-3} is

$$\begin{aligned}\text{density}(SiO_2) = N &= 2.27\text{ gm cm}^{-3} * \frac{\text{Avogadro's number}}{\text{\# of gms per mole for } SiO_2} \\ &= 2.27\text{ gm cm}^{-3} * \frac{6.02 \times 10^{23}\text{ molecules/mole}}{60\text{ gms/mole}} \\ &= 2.3 \times 10^{22}\text{ molecules cm}^{-3}\end{aligned}$$

Therefore the deposition rate on the flat, unobstructed surface is

$$\begin{aligned}\text{rate} = \frac{S_c F_d}{N} &= \frac{0.3 * 3 \times 10^{15}\text{ molecules cm}^{-2}\text{ sec}^{-1}}{2.3 \times 10^{22}\text{ molecules cm}^{-3}} \\ &= 3.9 \times 10^{-8}\text{ cm sec}^{-1} = 0.023\ \mu\text{m min}^{-1}\end{aligned}$$

For deposition on nonflat or obstructed surface locations, on sidewalls of trenches, for example, the local deposition rate can be less than this. The same expression is used but the local flux, F_d, can be less at these locations. Figure 9–46 to be discussed later illustrates LPCVD simulation on more complex topography.

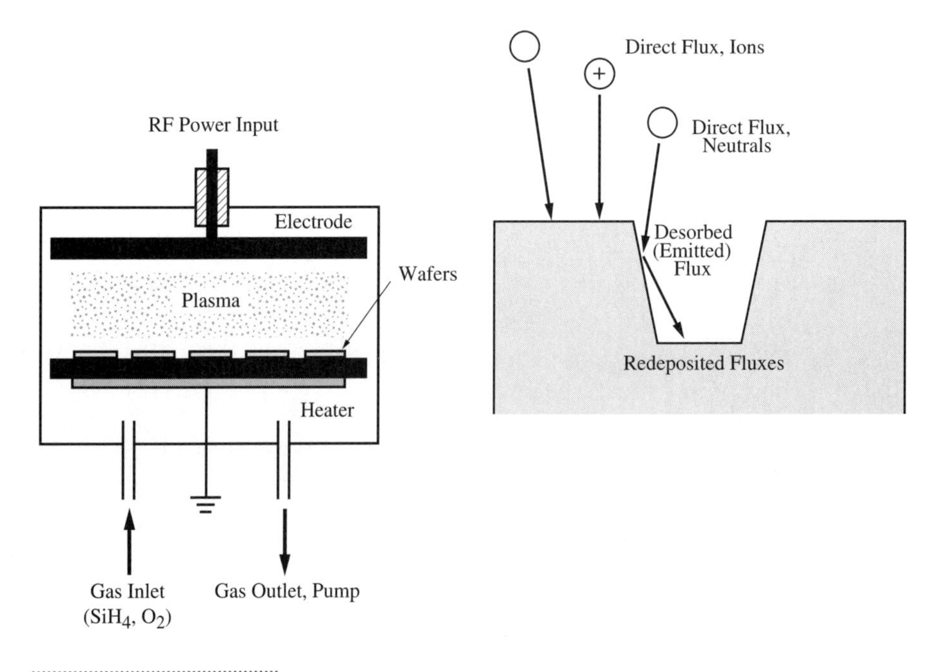

Figure 9–42 PECVD system and relevant fluxes needed to model this type of deposition.

For *PECVD deposition* there is an ion flux onto the wafer which can accelerate the deposition process. Figure 9–42 shows a PECVD system and the relevant fluxes needed to model this type of deposition. As in LPCVD there is a direct flux of neutral species and the emission and redeposition of those species. Also shown is the direct flux of ions, accelerated across the plasma sheath toward the wafer, which can enhance the deposition. The ion energy in this type of system is assumed low enough that sputtering is not significant and direct deposition of ions is also not appreciable. Again surface diffusion is not considered important.

Thus the ion-induced enhancement term, Eq. (9.50), is included in the rate equation, which becomes

$$\text{rate} = \frac{(S_c K_d F_d) + (K_i F_i)}{N} \tag{9.54}$$

K_d and K_i are relative rate constants for the non-ion-enhanced component and the ion-enhanced component, respectively. F_i is the net local ion flux, or F_{ion} as given above. N is the film density. Surface diffusion is not explicitly modeled here; however a low value of S_c can have a similar effect, as discussed earlier, and has been used in SPEEDIE in modeling PECVD oxide deposition [9.4, 9.5, 9.34, 9.36]. Both the non-ion-enhanced and the ion-enhanced terms are important in PECVD depositions [9.5, 9.36].

For *standard PVD*, the same fluxes and terms are used as for LPCVD. Figure 9–43 shows a PVD system, a standard DC sputtering system in this case, and the relevant fluxes needed to model PVD deposition. The rate equation is thus

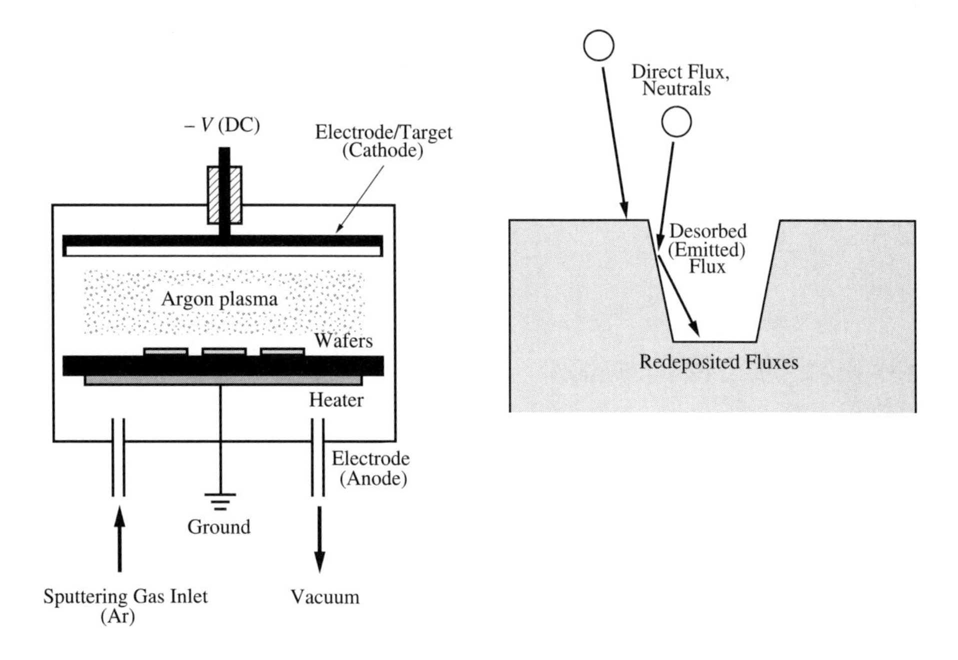

Figure 9–43 PVD (sputter deposition) system and relevant fluxes needed to model this type of deposition. The specific system illustrated here is a DC sputtering system.

$$\text{rate} = \frac{S_c F_d}{N} \tag{9.55}$$

However, different values for the sticking coefficient and the arrival angle distribution would be used for PVD versus CVD methods, as discussed below. There is no significant ion bombardment onto the wafer surface for standard sputter deposition systems, either DC or RF based, as described earlier. This model would also be applicable to collimated and long throw sputter deposition systems, but a narrower arrival angle distribution would be used than for standard sputtering systems. In addition, evaporation can be modeled by this model.

For *high-temperature PVD*, the relevant fluxes are the same as those illustrated in Figure 9–43, except that we now add the surface diffusion flux term, Eq. (9.44), to the rate equation for standard PVD, giving

$$\text{rate} = \frac{S_c F_d + \dfrac{D_s}{kT}\gamma_s \Omega \upsilon \dfrac{\partial^2 K}{\partial s^2}}{N} \tag{9.56}$$

For *ionized PVD*, there are several fluxes in addition to those in the standard PVD model. Figure 9–44 shows an ionized sputtering system and the relevant fluxes. In addition to the direct flux of neutral species, there is a significant flux of ionized species—both ionized Ar atoms and ionized precursor species (Al^+ or Ti^+, for example). These

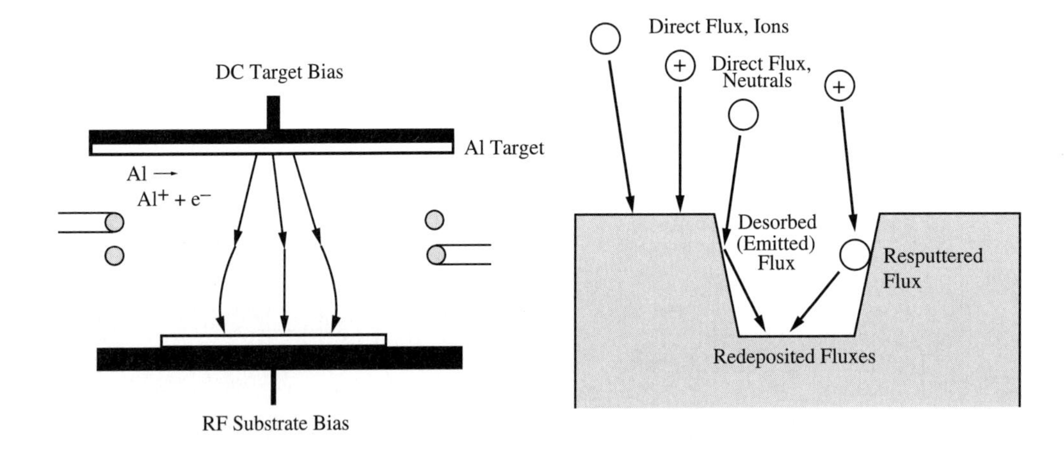

Figure 9–44 Ionized PVD system and relevant fluxes needed to model this type of deposition.

ionized species can be deposited as well as sputter surface atoms on the wafer. Therefore, for ionized PVD, several terms are added to the rate equation for PVD deposition: the term due to direct flux of precursor ions, $F^{i}_{\text{direct(ions)}}$; the ion-induced enhancement term [Eq. (9.50)]; and the sputtering and redeposition terms [Eqs. (9.48) and (9.49)]. The direct deposition of precursor ions and the ion-induced enhancement terms are combined into one term, equal simply to F_i, the total ion flux. This is done in SPEEDIE partly because SPEEDIE does not currently distinguish between Ar ions and ionized precursor species.

This leads to the expression given for the rate to be

$$\text{rate} = \frac{(S_c F_d) + F_i - (K_{\text{sp}} Y F_i) + (K_{\text{rd}} F_{\text{rd}})}{N} \tag{9.57}$$

Here F_{rd} is the flux given by Eq. (9.49) for redeposition of sputtered material. K_{SP} and K_{RD} are relative rate constants, used mostly as fitting parameters. A term for reflected Al ions may also be important for coverage issues and may be added in future models. (A model for bias sputtering would be similar to this, but the ions would be mostly Ar and not the deposited species.)

Similarly, for *high-density plasma (HDP) CVD* the sputtering and redeposition terms are added to the PECVD case, without any non-ion direct term. Figure 9–45 shows a HDP CVD system and the relevant fluxes used to model this deposition. This gives the following expression for the rate:

$$\text{rate} = \frac{(K_i F_i) - (K_{\text{sp}} Y F_i) + (K_{\text{rd}} F_{\text{rd}})}{N} \tag{9.58}$$

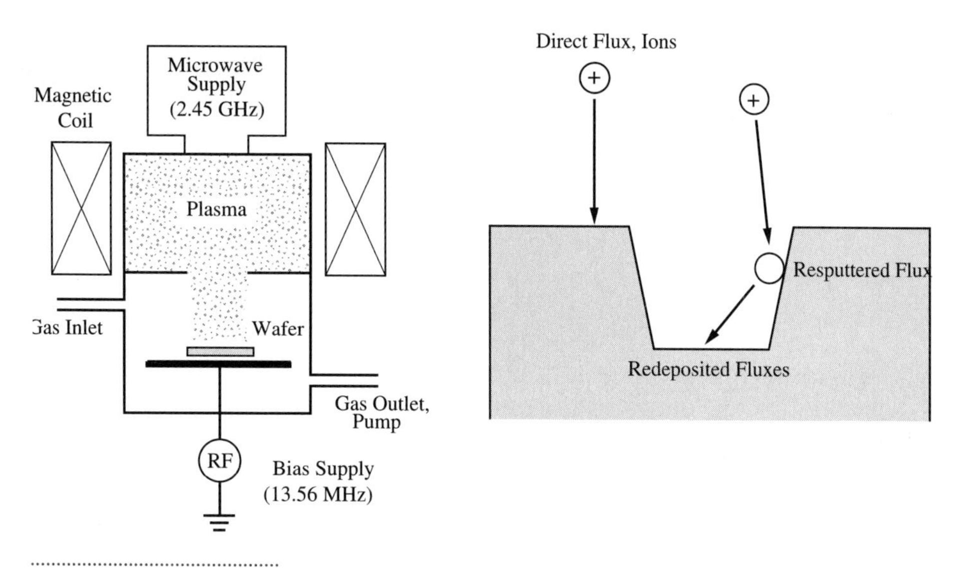

Figure 9–45 HDPCVD system (with a microwave ECR source) and relevant fluxes needed to model this type of deposition.

similar to that for ionized PVD. The ion flux would be quite high in these systems, about 1×10^{17} cm^{-2}. The non-ion (neutral) direct term is not included here because its flux is often too low at these low pressures to be important on its own, that is, when not enhanced by the ions. (However, more recent SPEEDIE models include other terms such as the neutral flux as secondary effects.) There could also be direct deposition of ionized precursor species; this is included in the ion-enhanced term for simplicity.

9.5.1.3 Comparing CVD and PVD and Typical Parameter Values

Before presenting some simulation results, we first want to make some general comments regarding some of the values used for CVD and PVD models. This will be done in terms of the standard models for low-pressure systems, that is, most CVD and PVD systems used today. The discussion will center around the parameter values summarized in Table 9–2.

In CVD deposition systems, the arrival angle distribution for neutral species is basically isotropic, while for PVD systems the arriving flux of neutrals is often more anisotropic and directed. This is due to the different types of sources and the different pressures.

In CVD systems the source gas fills the whole chamber and arrives at the wafers from many directions. This is partly due to injection systems and cages that may be used, as well as gas-phase reactions that may occur. More importantly, the precursor species in the gas phase in CVD systems undergo significantly more collisions than in PVD depositions before the species strike the wafers. This is due to the much higher gas pressure in CVD systems, even for low-pressure CVD systems, compared to PVD systems

Table 9–2 Typical values of modeling parameters for various PVD and CVD depositions

	n (exponent in cosine arrival angle distribution)	S_C (sticking coefficient)
Sputter deposition		
standard	~1.0–4	~1
ionized or collimated	8–80	~1
Evaporation	3–80	~1
LPCVD silicon dioxide		
silane	1	0.2–0.4
TEOS	1	0.05–0.1
LPCVD tungsten	1	0.01 or less
LPCVD polysilicon	1	0.001 or less

(HDPCVD systems with its very low gas pressure being the notable exception). More collisions result in a shorter mean free path and a wider arrival angle distribution. As a result, the arrival angle distribution can be assumed to be isotropic in most CVD systems. This means a value of 1 in the $\cos^n\theta$ arrival angle distribution given by Eq. (9.43) for the direct flux of deposition species, as shown in Table 9–2. (Higher values for n would be used for the ionic species in plasma CVD systems, where the ions are accelerated and directed toward the wafer surface.)

For PVD depositions, the depositing material comes off a remotely located and finite area source or target, and due to geometrical considerations often arrives at the wafers in a more directed manner. In addition, fewer collisions occur during the transport, as mentioned above, because of the much lower pressured used—usually in the 1- to 10-mtorr range for sputtering and even lower for evaporation, as compared to 0.25 to 2.0 torr for LPCVD. As a result of all this, the arrival angle distribution for PVD depositions can be less isotropic and the atoms arriving at the wafer surface can therefore be more directed. For standard sputter PVD the value of n in the $\cos^n\theta$ arrival distribution will often be greater than 1, representing a more directed distribution arriving from above. The exact value will depend on the system geometry (e.g., target size, target-to-wafer distance, rotation of substrate), the operating conditions (e.g., pressure) and the depositing material. Typical values range from very close to 1 (virtually isotropic) to about 4 (fairly directed), as shown in Table 9–2, with higher pressures, larger target sizes, and smaller target-to-wafer distances giving the lower n values.

For ionized species (most of the depositing species in ionized PVD systems and some of them in a plasma CVD system) as well as neutral species in collimated PVD systems, the species are very directed. The n value can be from about 8 to 80 or even higher, depending on the system and the plasma conditions.

The sticking coefficient is also generally different for CVD and PVD systems. For CVD systems, the sticking coefficients used in modeling are almost always less than one, as shown in Table 9–2. Typical values would be 0.05 to 0.1 for TEOS-based CVD of SiO_2, and somewhat higher—up to about 0.4—for silane-based CVD. Similar values would apply to the neutral component in PECVD systems. The value for CVD W (via hydrogen reduction) and polysilicon is even lower, 0.01 or less. Surface reactions are important for CVD depositions. The species can desorb before the reactions required for deposition can take place. Another precursor required for the reaction may not be present at that spot at that time. In addition, competing reactions and site occupation by other species and byproducts can occur. These all contribute to the effective sticking coefficient for CVD depositions being low. The species not reacted and deposited are desorbed, or emitted, and are usually assumed to have a diffuse emitted angle distribution, as opposed to a specular emission.

For conventional PVD, where physical processes dominate, the atoms generally attach and then stay attached, without desorbing. No surface reactions occur other than simple condensation. The sticking coefficient is therefore usually assumed to equal 1, or close to it, for PVD depositions. (One exception to this may be PVD of Ta, which seems to have a somewhat lower sticking coefficient.) For the ionized species in either PVD or CVD systems, the sticking coefficient is often assumed to equal one.

In PVD and CVD systems where large fluxes of ions are present, such as in ionized PVD and high-density plasma CVD, sputtering of deposited material can occur. This, like desorption, leads to redeposition of species elsewhere. The angular distribution for sputtered atoms is usually assumed to be perfectly diffuse, with n equal to 1, but is sometimes assumed to be specular. For example, sputtered Al is often modeled with specular redeposition with n equal to 2 or more for a cosine distribution that is directed away from the incident angle. HDPCVD deposition is dominated by the highly directional ion flux and actually acts more like PVD deposition rather than other CVD systems in regards to the sticking coefficient (which is effectively equal to one since no neutral species are considered) and arrival angle distribution. It is its angle-dependent sputtering and redeposition action as well as its very directed ion deposition, at the very low pressures, that give HDPCVD its good filling and planarization abilities.

We did not discuss models for evaporation deposition. However, by using a very directed angular arrival distribution (n equal to 15 or higher in the $\cos^n\theta$ distribution) for a stationary substrate or a less directed distribution for a rotated substrate, and using a sticking coefficient equal to one, one could simulate the evaporation deposition processes using the equations given above for conventional PVD.

Based on these generalizations we can now understand why CVD depositions usually give more conformal coverage than PVD depositions in these low pressure systems. An isotropic arrival distribution may lead to better step coverage. More importantly, a lower sticking coefficient, allowing more desorption and redeposition occurrences, leads to better step coverage, and a lower sticking coefficient is usually more important than the arrival angle in obtaining good coverage. Whatever the arrival angle distribution, a low sticking coefficient can lead to good coverage (even in a deep hole) since the deposition species, wherever they land, will bounce around and deposit on all sides of a structure. Thus CVD generally gives much more conformal coverage than PVD.

Having said that CVD techniques generally deposit films with better step coverage, it should be reiterated that a low sticking coeffecient and good step coverage are not always required. This is the case in applications like covering the bottoms of deep, narrow contact or via holes with materials like Ti or filling narrow spaces with SiO_2 or metal. While a low sticking coefficient can greatly help in filling or lining holes, such as with

CVD W or TiN, there is another approach. The idea behind collimated and ionized PVD techniques, and even in HDPCVD with its strong ion component, is to deposit material from the gas phase in a very vertical direction. In this case a narrow arrival angle distribution is desired, not a wide distribution associated with good step coverage, and a low sticking coefficient is not required. Step coverage per se may not be great, but the bottoms of vias will be covered. In addition, good filling of holes or gaps can be achieved by the use of directed ions and sputtering action—filling up the holes from the bottom and sputtering away any overhang that may develop. In addition, the resputtering may help with sidewall covering. Directed ions and sputtering are the keys to ionized PVD and HDPCVD. Of course, CVD techniques with very low sticking coefficients are also good at covering the bottoms of deep vias and filling holes and gaps. But viable CVD techniques have not been developed for some materials, and these other techniques have been shown to do a good job at achieving bottom coverage and gap filling.

9.5.2 Simulations of Deposition Using a Physically Based Simulator, SPEEDIE

We now describe a series of deposition simulations using the SPEEDIE simulator and the equations and ideas presented above. These simulations will be used to demonstrate and further explain some of the concepts covered earlier in this chapter. The main focus will be on issues of film coverage and filling the underlying topography.

The first example is a simple simulation of LPCVD deposition of SiO_2 following Eq. (9.53). We will use parameter values in some cases that may not be realistic for LPCVD deposition but are more appropriate for PVD deposition. We do this to illustrate some of the important concepts of the models.

The initial topography is a wide trench—3 μm wide and 1 μm deep—in underlying Si (Figure 9–46). 0.5-μm-thick SiO_2 layer is deposited over this topography. A $\cos^n\theta$ distribution for the arrival angle distribution [Eq. (9.43)] is used, with $n = 1$ in the first simulation. This corresponds to a uniform or isotropic distribution of arrival angles, that is, molecules coming from all directions equally. This would be the case when many collisions occur in the gas phase so that the mean free path is very short and the direction of molecules becomes randomized. As we mentioned above, an n value of 1 is used for most CVD depositions. The other important parameter is the sticking coefficient, S_c, and a value of 1 is used here. This means that there is no reemission or redeposition of depositing species once they strike the surface. This is unrealistic for most CVD processes, as discussed earlier, but we will use it here for illustrative purposes. Later we will use lower values for S_c.

Figure 9–46(a) shows the SPEEDIE simulation of this simple LPCVD simulation. The different contour lines of the deposited SiO_2 represent different time intervals, which makes the deposition process easier to follow. It is apparent that the thickness is reduced on the sidewalls and corners by about 50% or more, even for an isotropic arrival angle distribution. This is because the species are arriving from one side only to each wall (a 90° maximum view angle on the side versus 180° on top). Also the sidewall deposition is sloped inward, which could cause problems for the deposition of subsequent layers.

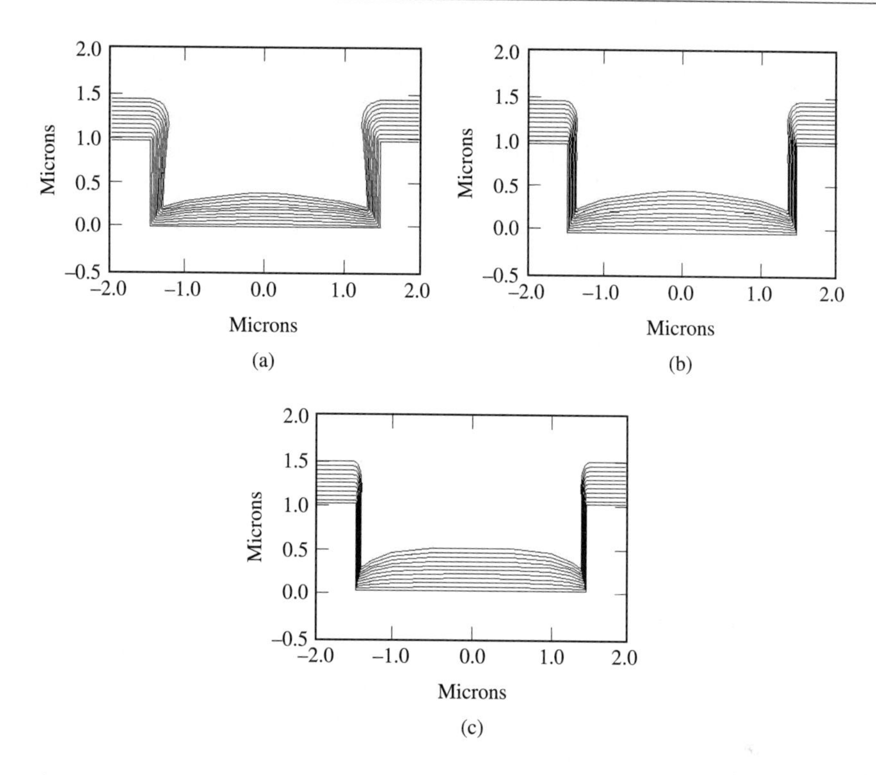

Figure 9–46 SPEEDIE simulations for LPCVD deposition of SiO_2 with $S_c = 1$ (which is more typical of PVD than LPCVD) and varying values of n, the arrival angle distribution factor: (a) $n = 1$; (b) $n = 3$; (c) $n = 10$. Worse step coverage results as n increases (the arrival angle distribution narrows).

The next simulation, shown in Figure 9–46(b) is the same as the previous one, except that the angular distribution of arrival atoms is changed. The value of n used in the $\cos^n\theta$ distribution is 3 here, compared to 1 in the previous simulation. This means that the arrival angle distribution is narrower, with more material coming in closer to the vertical direction. This might be the case when the gas pressure is lower and fewer gas-phase collisions occur, resulting in a longer mean free path. There is even less material deposited on the side walls and corners, as expected. Figure 9–46(c) shows a similar simulation, except with $n = 10$. (Again, this would be unrealistic for CVD processes, but is still illustrative since the same basic model is used for PVD where n can vary greatly—from close to 1 to very large values.) Here the sidewalls receive much less deposition. If the material deposited were a metal conductor, one can see that a narrow arrival distribution could cause problems with conduction of the interconnect line when it travels over steep topography. From these first three simulations we demonstrate the importance of the arrival angle distribution.

In the next example a narrower trench is utilized in the underlying layer (Figure 9–47). This corresponds to a higher aspect ratio (about 1.25 in this example compared to about 0.33 in the previous one). The same model (LPCVD) and parameters are used as

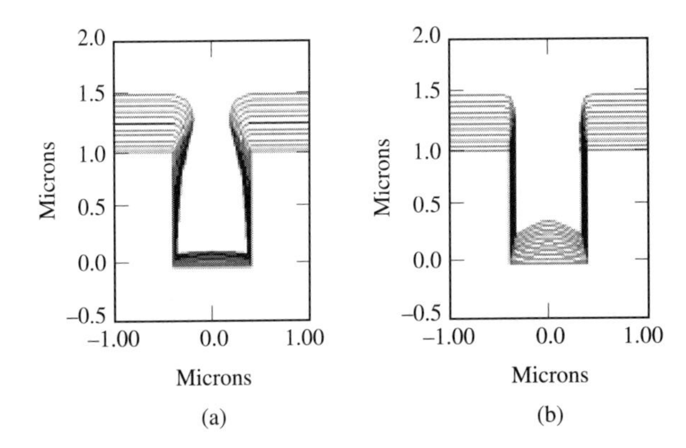

Figure 9–47 SPEEDIE simulations for LPCVD deposition of SiO_2 with $S_c = 1$ (again, more typical of PVD than CVD) and varying values of n, the arrival angle distribution factor, but for a narrower trench: (a) $n = 1$; (b) $n = 10$. Less deposition on sidewalls again results as n increases (the arrival angle distribution narrows), but better bottom filling is achieved due to more vertically directed deposition and less overhanging and shadowing at top corners.

in the previous simulations. Figure 9–47(a) shows the simulation results for the case of $n = 1$, a wide arrival distribution. Here the sidewalls and bottom of the trench have much less SiO_2 deposited on them as compared to Figure 9–46(a), which also had $n = 1$. Clearly geometry and shadowing effects came into play here. Those molecules arriving at large angles to the vertical cannot reach the inside of the trench. Instead they are blocked by the top corners of the trench. Another way to look at it is in terms of the view angle: For locations near the top of the trench the view angle is much larger than for points at the bottom, and more deposition occurs at the top corner and less at the bottom. This becomes even worse as the corners build up due to further deposition, leading to large overhangs. Eventually the top part will seal off, leaving a void in the trench. This angular-dependent blocking effect is called shadowing, for obvious reasons.

In Figure 9–47(b) the value of n is changed to 10. With the more directed incoming molecules, there is less deposition on the top part of the sidewalls. However, there is much more deposition on the bottom of the trench compared to when $n = 1$ [Figure 9–47(a)]. This is because there are more molecules coming vertically into the trench which are not blocked by the top corners or overhangs. Eventually the whole trench could be filled without the development of overhangs or voids.

We see from these examples where the sticking coefficient is unity, and therefore no reemission and redeposition occur, that geometry and line-of-sight considerations are very important. This would be the case for PVD depositions, where the sticking coefficients are usually assumed to be close to one.

We now change the value of the sticking coefficient, S_c, to see its effect. In the previous simulations it was set to 1. Next we set it to 0.1. This means that only one-tenth of the deposition species stay at each arrival point. The rest are reemitted and can be deposited elsewhere. In fact, each redeposited species also has a sticking coefficient

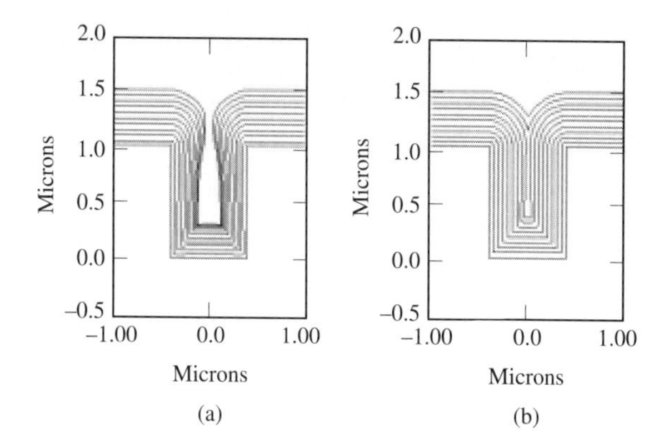

Figure 9–48 SPEEDIE simulations for LPCVD deposition of SiO_2 in a narrow trench with the same isotropic arrival angle distribution (n = 1) but with different values of the sticking coefficient: (a) $S_c = 0.1$, and (b) $S_c = 0.01$. Lowering the sticking coefficient from 1 to 0.1 results in much more conformal coverage. (a) has model parameters typical of CVD SiO_2 depositions, while (b) is typical of CVD W depositions.

of 0.1, so the effect is compounded. The net result is that the species bounce around a lot within the topographical features, giving much improved coverage.

Figure 9–48(a) shows the results for $S_c = 0.1$ and $n = 1$. In this case, these would be realistic parameters for LPCVD SiO_2. Comparing this with Figure 9–47(a), we see that much more uniform deposition occurs, with much more material deposited on both the sidewalls and the bottom. In fact better overall coverage occurs here than in any of the previous simulations (where S_c was set to one in all of them and n was varied), indicating that the sticking coefficient has a larger impact on the profile than the arrival angle distribution. Lowering the sticking coefficient improves both the step or sidewall coverage and the filling ability, and a low sticking coefficient can compensate for orientation and shadowing effects to a very large degree. Figure 9–48(b) shows the simulation results for an even lower value of $S_c = 0.01$, such as would be typical of W or polysilicon depositions, again with $n = 1$. Even more uniform coverage and better filling result.

Figure 9–49 shows the results of some SPEEDIE simulations in which the angle of the sidewall is varied. For all three simulations shown, a sticking coefficient of 0.2 and an n value of 1 are used. One can see that better filling is obtained as the slope is changed from completely vertical (90°) to slightly sloped. Contact and via holes are often sloped slightly to enhance filling. Sloping a step also helps sidewall step coverage.

While the above series of simulations utilized the LPCVD model in SPEEDIE, the same results and trends would occur with the standard PVD model since the same equations are used. Only the values used for the sticking coefficient and the arrival angle distribution would be different. As discussed earlier, CVD processes have sticking coefficients in the 0.001 to 0.3 range and an n value of 1. PVD processes generally have sticking coefficients close to 1, while n is often greater than 1. The above simulations help illustrate the difference between CVD and PVD by varying those parameter values.

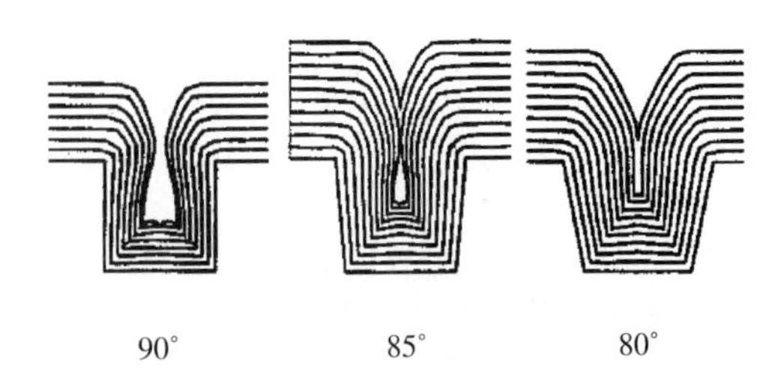

Figure 9–49 Results of SPEEDIE LPCVD simulations in which the sidewall angle is changed. Decreasing the angle from 90 to 80°C greatly improves the trench filling. (After [9.37])

We next compare the methods of LPCVD and HDPCVD. In the latter case there is a strong ion component that not only leads to good filling of holes (since the effective n value of the species would be high) but also causes angle-dependent sputtering of the surface. This causes sloped surfaces to etch away faster than flat surfaces, which can lead to more planar surfaces when depositing material over nonplanar underlying topography. We shall now demonstrate this with SPEEDIE simulations. We first show a simulation using the LPCVD model. The initial topography is a small, flat rectangle on a flat surface, such as would be the case for a polysilicon or metal interconnect line on a flat underlayer (Figure 9–50). We now deposit LPCVD SiO_2 on top. A cosine arrival distribution with $n = 1$ is used, and a sticking coefficient of 0.1 is specified, typical for LPCVD SiO_2 using TEOS. The simulated results are shown in Figure 9–50(a). One sees the very conformal coverage due to the isotropic arrival and, more importantly, the low sticking coefficient [compare this to Figure 9–46(a), which has isotropic arrival but $S_c = 1$]. Conformal coverage is good for obtaining a uniform thickness everywhere, but bad for planarizing the structure.

Next we simulate the same situation, but with the HDP model and typical parameters for that method. A very large and very directed ion flux with a high n value in the arrival angle distribution is used, typical for HDP systems. Sputtering and redeposition of material occur, with a maximum sputtering yield at 62° relative to the surface. This causes sloped surfaces, such as at corners, to be sputtered faster than vertical or horizontal surfaces. The simulation results are shown in Figure 9–50(b). One sees the characteristic pyramid shape that starts to form due to these effects, which then gets reduced to a small bump on the surface. The final topography is more planar than the final topography in the standard LPCVD case. For wider features in the topography, wider and taller pyramidal shapes would form and a thicker HDP oxide layer would have to be deposited for planar topography to be achieved. For this reason, other planarizing techniques, such as CMP, are often used in conjunction with HDP depositions to completely planarize the topography over all the features.

The ability of HDP deposition to fill spaces and to avoid the formation of voids, usually the main reasons for using HDPCVD, are demonstrated in the next two simulations. First in Figure 9–50(c) we show LPCVD deposition in a trench, similar to that described earlier in Figure 9–47(a). The sticking coefficient is still 0.1 and the angular distribution factor, n, is still 1, but the maximum deposition flux is increased a little more to try to fill the space. One sees that a void is formed in the narrow trench, even with a fairly small sticking coefficient. While low sticking coefficients of CVD processes help with filling, the shadowing effects are still important and voids can still form for high-aspect

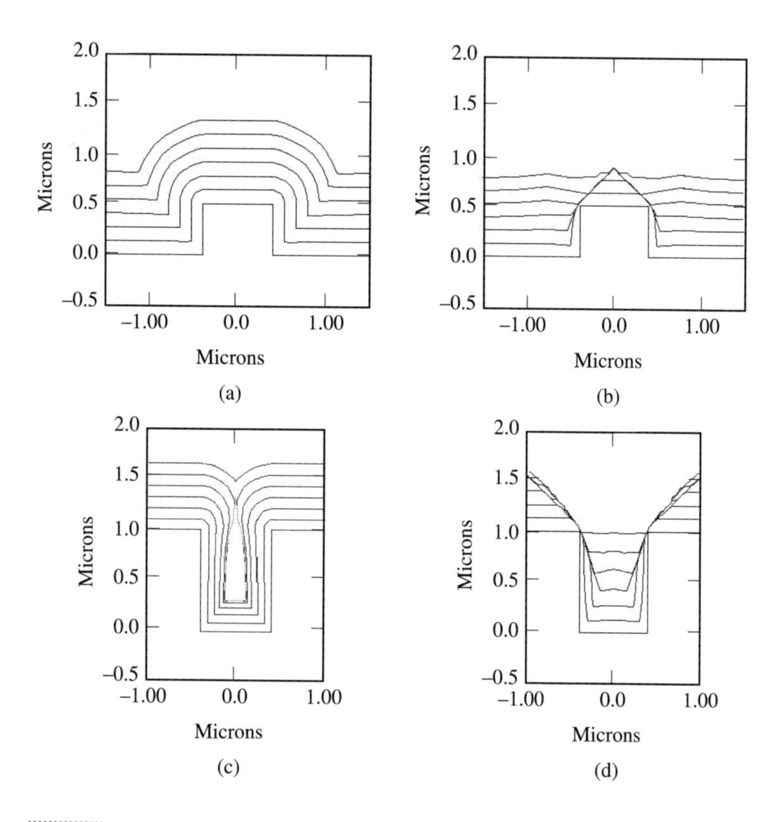

Figure 9–50 SPEEDIE simulations comparing LPCVD and HDPCVD depositions. (a) LPCVD deposition of SiO_2 over rectangular line. (b) HDPCVD deposition, with directed ionic flux and angle-dependent sputtering, over rectangular line showing much more planar topography. (c) LPCVD deposition in trench, showing void formation. (d) HDPCVD deposition in trench, showing much better filling.

ratio structures. The use of standard PECVD oxide deposition can help with the filling of gaps and spaces. With its directional ion component [Eq. (9.54)] which can be approximately equal in magnitude to the purely chemical component for oxide deposition [9.34], a little better filling of the gap occurs as compared to LPCVD deposition. But a void still results for this aspect ratio gap (though slightly higher up in the gap) and gets worse as the aspect ratio increases (see Figure 9–3). Using TEOS/O_3 films or the dep/etch/dep method can also improve the filling.

In Figure 9–50(d) we show how HDP deposition completely fills the gap, doing the same simulation with the trench structure but with the HDP model. No voids are formed. This is due to a combination of the highly directed ion flux component of deposition and the angle-dependent sputtering action. The deposition is very directed, and any overhang that does develop on the top corners is sputtered away, preventing any shadowing due to an overhang. Redeposition of sputtered material also helps with coverage and preventing voids. This is obviously a very attractive technique for filling narrow spaces with dielectric material. Simulations show that void-free depositions can result even for aspect ratios of 3:1 and higher [9.4]. Actual SEM images of HDP deposition of SiO_2 were shown earlier in Figure 9–34 illustrating the filling and planarizing abilities of HDP deposition.

We next describe some PVD simulations. The standard PVD deposition SPEEDIE model uses Eq. (9.55). This is identical to that used for LPCVD, but usually different values for the sticking coefficient and the arrival angle distribution are used, as discussed earlier. In the first simulation we deposit Al onto a very narrow SiO_2 via structure with an aspect ratio of about 3, indicative of more advanced technology. We use parameter values more typical of PVD (sputter deposition) here. For S_c, we use 1. For the arrival angle distribution, we assume a $\cos^n\theta$ distribution with $n = 4$ (at the high end for standard sputter depositions), giving a more directed incoming flux than LPCVD systems. In this case, we specify that the hole is a via (a cylinder) rather than a trench, as was the case in the LPCVD simulations shown earlier. SPEEDIE calculates slightly different normalized direct fluxes because of this, and a via is generally harder to fill than a trench. The simulation results are shown in Figure 9–51(a). Very little Al is deposited inside the narrow via. Even though the flux is somewhat more directed than in LPCVD systems, the shadowing effect and the absence of any reemission (or resputtering) and redepositing of material allow very little material to be deposited in and on the bottom of such high-aspect ratio vias.

We next simulate ionized PVD, or IPVD, of Al. We assume that 80% of the Al atoms being deposited are ionized. For the un-ionized atoms, we assume a $\cos^n\theta$ distribution with $n = 4$. But for the ionized Al, we use a $\cos^n\theta$ distribution with n equal to 80. Eq. (9.57) is used for the local deposition rate, similar to the HDPCVD case [Eq. (9.58)]. We use typical parameter values for PVD, such as a sticking coefficient of 1. The same sputtering yield dependence is used as was used in the HDPCVD simulation, that is, with a

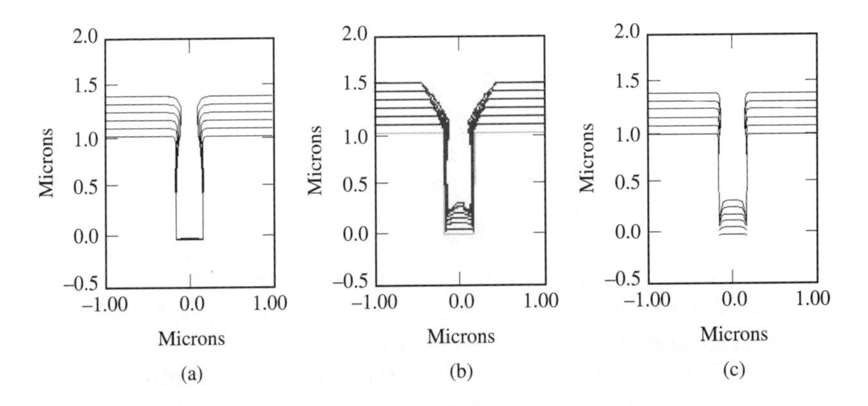

Figure 9–51 SPEEDIE simulations for sputtering (PVD) and ionized sputtering (IPVD) deposition of Al. (a) conventional PVD deposition with $S_c = 1$ and $n = 4$. (b) IPVD deposition with 80% of Al atoms being ionized (with near vertical arrival angles) and angle-dependent sputtering yield, showing much better filling of narrow via. (c) IPVD with no resputtering.

maximum sputtering yield at 62°. The simulation is shown in Figure 9–51(b). Two differences from the standard PVD simulation are evident. First, the bottom of the via gets filled much more than the standard PVD case. This is due to the very narrow (and vertical) ion angle distribution and is the reason why ionized PVD is an attractive alternative to standard PVD for some applications, such as for Ti or TiN deposition in today's deep contacts and vias. The second difference is the sloped sides at the top corners. This is due to the resputtering action, which not only bevels the corners but also redeposits material elsewhere. Resputtering from the bottom also occurs.

To see the effect of the resputtering and redeposition, another simulation is done. Everything is the same as in the first IPVD case except that the sputtering is turned off. The results are shown in Figure 9–51(c). With the very directed Al ion flux, a good amount of Al gets deposited down into the hole. But without the sputtering, the top corners are no longer sloped. The shadowing from the top corners and the lack of redeposition result in virtually no coverage on the sides of the via. Coverage on the side of a via or trench is often important, for example when depositing a TiN liner in a via, and the sputtering and redeposition action in IPVD is seen to help with this, especially at higher ion energies [9.14, 9.35].

In the final SPEEDIE simulations, High-Temperature PVD (or HTPVD) of Al in a trench is simulated. Eq. (9.56) is used in the HTPVD model. This includes the flux term that is due to surface diffusion driven by surface energy reduction, causing reflow during the deposition. For comparison we first show a standard PVD deposition into a trench, equivalent to setting the surface diffusivity in the HTPVD model to zero, in Figure 9–52(a). Next we do a HTPVD deposition with the deposition temperature specified to be 400°C, which determines the surface diffusion coefficient. The surface diffusivity and energy are taken from [9.38]. The resulting SPEEDIE simulated profile is shown in Figure 9–52(b).

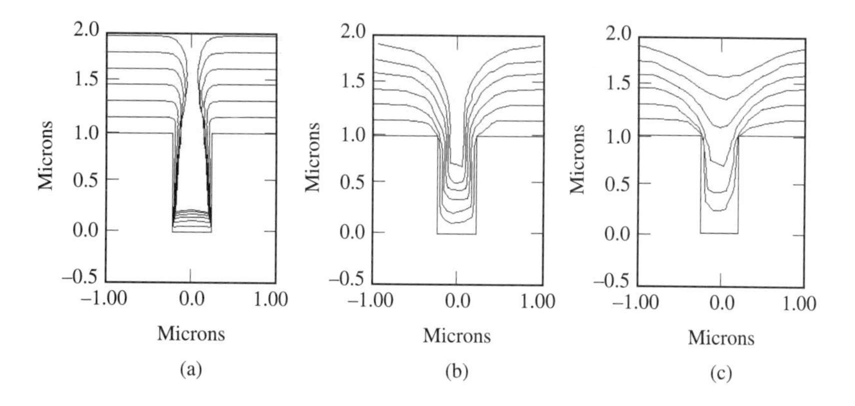

Figure 9–52 SPEEDIE simulations for High-Temperature PVD (HTPVD). (a) Standard PVD deposition with $S_c = 1$, $n = 4$, for comparison, showing poor filling. (b) HTPVD with surface diffusion at a deposition temperature of 400°C. Better filling is seen with the HTPVD. (c) HTPVD again but at a higher deposition temperature of 550°C, showing even more reflow during deposition than in (b), and even better filling and a smoother topography.

One can see that with the surface diffusion, much better filling of the hole and better step or sidewall coverage occur. Next we raise the deposition temperature even more to 550°C, resulting in a higher surface diffusivity, and the results are shown in Figure 9–52(c). The hole is completely filled, and much better planarization of the metal layer results. One can see from these simulations the advantages of high-temperature PVD deposition. More simulations involving surface diffusion driven reflow will be presented in Chapter 11. In that case, reflow of the metal after deposition will be simulated.

9.5.3 Other Deposition Simulations

We now describe some simulations done with a commercially available simulation tool. Here we use Silvaco's ATHENA simulator (using the ELITE topography tool) to simulate deposition of CVD SiO_2 and sputtered Al. While most of Silvaco's front-end simulation models for diffusion, oxidation, and so forth, are directly based on SUPREM IV models, the deposition and etch models used here and in the next chapter from ATHENA (many based on models originally in the SAMPLE simulator [9.39]) are more empirical in nature than SPEEDIE's models, and more user friendly. For example, instead of the user specifying the various fluxes, the user specifies the deposition rate and various parameters to obtain the shape and type of deposition profile.

First the ATHENA CVD deposition model is illustrated. Here the deposition rate, time, and step coverage are the input parameters. In the first simulation where we deposit oxide into a trench, the step coverage parameter is designated to be 1. This means that the same thickness is deposited everywhere. The resulting profile is shown in Figure 9–53(a). Next the step coverage is set to 0.2 instead of 1. The deposition rate, R, for the CVD model is given by:

$$R = dep.rate((1 - step.cov)\cos\theta + step.cov) \tag{9.59}$$

where θ is the angle between the surface segment and the horizontal. For a *step.cov* term less than 1, this results in the full deposition rate on horizontal surfaces (where $\theta = 0$),

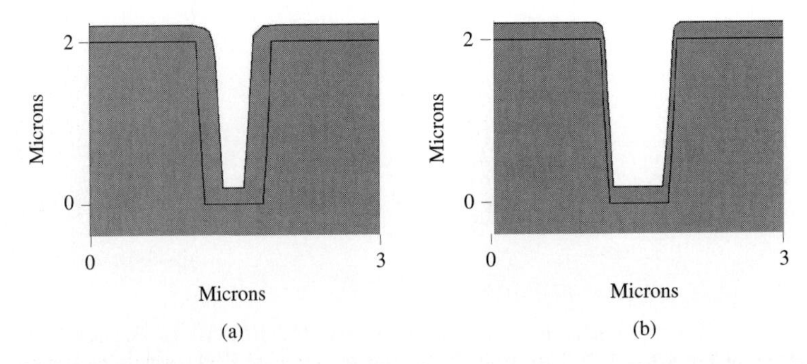

Figure 9–53 Silvaco's ATHENA [9.40] topography simulation of SiO_2 CVD deposition in a via for different values of the step coverage parameter, step.cov, selected by the user: (a) step coverage parameter = 1; (b) step coverage parameter = 0.2.

but less deposition on nonhorizontal surfaces. The result for the step coverage parameter equaling 0.2 is shown in Figure 9–53(b), exhibiting nonconformal coverage. Similar trends in step coverage using SPEEDIE were obtained by varying the value of the sticking coefficient in Figures 9–47(b) and 9–48(b).

The next example simulates the deposition of sputtered or evaporated Al using one of the Silvaco PVD models, the hemispheric deposition model. Here the incoming material flux arrives within a range of directions, coming from an extended, but limited, source such as in a planar sputtering system. The two angles designated by the user are the limits within which the flux is uniformly distributed. In this first case, the flux arrives at angles from 10 to -10 degrees from the normal to the substrate. The growth rate at each point is calculated after [9.41] by

$$R = C(\cos\omega_1 - \cos\omega_2)i + C(\sin\omega_1 - \sin\omega_2)j \tag{9.60}$$

where C is the deposition rate of an unshadowed surface normal to the flux direction, ω_1 and ω_2 are the upper and lower bounds of angles, and i and j are the unit vectors in the x and y directions, respectively. Figure 9–54(a) shows the simulation for such a deposition. One can see the directed deposition with most of the film being deposited on the horizontal surfaces. This is different from the ATHENA CVD model with a low step coverage value shown in the previous example in that now shadowing, overhangs, and cusping are observed on the corners. Figure 9–54(b) shows the result when the upper and lower angles are 45 and -45 degrees. More uniform deposition is observed, with more film deposited on the sidewalls, and less on the bottom of the trench. This model is similar to the SPEEDIE PVD model in which the distribution of arrival angles is controlled by the n term in the $\cos^n\theta$ distribution. However, unlike the SPEEDIE model, the sticking coefficient cannot be specified. The upper and lower bounds of angles used will depend on machine specifications, such as source and wafer geometry and characteristics, and operating pressure.

With this model one could also simulate asymmetric depositions such as might occur at the edge of a wafer in an evaporation system with a small source or in a sputtering

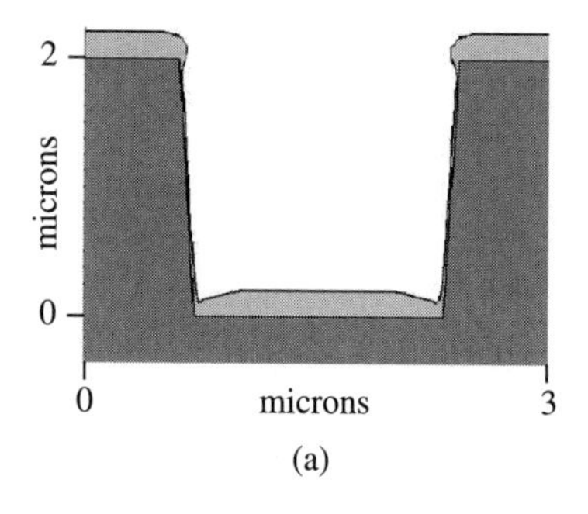

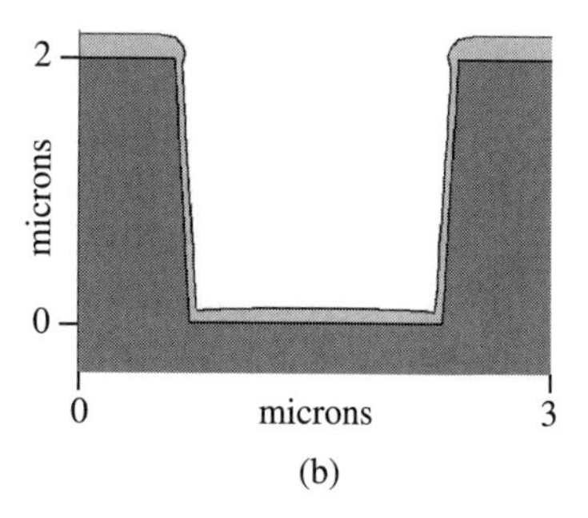

Figure 9–54 Silvaco's ATHENA [9.40] topography simulation of Al PVD deposition in a wide trench using the hemisphere model for different ranges of arrival angles: (a) the arrival angles are from -10 to $+10°$; (b) the arrival angles are from -45 to $+45°$. The wider angle range results in better step coverage, similar to a low n value in SPEEDIE's arrival angle distribution function.

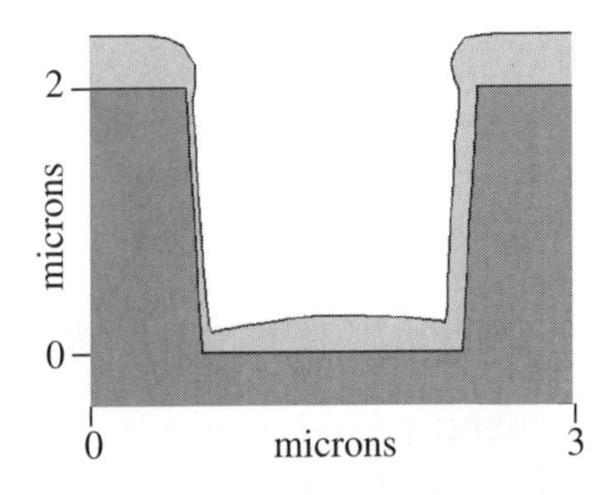

Figure 9–55 Silvaco's ATHENA [9.40] topography simulation of Al PVD deposition in a wide trench using the hemisphere model for asymmetric arrival angles: −25 to +45°. Asymmetric deposition is seen, as might be the case for the right side edge of a wafer in a PVD system with a small source or target.

system with a relatively small target, such as in a long-throw collimation system. In that case the absolute value of the two angles in the hemispheric deposition model could be different. Figure 9–55 shows an ATHENA simulation in which the upper angle is 45° and the lower angle is −25°. Asymmetric deposition is clearly seen in the profile.

The advantages of these models are their ease of use, as well as the ease of calibrating them. For a certain piece of deposition equipment, a given material to be deposited, and specific deposition conditions, one matches the profiles of some test structures to the simulations by varying the model parameters. One can then build up a library of deposition equipment, materials, and normal deposition conditions to use in simulations. Model parameter libraries of various commonly used pieces of deposition and etch equipment with model parameters for various films and normal operating conditions are often included with these simulators [9.40]. One can easily use these models to optimize the deposition process without worrying about all the details of the process.

The advantage of the SPEEDIE-type models is that they are more physically correct and the parameters are more closely linked to actual processes and mechanisms. One inputs the actual flux information in terms of flux rate, type, angular distribution. In addition one specifies physical properties such as sticking coefficients, surface diffusivities, sputtering and reemission coefficients, and the like. The models then calculate the combined effects of the various processes and phenomena in a 2D/3D structure. Obviously, these types of models are more apt to be valid for conditions outside those for which they are calibrated and tested. It should be noted that Silvaco and other commercial simulation tool vendors such as Avant! [9.42] also now offer other deposition and etch models which are less empirical and more physically based, such as those using Monte Carlo calculations. Avant!, for example, in their commercially available TAURUS-TOPOGRAPHY deposition and etch simulator, offers both the simpler, more empirical models as well as models and algorithms similar to those in SPEEDIE involving actual direct and indirect flux calculations. Silvaco has developed such models as well.

Models have also been developed for deposition processes that take into account the specific chemical reactions in CVD systems and the mechanisms for how ion bombardment enhances the deposition rate in plasma systems (see [9.43] to see this how all this has recently been done for HDPCVD of SiO_2, which considers 167 gas-phase reactions and 96 surface reactions!). These, or parts of these models, are sometimes incorporated into physically based simulators to make them even more complete.

9.6 Limits and Future Trends in Technologies and Models

A major problem that process developers face as the technology advances is the ever-increasing aspect ratios of the features. Depositing into smaller, deeper holes and spaces will only get more difficult. The NTRS roadmap [9.44] projects that the aspect ratios of metal lines, the spaces between the lines, and the via and contacts holes will all continue to increase over the next generations. (This is primarily due to the metal thicknesses not shrinking as fast as the lateral dimensions.) This means that the spaces and holes will get smaller and relatively deeper. We saw in this chapter how good coverage and filling are more difficult as the aspect ratio increases. High-density plasma deposition systems have proven successful in filling spaces between metal lines with oxide, and continued use and development of these types of systems are likely. New processes such as dual damascene described in Chapter 11, could place less importance on filling spaces with dielectrics in the future. Most metal films are still being deposited by sputtering techniques. The trend has been to try to use CVD because better filling and conformal step coverage are often achieved by CVD. However there are still problems with CVD deposition of metals which must be solved. These include contamination (impurities, such as carbon, from the precursors mostly) and difficulty with alloys (Al with Cu, for example). A PECVD process for Ti using $TiCl_4$ for filling small holes has recently been announced by one of the equipment manufacturers. New sputter techniques such as ionized, collimated, and hot-sputter depositions have been developed for metal deposition in high aspect ratio features. Future processes may use electroplating and spin-on methods for metals and dielectrics respectively. A potentially new type of deposition involves layer by layer adsorption and reaction of reactant species on the surface, utilizing sequentially pulsed precursors and self-limiting reactions for example. Commonly called Atomic Layer Deposition, or ALD, this can result in extremely conformal coverage of very thin layers.

A trend in deposition equipment is the use of cluster tools. Here various deposition (and etch) steps are performed sequentially with the wafers passed automatically from one process chamber to another, without breaking vacuum. As a result multiple deposition and etch steps can be done without exposing the wafers to the atmosphere between steps. This minimizes exposure of the wafers to ambient particulate contamination and surface oxidation. It also minimizes wafer handling as well as increases throughput. Both PVD and CVD chambers can be connected sequentially, as well as plasma etch chambers. Most of these tools are single-wafer, as opposed to batch, systems. More control over each wafer is possible, but the deposition rates must be high since each wafer must be processed individually. Depositing films on one wafer at a time does give a little more flexibility in choosing deposition conditions. For example, one can operate in the mass transfer regime in CVD deposition since gas-phase mass transfer is easier to control in a single wafer system.

In regards to modeling and simulation, we have been mostly concerned in this chapter with topology. That is, we discussed models and simulations that predict the shape of the deposited films over nonplanar underlying topography—over steps or in vias for example. These have been useful in explaining some of the basic concepts of deposition and the different types of equipment. However, there are other important properties of the deposited films, such as grain structure, composition, density, mechanical properties, and stress. It is important to model these physical and compositional properties as a function of deposition technique and conditions, as these will affect the film behavior and performance during subsequent processing and operation.

There have been deposition models and simulators developed for physical and compositional properties. An example is the SIMBAD/GROFILMS [9.45, 9.46] group that simulate as-deposited film structure. In SIMBAD, two-dimensional discs rather than atoms or molecules are used in simulating deposition, with each disc representing about 1000 atoms. In these Monte Carlo simulations, regions of dense, closely packed discs form and evolve into a columnar grain structure—the grains separated by the less dense grain boundaries. The exact structure depends on the amount of surface diffusion and flux shadowing, consistent with Thorton's zone model for microstructure evolution [9.47]. (For a good discussion of zone models for microstructure, see [9.48].) GROFILMS extends this modeling to include other processes that can occur during deposition such as wetting, reflow, grain boundary grooving, and crystal facetting. Many of these processes will be discussed in Chapter 11. Deposition simulators that include modeling the physical structure and composition of thin films will be increasingly important in the future.

Making the models more physically correct by including the chemistry and physics of specific deposition systems is important. The use of atomic-level models and simulators could also greatly help in developing more physically correct models. Simulations using Monte Carlo or Molecular Dynamics (MD) calculations, based on atomic-level, first principles models, have already revealed new insights into the deposition processes, as they have in oxidation, diffusion, and implantation modeling. The goal is to make these simulations more efficient and scalable to realistic dimensions and number of atoms. In addition they need to be linked to higher-level, continuum-type simulation tools to make their results more easily accessible.

9.7 Summary of Key Ideas

In this chapter we have examined how thin films are deposited as part of the fabrication of integrated circuits. Important issues in thin film deposition include the physical and chemical properties of the film, and coverage of nonplanar underlying topography, including step coverage and the filling of holes or spaces. Coverage and filling issues are especially important with the ever-decreasing lateral feature sizes, as well as with the increasing use of multilayer film structures.

The two main deposition techniques are Chemical Vapor Deposition (CVD) and Physical Vapor Deposition (PVD). CVD depositions are mostly done at elevated temperatures and are chemical reaction based. In the simple model for CVD presented, the deposition process is seen to be limited by the surface reactions or by mass transfer through a gas-phase boundary layer depending on the temperature, pressure, and system chemistry. At low pressures, mass transfer through the boundary layer is not a limiting step, and the surface reactions become rate limiting, allowing for fewer constraints on reactor geometry. However, shadowing by surface topographical features must still be considered to model coverage and fill profiles. In PVD, the processes are physically, rather than chemically, based. Arrival angle distribution of the source material at the wafer surface is important. There are fewer gas-phase collisions between the source and the wafer and virtually no reactions on the surface, so the species can arrive more vertical to the wafer from the source and stick where they hit without desorbing and redepositing. Shadowing by topographical features can be very important in PVD depositions. Many different types of both CVD and PVD systems have evolved and are still being used for different applications and different types of films. Other deposition techniques include spin-on techniques for dielectrics and electrolytic deposition of metals.

Most simulation of thin film deposition is based on topography modeling, that is, predicting the shape of the deposited film over nonplanar topography. SPEEDIE is one such topography simulator for both CVD and PVD. Both direct and indirect fluxes of neutral and ionic species are used to model the deposition process in low pressure systems. The direct fluxes are modeled by the arrival angle distribution. Indirect fluxes are due to surface or near-surface processes, such as surface diffusion or reemission and resputtering of surface species with subsequent deposition elsewhere. The sticking coefficient is used to model the reemission process. CVD processes, used mostly for dielectrics, in general have a low sticking coefficient and isotropic arrival angle distribution, leading to good step coverage. A low sticking coefficient also leads to better filling of holes. PVD processes, used more for metals, have a high sticking coefficient. A narrower arrival angle distribution, more characteristic of PVD processes leads to worse coverage over a step but can result in better filling of the bottoms of holes. Concurrent sputtering and redeposition of material along with the directed deposition of ionized species can lead to good gap or hole filling of relatively high aspect ratio features in either PVD or CVD systems, such as in ionized sputtering or HDPCVD. Simulations show the importance of different components and different parameters, especially in terms of arrival angle, sticking coefficient, angle-dependent sputtering, and coverage and filling issues.

9.8 References

[9.1]. F. C. Eversteyn, "Chemical-Reaction Engineering in the Semiconductor Industry," *Philips Res. Rep.*, vol. 29, p. 45, 1974.

[9.2]. A.S. Grove, *Physics and Technology for Semiconductor Devices*, John Wiley & Sons, 1967, p. 12.

[9.3]. T. J. Rogers, "Advanced Integrated Circuit Technology for Micropower Integrated Circuits," Ph.D. thesis, Stanford University, 1975.

[9.4]. J. Li, "Topography Simulation of Intermetal Dielectric Deposition and Interconnection Metal Deposition Processes," Ph.D. thesis, Stanford University, 1996.

[9.5]. J. Li, J. P. McVittie, J. Ferziger, K. C. Saraswat, and J. Dong, "Optimization of Intermetal Dielectric Deposition Module Using Simulation," *J. Vac. Sci. Tech. B*, vol. 13, p. 1867, 1995.

[9.6]. M. Ohring, *The Materials Science of Thin Films*, Academic Press, 1992, p. 90.

[9.7]. *Handbook of Thin Film Technology*, L. I. Maissel and R. Glang, eds., McGraw-Hill, 1970.

[9.8]. M. Knudsen, "Die Verdampfung von Kristalloberflachen," *Ann. Physik*, vol. 52, p. 105, 1917.

[9.9]. R. Siegel and J. R. Howell, *Thermal Radiation Heat Transfer,* 3d ed., Hemisphere Pub. Corp., 1992.

[9.10]. S. A. Campbell, *The Science and Engineering of Microelectonic Fabrication*, Oxford University Press, 1996, p. 284.

[9.11]. B. N. Chapman, *Glow Discharge Processes*, John Wiley & Sons, 1980.

[9.12]. M. A. Lieberman and A. J. Lichtenberg, *Principles of Plasma Discharges and Materials Processing,* John Wiley and Sons, 1994.

[9.13]. A. A. Mayo, S. Hamaguchi, J. H. Joo, and S. M. Rossnagel, "Across-Wafer Nonuniformity of Long Throw Sputter Deposition," *J. Vac. Sci. Tech. B.*, vol. 15. p. 1788, 1997.

[9.14]. S. Hamaguchi and S. M. Rossnagel, "Liner Conformality Ionized Magnetron Sputter Metal Deposition Process," *J. Vac. Sci. Tech. B*, vol. 14, p. 2603, 1996.

[9.15]. S. M. Rossnagel, "Ionized Magnetron Sputtering for Lining and Filling Trenches and Vias," *Semiconductor International,*" February 1996, p. 99.

[9.16]. G. A. Dixit, M. F. Chisholm, M. K. Jain, T. Weaver, L. M. Ting, S. Poarch, K. Mizobuchi, R. H. Havemann, C.D. Dobson, A. I. Jeffryes, P. J. Holverson, P. Rich, D. C. Butler, and J. Hems, "A Novel High Pressure Low Temperature Aluminum Plug Technology for Sub – 0.5 Micron Contact/Via Geometries," *IEDM Technical Digest*, 1994, p. 105.

[9.17]. T. Kamins, *Polycrystalline Silicon for Integrated Circuit Applications,* 2d ed., Kluwer Academic Publishers, 1998.

[9.18]. P. Joubert, "The Effect of Low Pressure on the Structure of LPCVD Polycrystalline Si Films," *J. Electrochem. Soc.*, vol. 134, p. 2541, 1987.

[9.19]. R. Falckenberg, E. Doering, and H. Oppolzer, "Surface Roughness and Grain Growth of Thin P-Doped Polycrystalline Si-Films," *Proc. of Fall 1979 Electrochem. Soc. Meeting* (Los Angeles, October 1979), abstract 570, p. 1492.

[9.20]. H. J. Kim and C.V. Thompson, "Kinetic Modeling of Grain Growth in Polycrystalline Silicon Films Doped with Phosphorus or Boron," *J. Electrochem. Soc.*, vol. 135, p. 2312, 1988.

[9.21]. M. M. Manduarh, K. C. Saraswat, and T. I. Kamins, "Phosphorus Doping of Low Pressure Chemically Vapor-Deposited Silicon Films," *J. Electrochem. Soc.,* vol. 126, p. 1019, 1979.

[9.22]. S. Robles, K. Russell, M. Galiano, V. Siva, V. Kithcart, and B. C. Nguyen, "Gap Fill and Film Reflow Capability of Subatmospheric Chemical Vapor Deposited Borophosphosilicate Glass," *J. Electrochem. Soc.*, vol. 143. p. 1414, 1996.

[9.23]. L. Q. Xia, E. Yieh, P. Gee, F. Campana, and B. C. Nguyen, "Process Characteristics for Subatmospheric Chemical Vapor Deposited Borophophosilicate Glass and Effect of Carrier Gas," *J. Electrochem. Soc.,* vol. 144. p. 3208, 1997.

[9.24]. E. Kondoh, Y. Kawano. N. Takeyasu, T. Katagiri, H. Yamamoto, and T. Ohta, "Interconnection Formation by Simultaneous Cu Doping in CVD Al (Al-Cu CVD)," *IEDM Technical Digest*, p. 277, 1993.

[9.25]. D. Pramanik and V. Jain, "Barrier Metals for ULSI: Deposition and Manufacturing," *Solid State Technology,* January 1993, p. 73.

[9.26]. R. Liu, "Metallization," in *ULSI Technology*, ed. C.Y. Chang and S. M. Sze, McGraw-Hill, NY, 1996, p. 388.

[9.27]. J. Li, T. E. Seidel, and J. W. Mayer, "Copper-based Metallization in ULSI Structures," *MRS Bulletin*, vol. 19, no. 8, p. 15, 1994.

[9.28]. Y. Shacham-Diamand, V. Dubin, and M. Angyal, "Electroless Copper Deposition for ULSI," *Thin Solid Films*, vol. 262, p. 93, 1995.

[9.29]. SPEEDIE 3.0 Manual, Stanford University, 1995.

[9.30]. K. Watanabe and H. Komiyama, "Micro/Macrocavity Method Applied to the Study of the Step Coverage Formation Mechanism of SiO_2 Films by LPCVD," *J. Electrochem. Soc.*, vol. 137, p. 1222, 1990.

[9.31]. H. C. Wulu, K. C. Saraswat, and J. P McVittie, "Simulation of Mass Transport for Deposition in Via Holes and Trenches," *J. Electrochem. Soc.*, vol. 138, p. 1831, 1991.

[9.32]. J. C. Rey, L. Y. Cheng, J. P. McVittie, and K. C. Saraswat, "Monte Carlo Low Pressure Deposition Profile Simulations," *J. Vac. Sci. Tech. A*, vol. 9, p. 1083, 1991.

[9.33]. L. Y. Cheng, J. P McVittie, and K. C. Saraswat, "New Test Structure to Identify Step Coverage Mechanisms in CVD of Silicon Dioxide," *Appl. Phys. Lett.*, vol. 58, p. 2147, 1991.

[9.34]. C. Y. Chang, "Experiments and Simulation of Plasma Deposition and Sputter Etching Processes," Ph.D. thesis, Stanford University, 1995.

[9.35]. David Bang, "Modeling and Simulation of Physical Vapor Deposition Systems for VLSI Metallization," Ph.D. thesis, Stanford University, 1997.

[9.36]. C. Y. Chang, J. P McVittie, J. Li, K. C. Saraswat, S. E. Lassig, and J. Dong, "Profile Simulation of Plasma Enhanced and ECR Oxide Deposition and Sputtering," *IEDM Technical Digest*, p. 853, 1993.

[9.37]. J.C. Rey, L.Y. Cheng, J.P. McVittie, and K.C. Saraswat, "Numerical Simulation of CVD Trench Filling Using a Surface Reaction Coefficient Model," *Proc. of Seventh Int'l. IEEE Multilevel Inter. Conf.*, Santa Clara, CA, June 1990, p. 425.

[9.38]. T. S. Cale, M. K. Jain, D. S. Taylor, R. L. Duffin, and C. J. Tracy, "Model for Surface Diffusion of Aluminum-(1.5%) Copper during Sputter Deposition," *J. Vac. Sci. Tech. B*, vol. B11, p. 311, 1993.

[9.39]. W. G. Oldham, An. R. Neureuther, C. Sung, J. L. Reynolds, and S. N. Nandgaonkar, "A General Simulator for VLSI Lithography and Etching Processes: Part II—Application to Deposition and Etching," *IEEE Trans. Elec. Dev.*, vol. ED-27, p. 1455, 1980.

[9.40]. ATHENA is a process simulator from Silvaco Inc.

[9.41]. I. A. Blech, "Evaporated Film Profiles Over Steps in Substrates," *Thin Solid Films*, vol. 6. p. 113, 1970.

[9.42]. TAURUS-TOPOGRAPHY is a topography simulator from Avant! Inc.

[9.43]. E. Meeks, R. S. Larson, P. Ho, C. Apblett, S. M. Han, E. Edelberg, and E. S. Aydil, "Modeling of SiO_2 Deposition in High Density Plasma Reactors and Comparisons of Model Predictions with Experimental Measurements," *J. Vac. Sci. Tech. A*, vol. 16, p. 544, 1998.

[9.44]. "National Technology Roadmap for Semiconductors," SIA, 1997.

[9.45]. S. K. Dew, T. Smy, and M. J. Brett, "Simulation of Elevated Temperature Al Metalization Using SIMBAD," *IEEE Trans. Elec. Dev.*, vol 39, p. 1599, 1992.

[9.46]. L. J. Frederick, S. K. Dew, M. Brett, and T. Smy, "Thin Film Microstructure Modelling Through Line-Segment Simulation," *Thin Solid Films*, vol. 266, p. 83, 1995.

[9.47]. J. A. Thorton, "Influence of Apparatus Geometry and Deposition Conditions on the Stucture and Topology of Thick Sputtered Films," *J. Vac. Sci. Tech.*, vol. 11, p. 666, 1974.

[9.48]. M. Ohring, *The Materials Science of Thin Films*, Academic Press, 1992, p. 223 ff.

9.9 Problems

9.1. What would you expect would happen to the threshold voltage of a MOS transistor if the gate oxide were deposited using $SiH_4 + 2O_2 \rightarrow SiO_2 + 2H_2O$ rather than thermally grown?

9.2. What are the two commonly observed rate limiting steps in silicon epitaxial growth? Under what conditions do they normally dominate the overall deposition rate?

9.3. In an epitaxial deposition, under mass transfer limited conditions, is it more important to control the reactor temperature or the source gas composition in the gas stream to obtain reproducible results? Why?

9.4. In a reactor used for epitaxial growth, the wafers are normally placed flat on the susceptor, and epi grows on the top side only. If the same reactor were used to oxidize wafers, by introducing O_2 rather than SiH_4 (or another Si gas source), SiO_2 would grow on both sides of the wafer. Explain why SiO_2 grows on both sides and epi grows only on the top side.

9.5. For CVD deposition of a film, it is found that the mass transfer coefficient $h_G = 10$ cm sec^{-1} and the surface reaction rate coefficient $k_S = 1 \times 10^7 \exp(-1.9 \text{ eV}/kT)$ cm sec^{-1}. For a deposition at 900°C, which CVD system would you recommend using: (a) a cold-walled, graphite susceptor type: or (b) a hot-walled, stacked wafer type? Explain your answer.

9.6. Calculate the deposition rate for an LPCVD system with the same parameter values given in the example following Eq. (9.10), but at a reduced total pressure so that h_G is increased by 100 times. Assume that the partial pressure of the incorporating species, P_G, remains the same, and C_T decreases by the same factor as the total pressure.

9.7a. Plot the deposition rate (on a log scale) versus $1/T$ (Kelvin), for 600–1200°C, for a CVD system with the following parameter values:

$h_G = 0.5$ cm sec^{-1}

$k_S = 4 \times 10^6 \exp(-1.45 \text{ eV}/kT)$ cm sec^{-1}

Partial pressure of incorporating species = 1 torr

Total pressure = 1 atm

$C_T/N = 1/10{,}000$

Identify the reaction and mass transfer limited regimes.

b. Redo the problem when the total pressure is decreased to 1 torr, so that h_G increases by 100 times. Assume that the partial pressure of the incorporating species remains the same, and C_T decreases by the same factor as the total pressure.

9.8. Show that placing the source in an evaporation system at the inside surface of a sphere facing the center, with the wafers also at the inside surface of the sphere facing the center, leads to uniform deposition wafer to wafer, assuming a small planar surface source.

9.9. Calculate the deposition rate for a small planar surface evaporation source in which $\theta_i = 30°$, $\theta_k = 45°$, the evaporation rate is 1×10^{-3} gm sec^{-1}, the distance from the source to the wafer is 5 cm, and the density of the material being deposited equal 5 gm cm^{-3}.

9.10. The new deposition engineer installed the company's new evaporation system. Hoping to get uniform depositions on all the wafers mounted on the inside of the spherical wafer holder, he installed the evaporation source crucible at the center of the sphere. If the evaporation source behaves like an ideal small-area planar source, what will be the deposition rate as a function of θ, as defined below? (Let the evaporation rate equal 3×10^{-3} gm sec^{-1}, radius r_o equal 10 cm, and the density of the material being deposited equal 10 gm cm^{-3}.) Sketch a plot of d versus θ for θ from $-90°$ to $+90°$, and specify the deposition rate at a point directly facing the planar source (at $\theta = 0°$) and at $\theta = 90°$. Will uniform depositions result?

9.11. Calculate the mean free path of a particle in the gas phase of a deposition system

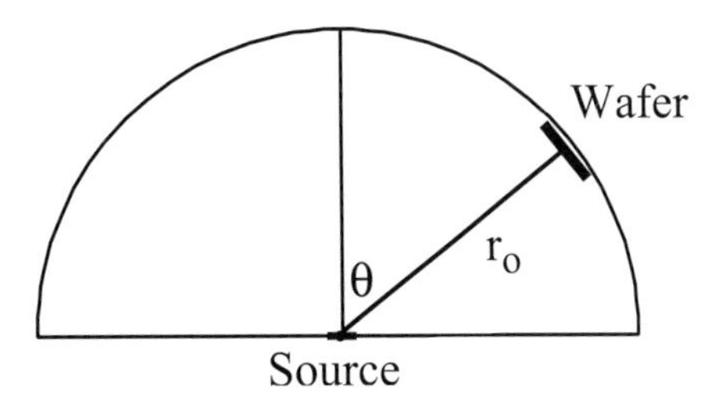

and estimate the number of collisions it experiences in traveling from the source to the substrate in each of the cases below. Assume that in each case the molecular collisional diameter is 0.4 nm, the source-to-substrate distance is 5 cm, and that the number of collisions is approximately equal to the source-to-substrate distance divided by the mean free path.

a. An evaporation system in which the pressure is 10^{-5} torr and the temperature is 25°C.

b. A sputter deposition system in which the pressure is 3 mtorr and the temperature is 25°C.

c. An LPCVD system in which the pressure is 1 torr and the temperature is 600°C.

d. An APCVD system in which the pressure is 1 atm and the temperature is 600°C.

9.12. a. Using schematic diagrams, show qualitatively how changing the gas pressure in a standard PVD system (using an appropriate S_c value for this type of system) can affect the deposition profile when depositing a material on a narrow trench structure.

b. In a similar fashion, show how changing the sticking coefficient affects the deposition profile when depositing a material on topography with a step.

9.13. How does the ability to fill the bottom of a narrow trench using sputter deposition change as the target is moved further away from the wafer? Neglect any gas phase collision effects.

9.14. Explain how asymmetric depositions can occur on a wafer in a sputter deposition system. Asymmetric deposition means that thicker deposition occurs on one side of a feature (a step or side of a trench, for example) than the other. Also suggest a way to decrease the asymmetry. Use schematic diagrams in your explanations.

9.15. What value of n in the arrival angle distribution is desired for good step coverage over a step in topography? For good bottom filling of a via? Explain with schematic diagrams. What value of S_C, the sticking coefficient, do you want in each case? Explain with diagrams.

9.16. We have seen how conformal coverage in low pressure systems results from a low sticking coefficient, which causes multiple reemission and redeposition processes within the feature topography. Describe how in atmospheric CVD systems, gas phase collisions by the reactants within the topograhical features can lead to good coverage and filling.

Etching

10

10.1 Introduction

After thin films are deposited on the wafer surface, they are usually selectively removed by etching to leave the desired pattern of the film on the wafer surface. This process was used many times in the CMOS process flow in Chapter 2 and is summarized in Figure 10–1. In addition to deposited films, parts of the silicon substrate itself may be etched, such as in creating trenches in isolation structures. The masking layer may be photoresist, or it may be another thin film such as silicon dioxide or silicon nitride. Oxide or nitride masks stand up better to etching conditions than photoresist and are often called hard masks. But they themselves must be selectively etched, usually using lithographically defined photoresist as the masking layer. The etching of a thin film is usually done until a different layer is reached underneath. Etching only partway through a layer without reaching an underlying material is sometimes done but can be difficult to control uniformly over the whole wafer. Multilayer structures can be etched sequentially using the same masking layer.

Etching can be done in either a "wet" or "dry" environment. Wet etching involves the use of liquid etchants. The wafers are usually immersed in the etchant solution and the exposed material is etched mostly by chemical processes. While such processes are not common in modern VLSI processing for reasons we shall see, they are sometimes used, as in Figure 2–34 in Chapter 2. Dry etching involves the use of gas-phase etchants in a plasma. Here the etching usually takes place by a combination of chemical and physical processes. Because a plasma is involved, dry etching is often called "plasma etching." This is normally the etching method today and was used many times in Chapter 2 (Figure 2–4 for example).

The ideal etch profile in Figure 10–1 has perfectly straight sidewalls exactly under the edge of the mask. What can happen in reality is shown in Figure 10–2. In Figure 10–2(a) the etching is both vertical and lateral. This leads to undercutting of the photoresist mask and nonvertical sidewalls in the film. In Figure 10–2(b) the photoresist is not perfectly rectangular, with rounded top corners and sloped sides. In addition, the etch rate of the photoresist is nonzero, and the mask itself is etched, or eroded, to some degree. This occurs both on its top and on its sides. This leads to even more lateral etching of the film since the photoresist mask gets narrower as the etching continues. If the substrate is attacked by the etchant as well, then its profile will change. Figure 10–2(b) also illustrates this issue, which is related to the selectivity of the etching process.

Etch selectivity is the ratio of the etch rates of the different materials in an etch process. When the etch rates of the mask and the underlying substrate are near zero,

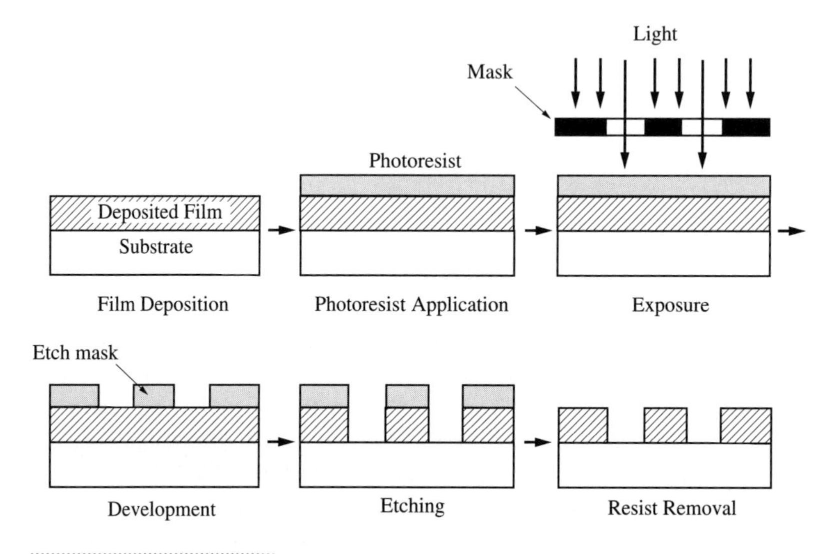

Figure 10–1 General process used in integrated circuit fabrication to define patterned films.

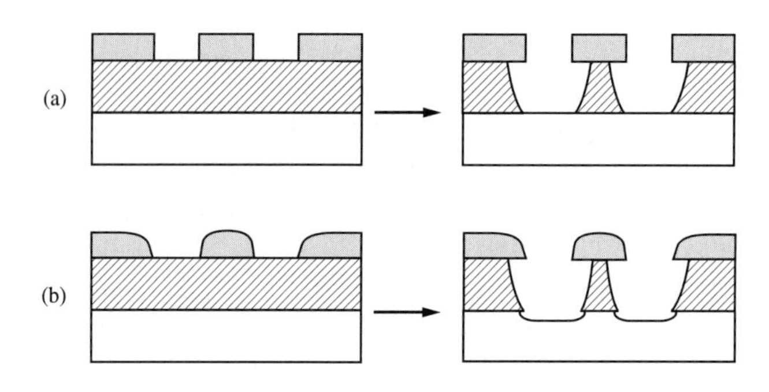

Figure 10–2 Actual etch profiles that can occur. (a) Lateral etching under mask. (b) Rounded photoresist which is further eroded during etching, leading to even more lateral etching. (b) also illustrates etch selectivity.

while the etch rate of the film is appreciable, then the etch selectivity of the film with respect to both the mask and the substrate is high. This is normally a desired situation. If the etch rate of the mask or substrate is significant, then the selectivity is poor. Selectivities, or etch rate ratios, in the range of 25–50 are usually considered reasonable. Different materials have different etch rates usually because of the chemical effects involved with etching, as opposed to the physical effects. Chemical reactions can be very selective whereas physical processes like sputtering tend to be similar for most materials.

Etch directionality is a measure of the relative etch rates in different directions, usually vertical versus lateral, as illustrated in Figure 10–3. Isotropic etching occurs when

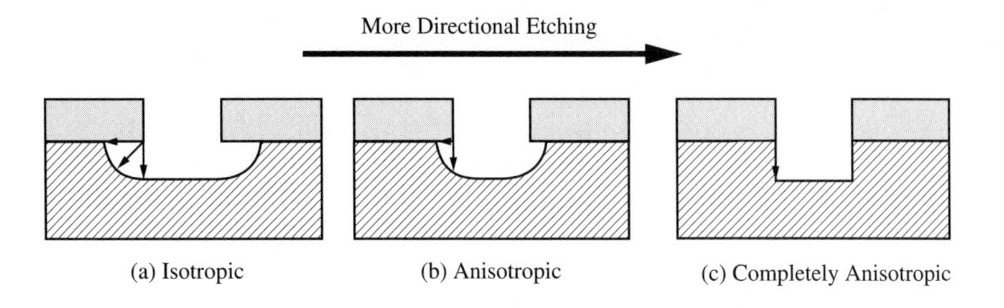

Figure 10–3 Etch profiles for different degrees of anisotropic, or directional, etching: (a) purely isotropic etching; (b) anisotropic etching; (c) completely anisotropic etching.

etch rates are the same in all directions, as in Figure 10–3(a). The etch distance laterally under each side of the mask is the same as vertically under the mask opening. As the opening under the mask approaches zero, the etch profile would approach a perfect semicircle. Figure 10–3(b) shows anisotropic etching, where less etching occurs laterally. Figure 10–3(c) shows completely anisotropic etching, with no etching at all in the lateral direction. Etch directionality is usually related to physical effects in etching such as ion bombardment and sputtering. As we shall see, the more physical an etch process is, the more directional and the less selective it generally is. On the other hand, the more chemical an etch process is, the more selective and the less directional it generally is.

Directionality is often desired in an etch process. Vertical etching maintains lithographically defined feature sizes as they are transferred by etching into underlying films. Vertical etching is also utilized in special applications such as sidewall spacer formation. (Recall Figure 2–30 in the CMOS process flow in Chapter 2.) However, vertical structures that result from vertical etching may also cause problems in subsequent processing. Depositing another layer on top of a structure with vertical steps may cause step coverage problems, as we discussed in Chapter 9. Less steep steps, obtained with less directional etching, would make it easier to obtain good step coverage and would allow easier filling in later deposited layers. Because of shrinking feature sizes, however, modern fabrication methods tend to employ directional etching and vertical steps with little undercutting, and use deposition techniques that achieve good filling and step coverage even for near-vertical structures.

Selectivity is also a requirement. This means that the etch rate of the layer to be etched should be fast compared to the etch rate of the mask and etch rate of the substrate or layer below. Achieving good selectivity and directional etching at the same time is sometimes quite difficult. Other requirements for an etch process are that the gases and liquids used for the etching must be able to be transported to the wafer surface, and the byproducts of the etch process must be transported away easily. The latter means that soluble byproducts are produced in wet etching, and that gaseous or volatile byproducts are produced in dry etching. The etch process should be uniform, safe to use, and should cause minimal damage to structures on the chip. Finally, the etching process should be clean, with low particulate production and little film contamination, and should be cost effective.

10.2 Historical Development and Basic Concepts

There are two main methods of etching used in the semiconductor industry: wet etching and dry, or plasma, etching. In the early days of the industry, wet etching was used exclusively. It was a well-established, simple, and inexpensive technology. Wet etching can also be very selective. Eventually, however, the need for smaller linewidths and more vertical structures required new techniques. Plasma etching methods were developed for integrated circuit fabrication and are used for most etching steps today.

In this section we will describe the basic concepts involved in both of these techniques. We will start with wet etching, which we will use to introduce concepts such as selectivity, overetch, etch bias, and anisotropy that are applicable to both wet and dry etching.

10.2.1 Wet Etching

The first etchants used in the integrated circuit industry were simple wet chemical etchants. By immersing the wafers into baths of liquid chemicals, the exposed films could be etched away, leaving unetched those regions of the film that were masked with photoresist or other films. Wet etches were developed for all steps in the fabrication process. A common wet etch for SiO_2 is hydrofluoric acid, HF. The overall reaction is

$$SiO_2 + 6HF \rightarrow H_2SiF_6 + 2H_2O \tag{10.1}$$

Wet etchants work through chemical processes rather than physical processes. In general, wet etchants work by chemically reacting with the film to form water-soluble byproducts or gases, such as the H_2SiF_6 byproduct which is a water-soluble complex in the above example.

In some cases the etching occurs by first oxidizing the surface of the film or material and then dissolving the oxide. For example, a common etchant for silicon is a mixture of nitric acid (HNO_3) and HF. The nitric acid partially decomposes to nitrogen dioxide, NO_2, which then oxidizes the surface of the silicon by the reaction

$$Si + 2NO_2 + 2H_2O \rightarrow SiO_2 + H_2 + 2HNO_2 \tag{10.2}$$

The HF then dissolves the SiO_2 by the reaction given in Eq. (10.1). The overall reaction is

$$Si + HNO_3 + 6HF \rightarrow H_2SiF_6 + HNO_2 + H_2O + H_2 \tag{10.3}$$

Buffering agents are often added to the etch solutions to keep the etchants at maximum strength over use and time. For example, ammonium fluoride (NH_4F) is added to HF to help prevent depletion of the fluoride ions in the oxide etch. This is called "Buffered HF" or BHF, or more commonly BOE for "Buffered Oxide Etch." The addition of ammonium fluoride also decreases the etch rate of photoresist and helps to minimize lifting of the resist during oxide etching. Acetic acid, CH_3COOH, is often added to the nitric acid/hydrofluoric acid silicon etch to limit the dissociation of the nitric acid.

Wet etches can be very selective because they depend on chemistry. The limiting steps in most etch processes are usually the chemical reactions in which the etch species react with the film, forming the soluble byproducts. The selectivity, S, of an etch process between two materials, 1 and 2, is simply the ratio of their etch rates, r, in that etchant, or

$$S = \frac{r_1}{r_2} \tag{10.4}$$

Material 1 is usually the film being etched, and material 2 is either the masking material (photoresist or perhaps silicon dioxide) or the material below the film. We often speak of an etch process for material 1 having a certain selectivity over (or "with respect to," or just "to") material 2. For a large selectivity ($S>>1$) we say that the etch process for material 1 has good selectivity over material 2.

Selectivity is important for a number of reasons. First, the selectivity for the material to be etched with respect to the mask determines how thick the mask material must be so that the mask is not completely removed during the etching process. Second, all etch processes generally employ some amount of overetching in order to ensure that the desired etching process has gone to completion. Thus underlying films are normally subjected to the etchant for some period of time toward the end of the etch period. The selectivity for the material being etched with respect to the underlying material determines how much etching of the underlying materials occurs.

Example 1 μm of SiO_2 is being etched on top of a Si substrate. The etch rate of the oxide is 0.40 μm min^{-1}, and the etch selectivity of the oxide with respect to the silicon is 25-to-1. If the etch is done for three minutes, how much of the underlying Si is etched?

Answer From Eq. (10.4), the etch rate of the Si can be calculated:

$$S = \frac{r_1}{r_2} \Rightarrow 25 = \frac{0.40\ \mu\text{m min}^{-1}}{r_{\text{Si}}} \Rightarrow r_{\text{Si}} = 0.016\ \mu\text{m min}^{-1}$$

The Si is only exposed to the etch after the overlying oxide is completely etched off. The time required to etch away the oxide equals 1 μm/0.40 μm min^{-1}, which equals 2.5 minutes. Therefore, the Si is etched for 0.5 minutes. Hence, the amount of Si etched is 0.016 μm min^{-1} * 0.5 min, which equals 0.008 μm, or 8 nm.

Most wet chemical etchants etch isotropically. The exceptions to this are those which are sensitive to crystallographic orientation. For example, some etchants etch much slower in the <111> direction in crystalline silicon as compared to the other directions. But most commonly used wet etches etch equally in all directions. In Figure 10–3(a) we saw how isotropic etching results in etching underneath the edge of the mask. The amount of undercutting is called the "etch bias." This is shown in Figure 10–4(a). Here we assume that the selectivity of the etch with respect to both the mask and the substrate is infinity (i.e., no etching at all of those materials). The etch thickness or depth is

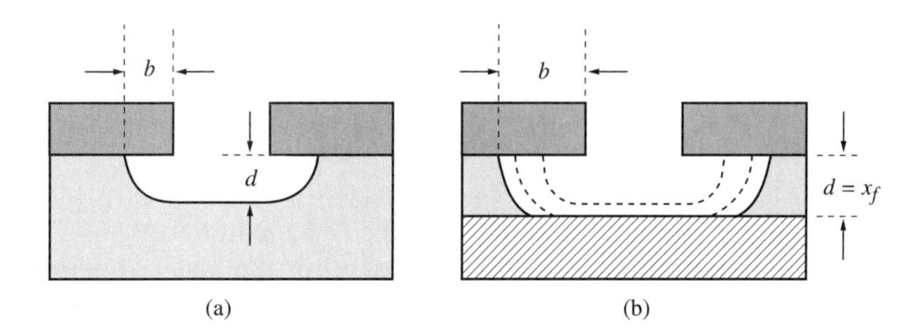

Figure 10–4 Illustration of etch bias and overetch. In (a) the etch bias, b, is shown for a given etch depth, d. In (b), overetching is illustrated where etching is continued even after the etch depth, d, equals the film thickness, x_f, with the result that the etch bias increases.

d and the bias is b. For perfectly isotropic etching b would equal d, but only if etching is stopped before the bottom of the film is reached.

As mentioned earlier, some overetching is normally part of every etch process. If each layer were of uniform thickness, and the etch were perfectly uniform through time and space, then overetching would theoretically not be needed. The etch time required would be based on the previously determined etch rate or on other endpoint detection methods, to be discussed later. It would not even matter what the etch selectivity over the layer beneath is in that case. However, the thickness of films is not perfectly uniform, and they do not always etch exactly uniformly. So some overetch is always done in manufacturing to ensure that the etch goes to completion everywhere. This is illustrated in Figure 10–4(b). In this figure we again assume that the selectivity with respect to the mask and substrate are infinite and that the etching is purely isotropic. The bias b now increases with time as the overetch continues. The amount of overetching needed, usually measured in terms of time or % time, can be determined by estimating the uncertainties in etch rates and in the nonuniformities of the thicknesses and then calculating the worst case etch time needed. Ten to twenty percent overetches are common. This ensures that while some of the structures may be overetched, none are underetched. We will see later that when the etching is anisotropic, overetching is also required to remove residual film from steps in the topography.

Example A 0.5-μm layer of silicon dioxide on a Si substrate needs to be etched down to the Si. Assume that the nominal oxide etch rate is r_{ox} (in μm min^{-1}). There is a ± 5% variation in the oxide thickness and a ± 5% variation in the oxide etch rate. (a) How much overetch is required (in % time) in order to ensure that all the oxide is etched? (b) What selectivity of the oxide etch rate to the Si etch rate is required so that a maximum of 5.0 nm of Si is etched? (Assume the overetch calculated in part (a) is done.)

Answer (a) The nominal etch time = x/r_{ox} = $0.5/r_{ox}$ (x = thickness in μm.) The overetch is done to make sure all the oxide is etched for the worst case condition; that means for the thickest oxide and the slowest etch rate. The thickest oxide =

$0.5 * 1.05 = 0.525$ μm. The slowest etch rate $= r_{ox} * 0.95$ μm min^{-1}. The time to etch the worst case $= x/r = 0.525/(r_{ox} * 0.95) = 0.553/r_{ox}$ min. The amount of overetch, in % time, is just the worst case etch time divided by the nominal etch time $= (0.553/r_{ox})/(0.5/r_{ox}) = 1.106$ or 10.6% overetch.

(b) The maximum amount of Si that will be etched will occur under the thinnest oxide being etched at the fastest etch rate. The thinnest oxide is $0.95 * 0.5$ μm $=$ 0.475 μm. The fastest etch rate is $r_{ox} * 1.05$ μm min^{-1}. The time to etch through that oxide is $x/r = 0.475/(r_{ox} * 1.05) = 0.4523/r_{ox}$ min. The time that the Si is exposed to the etch is equal to the total etch time ($0.553/r_{ox}$, as calculated in part (a)) minus the time it took to etch the thinnest oxide, etching at the fastest rate, or

$$(0.553/r_{ox}) - (0.4523/r_{ox}) = 0.1003/r_{ox} \text{ min}$$

We want to etch 0.005 μm or less of the Si, so

$$r_{Si} = x/\text{time} = 0.005/(0.1003/r_{ox}) \ \mu\text{m min}^{-1}$$
$$= 0.050 * r_{ox} \ \mu\text{m min}^{-1}$$

The selectivity of oxide etch rate to Si etch rate is therefore:

$$r_{ox}/r_{Si} = r_{ox}/(0.050 * r_{ox})$$
$$r_{ox}/r_{Si} = 20{:}1$$

Since overetching is usually done, it is important that the selectivity with respect to the layer below be as high as possible or else some etching of that layer will occur during the overetch. On the other hand, if the selectivity is very large, one cannot indiscriminately overetch. This would cause unwanted undercutting or bias.

The above examples assume infinite etch selectivity of the film with respect to the mask; that is, the etch rate of the mask is zero. But there will be some finite etch rate of the mask, which is usually photoresist. What will happen? Obviously the mask will etch at some rate during the etching of the film. This is shown in Figure 10–5(a) for the case of isotropic etching and a rectangular-shaped mask. Here Δm is the amount of mask etched, the same in all directions in this case. This is called mask erosion. Obviously the extent of lateral etching will increase beyond what would be expected without any mask erosion. For completely anisotropic (vertical) etching, etch erosion should not be a problem as long as the mask is perfectly rectangular in shape. The etch will only occur from the top. Only if the mask is etched all the way through would any difficulties arise.

In fact, the mask shape is usually not perfectly rectangular but often has rounded corners or sloped sides. Mask erosion leading to extra undercutting can occur even for completely anisotropic etching, as illustrated in Figure 10–5(b). With a finite etch rate for the mask, there will be equal vertical etching at all points of the mask. At the sloped edge, a finite amount of the mask will be etched away. This will allow lateral erosion of

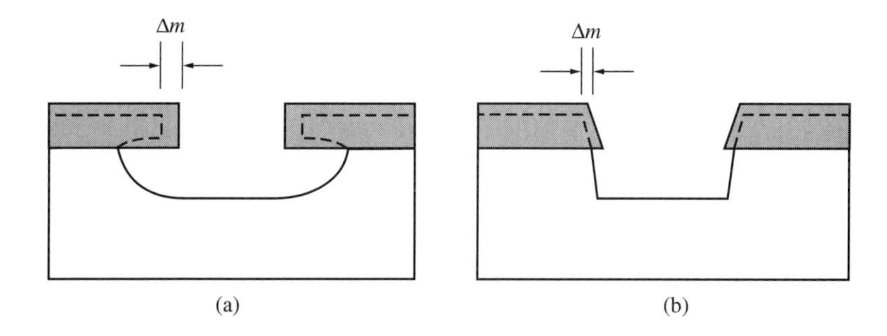

Figure 10–5 Illustration of mask erosion. In (a), there is an idealized rectangular mask and isotropic etching of the mask and the substrate. In (b), there is a sloped mask and anisotropic etching. In both cases more lateral etching of the substrate occurs as a result of the mask etching, or erosion.

the mask, shown by Δm in the figure, and etching of the film in this thin region will occur. This will result in undercutting with respect to the original mask edge, even for perfectly anisotropic, or vertical, etching.

Etching is often neither perfectly anisotropic nor perfectly isotropic, as was shown in Figure 10–3(b). We can define the degree of anisotropy of a film, A_f, as

$$A_f = 1 - \frac{r_{\text{lat}}}{r_{\text{ver}}} \tag{10.5}$$

where r_{lat} and r_{ver} are the etch rates in the lateral and vertical directions, respectively. In Figure 10–4, this would correspond to

$$A_f = 1 - \frac{b}{d} \tag{10.6}$$

Isotropic etching [Figure 10–3(a)] would have an anisotropy of 0, completely anisotropic etching [Figure 10–3(c)] would have an anisotropy of 1, and general anisotropic etching [Figure 10–3(b)] would have an anisotropy between 0 and 1. For a structure etched exactly to the bottom of the film, with no overetch, the anisotropy would be

$$A_f = 1 - \frac{b}{x_f} \tag{10.7}$$

where b is the bias and x_f is the film thickness.

Example Consider the structures shown in Figure 10–6. A 0.5-μm-thick oxide layer is etched to achieve equal structure widths and spacings (S_f). The etch process produces

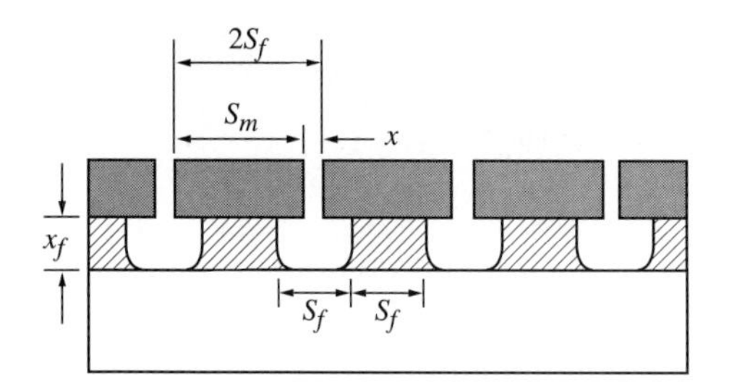

Figure 10–6 Structure and dimensions needed to fabricate features with equal widths and spaces (S_f) for a mask size of S_m, film thickness of x_f, and degree of anisotropy of A_f. x is the spacing between the masks and is usually the minimum lithographic feature. (After [10.1].)

a degree of anisotropy of 0.8. If the distance between the mask edges, x, is 0.35 μm, what structure spacings and widths are obtained? Neglect any overetch.

Answer To obtain equal widths and spacings, S_f, the mask width, S_m, must be made larger to take into account the anisotropic etching. Since

$$S_m = S_f + 2b$$

where b is the bias on each side, and using Eq. (10.6) we can now rewrite S_m as

$$S_m = S_f + 2x_f(1 - A_f)$$

which is the dimension of the mask needed. [This makes sense. For isotropic etching ($A_f = 0$), S_m is a maximum, and for completely anisotropic etching ($A_f = 1$), S_m is a minimum and equal to S_f.] The distance between the mask edges, x, is usually the minimum feature size that can be lithographically resolved. Since

$$x = 2S_f - S_m$$

x can be rewritten, using the expression above for S_m, as

$$x = S_f 2x_f(1 - A_f)$$

Rewriting this in terms of S_f gives

$$S_f = x + 2x_f(1 - A_f) \tag{10.8}$$

Plugging the above numbers into Eq. (10.8) gives

$$S_f = 0.35\mu m + 2(0.5\mu m)(1 - 0.8)$$
$$= 0.55\ \mu m$$

Eq. (10.8) shows that the structure size approaches the minimum lithographic dimension only when the film thickness gets very small (not always practical) or as the anisotropy gets close to 1. This means completely vertical etching. Unfortunately, wet etching does not result in vertical etching, but rather isotropic etching where A_f is a minimum. These considerations give some insight into the reasons wet chemical etching is not very commonly used in chip fabrication today.

Table 10–1 Common wet chemical etchants for various thin films used in IC fabrication

Material	Etchant	Comments
SiO_2	HF (49% in water) "straight HF"	Selective over Si (i.e., will etch Si very slowly in comparison). Etch rate depends on film density, doping.
	NH_4F:HF (6:1) "Buffered HF" or "BOE"	About $^1/_{20}$ th the etch rate of straight HF. Etch rate depends on film density, doping. Will not lift up photoresist like straight HF.
Si_3N_4	HF (49%)	Etch rate depends strongly on film density, O, H in film.
	H_3PO_4:H_2O (boiling @ 130–150°C)	Selective over SiO_2. Requires oxide mask.
Al	H_3PO_4:H_2O:HNO_3:CH_3COOH (16:2:1:1)	Selective over Si, SiO_2, and photoresist.
Polysilicon	HNO_3:H_2O:HF (+ CH_3COOH) (50:20:1)	Etch rate depends on etchant composition.
Single crystal Si	HNO_3:H_2O:HF (+ CH_3COOH) (50:20:1)	Etch rate depends on etchant composition.
	KOH:H_2O:IPA (23 wt. % KOH, 13 wt. % IPA)	Crystallographically selective; relative etch rates: (100): 100 (111): 1
Ti	NH_4OH:H_2O_2:H_2O (1:1:5)	Selective over $TiSi_2$.
TiN	NH_4OH:H_2O_2:H_2O (1:1:5)	Selective over $TiSi_2$.
$TiSi_2$	NH_4F:HF (6:1)	
Photoresist	H_2SO_4:H_2O_2 (125°C)	For wafers without metal.
	Organic strippers	For wafers with metal.

Before we describe techniques which do result in more anisotropic etching, we will look at some of the wet etch solutions that have been used, and are still used to some extent, in the Si integrated circuit industry. Table 10–1 gives a brief sampling of some of the common solutions and compositions.

The etch rate of a material in a particular etchant depends on the specific composition of the etch solution, and the etch rate can vary by orders of magnitude for different compositions of the same constituents. The rates of chemical reactions are strong functions of temperature, so the etch rates using wet, or chemical, etchants should be functions of temperature as well. For example, the etch rate of silicon dioxide in a 6:1 Buffered Oxide Etch (BOE) can change by a factor of two for a 10°C change in temperature [10.2].

Etch rates also depend on the composition and density of the films. For example, the etch rate of undoped, undensified CVD silicon dioxide in BOE is about 5 nm sec^{-1}, while the etch rate of phosphorus doped (8 atomic %) CVD silicon dioxide is about 9 nm sec^{-1}. On the other hand, the etch rate of densified (annealed at 800–1000°C), undoped CVD silicon dioxide is only about 1.5 nm sec^{-1}, the same as for thermal oxide. Clearly, the composition of the etchant and film, the density of the film, and the etch solution all affect the wet etch rates significantly.

The etch rate can also depend on the crystallographic orientation in some cases. In Table 10–1, the etch rates for two crystallographic directions in Si using KOH are given.

One sees that the etch rate for this etchant in the [100] direction is much faster than in the [111] direction, because the (111) planes are the most closely packed and etch more slowly. This can be used to form v-grooves on the surface of a (100) Si wafer because the {111} planes intersect the surface at a 54.7° angle.

10.2.2 Plasma Etching

While wet chemical etching was successfully used in the early days of integrated circuit manufacturing, it has been largely replaced by plasma, or dry, etching. There are two main reasons for this.

The first reason is that very reactive chemical species are produced in a plasma which can often etch more vigorously than species in a nonplasma environment. One of the first widespread uses of plasma etching was in the early 1970s to etch PECVD silicon nitride, used as the final passivation layer in integrated circuits. This film is difficult to etch with wet chemical etchants. Wet HF can etch it, but the etch rate is quite low, and the process is not selective with respect to SiO_2 which is often underneath. Boiling phosphoric acid was commonly used instead. But this etchant often lifts off photoresist masks so that a mask of SiO_2 has to be used, requiring its own masking and etching steps. A better etch process was sought. It was soon discovered that by using a CF_4/O_2 gas mixture in a plasma atmosphere, atomic fluorine is produced which can etch the nitride film much more easily. In addition, a photoresist mask is not lifted off in this process, making the process much simpler.

The second, and more important, reason why plasma etching has supplanted wet etching is the fact that directional or anisotropic etching is possible with plasma etch systems. Directional etching is needed to minimize underetching and etch bias, which then allows smaller and more tightly packed structures. This directional etching is due to the presence of ionic species in the plasma and the electric fields that direct them normal to the wafer surface.

Plasma etch systems can be designed so that either the reactive chemical components or the ionic components dominate. In many cases, a combination of ionic and reactive chemical species, usually acting in a synergistic manner, are utilized. The net etch rate can be much faster than the sum of the individual etch rates when they are acting alone. In addition, by utilizing both components this way, directionality can be achieved while maintaining an acceptable degree of selectivity.

A basic plasma etch system is shown schematically in Figure 10–7. This is similar to the PECVD and RF sputtering systems shown earlier in Figures 9–14 and 9–28. In these etch systems a low-pressure (1 mtorr – 1 torr) gas is used in the chamber. By applying a high electric field across two electrodes, some of the gas atoms are ionized, producing positive ions and free electrons and creating a plasma, as discussed in Chapter 9. In plasma etching systems, the energy is supplied by an RF generator, usually operating at 13.56 MHz. As we saw in Chapter 9, a voltage bias develops between the plasma and the electrodes. This is due to the difference in mobility of the electrons and the ions. Initially, the more mobile electrons are lost to the electrodes at a faster rate than the slower ions. This results in the plasma being biased positively with respect to the electrodes. For a symmetric RF plasma system, with the two electrodes of equal area, the

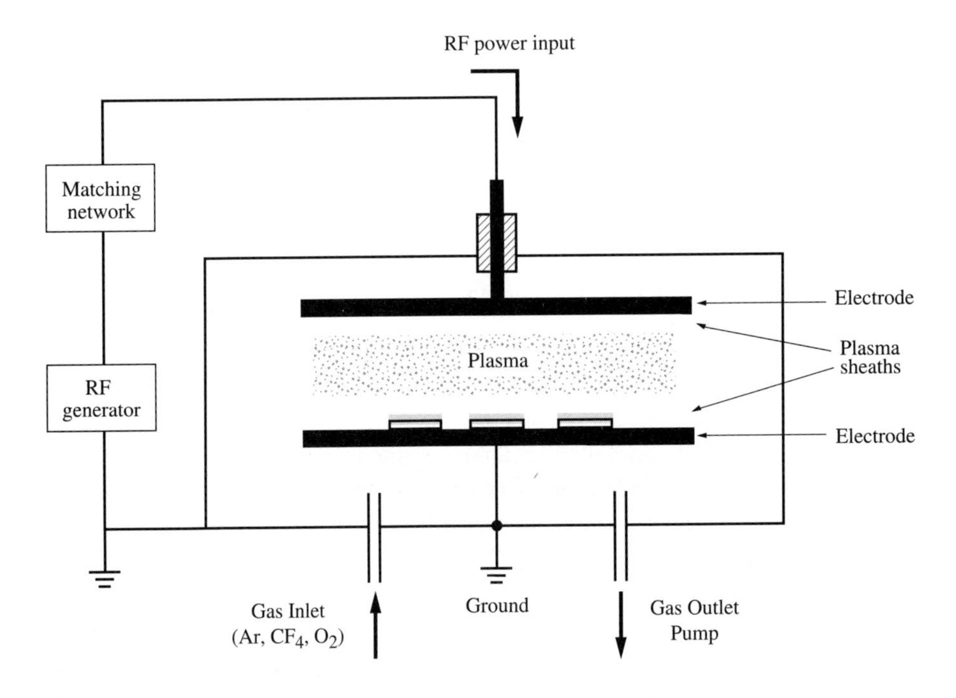

Figure 10–7 Schematic diagram of an RF-powered plasma etch system.

voltage distribution that develops is shown by the solid curve in Figure 10–8 (repeated from Figure 9–29). The sheaths are the regions next to each electrode where the voltage drops occur and correspond to the dark regions of the plasma.

The sheaths form to slow down the electron loss so that it is equal to the ion loss per RF cycle and so the average current to the electrodes is zero. Whereas the heavy ions respond to the average sheath voltage, the light electrons respond to the instantaneous voltage. However, due to the self-biasing, they only cross the sheath during a short period per cycle when the sheath voltage and thickness are near their minimum. During most of the RF cycle the electrons are turned back at the sheath edge, resulting in the sheaths, on the average, being deficient or depleted of electrons. This depletion of electrons in the sheath results in the sheath being dark because of the lack of electron/atom collisions and subsequent relaxation by light emission. In the bulk of the plasma, both ionization and excitation events occur, the latter producing the characteristic glow of the plasma. The lack of electrons in the sheath also increases the impedance of the sheath compared to the plasma bulk resulting in the main voltage drop being across the sheaths. If one of the electrodes is made much smaller in area, then the voltage distribution becomes asymmetric with a much larger voltage drop occurring from the plasma to the smaller electrode, as shown by the dashed curve in Figure 10–8. As described in Chapter 9, this happens because the RF current density must be much higher at the smaller electrode in order to maintain current continuity throughout the system. Therefore the fields must be higher at the smaller electrode.

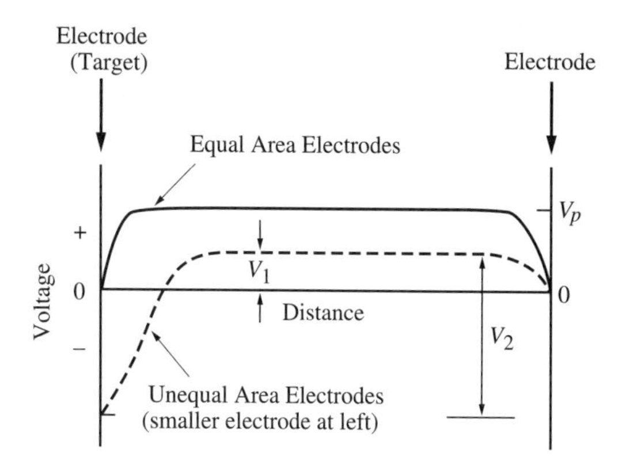

Figure 10–8 Steady-state voltage distribution in RF-powered plasma etch systems. (See Figure 9–27 and the associated text for a more complete discussion of this figure.)

For etching materials other than photoresist (for which O_2 is used) the reactant gases in the plasma are usually halide containing species, such as CF_4, Cl_2, and HBr. Sometimes small amounts of other gases, such as H_2, O_2, and Ar are also added. The high-energy electrons in the plasma can cause a variety of reactions to occur with the reactant gases, including electron-induced ionization, dissociation, recombination, and excitation reactions, as illustrated in Figure 10–9. The plasma will thus contain free electrons, ionized molecules, neutral molecules, ionized fragments of broken-up molecules, and free radicals. For example, in a CF_4 plasma, there will be electrons, CF_4, CF_3 (and other CF_X fragments), CF_3^+ and F. CF_3 and F are free radicals—very reactive species. Typically there will be about 10^{15} cm^{-3} neutral species (1 to 10% of which may be free radicals) and 10^8–10^{12} cm^{-3} ions and electrons. The actual numbers of the different species will depend on the balance between generation and loss or recombination reactions for each.

In standard plasma etch systems, the plasma density (the concentration of ions or electrons in the main plasma, which are virtually equal) and the ion energy as it travels across the sheath to strike the wafer are closely coupled. As the RF power increases, more ions are created, increasing the density, and the sheath voltage increases as well, increasing the ion energy. This coupling comes about because of the capacitive nature of the coupling between the RF current and the plasma [10.3].

10.2.2.1 Plasma Etching Mechanisms

The two main types of species involved in plasma etching are the reactive neutral chemical species and the ions. It is the reactive neutral species—free radicals in many cases, but sometimes other reactive species such as Cl_2—which are primarily responsible for the chemical component in plasma etch processes. It is the ions that are responsible for the physical component. They can work independently, or as we will see, they can work

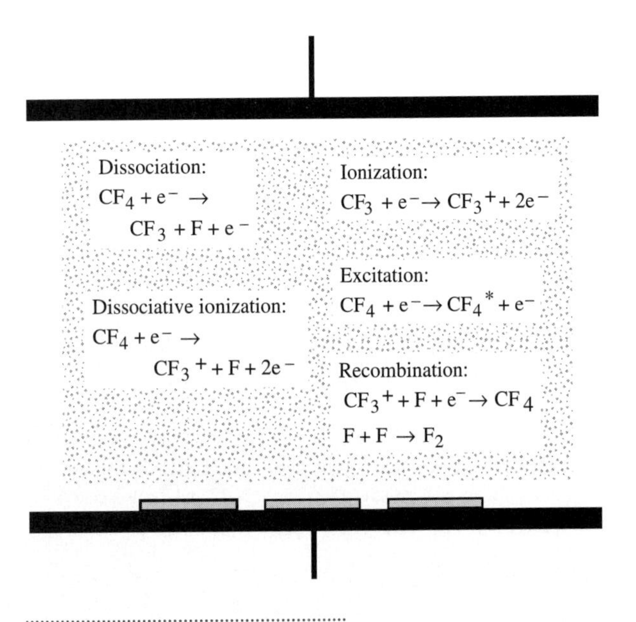

Figure 10–9 Typical reactions and species present in a plasma used for plasma etching.

together in a synergistic manner. When the reactive neutral species act by themselves, the process or mechanism is called chemical etching. Ions acting by themselves can result in physical etching, or sputtering. When the reactive neutral species and ions act in a synergistic fashion, this is called ion-enhanced etching. We will now describe each of these mechanisms.

Chemical Etching Chemical etching of materials in plasma systems is commonly done by free radicals. Free radicals are electrically neutral species that have incomplete bonding; that is, they have unpaired electrons. Examples are the fluorine free radical, F, and the neutral CF_3 free radical. Both of these can be produced by the reaction between free electrons in the plasma and CF_4, for example,

$$e^- + CF_4 \rightarrow CF_3 + F + e^- \tag{10.9}$$

Because of their incomplete bonding structure, free radicals are highly reactive chemical species. Free fluorine, with seven electrons in its outer shell instead of the energetically favorable set of eight, would much rather be bonded to other atoms so that all electrons are paired. It will therefore react quickly with other species to achieve that bonded state. The idea in plasma etching is for the reactive neutral species to react with the material to be etched, Si for example. The byproduct should be a volatile species

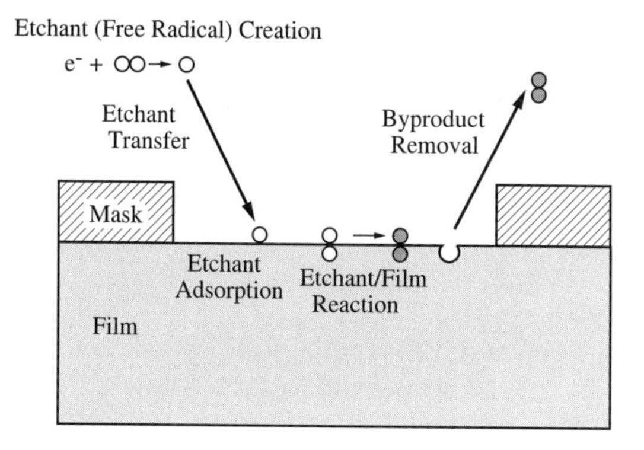

Figure 10–10 Processes involved in chemical etching during plasma etch process.

(that is, easily vaporized or evaporated into the gas phase) that leaves the surface, exposing more Si to be etched. This is illustrated in Figure 10–10. In fact, the fluorine free radical will react with Si via the reaction

$$4F + Si \rightarrow SiF_4 \tag{10.14}$$

to produce the gas SiF_4 (although there may be intermediate steps and species in that reaction). Thus a CF_4 plasma can be used to etch Si. It is important in etch processes that the byproducts of the etch, as well as any unreacted etchants, be removed from the surface for the etching to continue. Figure 10–10 shows a simple etch process, but more complex reactions may occur, involving multiple species and steps.

Gas additives can be used to increase the production of the reactive etch species and thereby increase the chemical etching rate. For example, oxygen is often added to a CF_4 plasma. The oxygen reacts with dissociated CF_4 species (CF_3 or CF_2, for example), which reduces the recombination of those species with F, thereby increasing the amount of free F. This enhances the chemical etching. However if too much O_2 is added, the etchant becomes too diluted or the surface is oxidized by the O_2, and the etching decreases.

We saw earlier that wet chemical etching occurs isotropically. The chemical component of plasma etching, when acting by itself, also occurs isotropically. Two factors lead to this behavior: an isotropic arrival angle distribution and a low sticking coefficient, with the latter usually more important. When we model and simulate plasma etching later in this chapter, we will closely follow the approach we used for deposition processes. That is, we will consider the incoming fluxes of species from the plasma to the wafer surface including the angular distribution of the various fluxes. This will be quantified by the $\cos^n\theta$ distribution, where a value of 1 for n describes an isotropic distribution (that is, coming in at all angles equally so that the normal component to the surface follows a $\cos\theta$ distribution) and a value of n larger than 1 describes a more directed distribution toward the surface. As in the deposition models we assume that all un-ionized chemical species arrive at the wafer surface at all angles. Since the free radicals are neutral species, the flux of the chemical component of plasma etching has an isotropic arrival angular distribution, or n equals 1.

We also consider the sticking coefficient of the species, as defined by Eq. (9.25), and repeated here.

$$S_c = \frac{F_{\text{reacted}}}{F_{\text{incident}}} \tag{10.11}$$

A high sticking coefficient (equal to 1) means that the reaction, and etching, occur the first time the species strikes the surface. A lower sticking coefficient means that before the species reacts, it can leave the surface—usually assumed to occur at a random angle —and strike the surface somewhere else. One might guess that free radicals would have very high sticking coefficients, since they are so reactive. However, as in deposition processes, the chemical reactions that occur in chemical etching often require multiple steps, and multiple atoms or species, all in the right proportions. In addition, the availability of suitable sites on the surface, competing reactions, and surface recombination of species can be issues. These issues result in most free radicals having effective sticking coefficients that are low, on the order of 0.01 to 0.05 for F etching of Si, for example. Thus the chemical etch species bounce around a lot and tend to maintain random angles of flight even under masks and other surface features. The fluxes for chemical species are illustrated in Figure 10–11(a).

These two properties of the reactive neutral species in plasma systems—isotropic arrival angles and low sticking coefficients—result in the fact that purely chemical etching acts in an isotropic or near-isotropic manner. Only if the sticking coefficient is relatively large would shadowing by the topography and etch mask become important. (Sticking coefficients on the order of 0.1 may actually occur for some purely chemical

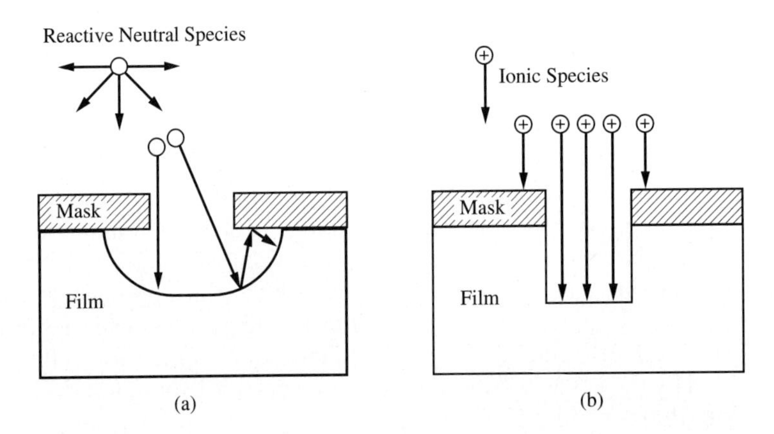

Figure 10–11 Fluxes of species in plasma etching: (a) fluxes of reactive neutral chemical species (such as free radicals), with a wide arrival angle distribution and low sticking coefficient; (b) fluxes of ionic species, with a narrow, vertical arrival angle distribution and high sticking coefficient (assumed equal to 1).

plasma etching cases [10.4].) In that event somewhat more anisotropic etch profiles can result. In general, though, pure chemical plasma etching results in isotropic or near-isotropic etching. We must reiterate that this is only for the chemical component acting independently, or for a purely chemical etch process. As we shall see shortly, the reactive chemical species and the ions can work in a synergistic manner so that the etching is not isotropic at all.

Since free radicals etch by chemically reacting with the material to be etched, the process can be very selective, as discussed earlier for wet chemical etching. Thus any chemical component to plasma etching will be relatively selective, as compared to the physical component.

In some cases, reactive neutral species other than free radicals may be involved in chemical etching. An example is in the plasma etching of Al by the Cl_2 molecule. For the same reasons given above, these reactive neutral species would have the same etching properties as the free radicals, namely isotropic profiles and selective chemical etching.

Physical Etching The other main species that participate in plasma etching are the ions that are present. Because of the voltage drop between the plasma and each electrode and the resulting electric field across each sheath, positive ions will be accelerated toward each electrode. Since the wafers are placed on one of the electrodes, then the ionic species such as Cl^+ (or Ar^+ in a purely physical sputter etch system) will be accelerated to the wafer surface. This striking of the wafer surface results in the more physical component of etching. The flux of ions toward the wafer surface is much more directional than the flux of neutral free radicals because of the directionality of the electric field from the plasma to the surface of the wafer. Thus the etching will be much more directional and more anisotropic. In fact it is usually assumed that all the ions arrive normal to the wafer surface, as shown in Figure 10–11(b), meaning that n is very large in the $\cos^n\theta$ distribution. Because the ions etch by more physical processes, rather than chemical, the etching will be much less selective. It is also assumed that once each ion strikes the surface, it does not strike the surface again somewhere else (or if it does, it does not have enough energy to do anything). This means that the sticking coefficient is effectively one. This also leads to more anisotropic behavior.

Ions can etch material in plasma systems by physical sputtering. Sputtering was discussed in Chapter 9, where we saw how sputtering of elemental, compound, or alloy targets was utilized to deposit material on the surfaces of wafers. We also saw how sputtering of the wafer itself could be done during a simultaneous deposition of material in order to planarize or fill features. Sputtering occurs by ions, accelerated by an electric field, striking the atoms on the surface of a material and physically dislodging them. The sputtering process is often described by a sputtering yield defined in Chapter 9 as the number of atoms or molecules ejected from the target per incident ion and is a measure of the sputter efficiency. As discussed in Chapter 9, the sputter yield is a function of incident angle, and it is this property that allows for planarization and filling in bias-sputtering deposition techniques. Because of the physical nature of sputtering by ion species arriving normal to the wafer surface, very anisotropic etching occurs, with profiles similar to that shown earlier in Figure 10–3(c).

When ionized reactive species such as Cl^+ and CF_3^+ are involved in sputtering, chemistry can also be important in determining the effective sputtering yield since these ions do have the potential of reacting chemically with surface atoms. Such effects can enhance the sputtering yield compared to Ar^+ sputtering, although the magnitude of these effects is usually small compared to ion-enhanced etching, which involves both neutral and ionized species and which we describe next.

Ion-Enhanced Etching Another way that ions participate in plasma etch processes is through ion-enhanced etching. It was recognized many years ago that the ions and reactive neutral species do not always act independently in an etch process. This was easily deduced when it was observed that the etch rate measured is not always just the sum of the two components acting independently; in many cases it is much higher. As a classic example of ion-enhanced etching, Figure 10–12 shows the etch rate of silicon as XeF_2 gas and Ar^+ ions are introduced to the surface. First XeF_2 gas (not a plasma, so there is no physical component at all) is introduced into the chamber and very little etching occurs. Then an Ar^+ ion beam is directed toward the surface and the etch rate increases ten times. Finally the XeF_2 gas is turned off so that only ion sputtering occurs, and the etch rate becomes almost zero. The chemical and physical species are obviously working in a synergistic manner.

This synergistic process is also demonstrated in the shape of the etch profiles that result. In ion-enhanced etching, both chemical and physical components are acting, but the profiles are not just a linear combination of isotropic chemical etching and anisotropic physical etching as illustrated in Figure 10–3(b). Instead, the profile for ion-enhanced etching is much more like the case for physical etching acting alone, as in Figure 10–3(c). If the chemical component in the etch system is increased, the vertical etching is increased but not the lateral etching, which is not what would be expected from chemical etching. In addition, the etch rate in many cases is much higher (>10 times) than that calculated from the measured ion flux assuming normal sputtering yields in the absence of neutral species; hence it is not likely that the observed plasma

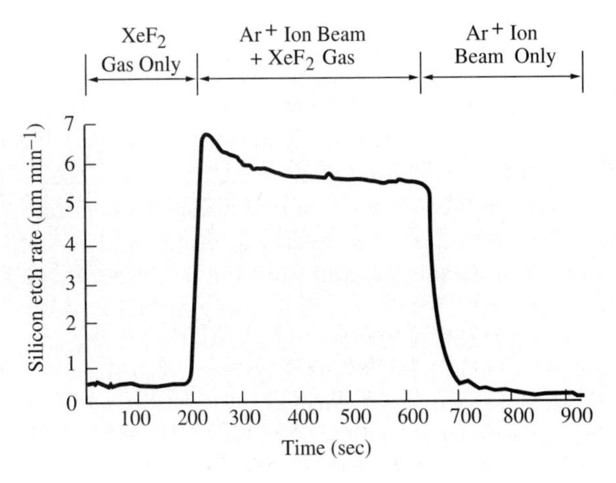

Figure 10–12 Etch rate of silicon as XeF_2 gas (not plasma) and Ar^+ ions are introduced to the silicon surface. Only when both are present does appreciable etching occur, illustrating synergistic etching behavior between chemical and ionic species. (After [10.5, 10.6].)

etch behavior in these cases is due simply to an ionized chemical species, such as CF_3^+. Observed saturation effects, which we will describe later, also support this dual component model involving both neutral and ion species.

In this type of etch process, the chemical components (the free radicals or other reactive neutral species) and the physical components (the ions) in the plasma somehow work together to etch the material, with both components required at each point for the process to work. In addition, because of the required chemical component and the chemical processes that occur, good selectivity can be obtained. So not only can one achieve very anisotropic etch profiles, but also a high degree of selectivity as well. This is something that is very difficult to achieve when the two components work independently. In addition, high etch rates can be achieved. Thus gas chemistries and etch conditions are usually chosen to promote ion-enhanced etching and to suppress independent chemical and physical etching.

There have been many explanations and mechanisms proposed for this type of cooperative etch process. In most of the models the ion bombardment enhances one of the steps of the chemical etch process, such as surface adsorption, etching reaction and formation of byproduct, or removal of byproduct or unreacted etchant. For example, the ion bombardment causes damage (breaking bonds, etc.) which makes the surface more apt to chemically react with the radical. Or the ion bombardment accelerates the formation of volatile byproducts. Or the ion bombardment may dislodge or sputter away etch byproducts which would otherwise tend to stay on the surface and impede the etch process. The removal of byproducts can also include secondary, or indirect, byproducts. It has been found that a chemically inert residue is often formed from etching or sputtering photoresist. In addition, species from the plasma may deposit on the surface. These layers that are formed or deposited, whatever their source, inhibit chemical etching either by physically blocking the chemical etch species or by reacting with them and depleting them. But the inhibitors can be removed, or prevented from forming, by ion bombardment, leading to anisotropic etching. In fact, these inhibitors are often intentionally produced on the surface by providing sources in the gas which enhance their formation so that more directional etching is achieved. In a particular ion-enhanced etch process, one or more of the above mentioned mechanisms (damage induced, inhibitor removal, etc.) may be occurring.

Whatever the exact mechanism for ion-enhanced etching, and it is often difficult to distinguish between them, directional etching occurs because of the directionality of the ions. The enhancement of the process, whether of enhancement of etch reaction or of inhibitor removal, occurs only where the ions strike the surface. Since the ions are striking normal to the wafer surface, the enhancement will occur normal to the wafer surface. This directional enhancement will result in directional, anisotropic etching. This is illustrated in Figure 10–13(a) for the case when the chemical etch reaction is enhanced by ion bombardment. It is assumed in this figure that etching by the neutral (radical) species alone without ion bombardment, the so-called "spontaneous chemical etching," is negligible, leading to no lateral etching at all. In Figure 10–13(b) the process of inhibitor formation and removal is illustrated, which also results in anisotropic etching. Ion bombardment on the horizontal surfaces removes the inhibitor there but leaves the sidewall inhibitor to protect against lateral chemical etching.

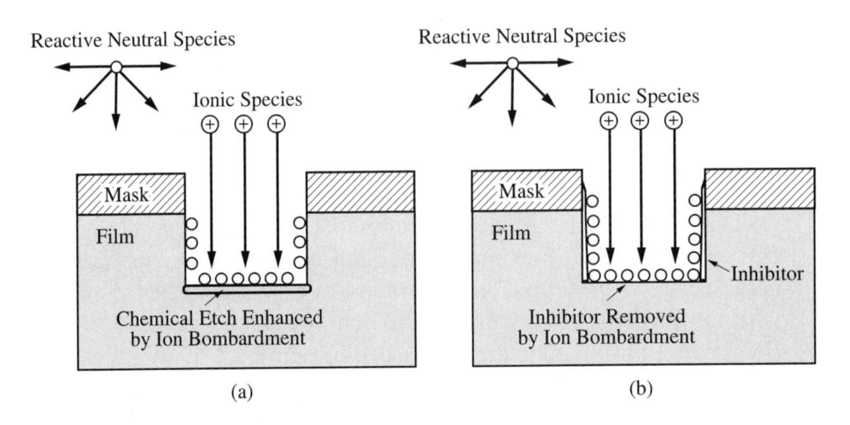

Figure 10–13 Illustration of ion-enhanced etching. In (a) the chemical etch reaction is enhanced by ion bombardment. In (b) an inhibitor is formed which is removed by ion bombardment, allowing chemical etching to proceed. In both cases, anisotropic etching results.

Even with ion-enhanced etching and no spontaneous chemical etching, the slope of the resulting sidewall may not always be exactly vertical. For example, the ion flux may not always be perfectly normal to the wafer surface and can result in slightly bowed sidewalls. Also, when inhibitors form or are deposited during etching, sloped sidewalls can result if the inhibitor formation or deposition rate is very high relative to the etch rate of the inhibitor and substrate, as demonstrated in Figure 10–14. Changing the relative deposition/etch rates by changing the etch chemistry or plasma conditions can be used, in fact, to tailor the desired slope if less than vertical sidewalls, without any undercutting, are desired in specific applications. But the important point still is that very anisotropic etching can be achieved when ion-enhanced etching is occurring.

Selectivity occurs in ion-enhanced etching because chemical reactions are involved in this type of etch process, and chemical reactions are by nature selective. To achieve the needed selectivity, one must choose the proper etchant gas (either F, Cl, or Br based, with or without oxygen or other species added, for example) and other etching conditions which favor the etching of the film over the mask material and the underlying films. With ion-enhanced etching, one can achieve good etch selectivity while still obtaining very directional etch profiles.

10.2.2.2 Types of Plasma Etch Systems

Different types of plasma etch systems and modes of operation have been developed to etch films in semiconductor structures which take advantage of the different species present in a plasma and the different etch mechanisms that can operate. We will now describe these different etch systems or modes, focusing on the advantages and disadvantages of each.

Plasma Etching in Barrel Etchers One of the earliest plasma systems developed was the barrel etcher, named because of its shape, and is shown in Figure 10–15. In this

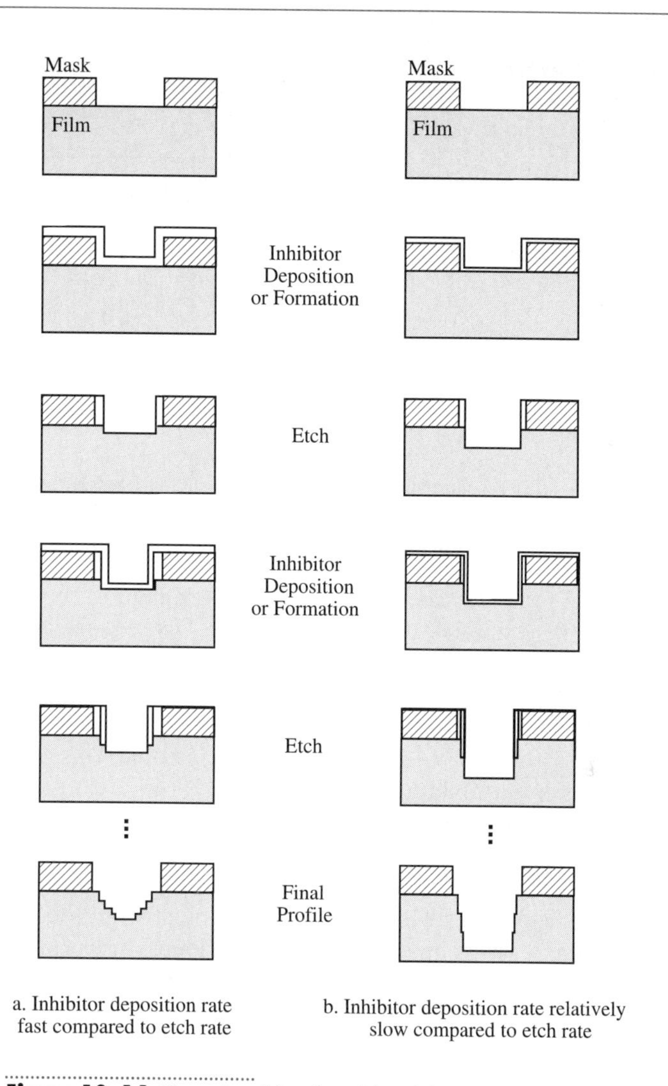

Figure 10–14 Illustration of the effect of the inhibitor deposition rate-to-etch rate ratio on the resulting sidewall slope. The different relative rates of inhibitor deposition and etch rate lead to different slopes of sidewall [10.4].

configuration, the electrodes are curved, wrapping around the quartz tube and the wafers are placed vertically in a substrate holder which sits in the middle of the tube. After evacuating the tube, reactant gases are introduced and RF power is applied to the electrodes. A plasma is generated but is kept away from the wafers themselves by the use of an etch tunnel, a perforated metal shield between the wafers and the electrodes. Reactant chemical species, such as F, diffuse from the plasma where they are generated, through the shield and to the wafers. There they can etch the wafers. Because the plasma and ions are kept away from the wafers by the shield, and the wafers do not sit

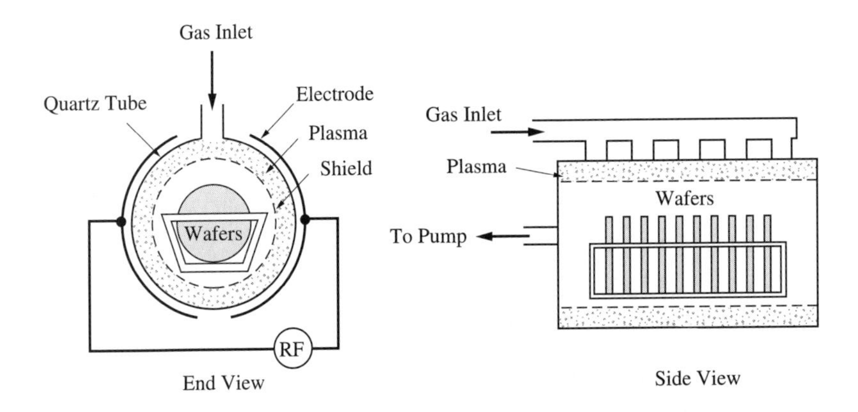

Figure 10–15 Schematic illustration of barrel etch system, in which purely chemical plasma etching occurs.

on either of the electrodes, no ionic bombardment of the wafers occurs. Thus the etching is purely chemical.

Because the etching is purely chemical, it can be very selective. It also causes very little damage to the surface because of the lack of ion bombardment. Also, it is a rather simple process and the throughput can be high with the closely stacked wafers. But because the etching is purely chemical, it is isotropic. This results in significant undercutting or mask bias. In addition, the etch uniformity across each wafer is not very good, especially from the outside of each wafer to the inside, because of the long diffusion path for the reactive species between the wafers.

As a result of the isotropic etching and nonuniformities, barrel etchers are used only for noncritical etch steps. In fact they are mostly limited to photoresist removal, using an O_2 plasma, where masking is not even done. This is called photoresist ashing, or just ashing, since the reaction between the oxygen and the hydrocarbon-based photoresist is the same as burning, producing CO_2 and H_2O. A long overetch is usually done in barrel etchers to compensate for the nonuniformities. This is allowable because of the high selectivity of the chemical etching processes used in these systems.

Similar to barrel etchers in principle but a little different in configuration are "downstream plasma etchers." Microwave or RF power can generate a plasma upstream in one chamber, while the wafers are placed in a separate but connected chamber "downstream" from the plasma. The neutral reactive chemical species can diffuse from the plasma in one chamber to the wafers in another, while the ions do not. Hence purely chemical etching occurs, resulting in good selectivity and little ion bombardment damage, but in isotropic etching. These are also called "afterglow etchers." These are also used for nonmasked etching steps, such as removing silicon nitride masks used for LOCOS processes.

Plasma Etching in Parallel Plate Systems—Plasma Mode Parallel plate etch systems, as shown earlier in Figure 10–7, are commonly used for plasma etching of films. This is very similar to the PECVD system described in Chapter 9, except that etch gases are used instead of deposition gases. Having this configuration with the wafers sitting on one of the electrodes and directly facing the other electrode gives much better etch uniformity than the barrel etcher design. In addition, it allows for the bombardment of ions on the wafer surface. The voltage distribution that develops from the RF source was shown in Figure 10–8. The voltage distribution is symmetric for equal area electrodes, with voltage drops across each sheath to the electrodes in the range of 10–100 V. As discussed earlier, this voltage drop accelerates the ions to the surface of the wafer, which is sitting on one of the electrodes. This results in a physical component to etching due to ion bombardment, as well as a chemical component due to the neutral reactive species. The physical component means that anisotropic etching is possible.

In symmetric parallel plate systems, with a gas pressure from 100 mtorr to 1 torr, the physical etch component is usually not very significant compared to other parallel plate configurations. In fact, the ion bombardment is even less since the bottom electrode is the grounded electrode in this setup. Since the chamber walls are also usually grounded and thus electrically connected to the bottom electrode, this effectively increases the size of that electrode. This means that the voltage drop from the plasma to that electrode is even smaller, as was shown in Figure 10–8 (the wafers would sit on the right side electrode for the dashed curve in that figure), and weaker ion bombardment would occur. One problem with etching in this mode is that with the large voltage drop to the top electrode, significant sputtering of that electrode can occur, causing contamination problems.

When the electrodes themselves are of equal area and the bottom electrode on which the wafers sit is grounded, making the effective size of the bottom electrode larger, then the etching is said to be operating in the plasma mode. Both chemical and physical components of etching are present in this mode, but as stated earlier the physical component is often rather weak, and highly directional etching is hard to achieve. However, the etching is still rather selective, and better uniformity and etch directionality are achieved compared to barrel etchers.

Plasma Etching in Parallel Plate Systems—Reactive Ion Etching Mode The parallel plate etch system can be modified to enhance the physical component of the etching by increasing the energy of the ions bombarding the wafers. This is achieved by having the electrode on which the wafers sit be smaller than the other electrode. Not only can the lower electrode be made physically smaller than the upper electrode, but the upper electrode can be the one that is grounded and electrically connected to the chamber walls. This makes the upper electrode effectively much larger. The bottom electrode is now much smaller than the upper electrode, and the voltage distribution is as shown in Figure 10–8, with the wafers on the left-hand side in this case. A much larger voltage drop occurs from the plasma to the wafers, in the 100–700 V range, resulting in more energetic ion bombardment of the wafer. With stronger ion bombardment, more directional etching can be achieved.

When the wafers sit on a smaller electrode, the etching is said to be operating in the Reactive Ion Etching or RIE mode. A better name for this might be "reactive and ion etching," since two types of species, the neutral reactive species and the ion species, are involved. In the RIE mode, both the physical ion component and the chemical reactive neutral component are important. They can act separately, but as we described earlier, gas chemistries and etch conditions are usually chosen so that they act together in a synergistic manner.

Even more directional etching can be attained by lowering the gas pressure. A lower pressure means fewer ion collisions during transit across the sheath in the gas phase, resulting in a more directed ion flux toward the wafer. Decreasing the pressure also increases the sheath voltage (that is, the voltage drop from the plasma to the wafer), which increases the ion energy. But decreasing the pressure can also decrease the plasma density (fewer gas atoms available to be ionized or converted into radicals), so that the pressure cannot be lowered too much. Reactive ion etch systems generally operate in the 10–100 mtorr range.

RIE systems can look very much like parallel plate plasma mode etchers (Figure 10–7) except that the RF power is supplied to the other electrode (to the bottom wafer holding electrode so that the top electrode is grounded with the chamber), and the size of the bottom electrode in the RIE case may be somewhat smaller. Single-wafer systems are often used for better control over each wafer. To increase the batch size other configurations have been used historically, such as with several electrode pairs stacked vertically above one another in a single chamber. Magnetic fields are often added to enhance plasma density and lower operating pressures.

Vertical RIE systems have also been developed. Here the wafers sit vertically against the inside electrode, which is often hexagonally shaped—hence the name, hexode batch etcher. The outside barrel chamber acts as the outer electrode. With its large size compared to the inner electrode, etching in the RIE mode can occur. Triode systems have also been developed. These are similar to the bias-sputtering systems discussed in Chapter 9, and add a second separate RF power supply to control the bias of the wafers. This separates plasma generation from ion energy, the latter being determined by the wafer bias. However, this independent control is only partially achieved using this technique with two capacitively coupled sources, and the plasma can suffer from nonuniformity. Also, the additional internal electrodes can cause contamination problems.

Operating in the RIE mode results in stronger ion bombardment than in the plasma mode, and a more physical component in the etching. While this leads to more directional etching, the higher enegy ions striking the surface can cause radiation or lattice damage, charging, and trenching. These will be discussed in more detail later. In addition, the higher physical component can lead to less selectivity. However, by choosing proper etch chemistries and utilizing ion-enhanced etching, an acceptable degree of selectivity can be achieved in these systems while still being able to etch material with excellent dimensional control. As a result, RIE etching is used extensively in the integrated circuit industry.

Etching in High-Density Plasma Systems A new type of plasma etch system that is becoming more popular is the High-Density Plasma (HDP) etch system. Like triode RIE etchers, these systems separate the plasma density and ion energy by using a second excitation source to control the bias voltage of the wafer electrode. But instead of using two capacitively coupled RF sources as in the triode systems, a different type of source for the plasma is used. The plasma generation source is non-capacitively coupled and produces a very high density plasma ($10^{11} - 10^{12}$ ions cm^{-3}) without itself generating a large sheath bias, utilizing a variety of methods. These include Electron Cyclotron

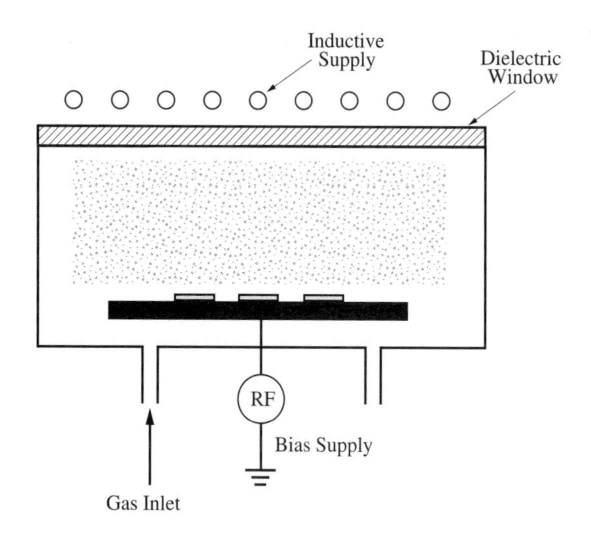

Figure 10–16 Schematic diagram of High-Density Plasma (HDP) etch system. This configuration is powered by an Inductively Coupled Plasma (ICP) source which produces and controls the high-density plasma. The RF wafer bias independently controls the ion energy.

Resonance (ECR) and Inductively Coupled Plasma (ICP) sources. The ICP method is becoming popular due to its much simpler design and equipment. A schematic diagram of an ICP high-density etch system is shown in Figure 10–16.

HDP etch systems are similar to the HDPCVD deposition systems described in Chapter 9. In those systems, the high-density plasma is produced using the same type of power sources, producing the reactive species for deposition as well as ionic species. A separate power source is used to bias the wafer in order to control the ion bombardment on the surface that is used for simultaneous biased sputtering. In Figure 9–45 in Chapter 9 we illustrated an ECR-powered HDPCVD system, which would be similar to an ECR HDP etch system. Similarly, an ICP high-density plasma CVD system would be very similar to the etch system shown in Figure 10–16.

In HDP etch systems, very high plasma densities are produced compared to standard RIE etch systems. Therefore lower pressures can be utilized, in the 1–10 mtorr range, while still achieving high ion fluxes and etch rates. A lower gas pressure means that even more directed etching can be achieved because of fewer gas-phase collisions in the sheath. In standard RIE systems, increasing the power increases the plasma density (and ion flux), allowing for higher etch rates, but also increases the sheath bias and ion energy, leading to more substrate damage. One could raise the pressure in standard RIE systems to produce a higher ion density while keeping the ion energies low, but the etching would become more isotropic due to more gas phase collisions in the sheath. In HDP systems, with the decoupling of the plasma density and ion energy, many ions can be produced at low pressures with low ion energies. As a result, ion bombardment damage can be kept low while maintaining high etch rates and good anisotropic etching. In addition, a lower ion energy usually gives better selectivity than higher ion energy.

Etching in HDP systems is similar to etching in the RIE mode, with a large physical component due to the ions combined with a chemical component involving the reactive neutrals (although the ionized species may themselves also contribute an appreciable chemical component to etching in these systems [10.6]). Therefore both directional etching and reasonable selectivity are possible. But in the HDP systems, the ion flux is even higher than in standard RIE systems, resulting in higher etch rates at lower pressures. And the higher ion flux, along with the lower pressures, leads to even more directional etching. The separate power sources allow independent control of ion density and ion energy, providing more flexibility in the etch process.

Sputter Etching and Ion Milling The sputter etching and ion milling techniques are at the other end of the spectrum from purely chemical systems; these are purely physical etching methods. We discussed sputtering in detail in Chapter 9, in which sputtering of a target was done to produce species for deposition. We also described how simultaneous sputtering of a film being deposited can be done to help with planarization of the film as well as filling in high aspect ratio spaces or holes. In sputter etching, physical bombardment of films with chemically inert ions, such as argon ions, produced in a plasma is used to etch the film. Figure 10–17 shows an RF sputtering system. The size of the cathode is minimized relative to the anode, which includes the chamber walls, to maximize the ion bombardment. The ion energies in these systems are large, greater than 500 eV, in order to get appreciable etching of films. While these systems are not normally used to etch thin films today, they do illustrate some important points about physical etching, and they have been used in the past.

The main advantages of sputter etching are that all materials can be etched this way and the etching is very directional, or anisotropic. The principle disadvantage is that selectivity is poor because little or no chemistry is involved. The sputtering rate, which is the same as the etch rate, depends on the sputtering yield. This is the efficiency of dislodging or removing an atom from the sputtered material by each impinging ion. The sputter yields of most materials by argon ions are fairly similar. This means that most materials can be sputter etched with about the same efficiency and that this method can often be used when other etch methods do not work. But this also means that the selectivity will not be good. The best selectivity ratios achievable are only about two-to-one. The sputtering yield is usually a function of incident angle. This can lead to faceting, which can be good or bad depending on the desired topography. The fact that

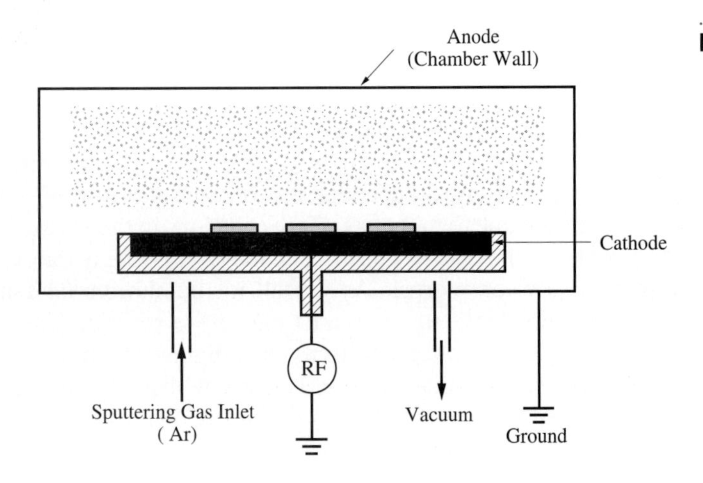

Figure 10–17 Illustration of sputter etch system.

all the etching is done by the highly directional ions means that highly directional etching can occur.

There are a few other problems associated with sputter etching. These would also be problems with any other method that utilizes energetic ion bombardment, such as reactive ion etching, but they are worse for sputter etching which is purely physical. One of these problems is called trenching, or "microtrenching." Along the sides of masking layers, some of the ions will glance off the sides and strike the films at the bottom corner. Hence these corner regions will receive a higher ion flux than if the sidewall were not there. This causes enhanced etching at the edges, resulting in trenches, as illustrated in Figure 10–18(a). Another problem is in redeposition. In a nonselective physical process other layers will be sputtered as well. These sputtered materials can be redeposited elsewhere, including in the region that is being etched. This is illustrated in Figure 10–18(b).

A third problem is lattice or radiation damage. During sputtering, the surface is subjected to bombardment of energetic ions, electrons, and photons. Ion bombardment can lead to displaced atoms and implanted atoms below the surface. Radiation damage can lead to electron traps being produced in gate oxides. Another problem is surface charging. This is associated with the bombardment of the wafer surface with charged ions and electrons. Because of nonuniformities that can exist in the plasma, dielectric materials can be charged by the local differences between ion and electron fluxes. This can lead to tunneling current damage to thin dielectrics. It can also lead to etch profile distortion. This is because the paths of the incoming charged ions will be affected by the presence of the charged regions, either positive or negative, as shown in Figure 10–18(c), and lead to uneven etching.

In ion milling, some of the problems associated with charged species are eliminated. In this technique, a confined plasma is used to generate a broad beam of Ar^+ ions. This is done by using a set of grids to extract and accelerate ions from the plasma chamber toward the target wafer to be etched. A separate electron source is used to supply electrons to neutralize the ion beam. This setup allows for more independent control over

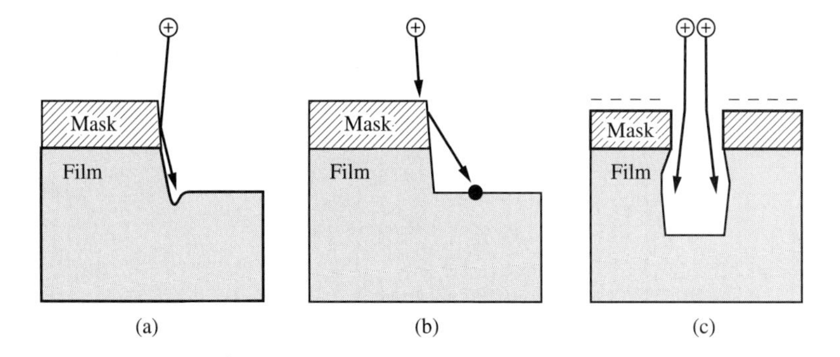

Figure 10–18 Problems associated with sputter etching (or any etching that has a high degree of physical/ionic etching): (a) trenching at bottom of sidewalls; (b) redeposition of photoresist and other material; (c) charging and ion path distortion.

the ion energy and ion density, which are usually closely coupled in a normal plasma system. An amount of reactive species may also be added to, or replace, the Ar in ion milling systems. These species may include CF_4, CCl_4, or O_2. This will add some amount of selectivity to the process. This method is called "Reactive Ion Beam Etching," or RIBE.

Ion beams can also be focused and then used to sputter, or etch, very small areas. This is called the Focused Ion Beam (FIB) technique. It can be used in advanced lithography applications to expose/etch resist instead of electron beams. It is commonly used to repair masks. It can also be used to cut or etch regions of films and substrates to expose cross sections for observation. The ions in this are often He^+, N^+, Ar^+, Xe^+, and most commonly Ga^+.

10.2.2.3 Summary of Plasma Systems and Mechanisms

Figure 10–19 summarizes the different types of plasma etch systems in terms of some of the operating and etch properties. Of course there are wide variations in the properties for different types of systems, and overlaps occur between the different types of etching. For example, the ion energy in HDP etch systems can be the same or lower than in RIE systems, and the selectivity can be better as well. And the selectivity in both HDP and RIE systems can be very good while still achieving anisotropy by choosing the right etch chemistries and utilizing ion-enhanced etching. But the basic trends shown are useful in understanding the differences in the various types of plasma etching systems.

Figure 10–20 summarizes some of the different etch processes that occur in plasma etching which affect the two-dimensional etch profile. Not all the processes would occur simultaneously of course—inhibitor formation and trenching would not just occur on one side with undercutting on the other, for example, but the figure does illustrate the many complex phenomena that can occur during plasma etching.

We have described the similarities between etching and deposition systems several times. PECVD systems are similar to parallel plate etch systems operating in the plasma

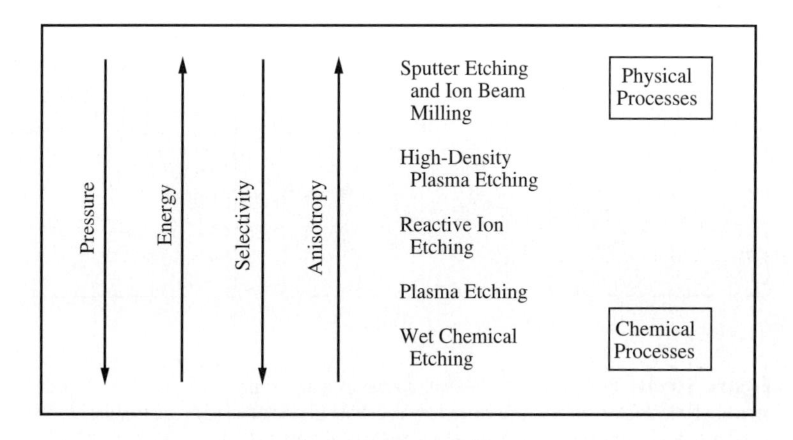

Figure 10–19 Summary of trends of different etch systems.

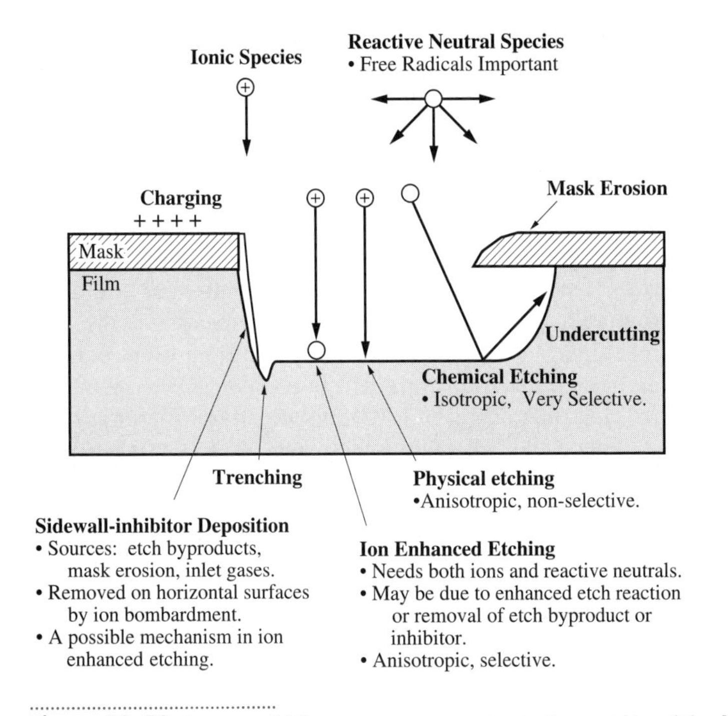

Figure 10–20 Summary of different processes occurring in plasma etching. (After [10.4].)

mode. There are reactive neutral species for either deposition or etching, with a minimum of ionic bombardment in either case. There are also similarities between deposition systems that utilize wafer sputtering, such as bias-sputtering and HDPCVD systems, and reactive ion and HDP etch systems. Bias-sputtering and HDPCVD deposition systems combine deposition of materials and sputter etching of the surface. Both of these processes also occur in reactive ion etching and HDP etching systems. Etching of the wafer surface is done using ion bombardment as well as chemical processes. But "deposition" is also commonly done in these etch systems in which inhibitor layers are "deposited" on the surface to promote anisotropy. These inhibitors form from byproducts of the etch process and the chemistry of the etch gases is often chosen to enhance their formation. This is called inhibitor deposition. So both deposition and etching occur in these deposition systems and etch systems. It is only the degree and type of deposition or etch that is different in specific systems. Many of the same concepts and models apply to both.

10.3 Manufacturing Methods

In this section we will describe some of the specific manufacturing methods used in plasma etching and some of the important issues related to manufacturing. We will limit ourselves to plasma etching here because of its dominance in current integrated circuit manufacturing. Limited information on wet chemical etching was given in Table 10–1. Most films in current semiconductor manufacturing are etched using parallel plate plasma systems in the RIE mode or using HDP systems.

10.3.1 Plasma Etching Conditions and Issues

The main parameters that can be directly controlled during plasma etching in standard parallel plate etch systems are RF power, pressure, gas compositions, and flow rates. (Some systems allow control of the self-bias, or sheath voltage, and the RF power is adjusted so that a particular bias is achieved.) Power densities of 0.1 to 5 W cm^{-2} are commonly used in parallel plate, capacitively coupled RF plasma systems, usually at 13.56 MHz with excitation voltages of 100–1500 volts RMS. Increasing the RF power increases the plasma density. In standard parallel plate systems, increasing the RF power also increases the self-bias or sheath voltage, which is the voltage drop between the plasma and the electrodes. This increases the ion energy. Ion energies produced are in the 10- to 700-eV range. Higher ion energy results in a higher sputtering yield which results in a higher physical component of etching but can also result in more surface damage.

In HDP systems, with separate power sources for the plasma and wafer bias, one can achieve high plasma densities and high fluxes, without necessarily getting high ion energies. In those systems, the power density on the wafer is in the 0.1–3 W cm^{-2} range. The resulting ion energies can range from 10 to 500 eV. A higher source power is used to generate the plasmas, in the 3- to 10-W cm^{-2} range.

The pressure in plasma etching systems ranges from 1 mtorr to 1 torr, with standard RIE systems operating in the 10- to 100-mtorr range and HDP systems in the 1- to 10-mtorr range. Increasing the pressure causes more gas-phase collisions to occur, decreasing the directionality of the etching. Increasing the pressure also increases the plasma density (since there are more atoms or molecules to begin with), but only up to a point. Above a certain pressure, depending on the etch system and operating parameters, the collisions between the gas molecules and electrons limit the energy of the electrons and thereby limit the ionization rate. Thus the plasma density decreases at higher pressures. In addition, increasing the pressure lowers the sheath voltage [10.7], thereby lowering the ion energy.

The etch rate, to first order, is proportional to the flux of active species, which would be the neutral chemical species and the ionic species. The flux of ionic species equals its concentration times its velocity. In plasma systems, increasing the power increases the plasma density and therefore increases the ion concentration in the plasma. The ion velocity in the plasma (by the electron temperature in the plasma) does not change to first order with a change in power at the sheath edge and determined. (The velocity across the sheath does increase as the power is increased in a parallel plate system, or as the wafer bias power is increased in a high-density plasma system. But the concentration of ions decreases proportionally across the sheath, so as to keep the flux constant across the sheath [10.11].) Thus the ion flux, being equal to the product of the ion concentration and velocity in the plasma at the sheath edge, would increase with power. The effect of increasing the pressure on the ion flux is less clearcut, and different systems show different relationships.

The etch rate due to the ion component would be proportional to the ion flux, as well as to the sputtering yield, or the effective sputtering yield in ion-enhanced processes as we will discuss later. The effective sputtering yield itself can be dependent on ion energy (approximately proportional to the square root of the energy), which for parallel plate systems would be dependent on the RF power. In parallel plate systems, increasing the RF power increases the ion energy which increases the sputtering yield. Likewise, increasing the pressure can decrease the ion energy and sputter yield, decreasing the etch rate with pressure. In HDP systems, one can change the ion energy and thus the sputtering yield, independent of the plasma density and flux, by changing the separate bias voltage control. One can thus increase the physical etch rate by directly increasing the bias voltage.

One might assume that the chemical flux would be increased by increasing the power, which would increase the plasma density, and the generation of reactive neutral radicals. However, perhaps due to the complex chemistry occurring, this is not often observed. Generally the chemical flux increases with pressure. Thus the etch rate which depends on this flux generally increases with pressure. The behavior of the overall etch rate as a function of pressure can get quite complicated when the etching depends on both the chemical and ion components. A more detailed examination of chemical and ion fluxes and how they relate to the etch process will be given in the models and simulation section. In general, decreasing the pressure too far—below about 10 mtorr for standard RIE systems and about 1 mtorr for HDP systems—will result in too low a plasma density and too low an etch rate for practical purposes.

The gas composition—which gases are used and in what proportions—and flow rates can also be controlled and are used to help achieve the desired etch properties. We will discuss different gas compositions used to etch various films below. The flow rate often has a minor effect on etch rate. Increasing the flow rate will initially increase the etch rate by producing more reactive species. But the actual supply of reactant species depends on the balance between generation and loss of species in the plasma, and a steady state is reached where the etch rate will become independent of gas flow. If too high a flow rate occurs, the etch rate may actually decrease since the residence time of the gas may become less than the lifetime of the active species produced in the plasma.

Usually the temperature of the etch system, including the wafer, is not intentionally raised during etching. The plasma supplies the energy for the etch process and heating the gas or wafer would not significantly increase the etch rate or improve the process. An exception to this is in aluminum etching in which the system, including the chamber walls, is heated to 35–65°C to help keep the species volatile and assist in the removal of the byproducts. Without intentional heating, the wafers may still heat up due to the plasma processes and ionic bombardment—temperatures of 90–100°C can be encountered on wafer surfaces. It is important to control and minimize the temperature rise on the wafers. Sidewall inhibitor deposition actually decreases as the temperature goes up in most cases, resulting in less directional etching. The trend in recent years is for better control of temperature and removal of heat from the wafers by developing better wafer chuck systems, including electrostatic chucks, which uniformly extract heat from the wafers.

At the beginning of this chapter we mentioned several desired properties or qualities of etch processes. These included selectivity, etch profile control, uniformity, minimal substrate damage, and low contamination. We now consider how these issues relate to manufacturing concerns.

Selectivity involves the chemical component of etching. It is achieved primarily by choosing the particular chemical reactants, in the proper proportions, that favor the etching of one material over another. Changing the plasma conditions, such as the wafer bias and sheath voltage, can also affect selectivity in some cases. Achieving selectivity will be discussed later in the context of some common etch chemistries used for films in integrated circuit fabrication.

Etch profile control means obtaining the desired shape of the etch profile. For most applications in today's technology this means obtaining vertical, or near-vertical, sidewalls. Directional etching, either with ion-enhanced mechanisms or physical sputtering, is basically due to the ion or physical component and can be enhanced by increasing the ion directionality (by decreasing the pressure, for example), increasing the ion flux (by increasing the RF power, for example), or by increasing the effective sputtering yield (by increasing the RF power or bias voltage, for example). Less vertical or more sloped sidewalls may sometimes be desired—adequate filling or conformal deposition of subsequent layers may require a slightly sloped underlying topography. Producing less vertical sidewalls could be accomplished by reversing the above mentioned parameter trends. Sloped sidewalls can also be produced by allowing a certain amount of mask erosion to occur and using a tapered mask. While this allows the slope to become less vertical, it does so by increasing the width of the etched region, as we will show later in a simulation.

The etch profile can also be altered by changing the etchant gases. More vertical sidewalls can be obtained by using etchant gas species that have a lower spontaneous chemical component and which have appreciable etching only where there is ion bombardment, such as by ion-induced damage or byproduct removal mechanisms. One can also choose a chemistry that favors inhibitor formation. The inhibitor layer obstructs the spontaneous chemical etching and allows for ion-enhanced etching, resulting in very vertical etching. If the inhibitor forms too quickly relative to the etch rate, nonvertical sidewalls can result, as discussed earlier and illustrated in Figure 10–14. Figure 10–21 shows how the sidewall angle can be changed by changing the relative composition of C_2H_6 in the Cl_2/C_2H_6 etchant chemistry to etch polysilicon. Adding C_2H_6 increases the sidewall polymer formation (or "deposition") relative to the etch rate, causing the sidewall to be less vertical. In this manner, the etch profile can be tailored to the desired shape.

It is interesting that while plasma etching is rather insensitive to temperature, the deposition of an inhibitor layer often shows a negative activation energy with respect to temperature. In a plasma, the bond breaking and forming, which often limit film deposition, is rather temperature insensitive since most of the energy for this is supplied by the plasma energy and not thermal energy. However, the desorption of the deposited inhibitor layers increases with temperature, so that the net temperature dependence of inhibitor deposition is actually negative.

Etch uniformity means uniform etch rates across a wafer and from wafer to wafer. In batch systems, wafer-to-wafer uniformity involves the proper design of equipment so that the plasma and gas flows are uniform across the wafers in the system. Single-wafer systems have been developed to achieve better control over each wafer and to elimi-

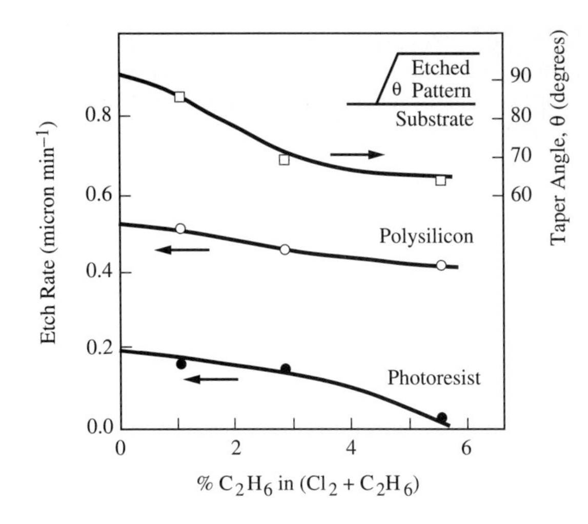

Figure 10–21 Etch rate of polysilicon and photoresist, and resulting taper angle as a function of C_2H_6 in Cl_2/C_2H_6 etch chemistry. More C_2H_6 results in more sidewall inhibitor formation and deposition relative to etching. (After [10.8].)

nate the wafer-to-wafer problems. Uniformity across a single wafer can still be a problem. Sometimes wafers develop "bulls-eye" patterns where the outside etches faster than the inside. This is usually due to depletion effects as the gas flows from the outside of the wafer to the inside.

Another kind of problem related to etch uniformity is called the "loading effect." There are two types of loading effects: macroscopic loading and microscopic loading. Macroscopic loading refers to the phenomenon in which more wafers in a chamber or more area exposed on a wafer to be etched results in a slower etch rate. This occurs because of the depletion of etchant species that occurs as the material is being etched. It is hard to predict to what extent this will occur due to the complex balance between species in the plasma and on the wafer surface. For the same reasons it is often difficult to control—increasing the flow rates does not always help.

Microloading occurs when etch rates vary over small distances on the surface of the wafer. This can occur when differences in the density of the unmasked area occur over small distances, resulting in differences in etch rates, just as in macroscopic loading. Microloading can also occur due to differences in aspect ratios. This effect is known as "Aspect Ratio Dependent Etching" or ARDE. It is also known as RIE "lag." As shown in Figure 10–22, the etch rate is different for different aspect ratios, with a lower etch rate for higher aspect ratio (smaller width) trenches. Different mechanisms have been suggested to explain this, each of which may be important under certain conditions. These include (1) depletion or trapping of the reactant species, or other conductance limitations, as the species travel to the bottom of the trench; (2) distortion of ion paths due to charging; and (3) shadowing effects involving either neutrals or ions. In the last case, collisions in the sheath may cause ions to be off-axis so that the number which reach the bottom is reduced due to simple geometrical shadowing. In each case, a narrower width decreases the chance that the reactant species, either ionic or reactive neutral, makes it to the bottom, thereby reducing the etch rate at the bottom. Etching at a lower pressure would reduce this effect if the shadowing mechanism were important, since reducing

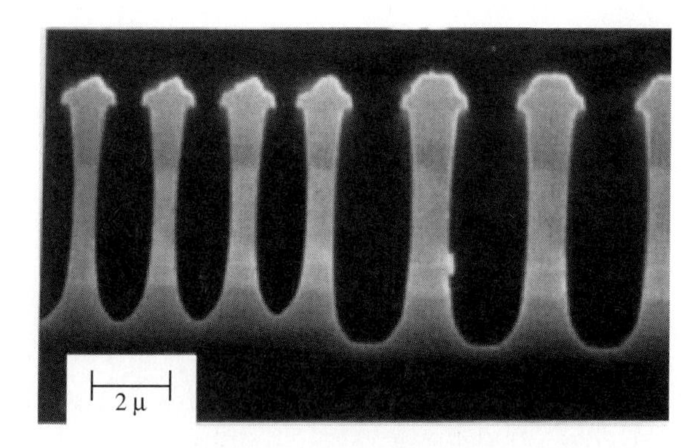

Figure 10–22 Example of Aspect Ratio Dependent Etching (ARDE) in silicon trench etching. The depth of etching decreases as the lateral feature size decreases [10.10].

the pressure would decrease the collisions in the gas phase and hence reduce shadowing effects. This is seen to be true experimentally [10.9] for some conditions, and we will simulate this later in the chapter.

Other uniformity issues involve differences in etching due to local variations in the film itself. The etch rate is a function of the density of the film, as one would expect, but also of the doping of the film [10.11]. Since these can vary locally across the film, the etch rate will vary as well.

Because of nonuniformities in the etch rate, and because the film itself may be of nonuniform thickness across the wafer or wafer to wafer, a certain amount of overetching is done to ensure that complete etching is achieved everywhere on the wafer. This is often 10–20%, in terms of time, past the endpoint detection. (*In situ* measurement and monitoring techniques, including endpoint detection, will be discussed in the measurement techniques sections.) Even more overetching may be required when anisotropic etching is done over nonplanar topography. Figure 10–23 illustrates this for purely vertical anisotropic etching of a conformally deposited film, where an additional time would be required to etch away the corner region. "Stringers" can results if strings of the material are left unetched at the bottom of the corner. Of course, this phenomenon can be taken advantage of in order to produce self-aligned spacers, as we discussed in Chapter 2 (Figure 2–30). In that case, no extra overetch would be done and the remaining oxide at the corner would be left as a spacer. The structure shown in the right side of Figure 10–23 would result, with the very narrow self-aligned spacer having a width approximately equal to the deposited film thickness.

Contamination and particulates can be reduced by reducing the pressure. Fewer contaminants are in the system and there is reduced polymerization of some etch species at lower pressures. Unwanted residues are often due to polymeric byproducts of the etch process. These can often cause problems with incomplete etching. If residues are left in contacts (or vias) after etching the contacts in a dielectric, high contact resistance can result. Reducing residue formation can be done by the proper choice of reactant gases. However, often polymeric formation is desired in order to achieve etch anisotropy, as discussed earlier, and gases are selected to promote such polymeric formation. In that case it is important to eliminate any unwanted residues from the etched surface following the etch process. Overetching can help remove residues in some situations. But in the

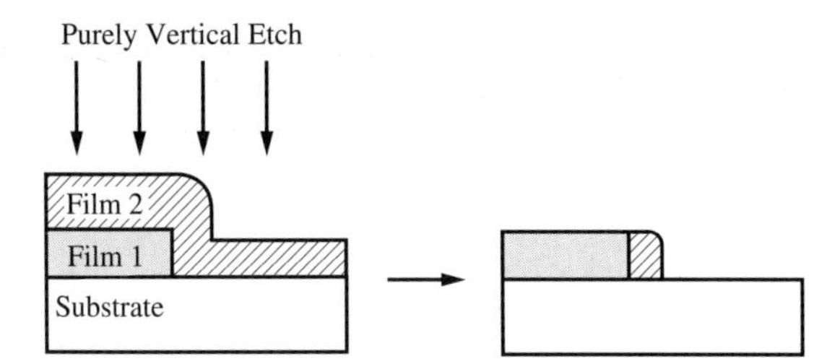

Figure 10–23 Overetching of a film over a step would be required to remove material at corner. In this example, completely anisotropic etching is assumed to emphasize this concept. This phenomenon can be used in producing self-aligned oxide spacers, in which no extra overetching is done so as to intentionally produce the structure at the right.

case of via etching, it may make it worse since sputtering of the underlying metal onto the sidewalls makes the sidewall residue harder to remove. One safe way to remove etch residues is by using a selective chemical etch after the plasma etch.

10.3.2 Plasma Etch Methods for Various Films

Most reactant gases for plasma etching contain halogens, generally Cl and F, and sometimes Br. Free radicals of these species can easily be produced in a plasma which can efficiently etch many films, and volatile etch products commonly result with these species. The exact choice of reactant gases to etch a specific film depends on a variety of factors, the most important being (1) etch selectivity to underlying films; (2) anisotropic etching; and (3) volatility of main etch byproducts.

Since in an etch process it is necessary to remove the byproducts from the surface, keep them off the wafer and pump them out of the system, the volatility of the main byproducts is an important consideration in choosing the gas chemistry. The volatility, or tendency to evaporate, depends on how tightly bound the species is to the surface. Table 10–2 lists the boiling points of typical etch products. The boiling point is an indicator of the volatility of a species—the lower the boiling point, the lower the surface binding energy and the higher the volatility. One can see that if Al is etched with a fluorine chemistry, AlF_3 would be the main byproduct. But the boiling point of AlF_3 (actually the sublimation temperature since it transforms directly from solid to gas without going through a liquid phase) is quite high at 1291°C. This means that the etch byproduct will be tightly bound to the surface with a very low vapor pressure, and even with ion bombardment it would be difficult to remove and keep off the surface. On the other hand, the byproduct of a chlorine-based etchant would be $AlCl_3$ with a boiling point (sublimation temperature again) of 177.8°C. This indicates looser bonding to the surface and a much more volatile species, so that a chlorine-based etchant would be a much better choice to etch Al. Having a volatile, weakly bound main etch byproduct is important when choosing an etch chemistry for a particular film. It is important to note that other, sometimes intermediate, byproducts may form during the etch process, and their removal or conversion to a more volatile species can be a rate limiting step in the etch process.

Table 10–3 lists some common chemistries used in plasma etching films in integrated circuit fabrication. These etchants are chosen mostly based on issues associated with byproduct volatility, etch selectivity, and etch profiles. The exact etch profiles and

Table 10–2. Boiling points of typical etch products (After [10.12]).

Element	Chlorides	Boiling Point (°C)	Fluorides	Boiling Point (°C)
Al	$AlCl_3$	177.8 (subl.)	AlF_3	1291 (subl.)
Cu	CuCl	1490	CuF	1100 (subl.)
Si	$SiCl_4$	57.6	SiF_4	− 86
Ti	$TiCl_3$	136.4	TiF_4	284 (subl.)
W	WCl_6	347	WF_6	17.5
	WCl_5	276	WOF_4	187.5
	$WOCl_4$	227.5		

selectivities will depend on the specific system and plasma conditions. We will next discuss the plasma etching of three films, silicon dioxide, polysilicon, and aluminum, in a little more detail. In doing so we hope to illustrate some of the major issues involved in plasma etching and in choosing the etch chemistries.

10.3.2.1 Plasma Etching Silicon Dioxide

Fluorine-based chemistries are usually used to etch silicon dioxide. The volatility of the main etch product, SiF_4, is very high as indicated by its low boiling point in Table 10–2 and thus the SiF_4 can easily leave the surface via thermal desorption. Fluorine can etch the SiO_2 by reaction of the fluorine free radical, with the overall reaction given by

$$4F + SiO_2 \rightarrow SiF_4 + O_2 \tag{10.12}$$

CF_2 and CF_3 free radicals may also be directly involved in the case of fluorocarbon etchants, in which case CO-containing byproducts would also be produced.

Etching with a significant isotropic component can result using source gases such as NF_3, SF_6, CF_4, or CF_4/O_2 mixtures. CF_4 dissociates to form free F in a plasma via the reaction given in Eq. (10.9). As mentioned earlier, adding O_2 to the CF_4 gas significantly increases the F free radical production and hence increases the etch rate as well as makes the etch profile more isotropic. Too much oxygen, though, can decrease the etch rate due to dilution [or by reversing the reaction in Eq. (10.12) and redepositing oxide on the surface]. These gas sources with relatively high free F concentrations will etch the oxide; however, depending on the conditions, the etching can result in undercutting. In addition, the etch selectivity over silicon or polysilicon, which is often underneath the oxide, is poor. The anisotropy can be enhanced by increasing the ion bombardment and lowering the pressure [10.14], but the selectivity over silicon is still generally poor with these chemistries.

The key to making the etching of silicon dioxide very anisotropic as well as much more selective over Si is to reduce the amount of F free radical production and increase the carbon content. Doing so will decrease any spontaneous isotropic etching by free

Table 10–3. Typical or representative plasma gases for films used in IC fabrication (After [10.1, 10.4, 10.13, 10.14].)

Material	Etchant	Comments
Polysilicon	SF_6, CF_4	Isotropic or near isotropic (significant undercutting); poor or no selectivity over SiO_2.
	CF_4/H_2, CHF_3	Very anisotropic; nonselective over SiO_2.
	CF_4/O_2	Isotropic or near isotropic; more selective over SiO_2.
	HBr, Cl_2, $Cl_2/HBr/O_2$	Very anisotropic; most selective over SiO_2.
Single-crystal Si	same etchants as polysilicon	
SiO_2	SF_6, NF_3, CF_4/O_2, CF_4	Can be near isotropic (significant undercutting); anisotropy can be improved with higher ion energy and lower pressure; poor or no selectivity over Si.
	CF_4/H_2, CHF_3/O_2, C_2F_6, C_3F_8	Very anisotropic; selective over Si.
	$CHF_3/C_4F_8/CO$	Anisotropic; selective over Si_3N_4.
Si_3N_4	CF_4/O_2	Isotropic; selective over SiO_2 but not over Si.
	CF_4/H_2	Very anisotropic; selective over Si but not over SiO_2.
	CHF_3/O_2, CH_2F_2	Very anisotropic; selective over Si and SiO_2.
Al	Cl_2	Near isotropic (significant undercutting).
	$Cl_2/CHCl_3$, Cl_2/N_2	Very anisotropic; BCl_3 often added to scavenge oxygen.
W	CF_4, SF_6	High etch rate; nonselective over SiO_2.
	Cl_2	Selective over SiO_2.
Ti	Cl_2, $Cl_2/CHCl_3$, CF_4	
TiN	Cl_2, $Cl_2/CHCl_3$, CF_4	
$TiSi_2$	Cl_2, $Cl_2/CHCl_3$, CF_4/O_2	
Photoresist	O_2	Very selective over other films

fluorine. The etching that then occurs involves other fluorine species and is strongly ion enhanced. In addition, polymer inhibitor formation will be increased, also suppressing lateral etching. Furthermore, selectivity over Si will be greatly enhanced.

One way to reduce the relative amount of F free radicals is by adding H_2 to the CF_4 gas. The hydrogen reacts with the fluorine to produce HF which reduces the amount of atomic F. Another possibility is to use more fluorine-poor and more carbon-rich gas species, such as CHF_3, C_3F_8, or C_2F_6. With fewer F free radicals, any spontaneous (non-ion-enhanced) chemical etching by these species is reduced. Appreciable etching happens only where ion bombardment occurs, perhaps involving an ion-induced damage or bond-breaking process, leading to anisotropic etching. CF_2 or CF_3 free radicals, rather than free F, are believed to be involved in the etch mechanism in these fluorine-deficient gas mixtures [10.14]. Increasing the carbon-to-fluorine ratio with these etchants also increases the amount of polymer inhibitor formed, or deposited, during the etching [10.6]. With a CF_4 or CF_4/O_2 gas, little or no polymer forms on the surface. However with a higher carbon concentration relative to fluorine in the gas mixture, more polymer formation will occur relative to etching. With a thick polymer inhibitor layer present, etching can not occur on vertical surfaces where there is little ion bombardment to remove the polymer inhibitor layer. Any lateral etching is suppressed, and near vertical sidewalls can result.

Of course, as even more carbon is added to the system and the deposition of the polymer becomes faster relative to the etching of the polymer and film, then sloped sidewalls (without mask undercutting) can result, as discussed earlier and illustrated in Figures 10–14 and 10–21. CHF_3 has a higher ratio of C to F than CF_4 does so that more polymer forms, in fact enough so that sloped sidewalls often result. If pure CHF_3 produces excess inhibitor deposition for particular plasma conditions, then O_2 could be added to react with the carbon and reduce the polymer deposition and change the etch profile. Other species such as CO_2 or CF_4 may also be added to CHF_3 for this purpose. Figure 10–24 conceptually illustrates the different etch profiles in SiO_2 that could result when different amounts of inhibitor formation occur.

Reducing the fluorine-to-carbon ratio also greatly improves the etch selectivity of SiO_2 over Si. This is because polymer formation preferentially occurs on Si surfaces compared to SiO_2 surfaces during the etch process. This may be due to the fact that carbon in the polymer reacts with the oxygen from the oxide, forming carbon monoxide, which results in much less accumulation of polymer on the oxide surface. With more polymer on the Si, its etching is slower, resulting in a higher SiO_2 to Si etch selectivity. Figure 10–25 shows how the etch rates of Si and SiO_2, and hence the selectivity, vary as H_2 is added to a CF_4 gas mixture [10.15]. The etch selectivities of oxide over $TiSi_2$ and TiN, which are important when etching contact or via holes in multilayer structures, are enhanced in this same manner by adding H_2 to the fluorocarbon etchant.

Changing the etchant chemistry may also change the etch rate of the mask. As seen in Figure 10–25, the etch rate of photoresist changes significantly as the H_2 content in the H_2/CH_4 gas mixture changes, with a lower H_2 content (and less F production) resulting in a higher etch rate. Adding O_2 to a CHF_3 mixture similarly increases the etch rate of the photoresist. The resulting mask erosion can cause the etch profile of the SiO_2 to change, as we will illustrate in the models and simulation section (Figure 10–33), and may alter the profiles shown above in Figure 10–24.

A relatively large bias voltage is often used for SiO_2 etching (in the 400- to 500-V range). This is needed to help remove the polymers. After the SiO_2 etching is complete, including a suitable overetch, any remaining polymer residue must be removed, espe-

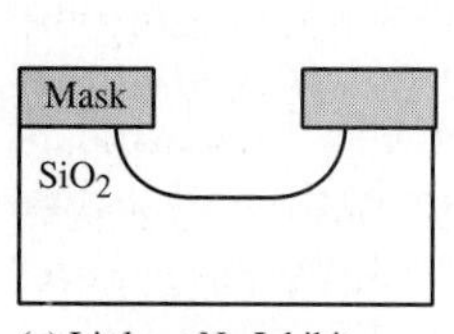

(a) Little or No Inhibitor Deposition (e.g. $CF_4 + O_2$)

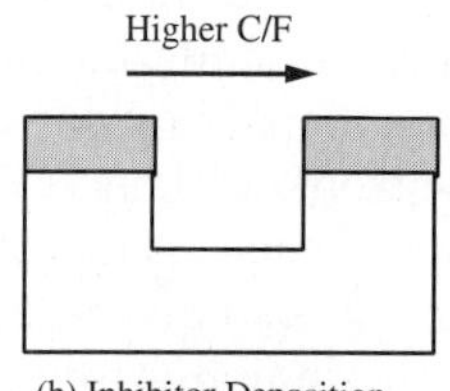

(b) Inhibitor Deposition (e.g. $CF_4 + H_2$, or $CHF_3 + O_2$)

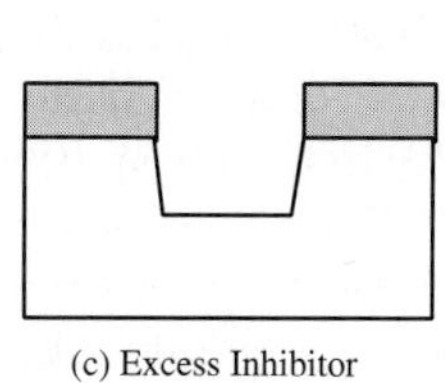

(c) Excess Inhibitor Deposition (e.g. CHF_3)

Figure 10–24 Effect of inhibitor deposition on resulting etch profile. The profiles shown assume no mask erosion, which may occur for different etch chemistries. The actual profiles obtained will also depend on the specific etch system and plasma conditions.

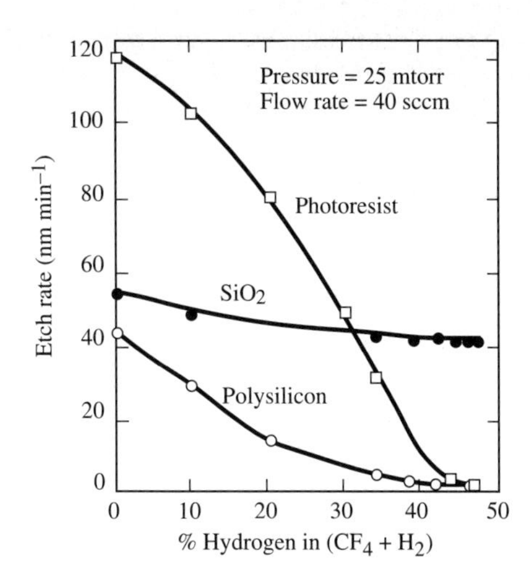

Figure 10–25 The etch rates of Si and SiO_2 (and photoresist) as H_2 is added to a CH_4 gas mixture. (After [10.15].)

cially in contact holes. The polymer can be removed by an O_2 or CF_4 plasma treatment. CF_4 is better at removing all the polymer and even some damaged substrate, but it cannot be over done since it has poor selectivity over Si and there can be lateral etching. A lower energy is used for the cleanup step so as not to damage the exposed material below. Also helpful is an anneal treatment; the polymer appears to break down at temperatures higher than $\approx 280°C$.

It should be clear from the discussion in this section that there are many details and subtleties associated with developing a particular manufacturing recipe for plasma etching. We will return to some of these issues in the models and simulation section.

10.3.2.2 Plasma Etching Polysilicon

The choice of etch chemistry for polysilicon depends on the same factors as etching silicon dioxide: byproduct volatility, selectivity, and anisotropy. Another issue is the presence of the ubiquitous native oxide layer on the film's surface, requiring an initial "breakthrough" etch step to remove it.

F-based etchants could be used for polysilicon etching because of the volatility of SiF_4. However, etching polysilicon with SF_6, CF_4, or CF_4/O_2 has a relatively large isotropic component due to the high concentration of F free radical species produced in such plasmas combined with little polymer formation. We saw that with etching SiO_2, anisotropy can be enhanced by reducing the relative F component and increasing the carbon component, thus decreasing the spontaneous etching, increasing polymer formation, and enhancing ion-induced etching. Adding H_2 or using CHF_3 can accomplish this. But doing so also increases the etch rate of SiO_2 relative to Si by preferentially forming a polymer on the Si. This is good when etching SiO_2 but bad when etching polysilicon when a high selectivity over the underlying SiO_2 is required. (Recall the structure in Figure 2–26 in the CMOS process flow in Chapter 2 for an example of why good selectivity over SiO_2 might be important.) Thus with a fluorine chemistry it is difficult to achieve both anisotropic etching and good selectivity of polysilicon over silicon dioxide at the same time.

If anisotropy is not important, then adding O_2 to CF_4 allows etching polysilicon selectively over silicon dioxide since the etch rate of the Si is increased by O_2 much more than that of SiO_2. But the etch will be fairly isotropic. One approach with fluorine chemistry when both anisotropy and selectivity with respect to an underlying oxide are desired is to switch the gas chemistry during the etching. One would start with an anisotropic etch, with a CF_4/H_2 mixture for example, and then when the etch is almost done, switch to an etch chemistry that is selective over SiO_2, using CF_4/O_2 for example. This will, however, result in some undercutting of the polysilicon.

Anisotropic and selective etching of polysilicon can be achieved simultaneously using Cl-based etchants. The byproduct volatility is a little lower with Cl than with F, but is still acceptable. Cl_2, HCl, or $SiCl_4$ can be used. These have a lower purely chemical component to etching than the F-containing etchants, and less lateral etching of Si occurs than with F. The etch rate in the vertical direction is significantly increased by ion bombardment, perhaps by surface bond breaking or by enhancing byproduct removal. Thus the etching of Si with Cl can be fairly anisotropic even without a polymer inhibitor layer present. Along with being anisotropic, the etch selectivity of Si to SiO_2 is high. For one thing, there is no polymer inhibitor layer that may form preferentially on the Si, as in the fluorine case, and degrade selectivity. Also, chlorine etches SiO_2 rather slowly. Furthermore, removing or minimizing the carbon in these systems is seen to significantly lower the etch rate of SiO_2 by chlorine—carbon evidently plays a role in the SiO_2-Cl etch reaction and enhances the etching at low carbon concentrations. Therefore the etch selectivity of Si to SiO_2 can be quite high, typically over 100, for these anisotropic, chlorine-based etchants. The anisotropy can be enhanced even more by adding a small amount of O_2. The O_2 reacts with the Si film, or with etch reaction byproducts that have adsorbed on the sidewall to form a nonpolymer, SiO_2-based inhibitor layer. The O_2 also helps with selectivity over oxide by removing any carbon that comes from photoresist erosion. Keeping the wafer temperature low, by providing helium backside heat conduction for example, also improves the anisotropy by enhancing inhibitor deposition.

Cl-based etchants exhibit a large doping sensitivity. High n^+ levels can increase the polysilicon etch rate by up to 25 times, and can increase the spontaneous etching and undercutting. An SiO_2-based inhibitor can block this. Cl-based chemistries etch the polysilicon slower than F-based chemistries, and mixtures of the two types have been used. The addition of SF_6 also reduces trenching. Trenching at gate edges can be a problem with chlorine etching, with the underlying gate oxide being damaged. Chlorinated flourocarbons, such as C_2ClF_5, have also been used for etching polysilicon but are out of favor since they are believed to cause environmental damage by depleting the ozone layer.

The most popular etchants used currently for polysilicon are chemistries based on bromine, the next halogen after F and Cl in the periodic table. HBr and Br_2 are commonly used. These act in a similar fashion to the Cl-based etchants, etching with a low purely-chemical component and without a polymer inhibitor, and are even more anisotropic and selective over oxide. Trenching of the underlying oxide is less of a problem as well. But the etch rates of Br-based chemistries are even slower than Cl-based chemistries, and they are often used in a mixture with Cl_2 in current polysilicon etch processes. As with etching with Cl, adding O_2 in these noncarbon containing gases promotes inhibitor formation, perhaps by forming SiO_2 from the Si film, and thereby increases the anisotropy. The O_2 also helps with selectivity over oxide by removing any carbon that might result from photoresist erosion. One drawback to the use of HBr and Cl_2 is their high toxicity which puts more stringent requirements on equipment and gas handling systems.

Polysilicon, like single-crystal silicon, usually has a small native oxide layer present on the surface, even after cleaning. This must be removed prior to etching. Since the etchants used for the main polysilicon etch have low-oxide etch rates, the etch must be initially modified to increase the oxide etch rate. This is called a breakthrough step. During the first 5 to 10 seconds of the poly etch, one can lower the selectivity with respect to oxide by adding an etchant such as CF_4 or by increasing the RF power to enhance the physical component of etching and etch the thin oxide layer from the surface.

An overetch step after the main etch is also important for polysilicon etching. This not only allows for deposition and etch nonuniformities, but also for the presence of stringers at steps, as discussed earlier and illustrated in Figure 10–23. This overetch step is often done at a lower RF power to increase the selectivity over oxide. A final postetch "cleanup" step is done to remove any sidewall layer material. While polymeric (carbon containing) layers would need an O_2 plasma strip, followed by an HF dip, inorganic layers usually need only an HF dip.

To produce shallow trench isolation structures, etching of the silicon is a critical process step as described in Chapter 2 (Figures 2–6 to 2–9). Achieving the desired etch profile and selectivity to mask layers is important, and many of the same ideas regarding polysilicon etching would apply. Using a Cl- or Br-based etchant can give good selectivity over silicon dioxide or silicon nitride mask layers and provide good anisotropy, as described above. Using Cl etchants alone can result in harmful ion-induced trenching at the bottom corners, so Br etchants are often used—either by themselves or in combination with Cl etchants. The slope of the etch profile can be tailored by including gas additives, such as O_2, to promote inhibitor deposition, and multistep etch processes may be utilized to achieve the desired profile.

10.3.2.3 Plasma Etching Aluminum

Plasma etching of aluminum interconnect lines has been a challenge for process engineers, but successful strategies have been developed to overcome the many problems associated with this film. Again, byproduct volatility, selectivity, and anisotropy are issues, as well as native oxide on the surface. In addition, a potential corrosion problem as well as Cu doping in the film lead to more difficulties.

Because of the presence of a native oxide, Al_2O_3, on the Al film surface, an initiation or breakthrough etch step must be done before the main Al etch step. Ion bombardment, or sputtering, is usually done to remove this film in conjunction with chemical scavenging. Argon sputtering can be used, but gases such as BCl_3, $SiCl_4$, CCl_4, or BBr_3 are often used to scavenge the O_2 and H_2O and remove Al_2O_3 on the Al surface by both physical and chemical means. A load lock system is required to control the H_2O level.

The byproduct of etching Al with F-based chemistries, AlF_3, is not very volatile as discussed earlier, so that a Cl-based chemistry is most often used for the main Al etch step. Cl_2 is commonly used, and Cl_2 (not a free radical, but still a reactive neutral species) can directly etch the Al. However Cl_2 etches Al isotropically, producing an undercut, and ion bombardment has little effect on the etch rate (unlike the etching of Si by Cl_2). To suppress lateral etching of the Al and obtain vertical profiles, sidewall inhibitor formation is needed. Therefore inhibitor sources or promoters are often added to the gas mixture. These include $CHCl_3$, $CFCl_3$, CCl_4, and N_2. Resist erosion plays a significant role in supplying inhibitor material in Al etching, and N_2 enhances the inhibitor formation from photoresist, perhaps forming a CN polymer. BCl_3 also seems to promote inhibitor formation. The etch rate and selectivity over silicon dioxide are acceptable for Cl-based chemistries.

Al interconnect lines usually contain Si and Cu, which can complicate the etching. While Si is readily etched by Cl, Cu is not (the volatility of the Cu byproducts by halogen etching is quite low). Ion bombardment and often higher temperatures are needed. We will describe in Chapter 11 how Ti and/or TiN layers are often used above and below Al layers in the interconnects. These are usually etched at the same time as the Al, and Cl-based chemistries can readily etch them as well.

An overetch step is especially important for Al etching to remove the residues, both from the inhibitor layers and the Cu precipitates that can remain. The difficulty in Cu precipitate and residue removal depends on the Al deposition conditions, with a higher deposition temperature giving larger precipitates and more residues.

Corrosion of the etched Al line can be a problem when it is exposed to the ambient. Residual chorine on the sidewall and in the resist can react with water to form HCl. The HCl can then etch the Al. Cu in the films enhances this electrochemical reaction. It is important to passivate the Al film after the etching and before it is exposed to air. The wafer can be heated to 100°C or 150°C to drive off the Cl. Or the Cl can be buried under a CHF_3 polymer, which is then wet etched. But the common method has been to expose the wafer to an F-containing plasma, such as a CF_4 plasma. The chlorine is replaced by fluorine on the Al surface, passivating it. An O_2 plasma then removes the photoresist, and a deionized H_2O bath removes any remaining chlorine. A wafer rinse may also be done before the ashing to help remove the water-soluble chlorides before they are converted by the ashing to insoluble metal oxides [10.16]. A newer process uses an H_2O plasma to both pacify the surface and to remove the resist.

We end this section with a short comment regarding the use of freons, or fluorocarbons. Chlorinated flourocarbons without any hydrogen, such as C_2ClF_5 or $CClF_3$, are believed to deplete the ozone layer in the upper atmosphere. There has been a trend to replace these with safer source gases in the semiconductor industry.

10.4 Measurement Methods

Measurement techniques for etching can be separated into two types: post-etch measurements and *in situ* measurements. Post-etch measurements are generally performed outside the etch chamber. *In situ* measurements are done inside the chamber as the etching is occurring for diagnostic and monitoring purposes. The most important type of monitoring is that done for endpoint detection.

Post-etch measurements for etching are performed to characterize the etch process. The resulting line width can be measured using an optical microscope. Observing the wafer under a microscope can also indicate whether some of the film still remains in the patterned areas due to underetching. However optical observations and measurements are difficult for submicron lines. A much more accurate method for line width measurement is the Scanning Electron Microscope (SEM), discussed in earlier chapters. More automated versions of SEMs have been especially designed for linewidth observation and measurement for both lithography and etching. Measurements from above the wafer looking down assume that the sides of the etched film are vertical. Obviously this may not be so. To observe and measure the actual profile of the etched film, cross-sectional SEM images are used. An example was shown in Figure 10–22. This method requires cleaving the sample and is done on test wafers, usually when developing the process. Linewidth measurements of etched films using electrical testing methods were discussed in Chapter 5.

Other post-etch measurement techniques include composition and contamination measurements. Small amounts of polymeric residues may remain which can have detrimental affects on later processing and circuit behavior. Surface analysis techniques such as Auger Electron Spectroscopy (AES) and X-ray Photoelectron Spectroscopy (XPS) can be used to detect and measure chemical species left on the film or in the near-surface region. XPS is often used to give bonding information and can distinguish whether carbon detected on the surface is bonded to fluorine in $C\text{-}F_2$ structures or to the silicon in the substrate with C-Si bonding, for example. This helps to determine the actual source of the contaminant or residue and the mechanism for its production.

Measuring damage induced by plasma processing is important. Physical damage, in terms of dislocations, trenching, and surface roughening, can be measured by TEM or SEM. Electrical damage, including charging and electron traps, is measured using device or electrical measurements, often using MOS capacitors as discussed in Chapter 6.

In situ measurements are performed inside the etch chamber while the etch process is taking place. The most important type of *in situ* measurement is that done for endpoint detection. Due to the physical component in most plasma etching, selectivity is not 100 percent. Therefore it is important to end the etching soon after the film has been etched to the bottom (allowing for a certain amount of overetch, of course). Some sort of *in situ* measurement is required to do this.

One way to detect the endpoint is to measure the thickness of the film as it is being etched. If one does not want to etch all the way through the film, the endpoint thickness may be some finite value. This method would also give etch rate information as well. An *in situ* thickness measurement technique for optically transparent films, such as silicon dioxide, is interferometry. This method determines the thickness of the film by measuring the interference of optical beams—using either light from a laser or from the plasma itself—reflected from the top and bottom of the etched layer. As the material is etched, oscillations in the reflected signal occur as constructive and destructive interference occurs. The period of oscillation is related to the change in film thickness, x_f, via the relationship

$$\Delta x_f = \frac{\lambda}{2n} \tag{10.13}$$

where λ is the wavelength of the laser light and n is the refractive index of the film. Therefore, for each complete cycle in the reflected signal, the film has been etched Δx_f. When the film has been etched completely, the oscillations cease. For nontransparent films, such as metals, techniques using reflectivity differences between the film and the layer underneath can be used. A major disadvantage in film thickness techniques is that the information is obtained from only a small area of the wafer which may not be fully representative of other regions. Recent single-wafer systems use an array of sensors to measure the thickness change at many points on each wafer. One advantage to these systems is that they can accurately measure the ongoing etch rate during an etch process, which can be valuable information concerning the process.

The most common methods for endpoint detection are those which monitor the reacting species or reaction products of an etch process. Optical spectroscopy or mass spectroscopy can be used, but the former is more common. In optical emission spectroscopy a photosensor detects and measures the emitted radiation, through a window into the chamber, from the various species in the plasma as a function of wavelength. In a plasma, light is emitted by exited atoms and molecules as electrons relax from one energy state to another (which is why the plasma glows). Each species emits light in a characteristic spectrum which can be used to identify the particular atom or molecule. (See Figure 4–18.) For example, the fluorine free radical emits light at 703.7 nm (among other wavelengths) as it relaxes from a plasma-induced excited state. Monitoring this wavelength can be used to determine the relative concentration of the fluorine free radical in the plasma. Endpoint detection is done by either monitoring the reacting species or the reaction products.

As an example, consider the etching of SiO_2 on Al by CF_4 chemistry. The main etch reaction occurring here involves the fluorine free radical which is produced in the plasma. As the etching begins, F is consumed by the etch process, forming SiF_4. Therefore the signal from F emission is decreased. When the etching finishes, the concentration of F increases, and its signal goes back up. The endpoint is thus indicated by the increase of the reactant species. Alternately, the endpoint can be indicated by the increase or decrease in the emission signal of an etch product. For example, in etching SiO_2 by CHF_3, one reaction that can occur is between the carbon on the SiO_2 surface and oxygen, producing CO. Monitoring CO at its characteristic 483.0-nm wavelength can be used to detect the presence of CO. When the CO signal decreases below a certain point, the etch is determined to be over. This method, in contrast to thickness measurements, takes its information from the gas phase and thus averages over a much larger region. Therefore, a more average endpoint is determined. Loading effects can occur, since the signal from either the reactants or products will depend on how much material is being etched. In addition, the exact quantification of the signal to concentrations is difficult and some calibration is necessary to determine at what point the etch is completed. However, this method is relatively simple and usually a good indicator of when the etching is complete, and is the most common method in current technology.

The technique of optical emission spectroscopy, in addition to being used as an end-point determination method, is also used in diagnostics of plasma etch processes. By following the emission signals, the relative concentrations of the various species present during the etching process can be measured throughout the etch process. This can give valuable information concerning the various mechanisms occurring and the roles of the different species.

In situ measurements can also be utilized for process control applications. For example, loading effects could be monitored and changes in equipment parameters could be made automatically and instantaneously, based on the feedback from such measurements. Such measurements could also be used to determine when chambers must be cleaned due to buildup of etch residues on the chamber walls.

10.5 Models and Simulation

We have described the different types of underlying mechanisms important for plasma etch processes: chemical etching by reactive chemical species; physical etching by bombardment or sputtering of ionic species; and ion-enhanced etching involving both types of species acting in a synergistic manner. As in Chapter 9, we will describe physically based models that predict the shape, or topography, that results from specific etching technologies. These models are implemented in a variety of simulation tools including SPEEDIE [10.17], TAURUS-TOPOGRAPHY [10.18], and ATHENA [10.19], as well as other topography simulation tools mentioned in the previous chapter. We will show examples from all three of these simulators. In this section we will first describe how physically based simulators model plasma etching. Since there are a number of similarities to the models described in Chapter 9 for simulating deposition of thin films, we will refer the reader to that chapter for some of the specific details.

10.5.1 Models for Etching Simulation

As in the simulation of deposition, plasma etching can be simulated by considering the fluxes of species that come from the plasma and strike the surface of the wafer. In Figure 10–20 we schematically illustrated the fluxes of species coming from the plasma and the various processes that occur on the wafer surface during etching of the films. In physically based topography simulators, the flux of each type of species is calculated, in particular the component of the incoming flux normal to the surface at each point. Because of the relatively low pressures used in etch systems and large mean free paths compared to the feature size on the wafer surface, it is usually assumed that free molecular flow is the dominant gas-phase transport mechanism near the surface, that is, there is no boundary layer diffusion process. The net etch rate at each point is then calculated using an expression that relates the etch rate to the different fluxes. The exact form of that expression depends on the model that is used. We will describe some of these models and expressions in the next section. With the etch rate determined at each location, the appropriate amount of material is removed, the boundary is moved, and the profile can evolve as the etching continues. The etch rate at each location can change with time as the etching progresses because the fluxes that reach each location on the surface can change due to changing geometrical effects, such as flux shadowing.

As in deposition modeling, the flux of species arriving from the plasma and striking the wafer surface can be calculated using Monte Carlo techniques. For example, the distribution of ions in terms of arrival angle at the surface and of energy can be calculated as a function of system parameters, such as gas pressure, composition, and RF settings. This explicitly takes into account the collisions that occur in the plasma and in the sheath, and the acceleration across the sheath to the wafer. There have been several simulation tools developed, including a version of SPEEDIE, that take this approach. However, we again will utilize a simpler approach and define the incoming fluxes analytically on a plane just above the surface. We specify the maximum, unobstructed flux of each species—ions or chemical, for example—and the angular distribution of each.

The angular distribution is assumed to be of the form

$$F_{\text{direct}}(\theta) = F^{\circ} \cos^{n}\theta \tag{10.14}$$

where F_{direct} is the normal component of the flux coming in at angle θ, F° is the flux at $\theta = 0$ degrees, and θ is the angle from the vertical direction. By adjusting n from 1 to large numbers, one can obtain isotropic to anisotropic distributions of arrival angles, respectively. This was illustrated in Figure 9–25 in Chapter 9. With $n = 1$, the distribution is isotropic, with fluxes coming from all directions equally. Higher pressure, more collisions in the gas phase, and shorter mean free path would all lead to a more isotropic arrival distribution. In etching, neutral chemical species are usually assumed to arrive at the top surface isotropically, and $n = 1$ is usually used. For $n > 1$, a tighter distribution of arrival angles would occur. This means that the fluxes arriving at each point on the surface are more directed, or more anisotropic. In etch models, the ionic species—accelerated across the sheath to the wafer surface due to the electric field—are assumed to arrive at the surface approximately perpendicular to the wafer and very anisotropically, and $n = 10$ to 80 is usually used.

Figure 10–26 illustrates the species and fluxes that occur in plasma etching that are included in physically based etch simulators. This is analogous to the fluxes used in deposition modeling (see Figure 9–35). The ionic species are involved in the physical component of etching, and the reactive neutral species would include those species involved in the chemical component of etching, and would primarily be the free radicals. Another type of species is the deposited, or deposition, species. These would include material that is deposited in the form of inhibitor layers, often carbon polymeric material. These would be analogous to the neutral species that deposit in the deposition models. As we mentioned earlier in this chapter, the same processes (deposition, chemical etch, ion bombardment, etc.) often occur in both deposition and etch processes.

As in deposition modeling, the total flux of each type of species arriving at each position will be the sum of that coming directly from the plasma (a direct flux) plus that coming from somewhere else on the surface of the wafer (an indirect flux). The indirect fluxes may be a result of reemission or resputtering from another location. In Chapter 9 many of those processes and the equations used to describe them were presented.

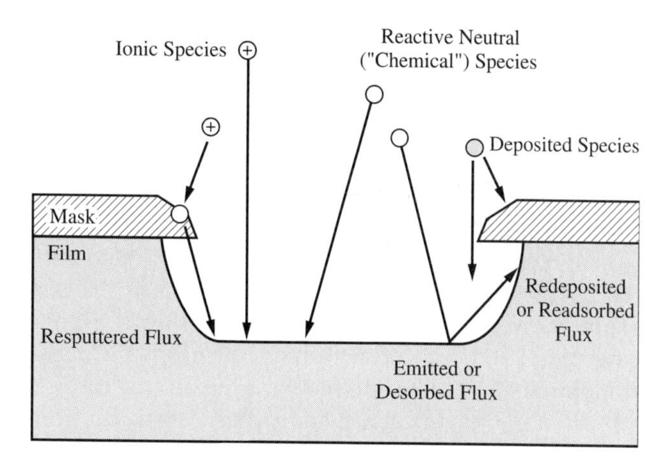

Figure 10–26 Illustration of fluxes, both direct and indirect, that are used in physically based etch simulations.

One of the important sources of indirect flux is that due to reemission of the etch reactant before it can react and etch. This is described by the sticking coefficient. The sticking coefficient is defined, as in Chapter 9 and earlier in this chapter, as the ratio of the flux of species that actually deposit or react at each location on the surface, to the flux of incident species:

$$S_c = \frac{F_{\text{reacted}}}{F_{\text{incident}}} \tag{10.11}$$

Therefore S_c times the chemical flux hitting the surface at each point is the net flux that actually etches, and $(1 - S_c)$ is the fraction of the flux that is reemitted. These reemitted atoms or molecules can then travel to other locations on the surface and etch material there. If S_c is set to a low number ($S_c << 1$) for the chemical species, as is usually the case, then isotropic etching can occur for purely chemical etch processes. Most of the chemical species move in all directions from place to place, as was illustrated in Figure 10–11(a), with a net result that etching is isotropic.

It is usually assumed that the angular distribution of the desorbed or emitted flux follows an ideal cosine distribution ($n = 1$ in $\cos^n\theta_i$ emitted distribution, where θ_i is the angle relative to the surface normal); that is, the emitted species are emitted in an ideal fashion from a small area on the surface. In SPEEDIE it is currently assumed that only the neutral species can be emitted from the surface; for ionic species the sticking coefficient is assumed to be one. This does not mean that all ionic species are successful in etching, or sputtering, an atom or atoms from the surface. It just means that the ions that do not etch any material are not reemitted to etch elsewhere.

In Chapter 9, we described how it has been experimentally determined that surface diffusion for SiO_2 deposited by both LPCVD and PECVD methods was not important—the results could be modeled better with the reemission and redeposition process. A similar experiment has been done to distinguish between the two processes in plasma etching of silicon [10.20, 10.21]. By modeling the undercut profiles, it was determined that using the reemission/readsorption model, with a low sticking coefficient, works better than using the surface diffusion process in the simulation. Thus surface diffusion of the species is often not included as a model in etch simulators.

Physical etching occurs by sputtering when ions strike the surface. Sputtering occurs when the incoming ion transfers enough energy to the wafer surface to break the bonds holding a surface atom in place. The sputtering yield, Y, is defined as the number of atoms or molecules ejected from the target per incident ion and is a measure of the sputtering efficiency. Therefore Y times the ion flux striking the surface at each point determines how much physical etching occurs for a given ion flux .

The sputter yield, Y, is a function of ion energy, the mass of the incoming ion and the target material (the wafer surface material, in this case), and the incident angle, θ, at point i, with a normal incidence being 0°. As we discussed in Chapter 9, ions coming in at low angles are reflected from the surface and do not transfer significant energy to the surface atoms, while ions coming perpendicular to the surface knock surface atoms further into the film and not off. The maximum sputtering yield occurs usually at somewhere from 40–70°. This is usually modeled as was described in Figure 9–39.

In some of our models we will use K_i, the ion-induced etch yield, or the effective sputtering yield. Like Y, it is a measure of how many atoms or molecules of substrate are etched per incident ion but can include the synergistic effects with the chemical component, resulting in higher values for it than normal physical sputtering yields. K_i generally has similar properties as Y, angle and energy dependencies for example. For cases of purely physical sputtering, K_i would just equal Y.

All of the geometrical issues involved in the etching process are taken into account in physically based etch simulators. That is, the net flux of each type of species at each point on the surface is calculated based on the relative orientation of that point to all sources of fluxes. This includes fluxes from the plasma source (the direct flux) and from all other points on the surface (the indirect fluxes). The view angles to all other sources of fluxes, as well as the angular distribution emitted from each source, are taken into account in the calculation of the arriving flux at each point.

Once the net flux of each type of species is calculated at each point on the surface, the etch rate can then be calculated at each point. This is determined by the specific etch model used in the simulation. We will next consider some of the models and corresponding etch rate expressions that etch simulators use to model plasma etching.

10.5.2 Etching Models — Linear Etch Model

Different types of etch models have been developed and are available in simulators. Some of these models are for specific types of etching equipment—for high-density plasma etch systems or for sputter etch systems, for example. However, there are also some more general-purpose models. These were developed to model the different types of mechanisms that occur during plasma etching: physical, chemical, and ion-assisted etching, and which can occur in any of the plasma etch systems. We will concentrate on those models, and two in particular: the linear etch model and the saturation/adsorption etch model, both of which are used in the SPEEDIE simulator.

The simplest model for etching assumes that the chemical and ionic components act independently of each other and combine in a linear fashion. This is the basis of the linear etch model in SPEEDIE. Other simulators include similar models. It is assumed in this model that the etch rate due to each component is linearly proportional to the flux of that component. Studies of chemical etching do show a linear dependence of etch rate on the chemical flow rate or flux for certain conditions [10.5, 10.22]. Likewise, the etch rate in the presence of ionic bombardment is seen to be linearly dependent on the ion current or flux over a range of conditions [10.23]. The two terms are then added together, so that

$$\text{Etch rate} = \frac{(S_c K_f F_c + K_i F_i)}{N} \tag{10.15}$$

The density, N (in cm^{-3}), is that of the film being etched. F_c is the chemical (reactive neutral, free radical) flux and F_i is the ion flux at each point on the surface. S_c is the sticking coefficient, which is between 0 and 1. K_f and K_i are the relative rate constants for the two processes and can include any stoichiometric factors. In practice, K_f is often used as a fitting parameter for the purely (non-ion-enhanced or "spontaneous") chemical etching. As described above, K_i is the ion-induced etch yield and is related to the number of ions needed to remove one atom or molecule for the material being etched. It is essentially equivalent to the physical sputtering yield, Y, but can be greater than Y in some cases as we will discuss. K_i can be a function of incident angle and ion energy. Like K_f, it is often used as a fitting parameter.

One can see that the net etch rate at each point is just the linear combination of purely chemical etching and ion-driven etching, with each term linearly dependent on the appropriate flux. The etch profile would likewise be a linear combination of the two components, with chemical etching occurring equally in all directions plus the physical, ion-driven etching occurring primarily in the vertical direction.

While being simple, with no coupling between the components, the model may be appropriate for certain conditions. It would be valid when the etch process is purely chemical, in which case the ion flux would be zero, and the etch rate is simply proportional to the chemical flux. Purely chemical etching would occur in a barrel etcher or in an after-glow system, for example, where the ions are prevented from striking the wafer surface. It could even occur in a parallel plate system if little or no inhibitor layer is formed and there is a very high concentration of free radicals in the plasma and only spontaneous chemical etching occurs. For purely chemical etching, the etch profile would be completely isotropic and look like Figure 10–3(a). This model would also be valid when the etch process is only dependent on the ion flux, as in solely physical etching, in which case the first term would be zero. This would occur, for example, in a sputter etch system where only high-energy, chemically inert Ar^+ ions are used. When the etch rate is simply proportional to the ion flux with no chemical term, the profile would look like Figure 10–3(c), with vertical or near-vertical etching and no undercutting.

The model would also be applicable when the etch process does have both chemical and physical etching components, but the two act independently of each other. Or at least they each appear as if they are independent in that they do not limit the action of the other for a given range of conditions. For example, the physical, ionic component in this model (the second term in the rate expression) does not, in fact, have to be due to purely physical sputtering. It could actually be ion-enhanced etching, but operating in a regime where the chemical component in that mechanism is high enough, due to a relatively high flux of neutrals, for example, and is not limiting the ion-driven etching, as we will describe later. In that regime the ion-enhanced etching would act as if it were purely physical and not dependent on the chemical flux, that is, simply proportional to the ion flux. In that case, K_i is often much greater than the normal physical sputtering yield. [And if there is no spontaneous chemical etching, the profile would look like that for purely physical etching, Figure 10–3(c).] In addition, any adverse effect the ion bombardment might have on the spontaneous chemical etch term, by depleting the surface chemical species for example, may not be significant at lower ion fluxes or higher neutral fluxes [10.21]. When two (seemingly) independent etch components are present, isotropic chemical and directional ionic, the etch profile would look like Figure 10–3(b), a linear combination of the profiles for spontaneous chemical etching and ion-driven etching. So in general, the simple linear etch model would be appropriate when one or two independent, or seemingly independent, etch components are present, resulting in a range of etch profiles.

Example Silicon is plasma etched for 5 minutes and the process follows the linear etch model. The flux of chemical species, F_c, on an unobstructed flat surface is equal to 2.5 $\times 10^{18}$ atoms cm^{-2} sec^{-1}, the sticking coefficient is 0.01, and K_f is 0.2. The flux of ionic species, F_i, on a flat surface is equal to 1×10^{16} atoms cm^{-2} sec^{-1} and K_i is 1. The density of Si is 5.0×10^{22} atoms cm^{-3} A photoresist mask is used so that a wide trench is etched in the Si. (There is no etching of the photoresist.) How far is the Si etched in the vertical direction (away from the mask edge), and how far is the Si etched in the lateral direction right under the mask for these conditions?

Answer For the linear etch model, Eq. (10.15):

$$\text{Etch rate} = \frac{(S_c K_f F_c + K_i F_i)}{N}$$

In the vertical direction, there would be both chemical and ion fluxes, and the total etch rate in this model would simply be the sum of those components. Away from the mask edge we assume no shadowing effects, so F_c and F_i are the unobstructed chemical and ion fluxes, respectively, given above. Therefore

$$\text{Etch rate(vert)} = \frac{(0.01 * 0.2 * 2.5 \times 10^{18}\text{cm}^{-2}\text{sec}^{-1} + 1 * 1 \times 10^{16}\text{cm}^{-2}\text{sec}^{-1})}{N}$$

$$= \frac{1.5 \times 10^{16}\text{cm}^{-2}\text{sec}^{-1}}{N}$$

The density of Si, N, is 5.0×10^{22} atoms cm^{-3}, so the Si etched in the vertical direction is

$$\text{Etch depth(vert)} = \frac{1.5 \times 10^{16}\text{cm}^{-2}\text{sec}^{-1}}{5.0 \times 10^{22}\text{cm}^{-3}} * 300\text{ sec} = 9.0 \times 10^{-5}\text{cm} = 0.9\mu\text{m}$$

In the lateral direction, right under the mask edge, there is virtually no ion flux ($F_i \approx 0$). Therefore only the chemical flux term is used in the etch rate expression and it is assumed that the chemical flux is the same in all directions (due to the isotropic arrival distribution and, especially, the low S_c), so that

$$\text{Etch depth(lat)} = \frac{(0.01 * 0.2 * 2.5 \times 10^{18}\text{cm}^{-2}\text{sec}^{-1} + 0)}{5.0 \times 10^{22}\text{cm}^{-3}} * 300\text{ sec}$$

$$= 3 \times 10^{-5}\text{cm} = 0.3\ \mu\text{m}$$

There is more etching in the vertical direction than in the lateral direction, and a profile such as that in Figure 10–3(b) occurs in this case.

This model has been used to accurately simulate the etching of Si under certain conditions. For example, Singh and colleagues [10.20] etched Si using a CF_4/O_2 plasma. As we noted earlier, this can result in isotropic etching, with a very strong chemical component. They used the etch system in the plasma mode, with symmetric electrode areas, which minimizes any ion bombardment. In addition, an oxide etch mask was used rather than photoresist so that the formation of a carbon-containing inhibitor layer was minimized. The etch profiles obtained were virtually isotropic and they were able to model them with the linear etch model in SPEEDIE and assuming no ion component. A value of 0.04 was used for S_c.

This same group [10.21] etched Si using an SF_6 plasma, but now observed a mixture of chemical and physical etching. Etch profiles similar to that in Figure 10–3(b) were obtained, with notable undercutting but not completely isotropic. They were able to accurately model the profiles again with the linear etch model, with a chemical-to-physical component ratio of 2:1. They actually identified the physical component as an "ion-assisted mechanism" as opposed to purely physical sputtering but modeled it with a simple linear dependence on ion flux, independent from the isotropic chemical flux. Ulacia and colleagues [10.24] did similar experiments etching Si using a SF_6/C_2ClF_5 plasma and modeled it with the linear etch model. (Again the physical component was identified as ion-enhanced, but following a linear relationship with ion flux.) They were able to vary the chemical-to-physical ratio from 4:1 (near-isotropic) to approximately 1:1 and then to 1:20 (almost perfectly anisotropic) by changing the $SF_6:C_2ClF_5$ ratio and the amount of carbon in the system, and model the resulting etch profiles quite well with the linear etch model for a specific set of conditions.

We now describe a series of plasma etch simulations using the SPEEDIE simulator and the linear etch model just described. As with the SPEEDIE deposition simulations in Chapter 9, we will use analytical $\cos^n\theta$ distributions for arrival angles (as opposed to Monte Carlo calculations of gas-phase processes). A value of n equal to 1 results in an isotropic arrival angle distribution, relative to the vertical direction. A value of n higher than 1 results in a more anisotropic arrival distribution, with a more directed downward distribution such as occurs with ionic species. In all the simulations presented in this section, we etch a silicon substrate using a photoresist mask. The top layer is 1-μm thick photoresist, with a slightly sloped window defined in it.

The first simulation uses the linear etch model, and Eq. (10.15) to govern the etch rate at each point. Pure chemical etching is illustrated first in Figure 10–27(a). The simulation time is 240 seconds, and each of the contours corresponds to a 30-second time step in the etching. The arrival angle distribution parameter, n, for chemical is set to one, indicating an isotropic arrival angle distribution. The maximum unobstructed direct flux of neutral species is set to 5×10^{18} cm^{-2} sec^{-1}. This corresponds to the total integrated direct flux of chemical species arriving from all directions and hitting a flat, unobstructed surface. Knowing the angular distribution of arriving atoms and the geometry of the surface, SPEEDIE can convert this to the direct chemical flux normal to the surface, $F_{c(direct)}$, at each point. The value of the maximum direct chemical flux used in the simulations is usually determined by knowing the chemical rate on a flat surface, in which case it is directly equal to F_c, or is determined by fitting experimental profiles to the simulations. The ion flux is set to zero in this simulation, so that the etch is purely chemical. A low value for the sticking coefficient, S_c, is used for the chemical species, equal to 0.01, ensuring that F_c is equal everywhere and the chemical component to etching occurs isotropically. A value of 0.2 is used for K_f. Negligible etching of the photoresist occurs in these simulations.

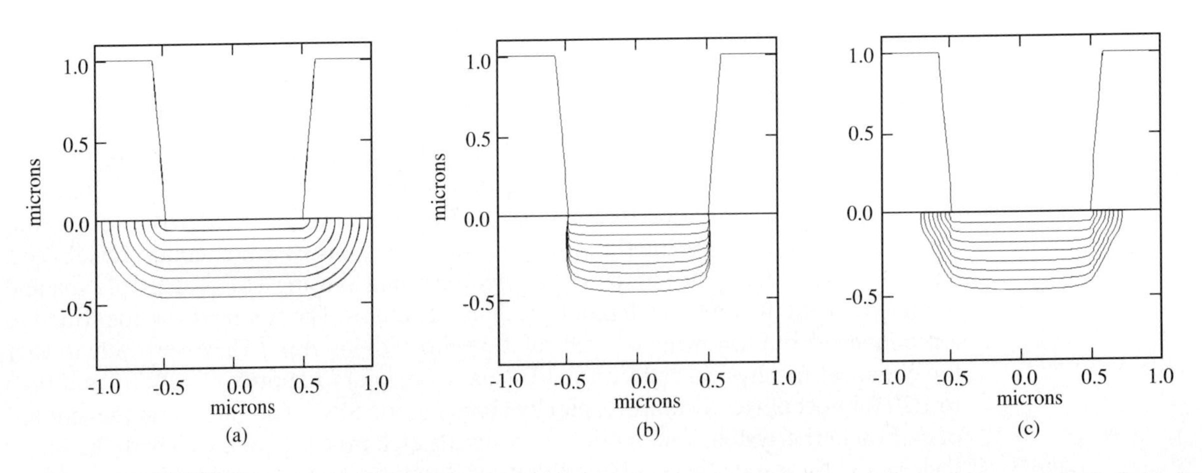

Figure 10–27 SPEEDIE simulations for etching of Si with linear etch model: (a) all chemical etching, showing isotropic etching; (b) all physical or ionic etching, showing very anisotropic etching; (c) half-chemical, half-ionic etching, showing a combination of isotropic and anisotropic etching. The different curves correspond to different times in the etch simulation.

Next only physical, ionic etching is illustrated using the same linear etch model. The chemical flux is set to zero while the maximum ionic flux is set to 1×10^{16} cm^{-2} sec^{-1}. Setting $n = 80$ means that nearly all the ionic flux will arrive from the vertical direction. K_i is set to 1. Figure 10–27(b) shows the results. Very anisotropic etching results as expected. Purely physical etching would occur in a sputter etch system (although one would expect etching of the resist as well in that case). This etch behavior could also occur, and be modeled in the same manner, for an ion-enhanced mechanism for conditions where the chemical component is not limiting the ion-driven etching anywhere in the structure, and where there is no spontaneous chemical etching.

Now we combine both chemical etching and physical/ionic etching in the linear etch model. As we discussed this model assumes that the two components are acting independently, or else in a regime where neither is limiting the action of the other. Here we use 2.5×10^{18} cm^{-2}sec^{-1} for the chemical maximum flux and 0.5×10^{16} cm^{-2}sec^{-1} for the ionic maximum flux, and the same values for S_c, K_f, and K_i we used above. This results in relatively equal contributions of the ionic and chemical components since the $S_cK_fF_c$ and K_iF_i products [see Eq. (10.15)] are equal. The resulting etch profile is shown in Figure 10–27(c). Different degrees of anisotropy can be achieved by varying the relative amounts of the two components. This behavior could occur in a plasma system in which there is both chemical etching and ionic sputtering acting separately. It could also occur where there is some spontaneous chemical etching, not affected by ion bombardment, as well as ion-enhanced etching for conditions in which the chemical component is not limiting the etching.

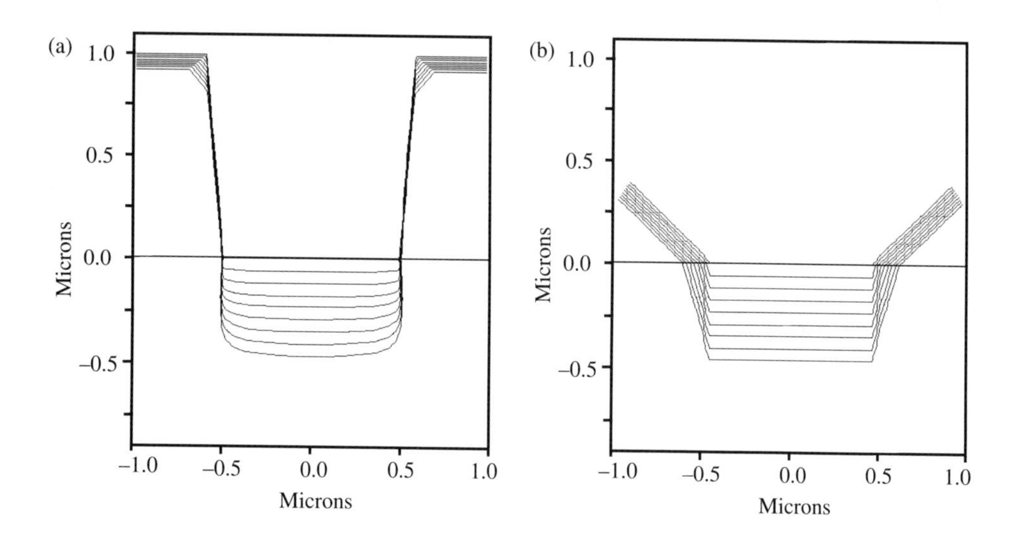

Figure 10–28 SPEEDIE simulations for etching of Si with linear etch model for physical-only etching with etching of photoresist included: (a) angle-dependent sputtering of photoresist included, showing faceting; (b) initial taper of photoresist changed, allowing for mask erosion due to vertical physical etching. A wider area of silicon is etched, and sloped sidewalls in the Si result.

Next we allow for some physical etching of the photoresist. We first allow for some angle-dependent physical sputtering of the photoresist during physical-only etching. We do this by increasing the value of K_i for the photoresist from 0 to 0.3. In Figure 10–28(a) we see the faceting that occurs at the top corners. Next we change the initial shape and thickness of the photoresist mask. We start with a thin mask, only 0.4 μm thick at the sides, which slopes diagonally to the opening. When physical etching occurs, the edge of the mask will be etched away, illustrating the phenomenon of mask erosion. Figure 10–28(b) shows the result. The etching away of the mask results in a wider etched area in the silicon, and nonvertical sidewalls. Changing the etch chemistry to change the amount of mask erosion can be utilized to obtain a desired etch profile.

We next illustrate the concept of Aspect Ratio Dependent Etching (ARDE). As discussed earlier this is the phenomenon in which the depth of etching decreases as the aspect ratio increases. One possible mechanism for this is that ion-neutral collisions in the sheath cause ions to be off-axis, making their arrival angle distribution wider. The less directed flux means that fewer ions reach the bottom of the etched trench due to view angle or shadowing considerations. With fewer ions getting to the bottom for the narrower openings, less vertical etching occurs, whether it is purely physical etching or ion-enhanced etching. This is simulated in the following two figures using the linear etch model. First we repeat the physical-only etching of Figure 10–27(b), except that we change the arrival angle distribution factor, n, for ions from 80 to 10, as might occur if the gas pressure were higher and more gas phase collisions take place, for example. This widens the arrival angle distribution a little, but the ions are still fairly directed downward. Figure 10–29(a) shows the result. More bowing of the sides results as compared to the $n = 80$ example in Figure 10–27(b), and this type of profile is seen in some etch

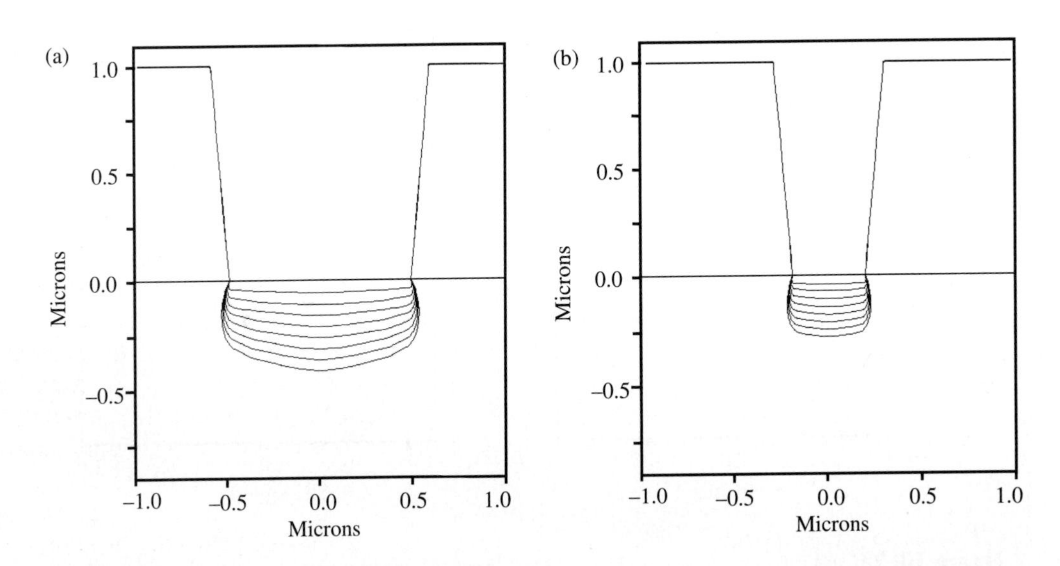

Figure 10–29 SPEEDIE simulations for etching of Si with the linear etch model illustrating Aspect Ratio Dependent Etching (ARDE). Physical-only etching (with arrival angle distribution factor $n = 10$) is done for two different mask opening widths: (a) mask opening = 1 μm; (b) mask opening = 0.4 μm. Deeper etching occurs for the wider mask opening.

systems. Now we decrease the window in the photoresist down to 0.4 μm. The resulting etch profile is shown in Figure 10–29(b). The depth of etching is clearly reduced. (The same effect is not seen if n were left at 80 for the two widths.) With the slightly wider angular distribution of arrival angles for the ions, the etch depth is less for the narrower mask opening than the wider opening even though all the other etch conditions are the same. Therefore, the etching could be different for different feature sizes on the same wafer, even if the features are right next to each other.

Interestingly enough, in some etch systems and under certain conditions, a reverse ARDE effect is sometimes observed where wider etch features etch less than narrower ones. Both forward and reverse ARDE has been simulated in SPEEDIE using the "Simuletchdepo" model, to be described later, which includes a modified saturation/adsorption etch term combined with a polymer deposition term [10.25]. In that modeling, the transport of the neutral species down the trench is important for the aspect ratio dependence.

In summary, the linear etch model is relatively simple, combining the chemical and physical components in a linear fashion. It can be used in a physically based simulator such as SPEEDIE to simulate etch profiles with different degrees of anisotropy, for a variety of etch systems. It can also model effects such as ARDE and mask erosion. While simple, the model may in fact be adequate for particular plasma etch situations, even for ion-enhanced etching under limited conditions. But it does not model the coupling between the chemical and physical components that can occur, particularly the synergistic interactions in ion-enhanced etching.

10.5.3 Etching Models — Saturation/Adsorption Model for Ion-Enhanced Etching

To account for the physical and chemical components acting together, and not independently, another model is needed. As was described earlier, the etching is often not just simply the sum of the two individual components, as in the linear etch model. In ion-enhanced etching the two components act in a synergistic manner, and the etch rate can be much higher than the sum of the two separate rates. Likewise, the etching can be limited by the deficiency or lack of either of the two components. Ion-enhanced etching can be due to a variety of mechanisms. Any one of the steps of the chemical etch process may be enhanced by ion bombardment, such as the reaction of the etchant and the surface material, or the removal of etch byproducts. Inhibitor layers, formed as a result of the etch process, may require ion bombardment to remove them.

What is needed in the model is an expression that allows for the etch rate to be larger than the sum of the two components acting independently. In fact, it may be the case that the presence of both components is needed for the etching to occur. Without any ion bombardment, for example, a byproduct layer may not be removed and no chemical etching can proceed. Without any chemical processes, the ion sputtering alone may be negligible. This means that the two components are acting in series, as opposed to in parallel. It also means that the deficiency of one component can limit the total etch rate, even as the other component is increased. This leads to saturation effects—increasing the flux of one of the components will increase the etch rate to a point, but then the rate will saturate due to the lack of enough of the other component. These results have all been observed experimentally [10.6, 10.23, 10.26, 10.27, and 10. 28].

A model for ion-enhanced etching that captures the above behavior is the saturation etch model. This model is also commonly called the Langmuir adsorption or the saturation/adsorption etch model and includes surface coverage issues involving species adsorbing on and leaving the surface in its formulation. While we will derive a simple expression below based on one type of ion-enhanced etching mechanism (ion-enhanced byproduct removal), its results are generally applicable to many different mechanisms in which ion bombardment enhances one or more of the steps in the etch process. It is really a phenomenological model which can incorporate many simultaneous reactions and kinetics into its simple form. Many versions of this basic model have been developed to include a variety of processes and chemistries, but they are all similar in idea and approach [10.26, 10.28, 10.29, 10.30, 10.31, and 10.32].

For this simple analysis we consider both reactive neutral species and ions striking a surface during an etch process. The neutral species are adsorbed on the surface and chemically react with the surface material, forming etch products which contain both reactant species and film atoms. The ions striking the surface can enhance the removal of the etch byproducts from the surface, perhaps by sputtering or dislodging the loosely held byproducts or by inducing their conversion to more volatile species which then spontaneously desorb [10.6, 10.32]. A steady state will develop when the net flux of the neutrals to the surface is zero, or equivalently when the rate of byproduct formation equals the rate of byproduct removal. The idea is that the number of neutral species absorbed and reacted on the surface per time, according to simple Langmuir adsorption behavior, is proportional to how many sites are available: one minus the surface coverage. And the number of sites available depends on the neutral flux and on the ion bombardment which removes the byproducts and increases the sites for reactive neutral species adsorption. At steady state, the etch rate is then just proportional to the removal rate of byproducts, or equivalently to the neutral species adsorption rate, and depends on both the neutral and ion fluxes in a synergistic manner.

According to Langmuir adsorption theory, the number of reactive neutral species that adsorb (per unit time per area) on the surface to react with the surface material is

$$\#\text{ reactive neutrals adsorbed per time per area} = S_c(1 - \Theta)F_c \qquad (10.16)$$

where S_c is the sticking coefficient of the available area, Θ is the fraction of sites covered by the byproducts, so that $(1 - \Theta)$ is the fraction of sites available, and F_c is the flux of neutral species onto the surface. A chemical reaction constant, K, can be included, but it is just assumed to equal one here. We assume in this derivation that all neutral atoms that adsorb and stick on the surface will react quickly with the surface and form etch byproducts.

The reactive neutrals (in the etch byproducts) that are removed by ion bombardment per unit time per area from the surface is proportional to the byproduct coverage and equals

$$\#\text{ reactive neutrals (contained in byproducts) removed per time per area} = K_i\Theta F_i \qquad (10.17)$$

F_i is the incoming flux of ions and K_i is the ion-induced etch yield, or the effective sputtering yield (in general, a measure of how many atoms or molecules are removed per incident ion in a given process). K_i can be much larger than the normal sputtering yield of surface atoms—removing reaction products by ion bombardment may be much easier than removing film atoms by direct physical sputtering of the surface.

We assume a steady-state condition will develop in which the number of neutrals adsorbed equals the number removed. Thus equating Eqs. (10.16) and (10.17) gives

$$S_c(1 - \Theta)F_c = K_i\Theta\, F_i \tag{10.18}$$

$$\therefore \Theta = \frac{1}{1 + \dfrac{K_iF_i}{S_cF_c}} \tag{10.19}$$

The etch rate is then just the flux of removed species, equal to Eq. (10.17) [or equivalently, the flux of adsorbed and reacted species given by Eq. (10.16)], divided by the density of the film being etched, N. (Any stoichiometric coefficients needed to relate the ratio of film atoms to the neutral species in the reactant or byproduct molecules can be added or just included in S_c or K_i). Therefore by using Eq. (10.19) for Θ we obtain

$$\text{Etch Rate} = \frac{1}{N}\frac{1}{\left(\dfrac{1}{K_iF_i} + \dfrac{1}{S_cF_c}\right)} \tag{10.20}$$

By writing the etch rate expression in this form, the two components (analogous to electrical conductances) are seen to be acting in series rather than in parallel.

We plot Eq. (10.20) in Figure 10–30. For simplicity we assume the density, N, is unity. Here the x-axis is ion flux times the ion yield, or F_iK_i, and the equation is plotted for various values of the chemical flux times the sticking coefficient, F_cS_c. However, due to the symmetry, we could interchange F_cS_c and F_iK_i and obtain the same results. One sees that for no ion flux, the etch rate is zero, no matter what the chemical flux is. Similarly, for no chemical flux, the etch rate is zero, no matter what the ion flux is. One also sees that as the ion flux is increased for a given chemical flux, the etch rate initially increases linearly but eventually saturates. The value it saturates at, or approaches, is equal to F_cS_c/density. Similarly, when increasing the chemical flux at a constant ion flux, the etch rate increases linearly and then saturates. The process is limited by the slower of the two component processes.

The same type of saturation behavior is seen with respect to the effective sputtering yield term, K_i. Increasing the effective sputtering yield by increasing the ion energy will result in an increase in etch rate, which will then saturate as the ion energy is further increased.

The initial linear behavior is made clear by noting that when F_iK_i is small and F_cS_c is large, then by Eq. (10.20) the etch rate becomes approximately equal to just F_iK_i/density. This is the same as the physical term in the linear etch model and shows why the simple linear etch model can be used in some cases for ion-enhanced etching, as discussed earlier.

Since both ion bombardment and chemical reaction by the reactive neutral species are required in the saturation model, this ion-enhanced etching mechanism results in

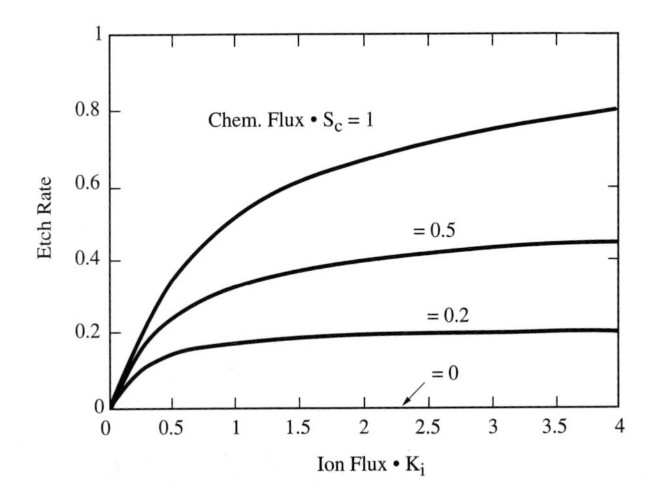

Figure 10–30 Etch rate versus ion flux for various values of the chemical flux, as calculated by Eq. (10.20). An identical plot can be obtained by interchanging $F_c S_c$ and $F_i K_i$.

mostly vertical etching. This is because the ion bombardment occurs mostly in the vertical direction, with no reemission. On sidewalls (vertical surfaces), F_i is close to zero, and hence the etch rate according to Eq. (10.20) would be close to zero in lateral directions.

Example Silicon is plasma etched for 5 minutes using a photoresist mask and this time the process follows the saturation/adsorption, or ion-assisted, etch model. The flux of chemical species, F_c, on an unobstructed flat surface is equal to 2×10^{18} atoms cm^{-2} sec^{-1} and the sticking coefficient is 0.01. The flux of ionic species, F_i, on an unobstructed flat surface is equal to 2×10^{16} atoms cm^{-2} sec^{-1} and K_i is 1. There is no etching of the photoresist, and no spontaneous chemical etching of the Si. How far is the Si etched in the vertical direction (away from the mask edge), and how far is the Si etched in the lateral direction right under the mask?

Answer In the vertical direction, away from the mask edge, there are both chemical and ion fluxes, and the total etch rate would be given by Eq. (10.20). The density of Si is 5.0×10^{22} atoms cm^{-3}. Therefore

$$\text{Etch Rate (vert)} = \frac{1}{5 \times 10^{22}\ \text{cm}^{-3}} \frac{1}{\left(\dfrac{1}{1 * 2 \times 10^{16}\ \text{cm}^{-2}\text{sec}^{-1}} + \dfrac{1}{0.01 * 2 \times 10^{18}\ \text{cm}^{-2}\text{sec}^{-1}}\right)}$$

$$= 2.0 \times 10^{-7}\ \text{cm sec}^{-1}$$

For a 5-minute etch, the Si etched in the vertical direction is

$$\text{Etch depth(vert)} = 2.0 \times 10^{-7}\text{cm sec}^{-1} \times 300 \text{ sec} = 0.6 \ \mu\text{m}$$

In the lateral direction, right under the mask edge, there is virtually no ion flux ($F_i \approx 0$), only chemical flux. Therefore the etch rate expression goes to zero. (And there is no spontaneous chemical etching.) Thus the Si etched in the lateral direction, right under the mask edge is virtually zero. A very anisotropic etch profile results.

The absence of lateral etching in this type of etching assumes that there is no spontaneous chemical etching, that is, no chemical etching without any ion bombardment. However, there may in fact be a degree of either spontaneous chemical or physical etching occurring in some systems. If the ion-enhanced etching occurs because the ion bombardment transfers energy to the surface atoms which speeds up the chemical reactions, there still may be appreciable etching without the enhancement. Or if the ion-enhanced etching is due to the presence of a byproduct layer whose removal is enhanced by ion bombardment, there may be significant spontaneous desorption of the byproduct layer. Likewise, there may be a finite component of spontaneous etching by ionic species for which neutral chemical species are not required, such as purely physical sputtering.

To account for any spontaneous etching, terms corresponding to pure chemical or pure physical etching can be included in the expression for ion-enhanced etching. In the simplest such model, terms the same as those used in the linear etch model are added to the ion-enhanced etching rate, with those terms scaled by some factor relative to the enhanced rate. For example, a ($S_C K_f F_c$/density) term can be added to Eq. (10.20) to provide for a spontaneous chemical etch component. Adding spontaneous terms would allow for some etching even if one of the two components were absent and could result in etch profiles that show some lateral etching in addition to the vertical etching [as in Figure 10–3(b)]. In more advanced models the spontaneous etch terms may be coupled with other terms, such as the surface coverage [10.26, 10.28, 10.30, 10.31, 10.32].

While Eq. (10.20) is a rather simple expression, and other more detailed versions of it have been developed, it captures the main features observed in ion-enhanced etching for many different mechanisms. Expressions the same as or very similar to this, most based on surface coverage or site considerations, have been used for a variety of ion-enhanced mechanisms. These include etching mechanisms where ion bombardment enhances the chemical etching by damaging the surface, where the sputtering yield of the surface is increased by the chemical reaction between the reactive neutral species and the surface atoms, as well as different byproduct removal mechanisms. (And it is often difficult to distinguish between the different mechanisms, both experimentally and conceptually.) In each of these cases, the analysis generally follows that as outlined above, with the ion bombardment term [Eq. (10.17)] corresponding to different ion-induced etch processes (damage creation, byproduct removal, etc.). But the end result is an expression for etch rate very similar to that given in Eq. (10.20), with the two components acting in series and in a synergistic manner. The saturation/adsorption model, or variations of it, has been used to model a variety of etch systems, including Si, SiO_2, and W thin films, under a variety of conditions and chemistries [10.26, 10.27, 10.28, 10.29, 10.30, 10.32, and 10.33].

Something that this expression does not account for is an inhibitor mechanism in which an inhibitor/byproduct forms or deposits independently of the main etch species and reaction, such as when etching Al with Cl_2 and a separate inhibitor component. Nor does it model thick or excess inhibitor formation and the highly sloped etch profiles that can result. Modeling which explicitly includes these processes will be described later.

We now describe some SPEEDIE plasma etch simulations using the saturation/adsorption etch model, as described by Eq. (10.20). Here the chemical components (neutral reactive species, such as free radicals) and physical components (ions) work together. Only when and where both are present does etching occur. In the first simulation, approximately equal contributions from the chemical and ionic etching are specified by having the K_iF_i and S_cF_c products equal. Figure 10–31 shows the simulation, with each etch contour representing a time increment of 30 seconds in the 240-second total etch time. As expected in this model, very anisotropic etching is achieved even with a strong chemical component. This is because ion bombardment is necessary in this ion-enhanced mechanism, and the ions only strike in a near-vertical direction. Etch chemistries are often chosen that produce this synergy between chemical and ionic components.

The shape of the etched sidewall can be changed in the saturation/adsorption model by changing the n factor for the ion arrival angle distribution. A smaller value for n (closer to 1), corresponding to a less directed flux, gives a more bowed sidewall. A less directed flux can occur for a higher pressure or a lower wafer bias.

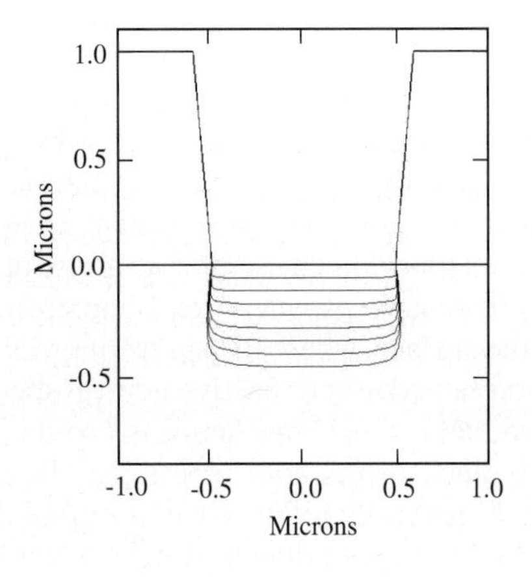

Figure 10–31 SPEEDIE simulations for etching of Si with saturation/adsorption etch model. Approximately equal components of chemical and physical etching are used.

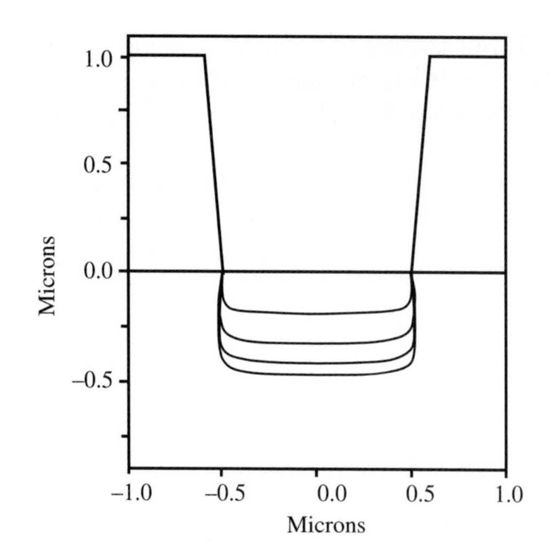

Figure 10–32 SPEEDIE simulations for etching of Si with saturation/adsorption etch model. The chemical flux is kept constant (at $2 \times 10^{18}\ cm^{-2}\ sec^{-1}$) while the ion flux is linearly increased from 0 to $1 \times 10^{16}\ cm^{-2}\ sec^{-1}$ in equal increments. Each contour here corresponds to the final etch profile for the different ion fluxes. The etch rate is initially linear with ion flux but then starts to saturate.

Next we do a series of simulations with this same model in which the chemical flux is kept constant, but the ion flux is increased. Figure 10–32 shows the simulation profiles. The maximum chemical flux is kept at $2 \times 10^{18}\ cm^{-2}\ sec^{-1}$ while the maximum ion flux is varied from 0 to $2 \times 10^{16}\ cm^{-2}\ sec^{-1}$ in equal increments. S_c and K_i equal 0.01 and 2, respectively. Unlike the plots in the previous simulation figures which showed the different time interval profiles, only the final 240-second etch profile is shown for each simulation in this figure. In this case the different profiles correspond to the different maximum ion flux values used. One can see that for zero ion flux, no etching at all takes place. As the ion flux increases, the etching increases. At first the etch rate is nearly linear with ion flux, but as the ion flux is increased more, the etch rate starts to saturate and the increase in the etch rate slows down. Eventually the etch rate will not perceivably increase at all with an increase in ion flux. This illustrates the saturation effect we discussed previously for this model and illustrated in Figure 10–30.

A result very similar to Figure 10–32 would be produced if the chemical flux were increased while the ion flux remains constant. With no chemical flux, no etching at all occurs. As the chemical flux increases, the net etch rate increases linearly at first, then not as fast, and eventually saturates. The etching of silicon and silicon dioxide is often done with a high chemical flux, operating in or near the ion-limited, chemical species saturated regime. However at the bottom of high aspect ratio features, chemical-limited etching may occur due to inadequate transport of the neutrals in some cases [10.25].

10.5.4 Etching Models — More Advanced Models

There are other models used in topography simulators—some of them variations of the saturation/adsorption model and some of them quite complex—which attempt to capture details of specific etch processes. Some of these more advanced models also try to directly address issues such as the sidewall inhibitor mechanism in ion-enhanced etching, and physical sputtering in sputter etch systems. We will not discuss these in detail but will briefly describe a few of them.

One such model in SPEEDIE attempts to separate the sidewall inhibitor effect from other ion-enhanced etch mechanisms in case two different effects may be dominating in different regions. For instance, there may be an ion-enhanced chemical reaction occurring at the bottom of the structure being etched where there is little inhibitor remaining, while the sidewall inhibitor may be affecting things on or near the sidewalls. This is implemented in the Sidewallpass model in SPEEDIE [10.17, 10.34] by modifying the saturation/adsorption model. The result is that the etch rate versus ion flux curve in Figure 10–30 is changed so that the left-hand portion, below some threshold level, drops faster than normal. The idea is that on or near the sidewalls, where the ion flux is low to begin with, it may be even lower due to the ions being consumed by the sputtering of a thin sidewall inhibitor layer. Zheng and McVittie [10.34] showed that in the case of etching polysilicon with a SF_6/Cl_2ClF_5 chemistry this model better matches the actual etch profile, with even less etching and bowing on the sidewalls where the ion flux is low. (However, this model does not explicitly account for thick or excess inhibitor formation, as we shall discuss below.) Other models have been developed which similarly consider multiple ion-enhancement mechanisms.

In other more advanced models, the formation and sputtering of a thick sidewall inhibitor layer are explicitly included. In these the sloped etch profiles due to excess inhibitor formation (as illustrated in Figure 10–14) are modeled, something that the simpler saturation models do not do. Examples are SPEEDIE's "Simuletchdepo Thick Sidewall Etch" model [10.17, 10.35] and Avant!'s TAURUS-TOPOGRAPHY's dry etch model [10.18], which include simultaneous deposition and etching of a polymer inhibitor layer. In SPEEDIE's model the polymer deposition is controlled by a CVD-like process with the inhibitor flux (the "deposited flux" in Figure 10–26) coming from the gas phase above the wafer, separate from the flux of reactive neutral etching species. Ion sputtering of the inhibitor layer then allows for etching of the substrate or film in the vertical direction. Such models can include ion-enhanced deposition and sputtering of the deposited material [like Eq. (9.58) in Chapter 9 for high-density plasma CVD deposition], as well as purely chemical etching of the inhibitor-free surfaces (for chlorine etching of Al, for example) or ion-enhanced chemical etching of the inhibitor-free surfaces (for etching of SiO_2 or Si, for example). Han and colleagues [10.35] have shown that this approach can model high-density plasma etching of silicon dioxide, using an ICP plasma source and C_2F_6 etchant gas. Ion-enhanced deposition and sputtering of the polymer with an ion-flux-dependent sticking coefficient, along with ion-enhanced etching of the SiO_2 (utilizing the saturation/adsorption expression), are used in this modeling.

Another advanced model similar to these was developed by Tuda and colleagues [10.36] for plasma etching of Si with Cl_2/O_2. This model includes passivation layer formation from surface oxidation and from etch byproducts arriving from the plasma as well as being directly redeposited from the bottom surface onto sidewalls. Other models include ion reflection, trenching, and localized surface charging. For HDP systems, a contribution from ionized chemical species to the chemical component of etching might also be included. All these advanced models can obviously be quite complicated, with many parameters.

Finally, advanced simulators may also include a separate model for pure physical etching, or ion sputtering, which includes redeposition of the sputtered material [10.37]. The expression used for this in SPEEDIE [10.17] is

$$\text{Etch rate} = \frac{K_{\text{sp}}Y(\theta)F_i - K_{\text{rd}}S_{\text{rd}}F_{\text{rd}} - S_{\text{cd}}F_{\text{d}}}{N} \tag{10.21}$$

The first term is due to the sputtering, and the sputtering yield can be angle dependent. The second and third terms are due to redeposition of sputtered material. In particular the second term is due to the direct redeposition from every other point on the structure where sputtering occurs. The third term is from material that is sputtered off the surface but goes into the plasma and then drops back down to the wafer surface. The third term can be very difficult to calibrate. N is the density of the film being etched.

10.5.5 Other Etching Simulations

As we mentioned in Chapter 9, commercial suppliers of integrated circuit simulation tools offer both empirical and more physically based models. Here we present examples of both types. The first is from Avant!'s TAURUS-TOPOGRAPHY simulator [10.18], utilizing the dry etch model with polymer deposition. This model is similar to SPEEDIE's physically based Simuletchdepo model described above. Using direct and indirect flux calculations similar to those in SPEEDIE, TAURUS-TOPOGRAPHY simulates the deposition, reemission, and sputtering of polymer material that occurs in the formation of a sidewall inhibitor layer. In the example described here, SiO_2 is plasma etched over Si using a photoresist mask.

Figure 10–33 shows the simulated results of the sidewall polymer etch model. Figure 10–33(a) shows the simulated results after 0.9 minutes of etching. One can see the sidewall polymer that has formed. This layer inhibits lateral etching of the oxide. No polymer layer is present on the trench bottom because of strong ion bombardment and sputtering there, and also because of less polymer deposition due to shadowing. Figure 10–33(b) shows the simulation after 1.8 minutes of etching. The sidewall layer is now thicker, affecting the etch profile as described earlier and illustrated in Figure 10–14. A sloped etch profile, with no etch bias, results due to the high-polymer deposition-to-etch ratio.

Finally, some commercially available simulation tools provide simpler, more empirical models. Silvaco's ATHENA simulator (using the ELITE topography tool) [10.19] is an example and we will use it here to simulate etching of silicon through a photoresist mask. In these simpler models, the user specifies the etch rates of the different components and various parameters to obtain the shape of the etch profile, rather than specifying fluxes. There is both a "wet etch model" and a "RIE model" in ATHENA. The wet etch model is completely isotropic, while the RIE model contains elements of both the linear etch and saturation/adsorption models. We will briefly describe the RIE model here and provide some examples.

In the RIE model in ATHENA, the etching process is separated into three adjustable etch rate components: the isotropic, the directional, and the chemical. Using the

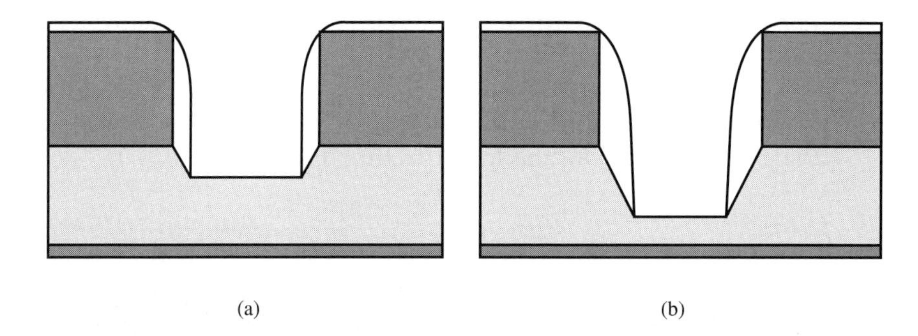

Figure 10–33 Avant!'s TAURUS-TOPOGRAPHY [10.18] simulation using their dry etch model with simultaneous polymer deposition. (a) shows the result of etching silicon dioxide over silicon with a photoresist mask after 0.9 minutes. Notice the sidewall polymer layer that has formed, inhibiting lateral etching. (b) shows the etch profile after 1.8 minutes. The sidewall layer is thicker and the etch profile in the oxide is sloped due to the high deposition-to-etch ratio.

first two is similar to using the linear etch model. The isotropic component, designated by r_{iso}, etches equally in all directions. The directional component, designated by r_{dir}, etches only in the vertical direction. For a sloped surface, where the etch rate normal to the surface is important, the etching due to r_{dir} is $r_{dir} * \cos\alpha$. Here α is the angle between the surface normal and the vertical direction. By using one or both of these two components, one can simulate purely chemical/isotropic etching, purely physical/directional etching, or a linear combination of the two. (As with the linear etch model, the physical component here may indeed be due to an ion-enhanced etching mechanism, but for which the chemical component is not limiting the process.) One can control the degree of etch anisotropy by changing the relative values of these two parameters, such that the degree of anisotropy is

$$A_f = \frac{r_{dir}}{r_{iso} + r_{dir}} \tag{10.22}$$

[One can show that this is equivalent to our definition of anisotropy in Eq. (10.5) if one observes that $r_{lat} = r_{iso}$ and $r_{vert} = r_{iso} + r_{dir}$).] No sticking coefficient is used, nor are arrival angle distributions. For these components, it is assumed that the etching is purely isotropic for the one component, and purely vertical for the other. One just specifies the etch rates for each component. The Taurus topography simulator from Avant! has a similar etch model in which one simply specifies the degree of anisotropy desired.

The third component of the ATHENA RIE model is called the chemical component. This implicitly assumes an ion-enhanced etch mechanism. When one specifies the chemical component etch rate in the RIE model, one must also specify the "divergence" parameter. The divergence parameter determines the standard deviation of the ion's Gaussian angular distribution function. It is assumed that this chemical etching only occurs where an ion strikes. In this simple way both the chemical and ionic components of the ion-enhanced mechanism are taken into account in this model; however saturation effects are not accounted for. By varying the divergence, different shaped sidewalls are obtained, very similar to changing the n factor in the $\cos^n\theta$ ion arrival angle distribution used earlier. In ATHENA, all three components—the isotropic, the directional, and the chemical—can be specified, resulting in almost any shaped profile imaginable.

In the first series of ATHENA etch examples, silicon is etched through a photoresist mask using each of the three RIE model components. Figure 10–34(a) shows the initial structure. For the first example the silicon is etched with a purely isotropic component. An isotropic etch rate, r_{iso}, of 5 nm per second is specified. The time of the etch is set at 2 minutes, which should etch the silicon 600 nm deep. The resulting profile is shown in Figure 10–34(b). In the next simulation, pure physical or directed etching is done. This is done by specifying r_{dir} to be 5 nm per second and r_{iso} to be zero. The simulated profile is shown in Figure 10–34(c). In the final simulation, the ion-enhanced chemical etching component is used. This is done by designating the chemical component to be 50 and the divergence to be 5. The resulting profile is in Figure 10–34(d). Changing the divergence parameter is similar to changing the arrival angle distribution (the n value) of ions in the earlier models, due to changes in gas pressure, for example.

The final series of ATHENA simulations are shown in Figure 10–35. Here different combinations of isotropic, directional, and chemical (ion-enhanced) components are

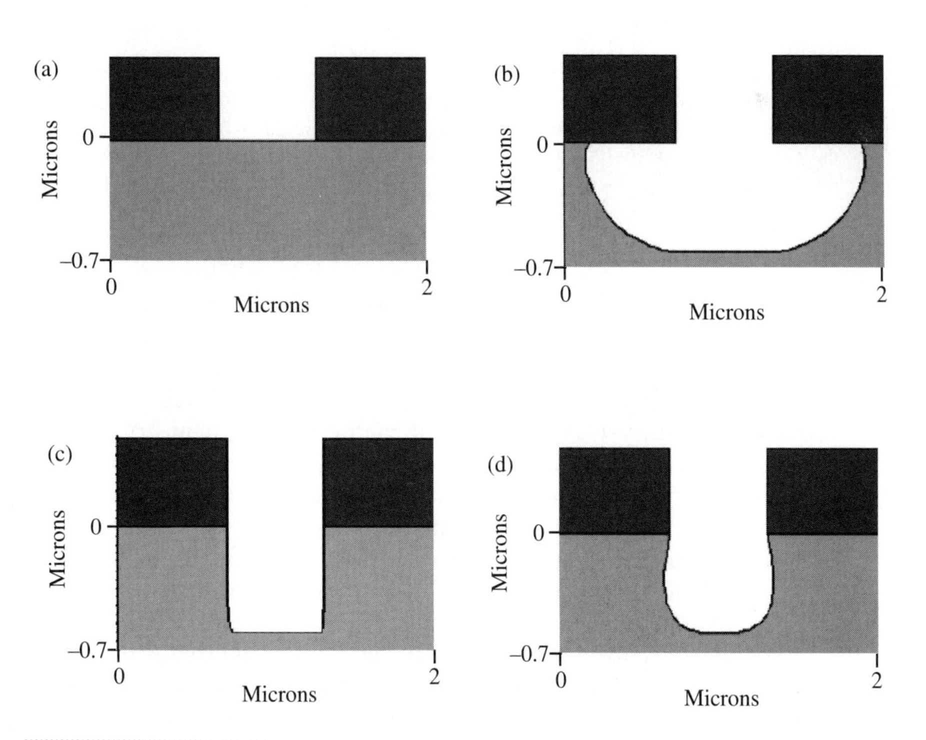

Figure 10–34 Silvaco's ATHENA [10.19] topography simulation of silicon etching using different etching components in the RIE model: (a) initial structure with photoresist mask over Si substrate; (b) purely isotropic etching; (c) purely directional; (d) ion-enhanced etching .

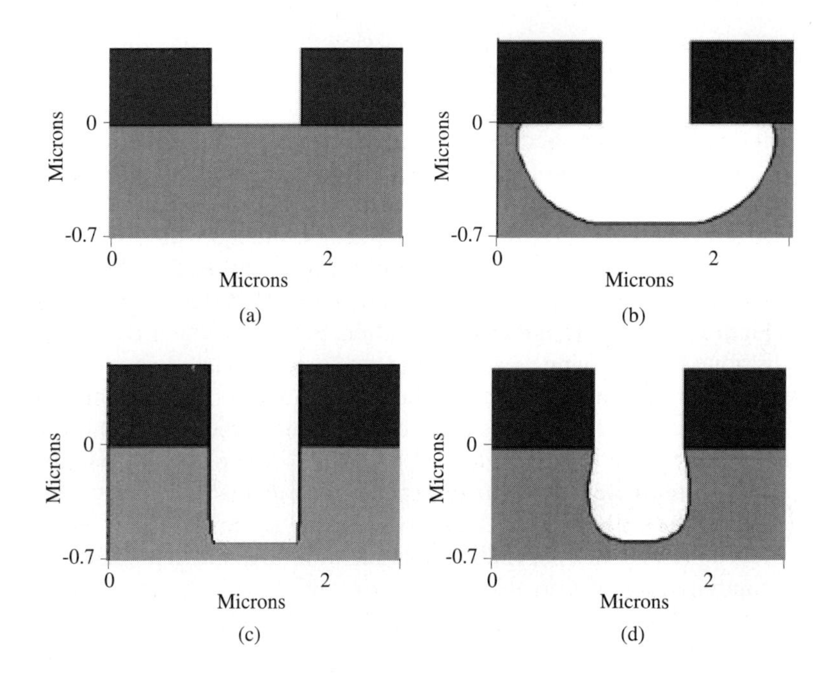

Figure 10–35 Silvaco's ATHENA [10.19] etch simulation using different etching component combinations in the RIE model: (a) chem = 50, div = 10, iso = 0, dir = 0; (b) chem = 30, div = 10, iso = 0, dir = 20; (c) chem = 30, div = 10, iso = 20, dir = 0; (d) chem = 30, div = 10, iso = 10, dir = 10. These illustrate the variety of etch profiles that are obtainable with this easy-to-use tool.

used to obtain a wide variety of etch profiles. These simulations demonstrate the usefulness of such simulation models. It is relatively simple to use them and calibrate them against actual etch profiles. These types of models are often used to characterize a particular etch system and etch chemistry used to plasma etch a particular film. One can build up a library of etch equipment, materials, etch chemistry, and plasma conditions to use in future simulations. This is sometimes done by commercial suppliers of these simulation tools and a model parameter library for various commonly used pieces of deposition and etch equipment with model parameters for various films and normal operating conditions is included with the simulator. One can then use these models and parameters to optimize an etch or deposition process without being involved with all the details. These types of simulations also run very quickly.

Of course the main advantage of the more physically based models is that they try to be more closely linked to actual physical processes. This is especially true for the models currently being developed which actually model the etch-enhancement mechanism, such as inhibitor layer formation and removal. As a result, these types of models are more apt to be valid for conditions outside those for which they are calibrated and tested, but both types of models are useful for different applications.

10.6 Limits and Future Trends in Technologies and Models

With the ever-decreasing feature sizes in future generations of integrated circuit technology, the challenges in etching will certainly continue. Etching features with smaller and smaller dimensions will obviously pose problems. Damage to the underlying films and active regions will also be issues as the dimensions decrease and plasma processing is used. High-density plasma etch systems will surely help in these regards. A high-density plasma at low gas pressures and the decoupling of the plasma density and ion energy mean that fast, anisotropic etching can be achieved while minimizing the ion-induced damage. Development of this type of etch technology will surely continue.

With ever-increasing wafer sizes in the future, uniformity and loading problems will be harder to control. Improvements in equipment design will have to continue to overcome these issues. More *in situ* control will be required. In addition to endpoint detection, automatic feedback will be needed to control equipment and process parameters such as gas flow, pressure, and power to the plasma sources.

As with deposition equipment, a trend in etch equipment will be the use of cluster tools. By connecting to multiple etch (and deposition) chambers and passing the wafers from one chamber to another, one can perform several processing steps sequentially without breaking vacuum. This minimizes exposure of the wafers to atmosphere, reducing particulate contamination and surface oxidation between steps. For example, one can have chambers to etch TiN and Al, do a fluorine passivation, and strip the photoresist. This becomes more important as the trend continues toward multilevel stack structures. One can also combine deposition and etch chambers in such a tool. Most of these tools are single wafer, as opposed to batch systems. More control over each wafer is possible, but the etch rates must be high since each wafer must be processed individually.

There will be more challenges in etching specific films as the dimensions decrease and aspect ratios increase. For example, in Al metal etching the issues of corrosion, resist and residue removal, Cu byproduct removal, loading effects (both macro and micro), and of course profile control and selectivity will have to be addressed each time the structure dimensions are decreased. As we have seen, there are many issues and considerations involved in developing an etch process for each film, and it will be harder and harder to satisfy all the requirements.

New plasma etching techniques may be used to meet the increasing demands as the technology progresses. Recently a new plasma etch process, called the Bosch process, has been developed in the MEMS (Micro-Electro-Mechanical Systems) industry for etching very deep Si trenches. This uses fluorine chemistry in a high-density plasma, and both excellent anisotropy and selectivity with respect to SiO_2 masks are reported [10.38]. In this process, polymer deposition and etching steps are sequentially alternated in an HDP etch system. Whether this can be adapted in the future for etching isolation structures or polysilicon gates in VLSI structures is unclear, but new plasma etching methods along these lines may be developed and used.

Etching and patterning processes other than plasma etching may be used more in the future. Chemical-Mechanical Polishing (CMP) has found widespread use in the past few years and is now a mainstream process. As described in the next chapter, this uses a combination of wet chemicals and mechanical grinding to polish or etch the top surface of a film, leaving a very planar surface. Dielectric films and W plugs are now often planarized by this technique. When CMP is combined with the "damascene" fill and etchback process, also described in the next chapter, materials such as copper that are difficult to plasma etch can be patterned to integrated circuit specifications.

New materials will be added in the future. As we discuss in the next chapter, new metal interconnect materials such as copper and new dielectrics such as low-k dielectrics will soon be required. There has already been extensive development on integrating these types of materials into the fabrication process, including the patterning of these films. Etching some of these films, especially Cu, has been found to be very difficult, so much so that other methods for patterning these films such as CMP are more attractive.

The models and simulation tools for etching processes will also undergo changes and improvements. As we mentioned earlier in the chapter, we need to model the actual processes more deeply, such as explicitly modeling the sidewall inhibitor formation and removal and phenomena such as ion reflection and charging. Work in these directions has begun. And as with the deposition models, physically based models and simulation tools need to be combined with user-friendly and efficient software tools.

10.7 Summary of Key Ideas

We have seen in this chapter how etching is used to pattern films by selectively removing material with the use of mask layers, usually photoresist but sometimes other thin films. Etching can be either wet or dry, the former using liquid chemical etchants and the latter using gas-phase, plasma-produced etch species. Some of the issues that are important in etching are selectivity with respect to masks and underlying films, directionality (anisotropic versus isotropic etching) for profile control, mask erosion, etch bias or undercutting, etch uniformity, residue removal, and damage in the underlying layers caused by etching.

In wet etching, chemical reactions dominate the etch process. This leads to very selective but isotropic etching. In dry or plasma etching, two types of species are present that are important in the etch process: reactive neutral chemical species (such as free radicals) and ionic species. The first etches by chemical processes and is isotropic or nearly isotropic and can be very selective, while the second etches by more physical processes and is very directional, or very anisotropic, but not very selective. The three main types of etch mechanisms that occur in plasma etching are chemical etching (involving the neutral chemical species), physical etching or sputtering (involving the ion species), and ion-enhanced etching (involving both in a synergistic way). Ion-enhanced etching can occur by the ions enhancing the chemical etch process or by removing inhibitor layers. Directional etching can be achieved in this manner, as well as selectivity, a combination usually desired in an etch process. Many types of plasma etching equipment have been developed that utilize the different etching mechanisms, including barrel etchers, plasma mode etchers, Reactive Ion Etching (RIE) systems, High-Density Plasma (HDP) systems, and sputter etching equipment. These systems range from purely chemical to purely physical etching, with many systems operating in between these two. Where both chemical and physical components are present, as in RIE and HDP systems, plasma conditions and etch chemistries are usually selected so that the two etch components act synergistcally, and ion-enhanced etching occurs giving directional etching and good selectivity.

Most simulation models focus on the two components of etching, the chemical and physical. Advanced simulators model the etch process based on the fluxes and surface processes of the chemical and ion species. As in deposition modeling, the ion species have a narrow arrival angle distribution (being very vertical to the wafer) and a high sticking coefficient. The chemical species have a wide arrival angle distribution and low sticking coefficient. The two components can act independently or synergistically. In the linear etch model, the chemical and physical components of etching are combined in an independent linear fashion, and a wide range of etch profiles can be produced for different plasma etch systems and for certain conditions. In the saturation/adsorption model for ion-enhanced etching, the two species act synergistically, as described by the expression for two processes acting in series. Very directional anisotropic etching results, along with saturation effects. Variations can occur, such as when some spontaneous, non-ion-assisted chemical etching occurs in parallel, multiple ion-enhanced mechanisms are present, or when excess inhibitor material forms, and modifications or additional models can be utilized to capture these features.

In the future, structures will get even smaller and new materials will be used. New etching tools and processes will also evolve. The models and simulation tools will evolve as well. As with deposition models, they will become based even more on the actual physical processes.

10.8 References

[10.1]. C. J. Mogab, "Dry Etching," in *VLSI Technology*, ed. by S.M. Sze, McGraw-Hill, 1983, p.307.

[10.2]. W. S. Ruska, *Microelectronic Processing*, McGraw-Hill, 1987, p. 206.

[10.3]. C. Chang, "Experiments and Simulation of Plasma Deposition and Sputter Etching Processes," Ph.D. thesis, Stanford University, 1996, p. 93.

[10.4]. J. P. McVittie, private communication.

[10.5]. J. W. Coburn and H.F. Winters, "Ion and Electron Assisted Gas-Surface Chemistry—An Important Effect in Plasma Etching," *J. App. Phys.*, vol. 50, p. 3189, 1979.

[10.6]. J. W. Coburn, "Surface-science Aspects of Plasma-assisted Etching," *Appl. Phys. A*, vol. A59, p. 451, 1994.

[10.7]. R. A. Morgan, *Plasma Etching in Semiconductor Fabrication*, Elsevier Science, 1985.

[10.8]. M. Kimizuka, Y. Watanbe, and Y. Ozaki, "Pattern Profile Control in Magnetron Reactive Ion Etching of Poly-Si," *J. Vac. Sci. Tech. B.*, vol. 10, p. 2192, 1992.

[10.9]. H. C. Jones, R. Bennett, and J.Singh, "Size Dependent Etching of Small Shapes" in *Proc. of the Eighth Symp. on Plasma Prcoessing*, G. S. Mathad and D.W. Hess, eds. the Electrochem. Soc., 1990, p. 45.

[10.10]. J. P. McVittie, unpublished data.

[10.11]. M. A. Leiberman and A.J. Lichtenberg, *Principles of Plasma Discharges and Materials Processing*, J. Wiley & Sons, 1994.

[10.12]. B. Gorowitz and R. J. Saia, "Reactive Ion Etching," in *Plasma Processing for VLSI*, N. G. Einspruch and D. M. Brown, eds., Academic Press, 1984, p. 307.

[10.13]. W. R. Runyan and K. E. Bean, *Semiconductor Integrated Circuit Processing Technology*, Addison-Wesley, 1990, p. 276.

[10.14]. D.L. Flamm, in *Plasma Etching, an Introduction*, D.M. Manos and D. L. Flamm, eds., Academic Press, 1989.

[10.15]. L. M Ephrath and E.J. Petrillo, "Parameter and Reactor Dependence of Selective Oxide RIE in $CF_4 + H_2$," *J. Electrochem. Soc.*, vol. 129, p. 2282, 1982.

[10.16]. P. Singer, "Plasma Etch: a Matter of Fine Tuning," *Semiconductor International*, December 1995, p. 65.

[10.17]. SPEEDIE is a 2D etch and deposition simulator developed at Stanford University.

[10.18]. TAURUS-TOPOGRAPHY is a commercially available topography simulator developed by Avant! Inc.

[10.19]. ATHENA and its ELITE topography simulator are commercially available from Silvaco Inc.

[10.20]. V. I. Singh, E. S. G. Shaqfeh, and J. McVittie, "Study of Si Etching in CF_4/O_2 Plasmas to Establish Surface Re-Emission as the Dominant Transport Mechanism," *J. Vac. Sci. Tech. B*, vol. B12, p. 2952, 1994.

[10.21]. V. I. Singh, E. S. G. Shaqfeh, and J. McVittie, "Simulation of Profile Evolution in Si Reactive Ion Etching with Re-Emission and Surface Diffusion," *J. Vac. Sci. Tech. B*, vol. B10, p. 1091, 1992.

[10.22]. D. L. Flamm, D. M. Donnelly and J. A. Mucha, "The Reaction of Flourine Atoms with Silicon," *J. Appl. Phys.*, vol. 52, p. 3633, 1981.

[10.23]. B. A. Heath, "Selective Reactive Ion Beam Etching of SiO_2 over Polycrystalline Si," *J. Electrochem. Soc.*, vol. 129, p. 396, 1982.

[10.24]. J. I. Ulacia and J. P. McVittie, "A Two-Dimensional Computer Simulator for Dry Etching Using Monte-Carlo," *J. Appl. Phys.,* vol. 65, p. 1484, 1989.

[10.25]. J. S. Han and J. P. McVittie, "Modeling of Aspect Ratio Dependent Etching in an Inductively Coupled Plasma," *Mat. Res. Soc. Symp. Proc.*, vol. 389, p. 197, 1995.

[10.26]. V. M. Donnelly, D. L. Flamm, W. C. Dautremont-Smith, and D. J. Weber, "Anisotropic Etching of SiO_2 in Low-frequency CF_4/O_2 and NF_3/Ar Plasmas," *J. Appl. Phys.*, vol. 55, p. 242, 1984.

[10.27]. R. Petri and D. Henry, "Tungsten Etching Mechanisms in Low-Pressure SF_6 Plasma," *J. Appl. Phys.*, vol. 72, p. 2644, 1992.

[10.28]. T. M. Mayer and R. A. Barker, "Simulation of Plasma-Assisted Etching Processes by Ion-Beam Techniques," *J. Vac. Sci. Tech.*, vol. 21, p. 757, 1982.

[10.29]. J. Pelletier and M. J. Cooke, "Microwave Plasma Etching of Si and SiO_2 in Halogen Mixtures: Interpretation of Modeling Mechanisms," *J. Vac. Sci. Tech.*, vol. B7, p. 59, 1989.

[10.30]. E. Zawaideh and N. S. Kim, "Plasma Etching Model Based on a Generalized Transport Approach," *J. Appl. Phys.*, vol. 62, p. 2498, 1987.

[10.31]. M. A. Lieberman and A. J. Lichtenberg, *Principles of Plasma Discharges and Materials Processing*, John Wiley & Sons, 1994.

[10.32]. D. C. Gray, I. Tepermeister, and H. H. Sawin, "Phenomenological Modeling of Ion-Enhanced Kinetics in Flourine-Based Plasma Etching," *J. Vac. Sci. Tech. B*, vol. 11, p. 1243, 1993.

[10.33]. J. P. Chang, A. P. Mahorowala, and H. H. Sawin, "Plasma-Surface Kinetics and Feature Profile Evolution in Chlorine Etching of Polysilicon," *J. Vac. Sci. Tech. A,* vol. 16, p. 217, 1998.

[10.34]. J. Zheng and J. P. McVittie, "Modeling of Side Wall Passivation and Ion Saturation Effects on Etching Profiles," *Proc. of IEEE Int'l. Mtg. Numerical Modeling of Process and Device for I.C.: NUPAD-V*, p. 37, 1994.

[10.35]. J. S. Han, J. P. McVittie, and J. Zheng, "Profile Modeling in High Density Plasma Oxide Etching," *J. Vac. Sci. Tech*, vol. 13, p. 1893, 1995.

[10.36] M. Tuda, K. Ono, and K. Nishikawa, "Effects of Etch Products and Surface Oxidation on Profile Evolution During Electron Cyclotron Resonance Plasma Etching of Poly-Si," *J. Vac. Sci. Technol. B*, vol. 14, p. 3291, 1996.

[10.37]. C. Y. Chang, J. P. McVittie, and K. C. Saraswat, "Backscattering in Ar Sputtering of Oxide," *Appl. Phys. Lett.*, vol. 63, p. 2294, 1994.

[10.38]. J. Bhardwaj, H. Ashara, and A. McQuarrie, "Dry Silicon Etching for MEMS," *Proc. of Symp. on Microstructures and Microfab. Sys.*, Electrochem. Soc., 1997.

10.9 Problems

10.1. Why might pure chemical etching, such as in wet etching, be adequate for patterning the silicon nitride layer used to define the field oxidation area in the CMOS process flow given in Chapter 2?

10.2. If the etch anisotropy is 0, what is the undercut or etch bias when etching a 0.5-μm thick film? What is the undercut when the anisotropy is 0.75? Assume no overetch in each case.

10.3. In a certain process, it is desired that the pitch of metal lines be equal to or less than 1.0 μm (the pitch equals one metal linewidth plus one spacing between metal lines, measured at top of features). Assume that the metal linewidth and spacing are equal (that is, 0.5 μm each). The height of such structures is also 0.5 μm, and the minimum lithographic dimension is 0.25 μm.

a. What minimum degree of anisotropy is needed in an etch process in order to produce such a structure?

b. What minimum pitch could be obtained for such a structure with *wet* etching? (Again with minimum lithograph dimension of 0.25 μm, thickness of 0.5 μm, and equal metal width and spacing.)

10.4. What are the advantages and disadvantages of reactive ion etching versus sputter etching? Cite a hypothetical example of when you might want to use sputter etching rather than RIE.

10.5. Explain how loading effects can affect endpoint detection.

10.6. It is found that a certain plasma etch chemistry in a certain RIE etch system produces vertical sidewalls with zero etch bias when etching a particular film. Adding chemical A to the etch chemistry results in nonvertical sidewalls, and an etch bias. Adding chemical B to the original etch chemistry results in nonvertical sidewalls, but with zero etch bias. Explain what may be going on.

10.7. a. In a particular etch process, if selectivity is the biggest concern, which type(s) of etch equipment should be used?

b. If the biggest concern is ion bombardment damage, which type(s) of etch equipment should be used?

c. If the biggest concern is obtaining vertical sidewalls, which type(s) of etch equipment should be used?

d. If the biggest concerns are selectivity *and* vertical sidewalls, which type(s) of etch equipment should be used?

e. What about selectivity *and* vertical sidewalls *and* damage, while maintaining reasonable etch rate?

10.8. It is observed that the sidewall slope in an etch process becomes more sloped as the temperature is reduced. Why?

10.9. If the anisotropy of an etch process is 0.45, sketch the etch profile. What percentage of the etch rate in the vertical direction is due to the chemical component and what percentage is ionic/physical, assuming a linear etch mechanism? State all assumptions.

10.10. For a particular plasma etch process in which the linear etch model is applicable, a degree of anisotropy of 0.8 or better is desired. If the unobstructed ionic flux on a flat surface is 1×10^{16} atoms cm^{-2} sec^{-1} (with K_i equal to 1), what unobstructed chemical flux would result in an anisotropy of 0.8? For this process S_C is 0.01 and K_f is 0.1.

10.11. We want to see how the etch rate in the vertical direction might depend on pressure assuming that the etch follows the saturation/adsorption model. Assume that for a particular etch system that the chemical flux is directly proportional to the pressure, while the ion flux is inversely proportional to the pressure. That is $F_c = F_c'{*}P$ and $F_i = F_i'/P$. (P is normalized to 1 atm and unitless.) Also assume that density $= 1$ atom nm^{-3}, and that $K_iF_i' = S_cF_c' = 1$ atom nm^{-2} sec^{-1}.

a. Plot the vertical etch rate versus pressure, P, from $P = 0$ to 10.

b. Repeat with $K_iF_i' = 40$ atoms nm^{-2} sec^{-1} and $S_cF_c' = 1$ atom nm^{-2} sec^{-1}.

10.12. In an etch process, there is a finite amount of purely chemical etching without any ion bombardment (i.e., spontaneous chemical etching). In addition, ion bombardment greatly increases the etch rate by facilitating the breaking up of the etch precursor. At high ion flux the etch rate saturates. No etching occurs when there is only ion bombardment with no chemical component.

a. Write a generalized etch rate equation that can describe this behavior.

b. Sketch an etch rate versus ion flux curve for this process for some nonzero chemical flux.

c. Sketch what the etch profile might look like for this process (i.e., etching through a window in a mask as in Figure 10–3).

Back-End Technology

11

11.1 Introduction

Back-end technology refers to the interconnect layers, contacts, vias and dielectric layers that wire the active devices into specific circuit configurations. Figure 11–1 is a schematic diagram taken from Chapter 2 showing these components in a typical integrated circuit structure. Figure 11–2 is a SEM micrograph of an IBM circuit showing the back-end structure with the dielectric layers etched away, revealing the interconnects, contacts, and vias. Another SEM of this same chip was shown in Figure 1–12. The relative importance of back-end structures has greatly increased in recent years because the circuit delays associated with interconnects have not kept pace with the faster device speeds provided by scaled technologies. Thus much recent effort has been devoted to improving back-end technology and it is widely believed that these efforts will only accelerate in the future.

Interconnects can be either local or global. In general, local interconnects are the first, or lowest, level of interconnects. They usually connect gates, sources, and drains in MOS technology, and emitters, bases, and collectors in bipolar technology. In MOS technology a local interconnect, polycrystalline silicon, also serves as the gate electrode material. Silicided gates and silicided source/drain regions and materials like TiN and W can also act as local interconnects. Local interconnects can tolerate higher resistivities than global interconnects since they are not very long. But they must also, in most cases, be able to withstand higher processing temperatures because they are deposited earlier in the process flow than global interconnects. Global interconnects, mostly made of Al, are generally all the interconnect levels above the local interconnect level. They often cover large distances between different devices and different parts of the chip and therefore are always low-resistance metals.

Ohmic contacts connect an interconnect with active regions or devices in the silicon substrate. A high-resistivity dielectric layer, usually silicon dioxide, separates the active regions from the first-level global interconnect, and electrical contact is made between the interconnect and the active regions in the silicon through openings in that dielectric layer. At the same time in the processing, contact can be made between the first-level global interconnect and the local interconnects, since they are also separated by that same dielectric layer. Connections between two levels of global interconnects are usually given a different name—vias. They are made through openings in the different levels of the intermetal dielectrics (IMDs), which separate interconnects from each other and from the active areas and devices. The bottom dielectric layer through which the contacts are made is usually called the first-level dielectric. Examples of these structures are shown in Figures 11–1 and 11–2.

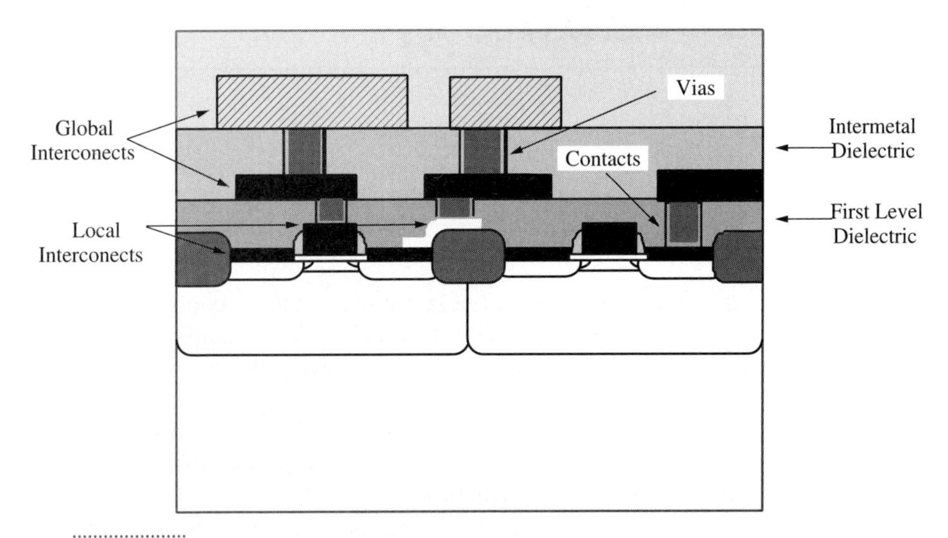

Figure 11–1 Schematic cross section of back-end structure, showing interconnects, contacts, and vias, separated by dielectric layers (cross-hatched regions).

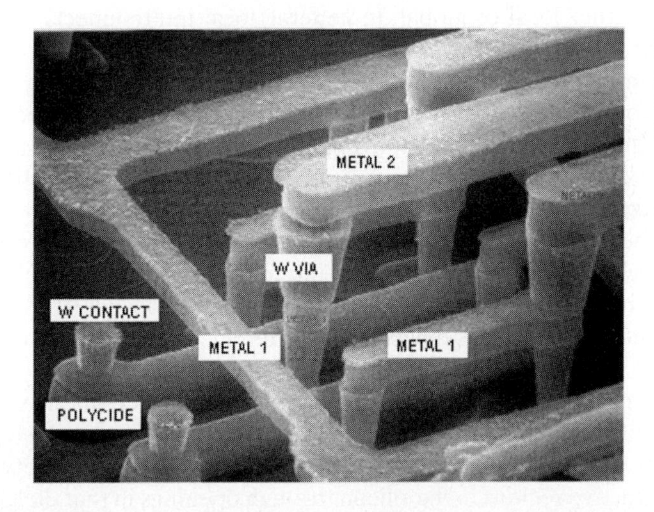

Figure 11–2 SEM micrograph of an IBM circuit showing the interconnects with the dielectric layers etched away. Photograph courtesy of Integrated Circuit Engineering Corporation.

It is easy to see why interconnect structures are becoming more important in overall chip performance. Consider the structure in Figure 11–3 [11.1]. The RC time delay of a signal propagating along such a line is to first order obtained by treating it as a distributed, unterminated transmission line. For such a system the time delay, τ_L, is approximately equal to $0.89RC$ where R is the line resistance and C is the total capacitance associated with the line [11.2]. A more accurate analysis would include such elements as the load capacitance, driver resistance, and line inductance [11.3, 11.4, 11.5]. However, the $0.89RC$ expression for the time delay which considers only the interconnect RC component is sufficient for our purposes.

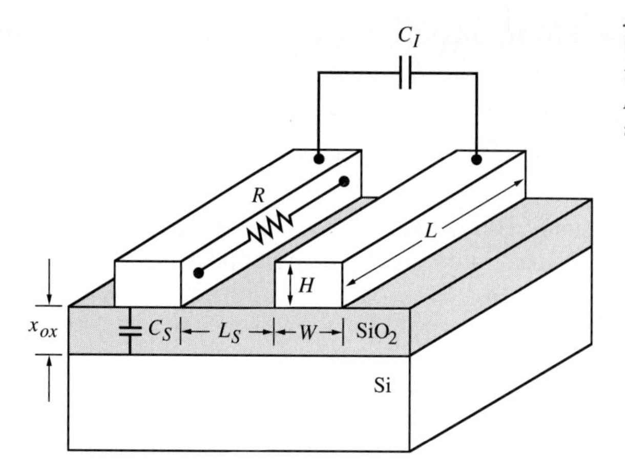

Figure 11–3 Interconnect structure for *RC* analysis. The two lines on top are the metal interconnects of dimensions *W*, *L*, and *H*, sitting on a SiO_2 layer. There is also SiO_2 between and above the metal lines. (After [11.1].)

The line resistance, in Ω, of one of the interconnects is given by

$$R = \rho \frac{L}{WH} \tag{11.1}$$

where ρ is the interconnect resistivity, and L, W, and H are the interconnect length, width, and height, respectively. The total capacitance associated with the line is

$$C = K_{\text{ox}}\varepsilon_o \frac{WL}{x_{\text{ox}}} + K_{\text{ox}}\varepsilon_o \frac{HL}{L_S} \tag{11.2}$$

where x_{ox} and K_{ox} are the oxide thickness and dielectric constant, respectively, and ε_o is the permittivity of free space. The first term represents the line to substrate capacitance, C_S, and the second term the coupling capacitance between adjacent lines, C_I. It is assumed that the lines are surrounded by oxide on all sides.

The total *RC* delay associated with the line is thus

$$\tau_L = 0.89 \cdot K_I K_{\text{ox}} \varepsilon_o \rho L^2 \left(\frac{1}{Hx_{\text{ox}}} + \frac{1}{WL_S} \right) \tag{11.3}$$

where K_I is added to empirically account for fringing fields and other interconnects above and below the line in multilayer interconnect systems. K_I is often taken to be ≈ 2.

Now we must consider what happens to the dimensions of the structure as the technology progresses. First, L_S and W are often close to the minimum feature size F_{min}. As the technology progresses, F_{min} gets smaller. The values of L_S and W may in fact be larger than the minimum feature size for some interconnect levels, but they still commonly scale with F_{min}. Both x_{ox} and H also shrink as F_{min} shrinks in this ideal scaling scheme, keeping the aspect ratio, H/W, constant. In the original analysis by Saraswat and Mohammadi [11.1], it was assumed that x_{ox} and H equaled $0.35\text{F}_{\text{min}}$ and $0.25\text{F}_{\text{min}}$, respectively. However, these thicknesses have not decreased as quickly as this in recent years, especially for the global interconnects. To keep the analysis simple, we assume that x_{ox} and H, as well as L_S and W, are all equal to F_{min}. Thus Eq. (11.3) with K_I equal to 2, becomes

$$\tau_L = 3.56 \cdot K_{ox}\varepsilon_o\rho \frac{L^2}{(F_{min})^2} \tag{11.4}$$

For local interconnects, L usually also shrinks as F_{min} shrinks. Therefore, the net result is that the RC time delay for local interconnects stays approximately constant according to this scaling scheme. However, for global interconnects the length usually increases rather than shrinks. This is because the chip area of each new technology generation usually keeps increasing, forcing the global interconnects to increase in length to connect all the devices. The average length of the longest global interconnect in a circuit can be approximated by [11.1]

$$L_{max} = \frac{\sqrt{A}}{2} \tag{11.5}$$

where A is the chip area. Inserting this into Eq. (11.4) finally leads to the following expression for the delay associated with global interconnects:

$$\tau_L = 0.89 \cdot K_{ox}\varepsilon_o\rho \frac{A}{(F_{min})^2} \tag{11.6}$$

Example Calculate the interconnect delay time according to Eq. (11.6) for the following conditions: Al interconnect ($\rho = 3.0 \times 10^{-6}\ \Omega$ cm), SiO_2 dielectric ($K_{ox} = 3.9$), area $= 100$ mm^2, and the minimum feature size of 0.35 μm.

Answer

$$\tau_L = 0.89 \cdot K_{ox}\varepsilon_o\rho \frac{A}{(F_{min})^2}$$

$$= 0.89 \cdot 3.9 \cdot 8.86 \times 10^{-14}\ \text{Fcm}^{-1} \cdot 3.0 \times 10^{-6}\ \Omega\ \text{cm} \frac{1\text{cm}^2}{(0.35 \times 10^{-4}\ \text{cm})^2}$$

$$= 7.5 \times 10^{-10}\ \text{sec} = 0.75\ \text{nsec}$$

As technology progresses, F_{min} shrinks and A usually gets larger. Both of these lead to an increase in the RC time delay in global interconnects. Even if A stays constant, the time delay will increase due to F_{min} shrinking. Physically this occurs because as the interconnect cross-sectional area decreases, R increases, but C does not decrease in proportion because the dielectric thicknesses surrounding the line also decrease. Hence RC

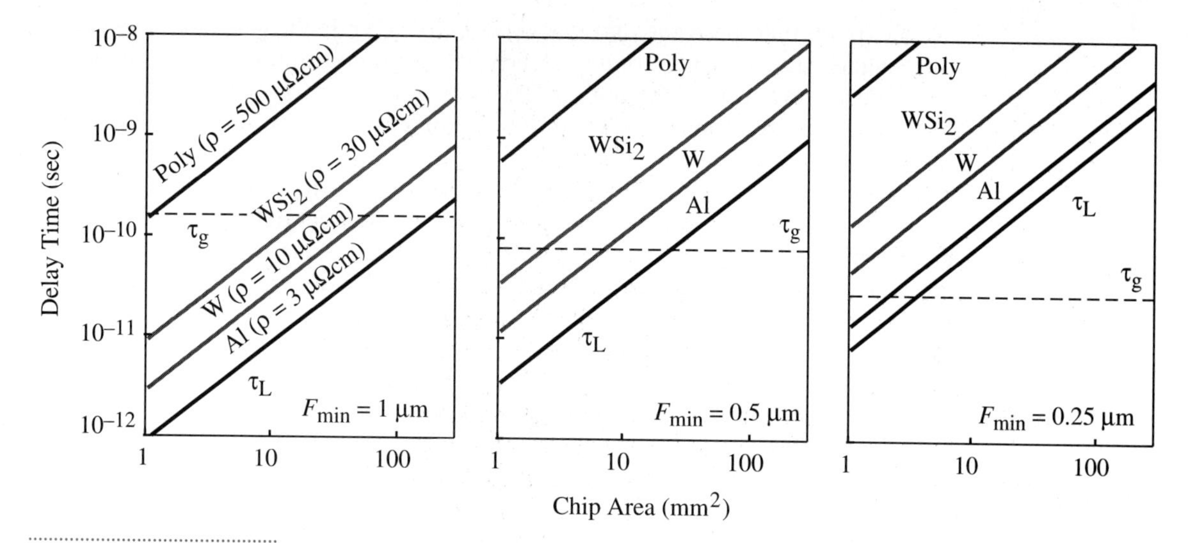

Figure 11–4 Global interconnect and gate time delay versus chip area and minimum feature sizes, F_{min}, for various interconnect materials. Interconnect delay corresponds to longest global interconnect in the circuit. (Updated from [11.1].)

increases. Having A increase only exacerbates this problem. Figure 11–4 plots Eq. (11.6) as a function of chip area for different values of F_{min} and different interconnect materials, updated from the original figure in [11.1] to use the new expressions for x_{ox} and H and to include the $F_{min} = 0.25$ μm case. Cu is also included as a possible interconnect material in the 0.25-μm technology. The interconnect delay here is based on the longest global interconnect using Eq. (11.6), with minimum feature size dimensions and assuming that the driver or load elements do not contribute significantly to the overall time delay. Also plotted for comparison is a typical gate delay, τ_g, for each minimum feature size, as measured in ring oscillator circuits. The gate delay is dependent upon F_{min} but not A and decreases as the minimum feature size decreases. It is obvious that for larger F_{min}'s, the gate delay is generally large relative to the delay for Al global interconnects. (And one can also see why one would not want to use polysilicon as a global interconnect.) But for smaller minimum features and larger chip areas, the global interconnect delay becomes quite large compared to the gate delay and can have a large impact on the circuit performance.

In 0.25 μm ($=F_{min}$) manufacturing technology, chip areas are typically 200–350 mm^2 (corresponding to a maximum global interconnect length of 7–9 mm), and gate delays as measured in ring oscillators are generally about 30–70 picoseconds. The RC delay of the longest global interconnect line, with minimum feature size dimensions, by this analysis is about 3–5 nanoseconds for Al lines, or about 80 times the gate delay. This does not necessarily mean that circuit performance is totally dominated by the interconnects in today's integrated circuits. The specific circuit architecture, the exact heights, widths and lengths of the interconnect lines on the different levels, the driver and load components, and other circuit factors will determine the speed of the circuit and the relative importance of the front-end and back-end elements. What is important are the trends that these and other analyses predict: While the gate delays will keep getting smaller, the local interconnect delays will stay about the same, and the global interconnect delays will get larger and have a larger impact on the circuit performance. Recent analysis by Bohr based on Intel's technology agree with the qualitative predictions of this simple analysis [11.6, 11.7].

Each new technology generation in the NTRS represents a $\sqrt{2}$ reduction in feature size. This corresponds to a 2x increase in RC interconnect delay per generation for a given line length [Eq. (11.4)]. However, the metal line aspect ratio is not typically kept constant but is increased with each technology generation. This is primarily due to the fact that the metal line thickness has stayed rather constant in recent times rather than shrinking in order to keep the resistance lower. This means that the interconnect delay does not increase quite as fast as Eq. (11.4) predicts, but it is still increasing while the gate delay is decreasing. It has been estimated [11.6, 11.8] that in current CMOS technology with Al lines the delay due to the interconnects can be about 30–40% of the total circuit delay, up from about 15–20% just a generation previously. In the next technology generations, the interconnect delay could be more than 50% of the total circuit delay, emphasizing the importance of the back-end structures.

As feature sizes shrink, the size of the contacts is also getting smaller. Since to first order the contact resistance, R_c, is inversely proportional to the contact area, the importance of the contacts increases as the circuit dimensions are shrunk.

The specific projections for back-end technology given by the NTRS are shown in Table 11–1. A number of the qualitative observations made earlier are apparent in this table. Note the increasing numbers of wiring levels in the future and the increasing aspect ratios associated with interconnect lines as well as contacts and vias. Finally, notice the decreasing metal resistivity requirement which cannot be met by aluminum in the future, and the decreasing dielectric constant required for intermetal dielectrics, which cannot be met by SiO_2. Clearly new materials will have to be introduced into back-end

Table 11–1 Future projections for back-end technology taken from the SIA NTRS [11.9]

Year of First DRAM Shipment	1997	1999	2003	2006	2009	2012
Minimum Feature Size, F_{min} (nm)	250	180	130	100	70	50
DRAM Bits/Chip	256M	1G	4G	16G	64G	256G
DRAM Chip Size (mm^2)	280	400	560	790	1120	1580
MPU Chip Size (mm^2)	300	360	430	520	620	750
Wiring Levels—Logic	6	6–7	7	7–8	8–9	9
Min Metal CD (nm)	250	180	130	100	70	50
Min Contact/Via CD nm	280/360	200/260	140/180	110/140	80/100	60/70
Metal Aspect Ratio	1.8	1.8	2.1	2.4	2.7	3.0
Contact Aspect Ratio (DRAM)	5.5	6.3	7.5	9	10.5	12
Via Aspect Ratio (logic)	2.2	2.2	2.5	2.7	2.9	3.2
Metal Resistivity (μΩ-cm)	3.3	2.2	2.2	2.2	<1.8	<1.8
Interlevel Metal Dielectric Constant	3.0–4.1	2.5–3.0	1.5–2.0	1.5–2.0	<1.5	<1.5

structures to meet these objectives. Cu interconnects and "low K" dielectrics are the likely answer to these requirements.

Metallization structures are also receiving increased attention because of failure and reliability issues. Failures are due to a variety of causes: stress-induced void formation in interconnect lines; hillock growth; unwanted chemical reactions and interdiffusion between layers; dopant diffusion and segregation; excessive roughening of films; corrosion; electromigration; and others. Many of these will be discussed in more detail later in the chapter.

Finally it should be pointed out that in the schematic figures in this section we illustrated each metal or dielectric level as simple single-layer structures. In practice, each level or layer is often a multilayered structure itself. The trends to multilayered back-end structures and the use of new processing techniques have been due to the ever-increasing demands on both processing stability and electrical performance as the technology progresses.

11.2 Historical Development and Basic Concepts

The earliest integrated circuits in the 1960s consisted of aluminum lines connecting active regions—transistors and resistors—in silicon. Silicon dioxide passivated the silicon surface and isolated the aluminum interconnects from those regions in the substrate where electrical contact was not wanted. Where contact was desired, openings in the oxide were made so that the aluminum could come in contact with the silicon. Figure 11–5 shows an early structure.

Pure aluminum was thus used for both the contact material and the interconnect. Why aluminum? First, it has a low electrical resistivity at room temperature. (See Table 11–2 for a listing and properties of commonly used interconnect materials). Second, it adheres well to silicon and silicon dioxide. Third, it makes good electrical contact to heavily doped Si. The latter two characteristics are related to the fact that the oxide of Al is very stable, more stable than SiO_2. This means that if Al is deposited on top of SiO_2, it will react with it even at low temperatures, forming a thin layer of Al_2O_3 at the interface. This forms a glue layer, binding the Al to the SiO_2. In the case of Al-to-Si contacts, the Al will reduce any native Si oxide on top of the Si. Without this reaction, the ubiquitous native oxide on the silicon could prevent ohmic contact. Fortunately, the Al_2O_3 that is formed allows Al to diffuse through it into the Si, so that good ohmic contact between the Al and Si is obtained. A fourth benefit of using Al is that its presence

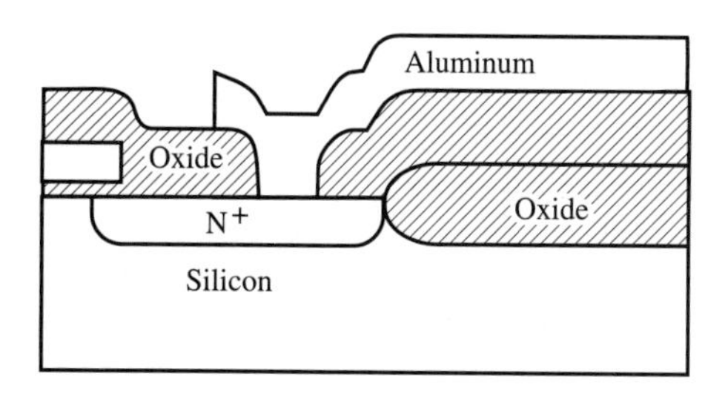

Figure 11–5 Early back-end structure with Al interconnect making contact to highly doped Si active region.

Table 11–2 Properties of interconnect materials

Material	Thin film resistivity (μΩcm)	Melting point (°C)
Al	2.7–3.0	660
W	8–15	3410
Cu	1.7–2.0	1084
Ti	40–70	1670
PtSi	28–35	1229
$TiSi_2$	13–16	1540
WSi_2	30–70	2165
$CoSi_2$	15–20	1326
NiSi	14–20	992
TiN	50–150	~2950
$Ti_{30}W_{70}$	75–200	~2200
polysilicon (heavily doped)	450–1000	1417

assists the annealing out of interface traps at the Si-SiO_2 interface, presumably by converting H_2O to free H, which passivates the traps. (See Chapter 6 where this process is described in more detail.) For all these reasons, contacts and interconnects made of aluminum were instrumental in the development of the first integrated circuits.

It was not long, though, before problems arose. As the circuits became more complicated, the structures became smaller, and the processing got more involved, new demands were placed on the metallization schemes. As a result, new metallization strategies, materials, and structures were developed. Even today the evolution continues, as evidenced by the changing requirements for interconnects in Table 11–1. We will now follow this evolution from the early days of integrated circuit fabrication, first with the contacts, then with the interconnects, and finally with the dielectrics.

11.2.1 Contacts

Contacts provide low-resistance connections between the metal interconnects and active device regions. Metal/semiconductor contacts can in general be rectifying (Schottky) or ohmic. Figure 11–6 shows the I-V characteristics and band diagrams for these modes of current transfer through a contact. Because of the work function difference between the metal and semiconductor, ϕ_B, a barrier exists at the interface. Nature provides a wide variety of metal work functions so in principle it should be possible to choose a metal which produces a small ϕ_B contact to silicon device regions. In practice, this is not generally possible, first because there are other requirements on which metals we may choose (resistivity, for example), and second, because surface states at the metal/semiconductor junction tend to pin the Fermi level deep in the silicon bandgap. This generally produces high ϕ_B contacts to N regions and relatively low ϕ_B contacts to p-type silicon.

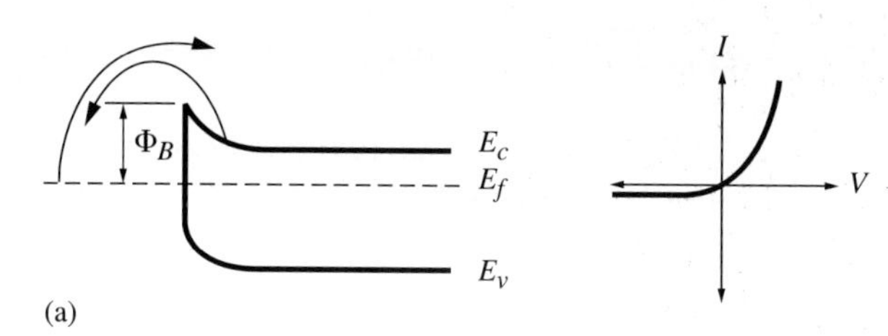

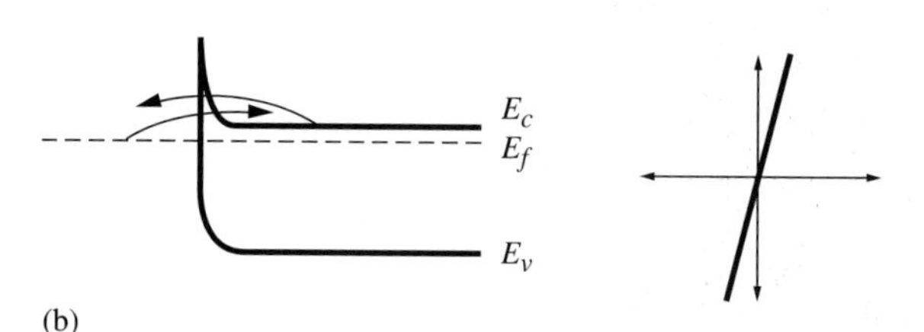

Figure 11–6 Band diagrams and I-V characteristics for metal/semiconductor junctions or contacts, illustrating different modes of current transfer: (a) Schottky or rectifying contact; (b) tunneling or ohmic contact.

Thermionic emission, shown in Figure 11–6(a), in which thermal energy allows the carriers to surmount the barrier, does allow some current to flow over a Schottky barrier. The basic properties of Schottky diodes operating in this mode are similar to the PN diode described in Chapter 1. However, for most metals the barrier is too high to n-type Si, resulting in rectifying behavior with high contact resistance for low to moderately n-doped contacts.

The other way for the carriers to get past the barrier is to tunnel though it [Figure 11–6(b)]. If the silicon is heavily doped, the width of the barrier, defined by the depletion region, x_d, becomes narrow enough that many of the carriers can quantum-mechanically tunnel through the barrier. Ohmic behavior, in which current can flow virtually unimpeded in both directions through a contact, can thus be achieved. This occurs when the doping is greater than about 6×10^{19} cm^{-3}.

The specific contact resistivity, ρ_c, is defined as

$$\rho_c \equiv \left[\frac{\partial V_{MS}}{\partial J}\right]_{V_{MS}=0} \tag{11.7}$$

where J is the current density across the metal/semiconductor interface and V_{MS} is the voltage across it. For a Schottky contact governed by thermionic emission over the barrier, the current density is given by

$$J_S = A^* T^2 \exp\left(\frac{-q\phi_B}{kT}\right)\left(\exp\left(\frac{qV}{kT}\right) - 1\right) \tag{11.8}$$

where A* is Richardson's constant. The specific contact resistivity, in Ω cm^2, is therefore

$$\rho_c = \frac{k}{qA^*T}\exp\left(\frac{q\phi_B}{kT}\right) = \frac{kT}{qJ_s} \tag{11.9}$$

For a tunneling contact, the analysis is somewhat more complicated, resulting in

$$J_s \propto \exp[-2x_d\sqrt{2m^*(q\phi_B - qV)/\hbar^2}] \quad (11.10)$$

where $\hbar$ is Planck's constant, m^* is the effective mass of the tunneling carrier, and x_d is the depletion layer through which the tunneling must occur, which is given by

$$x_d = \sqrt{\frac{2\varepsilon_s\phi_B}{qN_d}} \quad (11.11)$$

where ε_s is the semiconductor permittivity and N_d is the doping concentration in the semiconductor. When x_d is less than about 2.5 nm, tunneling can occur efficiently. Substituting Eqs. (11.10) and (11.11) into (11.7) leads to the contact resistivity, in Ω cm^2, for tunneling contacts:

$$\rho_c = \rho_{co} \exp\left(\frac{2\phi_B\sqrt{m^*\varepsilon_s}}{\hbar\sqrt{N_d}}\right) \quad (11.12)$$

where ρ_{co} is a constant dependent on the metal and semiconductor. The contact resistivity goes down as $\sqrt{N_d}$ goes up because x_d shrinks and tunneling becomes more efficient. For x_d to equal 2.5 nm or less in Si with an Al contact and result in ohmic behavior, N_d must equal $\approx 6 \times 10^{19}$ cm^{-3}. The contact resistance, in Ω, is the contact resistivity divided by the contact area A, assuming that J is uniform over the contact area.

Figure 11–7 shows experimental data for specific contact resistivity as a function of N_d, along with the theoretical prediction based on the preceding equations. At low doping, thermionic emission controls the process which is essentially independent of doping, while at high doping, ρ_c is dominated by tunneling which is a very strong function of the doping level. Measured ρ_c values may be higher than indicated in Figure 11–7 if a clean interface is not obtained, due to the presence of unetched material or etch residues in the contact hole, native oxide present at the metal/semiconductor interface, or other contaminants or reaction products. Another common reason for the contact resistivity being higher than expected is that there are fewer dopants in the Si at the surface than desired. This may be due to segregation of dopants into the contact materials above the Si.

Example The expression for specific contact resistivity for high doping levels where tunneling dominates, Eq. (11.12), can be written in the form

$$\rho_c = \rho_{co} \exp\left(\frac{\phi_B C_1}{\sqrt{N_d}}\right)$$

where $C_1 \approx 7.0 \times 10^{10}$ cm$^{-3/2}$ V^{-1} for Si. If $\phi_B = 0.6$ V and $\rho_{CO} = 1.0 \times 10^{-7}\ \Omega \cdot$ cm^2 for a Si-metal contact, how much does the specific contact resistivity decrease when the doping is increased from 1×10^{19} to 1×10^{20} cm^{-3}?

Answer At $N_D = 1 \times 10^{19}\ \text{cm}^{-3}$,

$$\rho_c = \rho_{co} \exp\left(\frac{\phi_B C_1}{\sqrt{N_d}}\right) = 1.0 \times 10^{-7} \exp\left(\frac{0.6 \cdot 7.0 \times 10^{10}}{\sqrt{1 \times 10^{19}}}\right)$$

$$= 5.9 \times 10^{-2}\ \Omega\ \text{cm}^2$$

At $N_D = 1 \times 10^{20}\ \text{cm}^{-3}$,

$$\rho_c = \rho_{co} \exp\left(\frac{\phi_B C_1}{\sqrt{N_d}}\right) = 1.0 \times 10^{-7} \exp\left(\frac{0.6 \cdot 7.0 \times 10^{10}}{\sqrt{1 \times 10^{20}}}\right)$$

$$= 6.7 \times 10^{-6}\ \Omega\ \text{cm}^2$$

which is about a factor of about 9000 lower. These numbers are in agreement with the values in Figure 11–7.

The general requirements for metal-to-silicon contacts are low contact resistance and good thermal stability. Low contact resistance means a high-dopant concentration

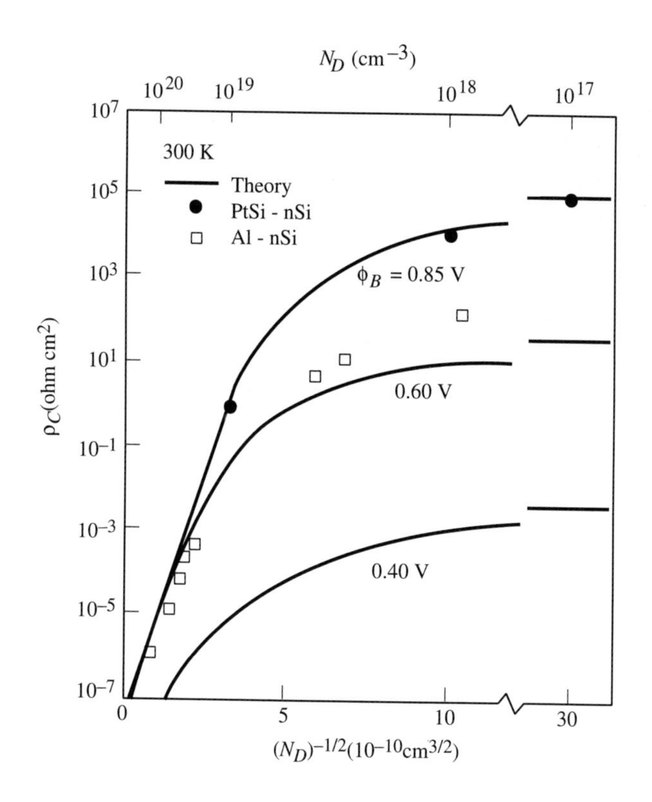

Figure 11–7 Contact resistivity (ρ_C) versus doping for three values of the metal/semiconductor work function. Both theoretical curves, based on Eqs. (11.9) and (11.12), and experimental data are plotted. (After [11.10, 11.11].)

at the Si surface and a good contact between the metal and silicon. Good contact requires an interface free of contaminants and residues. Good thermal stability means that the contact structure does not degrade during subsequent thermal processing, nor does it cause other areas to be adversely affected, such as active areas in the silicon underneath the contact.

A problem with thermal stability resulted in the first major change in the ohmic contact metallurgy. As mentioned previously, early integrated circuits used pure Al as the interconnect material, making direct contact to the Si substrate in heavily doped regions. Al makes a good contact to silicon by reducing the native oxide on the surface, which also removes any other contaminants on the surface. To ensure that the Al reduces the native Si oxide and that the Al is in good physical contact to the Si, a sintering anneal at about 450°C is done. This anneal, in a hydrogen ambient, is also done to anneal out interface traps at the Si-SiO_2 interface in the gates. Subsequent processing at about this same temperature can also occur, such as the deposition of an overlying dielectric or passivation layer.

However, the solubility of Si in Al is significant. At 450°C, the solubility is about 0.5 atomic percent, and at 500°C it is about 1 atomic percent. This means that pure Al in contact with Si will want to absorb the Si from the substrate up to its solubility level for that temperature. The only things limiting this process would be the diffusion of Si in the Al and the amount of Al acting as a sink for the Si. Unfortunately, the diffusivity of Si in polycrystalline Al is quite high, and the amount of Al nearby is large, so a significant amount of Si gets drawn up into the Al. This creates voids in the remaining Si, which are quickly filled by the overlying Al. If the Al penetrates uniformly into the substrate, typical processing conditions and contact/interconnect dimensions would result in about 0.2–0.3 μm of penetration. However, the situation is actually worse than that. That is because when the Al reduces the native oxide, it does so nonuniformly. Therefore the Al penetrates in localized spots. Al "spikes" occur in the Si substrate, penetrating in excess of 1 μm deep. Figure 11–8 illustrates this, showing the Al penetrating in some areas deeper than the diffused junction. This can short the junction. As a practical matter, pure Al contacts to Si cannot be used for junction depths of less than 2–3 μm.

One solution to the Al spiking problem is to use Al films that already have Si in them. Therefore the solubility requirement is already fulfilled. So Al films with approximately 1 atomic percent Si have been commonly used. This is the solubility of Si in Al at about 500°C, the highest temperature the Al sees during processing. The spiking problem is reduced, but another problem arises. When the contact structure is cooled down below

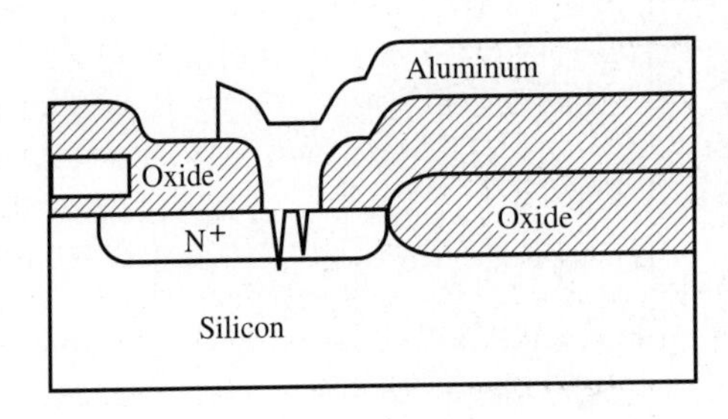

Figure 11–8 Si-Al contact region showing spiking of Al into Si active region. This is due to Si diffusing into the Al to satisfy the solubility requirement, with Al filling the resulting voids in the Si substrate.

500°C, or subsequent thermal steps are done at less than 500°C, the solubility of Si in Al is less. The now-excess Si precipitates out, usually at the interface where heterogeneous nucleation can occur, leaving Si nodules. In fact, there is enough Al dissolved in these nodules to make them p-type (Al is a p-type dopant in silicon), causing higher contact resistance to N^+ regions.

The use of Al(Si) to solve the spiking problem was adequate as long as the contact resistance was not limiting circuit performance. But as contact areas were reduced in size and the contact resistance did become an issue, another solution to Al-Si interaction and spiking was needed for contacts to small junctions. Barrier layers provided the answer. These layers are placed between the Al and Si to prevent or at least slow down any interaction. Such barriers need to be a barrier for chemical interdiffusion between Si and Al at processing temperatures (up to 450–500°C). They also need to be thermally stable. They should have low stress. This usually means that their coefficient of thermal expansion needs to be close to Si ($2.6 \times 10^{-6}\,°C^{-1}$). They need to adhere well to Si and Al, as well as SiO_2. This usually means that there is some interfacial reaction between the barrier and Si and Al. Finally, they should have good electrical conductivity and a low contact resistance to both Si and Al.

Barrier layers have been classified by Nicolet [11.12] into three types: passive barriers, stuffed barriers, and sacrificial barriers. The passive barriers would be chemically inert to both Si and Al and be good diffusion barriers as well. TiN is an example of this type. Some materials are chemically inert, but diffusion along their grain boundaries can be quite significant. However, it has been found that by "stuffing" the grain boundaries with other atoms or molecules, the diffusion of other species can be greatly reduced, making them diffusion barriers as well. The reduction of diffusion by stuffing the grain boundaries is a combination of a physical effect (physically blocking the diffusing species) and a chemical effect (the stuffed species, such as nitrogen or oxygen, chemically bond with the diffusing species, such as Al, stopping their diffusion). A Ti-W alloy with nitrogen stuffing the grain boundaries—achieved by sputtering the Ti-W in an N_2 ambient—is an example of a stuffed barrier. Sacrificial barriers are those in which the barrier material is "sacrificed" in order to prevent reaction between the Al and Si. The material, such as Ti, reacts with either the Al or Si or both, forming aluminides or silicides. But by doing so, it prevents the Al and Si from interacting since the reactions with the barrier material are favored both kinetically and thermodynamically over the reaction between the Al and Si. However, once the sacrificial barrier material is consumed, the barrier is gone, and so these types of barriers are only effective for limited processing temperatures and times.

One of the first barrier layers for contacts was platinum silicide. It is formed by depositing Pt on the wafer, and then annealing at low temperatures (250–350°C). Because the surface Si is consumed during the formation reaction, a new, clean interface is obtained, and very good electrical contact is made. It is also "self-aligned" because the silicide is only formed where the Si is exposed through the oxide contact opening (and the unreacted Pt is chemically removed from other areas). Therefore an extra mask is not needed and no alignment overlap is required. PtSi acts satisfactorily as a barrier between Al and Si, but only if subsequent processing is done at about 400°C or below, and junction depths underneath are greater than about 0.3 μm. That is because PtSi will react with Al, forming Pt-Al intermetallic compounds and eventually allowing the Al to spike into the Si substrate. Once junction depths got shallower than 0.3 μm and processing temperatures got above 400°C, another barrier was necessary.

Refractory metals by themselves have had limited use as barriers. Ti in particular is attractive since it reduces and breaks through any native oxide and adheres well to both Si and SiO_2. It forms very low resistive contacts, silicon diffusion through it is slow, and therefore it prevents the Si dissolving in the Al. However, it reacts with Al to form $TiAl_3$ at low temperatures. (Above 500°C, Ti will also react with the Si to form $TiSi_2$.) It thus acts as a sacrificial barrier, acting as a barrier only until it is consumed, which happens rather quickly above 400°C. So while Ti is a good contact/adhesion layer, it is not a very good barrier layer. Ti is thus often used in conjunction with a barrier layer on top.

Refractory metal silicides, such as $TiSi_2$, have also been used as barrier layers in contacts. They will also react with Al, but at a somewhat higher temperature (about 500°C for $TiSi_2$) than the noble metal silicides, such as PtSi. However, diffusion along their grain boundaries limits their effectiveness as barriers to below 400°C. Therefore, like Ti, refractory metal silicides are now usually used in contact structures as the adhesion/contact layer, with a better barrier layer on top. An advantage in using refractory metal silicides in contacts is the ability to form self-aligned contact structures. Ti can be deposited over both an oxide layer and into the openings in the contacts without a mask, but during an anneal it will only form a silicide in the contacts where Si is exposed. The unreacted Ti over the oxide can be etched off, leaving the silicide self-aligned to the contact.

In fact, the entire source and drain regions can be contacted by a refractory metal silicide this way, providing for local interconnects. By contacting the entire source and drain regions with silicide, rather than just in the contact holes, the contact resistance is also improved by providing a much larger contact area between the silicide and silicon. This is because the silicon/silicide contact resistance is much larger than silicide/barrier/metal contact resistances, and the net contact resistance thus depends on the silicon/silicide contact area.

As the backend processing temperatures were raised and junction depths decreased in later technology generations, the next commonly used barrier after PtSi Ti-W. This alloy, generally about 30 atomic percent, or 10 weight percent Ti, acts as a diffusion barrier between the Si and Al, especially when stuffed with nitrogen. While pure W is a good barrier itself, adding Ti helps it adhere to underlying layers and increases its corrosion resistance. Ti-W will react with Al at higher temperatures, about 600°C, while diffusion through the film limits its use to below 500°C. In addition, diffusion of Ti from the film into the Al at 400°C and above has been seen to raise the Al resistivity. Its contact resistance, however, is not as low as PtSi, possibly due to its difficulty in dissolving the native oxide on the Si surface. Thus a bilayer of PtSi and Ti-W has been generally used, taking advantage of the low contact resistance of the PtSi and the barrier properties of Ti-W. One problem with Ti-W is its relatively high stress. It is often very brittle, leading to cracking and peeling on the wafer and to flaking from chamber walls onto the wafer. [11.13] In addition, there is the problem of diffusion of Ti from the film into Al at 400°C and above, raising the resistivity of the Al interconnect line.

Refractory metal compounds, notably TiN, have become very popular barrier layers. These are commonly fine-grained structures, with grain sizes below 10 nm. Because of this, diffusion through them is very slow, making them impermeable to silicon and most other species. Incorporation of oxygen or nitrogen in these films makes them even better barriers. They are also chemically stable and chemically inert with most other layers. There may be some reaction with Al, forming some AlN and $TiAl_3$ at temperatures greater than 550°C. The electrical resistivity of TiN is low enough for use as both a contact material and a local interconnect. The contact resistance to Si is somewhat higher than that of PtSi, Ti, or $TiSi_2$. Therefore, TiN is usually used in a bilayer structure with TiN on top of Ti, with the Ti usually reacted to form $TiSi_2$ for a better contact. The best properties of both layers are utilized: the good adhesion and low contact resistance of the Ti or $TiSi_2$, and the good barrier properties of TiN. This is accomplished without much more processing, since the TiN can easily be deposited immediately after the Ti, just by adding nitrogen in the sputter deposition chamber. Or TiN can be formed on top of $TiSi_2$ by depositing Ti on top of the Si substrate in the contact opening, and annealing in a nitrogen ambient. The Ti reacts with the Si below it to form the silicide while simultaneously reacting with the nitrogen in the ambient to form TiN on top. This was in fact the process described in the CMOS process flow in Chapter 2 (Figures 2–3 to 2–33). The TiN can also be deposited by CVD.

Figure 11–9 shows a multilayer contact structure with $TiSi_2$/TiN contact/barrier layers. The $TiSi_2$ makes good electrical contact to the Si and provides good adhesion. The TiN serves as a barrier to interaction between the Al and both the $TiSi_2$ and Si. Table 11–3 lists commonly used contact barrier layers and compares their maximum processing temperature and modes of failure. It is clear that early contact structures have evolved from simple Al-on-Si structures to barrier-layer structures to multilayer structures. We will later see how W plugs are often used in contacts to improve step coverage and planarization.

11.2.2 Interconnects and Vias

Interconnects have similarly evolved as the technology has progressed and the requirements placed on interconnects have increased. The primary requirements on interconnects are low resistivity, good adhesion to underlying films, stability during processing and operation, and the ability to be deposited and etched.

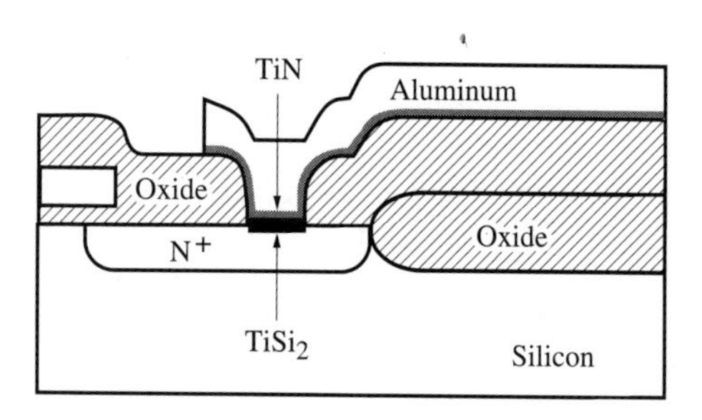

Figure 11–9 Multilayer contact structure with $TiSi_2$/TiN contact/barrier layers between the Si and Al.

Table 11–3 Barrier-layer properties [11.14, 11.15]

Structure	Failure Temperature (°C)	Failure Mechanism (Reaction products)
Al/PtSi/Si	350–400	Compound formation (Al_2Pt, Si)
Al/$TiSi_2$/Si	400	Diffusion ($Al_5Ti_7Si_{12}$, Si at 550°C)
Al/NiSi/Si	400	Compound formation (Al_3Ni, Si)
Al/$CoSi_2$/Si	400	Compound formation Al_9Co_2, Si)
Al/Ti/PtSi/Si	450	Compound formation (Al_3Ti)
Al/$Ti_{30}W_{70}$/PtSi/Si	500	Diffusion (Al_2Pt, $Al_{12}W$ at 500°C)
Al/TiN/$TiSi_2$/Si	550	Compound formation (AlN, Al_3Ti)

Aluminum, aluminum alloys, and aluminum containing multilayers have been the dominant interconnects in silicon technology to this point in time. Al has low resistivity (although not low enough to meet future NTRS specifications), adheres well to Si and SiO_2, can reduce other oxides, and can be etched and deposited using reasonable techniques. Its main shortcoming is its stability during processing and operation, which we will discuss. For early MOS technology, Al was used not only as the primary interconnect (i.e. global) but also as the gate electrode and a local interconnect. However the melting temperature of Al is low (660°C for pure Al), and it cannot withstand high processing temperatures. When self-aligned source and drain regions were needed to reduce gate-source and gate-drain capacitances, a new material was needed for the gate electrode that could withstand the 800–1000°C diffusion steps or implant anneals needed to dope the source and drain regions while the gate electrode material was present. Heavily doped polycrystalline silicon was the solution to this problem. Polysilicon can be utilized as an interconnect as well, although only as a local interconnect because of its resistivity.

The first modification to pure Al interconnects was the addition of Si at about 1 atomic percent. This prevents spiking of Al into the silicon substrate which is caused by silicon's relatively high solubility and diffusivity in Al. Even with the use of barrier layers such as TiN, Si is often still used in Al interconnects. This is because the presence of the Si reduces the driving force for interdiffusion and hence decreases the chance of barrier failure. Si also suppresses the reaction between Al and TiN.

Almost all the rest of the modifications made to the Al interconnect structure have been as a result of aluminum's low melting point and ease of deformation. Two phenomena that occur with aluminum which have caused significant problems and have required modifications in the Al interconnect are hillock growth and electromigration.

Hillock growth occurs when the Al thin film is subjected to high compressive stresses. Because of the polycrystalline structure of Al, coupled with its low melting point and resulting susceptibility to plastic deformation, the Al will deform under such stresses. High stresses can easily be generated due to Al's relatively high coefficient of thermal expansion ($23 \times 10^{-6}\ °C^{-1}$, while Si is $2.6 \times 10^{-6}\ °C^{-1}$ as shown in Table 11–4). If Al is deposited on a Si substrate (or even on another film, such as SiO_2, on a Si substrate) at low

Table 11–4 Mechanical properties of interconnect materials

Material	Thermal expansion coefficient (°C^{-1})	Elastic modulus, $Y/(1-\nu)$ (MPa)	Hardness (kg mm^{-2})	Melting point (°C)
Al (111)	23.1×10^{-6}	1.143×10^5	19–22	660
Ti	8.41×10^{-6}	1.699×10^5	81–143	1660
$TiAl_3$	12.3×10^{-6}	—	660—750	1340
Si (100)	2.6×10^{-6}	1.805×10^5	—	1417
Si (111)	2.6×10^{-6}	2.290×10^5	—	1417
SiO_2	0.55×10^{-6}	0.83×10^5	—	~1700

temperatures and the structure is heated, high compressive stresses in the Al can be generated. This is because the Al, which is tightly constrained to the wafer, will want to expand much more than the Si. To relieve the stress, portions of the Al are squeezed up, forming small hills or "hillocks." The movement of the Al occurs primarily along grain boundaries in the Al since diffusion is usually much faster along grain boundaries than through the interior of the grains. Whole grains of Al are often pushed or grow upward, forming hillocks about the size of the grains, 0.5 to 3 μm tall and wide.

Figure 11–10 shows schematically the process of hillock formation. Hillocks can result in electrical shorts between interconnect levels, as well as cause the surface topography to be rough, making lithography and etching more difficult. While the overlying films can help suppress hillock formation by acting as a mechanical barrier, this does not completely eliminate the problem. In fact, so much stress can build up that an overlying SiO_2 layer can crack. When this happens, the Al can protrude from the crack in long whiskers many microns long, increasing the chances of a short.

The addition of elements that have limited solubility in Al, such as Cu, has been found to suppress hillock formation. The excess atoms segregate and precipitate preferentially at the Al grain boundaries. This reduces the Al diffusion along the grain boundaries and suppresses hillock formation.

In a similar manner, voids can form when the Al is subjected to tensile stresses. Upon cooling, the Al will want to shrink more than the Si below it. (Unfortunately any hillocks that have formed during the previous heating do not significantly reverse themselves and disappear during the cooling.) Since the Si is more mechanically rigid than the Al, the stress is relieved by vacancy movement and agglomeration in the Al, with voids forming. This can greatly increase the interconnect electrical resistance and even cause open circuits. The addition of Cu to the Al can suppress void formation in Al as well as suppressing hillock formation.

Perhaps the biggest problem encountered with Al interconnects is that of electromigration. One of the requirements of an interconnect is that it be stable not only during processing, but also during circuit operation. Electromigration is a phenomenon that occurs during circuit operation and has very adverse effects. When an electrical current flows through aluminum (on the order of 0.1–0.5 MA cm^{-2}, which is commonly achieved in integrated circuits), the electrons can actually transfer enough momentum

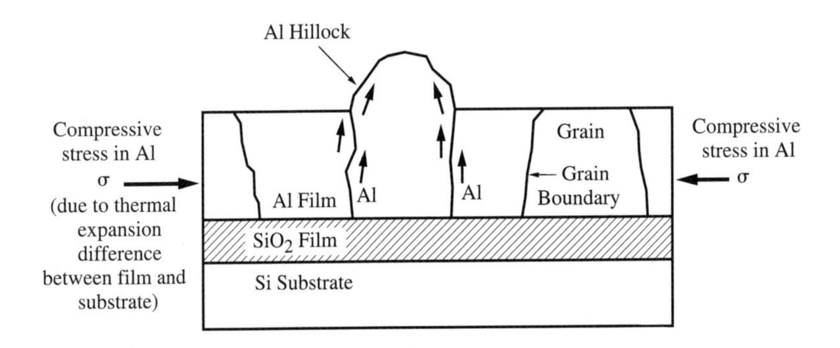

Figure 11–10 Schematic illustration of hillock formation due to compressive stress in an Al film. Al diffusion along grain boundaries is indicated.

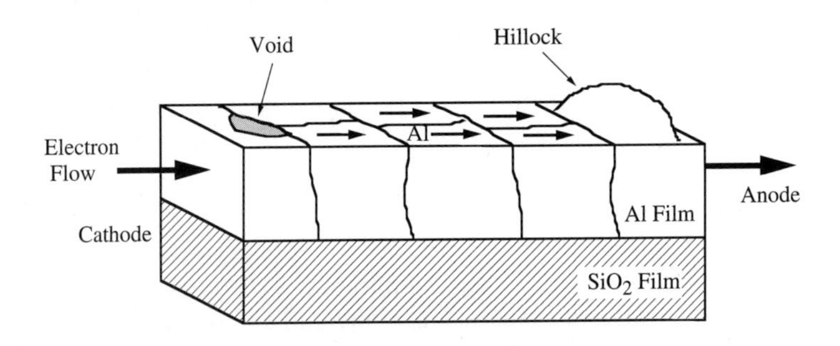

Figure 11–11 Schematic illustration of electromigration with resultant hillock and void formation. Diffusion of Al through grain boundaries is indicated.

to the Al atoms to cause them to diffuse. This diffusion is faster along grain boundaries, and it can cause a buildup of Al in some regions, resulting in hillocks, and can cause a depletion in other regions, resulting in voids. As a result shorts and opens in the interconnects can occur during the normal operation of the circuit. Figure 11–11 shows this process schematically, and Figure 11–12 shows a SEM of an actual circuit where this has occurred. Because most of the Al atoms and vacancies diffuse along the grain boundaries, electromigration is very dependent on the grain structure, including the size and crystallographic orientation of the grains. It also depends on over- and underlying layers, and on the processing history of the interconnects.

Substantial effort has been made to study and remedy this phenomenon. One of the early remedies for electromigration was to add Cu to the Al. As is the case in suppressing hillocks, adding Cu is believed to suppress grain boundary diffusion and hence slow down electromigration. Adding too much Cu, however, causes problems with etching of the interconnect as well as corrosion, and 4 weight percent Cu is the most that is usually added.

Thus, the first modifications to Al interconnects involved switching from pure Al to Al with about 1–2 weight percent Si and 0.5–4 weight percent Cu. Adding these elements to the Al increases the sheet resistivity of the interconnect by as much as 35%,

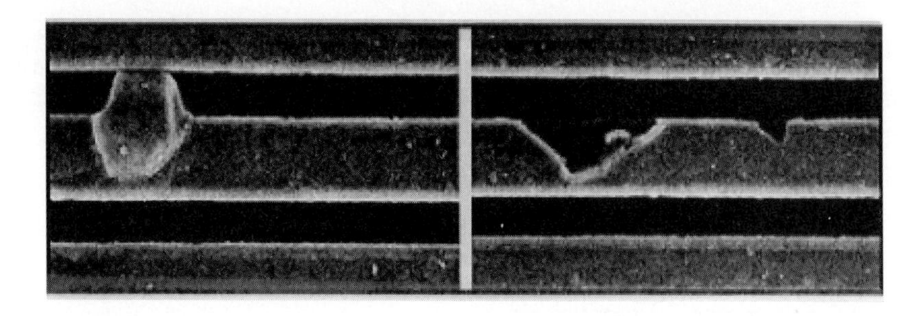

Figure 11–12 SEM top view of hillock and voids that have formed due to electromigration in an Al line [11.16]. Reprinted by permission of Materials Research Society.

but this was a necessary trade-off in order to prevent the failure of circuits due to electromigration and hillock and void formation. Other solutions, similar to those for contacts involving multilayer structures, were later developed and will be discussed later.

The next change to interconnects involved the local interconnects. Polysilicon has been used as the gate electrode since the mid 1970s. But as circuits got faster, the sheet resistivity of heavily doped polysilicon became a concern (Figure 11–4). In addition, the doped silicon in the source and drain regions has a fairly high resistivity (50–100 $\mu\Omega$-cm) which can add appreciable parasitic resistance to MOS transistors. Silicide materials can be used to reduce all these problems.

Silicides have been utilized as, or with local interconnects in three primary ways, as illustrated in Figure 11–13. On top of the polysilicon layer they form a "polycide" structure; on top of the source and drain regions they strap the doped silicon; and finally, they can be used as an independent local interconnect. All of these uses were illustrated in the CMOS process in Chapter 2 (Figure 2–33). In the polycide structure, the silicide decreases the sheet resistance of the polysilicon gate and local interconnect, while retaining the highly reliable polysilicon/SiO_2 interface. On top of the source and drain regions, the silicide reduces the resistance of the diffused layers. The silicide layer also provides a good contact to the silicon in the gate, source, and drain regions, while increasing the contact area. Silicides are also sometimes used as local interconnects by themselves, providing relatively low resistive paths below the lowest metal layers. Silicides are used because they offer low electrical resistivity (10–50 $\mu\Omega$-cm), they are stable at high temperatures, they provide good process compatibility with silicon, they are easy to plasma etch, they provide good contacts to other materials, and they do not exhibit much electromigration. Some of the common silicides used in silicon technology are listed in Table 11–5, along with some of their properties.

As discussed in Chapter 9, the formation of silicides can be accomplished in two ways: by direct deposition of the silicide and by the reaction between the metal and Si on the wafer to form the silicide. The direct deposition method can use sputtering from a composite target, cosputtering from two targets of the metal and Si, co-evaporation of the metal and Si, or Chemical Vapor Deposition (CVD). CVD is currently only done for WSi_2. The reaction method can be accomplished by two different techniques. The first technique is by depositing the metal and amorphous Si, both usually by sputtering, and

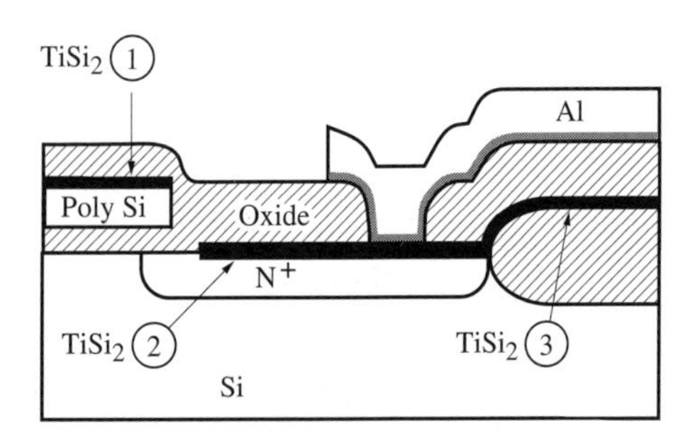

Figure 11–13 Uses of silicides in back-end structures: 1, on top of a polysilicon gate; 2, on top of source and drain regions; and 3, as a local interconnect.

Table 11–5 Properties of silicides (After [11.17])

Silicide	Thin film resistivity (μΩ-cm)	Sintering temp (°C)	Stable on Si up to (°C)	Reaction with Al at (°C)	nm of Si consumed per nm of metal	nm of resulting silicide per nm of metal	Barrier height to n-Si (eV)
PtSi	28–35	250–400	~750	250	1.12	1.97	0.84
$TiSi_2$ (C54)	13–16	700–900	~900	450	2.27	2.51	0.58
$TiSi_2$ (C49)	60–70	500–700			2.27	2.51	
WSi_2	30–70	1000	~1000	500	2.53	2.58	0.67
Co_2Si	~70	300–500			0.91	1.47	
CoSi	100–150	400–600			1.82	2.02	
$CoSi_2$	14–20	600–800	~950	400	3.64	3.52	0.65
NiSi	14–20	400–600	~650		1.83	2.34	
$NiSi_2$	40–50	600–800			3.65	3.63	0.66
$MoSi_2$	40–100	800–1000	~1000	500	2.56	2.59	0.64
$TaSi_2$	35–55	800–1000	~1000	500	2.21	2.41	0.59

patterning and selectively etching the amorphous Si. (The Si may be deposited and patterned either before or after the metal deposition.) The wafer is then annealed so that the metal and amorphous Si react to form the silicide, and the unreacted metal is selectively etched off. The second reaction method is similar but no amorphous Si is deposited. Instead, the metal is deposited on the exposed gate and/or source drain regions, all of which are silicon. The wafer is annealed and the silicide forming reaction occurs wherever the silicon and metal are in contact, that is, on the gate and source/drain regions. The unreacted metal is then selectively etched away. The first of these reaction techniques produces local interconnects independent of either gate or source/drain regions, while the second reaction method produces self-aligned silicide structures on the gate and/or source drains. This second technique is often called a salicide, for "self-aligned silicide." Figure 11–14 illustrates the salicide process.

A high-temperature anneal is required for either the direct deposition or reaction methods of silicide formation. In the reaction method, a high-temperature step is needed to react the metal with the Si to form the silicide and hence to achieve low re-

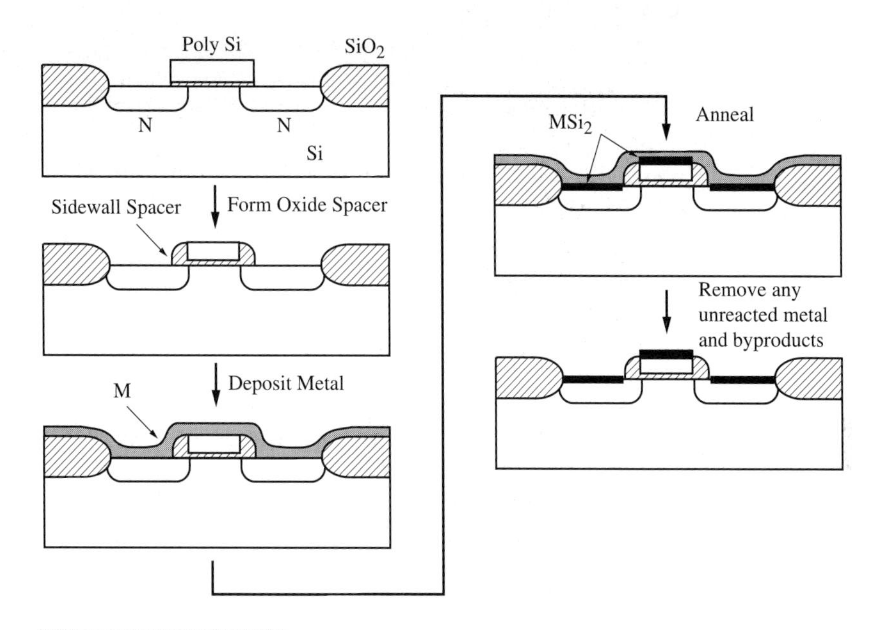

Figure 11–14 Salicide (self-aligned silicide) process. M represents a metal, such as Ti.

sistivity films. A high-temperature step is also required in the direct deposit methods. Depending on the exact deposition technique, the grain structure of the as-deposited film is either very fine, microcrystalline, amorphous, or even an unreacted multilayer structure. In any of these cases, annealing is needed to make the grains grow in size in order to achieve low-resistivity films. This is because in small-grain films there are more grain boundaries which scatter the carriers, reducing the electrical mobility. The final, or minimum, resistivity for various silicides is given in Table 11–5.

There have been several silicides used in silicon technology, including WSi_2, $TaSi_2$, $MoSi_2$, $TiSi_2$, and $CoSi_2$. Tungsten silicide has been used because a CVD deposition process is available for it, providing good step coverage and good process control. In addition, it can be oxidized rather easily, as long as a source of silicon is maintained below it. Therefore, a good thermal oxide can be formed over it rather than a deposited oxide. However, high stresses in WSi_2 often cause stability and adhesion problems. WSi_2, as well as $TaSi_2$ and $MoSi_2$, are not as easy to form through reaction with Si as $TiSi_2$ and $CoSi_2$ are, and therefore are not as attractive for salicide applications.

$TiSi_2$ is very popular due to its low resistivity, and its ability to reduce native oxides and to adhere well to most other materials. However, $TiSi_2$ has a high-resistivity phase ("C49") that forms at moderate temperatures. This must be transformed to a low resistivity phase by annealing, and this transformation becomes more difficult for narrow and thin lines. Also, the thin film has a tendency to agglomerate, or roughen up, at higher annealing temperatures.

$CoSi_2$ behaves better in regard to these particular problems. In addition, it generally shows less lateral encroachment during its formation reaction. Lateral encroachment means the silicide forms beyond the source, drain, and gate regions over the oxide (or

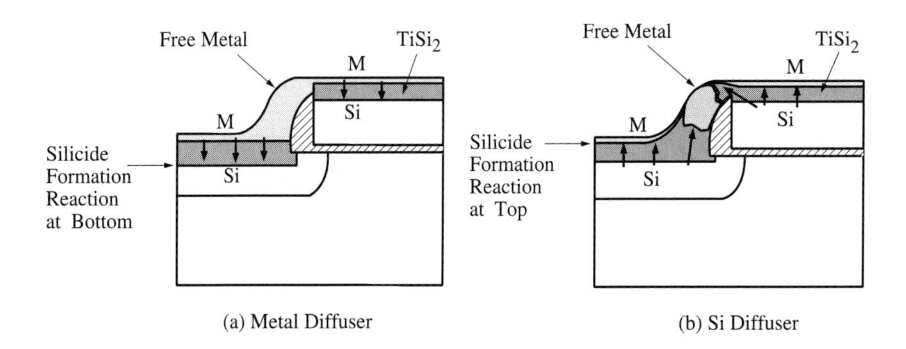

Figure 11–15 Schematic illustration of silicide formation for a silicide that forms by (a) diffusion of metal species and by (b) diffusion of silicon. In the latter case, lateral encroachment of the silicide over the oxide spacer can occur.

nitride) spacer, which can cause an electrical short between those areas. Encroachment is generally less for $CoSi_2$ because of its lower reaction temperatures, and also because the metal is believed to be the dominant diffusing species during silicide formation. This is shown schematically in Figure 11–15. However, the resistivity of $CoSi_2$ is slightly higher than $TiSi_2$, and it does not have as good adhesion and oxide reducing properties as $TiSi_2$. $CoSi_2$ is more sensitive to surface contaminants and oxides, which can lead to non-uniform silicidation and junction leakage.

TiN, as a byproduct of the $TiSi_2$ salicide process, can also be utilized as a local interconnect as was illustrated in the CMOS process flow in Chapter 2 (Figures 2–31 to 2–33). The reaction between Ti and Si in the salicide process is often done in a nitrogen ambient in a two-step anneal process, as will be discussed in the next section on processing techniques. Portions of the TiN that is formed can be masked and left on the circuit to act as a local interconnect. An advantage of using TiN as a local interconnect rather than polysilicon or a silicide is that TiN is a diffusion barrier for most dopants. TiN is commonly utilized as a local interconnect in SRAM cells, where small cell size is critical, connecting load drains with the input gate of the inverter.

Another material that has been used or considered for a local interconnect is tungsten. Selective deposition of tungsten over Si areas using CVD (see Chapter 9) has been used to form W/polysilicon gate and W/silicon source and drain structures. However, at temperatures above 600°C the W and silicon will react to form a silicide, eliminating the advantage of having a lower resistivity material strapping the gate, source, and drain regions. First-level dielectric processing is commonly done above this temperature, which would be a roadblock to utilizing W in this manner.

As circuits became larger and more complex, additional interconnect levels have been required (Table 11–1). Adding an additional level of global interconnect seems easy enough. The process could be as simple as opening a hole in the top dielectric level wherever a contact to the lower level is needed, depositing Al (with some Cu in it to inhibit electromigration), forming both the contact and the next level interconnect, fol-

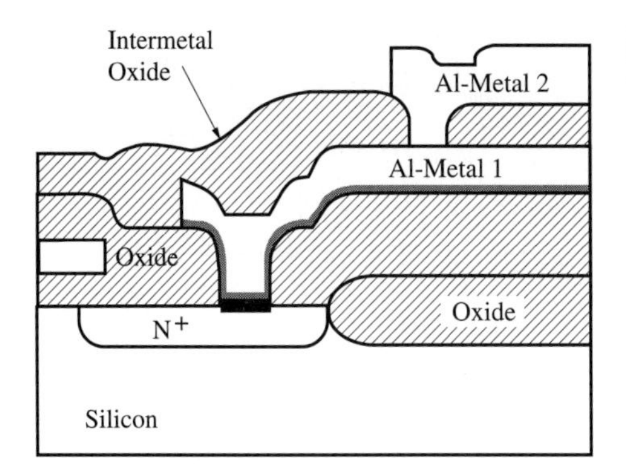

Figure 11–16 Illustration of early two-level metal structure.

lowed by patterning of the aluminum. Then the next level of intermetal dielectric material would be deposited. This structure is illustrated in Figure 11–16. This, in fact, is how the early multilevel interconnect structures were made. Looking at the contact, or via in this case, Al is now making contact to Al, so spiking into Si is not a problem. Good electrical contact between two layers of Al can be achieved if the interface is clean.

However, the topography gets less planar as more levels are added, as Figure 11–16 illustrates. A more planar topography is desired for two main reasons—lithography limitations and step coverage. The lithography limitations arise partly from the limited depth of focus of submicron lithography instruments. The maximum depth of focus is about $\pm$ 0.35 μm for state-of-the-art optical tools (see Chapter 5.). In addition, nonplanar topography results in nonuniform resist thickness, which can result in nonuniform exposure and development. Another lithography issue is that spurious UV light reflections can occur from the sides of metal as it goes over steep steps, again causing lithography problems. There are lithographic techniques that address these problems, such as using multilayer resist structures as discussed in Chapter 5, but these are not always effective or practical solutions.

Nonplanar topography also leads to problems with step coverage and filling of spaces with deposited films. We saw in Chapter 9 how step coverage and filling can be problems, especially for PVD deposited metal (see Figure 9–1, for example). Such problems lead to higher electrical resistance in the line, as well as potential reliability problems. To make matters worse, step coverage problems compound one another. A large step height on one level can lead not only to thinning of the next level on sidewalls, but also cusping and overhangs. This in turn leads to even worse coverage problems on the next level.

Reducing the step heights and achieving more planar topology through processing techniques is called planarization. The Degree Of Planarization (DOP) is defined as

$$\mathrm{DOP} = 1 - \frac{x^f_{\mathrm{step}}}{x^i_{\mathrm{step}}} \tag{11.13}$$

where x^f_{step} is the initial step height in the topography and x^f_{step} is the final step height after some sort of planarization is done. These step heights can refer to hole depths as

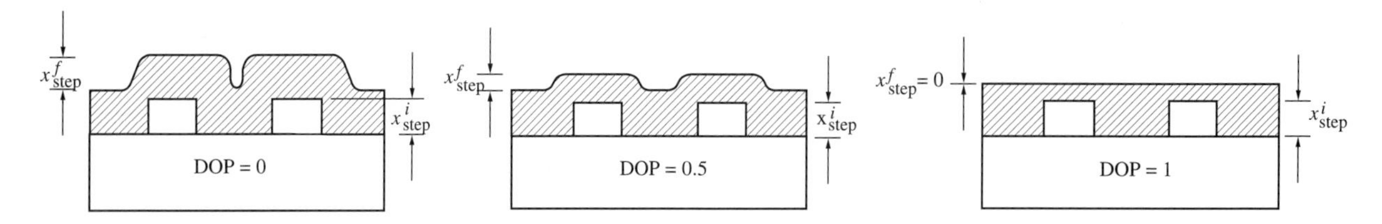

Figure 11–17 Demonstration of Degree Of Planarization (DOP).

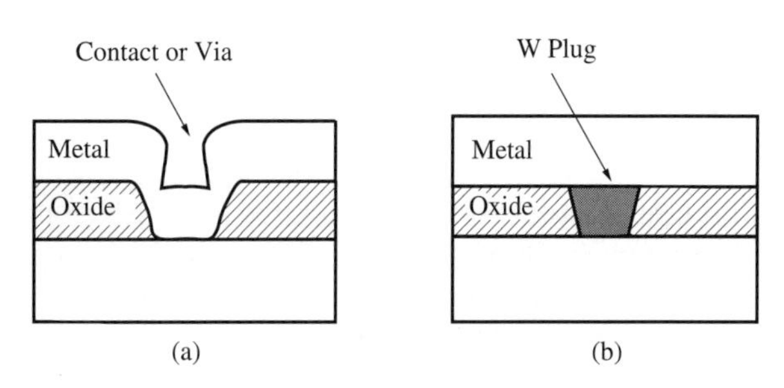

Figure 11–18 (a). Using Al as both the contact and the next level interconnect layer results in nonplanar topography. (b) Using a tungsten plug as the contact results in planar topography.

well. A DOP of 0 means that no planarization is achieved, while a DOP of 1 corresponds to complete planarization—the final step height is zero. Figure 11–17 shows different degrees of planarization. Several methods have been developed to improve the planarity of multilevel interconnect structures. Some involve the metals, which will now be discussed, while others involve the dielectric materials, which will be discussed later.

One way to help achieve planar metal layers is by using a W contact or via fill, also called a W plug. Figure 11–18(a) shows the topography above a contact or via which uses Al as both the contact material and the next level of interconnect. Not only might the step coverage of the Al be a problem, but the resulting topography over the contact can be very non-planar. Using a via fill or plug structure results in the structure in Figure 11–18(b). This can be accomplished in two ways. One method involves a selective W deposition into contact or via holes cut in the dielectric layer, which fills the contacts or vias without depositing any W over the top of the dielectric. The other, more common, method is using a blanket W deposition, which fills the contact or via as well as covering the dielectric. Then an "etchback" is done to remove the W over the top surface of the dielectric. This is illustrated in Figure 11–19. This process of filling holes or trenches in a dielectric level with the metal (usually followed by an etchback), rather than depositing, patterning, and etching the metal on top of a dielectric layer, is called the "damascene" method. Its name comes from the ancient practice of inlaying metal in wood or ceramics for decoration. It can be used for vias or interconnect layers, or both.

Using a W plug produces a much smoother topography over the contact or via, as shown in Figure 11–18(b), resulting in a near-planar contact or via level. The DOP approaches 1 here, where the initial step height corresponds to the height of the contact or via hole. Figure 11–2 illustrated such W contact plugs with an Al metal line on top. With a planar contact or via level, the problem with step coverage of sputtered Al is greatly reduced since there are few, if any, steps for the Al to cover. W is used for the

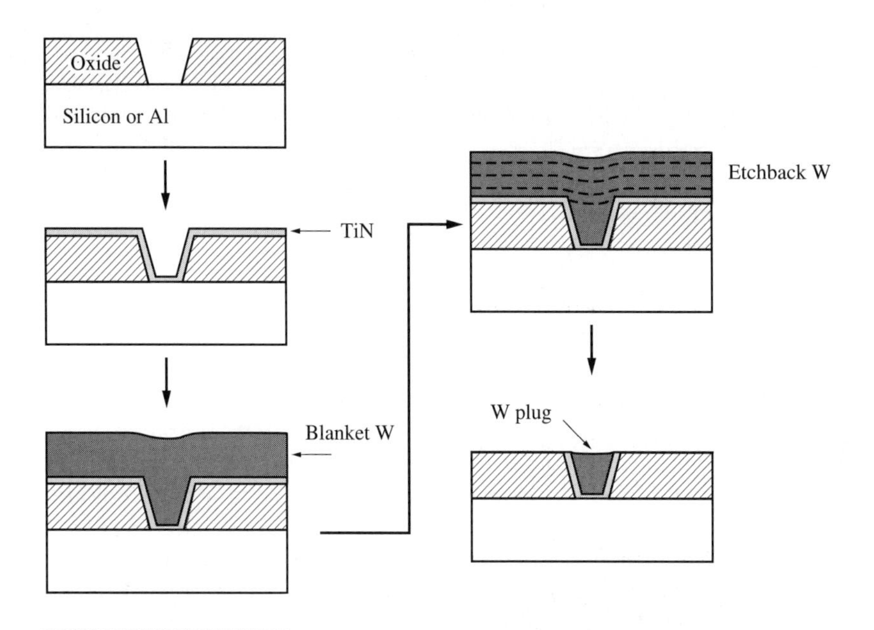

Figure 11–19 Schematic illustration of process to fabricate a W plug for a contact or via. TiN (or a Ti/TiN bilayer) is utilized as an adhesion and barrier layer. An etchback step is done to planarize the W and leave it only in the contact or via hole.

plug rather than Al because the deposition of W using the CVD technique gives much more conformal filling of the contact or via hole. Because of problems with CVD deposition of Al-Cu alloys, as discussed in Chapter 9, CVD Al processes are generally not used in manufacturing.

One planarizing technique under development that does utilize Al as the contact or via metal is called Al reflow. By heating the Al to 450–550°C either during the deposition or immediately afterward, the Al in a contact or via hole will flow and fill the hole, as well as help planarize itself. This is similar to reflow of dielectric materials which are heavily doped with B or P. With this technique, one could deposit the via (or contact) and interconnect levels in one step to obtain good filling of the contact and good step coverage and planarization of the interconnect level.

Just as contacts benefited from the use of multilayer structures, so have interconnects. This is due to a variety of reasons, most of them related to issues we have already discussed. First, electromigration has continued to be a problem that has hampered the reliability of silicon integrated circuits. While the addition of Cu to the Al has helped, it has not completely eliminated the problem. Other methods have been used to inhibit electromigration, or in some cases, negate its effect on the integrity of the interconnect lines. One method uses shunt lines. Another interconnect material is layered below, above, or within the Al layer, as shown in Figure 11–20. If electromigration does cause an opening in the Al line, the current can be shunted through the other material, maintaining the electrical integrity of that interconnect. The material does not have to have as low a resistivity as Al, since current will only flow through it for a short distance. But

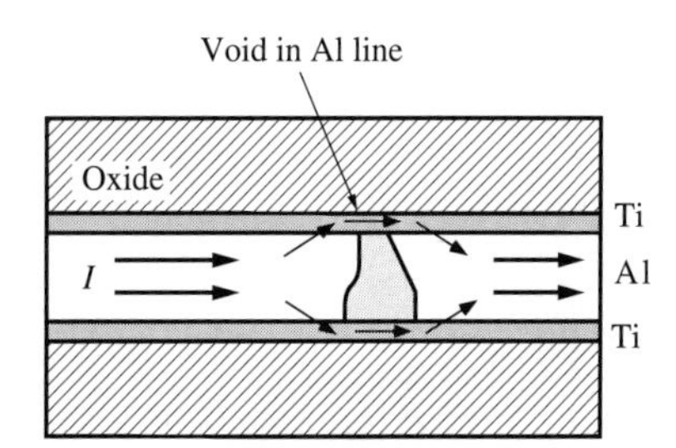

Figure 11–20 Illustration of shunt layers to minimize electromigration problems. Thin layers of metals, such as Ti, are used above and below the Al interconnect line. If a void should form, the current can be shunted around it and through these layers.

it should have good electromigration resistance, and good adhesion or barrier properties. Layers of Ti, Ti-W, TiN, or $TiSi_2$ can be used for this purpose.

These interlayers in interconnects help in electromigration protection for two other reasons. If they have high melting points and strong mechanical properties (see Table 11–4), they can be more rigid than the Al and act as physical or mechanical barriers to hillock and void formation. If Ti is used, it will actually react with Al to form $TiAl_3$, which is even harder mechanically than Ti, and will reduce the effects of electromigration. However, if too much $TiAl_3$ forms, it can increase the resistivity of the interconnect. If TiN is used, it is best to have excess Ti in it which will react with the Al to form $TiAl_3$. In addition, the electromigration of Al is very dependent on the grain texture of Al. The closer all the grains are to a single, usually (111), orientation in the vertical direction, the less electromigration occurs. The grain texture of the Al is very dependent on what underlayer it is deposited on. Al deposited on Ti exhibits much better grain texture (more grains closer to a single orientation) and electromigration behavior than on other films, such as Si, SiO_2, or TiN. If TiN is used between the Ti and Al, as a reaction barrier for example, the Al still has good grain texture. This is because the TiN takes on a pseudogranular structure, passing the Ti structure to the Al interface. Therefore, by using either Ti or Ti/TiN layers underneath the Al layers, electromigration is decreased due to grain texture considerations.

Interconnect and via structures made up of multilayers have been developed for barrier and adhesion reasons, just as with the contact structures. Ti can help with adhesion and electrical contact. TiN can serve not only as a good barrier, but as an adhesion layer as well, particularly in conjunction with W plugs. A TiN or Ti/TiN layer provides for good contact between Al and W and prevents any reaction between them. In addition, when CVD W is deposited in a via, a barrier layer must be used between the W and the underlying Al or else the fluorine in the WF_6 used in the CVD W deposition process will react with the exposed Al. (Similarly, in a contact a barrier is required to prevent the WF_6 from reacting with Ti or $TiSi_2$ layers or with Si.) Since the adhesion of W to dielectric layers is very poor, an adhesion layer is required and TiN (or Ti/TiN) is commonly used for this. A TiN layer can also be used in the interconnect stack to serve as a barrier between the Ti and the Al.

Another reason for using a multilayer interconnect structure is for lithographic purposes. The top Al surface is very reflective, and the reflection of light can adversely and unevenly affect the lithographic process. Therefore, an antireflective material is often deposited on top of the Al to minimize this. TiN again is usually used.

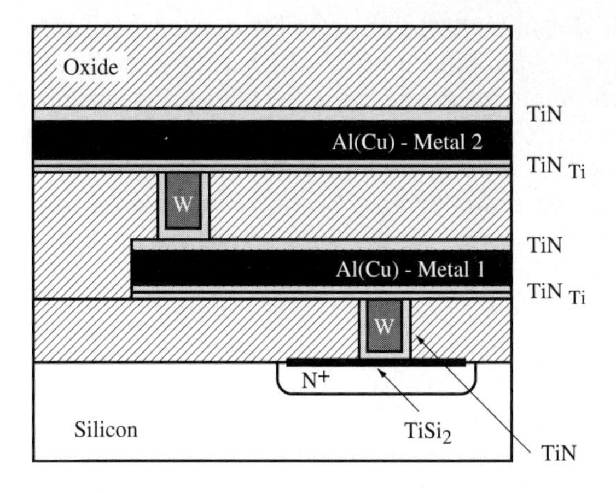

Figure 11–21 A typical metalization scheme used in current IC technology, showing the multilayer structures that have evolved.

For all these reasons, multilayer interconnect structures have been developed. One such structure is illustrated in Figure 11–21 and serves to summarize the issues we have discussed. A W plug is used in both the contact and the vias, resulting in good planarity. At the bottom of the contact, $TiSi_2$ is used to make good electrical contact to the Si, and also serves to strap the sources and drains, providing for lower sheet resistance along those paths. In both the contacts and the vias, TiN surrounds the W, promoting adhesion to the oxide. It also acts as a barrier to prevent attack of the underlying material by WF_6 during W deposition. The global interconnect structure, or "stack," in this example is Ti/TiN/Al(Cu)/TiN. Cu in the Al suppresses electromigration and hillock formation. Ti improves the grain texture of the Al for better electromigration protection and promotes adhesion. TiN is a barrier between the Al and Ti to limit $TiAl_3$ formation. The Ti/TiN and TiN layers on the bottom and top of each interconnect provide an electrical shunt in case of void formation in the Al. They also suppress hillock and void formation by providing mechanical barriers to plastic deformation. TiN on the top also acts as an antireflective layer for lithography. Many variations of this structure are used by different manufacturers, especially in the exact makeup and order of materials in the interconnect stack (the Ti or TiN is often omitted from the bottom of the stack, for example). But the basic idea of multilayer planar structures is very common.

11.2.3 Dielectrics

Dielectric layers are used to separate and electrically isolate conducting layers from each other. Two types of dielectric layers associated with metallization schemes were shown in Figure 11–1. The first-level dielectric is a deposited layer that separates the global (usually Al) interconnects from the diffused substrate areas, polysilicon, and local interconnects. The intermetal dielectrics (IMDs) are deposited dielectrics that separate the global interconnects. (The other common dielectric layers are the gate oxide and the field oxide, both of which are thermally grown and have been discussed in previous chapters.) Because the first-level dielectric is deposited before any Al is present, while the intermetal dielectrics are deposited after Al is present, they have different processing requirements and restrictions.

There are a number of general requirements for dielectric layers [11.18]. Good electrical isolation is paramount and includes properties such as a low dielectric constant so that interconnect capacitances are low; a high breakdown field strength (>5 MV/cm); and low leakage (bulk and surface resistivity should exceed 10^{15} Ω cm). In addition, dielectric layers should provide good adhesion to silicon, metals, and silicides; low intrinsic stress (50–100 MPa or less); thermal stability (up to 850–950°C for first-level dielectrics and up to 500°C for intermetal dielectrics); contain no moisture or metallic impurities (which can diffuse into the substrate and cause leakage current); low-defect density (pinholes and particulates); high-structural density (low porosity); contain no residual constituents that can outgas; and they should be permeable to hydrogen (so that passivation of the Si/SiO_2 interface states can take place). Table 11–6 lists several dielectric materials used or being considered for use in back-end structures.

Table 11–6 Materials used or considered for interlevel dielectrics (After [11.19])

Material class	Material	Dielectric constant	Deposition technique
Inorganic	SiO_2 (including PSG and BPSG)	3.9–5.0	CVD Thermal oxidation Bias-sputtering High-density plasma
	Spin-on-glass (SiO_2) (including PSG and BPSG)	3.9–5.0	SOD (spin-on-dielectric)
	Modified SiO_2 (e.g., fluorinated SiO_2 or hydrogen silsesquioxane—HSQ)	2.8–3.8	CVD/SOD
	BN (Si)	>2.9	CVD
	Si_3N_4 (only used in multilayer structure)	5.8–6.1	CVD
Organic	Polyimides	2.9–3.9	SOD/CVD
	Fluorinated polyimides	2.3–2.8	SOD/CVD
	Fluoro-polymers	1.8–2.2	SOD/CVD
	F-doped amorphous C	2.0–2.5	CVD
Inorganic/Organic Hybrids	Si-O-C hybrid polymers based on organosilsesquioxanes (e.g., MSQ)	2.0–3.8	SOD
Aerogels (Microporous)	Porous SiO_2 (with tiny free space regions)	1.2–1.8	SOD
Air bridge		1.0–1.2	

CVD silicon dioxide is the dominant dielectric material used in back-end structures. In the 1960s, it was found that if the CVD SiO_2 was doped with phosphorus, forming phosphosilicate glass, better properties for MOS technology were obtained (see Chapter 4, Section 4.2.3). Phosphosilicate glass (PSG) is made up of P_2O_5 and SiO_2. The phosphorus in the films allows the film to getter, or tie up, sodium ions, resulting in more stable MOS characteristics. It also reduces the built-in tensile stress often present in deposited SiO_2 films. In addition, the presence of phosphorus allows one to "reflow" the layer. By annealing the PSG in steam at a temperature from 950–1100°C, the dielectric layer flows in order to reduce surface energy, and any sharp corners are smoothed out. Undoped oxide does not flow nearly as much because of its higher viscosity. Reflowing also helps in filling spaces between closely spaced lines. Reflowing the dielectric results in better step coverage of subsequent layers and was one of the first planarization techniques. The amount of phosphorus incorporated in the films ranges from 4 to 8 wt. percent, with more phosphorus leading to more reflow. However, more phosphorus also enhances the film's absorption of water. Atmospheric moisture absorbed in the film can react with the phosphorus to form phosphoric acid, which can lead to corrosion of aluminum layers on top of and below the film. Absorbed water can also lower the dielectric constant of the film, and can outgas during heating, causing metal deposition problems. A sandwich structure is often used with layers of undoped SiO_2 below and above the PSG to help protect against these problems.

PSG has commonly been used as the first-level dielectric. Since Al is not present at this point in the processing, high-temperature densification and reflow can be used. If silicides are present, temperatures below 950°C are required for first dielectric-level processing since most silicides start to degrade at about 900°C. If boron is added to PSG, to form BPSG (borophosphosilicate glass), the reflow temperature is reduced to about 800°C. Reflowed BPSG is illustrated in Figure 11–22. BPSG, with 2–6 wt. percent boron and phosphorus, also traps sodium and reduces the stress in the film.

When two metal-level interconnect structures were first introduced, PSG or BPSG were initially used for the intermetal dielectric. But since the structures with Al layers could not be heated above 450°C, a reflow step could not be done, and these films had many problems. Because of the relatively high sticking coefficients (around 0.3 to 0.4) characteristic of silicon dioxide films formed by the oxidation of silane, conformal depositions were usually not achieved. This can lead to problems with step coverage and filling of spaces. These problems get worse as metal spacings shrink with each new

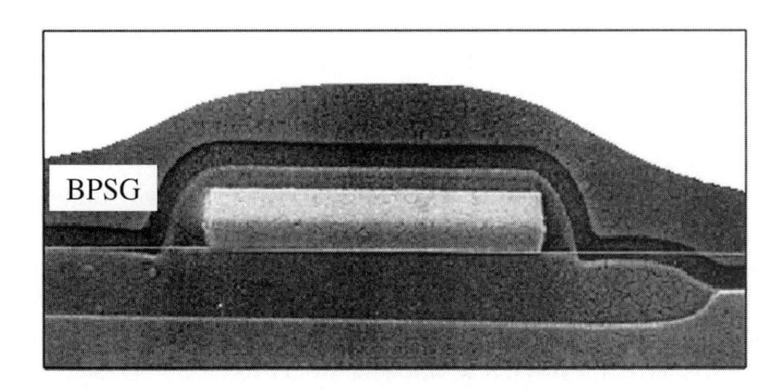

Figure 11–22 SEM image of BPSG oxide layer after 800°C reflow step, showing smooth topography over steps. Photo courtesy of VLSI Technology, Inc.

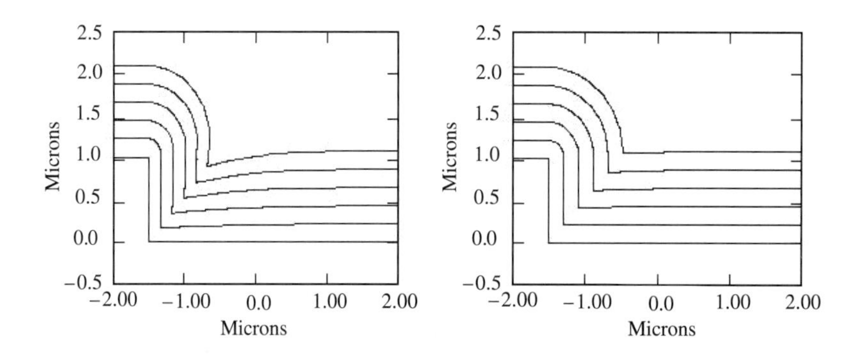

Figure 11–23 SPEEDIE simulations of silicon dioxide depositions over a step for silane deposition ($S_c = 0.4$) on left and TEOS deposition ($S_c = 0.1$) on right, showing less cusping in the latter case.

generation, especially if metal thicknesses do not shrink as fast. Without a reflow step to smooth out the films and fix the coverage and fill problems, failures in the interconnects can result. In addition, low-temperature SiO_2 films that are not annealed at higher temperatures are not as dense and not as good quality. Other deposition and processing techniques, as well as different materials, were needed for intermetal dielectrics.

Plasma-enhanced CVD techniques provide better oxide films for intermetal dielectrics. The energy from the plasma enhances the deposition reactions and provides for denser films and somewhat better coverage and filling at lower temperatures. Silicon dioxide films deposited by decomposing TEOS (tetraethooxysilane—$Si(OC_2H_5)_4$), rather than by reacting oxygen and silane, have also been developed. The reactant species in these depositions tend to have a low sticking coefficients, on the order of 0.1. This results in more conformal films than those produced from silane for both LPCVD and PECVD systems. Figure 11–23 shows SPEEDIE simulations of LPCVD silicon dioxide depositions over a step for silane deposition ($S_c = 0.4$) and TEOS deposition ($S_c = 0.1$). Less cusping occurs in the latter case, resulting in better conformality as well as filling ability. Even better conformality and filling ability at low temperatures is achieved by reacting the TEOS with ozone. Low-temperature deposition processes, using ozone or PECVD, allow the use of TEOS oxides as intermetal dielectrics. The non-plasma, TEOS/O_3 films are more porous than silane based or PECVD TEOS oxides and absorb more moisture. Often a thin layer of PECVD TEOS or silane oxide is used below and above TEOS/O_3 films. Bias-sputtering or a sequential deposition/etch/deposition process may also be used to help with filling. TEOS films are sometimes used in the first-level dielectric level as well. The TEOS films can be doped with P or B to help with Na gettering and reflow properties.

Planarization is important in multilevel back-end structures and can be divided into local planarization and global planarization. Local planarization occurs over submicron or micron (device) dimensions, while global planarization occurs over circuit or chip dimensions. Figure 11–24 illustrates this. Global planarization is usually desired, but local planarization is easier to achieve. An example of local planarization would be the reflow process, where the areas between closely spaced lines are filled in with the oxide during the reflow anneal, but larger spaces or areas outside are not.

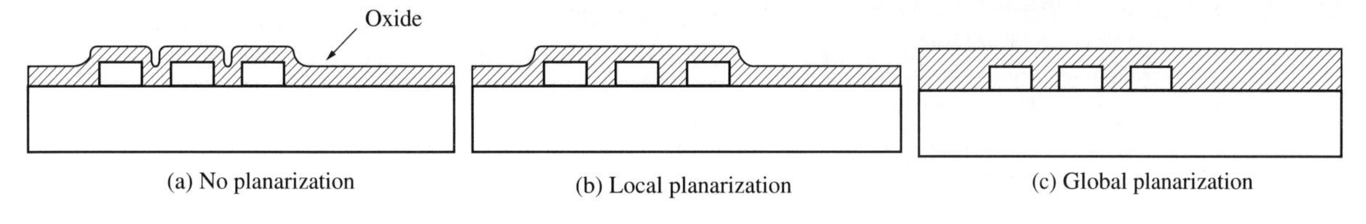

Figure 11–24 Schematic illustration of different types of planarization.

Example In Figure 11–24(b), approximately what degree of planarization has been achieved locally and what degree of planarization has been achieved globally?

Answer By Eq. (11.13), the degree of planarization is

$$\mathrm{DOP} = 1 - \frac{x^{f}_{\mathrm{step}}}{x^{i}_{\mathrm{step}}}$$

The initial step height is the height of the metal line and is some finite number. In regard to local planarization, the final step height corresponds to the step height in the region that was locally planarized, that is, the regions between or within the metal lines. The step height here is close to zero, so that the degree of planarization locally is close to 1. Globally, the final step height would correspond to the maximum step height on the surface. Here it would be close to the initial step height. Therefore, the degree of planarization globally is close to zero.

Another planarization method involves etchback. In this technique the dielectric is deposited, sometimes followed by the deposition of a sacrificial layer. The overall structure is then etched back to planarize it. The earliest such process used photoresist as a sacrificial etchback layer on top of oxide. The photoresist was deposited, or spun, over the oxide layer, filling up the spaces and ending up with a nearly flat top surface. After a hard-bake, an etch is done which etches both the oxide and photoresist, ideally at the same rate. When the bottom of the photoresist is reached, a nearly flat oxide is left behind. This is illustrated in Figure 11–25, and results in local planarization, but only limited global planarization. This can also be done without a sacrificial layer if the dielectric layer is deposited thick enough. This is because the thicker a material is, the smoother the local topography tends to become. Plasma etching, argon sputtering, or chemical-mechanical polishing can be used to etch back the dielectric layer, leaving a more planar topography.

An additional planarizing method is to use a Spin-On-Glass (SOG). This is similar to the photoresist etchback technique, but here the spun-on material is left behind and serves as an intermetal dielectric. SOG materials are initially liquids, containing organic siloxanes or inorganic silicates in an alcohol-based solvent. The liquid SOG is spun onto

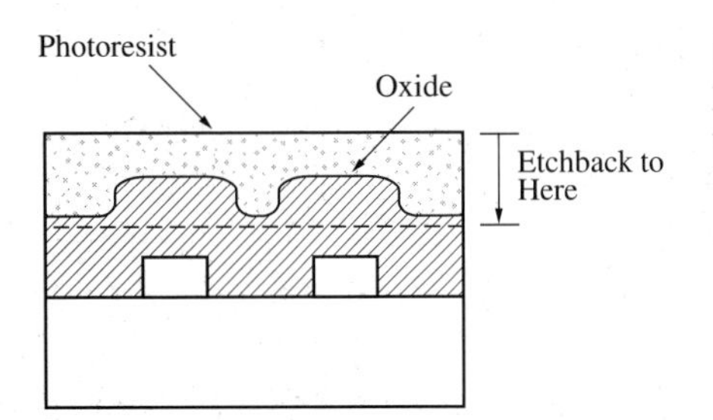

Figure 11–25 Illustration of photoresist etchback process. Photoresist is deposited over rough topography, then the structure is etched back, leaving a smooth top surface on the oxide.

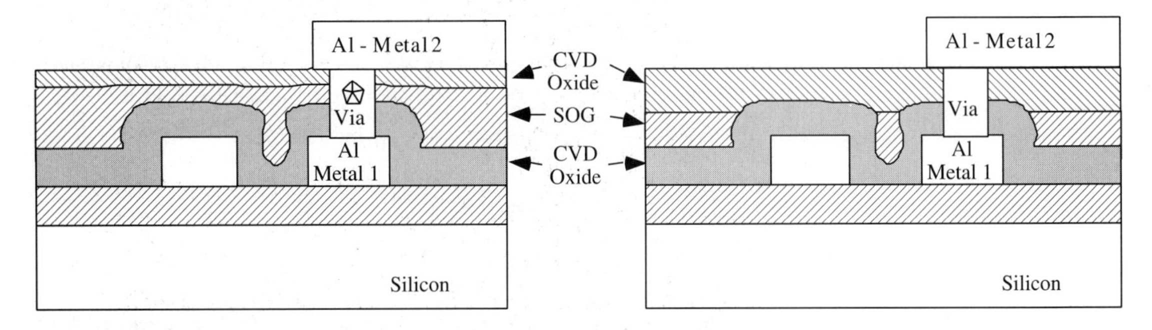

Figure 11–26 Back-end structure (left) without etchback step, showing poisoned via (star-shaped structure) where the via metal is in direct contact with Spin-On Glass (SOG) layer. The back-end structure on the right with an etchback step, does not have poisoned vias since the via metal is not in direct contact with the SOG layer.

the wafer like photoresist, filling the spaces between features. (It can also fill voids between lines as long as the voids are not completely closed off at the top.) Then the wafer is baked and cured, driving off the solvents and polymerizing the silicon-containing groups, resulting in the formation of Si-O-Si bonds. SOG is often sandwiched between layers of CVD SiO_2 in an intermetal dielectric structure, as shown in Figure 11–26. The SOG process is often combined with an etchback. After deposition and curing, the SOG is etchbacked so that no SOG remains over any metal region that will have a via made to it. This is so that when via holes are cut through the intermetal dielectric, they do not pass through any SOG, as also illustrated in Figure 11–26. If they did, residual gases and moisture from the SOG could contaminate the contacts or vias and cause large increases in contact or via resistance, so-called "poisoned vias." SOG films made from organic-based solutions, containing carbon, are more susceptible to this than those made from inorganic solutions. With SOG, local planarization and only very limited global planarization are achieved.

As alternatives to spin-on SiO_2 films, other Spin-On Dielectric materials (SODs) are being developed. These are either inorganic, organic polymer materials, or hybrid organic/inorganic materials (Si-O-C polymers). Table 11–6 lists some common materials. While providing good filling and local and some global planarization like SOG, they have the advantage of having lower dielectric constants than SiO_2. This means the intermetal capacitance is lower, and the *RC* delay of the interconnects is improved. The main problems with these low-*K* materials are thermal stability (i.e., they often decompose at moderate temperatures) and moisture absorption, both of which tend to degrade their electrical properties and adhesion. Sandwich layers with CVD SiO_2 are often used to mitigate these problems.

A more recently developed oxide deposition technique is called High-Density Plasma (HDP) deposition, and was described in Chapter 9. This high-density plasma results in a dense CVD oxide film at temperatures as low as room temperature. When a separate RF bias is applied on the substrate, the angular dependence of the sputtering yield of the ions is exploited, as in bias-sputtered deposition, resulting in more planar and void-free films. HDP oxides can be doped with phosphorus and boron when used as a first level dielectric, although boron is not usually used since reasonably planar and conformal films are obtained without the need of a high-temperature reflow step. Fluorinated oxides for low-dielectric constant material can also be deposited by HDP. While HDP deposition can planarize any topography if enough film is deposited, it is usually used in conjunction with other planarizing techniques and is mainly utilized for its excellent hole or gap filling ability.

A planarization technique that has recently become part of mainstream processing is Chemical-Mechanical Polishing, or CMP. With this technique, global or near-global planarization can be achieved. As its name implies, CMP is a combination of chemical and mechanical polishing or etching. Wafers are held face down against a spinning polishing pad (made of a roughened polyurethane plate), and a colloidal silica slurry is kept between the pad and the wafer. The chemical composition and pH of the slurry are important and depend on the material being polished. For planarizing an oxide layer, a high-pH alkali-based solution is often used, while a low-pH, oxidizer-based solution is commonly used for metals. In general the chemical reaction at the wafer surface makes the surface material susceptible to mechanical abrasion by the silica in the slurry. For silicon dioxide removal, it is believed that the potassium hydroxide in the slurry reacts with the oxide to form a hydrated silicate layer, which is then removed mechanically by abrasion. For metal removal, the solution oxidizes the surface which is then polished in a similar fashion to the oxide removal.

Figure 11–27 shows a cross section of the CMP pad in contact with the top of a wafer. A semirigid polishing pad is used to allow for any bowing or thickness nonuniformities

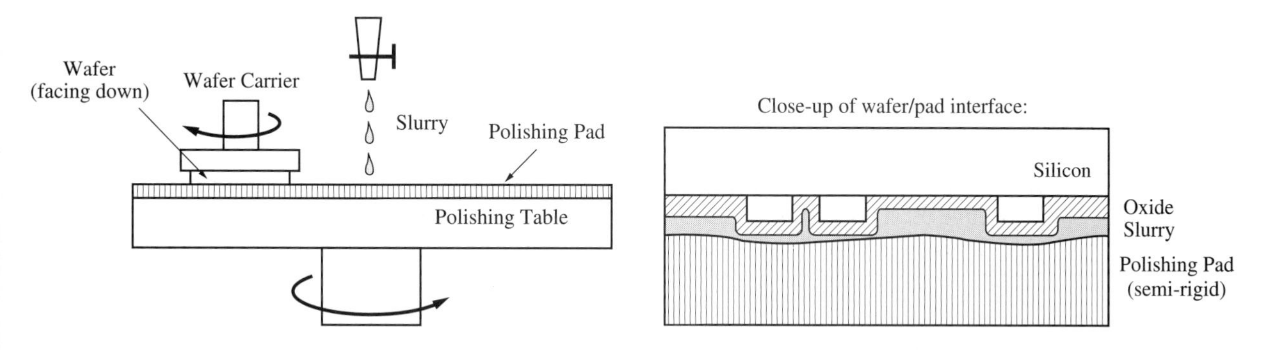

Figure 11–27 Illustration of Chemical-Mechanical Polishing (CMP) system. The right hand figure shows a close-up of wafer/pad interface.

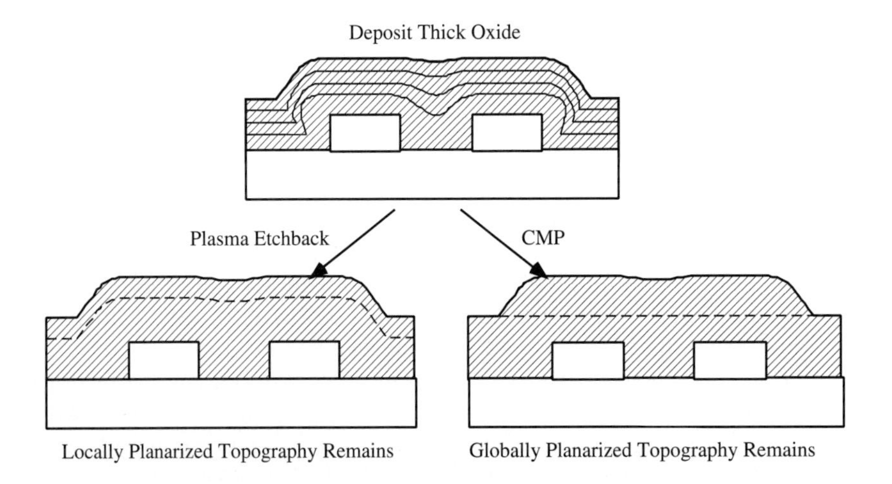

Figure 11–28 Illustrating the differences between using plasma etchback and chemical-mechanical polishing to planarize the dielectric.

in the silicon substrate. These would cause uneven etching if a perfectly rigid pad were used. The CMP process removes elevated features without much thinning of lower areas, thus planarizing the topography. CMP is used commonly for dielectric planarization, and is also being used for the W damascene process for the etchback of W (recall Figure 11–19). While standard plasma etchback processes achieve local planarization, global planarization is obtainable with CMP. Figure 11–28 illustrates this.

It should be pointed out that with all this effort at planarization, there is a drawback, other than just complicating the process. Without planarization, each layer is approximately uniform in thickness. The topography may go up and down, due to the presence or absence locally of features below it, but the vertical thickness of the layer is fairly constant (except just at the edges of features, of course). Therefore a process like etching holes in the layer is relatively straightforward since the depth one has to etch is constant from one area to the next. However, with planarization, local thicknesses of layers can vary significantly. As a result, one must etch different amounts in different locations to get to the level below. Fortunately this problem with planarization usually only occurs for the contact level. After the first dielectric level is planarized, the vias between consecutive interconnects in the upper planarized levels will have the same heights, as shown in Figure 11–1.

As with the contacts, vias, and interconnects, dielectrics have evolved from simple layers into more complex multilayered structures as the processing and circuit demands have increased. Low-temperature processing and planarization have been the two main driving forces in their evolution. Countless numbers of different structures and

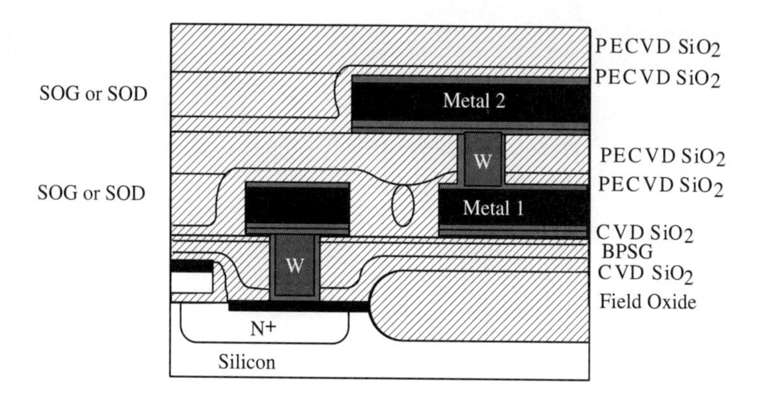

Figure 11–29 Schematic diagram of a back-end structure showing one possible dielectric multistructure scheme. Planarized topography is achieved. Other variations include HDP oxide or the use of CMP, either of which could reduce the number of sublayers—but the general structure would remain the same.

planarization schemes have been developed. Shown in Figure 11–29 is one possible, rather generalized, structure. It utilizes BPSG for the first-level dielectric, a W plug etchback, a Spin-On-Glass (SOG) or Spin-On-Dielectric (SOD) for the intermetal dielectric, and multilayer dielectric structures. The oxide layers could be either silane or TEOS based, using PECVD, bias sputtering, or HDP, and with or without an etchback or CMP. If an HDP oxide is used instead of BPSG or SOG/SOD, a moisture barrier below or above it may not be necessary. The intermetal dielectrics must be deposited and processed at temperatures less than 450°C, while the first-level dielectrics can often be done at temperatures up to 900°C or so.

Figure 11–30 shows SEM images of two current back-end structures. The first with three metal levels and 0.35-μm technology uses SOG and CMP, while the second one, a more advanced technology with five metal levels and 0.25-μm technology, uses HDP oxide and CMP.

11.3 Manufacturing Methods and Equipment

There are countless different structures and fabrication strategies for practical back-end structures, and we cannot hope to cover them all here. However, we will go through some representative processing steps and procedures used to fabricate CMOS integrated circuits. This discussion will provide some of the details that were left out in the CMOS process in Chapter 2. We will refer to that process throughout this section.

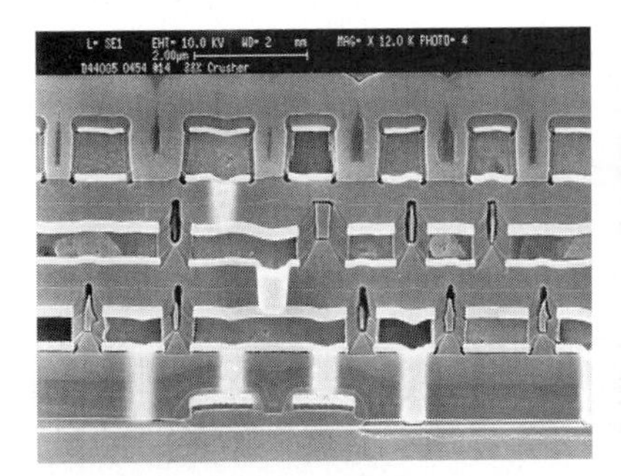

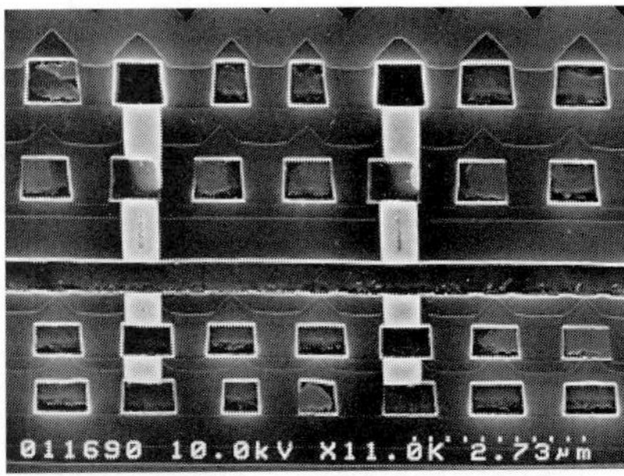

Figure 11–30 Two current back-end structures from VLSI Technology, Inc. The one on the left has three metal levels and uses encapsulated BPSG for the first-level dielectric, and SOG (encapsulated top and bottom with PECVD oxide) and CMP in the intermetal dielectrics. The multilayer metal layers and W plugs are also clearly seen. The SOG regions were deformed during SEM cleaving and erroneously look voidlike. The structure on the right, with five metal levels, uses HDP oxide (with PECVD oxide cap) and CMP in the intermetal dielectrics. Photos courtesy of VLSI Technology, Inc.

11.3.1 Silicided Gates and Source/Drain Regions

We start with a circuit that has been fabricated up to the gate and source/drain formation, with the source/drain N+ and P+ implants and anneals just finished (Figure 2–33 in Chapter 2). The next step is to silicide the source/drain regions and the polysilicon gate electrode to reduce their sheet resistances. $TiSi_2$, a common silicide for this process will be used here. Figures 2–34 to 2–37 show the process, and Figure 11–31 shows the silicide formation step.

After the SiO_2 is removed from the device source, drain, and gate regions, 50–100 nm of Ti is deposited by sputtering over the whole wafer. This is followed by a two-step anneal. The first anneal is at a low temperature, about 600 – 700°C for a time of 15–60 seconds. A low temperature is used to limit excess lateral growth and to minimize the reaction of the Ti with the SiO_2. Lateral growth refers to the $TiSi_2$ forming laterally out from the silicon contact regions, which could lead, for example, to shorting the gate to the source and drain. The anneal is done in a nitrogen ambient to further limit lateral growth. Where Si is exposed, the Si reacts with the Ti to form $TiSi_2$ at the bottom and N_2 reacts with the Ti to form TiN at the top. Over the SiO_2, TiN forms. This inhibits the formation of $TiSi_2$ over the oxide between the gate and source/drain regions. In addition, nitrogen is believed to stuff the grain boundaries of any unreacted Ti which slows down Si diffusion and helps in retarding lateral growth. The TiN, and any unreacted Ti, can then be selectively etched off using a solution of NH_4OH:H_2O_2:H_2O (1:1:5).

A second anneal is then required to lower the resistivity of the silicide. This is because below about 750°C, a metastable phase of $TiSi_2$ forms, called the "C49" phase, which has a higher resistivity (60–70 μΩ-cm). An 800°C anneal for 30–60 seconds is required to transform it to the equilibrium, "C54," phase, with its lower resistivity of 13–20 μΩ-cm. Going to a higher temperature and longer annealing times for either anneal leads to problems. As mentioned above, a longer time in the first anneal leads to lateral encroachment and reaction with the oxide. For the second anneal, higher temperatures

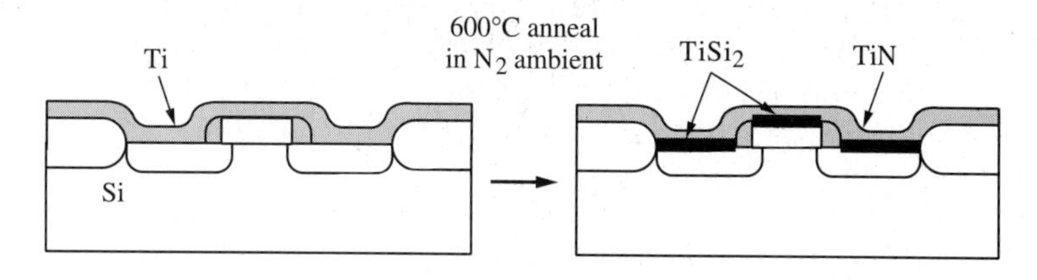

Figure 11–31 Formation of self-aligned $TiSi_2$ regions for gate, source, and drain. TiN also forms. After the formation anneal, the TiN may removed, and a second 800°C anneal is used to decrease the film resistivity.

and longer times lead to the silicide surface roughening up, or "agglomerating." A second problem is that dopants in the contacted Si substrate can diffuse up into the $TiSi_2$ because of their high diffusivities and solubilities in the polycrystalline silicide. So anneals at minimum temperatures and times required to form and transform the silicide are used. This means seconds to minutes for anneal times, necessitating the use of RTA equipment for both anneals.

One option during this process is to mask off some of the TiN area before the selective wet etch and plasma etch, leaving some TiN behind as a local interconnect. This was done in the CMOS process flow in Chapter 2 (Figure 2–37). The second, high-temperature anneal not only reduces the $TiSi_2$ resistance, but also the TiN sheet resistance. The TiN can also be left in the source/drain or gate areas to act as an Al/Si barrier layer for subsequent Al deposition on top. However if a TiN local interconnect, which requires an additional masking step, is not used, the TiN is etched away everywhere. New TiN would then be deposited later over the $TiSi_2$ in the contacts just before the contact metal (W, for example) is deposited.

The thickness of the $TiSi_2$ is dependent on how much Ti is deposited and the time and temperature of the anneals. For a 100-nm layer of Ti, and reaction of all 100 nm of the Ti with the underlying Si, 227 nm of the Si will be consumed, and 250 nm of $TiSi_2$ will be formed (the reaction ratios for $TiSi_2$ and other silicides are given in Table 11–4). This would give a film sheet resistance of approximately $15 \times 10^{-6}\ \Omega\ \text{cm} / 2500 \times 10^{-8}\ \text{cm} = 0.6\ \Omega/\text{square}$. But less silicide is produced if the first anneal is done in N_2, since the top part of the Ti reacts with the nitrogen to form TiN instead of the silicide. The actual silicide thickness in this case depends on the relative kinetics of the silicide and nitride formation reactions and will depend on anneal time and temperature. Typical final thicknesses for 100 nm of deposited Ti are about 150 nm of $TiSi_2$ and 75 nm of TiN on top, giving a silicide sheet resistance of about 1.2 Ω/square. The amount of Si consumed would be about 140 nm in this case. The TiN formed on top of SiO_2 and left as a local interconnect would be about 100 nm thick and have a final sheet resistance of about 10 Ω/square. As the diffused junction depth beneath the silicide decreases as the technology progresses, the silicide must also decrease in thickness so that the amount of Si consumed is not greater than the junction depth. In fact, it is typically desirable to leave about 50 nm between the bottom of the silicide and the junction, or else leakage current through the junction may become too large.

While Ti will reduce and break through any thin native oxide on the silicon or polysilicon surfaces, it is still important to clean the wafer surface before the Ti deposition. Polymers, usually C-F compounds, left over from previous dry etching must be removed. In addition, if the native SiO_2 is too thick (greater than about 2 nm), rough $TiSi_2$ surfaces can result. This is similar to the process that occurs in Al spiking into Si. In this case, the Ti will reduce the oxide at weak points first. The Si diffuses through these points and moves rapidly into the adjoining regions before the oxide in other areas is reduced. This leads to faster Si consumption in some areas, and slower consumption in others, resulting in a rough Si/$TiSi_2$ interface and a rough $TiSi_2$ surface. Only if the native oxide is thin will uniform reaction occur, giving smooth silicide films. To minimize the native oxide thickness, a wet HF clean is done immediately prior to loading the wafers into the sputtering equipment. In addition, an RF plasma sputter clean in the sputtering chamber can remove the native oxide and any polymer films. However, too harsh a sputter clean can damage the Si surface. It is also important to minimize any oxygen or water on the wafer surface or in the sputtering chamber since the Ti will react with these species and incorporate oxygen into the silicide film, increasing its resistivity. Minimizing oxygen in the RTA chamber is also important.

11.3.2 First-level Dielectric Processing

After silicide formation, the first-level dielectric layer is deposited. This corresponds to Figure 2–38 in Chapter 2. This physically and electrically separates the local interconnects from the global interconnects, the latter being Al-based metals. Since the topography is usually nonplanar at this stage, and there are many layers that follow which can suffer as a result, it is especially important to planarize the structure here.

The first-level dielectric is usually SiO_2, doped with P and B at 2–6 wt. percent, at a thickness of about 500 nm. This BPSG (borophosphosilicate glass) can be deposited by CVD using the silane reaction [Eq. (9.32)] or the TEOS reaction [Eq. (9.33)], as discussed in Chapter 9. Doping can be done using hydrides for the silane case and organometallic compounds for the TEOS case. The silane deposition can be done using either APCVD or LPCVD at temperatures from 380–500°C, or using PECVD at lower temperatures. The TEOS deposition can be done at 650–800°C, but this temperature can lowered to 400°C or less by using either PECVD or an ozone-enhanced reaction [Eq. (9.34)].

The TEOS films give more conformal coverage than the silane films. As mentioned earlier the TEOS/O_3 films, which can be very conformal, can be quite porous and absorb moisture. Absorbed water can have an adverse affect on electrical behavior and reliablity, as well as subsequent processing. Thin underlayers, and sometimes overlayers, of undoped CVD SiO_2 using silane or PECVD films using TEOS are often used as moisture barriers for TEOS/O_3 films, or as dopant buffer layers for either silane or TEOS films.

To obtain a smoother and more planar topography, a thermal reflow anneal is done after the PSG or BPSG deposition at 800–1000°C. (The lower temperature is appropriate for BPSG films; the higher temperatures are used for PSG films.) The reflow is often done in a steam environment. Doing so lowers the reflow temperature by about

70°C. It also leaches the dopants from the surface to avoid corrosion problems with the overlying Al, but this is not as important when buffer or sandwich layers of undoped SiO_2 are used.

The as-deposited PSG or BPSG is amorphous and not as dense as thermally grown oxide. A dense film is needed to improve both electrical and physical properties, so a densification anneal is done. This is usually done at temperatures from 600–1000°C, before the reflow anneal, but it can be done simultaneously with the reflow. The thickness of the film decreases as the arrangement of the SiO_4 tetrahedra becomes more regular.

Reflowing the PSG or BPSG is also often done after the contact holes are etched to round off the contact hole corners, resulting in better filling of the holes with the contact metal. This is done in an inert atmosphere so that the bottom of the contact is not oxidized and is done in a separate step from the steam reflow used to planarize the surface.

As an alternative to reflow, or in addition to it, an etchback step is sometimes done after first-level dielectric deposition. This can done either by resist etchback, direct etchback of the dielectric, or with Chemical-Mechanical Polishing (CMP). This was the process illustrated in Figure 11–28 and Figure 2–39 in Chapter 2. The latter provides more global planarization. If an etchback is done instead of a reflow, the film does not need to be doped with boron, but a phosphorus doped layer should be present somewhere in this level for Na gettering.

The recently developed method of High-Density Plasma (HDP) deposition of oxide is being more commonly used for the first-level dielectric as well as intermetal dielectric levels (see Figure 11–30). Silane is preferred since one can achieve planar and void-free films without having to use TEOS, with its inherent disadvantages over silane (carbon residue in films and a more difficult source to use, for example). Since the film is dense and a better moisture barrier than some TEOS-based CVD oxide films and spin-on-dielectrics, it might not need an additional dielectric layer deposited under it as the other planarizing films do. If HDP oxide is used, boron is not needed. Because of the sputtering of the wafer and the high-plasma density, heating of the wafer can occur, and cooling of the substrate via a thermal chuck must be used to cool the wafer and control the temperature. Often CMP is used in conjunction with HDP oxide deposition to achieve global planarization.

11.3.3 Contact Formation

The next step is to open up holes in the first-level dielectric level and form metal contacts to the silicided gate, drain, and source regions, as well as to any local interconnects. This step corresponds to Figure 2–40 in the CMOS process flow in Chapter 2. Anisotropic plasma etching, using CHF_3 for example, is commonly used to open up these areas. It is important to make sure that all of the dielectric material is removed with the etch so that a low-resistivity contact is made. In addition, any residues from the etching process must be removed. These include both organic residues, such as C-F containing polymers from the etch chemistry and photoresist, as well as inorganic residues, such as SiO_2 that have been resputtered from the sidewalls of the contact hole. Usually a cleanup process following the etch and photoresist strip is done which includes both a wet chemical resist clean and an O_2 plasma etch or "ash."

The contact etch is complicated by the differences in dielectric thickness from position to position, as illustrated in Figure 11–1. Because of the planarization techniques used, the thickness of dielectric layer that must be etched through to reach gates, source/drains, or local interconnects can vary by as much as a factor of two. All contact holes must all be etched simultaneously, requiring very selective etching, or else expensive additional mask levels must be used.

Before the contact metal is deposited, the contact/adhesion/barrier structure is formed (see Figure 2–41 in Chapter 2). If the gate and source/drain regions are already silicided, then that layer can act as the contact/adhesion layer. If not, then Ti can be deposited at this point by sputtering. (In many cases, Ti is deposited here in any case to reduce any oxide as well as help with adhesion.) The Ti can then be annealed to form $TiSi_2$ or it may form during a later heat step. An argon *in situ* sputter etch is often done just prior to Ti deposition to clean the surface. This etch must not cause too much damage, so a "soft etch" is done, with a DC bias of only 100–300 V. Usually a few tens of nanometers of Ti are deposited. It is important that the Ti cover the entire bottom of the contact hole, which is not an easy task for today's narrow but deep contact holes. Collimated or ionized sputtering may be used for this purpose.

Next several tens of nanometers of TiN is deposited. For Al contacts this serves as a barrier layer. For W contacts it serves as an adhesion layer between the W and the dielectric as well as a barrier to prevent WF_6 from reacting with the underlying Ti or $TiSi_2$ during the W deposition process. This TiN deposition can be done by sputtering (including ionized PVD), or by CVD. The TiN is needed on the bottom of the contact holes (to act as a barrier), and also on the sides of the contact hole and the top of the dielectric layer to help with W adhesion. CVD deposition usually provides better coverage or filling on the contact bottom and sidewalls than sputtering. After the TiN is deposited, it can be annealed in N_2 or O_2 at 400–500°C for 30 minutes to improve its barrier properties. The N_2 and O_2 stuff the grain boundaries, limiting diffusion by providing a physical barrier in the fast diffusion paths. There can also be a chemical effect, in which the oxygen bonds with any Al diffusing through the TiN, for example.

If a W plug is used as the contact metal, the W is now deposited. As discussed in Chapter 9, W can be deposited either by selective or blanket deposition. The selective process is very difficult to control, and so blanket W is more commonly utilized. This is the process illustrated in Figure 2–41 in Chapter 2. A one-step process, using either the hydrogen reduction reaction [Eq. (9.35)] or the silane reduction reaction [Eq. (9.36)], deposits W in the contact hole as well as on top of the dielectric. A two-step deposition process, rather than a one-step process, is commonly used. A silane reduction reaction is used to deposit the first few tens of nanometers of W and results in a film with good adhesion but with poor step coverage. Next, the hydrogen reduction reaction is used which is slower but has much better step coverage and also leads to less void formation. The disadvantage to the blanket W deposition method is that it deposits W everywhere, including on top of the first-level dielectric oxide where it is not wanted. However, the contact hole can be filled with a W plug by doing a thick blanket deposition and then doing an etchback in the damascene process. This process was illustrated in Figure 11–19 and is also the process illustrated in Figure 2–42 in Chapter 2. The etchback can be

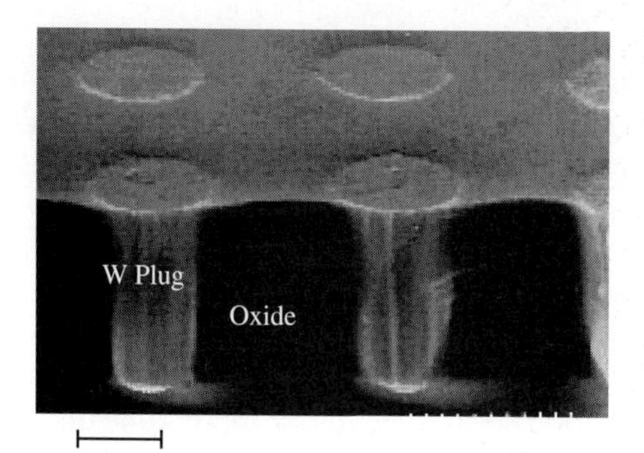

Figure 11–32 SEM image of W plugs after blanket CVD deposition and CMP. Photo courtesy of VLSI Technology, Inc.

done either by dry etching or CMP, although the latter is much more commonly used today. Figure 11–32 shows a SEM image of an array of W via plugs fabricated by blanket W deposition followed by CMP in this case. One can see that very planar topography is achieved.

W contact and via plugs are currently preferred over Al plugs because of more conformal filling by W and several years of experience with this process. There is an effort to develop manufacturable processes using Al with good filling properties, in which case Al could replace W in this step. The Al would be blanket deposited, perhaps with a reflow process during or after the deposition to ensure complete filling. This would be followed by an etchback step, dry etching or CMP, just like the W damascene process. An even more attractive alternative is to deposit the Al for contacts or vias and the interconnect in one step. Methods to do this are discussed in the next two sections.

11.3.4 Global Interconnects

The global interconnects are next deposited. This corresponds to Figure 2–43 in the CMOS process flow in Chapter 2. These are usually made of Al with 0.5–1 wt. percent Cu. Si is still often added, about 1 wt. percent, even though spiking of the Al through the substrate is not a problem if barrier layers are used. (Si may suppress reaction of the Al with Ti containing layers.) The Al layers are usually clad with thin Ti or TiN layers. Typical thicknesses for a Ti/TiN/Al/TiN (bottom to top) structure would be 40 nm/50 nm/500 nm/50 nm. Before deposition, the surface area of the wafer, especially the exposed contact regions, must be clean to ensure good electrical contact between the interconnect and the contact metal. To do this, wet and plasma cleans similar to those for contact deposition are done. Since many low-temperature oxides evolve some amount of water, it is often necessary to outgas the wafers in the sputtering chamber prior to metal deposition. The interconnect stack is then deposited, usually by sputtering. To minimize interface contamination the depositions are done one layer right after the other without opening the chamber.

As mentioned in Chapter 9, the microstructure of the deposited films are very dependent on the deposition conditions. In the case of sputter deposition, the grain size of the films will be dependent on the substrate temperature, the sputtering conditions (power, pressure, etc.), the vacuum integrity, the surface topography, and the underlying layers. The grain size of deposited Al ranges from 0.5 μm to about 2 μm. During any subsequent annealing, such as during the alloy anneal, the grains can grow (actually the large grains will grow at the expense of the smaller ones). They will grow until they reach a diameter equal to about two to three times the film thickness, so the average grain size of Al interconnects will be about 1 to 2 μm after annealing. The grain structure of deposited Al is normally columnar, with most of the grains spanning the entire thickness of the film with the <111> crystallographic direction oriented upward. The film's texture (crystallographic orientation) also depends on these same deposition conditions. Both grain size and texture influence many other properties of the films, including mechanical, electrical, and reliability properties.

To achieve both filling of deep holes as well as providing good step coverage and better planarization for the interconnect level, one could heat the aluminum, either during the deposition itself or right afterwards. The first method is called "hot aluminum deposition," using the high-temperature, or "hot-," sputter deposition technique. The substrate holder in the sputtering chamber is heated to 450–550°C during the deposition. In the second method, the wafer is heated to this temperature range immediately after the Al deposition, right in the sputtering chamber, and before any capping layer is deposited. In either case, the Al reflows, providing better filling of contact holds and smoother topography. Hot-sputtered Al deposition or deposition followed by reflow can also be used in an Al dual-damascene process where the contact and interconnect levels are again deposited in one step. These hot Al methods are still being developed.

Because reflow is a surface and interface controlled process, it is very dependent on ambient and interface conditions. For example, any oxygen in the chamber will form a thin Al oxide on the surface and inhibit reflow. When using hot Al deposition or doing an Al reflow, it is especially important to have a good barrier and adhesion layer between the Al and underlying layers. Thin Ti/TiN layers are usually used for this. Often a "cold/hot" Al deposition is done for this process. Right after the barrier/adhesion layer is deposited a thin Al layer is deposited at room temperature, often using collimated PVD. This acts as a continous "seed" or nucleation layer. CVD Al may also be used for this. Next the bulk of the Al is deposited by PVD at a higher temperature (400–500°C) for *in situ* reflow, with good adhesion and conformal filling in the contact hole, as well as good planarization and step coverage elsewhere. Topography simulations of reflow used during deposition were shown in Chapter 9 (Figure 9–52). CMP of the Al may still be done after the deposition/reflow but it is much easier and more efficient when the metal is already planarized to a degree.

To pattern the Al-based interconnect structures, a chlorine-containing plasma etch is used, usually in an RIE mode. Because chlorine and water or moisture in the air can corrode the Al, the wafers are passivated immediately after the chlorine etch and before they are removed from the etch chamber and subjected to the atmosphere. The Al surface is passivated by subjecting the wafers to a fluorine-containing plasma, such as CF_4, which replaces the residual Cl on the Al surface with F.

An alternative to etching the global interconnect is to use the dual damascene method to pattern the interconnect, which will be discussed in the next section.

11.3.5 IMD Deposition and Planarization

The intermetal dielectric (IMD) levels are deposited between the global interconnect levels, and some sort of planarization technique is usually used (see Figure 11–1). Currently most intermetal dielectric materials are SiO_2 based, often with multilayers utilizing different deposition techniques to obtain SiO_2 films with different properties. The total thickness of the level is around 0.5 to 1 μm. The SiO_2 films can be deposited at low temperatures (≤400°C) by CVD (including PECVD, LPCVD, HDPCVD, and AP/SACVD) using silane or TEOS, or can be spun on using spin-on-glass. The CVD methods were discussed earlier in Chapter 9.

Spin-on-glass (SOG) provides a way to fill spaces between features with a dielectric and to achieve local planarization. The starting material can contain either inorganic silicates or organic siloxanes. These are dissolved in an alcohol-based solvent, such as ethanol. The liquid is spun on the wafer like photoresist, with the thickness dependent on the spin speed: Faster spinning gives thinner layers. The wafer is then baked and cured, usually in a two-step process. The first anneal is at 150–250°C and the second anneal is at 350–450°C. The solvent is first driven off. Then the film condenses and polymerizes, forming Si-O-Si bonds to produce the SiO_2 layer. Water is produced by the polymerization reaction and must be driven off. Considerable shrinking of the film occurs during these processes, and high-tensile stress can result which can cause cracking of the film. The two types of SOG starting materials lead to different film properties. Some carbon is retained in the films made from siloxane materials and decreases the Si-O-Si polymerization. This decreases the film shrinkage and stress and increases the cracking resistance, but makes the film more porous and more susceptible to chemical attack. With either type of SOG, the final film quality is not as good as CVD SiO_2 due to its porosity, stress, and residual moisture content, and sandwich layers of CVD SiO_2 are usually used in conjunction with these films. The SOG films can be etched back, as was illustrated in Figure 11–26(b), to provide further planarization and to avoid poisoned vias. This is usually done with the organic, siloxane-based films since they are more prone to this problem.

Spin-on-dielectrics (SOD) other than SiO_2 are starting to be used. They not only provide planarization but also lower dielectric constants which reduce interconnect capacitances. Their processing is similar to that of SOG. Other low-K dielectrics, such as fluorinated SiO_2, are deposited by CVD. Some low-K dielectrics can be deposited by either spin-on techniques or CVD.

High-density plasma CVD oxides have gained popularity for this level as well as for the first-level dielectric. As with its use in that application, an additional dielectric layer deposited under it may not be needed, and CMP is still usually done in conjunction with HDP oxide deposition to achieve global planarization.

Other planarization techniques used on the intermetal dielectric level include etchback, Chemical-Mechanical Polishing (CMP), and the dual damascene process. In both the etchback and CMP cases, thick dielectric or photoresist layers are deposited which become more planar locally as the thickness increases. In the case of etchback, the film is then etched uniformly in thickness in a plasma etch system, resulting in a locally planar structure. With CMP, the structure is etched more or less uniformly in space across a horizontal plane, resulting in global planarization, as was illustrated in Figure 11–28.

Even better results can be obtained if "dummy" oxide or metal features are included in less dense areas to make the process more uniform across the entire circuit. Mechanical damage from the polishing as well as chemical and particle contamination from the slurry are concerns. But fairly successful procedures to minimize surface damage and to clean up the chemical residue have been developed. Endpoint detection can be difficult. Some systems detect the change in friction between the wafer and polishing pad when one layer is polished away and the layer below is contacted. Other methods include timed polishing or newly developed *in situ* film thickness measurement techniques. One such method is an *in situ* optical system which uses a window in the polishing pad and measures the interference patterns of reflected light [11.20]. CMP is now the dominant planarization technique in IC fabrication.

We saw earlier how the damascene process can be used for the contact level in which W is used to fill the contact hole. The damascene process could also be used for the interconnect level. In this process the interconnect metal, Al for example, is deposited at high temperature or by collimated or ionized sputtering (all to enhance filling) into interconnect openings in an intermetal dielectric level, then etched back or polished using CMP. This process is especially applicable for copper interconnects, which are beginning to replace Al in some cases. Cu is difficult to etch, and in the damascene process when CMP is used, etching of the metal is not required. In addition good filling of Cu in holes in trenches can be achieved using well-established Cu electroplating techniques.

A more advanced version of the damascene process provides both the via/contact and interconnect levels simultaneously. In this "dual damascene" process, both the openings in the IMD for the metal interconnect and for the contact or vias underneath are opened, one after the other. The metal is then deposited into both layers at once which is then followed by a CMP etchback. The dual damascene process is illustrated in Figure 11–33. An "etchstop" layer, such as a thin Si_3N_4 film, is usually deposited halfway through the thick intermetal dielectric (IMD) layer. When the etching is done for the interconnect trench in the top half of the IMD layer, the etching can easily be stopped when the nitride layer is reached, either due to the etch selectivity or by endpoint detection techniques, or both. This ensures that the interconnect trench is only etched halfway through the IMD.

11.3.6 Via Formation

Via formation is done the same way as the contact, as described above, with TiN used as an adhesion/barrier layer, followed by a W plug using the damascene/etchback method. Ti can be deposited under the TiN to help with adhesion and contact. However, if WF_6 from the W deposition process gets through the TiN, a volatile reaction can occur between it and the Ti. Al could be used as the via metal instead of W, just as was the case for the contacts. This requires good filling ability of the Al, which can be enhanced by using collimated or ionized deposition, hot Al deposition, or Al reflow, as discussed previously.

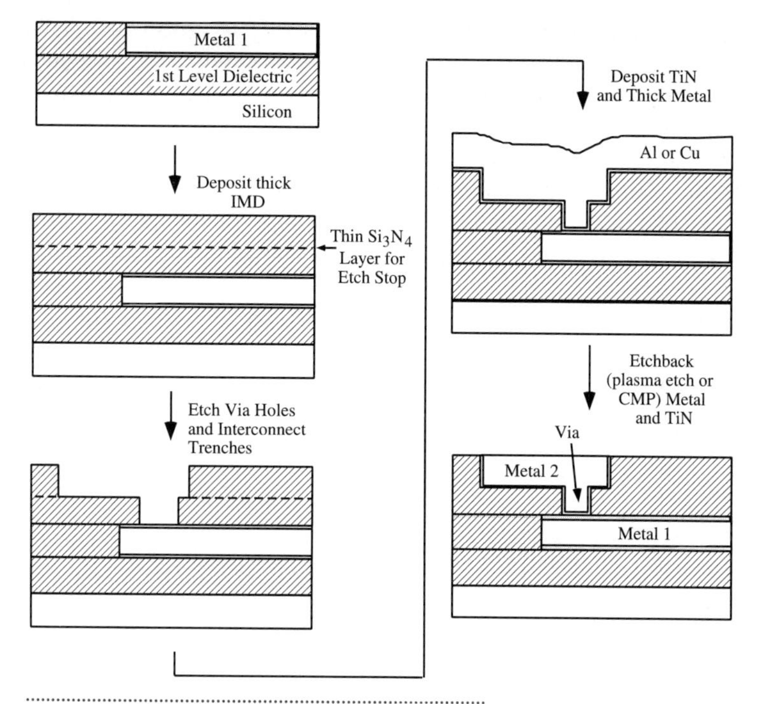

Figure 11–33 Schematic illustration of the dual damascene process.

11.3.7 Final Steps

It is now just a matter of repeating the global interconnect, intermetal dielectric, and via formation steps until the required number of metal layers are fabricated. Generally, the only difference is that as the upper levels of metals are added, the thickness and width of the metal lines often increase. More current can then be carried by the upper levels, with less probability of electromigration. Before bonding and packaging, a final passivation level is added. This would typically be a phosphorus-doped silicon dioxide layer, 500 nm thick, and a 1-μm thick silicon nitride layer. Both are deposited by PECVD at about 400°C. Bond pad openings are etched, and then a final alloy step is done at 400–450°C for 30 minutes in forming gas (10% H_2 in N_2). This alloys the metal contacts in the structure, reduces some of the electrical charges at the Si/SiO_2 interface, and reduces radiation damage in the gate oxide induced during sputtering processes.

11.4 Measurement Methods

A wide assortment of measurements are made on back-end layers and structures. These include morphological, electrical, imaging, chemical, structural, and mechanical measurements. The thickness of each layer is of course important, as are the electrical properties, especially the sheet and contact resistances of the interconnects. Also important is the reliability of the interconnects, including problems of electromigration and the formation of voids and hillocks. The electrical integrity of the dielectric layers is critical, as are their chemical and structural makeups. Imaging the structures, using electron and ion beam microscopy, is essential to diagnosing and solving problems that occur during their fabrication and use. Imaging techniques generally use standard optical microscopes, SEM or TEM methods (Figures 11–2, 11–22 and 11–30, for example), which have been extensively discussed in earlier chapters. We focus here mostly on measurement methods unique to back-end structures.

11.4.1 Morphological Measurements

The morphology of a material or structure refers to the thickness, surface roughness, and grain size. The thicknesses of dielectric layers are usually measured using the optical methods described in Chapter 6. The interconnect layers are commonly measured either by using the stylus/etch step method described in Chapter 6, or by electrical resistance measurements. The sheet resistance, ρ_S (in Ω/square), of the layer equals the sheet resistivity, ρ (in Ω cm), divided by the layer or film thickness, x_f:

$$\rho_s = \frac{\rho}{x_f} \tag{11.14}$$

Thus a measurement of ρ_s using a four-point probe, as described in Chapter 3, directly gives the layer thickness provided that ρ is assumed to be known as a basic material property. This measurement is generally done on test wafers on which the interconnect material is deposited at the same time as the device wafers. Other, more exotic, metal thickness measurement techniques involve acoustic or sonar measurements, including laser-generated sound wave and echo detection systems. Though more complicated, these measurements can be done nondestructively on metal lines and films without test structures or test wafers.

Surface roughness, or local nonuniformities in thickness, can be measured by either the stylus method, or by a related technique, Atomic Force Microscopy (AFM). Here an extremely sharp tip is raster-scanned over the sample surface, and its vertical deflection is measured very accurately generally using laser techniques or piezoelectric sensors. A 3D mapping of the surface topography can be acquired. The measurement sensitivity is so high that surface grain size can often be determined.

11.4.2 Electrical Measurements

The primary electrical measurements made on back-end structures are sheet resistance and contact resistance of the interconnects and breakdown voltage of the dielectrics. In addition, the reliability of the interconnects is often measured electrically by accelerated electromigration measurements.

The sheet resistances of the interconnects directly affect the electrical performance of the circuit. In addition, they can provide information about the film itself. The sheet resistances of the interconnects are often measured by four-point probe measurements or using resistor structures, and depend on layer thickness, chemical composition, and structure. The sheet resistivity of Al lines generally increases as the doping with Si and Cu increases. Also, the grain size of polycrystalline films affects the resistivity: the smaller the grain size the higher the resistivity due to more electrical scattering at the grain boundaries. In the case of $TiSi_2$, the crystal structure affects the resistivity, with the C49 phase having a higher resistivity than the C54 phase.

Specific contact resistivity was described earlier in connection with Figure 11–7. What is usually measured experimentally is the contact resistance, R_c, obtained by measuring the current through the contact for a given voltage across the contact interface. R_c is related to the specific contact resistivity by

$$R_c = \frac{\rho_c}{A} \tag{11.15}$$

where A is the contact area and R_c is in Ω. If the current flowing across the metal-semiconductor interface were uniform, then A would just be the actual area of the entire contact. One could measure V and I across a contact to get R_c, then multiply by the contact area to get ρ_c. However in actual contact structures, the current flow can be highly nonuniform.

Figure 11–34 shows the cross section of a simple Al-to-silicon contact. The current in this example is flowing from the left in the semiconductor, up through the contact, and to the right in the interconnect line. Since the electrical resistance in the N^+ silicon is much greater than in the interconnect line, the current preferentially takes the route of lowest resistance, leaving the semiconductor and entering the metal interconnect close to the left edge of the contact. Thus the current density is higher at the left edge of the contact as it flows up into the metal interconnect. This is called "current crowding." The effective area of the contact is thus decreased from the actual area.

A transfer length, ℓ_t, is defined by the equation

$$\ell_t = \sqrt{\frac{\rho_c}{\rho_s}} \tag{11.16}$$

where ρ_s is the sheet resistance of the N^+ doped silicon region in Ω/square. The transfer length is the length within which most of the current flows through the contact interface, as measured from the leading edge of the contact. (More precisely, it is the

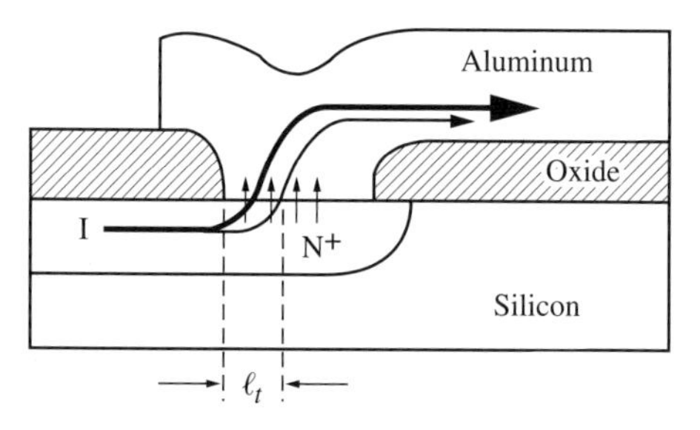

Figure 11–34 Schematic cross section of contact region, showing current crowding toward one end of the contact due to the higher resistivity of the silicon compared to the Al. The transfer length, ℓ_t, defined by Eq. (11.16) and within which most of the current flows, is also indicated in the figure.

distance from the edge of the contact at which the current density drops to $1/e$ of the density at the leading edge.) For ρ_c equal to $10^{-7}\ \Omega\ \text{cm}^2$ and ρ_s equal to 100 Ω/square, the transfer length, ℓ_t, is 0.3 μm. The voltage also varies across the contact since the current varies. So depending on how the actual measurement is made and how the contact structure is laid out, different values of R_c may result.

To take the nonuniform current flow into account, several test structures have been developed to measure contact resistance and resistivity. An excellent reference on this topic is Schroder's book [11.21]. In these structures, a measurement of voltage drop across the contact with current flowing through the contact is made. Then 1D or quasi-2D electrical models are used to relate those values to the actual contact resistivity. In each of these methods, it is assumed that the contact width—that is, the dimension of the contact into the page in Figure 11–34—equals the diffusion (N^+ region) width. This is not always a good approximation as we will discuss later. It is also assumed that the metal resistance is negligible compared to the N^+ region resistance, which is generally a reasonable assumption. Even if silicide layers, TiN barriers, and W plugs are used between the silicon and the metal in the contact hole as shown in Figure 11–21, the N^+ region will dominate the resistance in the lateral direction. Thus accurate measurement of the contact resistivity between the silicon and different contacting layers or multilayer structures can be made with this method.

While a number of test structures are utilized for measuring contact resistance [11.21, 11.22], the simplest and most common is the "cross-bridge Kelvin structure," shown in Figure 11–35. In this structure, the voltage is measured at right angles to the current flow, so that an "average" voltage is measured. In this case, Eq. (11.15) can be used directly, with R_c (called R_k in this case) equaling the measured V divided by the measured I. Thus the contact resistance is simply

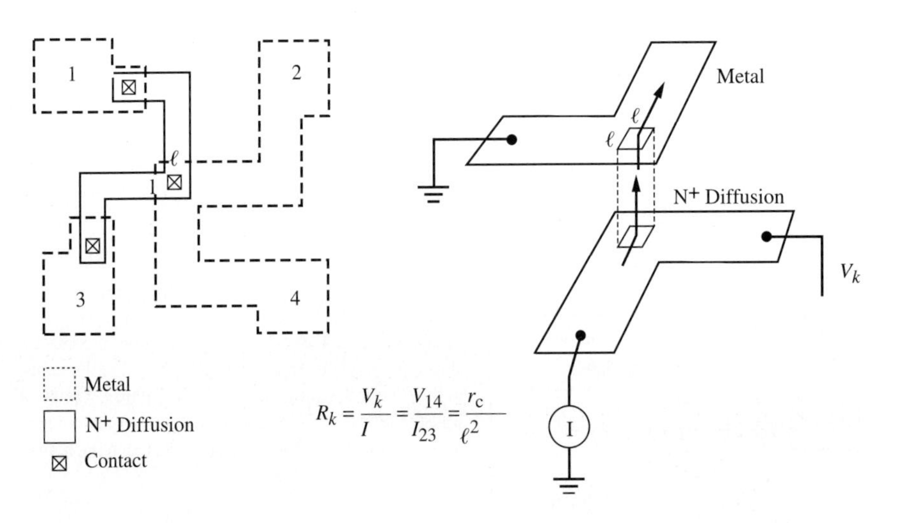

Figure 11–35 Cross-bridge Kelvin structure used to measure an average contact resistance, called R_K in the figure. (After [11.22].)

$$R_k = \frac{\rho_c}{\ell^2} \quad (11.17)$$

where ℓ is the size of the contact. Other more complex structures are described in detail in [11.21].

Example Using the cross-bridge Kelvin structure with a 1-μm-by-1-μm contact, it was found for that for a current of 10 μA through the contact (I_{23} in the structure), the voltage difference across the contact (V_{14}) was measured to be 320 μV. What is the specific contact resistivity for this contact?

Answer For the cross-bridge Kelvin structure, the average contact resistance, R_c (or R_k) is simply V_{14}/I_{23}. Then the specific contact resistivity, ρ_C, can be calculated from Eq. (11.17).

$$\frac{V_{14}}{I_{23}} = R_k = \frac{\rho_c}{\ell^2}$$

$$\frac{320\ \mu\text{V}}{10\ \mu\text{A}} = 32\ \Omega = \frac{\rho_c}{\ell^2}$$

$$\rho_c = 32\ \Omega(1 \times 10^{-4}\,\text{cm})^2 = 0.32\ \mu\Omega\text{cm}^2$$

Unfortunately, the current through the contacts may not only be nonuniform in the main direction of the current flow (shown in Figure 11–34), but can also be nonuniform and non-ideal in the lateral dimension, around the contact. This is because the contact width does not necessarily equal the N^+ diffusion region width, and two-dimensional current crowding and flowing around the periphery of the contact can occur, as shown in Figure 11–36. This results in an overestimation of ρ_c in experimental test structures which gets worse as the contact area gets smaller. Loh [11.22, 11.23] did extensive 2D computer simulations to take this into account. He plotted his results in a generalized, universal format which can be utilized to convert measured values of R_c to correct values of ρ_c.

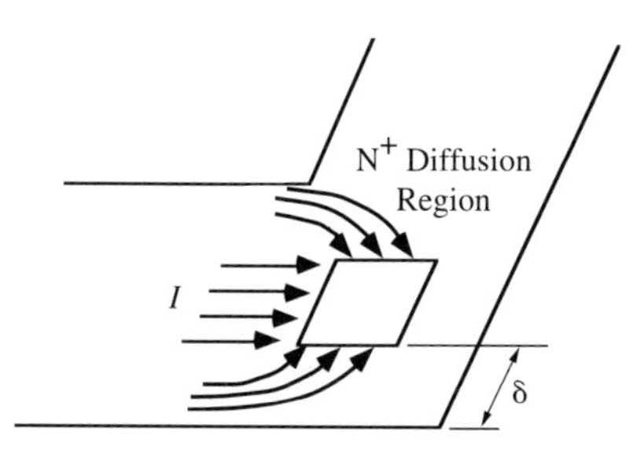

Figure 11–36 Current flow in lateral direction, showing current crowding and flowing around the periphery as it enters the narrower contact region. (After [11.23].)

It is important to note that in an actual circuit structure, the entire N^+ diffusion region is often strapped with silicide, as illustrated in Figure 11–1. This reduces the contact resistivity appreciably because the silicon-to-silicide contact area is significantly increased, with the contact area now defined by the silicide area and not the contact hole area. Using the test structure in Figure 11–35 with the silicide strapping the entire diffusion region would only measure the metal-to-silicide contact resistivity and not the silicide-to-silicon contact resistivity which usually dominates the contact resistance. One could use the silicide as part of a metal stack, forming it only in the contact hole, and use the Kelvin test structure to measure the silicide-to-silicon resistivity. However, this would involve structures and processing that would be different than those actually used in the circuit fabrication. Other test structures have been developed to measure self-aligned silicide contacts in which the silicide straps, or covers, the entire S/D regions [11.24]. These structures are more representative of the actual processes that are used in modern technologies.

As a process monitor, contact resistance is also measured in long contact chains. These are hundreds, sometimes thousands, of contacts that are in series with each other, located in the scribe streets or in test chips on the wafers. These contact chains pass over various topographies. A current is forced through each of these long chains, and the measured voltage is a measure of the average contact resistance. Via resistance is also monitored in this manner. These structures are used to monitor the contacts and vias as a function of processing conditions and structures, and to measure lot-to-lot variability. A high value of resistance in these structures could indicate a problem with incomplete etching, etch residue, poor metal deposition, stress-induced voids in contact regions, or other problems.

The quality of a dielectric layer is usually defined in terms of its breakdown voltage, or field strength, expressed in units of V cm^{-1}. In this measurement, a voltage is applied across the dielectric layer and is ramped up at a constant rate (see Figure 4–15). The voltage is monitored, and at a certain point, the voltage drops abruptly. This occurs when the dielectric "breaks down" and excessive current flows through it, discharging the applied charge. The physical mechanism for oxide breakdown may involve bond-breaking or hole trapping at defect sites, leading to changes in the structural and electronic properties of the material. These defects can include weak Si-O bonds, oxygen vacancies, surface roughness, local thinning, and sodium or metal contaminants in the film. An alternate test is the constant current test (as opposed to the voltage-ramp test). Here a current is passed through the dielectric at a constant level until the oxide is broken down. The charge-to-breakdown is measured, and is on the order of 10 C cm^{-2} for a good oxide. Other breakdown measurements include time-to-breakdown under constant voltage, and charge-to-breakdown under ramped current. Chapter 6 discusses some of these measurements in connection with thermal oxides.

The reliability of interconnects is measured by electrical tests. Common causes of failure of interconnect lines are void and hillock formation, either due to stresses on the lines or due to electromigration. Stress-induced voids can be detected simply by measuring the electrical resistance of the line. An open circuit would indicate a line-spanning void. When shunt layers such as TiN are used, a void which spans the entire Al layer would not cause an open circuit since current could still flow through the shunt line. In this case, a failure would be defined for a certain percentage increase in the line resistance, perhaps 20%. Stress-induced hillocks which crack overlaying dielectric layers and contact adjacent interconnect layers can be detected by short circuits. Failure due to electromigration—current-induced void and hillock formation—is measured using accelerated lifetime tests.

It would take too long to monitor the interconnects for electromigration under normal circuit operating conditions. Therefore, tests are done at elevated temperatures and higher than normal current levels, so-called accelerated lifetime tests. In these tests, current at elevated densities (about 1–2 MA cm^{-2}) and temperatures (200–225°C) is forced through an interconnect line. The voltage is monitored through taps to this line, and the resistance is measured. An open circuit, or even a partially open circuit, indicating void formation due to electromigration, is thus detected by an increase in the resistance. A second line adjacent to the line under test is monitored as well. A short circuit to this line indicates hillock formation and extrusion. Again, a certain percentage change in resistance (20% or so) defines a line failure. The time to failure for a number of lines is determined and statistically analyzed. This is done by plotting the cumulative percent that have failed versus time on a lognormal plot. The median time to failure, or t_{50}, is found by finding the time at which 50% cumulative failure occurs. The Median Time To Failure (MTTF) has been found to follow the general relationship:

$$\text{MTTF} = AJ^{-n}\exp\left(\frac{E_A}{kT}\right) \tag{11.18}$$

where J is the current density, n is typically close to 2, although values ranging from 1–3 have been reported, and A is a constant which depends on film structure (grain size, etc.) and processing. E_A is the activation energy for electromigration and is often associated with Al grain boundary diffusion. Its value ranges from 0.5 to 0.8 eV. Once the exact values for this expression have been determined experimentally at the elevated temperatures and currents for the particular structure and process, one can extrapolate down to the normal operating conditions to determine how long the interconnects will operate before failure occurs. This of course assumes that the failure occurs by the same mechanisms at the lower temperatures and current densities, which may not always be the case.

Example Under accelerated testing at 225°C and a current density of 1 MA cm^{-2}, the MTTF of an Al(Cu) interconnect line is found to be 200 hours. If n equals 2.0 and E_A equals 0.7 eV, what is the MTTF at operating conditions of 70°C and 0.1 MA cm^{-2}?

Answer Using Eq. (11.18), one can determine A, the MTTF constant for this case:

$$\text{MTTF} = AJ^{-n}\exp\left(\frac{E_A}{kT}\right)$$

$$200 \text{ hr} = A(1 \times 10^6 \text{Acm}^{-2})^{-2.0} \exp\left(\frac{0.7 \text{ eV}}{8.62 \times 10^{-5} \text{eVK}^{-1} 498\text{K}}\right)$$

Solving for A gives $A = 1.66 \times 10^7$ hr A^{-1} cm^2. Solving now for 70°C and 0.1 MA cm^{-2} gives

$$\text{MTTF} = 1.66 \times 10^7 \text{hr } A^{-1} \text{cm}^2 (0.1 \times 10^6 \text{Acm}^{-2})^{-2.0} \exp\left(\frac{0.7 \text{ eV}}{8.62 \times 10^{-5} \text{eVK}^{-1} 343\text{K}}\right)$$

$$= 3.18 \times 10^7 \text{ hrs} = 3620 \text{ years}$$

This may seem like a long time (and it is), but this time is the median time (t_{50}) to failure. Generally the goal is to have the earliest failures (where the first 0.1% or so lines fail) at not less than 10–20 years of service.

11.4.3 Chemical and Structural Measurements

Many techniques are utilized to obtain chemical and structural information from metallization structures. The chemical information relates to the chemical or compositional makeup of the films, including impurity concentrations and distributions. Structural information relates to microstructural, as opposed to macrostructural or morphological, attributes. This includes lattice spacings, material density, and crystallographic information. Most of the techniques to measure the chemical and structural characteristics have been discussed in earlier chapters, and we will only briefly discuss them here.

For compositional analysis of thin films, many techniques are available. In Auger Electron Spectroscopy (AES, see Chapter 4), elemental identification and mapping are done by generating Auger electrons by a focused electron beam and then analyzing the energy of the Auger electrons. Combining this with simultaneous sputtering of the surface leads to Auger depth profiling. A typical application of Auger depth profiling would be to investigate interdiffusion of elements between different interconnect layers.

Rutherford Backscattering Spectrometry (RBS, see Chapter 4), in which the yield and energy of backscattered helium atoms are measured, gives compositional information without the need of standards. This is especially useful for the measurement of hydrogen in thin films as a function of depth, which other techniques have difficulty measuring. In Fourier Transform Infrared Spectroscopy (FTIR, see Chapter 3), films are radiated with infrared radiation, exciting the molecular bonds. Measurement of the absorption spectrum leads to chemical bond identification in thin films. For example, one can measure Si-OH bonds in dielectric layers, determine relative water concentrations in SOG films, or measure B and P levels in BPSG. Electron Spectroscopy for Chemical Analysis (ESCA), also known as X-ray Photoelectron Spectroscopy (XPS, see Chapter 4), is used to identify surface constituents and to measure bond energies by irradiating a surface with a monoenergetic X-ray beam and analyzing the photoemitted electrons. Total X-Ray Fluorescence (TXRF, see Chapter 4) is used to measure contaminant levels on surfaces. This technique utilizes a low-divergence X-ray beam impinging at a glancing angle on a surface. Fluorescence X-rays are emitted by atoms on the surface and detected. Each element emits X-ray photons of a characteristic energy, allowing elemental identification of impurities. An example of its use is the measurement of contaminants left on the surface after a via etch. The most common technique to measure impurity atoms in thin films, as well as in the silicon substrate, is by Secondary Ion Mass Spectrometry (SIMS, see Chapter 4). By mass analysis of sputtered (secondary) ions as a result of bombardment with a focused beam of oxygen or cesium primary ions, very accurate measurement of low levels of impurity atoms can be obtained as a function of depth. Measuring the redistribution of dopant atoms into and out of silicides is an example of SIMS use in interconnect structures.

X-Ray Diffraction (XRD) is often used for structural measurements. By analyzing the constructive and destructive interference of X-rays scattered from thin films, one can measure lattice parameters and make phase identifications. One can also measure stress (as discussed in the next section), and measure preferred orientation, or texture. Crystallographic information can also be determined by utilizing the diffraction of backscattered electrons, rather than X-rays. In Electron Back-Scattering Diffraction (EBSD), a small electron beam is incident on the surface at a glancing angle of less than 45°. A phosphor screen is located near the specimen to collect the backscattered electrons. Diffraction patterns are generated on the screen, allowing one to determine the crystallographic orientation of the region where the beam is incident. In this manner, the crystallographic orientation of individual grains of an Al interconnect line can be determined. By using computer-automated diffraction pattern analysis techniques, one can map out the crystallography of entire interconnect lines, leading to analysis and understanding of reliability problems such as electromigration.

The dielectric properties, particularly the dielectric constants of films, are measured using optical techniques. Ellipsometry, discussed in Chapter 6, is primarily used for this purpose. The dielectric constant of a layer is not only useful to determine the electrical properties of a dielectric layer in an interconnect structure, but it also gives information regarding its structure and density. However other properties, such as composition and stress, also affect these parameters, and it is often difficult to separate them all out.

A rather crude, yet simple, measure of a film's density can be obtained by measuring the etch rate of the film. Buffered HF can be used to measure the relative etch rate of SiO_2 films, for example. Films that are less dense have higher etch rates. However, the film's stoichiometry, structure, and other impurities such as hydrogen can also affect the etch rate so one cannot unequivocally equate etch rate with film density. But such data still can give an indication of differences in films that have different deposition conditions, are processed differently, or are in different locations on the surface of the wafer. Measuring the etch rate of PSG films can also be used for a quick determination of the phosphorus concentration since there is a good correspondence between the two properties.

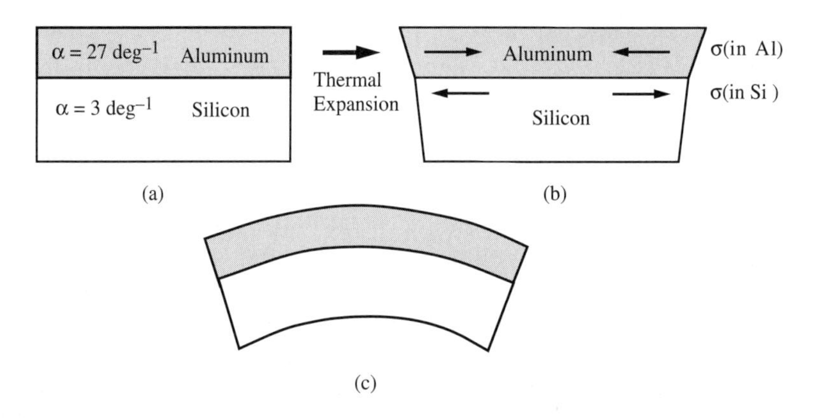

Figure 11–37 Thermal expansion differences between Al and Si, shown in (a), lead to stresses in the Al thin film and Si substrate, shown in (b). In this case, tensile stress develops on top of the Si substrate and compressive stress develops in the Al thin film. σ designates the normal, or direct, stress in each case. (c) shows the bending of the structure (exaggerated) that occurs due to these stresses.

11.4.4 Mechanical Measurements

Stresses that develop in interconnect layers and structures can greatly affect their physical integrity, leading to failures such as cracking and loss of adhesion, as well as to reliability problems such as void and hillock formation. A common source of stresses in thin films is differences in thermal expansion. If two films (or a film on a substrate) with different coefficients of thermal expansion, α, are in contact with each other, then upon heating or cooling one film will want to shrink or expand more than the other. If good adhesion between the films is maintained, then stresses (normal, or direct, stresses) will develop in the two films. Figure 11–37 illustrates this for an Al film on a Si substrate. Al has a much higher coefficient of thermal expansion than Si, as seen in Table 11–4. Upon heating, the Al film will want to expand more than the Si. If good interface contact is maintained, then the Al will pull out on the Si, inducing a tensile stress on the top of the Si. Likewise, the Si will pull in on the Al, causing a compressive stress on the Al film. (If another thin film such as SiO_2 is between an Al film and a thick Si substrate, it is the difference in thermal expansion coefficients between the Al and the much thicker Si that primarily determines the thermal stress in the Al.) To relieve this stress, plastic flow of the Al can occur. Hillock formation in Al thin films, illustrated earlier in Figure 11–11, can result from this.

Another type of stress in thin films is called "intrinsic" stress. This is the stress present after deposition, at the deposition temperature. This can be due to differences in lattice constants between the film and the layer it is deposited on, energetic ion bombardment during deposition, or gas or precipitation inclusion in the film. If the deposition is done at an elevated temperature, the stress measured afterwards at room temperature would include contributions from both the intrinsic stress and the stress due to differential thermal expansion.

A common way to measure stress in a thin film is by measuring how much the substrate bends after the film is deposited or processed. In the absence of any movement restraints, the structure in Figure 11–37(b) will in fact bend in order to balance the force moments caused by the stresses. This is shown in Figure 11–37(c). For the top film in compressive stress, as is the case in this example, the entire structure will bend with the edges downward relative to the middle. The interface stays constant in length, but the top film wants to expand and the bottom film wants to shrink, leading to the concave downward bending. The amount of bending is dependent on the internal mechanical properties of the film and substrate (specifically Young's modulus and Poisson's ratio), the thicknesses, and the stresses in the film and substrate. By measuring the amount of bending, and knowing the film thickness and mechanical constants, one can extract the stress in the film. If we assume that the film thickness is much smaller than the thickness of the substrate and that the film is in an isotropic biaxial stress state (i.e., $\sigma_z = 0, \sigma_x = \sigma_y$), then the biaxial stress in the film, $\sigma_f (= \sigma_x = \sigma_y)$, approximately equals

$$\sigma_f = \frac{1}{6R} \frac{Y_s x_s^2}{(1 - \upsilon_S) x_f} \tag{11.19}$$

Here R is the radius of curvature (i.e., a measure of the bending), Y_s is Young's modulus of the substrate, υ_s is Poisson's ratio for the substrate, x_s is the substrate thickness, and x_f is the film thickness. In practice the curvature is measured before and after the film is deposited (or before and after the film is processed in some way), since the wafer might not be flat to start with. Thus $1/R$ would be given by $(1/R_{\text{final}} — 1/R_{\text{initial}})$. The difference in curvature is then related to the stress induced by depositing or processing the film.

Example What is the stress in a 0.5-μm Al film on a 600-μm-thick (100) Si wafer if it induces a radius of curvature of 2.7×10^4 cm? (Assume $1/R_{\text{initial}} = 0$.)

Answer $Y_s/(1\text{-}\upsilon_s)$ is the bulk modulus of the substrate and given in Table 11–4 as 1.805×10^5 MPa, which equals $1.805 \times 10^5 \times 10^7$ dynes cm^{-2}. Substituting numbers into Eq. (11.19), we have

$$\sigma_f = \frac{1}{6R} \frac{Y_s x_s^2}{(1 - \upsilon_S) x_f}$$

$$= \frac{1}{6(2.7 \times 10^4 \text{cm})} \frac{1.805 \times 10^{12} \text{dynes cm}^{-2} (600 \times 10^{-4} \text{ cm})^2}{0.5 \times 10^{-4} \text{cm}}$$

$$= 8.0 \times 10^8 \text{ dynes cm}^2$$

Another technique used to measure stress in a thin film is with X-Ray Diffraction (XRD). The stresses in the film induce a change in the lattice parameter of the film, which can be measured by XRD techniques. For a crystalline or polycrystalline film with an isotropic biaxial stress, the film stress σ_f is

$$\sigma_f = -\frac{Y_f}{2\upsilon_f}\left(\frac{a_o - a_s}{a_s}\right) \tag{11.20}$$

where a_s is the lattice constant in the stressed film, a_o is the lattice constant in the unstressed film, Y_f is Young's modulus in the film, and υ_f is Poisson's ratio for the film. Conventional XRD measures the average stress over large areas. Blanket, unpatterned films are used in this case. However, recent advances in high brightness XRD, using synchotron X-ray sources, have allowed "microdiffraction stress analysis." With this technique the local stresses in patterned films can be measured.

X-ray diffraction methods are not well suited for amorphous films since they do not have well-defined lattice spacings. Instead, in addition to using wafer bending techniques, stresses in amorphous films are often measured by FTIR. In this technique bond angles are determined from the light absorption measured at different wave numbers. The bond angles are assumed to be stress dependent, and stress levels can thus be determined from the change in bond angles.

Figure 11–38 shows a measured stress-temperature curve, using X-ray diffraction, for an Al film on a SiO_2 coated Si substrate. The stress in the Al starts out tensile (by convention, a tensile stress is positive, a compressive stress is negative) at about 50 MPa. As the sample is heated, the difference in thermal expansion results in the stress in the Al becoming more compressive. The stress in the film due to differences in thermal expansion coefficients is

$$\sigma_f = (\alpha_S - \alpha_f)\Delta T \frac{Y_f}{1 - \upsilon_f} \tag{11.21}$$

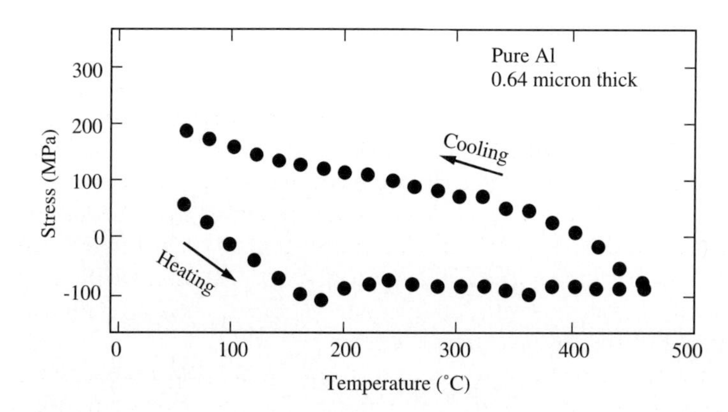

Figure 11–38 Stress-temperature curve of 0.64-μm-thick Al film on SiO_2. The lower points are for heating, while the upper points are for cooling. (After [11.25].)

where ΔT is positive upon heating and negative upon cooling. Thus the slope of the stress-temperature curve initially is approximately $\Delta\alpha\ Y_f / (1 - \upsilon_f)$. At about 200°C, the elastic behavior turns to plastic deformation as processes occur that relax the stress. This might involve grain boundary or dislocation movement as well as hillock formation. Instead of following the elastic curve, the stress remains fairly constant up to 450°C. Upon cooling, elastic deformation again occurs, with about the same slope in the curve as at the beginning. Then plastic deformation again occurs when the temperature is lowered below about 350°C. Film hardening is evident as the sample is cooled from about 200°C back to room temperature. Note that the final stress level in this example is significantly higher than the starting stress level because of the plastic deformation that takes place.

Another important thin film property is adhesion. Measurement of this property in a quantitative way is difficult. A simple, very crude technique to measure film adhesion is the "scotch tape method." A thin film is deposited on a substrate or on another thin film. Adhesive tape is attached to the top and then pulled off. The amount of film stripped off is a qualitative measure of the film's adhesion to the layer below. More quantitative tests of this type involve attaching a metal pin to the film with epoxy, then using a calibrated mechanical force to pull the pin at a specific rate and/or force. Another technique is to deposit an additional thin film on the top of the thin film/substrate couple. With prior knowledge of the top film's stress as a function of thickness, one can increase the stress applied to the lower thin film by increasing the thickness of the top film until the lower films loses adhesion to the substrate. Using stress simulation methods, one can determine the stress, or force, needed for the lower film to lose adhesion, thus quantifying the adhesiveness to some degree. This technique is often close in practice to the scenario in which thin films do lose their adhesion (i.e., when other stressed films are put on top).

11.5 Models and Simulation

Back-end processing involves the deposition and patterning of insulators and conductors. Because of this, the simulation tools described in Chapters 9 and 10 for deposition and etching are very useful in simulating back-end processes. In fact, many of the examples given in those chapters involved back-end processing issues. Thus tools like SPEEDIE [11.26], ATHENA [11.27], and TAURUS [11.28] are widely used for understanding and simulating back-end structures and process flows. Since deposition and etching were covered in those earlier chapters, we will focus here on a few additional simulation tools and simulation problems that are particularly useful in back-end structures. The first section deals with silicide formation which, as we have seen, is widely used to strap junctions and polysilicon lines to reduce their sheet resistances. The second section discusses models for CMP which is now a key technology for back-end structures. The next two sections deal with polycrystalline materials and describe modeling approaches for grain growth and diffusion in these materials. Such models are useful in polysilicon, but also more generally in other back-end materials used for interconnects, almost all of which are polycrystalline. We will find that the single-crystal models developed in earlier chapters for diffusion can be extended to polycrystalline materials, although because the properties of these materials vary with processing conditions and even with position on a given chip, the models are not as predictive as they are in the single-crystal case. Finally, we cover a problem unique to back-end structures. This is the electromigration failure mode which can cause catastrophic failure of interconnects, particularly aluminum lines. Sophisticated models have been developed to predict these types of failures and some simulation capability exists.

11.5.1 Silicide Formation

In Chapter 6 we saw how the thermal oxidation of silicon is modeled using the linear-parabolic Deal-Grove model. Oxygen diffuses through the growing SiO_2 layer and reacts with Si at the Si-SiO_2 interface. For short times and thin oxides, the reaction between Si and O limits the oxidation process, and the oxidation rate is linear with time. For long times and thick oxides, the diffusion of oxygen through the oxide limits the oxidation process, and the overall oxidation rate is parabolic in time (that is, proportional to $\sqrt{t}$). In small structures where 2D and 3D effects are important, it is necessary to include stress effects on the oxidation process due to volume expansion in constrained regions. Stress-dependent oxidation parameters and appropriate visco-elastic flow models are needed for these cases. This same linear-parabolic model was also used for silicide oxidation in Chapter 6. Silicide formation, the reaction of a metal with the underlying Si to form the silicide, can be modeled in a similar fashion. In fact, Cea and Law [11.29, 11.30] and others have used the same models used in SUPREM-IV for the oxidation of silicon to simulate the formation of $TiSi_2$. We will describe this approach here.

The formation of $TiSi_2$ occurs by the diffusion of Si through the forming $TiSi_2$ and the reaction between Si and Ti at the $TiSi_2$-Ti interface to form new $TiSi_2$. Figure 11–39(a) illustrates this. The similarity between this process and the silicon oxidation process is obvious. Either the diffusion of the Si or the reaction at the interface can dominate the

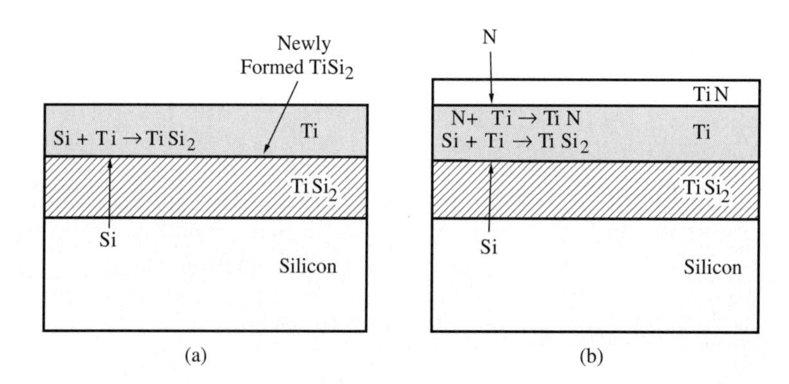

Figure 11–39 Illustration of $TiSi_2$ salicide formation: (a) $TiSi_2$ formation only, showing Si diffusion through silicide forming new silicide at the $TiSi_2$/Ti interface. (b) $TiSi_2$ formation in nitrogen ambient with simultaneous TiN formation on top. Nitrogen diffuses through the TiN layer, forming new TiN at the TiN/Ti interface.

overall formation kinetics depending on the conditions, leading to linear-parabolic behavior. For oxidation of silicon, there is a net increase in material volume, leading to a compressive stress. For $TiSi_2$ formation, one might expect the opposite to be true. This is because for every 1 nm of Ti consumed, 2.27 nm of Si are consumed producing 2.51 nm of silicide. Therefore for every $1 + 2.27 = 3.27$ nm of reactants, only 2.51 nm of product is formed, leading to a net volume reduction of about 23%. Hence tensile stresses should result in the $TiSi_2$ film. However, experimentally it is found that either compressive or tensile stresses can develop in silicide films depending on the conditions of formation. For the formation from codeposited thin multilayers of Ti and Si, tensile stresses are usually produced. But for a single, thicker layer of Ti deposited on a substrate of Si, compressive stresses often arise. Other factors can affect the stress development, such as differences in thermal expansion, relaxation processes, localized compressive stress at the $Ti/TiSi_2$ interface where the new $TiSi_2$ is forming, and incorporation of argon, oxygen, or excess silicon. These may dominate over simple, net volume reduction.

The linear parabolic model for SiO_2 growth [Eq. (6.27)] is also useful in describing silicide growth since the physical processes are similar. Thus

$$\frac{x_s^2}{B} + \frac{x_s}{B/A} = t + \tau \quad \text{or} \quad x_s = \frac{A}{2}\left\{\sqrt{1 + \frac{t + \tau}{A^2/4B}} - 1\right\} \tag{11.22}$$

where x_s is the silicide thickness, t is the time, τ is the effective initial time [given by Eq. (6.26)], and B and B/A are the parabolic and linear rate constants, respectively. When the parabolic term dominates, these expressions reduce simply to

$$x_s^2 \cong B(t + \tau) \tag{11.23}$$

Physically this corresponds to the diffusion process (Si in the $TiSi_2$) being the rate-limiting step. B is primarily determined by the Si diffusivity in $TiSi_2$. When the linear term in Eq. (11.28) dominates, the growth model reduces to

$$x_s \cong \frac{B}{A}(t + \tau) \tag{11.24}$$

Physically this corresponds to the interface reaction forming new $TiSi_2$ being the rate-limiting step. B/A is largely determined by the rate of this reaction.

Cea and Law [11.29, 11.30, 11.31] have simulated the formation of $TiSi_2$ in 2D using the FLOOPS process simulator [11.32]. FLOOPS simulates the silicidation process in the same way that SUPREM models silicon oxidation. To do this in 2D, and to be able to include stress effects which are functions of position, the various mechanisms in the silicidation process are modeled step by step. The diffusion of Si from its source (either the Si substrate or polysilicon layers) through $TiSi_2$ is used to calculate the concentration of free Si at the $TiSi_2/Ti$ interface. The velocity of the $Si/TiSi_2$ interface moving downward is determined by how many Si atoms leave the interface. The reaction of Si and Ti at the $TiSi_2/Ti$ interface is then modeled. The amount of Ti consumed and $TiSi_2$ produced is a linear function of the free Si concentration and B/A, the linear rate constant. The formation of $TiSi_2$ thus occurs only when Ti is on Si, or on $TiSi_2$ which is on Si.

Table 11–7 *B* and *B/A* values for $TiSi_2$ formation [11.29]

	B ($\mu m^2\ min^{-1}$)	B/A ($\mu m\ min^{-1}$)
(100) Si	$1.85 \times 10^{11} \exp\left(\frac{-2.5\ eV}{kT}\right)$	"large"
(111) Si	"large"	$8.9 \times 10^{11} \exp\left(\frac{-2.5\ eV}{kT}\right)$

For these simulations Cea used the experimental silicide thickness versus time data of Pico and Lagally [11.33] to extract values for *B* and *B/A* for $TiSi_2$. As discussed in Chapter 6 (Figure 6–17), plotting x_s versus $(t + \tau)/x_s$ gives $-A$ as the y-intercept and *B* as the slope. By this method, *B*, the parabolic rate constant, and *B/A*, the linear rate constant, can be easily extracted from experimental thickness-time data. Cea's values for *B* and *B/A* are given in Table 11–7. For (100) Si, *B/A* is "large" meaning that the Si/Ti reaction is very fast and the formation is limited by the diffusion of Si, as governed by the parabolic rate constant, *B*. Therefore, any sufficiently large value of *B/A* will work (and will have no effect on the outcome). Alternately, for (111) Si the formation is limited by the Si/Ti reaction, and the parabolic rate constant is "large."

Example $TiSi_2$ is formed by depositing 55 nm of Ti on a (100) Si substrate and annealing in an argon atmosphere. If the anneal is done long enough so that all the Ti is reacted, how thick is the $TiSi_2$ that is formed, and how much Si is consumed? Repeat the problem if the anneal is done at 700°C for 30 sec using Cea's values in Table 11–7 for *B* and *B/A*.

Answer When the annealing is long enough so that all the Ti is reacted, 2.51 nm of $TiSi_2$ is formed for each 1.00 nm of Ti, consuming 2.27 nm of Si. (Since the anneal is done in an inert, argon ambient, no TiN is formed.) Therefore

$$\text{Amount of } TiSi_2 \text{ formed} = 55\ \text{nm} \times 2.51 = 138\ \text{nm}$$

$$\text{Amount of Si consumed} = 55\ \text{nm} \times 2.27 = 125\ \text{nm}$$

For a 700°C, 30-sec anneal, not all of the Ti may have reacted. We must therefore use the Deal-Grove-like equations. For (100) Si, Table 11–7 shows that B/A = "large" and $B = 1.85 \times 10^{11} \exp(-2.5/kT)\ \mu m^2\, min^{-1}$. The "large" *B/A* value means that the growth is not limited by the Si surface reaction. Therefore using Eq. (11.23), and letting τ be zero, the silicide thickness x_o is given by

$$x_s = \sqrt{Bt}$$

At 700°C,

$$B = 1.85 \times 10^{11} \exp\left(- \frac{2.5 \text{ eV}}{8.63 \times 10^{-5} \text{ eVK}^{-1} 973\text{K}} \right) \mu\text{m}^2 \text{ min}^{-1} = 0.022 \ \mu\text{m}^2 \text{ min}^{-1}$$

Therefore x_s, the amount of $TiSi_2$ formed, is

$$x_s = \sqrt{0.022 \ \mu\text{m}^2 \text{ min}^{-1} * 0.5 \text{ min}} = 0.105 \ \mu\text{m} = 105 \text{ nm}$$

The amount of Ti needed to form this $= 105 \text{ nm} * \frac{1}{2.51} = 42$ nm, and, thus

Amount of Si consumed $= 42 \text{ nm} \times 2.27 = 95.3$ nm.

As with the oxidation models presented in Chapter 6, the B and B/A parameters may be affected by stress. There is some experimental evidence [11.30] that Si diffusion in $TiSi_2$ is in fact retarded by high-compressive stress levels, and this is incorporated in Cea's simulations by including a value of 1.3 nm^3 for V_D, the activation volume for the stress-dependent Si diffusivity in $TiSi_2$. This is utilized in Eq. (6.44), repeated here

$$D(\text{stress}) = D\exp\left(- \frac{PV_D}{kT} \right) \tag{11.25}$$

where P is the hydrostatic pressure (positive for compression) in the growing silicide. This will locally affect the value of B since $B = 2DC^*/N_1$ in the Deal-Grove model. In regions of high stress, or hydrostatic pressure, such as at corners, the diffusivity of the silicon through the silicide will be reduced and the silicide growth rate will be reduced.

Figure 11–40 shows a simulation in which 40 nm of Ti is deposited on top of a 2.0-µm-wide polysilicon gate structure. The left side of Figure 11–40 shows the initial structure. The structure is then annealed in an RTA for 30 sec at 650°C in an argon

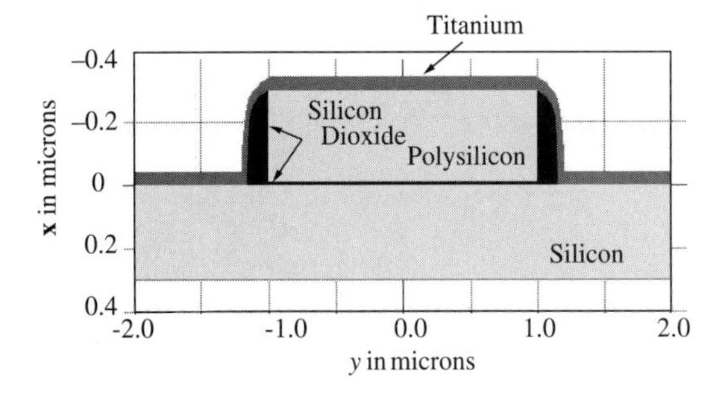

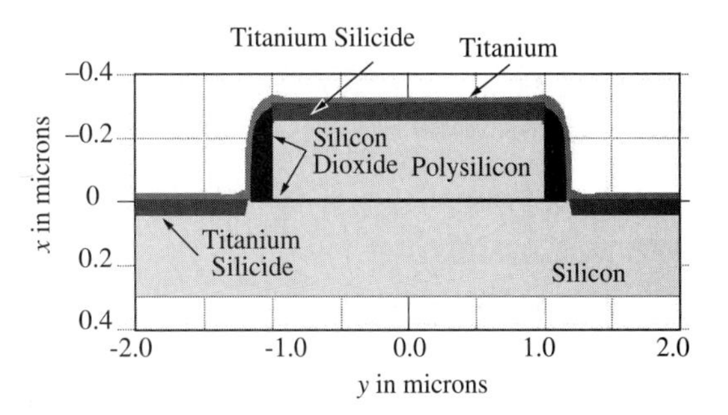

Figure 11–40 Simulation of $TiSi_2$ formation using FLOOPS [11.32] on a 2-µm-wide gate structure: left, before formation anneal step; right, after formation anneal step, 30 sec at 650°C in an argon atmosphere. $TiSi_2$ is formed everywhere the Ti is in contact or close to Si [11.31].

atmosphere, with the resulting structure on the right of Figure 11–40. The linear and parabolic rate constants used are those in Table 11–7 for (100) Si. As the $TiSi_2$ grows volumetric changes can cause stresses in the films. These are governed by the mechanical properties of each material, in particular the viscosity, Young's modulus, and Poisson's ratio. Values for the latter two were taken from the literature for the various materials (Si, oxide, polysilicon, Ti, and $TiSi_2$) in the structure. The viscosities for all the materials except $TiSi_2$ were taken to be high so that they behave elastically. The viscosity of $TiSi_2$ was set lower based on recent experimental measurements showing significant stress relaxation during the formation anneal [11.34]. As can be seen in the simulation, about 20 nm of the Ti remains, so that 20 nm reacted. Approximately 48 nm of $TiSi_2$ is formed, consuming about 43 nm of Si. This agrees reasonably well with the ratios given earlier for $TiSi_2$ formation (reaction of 1 nm of Ti consumes 2.27 nm of Si, forming 2.51 nm of $TiSi_2$). As one can see in the figure, the $TiSi_2$ forms only near where Ti is initially in contact with Si—in this case over the polysilicon gate and on the source/drain regions. The sidewall spacer prevents $TiSi_2$ formation from shorting the gate to the source and drain.

The formation of $TiSi_2$ is often done in a nitrogen ambient. As discussed previously, this causes TiN to form on top of the silicide and on top of the oxide spacer, inhibiting lateral encroachment of the $TiSi_2$, and perhaps serving as a local interconnect. The TiN forms at the expense of $TiSi_2$ and must be included in any simulation when the silicidation is done in a nitrogen ambient. The model for TiN formation is similar to $TiSi_2$ formation. In this case, nitrogen diffuses through the forming TiN, reacting with the Ti at the Ti/TiN interface, as illustrated in Figure 11–39(b). This reaction can also be modeled with the Deal-Grove linear-parabolic model. This requires simulating two reacting and moving interfaces simultaneously.

An example of $TiSi_2$ formation in a nitrogen ambient is shown in Figure 11–41. Here 40 nm of Ti is deposited on a 0.35 μm polysilicon gate structure, with adjoining source/drain regions. The structure is annealed for 30 seconds at 650°C in a nitrogen ambient. The model parameters are the same as in the previous simulation, except that

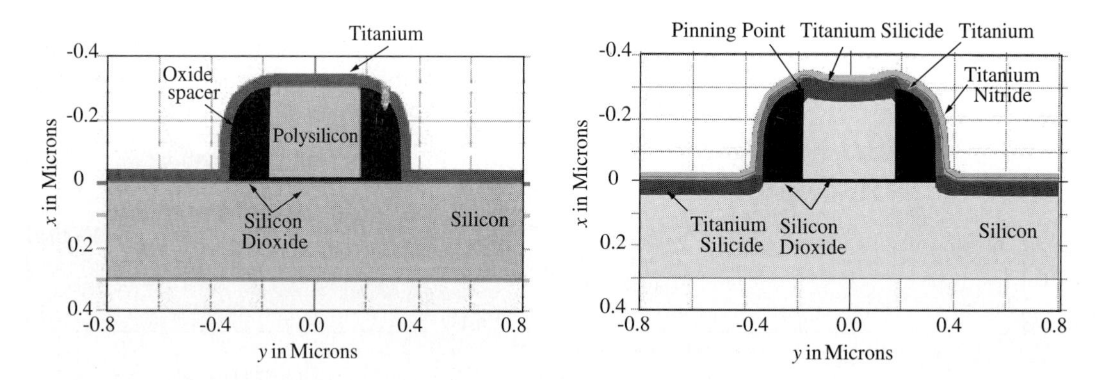

Figure 11–41 Simulation of $TiSi_2$ formation using FLOOPS [11.32] on a 0.35-μm-wide gate structure: left, before formation anneal step; right, after formation anneal step, 30 sec at 650°C in a nitrogen atmosphere. $TiSi_2$ is formed everywhere the Ti is in contact or close to Si. TiN is formed on top of the Ti layer. Bowing in the silicide on top of gate and the lateral encroachment are evident [11.31].

parameters for TiN have been added. Based on limited experimental data, the linear and parabolic rate constants for TiN growth were set to be 20% of the values for $TiSi_2$. The simulated structure after the RTA silicidation anneal in a nitrogen ambient is shown on the right in Figure 11–41. $TiSi_2$ forms as before over the polysilicon gate and Si source/drain regions, but in addition TiN forms over the entire structure. Not all of the Ti over the silicon is reacted, with about 7.5 nm remaining. Approximately 32.5 nm of Ti and 44 nm of Si are consumed, producing approximately 50 nm of $TiSi_2$ and 27 nm of TiN over the silicide. In the simulated structure, some lateral encroachment of the silicide over the oxide spacers is evident, as well as downward bowing of the silicide over the gate. Both of these features are characteristic of experimental $TiSi_2$ formation and are more pronounced in small-scale structures. The lateral encroachment is due to the Si diffusion through the silicide and over the oxide to react with the Ti there. The continued formation of TiN over the oxide spacer would block the lateral growth of $TiSi_2$ and prevent it from encroaching further. In addition, nitrogen is believed to stuff the grain boundaries of any unreacted Ti, slowing Si diffusion and helping to retard lateral growth—however this is not explicitly modeled here.

The bowing is believed to be due to the mechanical pinning of the bottom of the silicide at each end to the top of each oxide spacer [11.35, 11.36]. This pinning point is shown in Figure 11–41. As the $TiSi_2$ is formed, Si leaves the polysilicon at the $TiSi_2$/polysilicon interface, diffusing up to the $TiSi_2$/Ti interface where it forms more $TiSi_2$. The $TiSi_2$ then moves down to fill the space left from the vacant Si. If pinning of the silicide occurs at the top of the oxide spacers, consumption of Si to form the silicide can only occur in the middle of the gate and not the ends. All this leads to a bowed downward structure.

A final simulation example is shown in Figure 11–42. In this case the TSUPREM-IV simulation tool was used to simulate the formation of $TiSi_2$. 25 nm of Ti was deposited on a MOSFET structure similar to those in the previous examples. The oxide spacer was overetched prior to Ti deposition in this case. A 1.3 min anneal at 650°C formed 62.5 nm of $TiSi_2$. Finally, the remaining Ti on the sidewall spacers was etched off, resulting in the structure in Figure 11–42. The basic physical models are similar to those described above, producing the expected amount of silicide over the exposed silicon regions. .

These models and simulations should be applicable to other silicide formation processes, as well as to any reaction between adjacent layers which produces a new

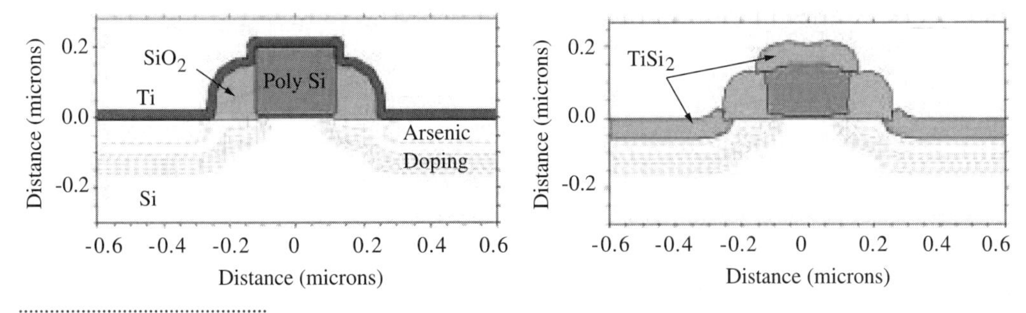

Figure 11–42 TSUPREM-IV [11.28] simulation of the formation of $TiSi_2$ on the gate and source-drain regions of a MOSFET: left, before silicidation anneal; right, after silicidation anneal and removal of unreacted Ti.

phase between them. These models can also be used for the silicides which form by the metal, rather than the Si, diffusing through the silicide.

11.5.2 Chemical-Mechanical Polishing

We have seen many examples throughout this chapter of how Chemical-Mechanical Polishing (CMP) is used to planarize films, utilizing a combination of chemical and mechanical polishing or etching. Models and simulation tools have been developed for this complex process. They are, however, mostly phenomenological in nature. The starting point for modeling polishing is the Preston equation [11.37]:

$$P = K_p p v \tag{11.26}$$

where P is the polish or etch rate. K_p is a constant (with units of pressure) and is a function of the mechanical and chemical properties of the film and pads and the composition and properties of the polishing slurry, p is the applied pressure between the wafer and the pad, and v is the relative velocity between the pad and wafer. The applied pressure, p, depends on the geometry or topography of the surface. Since the pads used are not perfectly rigid, they conform to the surface to a limited degree, but of course not exactly. As a result the pressure at each point varies, with protruding points receiving high pressure, and sunken or shadowed points receiving little or no pressure. Because of the semi-rigidity of the pads, the resulting profiles depend on both the stiffness of the pad as well as on the density and spacing of elevated features on the surface.

Most models for CMP attempt to determine the relative pressure at each point and then calculate the relative removal rate at each point assuming that it is linearly proportional to the local pressure, as given by the Preston equation. One such model was developed by Warnock [11.38], and is utilized in the commercially available process simulator ATHENA [11.27]. Here the local polish rate, P_i, is given by

$$P_i \propto \frac{K_i A_i}{S_i} \tag{11.27}$$

The three terms in this expression take into account the increases or decreases in pressure depending on the local topography as well as the rigidity of the polishing pad and wafer. K_i is called the kinetic factor at point i and is a geometrical factor that takes into account sloped surfaces by calculating an effective vertical component of the horizontal polish rate. A_i is an accelerating factor for points which protrude above neighboring points, while S_i is a shading factor for points that are lower than neighboring points so that the pressure, and hence polishing rate, is decreased. The three factors are calculated at each point and depend on the geometrical relationship of the point to its neighboring points through various mathematical-geometrical expressions. They are also dependent on the rigidity of the polishing pad. Most of the constants in these expressions are empirically determined.

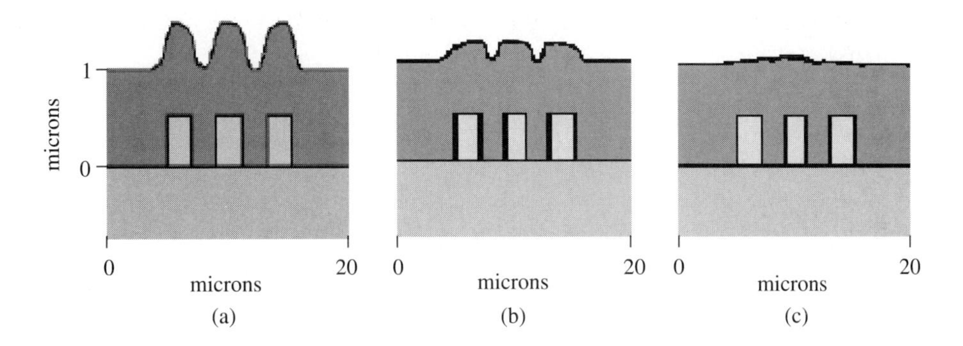

Figure 11–43 ATHENA [11.27] simulation of chemical-mechanical polishing of SiO_2 over Al lines: (a) before polishing; (b) after three minutes of polishing; (c) after six minutes of polishing. Nominal model parameter values are used, including *soft* = 25, *height.fac* = 0.02, *length.fac* = 4.2, and *kinetic.fac* = 10.

In Figure 11–43 an ATHENA simulation is illustrated. SiO_2 is deposited over three closely spaced Al lines, as shown in Figure 11–43(a). CMP is then simulated for three minutes and six minutes polishing time. The parameters used are given in the figure caption.

The *soft* parameter is the normalized polishing rate, equivalent to the proportionality constant implicit in Eq. (11.27). The *height.fac* parameter is the vertical deformation scale and measures how much the polishing pad will deform with respect to the height of the feature. The *length.fac* parameter is the horizontal deformation scale and describes the distance at which shadowing will be felt by a tall feature. Both are measures of the pad's flexibility and are used in calculating A_i and S_i at each point. The *kinetic.fac* parameter is just the proportionality factor for K_i. In Figure 11–43 we have used a nominal value for the height factor of 0.02 μm, where parts (b) and (c) show the profiles after three and six minutes, respectively. One can see that very good global planarization is achieved. In Figure 11–44, we repeat the simulations but use a smaller value for the height factor of 0.005 μm. This corresponds to a more rigid pad. One can see that even less rounding occurs, resulting in virtually perfect planarization here.

When the polishing rate is somewhat different for two different materials and the pad is not perfectly rigid, a phenomenon called "dishing" can occur. This would happen, for example, when CMP is done on metal for via formation in an oxide dielectric layer (see Figure 11–19). An overpolish, like an overetch, is done to ensure that all the metal is removed from on top of the oxide layer. But metals generally polish faster than oxide in the metal polishing slurry. (This would be worse for Al or Cu compared to W, since the latter is harder and etches slower.) Due to the semi-rigidity of the pad and the difference in polishing rates, this causes the metal in some places to be removed below the top of the oxide layer. The shape of the resulting metal surface is curved, or "dished." This is demonstrated in a simulation, shown in Figure 11–45. Having less selectivity between materials would reduce this, but would make it harder to stop the polishing without removing too much oxide. Having a more rigid pad would also help but could cause unequal polishing due to any bowing or thickness nonuniformities in the

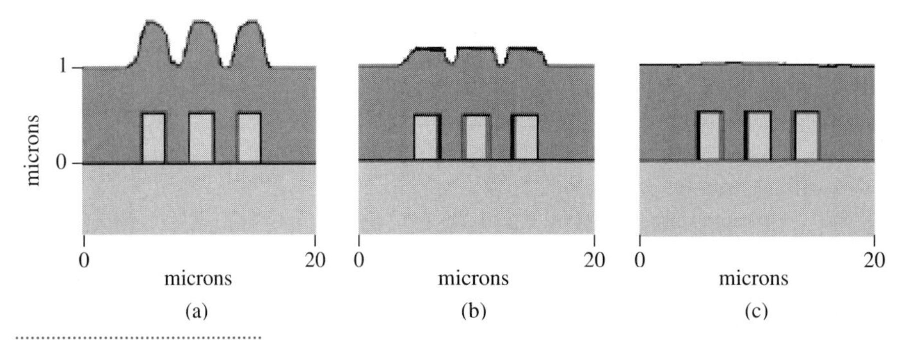

Figure 11–44 ATHENA [11.27] simulation of chemical-mechanical polishing of SiO_2 over Al lines: (a) before polishing; (b) after three minutes of polishing; (c) after six minutes of polishing. This time the *height.factor* = 0.005 μm, corresponding to a more rigid pad than in Figure 11–43.

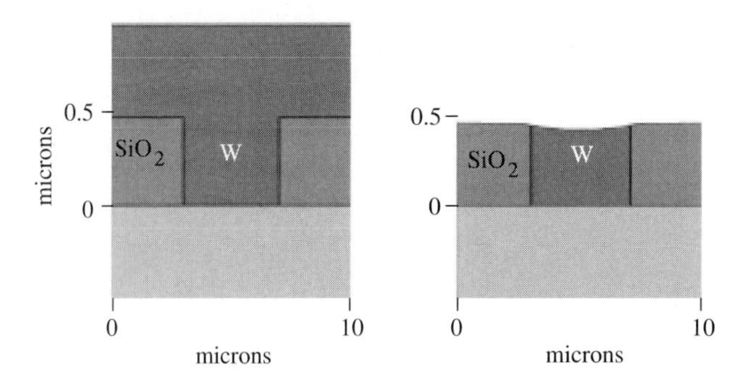

Figure 11–45 ATHENA [11.27] simulation of chemical-mechanical polishing of a tungsten via structure: Left, before polishing; right, after polishing. Due to the faster polishing of tungsten compared to silicon dioxide and the semirigid pad, "dishing" of the tungsten plug can result.

silicon substrate—the main reason that a nonrigid pad is used. Dishing in general is worse for wider structures, such as contact pads, but can still affect smaller features as well. Dishing effects can also result when an initially non-planar surface is polished and some "residue" of the original surface remains after polishing. Again this is a result of using semi-rigid pads.

One can also see in Figure 11–45 that the oxide layer is also slightly polished, especially at the edges. This is called "erosion" and refers to any excess removal of material during the over-polishing.

11.5.3 Reflow

Reflow is the smoothing of the topography of a layer during a thermal treatment. It is usually done intentionally, with the flow of the material causing sharp features to be flattened or smoothed, and valleys and trenches to be filled in. Reflow of PSG or BPSG layers is commonly done to smooth and planarize the first-level dielectric level. Reflow of metal layers such as Al, though not commonly done today, could be used to planarize and fill contacts and vias and is being investigated for future use. We also saw an example of photoresist reflow in Chapter 5 (Figure 5–50), where the purpose was similar. In that case reflow was used to minimize sharp edge features in the resist pattern associated with standing wave effects during the exposure process.

The reason reflow occurs is because it minimizes the total energy of the system. In this case, the surface energy of the structure is reduced. This occurs by minimizing the curvature of surface features. Surface energy arises because atoms at the surface are not completely surrounded by other atoms as they are below the surface, leading to either unsatisfied bonds with unpaired electrons (essentially broken bonds) or distorted bonds at the surface. (The unsatisfied bonds will in fact often stretch or distort in order to form some kind of bond to the neighboring atoms, but the energy is still higher than in the bulk due to the nonequilibrium interatomic spacings and angles.) A topography that is smooth has less surface area, and hence fewer unsatisfied or distorted bonds, than a topography that is rough and has steps, valleys, or sharp features. If the structure is heated and atoms have a chance to move around, they will preferentially move so that the surface becomes smoother and the surface energy is reduced. Another way to say this is that the atoms will move to regions of lower chemical potential, decreasing the total energy of the system.

W.W. Mullins [11.39, 11.40], who did much of the pioneering work on modeling reflow (and whose derivations we follow below), has mentioned four mechanisms by which atoms move at high temperatures to reduce the surface energy. These are surface diffusion, volume diffusion, evaporation/condensation, and viscous flow. Figure 11–46 illustrates these mechanisms. In the surface diffusion mechanism, atoms diffuse along the surface of the material to regions of lower chemical potential. New atoms are exposed, which can then diffuse along the surface. In the volume diffusion mechanism, the atoms move to reduce the surface energy by diffusing through the volume of the material. In the evaporation/condensation mechanism, the atoms preferentially evaporate from areas of high energy and preferentially condense in areas of low energy. For amorphous materials, viscous flow can also occur. This mechanism occurs when groups of atoms or

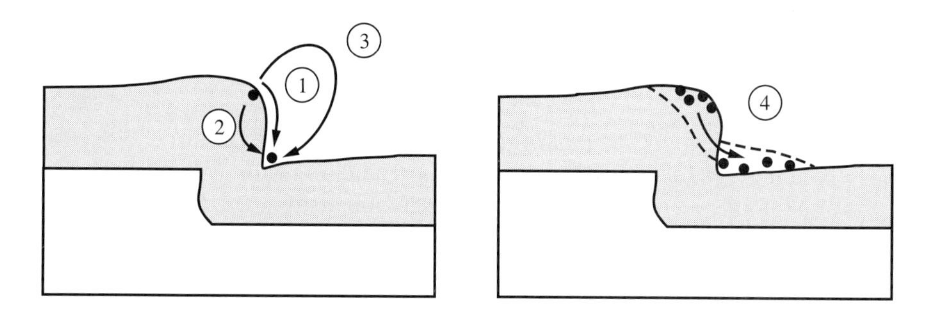

Figure 11–46 Illustration of high-temperature reflow mechanisms: (1) surface diffusion; (2) volume diffusion; (3) evaporation/condensation; and (4) viscous flow.

molecules in the solid slide past one another, breaking and reforming interatomic bonds, similar to motion in a liquid.

In all four cases the driving force is to reduce the total surface energy, and the forces involved in each are all proportional to γ_s, the surface energy per unit area (or surface tension). Which mechanism dominates for a given situation depends on the material, the temperature, and the topography. Mullins points out that for metals often the surface diffusion mechanism dominates near a metal's melting point for small feature sizes. Brain [11.41, 11.42], whose simulations we present below, argues that for thin film Cu reflow in integrated circuit structures, surface diffusion dominates over volume diffusion for normal reflow temperatures. For silicon dioxide reflow, viscous models are often used. Here we will concentrate mostly on surface diffusion models and show the results of simulating Cu reflow. At the end of this section we will show a simulation example of oxide reflow via viscous flow.

As with most models describing the motion of atoms or particles, we start with

$$v = M \cdot \text{Force} \tag{11.28}$$

in which v, the average velocity of a particle, equals M, the mobility of the particle, times the force acting on the particle. For the case of surface diffusion, v is the average velocity of a surface atom's diffusion along the surface. The force is determined from

$$\text{Force} = -\frac{\partial \mu}{\partial s} \tag{11.29}$$

where μ is the chemical potential, in this case the increase in chemical potential per atom that is transferred from a point of zero curvature to a point of curvature K on the surface. The unit length that it travels along the surface is s. The chemical potential is related to the curvature, K, and the per-area surface energy, γ_s, by

$$\mu(K) = K\gamma_s\Omega \tag{11.30}$$

where Ω is the atomic volume of the atom. Therefore

$$\text{Force} = -\frac{\partial \mu}{\partial s} = -\gamma_s\Omega\frac{\partial K}{\partial s} \tag{11.31}$$

This means that the higher that γ_s is for the material, the larger is the force acting on the atom. Also, the larger the gradient in K, the more force there is to move an atom from one point to another. The negative sign means that the force pushes the atom from an area of high K to an area of low K. As mentioned above, the curvature, K, is a measure of how "unsmooth" or how rounded the surface is at a point. In two dimensions, K is equal to the inverse of the radius of curvature, R, at that point

$$K = \frac{1}{R} \tag{11.32}$$

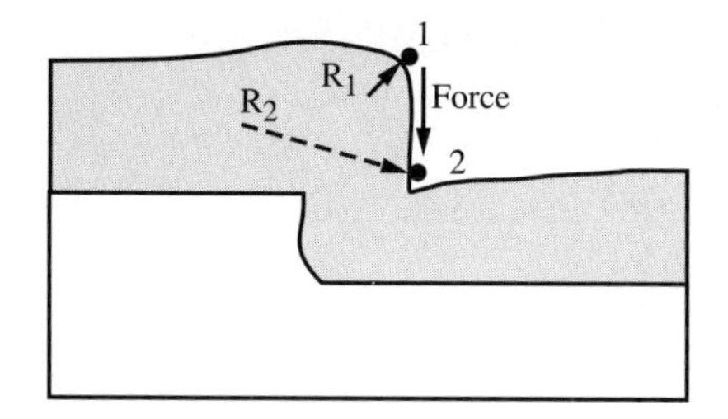

Figure 11–47 Illustration of differences in radii of curvature, R_1 and R_2 at points 1 and 2, respectively, causing a movement of an atom to a point of lower chemical potential (lower surface energy).

In three dimensions, K is given by

$$K = \frac{1}{R_x} + \frac{1}{R_y} \tag{11.33}$$

where R_x and R_y are radii of curvature in any two orthogonal directions. Figure 11–47 shows how the force acting on an atom due to surface energy minimization is in the direction away from a point of higher curvature to a point of lower curvature. R_1 is less than R_2 (so $K_1 > K_2$, and $\mu_1 > \mu_2$), so that the atom, given enough thermal energy, would move from point 1 toward point 2, causing a flattening of the topography. (In fact, right at the cusp the curvature is negative, as is the case for any concave surface, and the driving force to that point is even higher).

On an atomistic level, one can imagine that an atom sitting on the surface at a point of high curvature, such as point 1 in Figure 11–47, will be surrounded by and bonded to fewer atoms at equilibrium interatomic spacings than one at a point of low curvature, such as point 2 or even right in the cusp. Thus the atom will lower the total energy of the system by being at point 2. We will see a similar effect when we look at grain growth and see why grains grow "against" the curvature of the grain boundary to maximize the number of bonds and lower the total energy.

Substituting Eq. (11.31) into (11.38), and given that the mobility, M, is D_s/kT, where D_s is the surface diffusivity of the atoms, yields

$$\nu = -\frac{D_s}{kT}\gamma_s \Omega \frac{\partial K}{\partial s} \tag{11.34}$$

The surface current or surface flux of atoms, F_s (in atoms cm^{-1} sec^{-1}), equals

$$F_s = \nu \cdot \upsilon \tag{11.35}$$

where υ is the number of atoms per unit area, or the surface density. Therefore

$$F_s = -\frac{D_s}{kT}\gamma_s \Omega \upsilon \frac{\partial K}{\partial s} \tag{11.36}$$

One can see from this expression that a surface flux of atoms will occur along a surface down the curvature gradient, similar to diffusion down a concentration gradient.

Therefore atoms will move from a position of high curvature to low curvature, or from positive curvature to negative curvature.

Example Calculate the surface flux (F_s, in atoms cm^{-1} sec^{-1}) due to a surface curvature difference between points *a* and *b* for a copper film. The radius of curvature at point *a* is 0.5 μm, and the radius of curvature at point *b* is infinity (i.e., a flat surface). The two points are separated by a distance of 0.5 μm along the surface. Use the parameter values given in Table 11–8, with $T = 800$K. State which direction the atoms are moving (*a* to *b*, or *b* to *a*).

Answer The parameter values needed for Eq. (11.43) are

$T = 800\text{K}$

$D_s = 0.07 \exp(-0.82/kT)\ \text{cm}^2/\text{sec} = 0.07 \exp(-0.82/8.62 \times 10^{-5}\ \text{eV/K} / 800K)$
$= 4.80 \times 10^{-7}\ \text{cm}^2\ \text{sec}^{-1}$

$k = 1.381 \times 10^{-23}\ J/\text{K} = 1.381 \times 10^{-23}\ J/\text{K} \times 10^7\ \text{ergs}/J = 1.381 \times 10^{-16}\ \text{ergs/K}$

$\gamma_S = 1800\ \text{ergs cm}^{-2}; \Omega = 1.2 \times 10^{-23}\ \text{cm}^3; \upsilon = 1.43 \times 10^{15}\ \text{atoms cm}^{-2}$

$K_A = 1/R_A = 1/(0.5 \times 10^{-4}\ \text{cm}) = 2 \times 10^4\ \text{cm}^{-1}$

$K_B = 1/R_B = 1/\infty = 0\ \text{cm}^{-1}$

$s = 0.5\ \mu\text{m} = 0.5 \times 10^{-4}\text{cm}$

$$\frac{\partial K}{\partial s} = \frac{0 - 2 \times 10^4\ \text{cm}^{-1}}{0.5 \times 10^{-4}\ \text{cm}} = -4 \times 10^8\ \text{cm}^{-2}$$

Therefore

$$F_s\,(\text{from } a \text{ to } b) = -\frac{D_s}{kT}\gamma_s\,\Omega\upsilon\frac{\partial K}{\partial s}$$

$$= -\frac{4.80 \times 10^{-7}\ \text{cm}^2\ \text{sec}^{-1}}{1.38 \times 10^{-16}\ \text{ergs K}^{-1}\,800\text{K}}$$

$$\cdot\,(1800\ \text{ergs cm}^{-2})(1.2 \times 10^{-23}\ \text{cm}^3)(1.43 \times 10^{15}\ \text{atom cm}^{-2})(-4 \times 10^8\ \text{cm}^{-2})$$

$F_S = 5.4 \times 10^{10}$ atoms cm^{-1} sec^{-1} and the direction of the flux is from a (where the curvature is higher) to b (where the curvature is lower).

The negative of the change in surface current per change in s, $-\partial F_s/\partial s$, gives the increase is number of atoms per unit area per unit time for a given location. Multiplying this by the atomic volume, Ω, gives r_n, the speed of movement of the surface element along its normal (the "normal velocity"). Thus

$$r_n = \frac{D_s}{kT}\gamma_s\Omega^2\upsilon\frac{\partial^2 K}{\partial s^2} \tag{11.37}$$

Eq. (11.37) becomes the governing equation for the surface movement due to surface diffusion controlled reflow. This is usually abbreviated to

$$r_n = B\frac{\partial^2 K}{\partial s^2} \tag{11.38}$$

where

$$B = \frac{D_s}{kT}\gamma_s\Omega^2\upsilon \tag{11.39}$$

To model the reflow phenomenon, these equations can be applied at each point, at each time step using a finite element program. It is only by doing such simulations that one can see the net affect of the process on the topography and assess the validity of the model.

Such simulations have been done by R. Brain and colleagues [11.41, 11.42] for the reflow of Cu. As will be discussed in Section 11.6, Cu is being developed as a replacement for Al as the main interconnect metal in some applications due to its lower resistivity and better electromigration resistance. In order to improve the filling of contacts and vias with Cu, and to planarize the structure, a reflow of the Cu can be done. Like Al, this can be done either during the deposition of Cu itself, or afterwards in a separate anneal step.

Brain simulated the Cu reflow using the surface diffusion mechanism, that is, Eq. (11.39), using a finite element program to simulate the surface topography movement during an anneal. The surface diffusion mechanism was chosen after comparing relative rates for the other three mechanisms using typical literature values for the parameters. The parameter values Brain used are given in Table 11–8. The simulations of Cu reflow in trenches of various sizes are shown in Figure 11–48. The initial profile was taken from an actual as-deposited Cu film profile, with some asymmetry. For the widest trench, 1 μm wide, one can see that the trench gets filled in with the Cu during the course of the reflow anneal, and the topography becomes much smoother. For narrower trenches, hourglass shapes develop near the bottom of the trenches, with the sides thinning and Cu accumulating at the bottom. Also, Cu agglomerates at the top shoulders, producing overhangs. This illustrates how the geometry of the structure is very important for this process. For longer times, the Cu profile becomes smoother, even for the narrowest

Table 11–8 Cu reflow simulation parameters at 800K [11.42]

D_s	surface diffusivity	$0.07\exp\left(\frac{-0.82\text{ eV}}{kT}\right)\text{ cm}^2\text{ sec}^{-1}$
γ_s	surface energy per unit area	1800 ergs cm^{-2}
Ω	atomic volume	$1.2\times10^{-23}\text{ cm}^3$
υ	number of atoms per unit area, or surface density	$1.43\times10^{15}\text{ atoms cm}^{-2}$

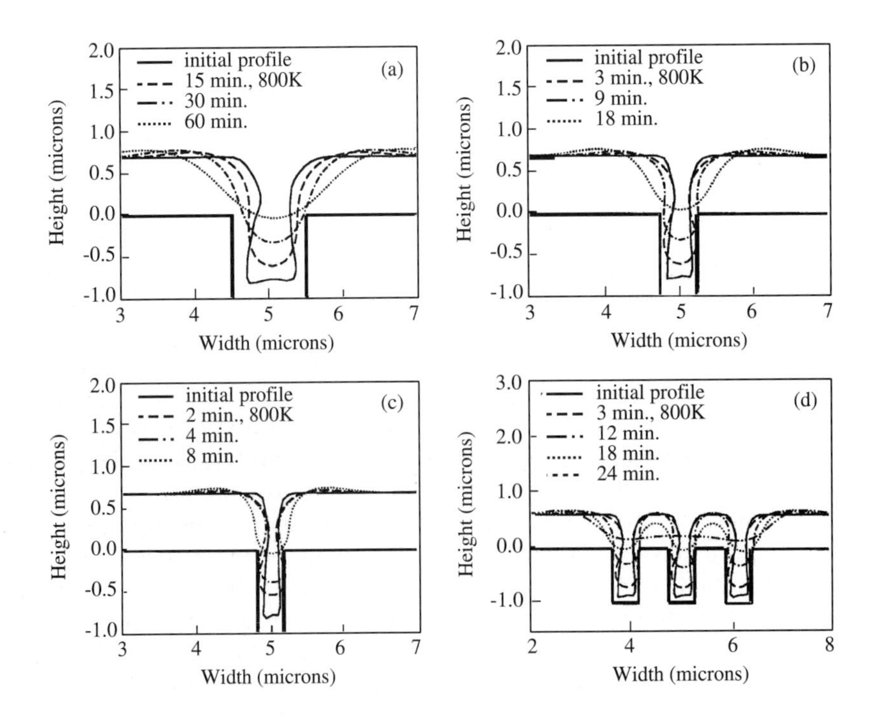

Figure 11–48 Cu reflow simulation for different trench sizes: (a) 1×1 μm; (b) 0.5×1 μm; (c) 0.33×1 μm; and (d) three 0.5×1 μm trenches spaced 0.5 μm apart. (After [11.41].)

structures simulated. For the multiple trenches, seen in Figure 11–48(d), similar behavior to the individual trenches is observed, indicating that the reflow process is more or less acting independently at each of the trenches and they do not interact.

However, experimental observations by Brain of this behavior indicate differences from the simulations shown above. For example, the extent of filling due to reflow varied along a trench, and this correlated to the position of grain boundaries. It was possible to qualitatively model this effect by placing the end of a grain boundary at various locations along the profile in a trench and including a grain boundary energy term, similar to the surface energy term. Also evident in the experimental observations were two prominent features: faceting of the Cu along crystallographic orientations during the reflow and nonsymmetric reflow behavior with agglomeration of Cu along one side wall and not the other. Brain proposed that these are due to an anisotropic surface energy. It was assumed in the initial simulations that γ_s is constant in all crystallographic directions. However, previous measurements indicate that this is not the case. The value of γ_s for Cu is not only different for the main directions (<100, 110, and 111>), but varies significantly for directions between those. Using this more advanced model for γ_s, Brain was able to better match actual experimental results [11.42].

Other types of reflow models are also used in simulators. In some situations, a viscous flow model, similar to that used in modeling 2D oxidation is more appropriate than the surface diffusion model described above. Viscous flow models are often used for silicon dioxide reflow, although surface diffusion models are sometimes used for computational convenience and can give similar results. An example using a viscous flow model is shown in Figure 11–49. In this case the ATHENA simulator is used to simulate PSG reflow over a polysilicon line. This situation might correspond to the first-level dielectric in Figure 11–1. In this case, much higher temperatures can be used for the reflow and the PSG behaves like a viscous incompressible fluid. Reducing surface energy is again the driving force for the reflow. The relevant model parameters in this case for the glass include the per area surface energy, the viscosity, Poisson's ratio, and Young's modulus. Default parameter values were used in the simulation in Figure 11–49.

The reflowing behavior can be very dependent on the specific surface structure and chemistry, such as any native oxide present on a metal film, which will affect the surface energy term. Reflow is also dependent on the bottom interface. Different underlayers can give different reflow results. This can be taken into account by including in the equations the interfacial energy between the reflowing layer and the layer beneath, analogous to the surface energy. For polycrystalline material, grain structure and grain growth also affect reflow. These are more difficult to include in the models.

11.5.4 Grain Growth

All of the materials used for interconnects are polycrystalline. This means that they are made up of regions of single-crystal material in which all the atoms line up perfectly in crystallographic positions, with the regions separated by grain boundaries. This is shown

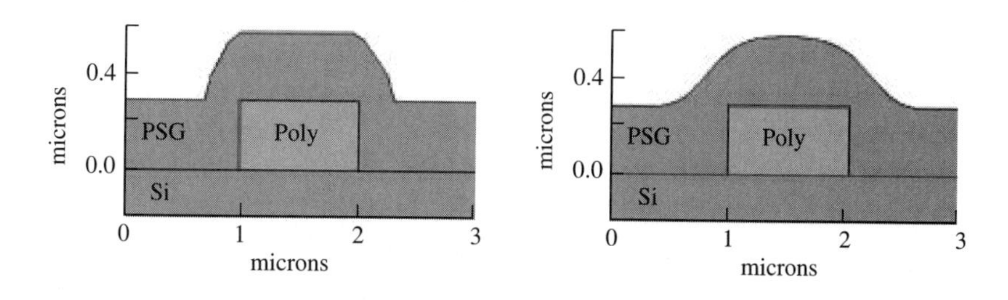

Figure 11–49 ATHENA [11.27] simulation of PSG reflow. The initial structure is on the left, the final structure on the right. The reflow heat cycle was 20 min at 950°C.

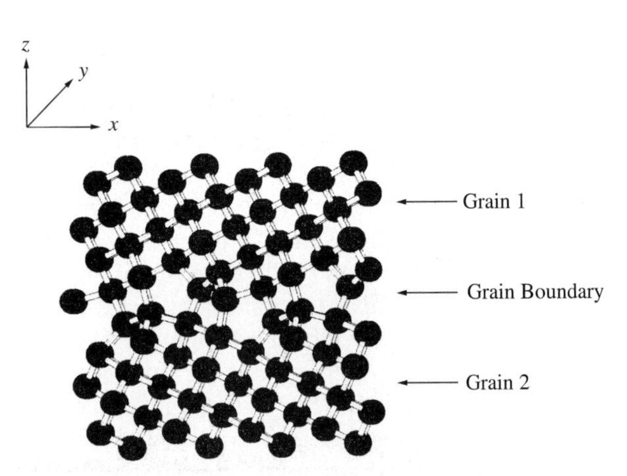

Figure 11–50 Illustration of two side-by-side grains of different crystallographic orientation. The region between them where the atoms cannot line up perfectly is called the grain boundary. This example is a low energy grain boundary in polysilicon. The structure is based on atomic-level calculations [11.43]. Reprinted with permission of the Electrochemical Society.

in Figure 11–50. Within the grains, the atoms are closely packed. Across the grain boundaries, however, the atoms cannot maintain the close packing because of the orientation differences between the grains. Therefore the grain boundary region is often less dense than the interior of the grain. In addition there may be unsatisfied or distorted bonds at the grain boundaries. Finally, charged defects may form preferentially at grain boundaries because these regions represent trapping sites for holes and electrons. These features give the grain boundary regions significantly different properties than the interior of the grains. We will describe simulations involving grains and grain boundaries in this section on grain growth, as well in the following sections on diffusion and electromigration.

When polycrystalline material is heated, grain growth usually occurs such that the average grain size increases. This is also termed grain coarsening. This occurs to minimize the energy of the system associated with grain boundaries. In fact, the lowest energy state of the material would be single-crystal without any grain boundaries at all. While this state is rarely achieved due to kinetic and metastability factors, this is the state the system is driven toward, with the average grain size getting larger. With silicides and polysilicon, especially when these films are deposited amorphous or highly doped, significant grain growth often occurs during annealing. With Al, less growth occurs because large grains are formed during its deposition due to its low melting point and high atomic mobility.

Grain growth is very similar to the process of reflow, as discussed in the previous section. The driving force is the minimization of the "surface" energy. In this case the "surface" is the surface of the grain, or the grain boundary. Since the grain boundaries have higher energies than the bulk or interior of the grains due to the unsatisfied or distorted bonds at the boundaries, the total energy of the system is decreased by reducing the relative amount of grain boundary area. This is done by increasing grain size. Locally, the driving force is the decrease in grain boundary curvature to increase bonding. Decreasing the local grain boundary curvature results in a shorter grain boundary length and a larger average grain size, leading to a lower total energy.

Thin film materials may be deposited as either polycrystalline or amorphous layers. In the latter case, single-crystal regions nucleate and grow during annealing, and eventually the grains will impinge on each other converting the material to polycrystalline material. Annealing of polycrystalline material will cause grain growth to occur to reduce the grain boundary energy. However, not all the grains can grow. For some grains to grow in a polycrystalline film, others must shrink. But overall, the average grain size will increase. We will now consider the models and equations for grain growth in polycrystalline thin films (assuming that the entire layer is composed of grains from the start) and then use simulations to help illustrate the key points. Excellent overview articles can be found in [11.44, 11.45].

We start with the same equation that we started with for reflow, relating the force on an object to its velocity, v:

$$v = M \cdot \text{Force} \tag{11.28}$$

The proportionality constant is the mobility, M. Here v refers to the velocity of the grain boundary, and F is the force on the grain boundary. Grain growth occurs by grain boundary movement or "migration" due to the force on each grain boundary.

To calculate the force on a grain boundary, we can use the fact that the force per area is equal to the pressure difference across the grain boundary between grains. The pressure difference, or force per area, is related to its curvature and surface energy [11.46]:

$$\text{Force per area} = \gamma_{gb} \cdot K \tag{11.40}$$

Here γ_{gb} is the grain boundary energy per unit area (in ergs cm^{-2}) and K is the curvature of the grain boundary at each point along it, defined such that the force is against the curvature, as we will discuss later.

The mobility, M, is usually related to the atomic diffusivity by $M = D/kT$, where D in this case would be the diffusivity of atoms across the grain boundary, or $D_{gb}^{\perp}$. However since we are dealing with force on a per unit area basis, we must multiply $D_{gb}^{\perp}/kT$ by A_{gb}, the atomic area of a grain boundary. (One could include the atomic area factor in the force term as was done in the reflow analysis or even leave it as a separate term, but we will include it at part of the mobility term to make it more consistent with treatments in the literature.) The atomic area of grain boundary, A_{gb}, can be written effectively as $\Omega/\lambda^{\perp}$ [11.47], where Ω is the atomic volume in cm^3, and $\lambda^{\perp}$ is the atomic jump distance across the grain boundary in cm (approximately an atomic diameter or lattice constant). A geometrical constant, g, dependent on the grain shape (and on the order of 0.5 to 3) may also be included in the area term. Combining $(D_{gb}^{\perp}/kT)$ and A_{gb} in the mobility term lumps terms such as $D_{gb}^{\perp}$, g, and $\lambda^{\perp}$ that are not easily determined into a single parameter. The grain boundary mobility, M_{gb}, is thus defined to be:

$$M_{gb} = \frac{D_{gb}^{\perp}}{kT} A_{gb} \tag{11.41}$$

and is in units of $\text{cm}^4\ \text{sec}^{-1}\ \text{erg}^{-1}$. One can think of the mobility in this form as being the grain boundary velocity per unit pressure [11.46], as opposed to the standard velocity per unit force definition of mobility. The velocity of the grain boundary is equal to the product of the mobility and force terms:

$$v = M_{gb}\,\gamma_{gb}\,K \tag{11.42}$$

Example If the grain boundary mobility, M_{gb}, is 1×10^{-15} cm^4 sec^{-1} erg^{-1}, the grain boundary energy is 300 ergs cm^{-2}, and the curvature, K, is 20 μm^{-1}, what is the grain boundary velocity due to the curvature?

Answer Substituting into Eq. (11.48), we have

$$v = M_{gb}\,\gamma_{gb}K = 1 \times 10^{-15}\ \text{cm}^4\ \text{sec}^{-1}\ \text{erg}^{-1} \cdot 300\ \text{ergs cm}^{-2} \cdot 20 \times 10^4\ \text{cm}^{-1}$$

$$= 6.0 \times 10^{-8}\ \text{cm sec}^{-1} = 0.6\ \text{nm sec}^{-1}$$

The diffusivity of atoms across the grain boundary, $D_{gb}^{\pm}$, follows an Arrhenius temperature dependence. The grain boundary mobility, M_{gb}, therefore depends strongly on temperature, with the exponential temperature dependence of the $D_{gb}^{\pm}$ term dominating over the T in the denominator of Eq. (11.41). In fact, the mobility is often written in the form

$$M_{gb} = M_o \exp\left(-\frac{E_a}{kT}\right) \tag{11.43}$$

where E_a is the activation for atomic diffusion across the grain boundary. M_o would include all the other terms in Eq. (11.41) except for the temperature dependence of $D_{gb}^{\pm}$. Therefore the grain boundary mobility and velocity, and thus the grain growth, increase with temperature.

For semiconductors, the diffusivity across the grain boundary and hence the mobility will also depend on the doping level of the polycrystalline material. This is possibly due to the increase in vacancy concentration with doping [11.48]. This is especially important for polysilicon, which shows a very strong dependence of grain growth on n-type doping concentration, and leads to a $(n/n_i)^m$ dependence of the mobility. The presence of nonelectrically active impurity atoms in a film, especially if they form precipitates, can decrease the grain boundary mobility due to mechanical pinning of the grain boundary. This is called the impurity or particle drag effect and is observed when Al is alloyed with Cu, with Cu precipitates slowing down the grain growth of the Al films.

In two dimensions the curvature, K, at each point is just the inverse of the radius of curvature, R, as given in Eq. (11.32), Shortly we will look at how the curvature varies around grains in a polycrystalline material, as well as the direction of the grain boundary velocity relative to the local curvature. For now, if we simply let the average radius of curvature of all the grain boundaries in a film be equal to the average grain size or radius, $\bar{r}$, we can derive approximate expressions for the average grain boundary velocity in a polycrystalline film as a function of grain size, and the average grain size as a function of time [11.49]. Letting $\bar{K}$ equal $1/\bar{r}$ in Eq. (11.42) gives the average velocity as

$$\bar{v} = M_{gb}\frac{\gamma_{gb}}{\bar{r}} \tag{11.44}$$

More rigorous derivations, including those based on the average curvature, those involving grain boundary energy per volume calculations, as well as statistical treatments based on grain size distributions, have all resulted in the same expression for the average velocity or growth rate [11.47, 11.50, 11.51, 11.52]. From this expression we see that as the average grain radius increases (and the grain boundary area per volume decreases), the average curvature gets smaller, leading to a lower driving force for growth and a lower average grain boundary velocity. Taking $\bar{v} = d\bar{r}/dt$ in Eq. (11.44) and integrating then leads to

$$\bar{r} = (\bar{r}_o^{\,2} + 2M_{gb}\gamma_{gb}t)^{1/2} \tag{11.45}$$

where $\bar{r}_o$ is the initial grain radius. Therefore the average grain radius, $\bar{r}$, by this model grows approximately as $t^{1/2}$, slowing down with time as the grain growth proceeds. This is quite close to experimental measurements for the average grain size during grain growth. It is also seen experimentally that the average grain size increases with anneal temperature. This is because M_{gb} increases exponentially with temperature.

Grains in a polycrystalline film cannot grow independently of one another—some grow larger while others grow smaller. This makes the analysis and modeling quite a bit more complicated. Figure 11–51 shows a large grain with many smaller grains around it. The curvature of each grain boundary is such that the boundaries are concave toward the smaller grains. This is so the grain boundaries meet at triple points with approximately equal angles of 120°. The movement of the grain boundaries occurs against the local curvature, and the larger grain grows at the expense of the smaller grain [11.53].

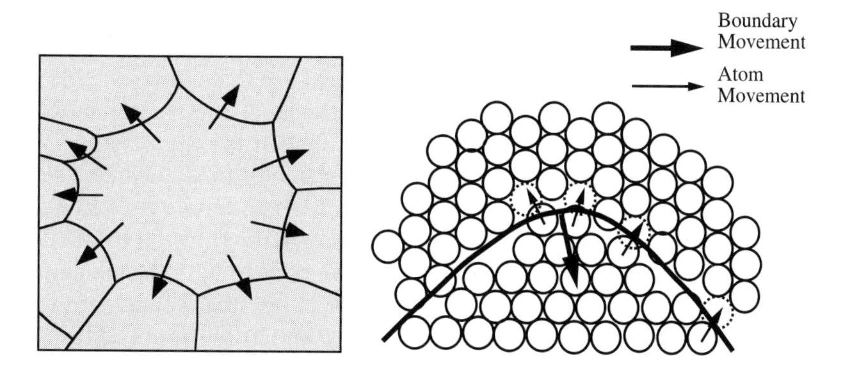

Figure 11–51 Left: Illustration of a large grain with smaller grains around it. The larger grains grow at the expense of smaller grains. Right: Atomic-level illustration of why movement of grain boundaries occurs against the curvature. (After [11.53].)

Figure 11–51 also shows what is happening on an atomistic scale and explains where the driving force originates. The atoms in the smaller grain, below, move across the grain boundary to the larger grain above. They are more stable there because, due to the curvature, they are surrounded by and bonded to more neighboring atoms at equilibrium interatomic spacings. This is very similar to the atomistic mechanism for reflow. In this way the grain boundary is shifted downward with the larger grain growing and the smaller grain shrinking. This movement reduces the curvature of the grain boundary and decreases the total grain boundary area. Eventually the smaller grains are annihilated.

M. Hillert [11.54] described this mathematically by using the idea of the critical size (used in dissolving and precipitating theory) with Eq. (11.42) for grain boundary movement to obtain

$$\frac{\partial r}{\partial t} = M_{gb}\,\gamma_{gb}\left(\frac{1}{r^{crit}} - \frac{1}{r}\right) \tag{11.46}$$

$\partial r/\partial t$ is the growth rate of an individual grain and r is the radius of the individual grain. Grains with a radius greater than r^{crit} will have a positive growth rate and grow, and grains with a radius smaller than r^{crit} will have a negative growth rate and shrink. What is r^{crit}? Because the sum of all $r\,\partial r/\partial t$ over all the grains must be zero in order to conserve the total size of the 2D system, it can be shown that r^{crit} must equal the average size or radius. Therefore Eq. (11.46) becomes:

$$\frac{\partial r}{\partial t} = M_{gb}\,\gamma_{gb}\left(\frac{1}{\bar{r}} - \frac{1}{r}\right) \tag{11.47}$$

Hillert also showed that these equations lead to an expression for the average grain size, growing as $t^{1/2}$, with an equation very similar to Eq. (11.44). The larger grains thus grow at the expense of the smaller grains, and the average grain size increases with time.

The above models and equations can be used to simulate simple grain growth, or "normal growth." This is in contrast to "abnormal" or "secondary" grain growth which we will briefly discuss later. Frost and colleagues [11.44, 11.55] have developed a two-dimensional computer simulation program for the growth of grains in a thin film polycrystalline layer after nucleation and growth to the polycrystalline state have occurred. Grain growth is modeled by calculating the local grain boundary velocity at each point. Figure 11–52 shows the simulation of normal grain growth using their program. In their algorithm, each grain boundary segment is described by a series of points. Triple points occur where three segments meet. The boundary segments move according to the local boundary velocity which is proportional to the local curvature, as given by Eq. (11.42). After each incremental movement of boundary segments, the triple points are shifted to locations at which the three boundary segment tangents meet at 120°. This sequence of boundary movement and triple point shifting is then continued throughout the simulation.

In Figure 11–52 one can clearly see the growth of grains, with the large grains growing at the expense of the smaller ones, with the latter eventually disappearing and the average grain size increasing with time. All this occurs in the simulation simply by having the grain boundary velocity proportional to the curvature at each point and by

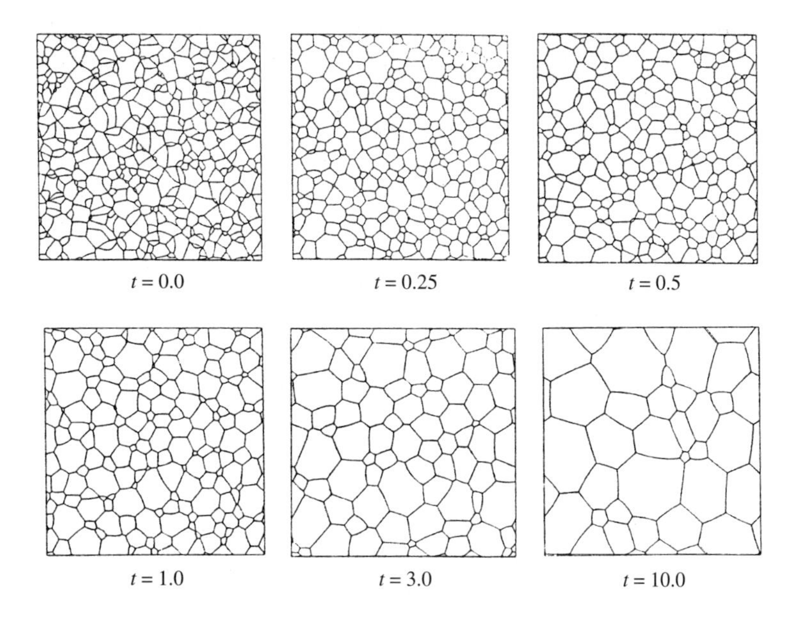

Figure 11–52 Simulation of normal grain growth. The initial structure contained approximately 400 grains of unit average area. τ is the normalized time [11.55]. Reprinted by permission of TMS.

maintaining equilibrium at the triple points. While the initial structure will affect the early growth, a steady-state regime is soon reached which is fairly independent of the initial conditions. In this steady-state regime, the average grain size is determined to be proportional to $t^{1/2}$ in these simulations, in agreement with our earlier treatment.

Walton, Frost, and Thompson [11.56] have also applied their simulations to grain growth in narrow lines, such as that encountered when annealing narrow lines of aluminum interconnects. The simulations are shown in Figure 11–53 which shows top views of a long, narrow film. The same simulation method and equations as above were used, with the additional boundary condition that all intersections between grain boundary segments and the line sidewalls must be at right angles. As the time steps progress, large grains grow again at the expense of smaller grains. Some of these traverse the entire line width, forming stable, rectangular "bamboo" segments. At intermediate times, one can see clusters of grains between the bamboo segments. These are relatively stable and are important in electromigration, as we shall see later. Eventually, though, they disappear and the final structure consists of rectangular bamboo grains of average length approximately 2.3 times the line width.

These simulations are two-dimensional and do not model what is happening in the z, or vertical, direction. This is often a reasonable approximation since many thin films have columnar structures. That is, the grains traverse the entire height of the film and the grain boundaries are constant in the z-direction. And those films that are not columnar as deposited often become columnar or near columnar during grain growth as the average grain size exceeds the film thickness. However, interfaces and surfaces—the boundaries in the third dimension—are still important in columnar structures.

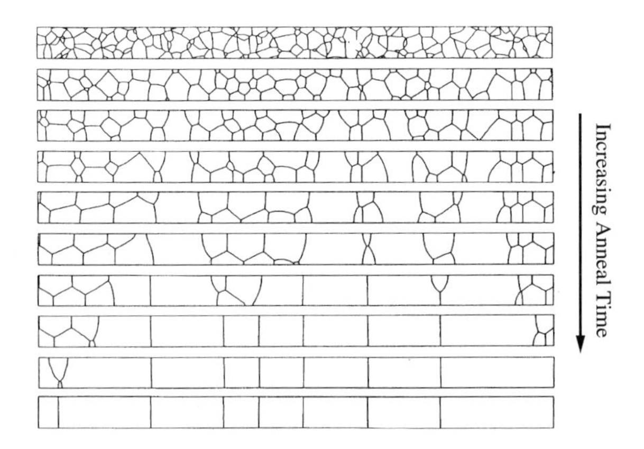

Figure 11–53 Simulation of grain growth within a strip. The grain growth leads to a bamboo structure where all the grains span the line [11.56]. Reprinted by permission of American Institute of Physics.

For many materials, normal grain growth of polycrystalline films proceeds until the average grain diameter is approximately two to three times the film thickness. At this point, normal grain growth stops, or "stagnates." This is believed to be due, at least partly, to a surface effect called grain boundary grooving, as proposed by Mullins [11.39]. Grooves form at the top surface where grain boundaries intersect the surface. This is due to the balancing of grain boundary and surface energies at that intersection. It is similar to triple points which form 120° angles, but this time they are in the vertical plane. Grooving occurs by surface diffusion of atoms in order to minimize the surface energy, such as we discussed in the reflow process, but now with the grain boundary energy also involved. If the force on the grain boundary due to its own curvature is not large enough to overcome the pinning force from the groove, then normal grain growth stops. This tends to occur when the grain diameter is approximately two to three times the film thickness [11.44]. In grain growth simulations, this effect has been included by setting the local grain boundary velocity to zero if the local curvature falls below a critical curvature [11.44].

It has been experimentally observed that the grain size distribution for a thin film that has undergone normal grain growth is often close to a lognormal distribution. A lognormal distribution means that if the natural log of the grain diameter, ln(d), is plotted against the fraction of grains within a range of sizes, a normal (that is, Gaussian) distribution curve results. This distribution is described by

$$f(d) = \frac{1}{\sigma_d \, d\sqrt{2\pi}} \exp\left[-\left(\frac{1}{\sigma_d\sqrt{2}} \ln\frac{d}{d_{50}}\right)^2\right] \tag{11.48}$$

where $f(d)$ is the fraction (in percent) of grains with diameter between d and Δd, d_{50} is the median grain diameter, and σ_d is the lognormal standard deviation, usually around 0.4.

An example is shown in Figure 11–54 in a variety of formats with $d_{50} = 1$ μm and $\sigma_d = 0.4$. In (a) the grain size is plotted on the x-axis, and the fraction (in percentage) of

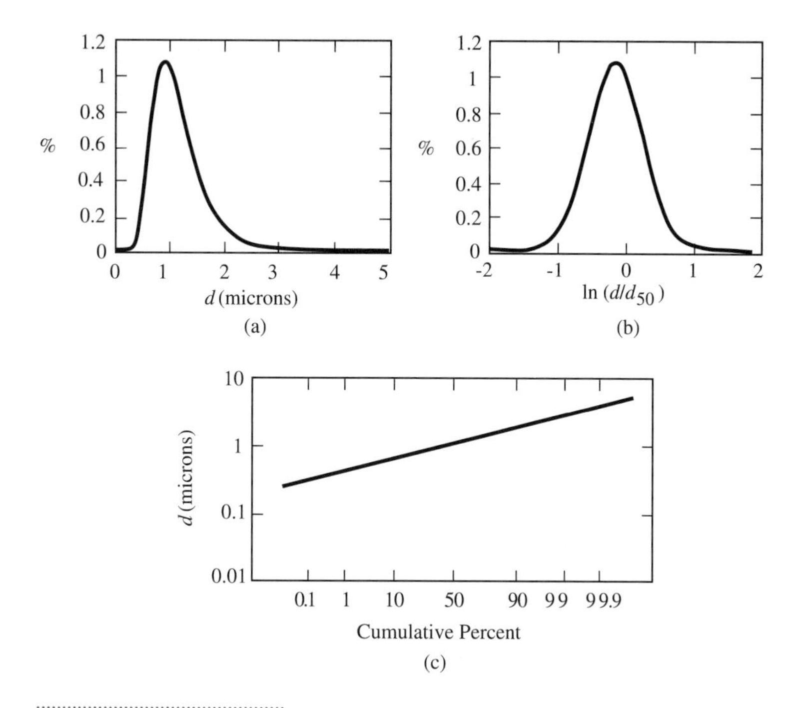

Figure 11–54 Theoretical grain size distribution [following Eq. (11.48) for a lognormal distribution, with median grain size, d_{50}, of 1 μm and σ_d of 0.4] plotted in a variety of formats: (a) percentage of grains with a given grain size, d, plotted versus d; (b) percentage of grains plotted versus $\ln(d/d_{50})$; (c) grain size (on a log scale) plotted versus the cumulative percent of those grains with size d or less.

the number of grains with that size is plotted on the y-axis. The distribution is somewhat skewed in this plot format. (The average grain size for this distribution is 1.08 μm, and the peak of the curve occurs at 0.85 μm). If we plot the fraction of grains with size d versus $\ln(d/d_{50})$, as in (b), we see a normal distribution. Finally we plot d versus the cumulative percentage of grains of size d or less (calculated by integrating the percent versus d curve up to each d value) on a lognormal scale. This shows a straight line, with the 50 percent cumulative percent being at $d = 1$ μm, as expected since that was selected as the median grain size. The slope of the curve is directly related to σ_d of the distribution.

After the normal grain growth stagnates, some grains do sometimes continue to grow. This is due to abnormal or secondary growth. If this happens, the few secondary grains grow quite rapidly until they impinge on one another and eventually all the normal grains are consumed. One reason for this is due to the fact that grains with different crystallographic orientations may have different surface energies. Those grains with lower surface energies will grow faster than, and preferentially to, grains with higher surface energies. When the grain size is on the order of the film thickness (when normal growth starts to stagnate), then the surface effects will become significant compared to the grain boundary effects, and secondary growth becomes important.

When secondary grain growth occurs, the grain size distribution will show a bimodal distribution, with two peaks in plots as in Figure 11–54(a). The first peak corresponds to the normal growth grains and the second peak corresponds to the secondary growth grains with their larger average grain size. Eventually when the secondary grains completely consume the normal grains, the distribution becomes a standard lognormal distribution again, with just the second peak.

11.5.5 Diffusion in Polycrystalline Materials

Diffusion can be important in back-end processes. For examples, dopants can diffuse from the source/drain regions into polycrystalline silicide layers, depleting the dopants in the silicon and degrading the contact resistance. Another important example is host (or matrix) atom diffusion, such as when Al diffuses during electromigration, reflow, and grain growth. In Chapter 7 we looked at diffusion of dopants in single-crystal silicon quite extensively. Most interconnect materials are polycrystalline.

The key to understanding diffusion in polycrystalline materials is the presence of grain boundaries and the fast diffusion paths that they provide. Figure 11–50 illustrated what a grain boundary might look like at the atomic scale, and one can imagine in a simple way why diffusion of atoms might occur more quickly along grain boundaries. These regions provide more open space, letting atoms move more quickly. Atoms in these regions also tend to be less tightly bound, with unsatisfied or stretched bonds, allowing for faster movement. Calculations show that grain boundaries provide low-energy sites for vacancy formation; therefore one would expect a high concentration of vacancies along grain boundaries. This also leads to faster diffusion as compared to diffusion in the interior of the grain. While the exact mechanisms and reasons are not completely understood, the diffusion along grain boundaries is generally faster and the activation energy lower than in the lattice. The mathematical models for diffusion in polycrystalline materials are based on such a picture of a material containing a mixture of fast diffusion paths along the grain boundaries and slow diffusion paths through the lattice, or the interior or the grains.

Modeling diffusion in polycrystalline materials follows the same basic approach used in single-crystal material, except that in the two types of regions—grain boundary and lattice—the diffusion coefficients are different. In addition, the atoms can move between the two regions depending on their local concentration and the segregation coefficient and transfer coefficient between the grain boundaries and lattice regions. The flux equations for any species in each path are simply

$$F_{gb} = -D_{gb}\left(\frac{\partial C}{\partial x}\right)_{gb} \tag{11.49}$$

$$F_{\ell} = -D_{\ell}\left(\frac{\partial C}{\partial x}\right)_{\ell} \tag{11.50}$$

where D_{gb} refers to the diffusivity in, or along, the grain boundary, and D_{ℓ} is the diffusivity through the lattice, or interior of the grain. These are just forms of Fick's first law, as presented in Chapter 7, for different regions of material.

The complexity in modeling diffusion in polycrystalline materials and variations in modeling techniques arise from the determination of how much transport occurs through each of the two types of regions. This depends on the geometrical layout of the grains, which may not be uniform or regular. It may also change with time because of grain growth. Various levels of mathematical treatment of diffusion in polycrystalline materials have been developed based on assumptions of the geometrical layout.

The simplest model assumes that there is an effective diffusion coefficient for a species that describes the net diffusion through a polycrystalline material. This D_{eff} is just the sum of the diffusion coefficients in each of the two types of region—grain boundary and lattice—each scaled by the relative cross sectional area of each region. The larger the relative cross sectional area of the region, the more atoms transport through that region, and the more weight is given to the diffusion coefficient of that region. Consider diffusion through a structure with square columnar grains of length ℓ, and grain boundary thickness δ, as shown in Figure 11–55, with $\ell >> \delta$. The cross sectional area of each grain is ℓ^2 and the area of the grain boundary (per unit grain), is $\ell \cdot \delta$. The ratio of grain boundary area to grain or lattice area is thus:

$$\frac{\text{gb area}}{\text{grain area}} = \frac{\ell\delta}{\ell^2} = \frac{\delta}{\ell} \tag{11.51}$$

The effective diffusion coefficient in this model is therefore

$$D_{\text{eff}} = \left(1 - \frac{d}{\ell}\right)D_\ell + \frac{\delta}{\ell}D_{\text{gb}} \approx D_\ell + \frac{\delta}{\ell}D_{\text{gb}} \tag{11.52}$$

Diffusion through the material is described simply by Fick's law:

$$F_{\text{net}} = -D_{\text{eff}}\nabla C \tag{11.53}$$

where F_{net} is the net or total flux through the material, D_{eff} is the diffusion coefficient described by Eq. (11.52), and C is the average concentration over both grain and grain boundary regions. This approach can give only a first-order estimate of diffusion profiles.

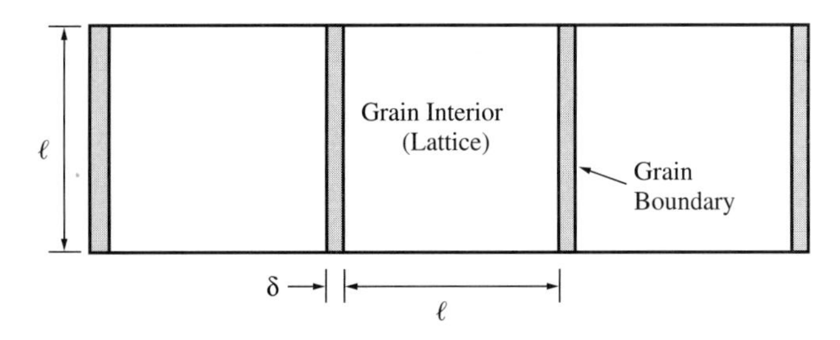

Figure 11–55 Simple representation of grains and grain boundary regions. This is a cross section of a columnar polycrystalline film with square grains. ℓ is the grain width and length and δ is the grain boundary width with $\ell >> \delta$. Diffusion from bottom to top is considered.

Example A columnar polycrystalline material has an average grain size, ℓ, of 0.1 μm and a grain boundary thickness, δ, of 0.001 μm. An impurity atom has a lattice diffusivity, D_ℓ, of 5.0×10^{-14} cm^2 sec^{-1}, and a grain boundary diffusivity, D_{gb}, of 5.0×10^{-11} cm^2 sec^{-1}. What is the effective diffusion coefficient?

Answer Using Eq. (11.52),

$$D_{eff} = D_\ell + \frac{\delta}{\ell} D_{gb} = 5.0 \times 10^{-14}\ \text{cm}^2\ \text{sec}^{-1} + \frac{0.001\ \mu\text{m}}{0.1\ \mu\text{m}} 5.0 \times 10^{-11}\ \text{cm}^2\ \text{sec}^{-1}$$

$$= 5 \times 10^{-14}\ \text{cm}^2\ \text{sec}^{-1} + 5 \times 10^{-13}\ \text{cm}^2\ \text{sec}^{-1} = 5.5 \times 10^{-13}\ \text{cm}^2\ \text{sec}^{-1}$$

Generally it is difficult to separate out the D_{gb} and δ terms from the $D_{gb}\delta$ product, the product equaling 5.0×10^{-18} cm^3 sec^{-1} in this example. One sees that the lattice diffusion adds only about 10% to the effective diffusivity.

Models much beyond this level of complexity require computer simulation techniques. We can illustrate some key ideas using TAURUS, a very flexible process and device simulator [11.28]. We assume two regions in the polycrystalline thin film, grain boundaries and grain interiors. We also assume a simple grain structure with two grains separated by a grain boundary perpendicular to the substrate, as shown in Figure 11–56(a). The grain boundary width is 0.03 μm, which is wider than actual grain boundaries but still illustrates the concepts we wish to demonstrate. We then use TAURUS to solve the coupled diffusion/continuity equations at each point in the mesh. Transport across the interior/grain boundary region is governed by simple segregation, with $k_o = C_{gb}/C_\ell$ equal to 1 in most cases. We do not include any grain boundary motion due to grain growth.

In Figure 11–56(a), the substrate below the two grains is doped at 1×10^{21} cm^{-3}. The segregation coefficient between the substrate and both the grain interior and grain boundary region is set to 100. This keeps the substrate/thin film interface concentration at 1×10^{19} cm^{-3} throughout the diffusion time. The assumed diffusivities in the grain boundary and grain interiors are given in the figure caption, with the diffusivity in the grain boundary 100 times larger than that in the grain interiors in (a). The simulation results after a 30-minute anneal are shown in the figure. (The temperature is not important in these simulations since we assume temperature-independent diffusivities here, although of course we could use Arrhenius expressions.) One can see that the dopant has diffused both up through the grain and up through the grain boundary region—much further in the latter case. One can also see where the dopant has diffused sideways from the grain boundary region into the grain interiors.

Figure 11–56(b) shows a second example in which the diffusion in the grain interior, or lattice, is only a factor of 10 slower than in the grain boundaries. More diffusion in the grains is seen, and more dopant spills into the grains from the grain boundary on

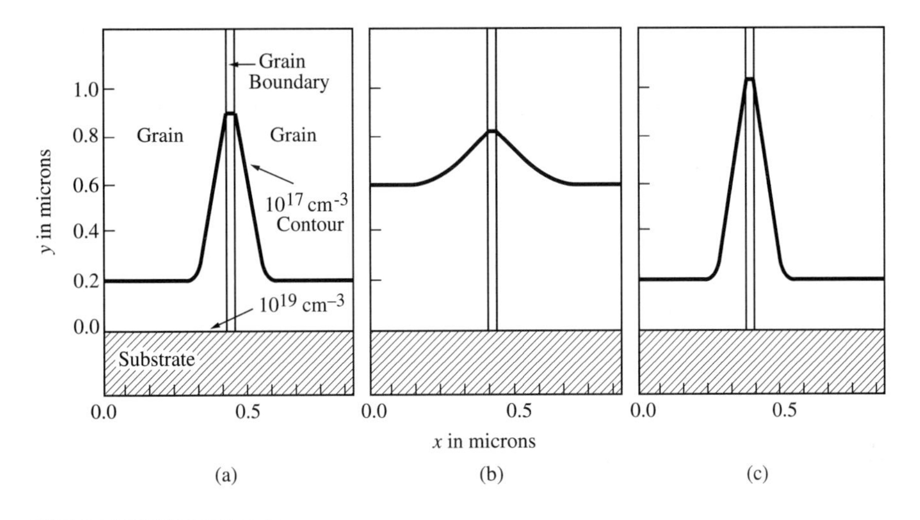

Figure 11–56 TAURUS [11.28] simulations of polycrystalline diffusion where a concentration of 1×10^{19} cm^{-3} is maintained at $y = 0$. Shown is the 1×10^{17} cm^{-3} contour after a 30 minute anneal in each case. (a) The diffusivities in the grains (or lattice) and grain boundary are 1×10^{-14} and 1×10^{-12} cm^2 sec^{-1}, respectively. (b) The diffusivity in the grains is increased to 1×10^{-13} cm^2 sec^{-1}, keeping the diffusivity in the grain boundary at 1×10^{-12} cm^2 sec^{-1}. (c) Same diffusivities as in (a), but the segregation coefficient between the grain boundary and grains is increased from 1 to 1.5.

the sides. Since the activation energy for lattice diffusion is usually greater than that of grain boundary diffusion, the relative importance of lattice diffusion increases with temperature and Figure 11–56(b) might be more representative of a high-temperature diffusion step.

If the segregation coefficient, k_o, between the grain boundary and grain regions is changed, the diffusion profiles change as well. Figure 11–56(c) shows the result when $k_o(\mathrm{gb}/\ell)$ is 1.5 instead of 1 for the same diffusion coefficients as in Figure 11–56(a). Compared to Figure 11–56(a), one sees that the dopant preferentially stays in the grain boundary and therefore diffuses further since the diffusivity in the grain boundary is higher. Changing the segregation coefficient between the grain boundary region and grain region thus has similar effects to changing the relative diffusivities.

It is also possible to include grain growth in these models by merging the models described in Section 11.5.4 with the grain boundary and grain diffusion ideas described here. This is more complex and generally requires numerical simulation.

11.5.6 Electromigration

The phenomenon of electromigration is one of the biggest problems in interconnect technology. Electromigration is the movement of atoms due to the presence of an electrical force. When high currents pass through relatively soft polycrystalline metals with high-atomic diffusivities, such as Al, the electrons can transfer some of their momentum to the metal atoms causing them to move. The force on the atoms is found to be

$$\text{Force} = Z^* q\varepsilon = Z^* q\rho J \tag{11.54}$$

Z^* is the effective ion valence or charge number, a negative number for electron conductors on the order of -4 to -8 for Al and usually empirically determined for polycrystalline films. ε is the electric field due to the current, ρ is the electrical resistivity of the metal, and J is the current density (A cm^{-2}). The atomic flux induced by the current (in the direction of the electron flow, or opposite to the current) equals the force times the mobility times the concentration and is thus

$$F = \frac{DC}{kT} Z^* q\varepsilon = \frac{DC}{kT} Z^* q\rho J \tag{11.55}$$

where D is the atomic diffusivity and C is the atomic concentration. D is related to the motion of atoms usually via vacancy mechanisms. It is thermally activated and of the form

$$D = D_0 \exp\left(-\frac{E_A}{kT}\right) \tag{11.56}$$

so that E_A is the activation energy for diffusion. The atomic diffusivity may also be dependent on the local stress level [11.57] but for simplicity it is often assumed that it is constant with stress. The diffusion of the metal atoms (or vacancies in the opposite direction) in polycrystalline materials predominately occurs along grain boundaries, which we have seen usually have much higher diffusivities than the grain lattice. Therefore D in the above equations usually relates to atomic or vacancy diffusion through the grain boundaries. (Surface and interface diffusion may also be important, but grain boundary diffusion often plays a dominant role, particularly for Al.) One would expect that grain structure, including grain size and the location of grain boundaries, would be important in electromigration behavior.

This current-induced diffusion can lead to void and hillock formation, as illustrated earlier in Figure 11–11. Void formation can lead to an open circuit, while a hillock which extends to make contact with another interconnect line can lead to a short circuit. Either of these will lead to circuit failure. As we discussed in Section 11.4.2, the failure rate is often modeled empirically, with the following equation for the Median Time To Failure (MTTF) repeated here:

$$\text{MTTF} = AJ^{-n} \exp\left(\frac{E_A}{kT}\right) \tag{11.18}$$

where J is the current density, n is typically close to 2, and A is a constant which depends on film structure (grain size, etc.) and processing. E_A is the activation energy for electromigration and is often associated with Al grain boundary diffusion as above; its value ranges from 0.5 to 0.8 eV (the activation energy of lattice diffusion in bulk Al films is about 1.4 eV). The parameters for this equation are usually determined under accelerated testing conditions—higher than usual current and temperature. Accelerated testing is also used to predict when shorts or opens occur in the interconnect lines or when the line resistance reaches a critical value.

The original theoretical basis for Eq. (11.18), especially in regard to the n dependence of the current density, was provided by Black [11.58], and the equation is often referred to as Black's equation. He argued that n should equal 2 based on the momentum exchange between the moving electrons and the metal atoms. Other justifications for n being equal to 2, or at least being in the range of 1–3, have been based on Joule heating considerations, critical vacancy [11.59] or stress [11.60] levels, and on void nucleation and growth models [11.61].

Many models, some rather empirical like Eq. (11.18) and some much more physically based, have been developed to explain and predict electromigration failure behavior, from the atomic level up to the circuit level. Here we will describe a model that explains how interconnect reliability in Al lines depends strongly on grain structure and interconnect dimensions, as well as current density and stress properties, largely following the work of Thompson and colleagues [11.62, 11.63, 11.64, 11.65, 11.66] and Korhonen and colleagues [11.60, 11.67]. This will also serve to tie together many of the concepts described earlier in this chapter.

A very interesting result occurs if Al electromigration failure, in terms of MTTF, is measured as a function of interconnect line width, w. As w decreases to a certain value while keeping all the other parameters and conditions constant, the time to failure decreases. But then as the line width decreases further, the MTTF bottoms out and then increases. The median time to failure can get quite high for narrow lines, which is a positive result for scaling. In fact, the same behavior is seen if MTTF is measured not just as a function of line width, but also of line width divided by the average grain size of the line, or w/d. As w/d decreases, the MTTF decreases. But then at some point—somewhere below w/d equaling one—the MTTF goes way up for small values of w/d. This is shown conceptually in Figure 11–57. So if the line width is kept constant, we see a strong relationship between MTTF and grain size, but it is not a simple relationship. Why does this occur?

As the line width decreases, one might expect that there is more chance for a void to span across the whole line resulting in an increase in line resistance or open circuit. This results in a lower MTTF as w decreases while keeping d constant but would not result in a higher MTTF as w is decreased further. Since electromigration occurs via diffusion along grain boundaries, one might expect that as $1/d$ decreases (i.e., the grain size increases), the metal diffusion would decrease since there are fewer fast diffusion paths available. This would result in a higher MTTF as $1/d$ decreases. These two trends in w

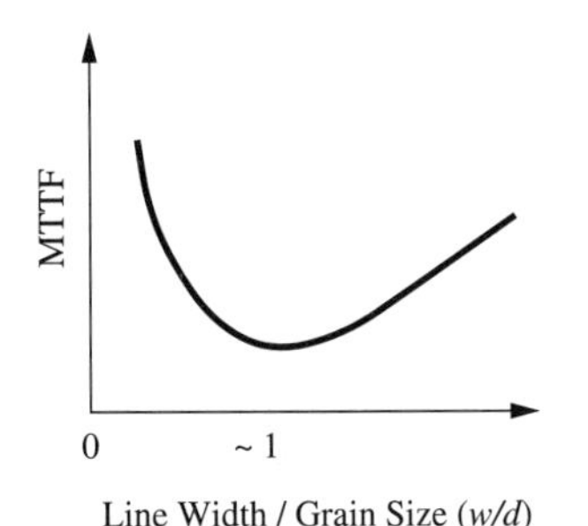

Figure 11–57 Observed relationship between Median Time To Failure (MTTF) due to electromigration versus the ratio of line width to grain size.

and $1/d$ would both be fairly linear relationships, yet in opposite directions. So when combining them, one would conjecture that the MTTF should be fairly independent of w/d. How do we then explain this behavior where the MTTF goes down and then goes up quite rapidly as w/d decreases? We start by going back to the grain growth simulations by Frost's and Thompson's groups that we presented in Section 11.5.4.

In Figure 11–52 we showed the simulation results of Frost and colleagues [11.44, 11.55] for the grain structure after grain growth in a polycrystalline layer. Figure 11–58 shows what happens to a blanket film if it is etched into straight lines of various widths. Shown are top views of lines of various values of w/d_{50} ranging from 1.30 down to 0.31. Some important features are noticed. For the narrowest line ($w/d_{50} = 0.31$), the structure is near-bamboo. When the width of the film and the median grain diameter are about the same (at $w/d_{50} = 1.30$ for example), grains that span the entire width are present. One such spanning grain is seen near the right side in the top line. For very wide lines ($w/d_{50} >> 1.30$ for example), no spanning grains would be present.

These spanning grains greatly affect electromigration behavior. Since electromigration occurs primarily by atomic diffusion along grain boundaries, the spanning grains define regions of atomic flux divergence. Figure 11–59 illustrates this. The flux of atoms will be from left to right in this case due to the electrons flowing left to right, or the current flowing right to left. This atomic flux will be greater in areas where there are no spanning grains due to the presence of grain boundaries there, and less or zero in the area of the spanning grain where there are no grain boundaries, as indicated in the figure. This results in a divergence of flux at the ends of each polygranular cluster, points A and B in the figure. Atoms will diffuse from point A to point B. But few atoms will diffuse to point A or out of point B. This means that metal atoms will be depleted at point A and will build up at point B. For lines that are wide enough so that there are no spanning grains, the only divergence of flux would occur at the ends of the lines. As long as the ends are large areas, such as bonding pads or large contact overlaps, they would not be affected very much by a depletion or buildup of material. (Although when the

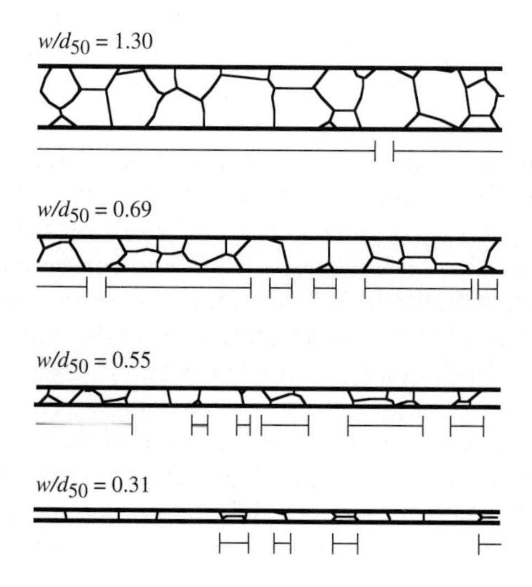

Figure 11–58 Grain structure in lines (top view) after patterning a blanket film, taking random strips of various widths so that w/d_{50} ranges from 1.30 down to 0.31 (w is the line width and d_{50} is the average grain size in the blanket film). Polygranular clusters (the regions between grains that span the entire line) are identified by the line segments below each line. One can see that as w/d_{50} decreases, the number of spanning grains increases and the average length of polygranular clusters decreases. (After [11.64])

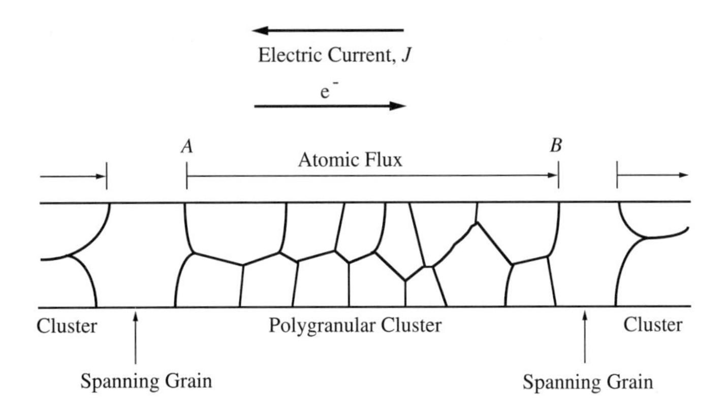

Figure 11–59 Illustration of polygranular cluster, the region between spanning grains. It is in these regions that the Al diffusion is high due to the high-diffusivity paths along the grain boundaries. A divergence of atomic flux will occur at the ends of polygranular clusters, causing metal atom depletion at point A and metal atom buildup at point B. (After [11.68].)

line ends in a tungsten via with a small contact overlap, problems can occur there, and electromigration failures at these points have become more important recently.) But in narrow lines where spanning grains are present, the depletion and buildup can lead to void and hillock formation at the ends of each spanning grain, ultimately leading to interconnect failure. Figure 11–12 showed an example of this.

The regions between the spanning grains are termed "polygranular clusters," since they contain multiple, not single, grains across the width at each point. The regions of polygranular clusters are indicated on the simulated lines in Figure 11–58. One can see that the number of spanning grains increases, and hence the average length of the polygranular clusters decreases, as the w/d_{50} value decreases. One might then expect that as the w/d_{50} ratio decreases, the chance of electromigration would get higher due to the increasing spanning grains and decrease the MTTF. It does, explaining one part of the w/d_{50} versus MTTF behavior. But then something else comes into play.

The additional effect is a back flux of atoms that opposes the forward flux. This back flux is due to a stress gradient that occurs due to the depletion and buildup of metal atoms at the flux divergence points. Figure 11–60 illustrates this. When the metal atoms diffuse due to the electromigration force, they get depleted at the start of a polygranular cluster region and build up at the end of the region. Because the metal line is constrained within the encapsulating dielectric materials, this creates a tensile stress at the start (point A in Figures 11–59 and 11–60) and a compressive stress at the end (point B). A stress gradient or field results that induces a back flux of the atoms from point B to point A. The excess atoms do not want to be where there is a compressive stress but would rather be where they are depleted. Therefore there is a flux term that opposes the original electromigration flux due to the stress gradient. (This is similar to an n/p junction in a semiconductor. The electrons and holes initially diffuse due to concentration gradients in the two carriers, but an electric field develops which wants to pull them

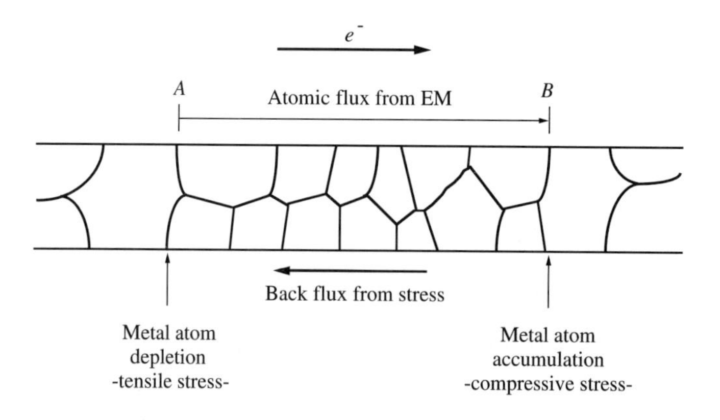

Figure 11–60 Polygranular cluster region showing stress buildup due to depletion and accumulation of the metal atoms at the ends of the region. This stress causes a back flux of the metal atoms which opposes the flux due to electromigration. (After [11.68].)

back. Ultimately a steady state is reached where the two fluxes balance each other.) The net flux due to these two opposing fluxes is now

$$F = \frac{DC}{kT}\left(Z^* q\rho J + \Omega \frac{\partial \sigma}{\partial x}\right) \tag{11.57}$$

where Ω is the atomic volume of the metal atom and σ is the stress, normal to the grain boundary. The first term in the equation is the original electromigration flux and the second term is due to the stress gradient and acts in the opposite direction.

We can solve for the steady-state condition where the net flux becomes zero and see what the stress, σ, is for that condition. To do this we set $F = 0$ in Eq. (11.57), leading to

$$\frac{\partial \sigma}{\partial x} = \frac{-Z^* q\rho J}{\Omega} \tag{11.58}$$

Letting $G = Z^* q\rho J/\Omega$, and integrating Eq. (11.58) gives

$$\sigma = -Gx + C \tag{11.59}$$

where C is the integration constant. If we assume that the stress gradient is symmetric around the center of the polygranular cluster segment of length L_p such that $\sigma = 0$ at $x = L_p/2$, we can solve for the constant, and the steady-state solution for the stress becomes

$$\sigma = G\left(\frac{L_p}{2} - x\right) = GL_p\left(\frac{1}{2} - \frac{x}{L_p}\right) \tag{11.60}$$

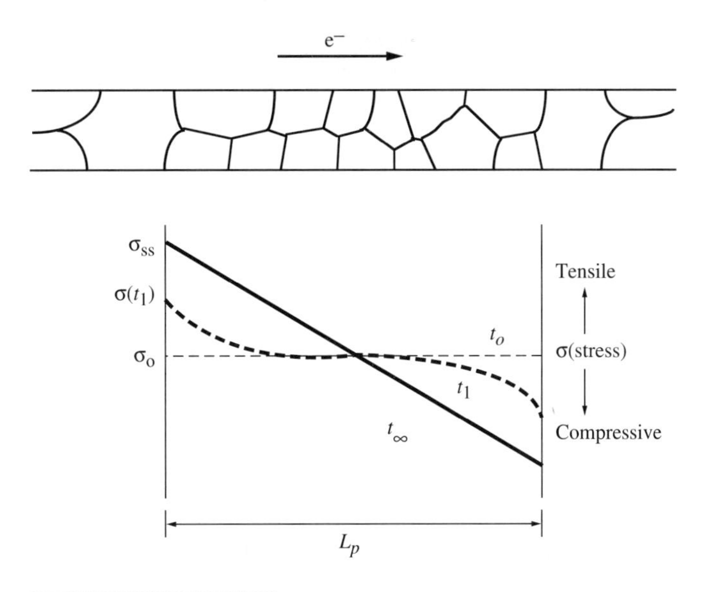

Figure 11–61 Schematic illustration of buildup of stress within polygranular cluster with time due to electromigration. In the bottom graph, stress (σ) is plotted versus distance along the cluster of length L_p for various times. Positive stress is tensile stress, and negative stress is compressive stress. Eventually (as $t \rightarrow t_\infty$), a steady-state is approached where the forward flux is equal to the backward flux due to stress. (After [11.68].)

This steady-state solution is shown in Figure 11–61.

Thus the flux due to electromigration causes depletion and accumulation of metal at the two ends of polygranular clusters, or the ends of lines in the extreme case. Stresses build up within the encapsulated metal which cause a back flux. Ultimately the back flux equals the forward flux, and no more electromigration occurs. This is the steady-state condition, and the steady-state stress of Eq. (11.60) is the stress that would be present at that time. If the metal, in its environment, can withstand and sustain this stress then failure or damage will not occur. But if it cannot, then failure is likely. The stress at which damage or failure occurs is called the critical stress, σ_{crit}. For an encapsulated metal line, which is usually the situation since metal interconnects are invariably surrounded by dielectric layers, this could correspond to the stress needed to rupture the encapsulating material. Or it could be the stress needed to initiate void formation. Not only are ruptures or voids formed, but this can also release the stress, and further electromigration of Al can occur. Even for an unencapsulated line, a stress develops which creates a back flux. The surface energy of the metal or the native metal oxide, as well as the substrate below it, will act as restraining forces. However, the critical stress in these cases would be less than for a thick dielectric layer encapsulation.

Therefore a criterion for failure of an interconnect under electromigration conditions could be if the steady-state stress is equal to or greater than some critical stress for plastic deformation, encapsulent rupture, large void formation, and so on. The maximum steady state stress would occur at $x = 0$ or $x = L_p$. Using Eq. (11.60), the stress at these points is

$$\sigma_{max} = \pm \frac{GL_p}{2} = \pm \frac{Z^* q\rho J}{\Omega} \frac{L_p}{2} \tag{11.61}$$

If failure occurs when $\sigma_{max} = \sigma_{crit}$, then

$$\sigma_{crit} = \pm \left(\frac{Z^* q\rho J}{\Omega} \frac{L_p}{2} \right)_{crit} \tag{11.62}$$

Since Z^*, ρ, and Ω are material constants, this defines a critical JL_p product, with magnitude:

$$|JL_p|_{Crit} = \left| \frac{\sigma_{crit} 2\Omega}{Z^* q\rho} \right| \tag{11.63}$$

If the actual $|JL_p|$ is less than this value, then the maximum stress that develops is less than the critical stress and no failure will occur due to electromigration. But if $|JL_p|$ is above this value, failure will occur. This means that for a certain polygranular cluster length, no electromigration damage will occur below a critical current density. (Some electromigration of Al will occur, but it will stop due to the back flux before any critical stress level for damage occurs.) Likewise, for a given current density, no electromigration damage will occur below a critical polygranular cluster length, $(L_p)_{crit}$. Figure 11–62 illustrates this, where the steady-state stress is shown for two polygranular clusters—one long and one short. For the long cluster, which is above the critical length for the given current density, the steady-state stress at the end is greater than the critical stress. For the short cluster, which is below the critical length, the steady-state stress is less than the critical stress. In an interconnect line, if all the polygranular clusters are shorter than $(L_p)_{crit}$, the stresses that develop will all be less than the critical stress, and the line should not fail by this mechanism.

We can now explain the behavior for Al lines described in Figure 11–57, and repeated in Figure 11–63. For very large w/d_{50} values, no spanning grains are present. If there are large contact or pad areas at the ends of the line, and no significant points of flux divergence present in the line, the time to failure can be relatively high. But as w/d_{50} decreases, some spanning grains occur. This would be the case for $w/d_{50} = 1.3$ as shown in Figure 11–58. This results in divergences in the flux, causing stress to develop that can be greater than the critical stress for failure (with $L_p > (L_p)_{crit}$ for most or all of the polygranular clusters). The lines would fail and the median time to failure would decrease. Now as w/d_{50} decreases more, more spanning grains are present, but the lengths of the polygranular cluster regions between them are shorter, many of them shorter than $(L_p)_{crit}$. The stresses that develop, which create the back fluxes and which in turn eventually stop the electromigration flux, are in many cases smaller than the critical stress. For small enough values of w/d_{50} (0.31 for example), bamboo or near-bamboo structures are present. The polygranular clusters are few, and for some lines, all the clusters are

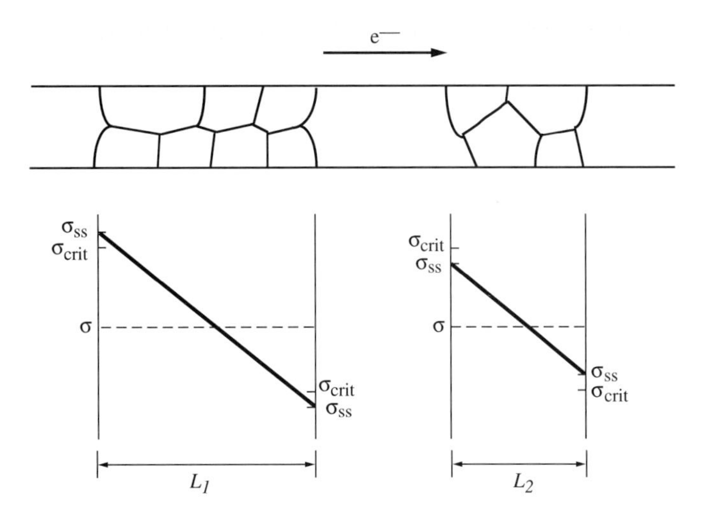

Figure 11–62 Steady-state stress distribution for two polygranular clusters of different lengths, L_1 and L_2. For the cluster of length L_1, the maximum steady-state stress (which occurs at the end of the cluster) is greater than some critical stress for line failure. For the cluster of length L_2, the maximum steady-state stress is less than the critical stress for line failure. Failure would occur in the first cluster, but not in the second. (After [11.68].)

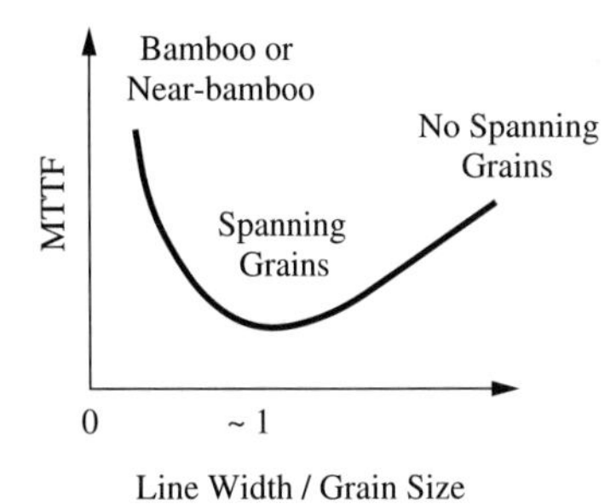

Figure 11–63 Relationship between MTTF due to electromigration versus the ratio of line width to grain size, with grain structure regimes indicated.

shorter than $(L_p)_{crit}$ and the lines will not fail by this mechanism. The MTTF thus increases dramatically. Simulations by Thompson and colleagues [11.62, 11.63, 11.64] based on this model have captured this behavior quite well.

An analysis very similar to that above was originally developed by Blech [11.69] back in 1976. He derived an expression equivalent to Eq. (11.63). (In Blech's analysis the stress is defined in terms of $\Delta\sigma$, the difference in stress between the two ends, which would be equivalent to 2σ in our analysis above.) Blech did not consider polygranular clusters, but just the entire interconnect length, L. In 1976 interconnect lines were usually not narrow enough to have many, if any, spanning grains. Without them, the whole line acts like a single polygranular cluster, and significant depletion and accumulation can occur at the two ends of each line. This depletion and accumulation can be noticeable if there are not large areas, such as bonding pads, at the ends to act as virtually infinite sources or sinks of Al. In Blech's derivation, L is therefore used instead of L_p, but with the same results. For a given current density, Eq. (11.63) can be rewritten in terms of a critical length as

$$(L_p)_{\text{crit}} = \left| \frac{2\sigma_{\text{crit}}\Omega}{Z^* q\rho J} \right| \tag{11.64}$$

and has become known as the Blech length. L_P can refer to the actual line length for wide lines without any spanning grains, as well as to polygranular cluster length for narrow lines. Wide lines (or polygranular clusters in narrow lines) shorter than the Blech length will not incur damage or failure due to electromigration. But for a wide line longer than this which does not have large areas at the ends to serve as sources and sinks, electromigration damage can occur, usually in the form of void formation and hillock growth at the two ends, with a significant transport of metal atoms from one end of the line to the other. Typical values for the Blech length would be 5–20 μm for an Al line and about 0.5 MA cm^{-2} current density, depending on the exact conditions. Classic experiments by Blech and Herring [11.69, 11.70] accompanying their analysis nicely confirmed the concepts of electromigration-induced stress, back fluxes, critical line lengths, and critical current densities.

Example A wide Al interconnect line (with no spanning grains and no large Al sources at the ends) is 10 μm long, and a current density of 0.3 MA cm^{-2} is passed through it. If the critical stress for failure is 0.4×10^9 dyne cm^{-2}, should this line fail due to electromigration?

Answer For a wide line with no spanning grains, the whole line can be considered as one polygranular cluster. Therefore, if the line length (or line length times the current density) is greater than some critical value, then the line should fail. Either Eq. (11.63) or (11.64) can be used. Using Eq. (11.63), L_p can refer to the polygranular cluster length for narrow lines with spanning grains, or to the actual line length for wide lines without any spanning grains. For Al, the atomic volume, Ω, is 16×10^{-24} cm^3, Z^* is on the order of -4 to -8, so we will use -6, and the resisitivity of Al, ρ, is about 3.0×10^{-6} Ω cm. Therefore $|JL_p|_{\text{crit}}$, where L_p is the line length in this case, is

$$|JL_p|_{\text{crit}} = \left| \frac{0.4 \times 10^9 \text{ dyne cm}^{-2} * 2 * 16 \times 10^{-24} \text{ cm}^3}{-6 * 1.6 \times 10^{-19}\text{C} * 3 \times 10^{-6}\ \Omega \text{ cm}} * \left(\frac{\text{J}}{10^7 \text{ dyne cm}} \right) \right|$$

$$= 444 \text{ A cm}^{-1}$$

The actual $|JL_p|$ equals 0.3×10^6 A cm^{-2} times 10×10^{-4} cm, which equals 300 A cm^{-1}.

Therefore $|JL_p| < |JL_p|_{crit}$ and the line will not fail.

One could also use Eq. (11.64) and compare the actual line (or polygranular cluster) length to the critical line length. Substituting in the numbers, or noting that $(L_P)_{crit}$ just equals $|JL_p|_{crit}$ divided by $|J|$, leads to

$$(L_P)_{crit} = 444 \text{ A cm}^{-1} / 0.3 \times 10^6 \text{ A cm}^{-2} = 1.5 \times 10^{-3} \text{ cm} = 15 \text{ μm}$$

Since the actual line length of 10 μm is less than the critical line length, the line should not fail. The stress that builds up for this length is less than the critical stress for failure.

Korhonen and colleagues [11.67] have taken the stress development even further. They have solved for the stress buildup as a function of time, with the following result:

$$\frac{\partial\sigma}{\partial t} = \frac{\partial}{\partial x}\left[\frac{D\Omega\kappa}{kT}\left(\frac{\partial\sigma}{\partial x} + \frac{Z^*J\rho q}{\Omega}\right)\right] \tag{11.65}$$

where κ is the modulus relating a change in atomic concentration with stress. Eq. (11.65) is then solved numerically for the stress, σ. One solution was shown schematically in Figure 11–61. Eventually the steady-state solution is reached, also shown in that figure. In other modeling work by Thompson and colleagues. [11.65, 11.66], the MTTF is calculated by determining the time it takes for the stress level to build up to a critical value in randomly picked interconnect lines from grain growth simulations. It has also been shown that nearby polygranular clusters can interact with each other and affect the electromigration behavior [11.66].

Also important in the modeling and prediction of reliability is the variation in MTTF, that is, the standard deviation. This is needed to predict the initial failures in an interconnect line. In fact, the standard deviation is seen to increase as bamboo or near-bamboo grain structure is approached due to a certain percentage of lines having polygranular cluster regions longer than the critical length. By using a statistically large number of randomly chosen lines from the grain structure simulation, the standard deviation of MTTF can also be predicted with this model.

The model presented above for electromigration based on stress and polygranular clusters does a good job of explaining the observed phenomena regarding electromigration, line dimensions, and grain structure. The model does not deal with the specific failure mechanisms, such as void formation, hillock formation, or dielectric cracking, other than saying that failure occurs when some critical stress is reached. There is much work today in developing models that account for specific failure mechanisms as well as other phenomena and aspects of electromigration.

For example, failure may not happen right when a critical stress is reached, but sometime later when a void grows and reaches a critical size. Joule heating can occur, especially in areas where voids form and the current density is increased locally. In fact, self-healing may occur due to temperature increases around voids. We have mentioned that Cu is added to Al lines to reduce electromigration, and Cu solutes and precipitates affect the Al diffusion along grain boundaries. Electromigration in Al(Cu) films usually occurs after an incubation period—the time it takes for the Cu itself to electromigrate from the anode side, thus depleting itself and allowing the Al to then electromigrate. Flux divergences at *W* vias can also be common failure sites. And in bamboo structures electromigration failure can still occur. In that case lattice, surface or interface diffusion can be important and must be considered.

Many models are being developed which address these and other issues. But the simple model presented above does serve to illustrate the basic concepts of electromigration, and it ties together a lot of ideas we discussed earlier in the chapter, including grain growth and grain structure, diffusion in polycrystalline materials, mechanical behavior, electrical behavior, and circuit reliability.

11.6 Limits and Future Trends in Technologies and Models

We have seen how back-end technology has evolved over the years, and it will certainly continue to change in the future. There are several driving forces for this change. One is the fact that the lateral dimensions will keep on shrinking in order to build more devices and more complex circuits per unit area. However, the vertical dimensions usually do not scale as quickly, resulting in an ever-increasing aspect ratio. This makes it harder to adequately fill spaces and planarize the topography. Another driving force is the trend toward lower thermal budgets, requiring lower processing temperatures for shorter times. Of course the overriding driving force is the need for faster circuit speeds, necessitating smaller interconnect delays. All these may require new structures, processes, and even new materials in back-end structures.

The back-end structures used in today's silicon-based integrated circuit technology have come a long way from the simple Al/SiO_2 system originally developed. Yet considering all the circuit and processing requirements and issues that have been encountered as the technology has progressed, the structures and processes have remained relatively simple. Part of this is attributable to the fact that a relatively few number of materials, Ti, $TiSi_2$, and/or TiN in particular, used in conjunction with Al(Cu) global interconnects and W contacts and vias, can be used to create very robust multilevel metallization systems. Another reason why the processing has remained relatively simple is that simple processing is in itself a goal. Over the years many solutions to problems have been proposed and even demonstrated but have not been adopted in manufacturing because they were too complex.

One possible change in the back-end structure is to replace the W contacts and vias with Al contacts and vias. This is consistent with the philosophy of fewer materials and types of processing. It also solves some problems associated with W contacts and vias. Electromigration problems in Al often occur in the vicinity of W contacts and vias. This may be partly due to mechanical stresses that can develop at W/Al interfaces which can enhance electromigration or void and hillock formation. But it is also because the different material in the contact or via serves as a point for flux divergence. Al also has a lower electrical resistivity than W which can be important especially in circuits where current flow between different metal layers is significant. Via alignment and overetching may also cause problems. Using Al as the contact or via material would reduce many of these problems. But the problems of Al contacts and vias that originally caused people to use W plugs for contact and vias would have to be solved. These problems are mostly related to filling of small, deep vias and contacts and planarized structures. Possible solutions to this are reflowing Al, either after deposition or during the deposition itself, or using ionized PVD Al deposition. Damascene processes, either single or dual, are being investigated and developed for Al in order to obtain planarized Al via and interconnect levels.

Smaller, deeper spaces and holes will be a problem for all back-end materials, not just Al. While many of these materials are still being deposited by sputtering techniques, especially the metals, the trend has been to try to use CVD. This is because better filling and conformal coverage are often achieved by CVD. However there are still problems with CVD deposition of metals which must be solved. These include contamination and difficulty with doping (Al with Cu, for example). New sputter techniques such as ionized and hot sputter depositions are also being developed, but they can be complicated processes or require a high temperature. New processes, such as the dual damascene, may put more emphasis on filling or covering spaces with metal, and less on filling with dielectrics.

CVD is being considered for silicides not only for better coverage, but for another reason as well. CVD deposition of silicides offers the advantage of little or no silicon consumption as compared with the common method of sputtering Ti and reacting it with the underlying Si. This is becoming important as junctions in the silicon are getting shallower. However, in order to obtain self-aligned silicide structures with the reactive method, silicon must be consumed. Some selective CVD techniques for silicides are being developed, but these also consume some Si. Another possible solution is the selective epitaxial deposition of Si in the source/drain regions prior to refractory metal deposition, with the epitaxial Si serving as the Si source for the silicidation process.

Another driving force in future process development is the lowering of the thermal budget. Less diffusion of dopants in the underlying Si is one reason for this. Another is the thermal stability of some of the new low-K dielectric materials being considered. Currently the highest back-end processing steps are the silicide formation anneal and the BPSG reflow anneal, both at about 800°C. For the latter, new dielectric deposition techniques are being used, notably High-Density Plasma (HDP) deposition of SiO_2, which eliminates the need for a reflow anneal. This technique is quickly replacing the normal CVD deposition and reflow of BPSG, in addition to being used for intermetal dielectric deposition. Chemical-Mechanical Polishing (CMP) methods for the dielectric layer are being used to obtain planar topographies, and more emphasis is being placed on this room-temperature process.

In $TiSi_2$ processing, a high-temperature step is needed to transform the high resistivity C49 phase to the low resistivity C54 phase. This transformation becomes even more difficult as the line thickness and width decrease to submicron dimensions. Several techniques or options are being investigated or considered to reduce this problem and allow lower processing temperatures. These include preamorphizing the Si surface by As or Ge implantation or implanting or depositing thin layers of W or Mo prior to Ti deposition. Another option is to use $CoSi_2$ instead of $TiSi_2$, sometimes with a Ti under- or overlayer. Other silicides being studied include PdSi and NiSi, which form low-resistivity silicides at low temperatures.

Multilayer interconnect structures will continue to be used, but again there will be a trade-off between simpler structures with fewer layers and more complex structures to address some of the emerging problems. For example, to reduce electromigration failures as lines become thinner one can sandwich a TiN layer in the middle of the Al layer [11.71]. This not only provides another shunt layer but also prevents any voids from spanning the whole line. Other shunt or barrier layers are also being considered in addition to the conventional Ti or TiN layers including Mo, Ta, W-Si-N layers.

Even with all the improvements being considered and developed for the Al/SiO_2-based interconnect system, there is still a crisis looming ahead which will require some major changes in back-end structures and processing. The speed of circuits is becoming more and more dominated by the back-end structure as technology progresses. For the next generations of circuits, the interconnect delay will be prohibitively large and new technology will be required [11.9].

To consider how one may improve the interconnect speed, we turn to the simple expression from Section 11.1 for the delay time for global interconnects

$$\tau_L = 0.89 \cdot K_I K_{ox} \varepsilon_o \rho L^2 \left(\frac{1}{H x_{ox}} + \frac{1}{W L_S} \right) \tag{11.3}$$

The goal is to decrease τ_L, or at least to keep it from increasing too much as some of the dimensions change. One can see that if the metal interconnect height, H, width, W, spacing, L_S, or oxide thickness, x_{OX}, are smaller, then the delay time increases. As we discussed at the beginning of the chapter, these dimensions have generally gotten smaller as the technology has evolved, leading to in increase in interconnect delay with each technology generation. One recent trend has been to keep the metal thickness H constant to minimize the reduction in resistivity while shrinking the lateral dimensions. This does slow down the increase in *RC* delay as the lateral dimensions are scaled. However, if the thickness is kept constant while the lateral dimensions decrease, the aspect ratios of the features increase making the deposition and etching more difficult. And the benefits to the *RC* delay diminish above aspect ratios of about 2 due to the increase in line-to-line capacitance [11.7]. The second term in Eq. (11.3) will eventually dominate and the increase in *RC* delay will again approach 2x per generation.

Another option is to actually increase the height, width, and spacing of those interconnects where the major delays occur. These would be the longest lines and would probably be the higher levels of interconnects. Such a scheme is commonly used today, with the higher-level interconnects kept thicker and wider. The intermetal spacing, L_S, is also kept larger, which decreases the line-to-line capacitance. One disadvantage of such "reverse scaling" is that fewer metal lines can be fabricated on any level where the line widths and spacings are larger, and additional metal levels may be needed to achieve the same functionality.

Additional strategies to reduce the relative interconnect delay time will be required as the active devices get smaller and the circuits gets faster. Perhaps L, the length of the global interconnect lines, can be shortened. This will require circuit architectural changes, perhaps using buffers or repeaters. Eq. (11.3) suggests another change that can be made: changing the physical constants of the materials, ρ and K_{ox}, the metal resistivity and the dielectric constant, respectively. By decreasing these, the interconnect *RC* delay will be decreased.

Replacing SiO_2 with dielectric materials which have lower dielectric constants is being aggressively studied and developed for future use. Decreasing the dielectric constant would decrease the interconnect delay by decreasing both the line-to-substrate and line-to-line capacitances. Decreasing the capacitance also minimizes interconnect cross talk. As shown in Table 11–6, many low-K dielectrics are being considered. These include fluorinated SiO_2, polymers, and inorganic/organic hybrid polymers, as well as aerogels (SiO_2 with holes in them) and air bridges (no dielectric material at all!). The main problems with many of these materials are thermal and mechanical stability: They tend to evaporate or melt when heated and crack easily when subjected to stresses.

Replacing Al with a metal conductor having a lower electrical resistivity is another way of decreasing interconnect delay. For long interconnect lines where the total delay is dominated by the interconnect RC product, Eq. (11.3) indicates a linear relationship between resistivity and delay time. However, shorter or thicker lines may not be enhanced as much by reducing the interconnect resistance if the driver and load terms dominate the delay [11.4, 11.72]. The line inductance may also limit how much improvement can be made by using low resistance interconnect materials [11.5]. Alternately, one may reduce the thickness of the interconnect by using a lower-resistance metal in place of Al, keeping the same net line resistance. While R would stay the same, this would decrease the line-to-line capacitance and the total delay. Cross talk would also be decreased with the thinner interconnects.

Three elements do have lower resistivities than Al: silver, gold, and copper. Silver has corrosion problems and poor electromigration resistance, and gold has just marginally lower resistivity than Al along with device contamination problems. Copper has a lower resistivity, 1.72 $\mu\Omega$-cm versus 2.7 for Al. Perhaps more importantly, Cu has much better electromigration resistance than Al, although more research must be carried out. Higher electromigration resistance also allows for circuit operation at higher current densities in the interconnects, resulting in potentially faster circuit speed. For these reasons, many manufacturers have been developing new processes that use Cu as an interconnect metal.

However, there are problems with using copper interconnects which have hindered its development. Copper is difficult to plasma etch since the byproducts, copper halides, are nonvolatile at low temperatures. Corrosion of copper is a problem, especially if the halides are not all removed. A damascene process, single or dual, is the obvious solution to this problem since the copper in this process does not have to be plasma etched, just polished back using CMP. Another problem with copper interconnects is that Cu is a harmful contaminant in Si devices, and Cu atoms can move quickly through SiO_2 and organic dielectrics. Cladding layers, of TiN, Si_3N_4 or Ta-based alloys, for example, must be used as barriers around the copper to prevent this. But this can reduce the effectiveness of using the lower-resistivity material if cladding layers of higher-resistivity material must be used on all sides of the interconnect, thus reducing the volume of the Cu. One alternative to this is to treat the surface of the dielectric, using NH_3 plasma for example, which creates a diffusion barrier out of the dielectric instead of out of the metal interconnect [11.73]. Another disadvantage of copper is that it is not self-passivating which can lead to corrosion problems, unlike Al which forms a thin protective Al_2O_3 skin in air.

Yet, as in the past with other new technologies, the problems with Cu are being solved and Cu will be common in many IC processes in the near future. These processes will make use of the damascene process, Cu electroplating, and CMP. But questions still remain. Will Cu be used only on upper metal layers or will it replace Al entirely, keeping with the "keep it simple" philosophy? Also, which circuits will truly benefit from Cu interconnects? Perhaps only high-performance logic circuits will. Memory chips may use Al interconnects for some time to come.

Even if new materials are used for interconnects and dielectrics, there is a limit to which they will help the circuit speed. Copper has only a 40% lower resistivity than Al so that the improvement in signal delay is a maximum of 40%—less if additional cladding is required. The lowest dielectric constant obtainable is 1 (that of air), so there is a limit to which this can be improved. So even by using Cu as the interconnect instead of Al, and air as the dielectric instead of SiO_2, the maximum decrease in signal delay is about 85%. Eventually another evolution is required if the progression to even faster integrated circuits is to continue. Other types of interconnects may be needed such as superconductors, optical interconnects, or RF transmitters to broadcast signals across chips. And other circuit architecture will probably be needed, with less dependence on long global interconnect lines.

Even though the technologies will evolve and the materials may change, the basic models and concepts as presented in the chapter should still apply. Whether the main global interconnect material is Al or Cu, the silicide is $TiSi_2$ or $CoSi_2$, the contact material is W or Al, or the dielectric material is SiO_2 or a low-K polymer, the basic models for silicide formation, CMP, reflow, grain growth, grain boundary diffusion, and electromigration will still be applicable.

11.7 Summary of Key Ideas

In this chapter we have looked at back-end technology—the structures and fabrication techniques to electrically connect devices to each other and to the outside world. As structures and devices get smaller and chips larger, the importance of interconnects and back-end structures increases—even dominates—over the active devices in terms of circuit performance. The back-end structures include a variety of components: contacts to active areas, local interconnects, global interconnects, vias between interconnect levels, first-level dielectrics, and intermetal dielectrics to physically and electrically separate the different interconnects, and finally a passivation layer to protect the entire circuit. We saw how the back-end structure has evolved considerably from the simple $Si/SiO_2/Al$ structures in the first integrated circuits. Today's technology is characterized by multilevel interconnects, each level itself made up of multilayer metal structures with multilayer dielectrics separating them. Adhesion, contact, barrier, and shunt layers are used in the interconnects, while barrier and planarization layers are utilized in the dielectric structures. There have been many driving forces at work in this development. Some of the most important include the need for additional interconnect levels, the need for planarized structures, lower processing temperatures, and the minimization of reliability problems. In addition, there has always been an effort to make the process as simple and cost effective as possible.

We described the typical processing steps that are commonly used in back-end technology. These include the formation of local interconnects such as silicide structures; the fabrication of the first-level dielectrics like reflowed BPSG; contact formation using tungsten plugs and the etchback process or Chemical-Mechanical Polishing (CMP); global interconnects with stacked multi-layer structures; intermetal dielectric deposition and planarization, using different combinations of PECVD oxide, spin-on-dielectrics, high-density plasma CVD gap-fill oxides, and CMP; via formation with either W or Al plugs; and final passivation with PECVD oxide/nitride layers.

Back-end structures and technology will continue to evolve as devices get smaller, processing temperatures decrease, and even higher performance is required. We will soon be switching to copper, low-K dielectric interconnect systems for many types of high-performance circuits, or to something even more radically different in the future. Nevertheless, many of the same basic processing concepts and ideas will be important.

11.8 References

[11.1]. K.C. Saraswat and F. Mohammadi, "Effect of Scaling of Interconnections on the Time Delay of VLSI Circuits," *IEEE Trans. Electron Dev.*, vol. ED-29, p. 645, 1982.

[11.2]. A. Wilnai, "Open-Ended RC Line Model Predicts MOSFET IC Response," *EDN*, p. 53, 1971.

[11.3]. G. K . Rao, *Multilevel Interconnect Technology*, McGraw-Hill, 1993, p. 24.

[11.4]. H.B. Bakaglu and J.D. Meindl, "Optimal Interconnection Circuits of VLSI," *IEEE Trans. Elect. Dev.*, vol. ED-32, p. 903, 1985.

[11.5]. T.Schreyer, Y. Nishi, and K.C. Saraswat, "A Complete RLC Transmission Line Model of Interconnect Delay," *Proc. of 1988 Symp. on VLSI Technology*, p. 95, 1988.

[11.6]. M.T. Bohr and Y.A. El-Mansy, "Technology for Advanced High-Performance Microprocessors," *IEEE Trans. Elec. Dev.*, vol. 45, p. 620, 1998.

[11.7]. M.T. Bohr, "Interconnect Scaling—the Real Limiter to High Performance ULSI," *IEDM Technical Digest,* p. 241, 1995.

[11.8]. A.K. Stamper, V. McGahay, and J.P. Hummel, "Intermetal Dielectrics—a Five Year Outlook," *Proc. of Diel. for ULSI Multilevel Inter. Conf.*, p. 13, 1997.

[11.9]. National Technology Roadmap for Semiconductors, SIA, 1997.

[11.10]. S. M. Sze, *Physics of Semiconductor Devices*, 2d ed., John Wiley & Sons, 1981, p. 305.

[11.11]. C.Y. Chang, Y.Y. Fang, and S.M Sze, "Specific Contact Resistance of Metal-Semiconductor Barriers," *Solid State Elect.*, vol. 14. p. 541, 1971.

[11.12]. M.A. Nicolet, "Diffusion Barriers in Thin Films," *Thin Solid Films,* vol. 19, p. 52, 1978.

[11.13]. S. Wolf, *Silicon Processing for the VLSI Era, Vol. 2, Process Integration*, Lattice Press, 1990, p. 126.

[11.14]. C.R.M. Grovenor, *Microelectronic Materials*, Institute of Physics Publishing, 1989, p. 278.

[11.15]. M. Wittmer, "Barrier Layers: Principles and Applications in Microelectronics," *J. Vac. Sci. Tech. A.*, vol. 2, p. 273, 1984.

[11.16]. S Bauguess, L.H. Liu, M.L. Dreyer, M. Griswold, and E. Hurley, "The Effects of Accelerated Stress Conditions on Electromigration Failure Kinetics and Void Morphology," *Mat. Sci. Soc. Symp. Proc.*, vol. 428, p. 93, 1996.

[11.17]. S.P. Maruarka, *Silicides for VLSI Applications*, Academic Press, 1983.

[11.18]. D. Pramanik, "CVD Dielectric Films for VLSI," *Semicond. Int'l.*, June 1988, p. 94.

[11.19]. C. H. Ting and T.E. Seidel, "Methods and Needs for Low K Material Research," *Mat. Sci. Soc. Symp. Proc.*, vol. 381, p. 3, 1995.

[11.20]. S.J. Fang, A. Barda. T.Janecko, W. Little, D. Outley, G. Hempl, S. Joshi, B. Morrison, G.B. Shinn, and M Birang, "Control of Dielectric Chemical Mechanical Polishing (CMP) Using An Interferometry Based Endpoint Sensor," *Proc. of the Inter. Interconnect Tech. Conf.*, 1998, p. 76.

[11.21]. D. K. Schroder, *Semiconductor Material and Device Characterization*, J. Wiley & Sons, 1990.

[11.22]. W.M. Loh, S.E. Swirhun, T.A. Schreyer, R. M. Swanson, and K.C. Sarswat, "Modeling and Measurement of Contact Resistances," *IEEE Trans. Elec. Dev.*, vol. ED-34, p. 512, 1987.

[11.23]. W.M Loh, "Modeling and Measurement of Contact Resistances," Ph.D. thesis, Stanford University, 1987.

[11.24]. W.T. Lynch and K.K. Ng, "A Tester for the Contact Resistivity of Self-Aligned Silicides," *IEDM Tech. Dig.*, p. 352, 1988.

[11.25]. R. Venkatraman, "Plasticity and Flow Stresses in Al Thin Films on Si," Ph.D. thesis, Stanford University, 1992.

[11.26]. SPEEDIE is a topography simulator developed at Stanford Univeristy.

[11.27]. ATHENA is a process simulator from Silvaco Inc.

[11.28]. TSUPREM-IV and TAURUS are process (and device) simulators from Avant! Inc.

[11.29]. S. Cea and M.E. Law, "Two Dimensional Simulation of Silicide Growth and Flow," *Proc. of IEEE Int'l. Workshop on Numerical Modeling of Processes and Devices for Int. Circuits, NUPAD V,* 1994, p. 113.

[11.30]. S. Cea, "Multidimensional Viscoelastic Modeling of Silicon Oxidation and Titanium Silicidation," Ph.D. thesis, University of Florida, 1996.

[11.31]. S. Cea, unpublished.

[11.32]. FLOOPS is a process simulator developed by Mark Law at University of Florida.

[11.33]. C.A. Pico and M.G. Lagally, "Kinetics of Titanium Silicide Formation on Single Crystal Si: Experiment and Modeling," *J. Appl. Phys,* vol. 64, p. 4957, 1988.

[11.34]. V. Svilan, J.M.E. Harper, C. Cabral, L.A. Clevenger, "Stress Evolution During the Formation and Transformation of Titanium Silicide," in *Thin Films: Stresses and Mechanical Properties V. Symposium*, S.P. Baker, editor, Materials Research Society, 1995, Pittsburgh, p. 167.

[11.35]. H. Norstrom, K. Maex, and P. Vandenabeele, "Thermal Stability and Interface Bowing of Submicron $TiSi_2$/Polycrystalline Silicon," *Thin Solid Films*, vol. 198, p. 53, 1991.

[11.36]. H. Norstrom, K. Marx, A. Romano-Rodriquez, J. Vanhellemont, and L Van den hove, "Formation of $CoSi_2$ and $TiSi_2$ on Narrow Poly-Si Lines," *Microelectron. Eng.*, vol. 14. p. 327, 1991.

[11.37]. F.W. Preston, "The Theory and Design of Plate Glass Polishing Machines," *J. Soc. Glass Tech.,* vol. 11, p. 214, 1927.

[11.38]. J. Warnock, "A Two-Dimensional Process Model for Chemimechanical Polish Planarization," *J. Electrochem. Soc.*, vol. 138, p. 2398, 1991.

[11.39]. W.W. Mullins, "Theory of Thermal Grooving," *J. Appl. Phys.*, vol. 28, p 333, 1957.

[11.40]. W.W. Mullins, "Flattening of a Nearly Plane Solid Surface Due to Capillarity," *J. Appl. Phys.*, vol. 30, p 77, 1959.

[11.41]. R.A. Brain, D.S. Gardner, D.B. Fraser, and H.A. Atwater, "The Effect of Grain Boundaries on Surface Diffusion Mediated-Planarization of Polycrystalline Cu Films," *Mat. Res. Soc. Symp. Proc.*, vol. 389, p. 107, 1995.

[11.42]. R.A. Brain, "Capillary-Driven Reflow of Thin Cu Films with Submicron, High Aspect Ratio Features," Ph.D. thesis, California Institute of Technology ,1996.

[11.43]. S.P. Chen, J.D. Kress, A.F. Voter, and R.C. Albers, "Electrically Inactive Poly-Silicon Grain Boundaries," *Electrochem. Soc. Proc.*, vol. 96-4, p. 359, 1996.

[11.44]. H.J. Frost, "Microstructural Evolution in Thin Films," *Materials Characterization*, vol. 32, p. 257, 1994.

[11.45]. C.V. Thompson, "Grain Growth in Thin Films," *Ann. Rev. of Mat. Sci.*, vol. 20, p. 245, 1990.

[11.46]. W.W. Mullins, "Two-Dimensional Motion of Idealized Grain Boundaries," *J. Appl. Phys.*, vol. 27, p. 900, 1956.

[11.47]. C.V. Thompson, "Secondary Grain Growth in Thin Films of Semiconductors: Theoretical Aspects," *J. Appl. Phys.*, vol. 58, p. 763, 1985.

[11.48]. H.J. Kim and C.V. Thompson, "Kinetic Modeling of Grain Growth in Polycrystalline Silicon Films Doped with Phosphorus of Boron," *J. Electrochem. Soc.*, vol. 135, p. 2312, 198

[11.49]. D.A. Porter and K.E. Eastering, *Phase Transformations in Metals and Alloys*, 2d ed., Chapman and Hall, 1992, p. 139.

[11.50]. W.W. Mullins, "The Statistical Self-Similarity Hypothesis in Grain Growth and Particle Coursening," *J. Appl. Phys.*, vol. 59, p. 1341, 1986.

[11.51]. J.E. Burke, "Some Factors Affecting the Rate of Grain Growth in Metals," *Trans. Amer. Inst. of Mining and Metall. Engineers,* vol. 180, p. 73, 1949.

[11.52]. S.K. Kurtz and F.M.A. Carpay, "Microstructure and Normal Grain Growth in Metals and Ceramics. Part 1, Theory," *J. Appl. Phys.*, vol. 51, p. 5725, 1981.

[11.53]. L.H. Van Vlack, *Elements of Materials Science and Engineering*, Addison-Wesley, 1989.

[11.54]. M. Hillert, "On the Theory of Normal and Abnormal Grain Growth," *Acta Metall.*, vol. 13, p. 227, 1965.

[11.55]. H.J. Frost and C.V. Thompson, "Computer Simulation of Microstructrual Evolution in Thin Films," *J. of El. Mater.*, vol. 17, p. 447, 1988.

[11.56]. D.T. Walton, H.J. Frost, and C.V. Thompson, "Development of Near-Bamboo and Bamboo Microstructures in Thin-Film Strips," *Appl. Phys. Lett.,* vol. 61, p. 40, 1992.

[11.57]. Y.J. Park and C.V. Thompson, "The Effects of the Stress Dependence of Atomic Diffusivity on Stress Evolution due to Electromigration," *J. Appl. Phys.*, vol. 82, p. 4277, 1997.

[11.58]. J.R. Black, "Electromigration—A Brief Survey and Some Recent Results," *IEEE Trans. El. Dev.*, vol. ED – 16, p. 338, 1969.

[11.59]. M. Shatzkes and J.R. Lloyd, "A Model for Conductor Failure Considering Diffusion Concurrently with Electromigration Resuling in a Current Exponent of 2," *J. Appl. Phys.*, vol. 59, p. 3890, 1986.

[11.60]. M.A. Korhonen, P. Borgeson, K.N. Tu, and C.Y. Li, "Stress Evolution due to Electromigration in Confined Metal Lines," *J. Appl. Phys.*, vol. 73, p. 3790, 1993.

[11.61]. J.R. Lloyd, "Electromigration Failure," *J. Appl. Phys.*, vol. 69, p. 7601, 1991.

[11.62]. C.V. Thompson and J.R. Lloyd, "Electromigration and IC Interconnects," *MRS Bulletin*, December 1993, p. 19.

[11.63]. C.V. Thompson, Y.C. Joo, and B.D. Knowlton, "Modeling of the Structure and Reliability of Near-Bamboo Interconnects," *Mat. Res. Soc. Symp. Proc.*, vol. 391, p. 163, 1995.

[11.64]. Y.C. Joo and C.V. Thompson, "Analytic Model for the Grain Structures of Near-Bamboo Interconnects," *J. Appl. Phys.*, vol 76, p. 7339, 1994.

[11.65]. B.D. Knowlton, J.J. Clement, R.I. Frank, and C.V. Thompson, "Coupled Stress Evolution in Polygranular Clusters and Segments in Near-Bamboo Interconnects," *Mat. Res. Soc. Symp. Proc.*, vol. 391, p. 189, 1995.

[11.66]. B.D. Knowlton, J.J. Clement, and C.V.Thompson, "Simulation of the Effects of Grain Structure and Grain Growth on Electromigration and the Reliability of Interconnects," *J. Appl. Phys*, vol. 81, p. 6073, 1997.

[11.67]. M.A. Korhonen, P. Borgeson, D.D. Brown, and C.Y. Li, "Microstructure Based Statistical Model of Electromigration Damage in Confined Line Metallizations in the Presence of Thermally Induced Stressses," *J. Appl. Phys.*, vol. 74, p. 4995, 1994.

[11.68]. C.V. Thompson, "Electromigration, Microstructure, and IC Interconnect Reliability: Metallurgy Meets TCAD," presented at Stanford University, Nov. 1995.

[11.69]. I.A. Blech, "Electromigration in Thin Aluminum Films on Titanium Nitride," *J. Appl. Phys.*, vol. 47, p. 1203, 1976.

[11.70]. I.A. Blech and C. Herring, "Stress Generation by Electromigration," *Appl. Phys. Lett.*, vol. 29, p. 131, 1976

[11.71]. D. Gardner, "Layered and Homogeneous Films of Al and Al/Si with Ti and W for Multilevel Interconnects," *IEEE Trans. Elect. Dev.*, vol. ED-32, p. 174, 1985.

[11.72]. S. Bothra, B. Rogers, M. Kellam, and C.M. Osburn, "Analysis of the Effects of Scaling on Interconnect Delay in ULSI Circuits," *IEEE Trans. on Elect. Dev.*, vol. 40, p. 591, 1993.

[11.73]. K. Mikagi, H. Ishikawa, T. Usami, M. Suzuki, K. Inoue, N. Oda. S. Chikaki, I. Sakai, and T. Kikkawa, "Barrier Metal Free Copper Damascene Interconnections Technology Using Atmospheric Copper Reflow and Nitrogen Doping in SiOF Film," *IEDM Technical Digest*, vol. 96, p. 365, 1996.

11.9 Problems

11.1. Replot the delay time versus chip area curve (Figure 11–4) for $F_{min} = 0.25$ μm, for the following cases (all on the same graph), assuming no driver or load elements.

a. With Al as the interconnect metal (assume the resistivity of Al is 3.0 μΩ cm) and SiO_2 as the dielectric (assume $K_{ox} = 3.9$).

b. With Al as the interconnect metal but with a new dielectric material, whose dielectric constant, K, is equal to 2.2.

c. With Cu as the interconnect metal (resisitivity is 1.7 μΩ cm) and a low-K dielectric material (K is equal to 2.2).

11.2. Calculate the percentage increase in the interconnect RC delay according to Eq. (11.3) if the thicknesses H and x_{ox}, remain constant while the lateral dimensions W and L_S scale with (and equal) F_{min}. Assume F_{min} is decreased from 0.5 to 0.35 μm and H and x_{ox} equal 0.5 μm. Also assume that the interconnect length L remains constant.

11.3. Al spiking of Si would not be a problem if the Si diffusion in Al were small and little Si diffused into the Al, leaving voids in the Si for the Al to fill. Just how much does the Si diffuse into the Al? If the diffusivity of Si in Al at 450°C is about 40 $\mu m^2\ min^{-1}$, calculate how far the Si will diffuse into the Al after 60 minutes at 450°C? (Calculate the distance in which the Si concentration falls to 50% of the surface concentration.)

11.4. For 0.35-μm technology, the junction depth (before silicidation) is about 100 nm. If you want to leave 50 nm of Si after silicidation to ensure low leakage current, how much $TiSi_2$ is formed and how much Ti is needed if all is consumed?

11.5. A source/drain implant is done with arsenic with a dose of $1 \times 10^{15}\ cm^{-2}$ and an energy of 40 keV. A titanium silicide layer is then formed on top of the source/drain regions to reduce the sheet resistance of those regions. This is done by depositing Ti on the surface and annealing. 55 nm of silicide is formed, which consumes the top surface of the Si in the source/drain regions and as a result reduces the amount of As dopant in the Si. What is the peak concentration of As in the Si in the source/drain regions after the silicidation process? (Assume that the implant is done directly into the Si with no oxide and that no dopant diffusion or segregation occurs during the silicidation.)

11.6. What are two reasons why the damascene process (single damascene version) might be used instead of the normal masked plasma etch process?

11.7. An oxide layer is deposited over 0.5-μm-thick metal lines, as in Figure 11–17. The resulting step height in the oxide layer is 0.4 μm. What is the degree of planarization?

11.8. 0.5-μm-thick Al lines are formed on a flat surface. A layer of SiO_2 (at least 1 μm thick) is then deposited over this. A Degree Of Planarization (DOP) of 1 is desired but the actual DOP obtained was 0.4. A CMP etchback of the oxide is then done to obtain a net degree of planarization of 1. If the CMP etch rate is 0.12 μm per minute, what is the minimum CMP etch time needed to obtain this net DOP of 1? Assume no variations in thicknesses or CMP etch rates.

11.9. A damascene process is used to fabricate a tungsten via through a SiO_2 dielectric layer. First the SiO_2 dielectric layer is deposited, with a thickness of 1 μm. A via hole is etched in the SiO_2, and W is blanket deposited by CVD. Right after the W deposition, the Degree Of Planarization (DOP) equals 1.0, and the thickness of the W directly above the dielectric layer is equal to 0.8 μm. A plasma etchback of the W layer is now done to remove the W that covers the top of the dielectric layer, and leaving the W only in the via hole. If the etch rate of the W in the etchback process is 5.0 nm sec^{-1}, and the etch selectivity of W with respect to SiO_2 is 4:1, what is the profile of the structure after 180 sec of etching? Specify the heights of the W and SiO_2 layers in nm. (Neglect any variations in thicknesses or etch rate.)

11.10. A SiO_2 layer is deposited by LPCVD over a single 1-μm-wide, 0.5-μm-high metal line. The deposition flux and time are such that 0.25 μm of SiO_2 would be deposited on a flat surface. The sticking coefficient for this process is 0.01 and the arrival angle distribution parameter n is equal to 1. Very conformal deposition is obtained, but the DOP is 0. Would changing n or S_C improve (increase) the DOP? Explain.

11.11. SiO_2 is deposited on a Si wafer at 800°C. How much stress is induced in the film due to the cooling of the wafer from 800°C to 25°C? Is the stress tensile or compressive? Assume no intrinisic stress in the film and no stress relaxation processes.

11.12. Consider a surface that has a region that is concave and as well as a region that is convex. During reflow, will atoms move from a concave region to a convex region, or from a convex region to a concave region? Explain both in terms of the force equations for reflow as well as in terms of the atomistic picture.

11.13. If the grain boundary mobility, M_{gb}, is 1×10^{-15} cm^4 sec^{-1} erg^{-1}, the grain boundary energy is 300 ergs cm^{-2}, and the curvature, K, is 20 μm^{-1}, calculate the average grain radius after 60 minutes of grain growth. Assume the initial grain size is zero.

11.14. An Al interconnect line has polygranular clusters that are all equal or less than 5 μm long, and a current density of 0.5 MA cm^{-2} is passed through it. If the critical stress for failure is 0.4×10^9 dyne cm^{-2} (and let Z^* equal -6), should this line fail due to electromigration? What is the critical current density below which electromigration failure will not occur for this line?

Appendices

A.1 Standard Prefixes

Prefix	Symbol	Value
peta-	P-	10^{15}
tera-	T-	10^{12}
giga-	G-	10^{9}
mega-	M-	10^{6}
kilo-	k-	10^{3}
milli-	m-	10^{-3}
micro-	μ-	10^{-6}
nano-	n-	10^{-9}
pico-	p-	10^{-12}
femto-	f-	10^{-15}

A.2 Useful Conversions

1 atm = 760 torr (exactly)
1 atm = 1.013×10^{5} Pa
1 Pa = 1 J m^{-3} = 10 dyne cm^{-2}, 1 MPa = 10^{7} dyne cm^{-2}
1 eV = 1.60219×10^{-19} J
1 cal = 4.184 J
1 J = 10^{7} erg
1 erg = 2.39×10^{-8} cal
1 N = 1 J m^{-1} = 10^{5} dyne
1 V = 1 ohm amp
1 J = 1 volt coulomb = 1 coulomb amp ohm
1 J = 10^{7} dyne cm
1 coulomb = 1 amp sec = 1 farad volt
1 amp = 1 farad volt sec^{-1}
1 nm = 10^{-3} μm = 10^{-7} cm = 10^{-9} m = 10 Å
T K = T°C + 273.15

A.3 Physical Constants

Quantity	Symbol	Value
Avogadro constant	N_{AV}	6.02204×10^{23} mole^{-1}
Boltzmann constant	k	1.38066×10^{-23} J K^{-1} = 8.617×10^{-5} eV K^{-1}
Electron charge	q	1.60218×10^{-19} C
Electron rest mass	m_o	9.1×10^{-28} g
Gas constant	R	1.987 cal mole^{-1} K^{-1}
Permittivity in vacuum	ε_0	8.854×10^{-14} F cm^{-1}
Planck constant	h	6.626×10^{-34} J sec = 4.136×10^{-15} eV sec
Reduced Planck constant	$\hbar$ $(=h/2\pi)$	1.055×10^{-34} J sec
Speed of light in vacuum	c	2.998×10^{10} cm sec^{-1}
Thermal voltage at 300 K	kT/q	0.0259 V

A.4 Physical Properties of Silicon

Property	Value
Band gap at 300K	1.107 eV
Electron majority carrier mobility at 300K	1500 cm^2 volt^{-1} sec^{-1}
Hole majority carrier mobility at 300K	450 cm^2 volt^{-1} sec^{-1}
Crystal structure	Cubic diamond
Melting point	1417°C
Density	2.328 gm cm^{-3}
Knoop hardness	950–1150 kg mm^{-2}
Thermal conductivity k_S at 300K	0.358 cal (sec cm °C)$^{-1}$
Latent Heat of Fusion	340 cal gm^{-1}
Emissivity at high temperatures	≈ 0.55
Linear thermal expansion coefficient $\Delta L/L\Delta T$	2.6×10^{-6} °C^{-1}
Young's modulus	$Y_{100} = 1.3 \times 10^{12}$ dyne cm^{-2} $Y_{111} = 1.9 \times 10^{12}$ dyne cm^{-2}
Lattice constant	0.543095 nm
Specific heat	0.7 Joule gm^{-1} °C^{-1}
Thermal diffusivity	0.92 cm^2 sec^{-1}
Atomic density	5×10^{22} cm^{-3}
Atomic weight	28.09
Breakdown field	$\approx 3 \times 10^5$ V cm^{-1}
Effective density of states (valence band) N_V	1.04×10^{19} cm^{-3}
Effective density of states (conduction band) N_C	2.8×10^{19} cm^{-3}
Density of states effective mass of electrons m_e^*	1.08 m_o ($m_o = 9.1 \times 10^{-28}$ g)
Density of states effective mass of holes m_h^*	0.81 m_o
Peak electron velocity v_{SAT}	1×10^7 cm sec^{-1}
Peak hole velocity v_{SAT}	1×10^7 cm sec^{-1}
Electron affinity χ	4.05 eV
Intrinsic carrier concentration n_i at 300 k	1.45×10^{10} cm^{-3}
Intrinsic resistivity at 300 k	2.3×10^5 Ωcm
Relative permittivity ε_r	11.9

A.5 Properties of Insulators Used in Silicon Technology

	SiO_2	Si_3N_4	SiO_XN_Y
Structure	Amorphous	Amorphous	Amorphous
Resistivity (Ωcm)	$10^{14}-10^{16}$	$\approx 10^{14}$	
Density (gm cm^{-3})	2.27	3.1	
Dielectric constant, K	3.8 – 3.9	7.5	5 – 6
Dielectric strength (V cm^{-1})	$5–10 \times 10^6$	$\approx 10^7$	$\approx 5 \times 10^6$
Energy gap (eV)	≈ 9	≈ 5	
Expansion coeff. (°C^{-1})	5×10^{-7}		
Refractive index	1.46	2.05	1.6 – 1.9
Thin film stress (dyne cm^{-2})	$2–4 \times 10^9$	$9–10 \times 10^9$	$1–6 \times 10^9$
Thermal conductivity (W/cm°C)	0.014		
Infrared absorption peak (μ)	9.3	11.5 – 12	9 – 12
Etch rate in buffered HF (nm min^{-1})	100	0.5–1	2–40
Melting point (°C)	≈ 1700		
Electron mobility (cm^2 volt^{-1} sec^{-1})	20–40		
Hole mobility (cm^2 volt^{-1} sec^{-1})	$\approx 2 \times 10^{-5}$		
Surface conductivity (Ω/sq)	$10^{16}–10^{19}$		

A.6 Color Chart for Deposited Si_3N_4 Films Observed Perpendicularly under Daylight Fluorescent Lighting

Film Thickness (nm)	Color	Film Thickness (nm)	Color
10	Light brown	95	Light blue
17	Medium brown	105	Very light blue
25	Brown	115	Light blue-brown
34	Brown-pink	125	Light brown-yellow
35	Pink-purple	135	Very light yellow
43	Purple	145	Light yellow
53	Very dark blue	155	Yellow
60	Dark blue	165	Bright yellow
70	Medium blue	175	Intense yellow

A.7 Color Chart for Thermally Grown SiO_2 Films Observed Perpendicularly under Daylight Fluorescent Lighting [6.7]

Film Thickness (nm)	Color	Film Thickness (nm)	Color
50	Tan	630	Violet-red
70	Brown	680	"Bluish"
100	Dark violet to red violet	720	Blue green to green
120	Royal blue	770	"Yellowish"
150	Light blue to metallic blue	800	Orange
170	Metallic to light yellow green	820	Salmon
200	Light gold or yellow	850	Light red-violet
220	Gold with slight yellow orange	860	Violet
250	Orange to melon	890	Blue
270	Red-violet	920	Blue-green
300	Blue to blue-violet	950	Dull yellow-green
310	Blue	970	Yellow
320	Blue to blue-green	990	Orange
340	Light green	1000	Carnation pink
350	Green to yellow-green	1020	Violet-red
360	Yellow-green	1050	Red-violet
370	Green-yellow	1060	Violet
390	Yellow	1070	Blue-violet
410	Light orange	1100	Green
420	Carnation pink	1110	Yellow-green
440	Violet-red	1120	Green
460	Red-violet	1180	Violet
470	Violet	1190	Red-violet
480	Blue-violet	1210	Violet-red
490	Blue	1240	Carnation pink to salmon
500	Blue-green	1250	Orange
520	Green	1280	"Yellowish"
540	Yellow-green	1320	Sky blue to green-blue
560	Green-yellow	1400	Orange
570	Yellow to "yellowish"	1450	Violet
580	Light orange or yellow to pink	1460	Blue-violet
600	Carnation pink	1500	Blue

A.8 Irvin's Curves

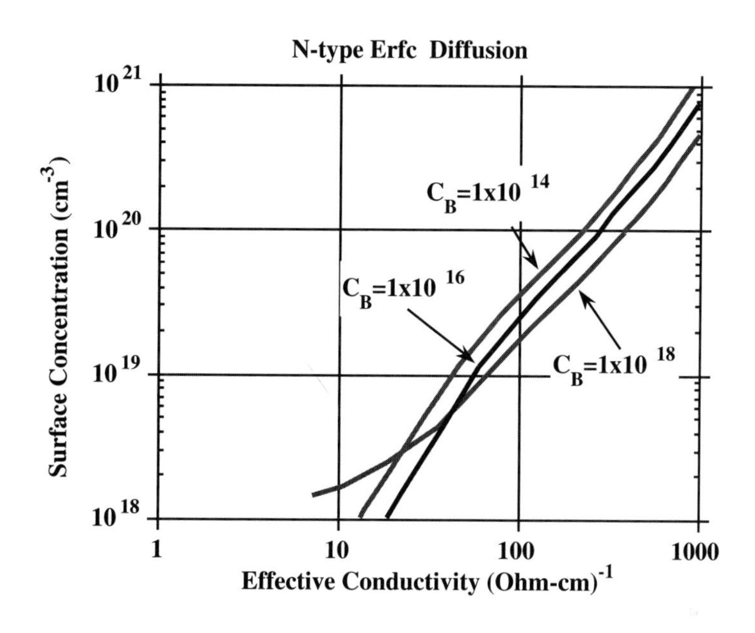

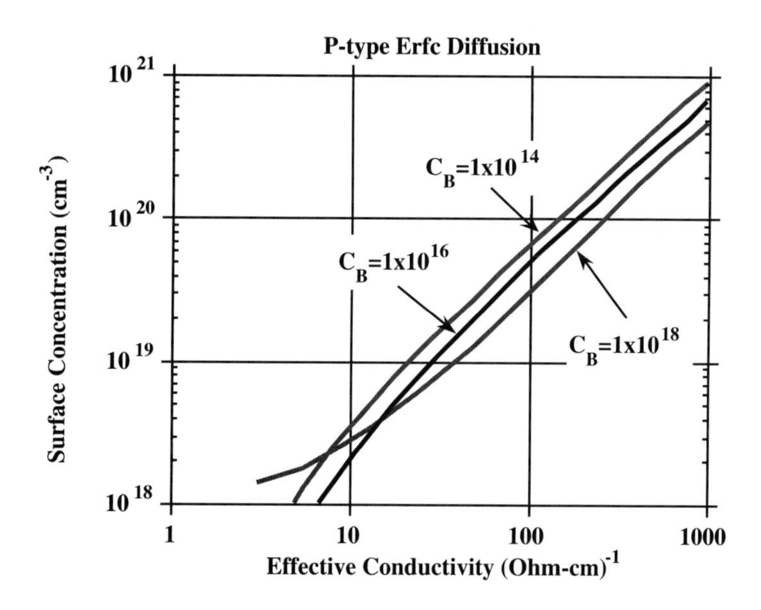

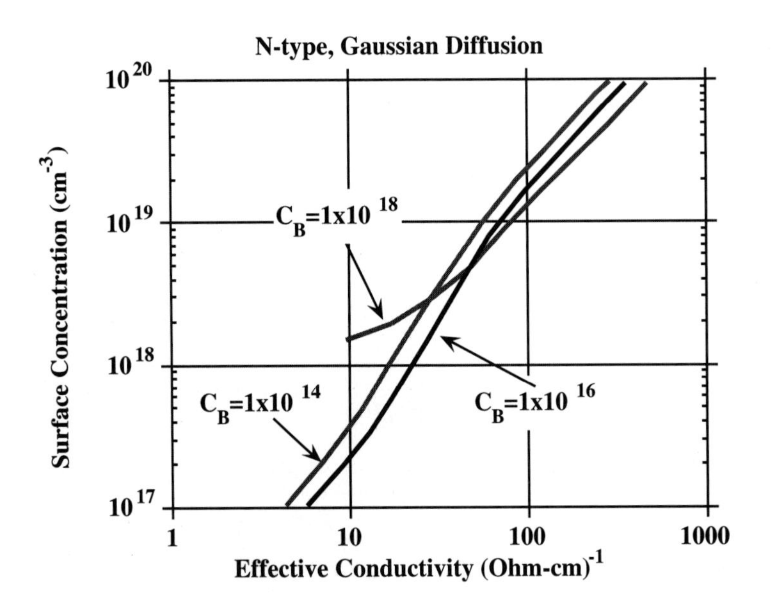
N-type, Gaussian Diffusion
Surface Concentration (cm^{-3})
Effective Conductivity (Ohm-cm)$^{-1}$
C_B=1x10 ^{18}
C_B=1x10 ^{14}
C_B=1x10 ^{16}
10 ^{20}
10 ^{19}
10 ^{18}
10 ^{17}
1
10
100
1000

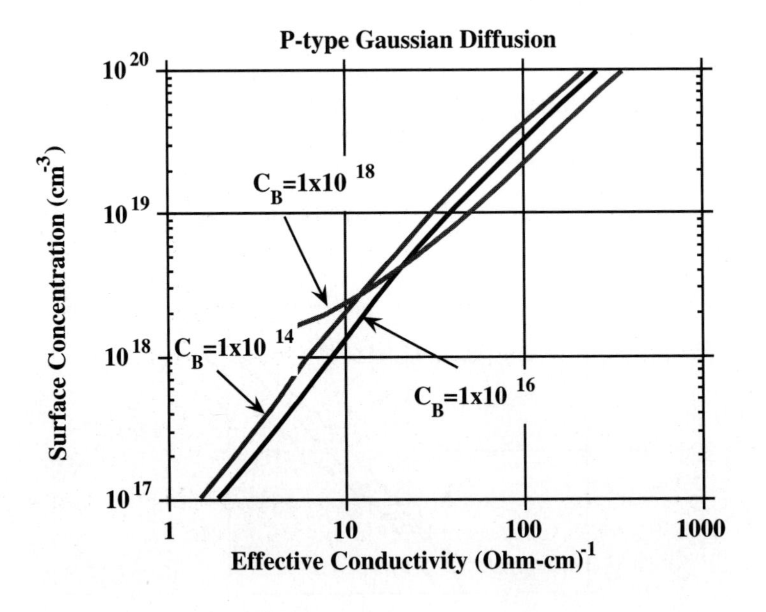
P-type Gaussian Diffusion
Surface Concentration (cm^{-3})
Effective Conductivity (Ohm-cm)$^{-1}$
C_B=1x10 ^{18}
C_B=1x10 ^{14}
C_B=1x10 ^{16}
10 ^{20}
10 ^{19}
10 ^{18}
10 ^{17}
1
10
100
1000

A.9 Error Function

Properties

The error function is defined by

$$\mathrm{erf}(z) = \frac{2}{\sqrt{\pi}} \int_0^z \exp(-\eta^2) d\eta$$

so that

$$\mathrm{erfc}(z) = 1 - \mathrm{erf}(z) = \frac{2}{\sqrt{\pi}} \int_z^\infty \exp(-\eta^2) d\eta$$

The error function is an odd function:

$$\mathrm{erf}(-z) = -\mathrm{erf}(z)$$

which also means

$$\mathrm{erf}(0) = 0$$

The limit as $z \to \infty$ is

$$\mathrm{erf}(\infty) = 1$$

which also means

$$\mathrm{erf}(-\infty) = -1$$

The derivative of the error function is

$$\frac{d}{dz}\mathrm{erf}(z) = \frac{2}{\sqrt{\pi}} \exp(-z^2)$$

A useful approximation with better than 4% accuracy:

$$\mathrm{erfc}(z) \approx \frac{1.1 \exp(-z^2)}{\left(|z| + \sqrt{z^2 + 1.21}\right)}$$

(from the NBS Applied Math Series 55–1964, "Handbook of Mathematical Functions with Formulas, Graphs and Mathematical Tables.")

Asymptotic approximations:

$$\mathrm{erf}(z) \to \frac{\exp(-z^2)}{z\sqrt{\pi}} \text{ for } z \gg 1$$

$$\mathrm{erf}(z) \to \frac{2z}{\sqrt{\pi}} \text{ for } z \ll 1$$

z	**erf(z)**	z	**erf(z)**	z	**erf(z)**
0.00	0.00	0.34	0.369365	0.68	0.663782
0.01	0.011283	0.35	0.379382	0.69	0.670840
0.02	0.022565	0.36	0.389330	0.70	0.677801
0.03	0.033841	0.37	0.399206	0.71	0.684666
0.04	0.045111	0.38	0.409009	0.72	0.691433
0.05	0.056372	0.39	0.418739	0.73	0.698104
0.06	0.067622	0.40	0.428392	0.74	0.704678
0.07	0.078858	0.41	0.437969	0.75	0.711156
0.08	0.090078	0.42	0.447468	0.76	0.717537
0.09	0.101281	0.43	0.456887	0.77	0.723822
0.10	0.112463	0.44	0.466225	0.78	0.730010
0.11	0.123623	0.45	0.475482	0.79	0.736103
0.12	0.134758	0.46	0.484655	0.80	0.742101
0.13	0.145867	0.47	0.493745	0.81	0.748003
0.14	0.156947	0.48	0.502750	0.82	0.753811
0.15	0.167996	0.49	0.511668	0.83	0.759524
0.16	0.179012	0.50	0.520500	0.84	0.765143
0.17	0.189992	0.51	0.529244	0.85	0.770668
0.18	0.200936	0.52	0.537899	0.86	0.776100
0.19	0.211840	0.53	0.546464	0.87	0.781440
0.20	0.222703	0.54	0.554939	0.88	0.786687
0.21	0.233522	0.55	0.563323	0.89	0.791843
0.22	0.244296	0.56	0.571616	0.90	0.796908
0.23	0.255023	0.57	0.579816	0.91	0.801883
0.24	0.265700	0.58	0.587923	0.92	0.806768
0.25	0.276326	0.59	0.595936	0.93	0.811564
0.26	0.286900	0.60	0.603856	0.94	0.816271
0.27	0.297418	0.61	0.611681	0.95	0.820891
0.28	0.307880	0.62	0.619411	0.96	0.825424
0.29	0.318283	0.63	0.627046	0.97	0.829870
0.30	0.328627	0.64	0.634586	0.98	0.834231
0.31	0.338908	0.65	0.642029	0.99	0.838508
0.32	0.349126	0.66	0.649377		
0.33	0.359279	0.67	0.656628		

z	**erf(z)**	z	**erf(z)**	z	**erf(z)**
1.00	0.842701	1.34	0.941914	1.68	0.982493
1.01	0.846811	1.35	0.943762	1.69	0.983153
1.02	0.850838	1.36	0.945561	1.70	0.983790
1.03	0.854784	1.37	0.947312	1.71	0.984407
1.04	0.858650	1.38	0.949016	1.72	0.985003
1.05	0.862436	1.39	0.950673	1.73	0.985578
1.06	0.866144	1.40	0.952285	1.74	0.986135
1.07	0.869773	1.41	0.953852	1.75	0.986672
1.08	0.873326	1.42	0.955376	1.76	0.987190
1.09	0.876803	1.43	0.956857	1.77	0.987691
1.10	0.880205	1.44	0.958297	1.78	0.988174
1.11	0.883533	1.45	0.959695	1.79	0.988641
1.12	0.886788	1.46	0.961053	1.80	0.989091
1.13	0.889971	1.47	0.962373	1.81	0.989525
1.14	0.893082	1.48	0.963654	1.82	0.989943
1.15	0.896124	1.49	0.964898	1.83	0.990347
1.16	0.899096	1.50	0.966105	1.84	0.990736
1.17	0.902000	1.51	0.967277	1.85	0.991111
1.18	0.904837	1.52	0.968413	1.86	0.991472
1.19	0.907608	1.53	0.969516	1.87	0.991821
1.20	0.910314	1.54	0.970586	1.88	0.992156
1.21	0.912956	1.55	0.971623	1.89	0.992479
1.22	0.915534	1.56	0.972628	1.90	0.992790
1.23	0.918050	1.57	0.973603	1.91	0.993090
1.24	0.920505	1.58	0.974547	1.92	0.993378
1.25	0.922900	1.59	0.975462	1.93	0.993656
1.26	0.925236	1.60	0.976348	1.94	0.993923
1.27	0.927514	1.61	0.977207	1.95	0.994179
1.28	0.929734	1.62	0.978038	1.96	0.994426
1.29	0.931899	1.63	0.978843	1.97	0.994664
1.30	0.934008	1.64	0.979622	1.98	0.994892
1.31	0.936063	1.65	0.980376	1.99	0.995111
1.32	0.938065	1.66	0.981105		
1.33	0.940015	1.67	0.981810		

z	**erf(z)**	z	**erf(z)**	z	**erf(z)**
2.00	0.995322	2.34	0.999065	2.68	0.999849
2.01	0.995525	2.35	0.999111	2.69	0.999858
2.02	0.995719	2.36	0.999155	2.70	0.999866
2.03	0.995906	2.37	0.999197	2.71	0.999873
2.04	0.996086	2.38	0.999237	2.72	0.999880
2.05	0.996258	2.39	0.999275	2.73	0.999887
2.06	0.996423	2.40	0.999312	2.74	0.999893
2.07	0.996582	2.41	0.999346	2.75	0.999899
2.08	0.996734	2.42	0.999379	2.76	0.999905
2.09	0.996880	2.43	0.999411	2.77	0.999910
2.10	0.997021	2.44	0.999441	2.78	0.999916
2.11	0.997155	2.45	0.999469	2.79	0.999920
2.12	0.997284	2.46	0.999497	2.80	0.999925
2.13	0.997407	2.47	0.999523	2.81	0.999929
2.14	0.997525	2.48	0.999547	2.82	0.999933
2.15	0.997639	2.49	0.999571	2.83	0.999937
2.16	0.997747	2.50	0.999593	2.84	0.999941
2.17	0.997851	2.51	0.999614	2.85	0.999944
2.18	0.997951	2.52	0.999635	2.86	0.999948
2.19	0.998046	2.53	0.999654	2.87	0.999951
2.20	0.998137	2.54	0.999672	2.88	0.999954
2.21	0.998224	2.55	0.999689	2.89	0.999956
2.22	0.998308	2.56	0.999706	2.90	0.999959
2.23	0.998388	2.57	0.999722	2.91	0.999961
2.24	0.998464	2.58	0.999736	2.92	0.999964
2.25	0.998537	2.59	0.999751	2.93	0.999966
2.26	0.998607	2.60	0.999764	2.94	0.999968
2.27	0.998674	2.61	0.999777	2.95	0.999970
2.28	0.998738	2.62	0.999789	2.96	0.999972
2.29	0.998799	2.63	0.999800	2.97	0.999973
2.30	0.998857	2.64	0.999811	2.98	0.999975
2.31	0.998912	2.65	0.999821	2.99	0.999976
2.32	0.998966	2.66	0.999831	3.00	0.999978
2.33	0.999016	2.67	0.999841		

A.10 List of Important Symbols

A—area, in units of cm^2
C—capacitance, in units of F or farads
C—concentration, in units of cm^{-3}
D—diffusivity (experimentally measured), in units of $cm^2\ sec^{-1}$
d—diffusivity of mobile species, in units of $cm^2\ sec^{-1}$
E—energy, in units of eV
F—flux, in units of $cm^{-2}\ sec^{-1}$
F_{min}—minimum feature size, in units of nm
I—current, in units of amps
I—optical intensity in units of $J\ cm^{-2}\ sec^{-1}$
I—interstitial (Si interstitial in Si crystal, unless otherwise designated)
I—number of impurities in crystal growth model
J—current density, in units of amps cm^{-2}
m—mass, in units of gm
M—particle or atomic mobility (D/kT), in units of $cm^2\ eV^{-1}\ sec^{-1}$
n—electron concentration, in units of cm^{-3}
n—index of refraction, unitless
N–density, in units of atoms cm^{-3}
P -pressure, in units of atm or torr
Q—dose, in units of cm^{-2}
R—resistance, in units of ohms or Ω
t—time, in units of sec
T—temperature, in units of K (unless noted by °C)
v—velocity, in units of $cm\ sec^{-1}$
v—deposition or etch rate (velocity of surface), in units of $cm\ sec^{-1}$
V—voltage or potential difference, in units of volts
V—volume, in units of cm^3
V—vacancy (in Si unless otherwise designated)
$\mathcal{E}$—electric field, in units of $V\ cm^{-1}$
ε—permittivity, in units of $F\ cm^{-1}$
μ—carrier mobility , in units of $cm^2\ volt^{-1}\ sec^{-1}$
σ—conductivity, in units of $S\ m^{-1}$
σ—stress, in units of dynes cm^{-2} or Pa
τ—lifetime, in units of sec
ρ—electrical resistivity, in units of ohm cm
ρ_S—sheet resistance, in units of ohms per square
ρ_C—specific contact resistivity, in units of ohm cm^2

A.11 List of Common Acronyms

AC—alternating current
A/C—amorphous/crystalline interface in Si
AES—Auger electron spectroscopy
AFM—atomic force microscopy
APCVD—atmospheric pressure chemical vapor deposition
AR—aspect ratio
ARC—antireflection coating
ARDE—aspect ratio dependent etching

BCC—body-centered cubic unit cell
BICMOS—bipolar and CMOS devices on the same chip
BJT—bipolar junction transistor
BOE—buffered oxide etch (same as BHF, buffered HF)
BPSG—borophosphosilicate glass

CVD–chemical vapor deposition
CZ—Czochralski crystal growth method
DC—direct current
DI—deionized, or very pure, water
DLTS—deep level transient spectroscopy
DNQ—diazonaphthoquinone, a resist material
DOF—depth of focus
DOP—degree of planarization
DRAM—dynamic random-access memory
DUV—deep ultraviolet

E-beam—electron beam
EBSD—electron back-scattering diffraction
ECR—electron cyclotron resonance
EGS—electronic grade silicon
EM—electromigration
EMP—electron microprobe
EOR—end of range defects
ERF—error function
ERFC—complementary error function
EUV—extreme ultraviolet

FC—float-zone crystal growing technique
FCC—face-centered cubic unit cell
FET—field effect transistor
FIB—focused ion beam
FTIR—Fourier transfrom infrared spectroscopy
FZ—float-zone crystal growth method

GOI—gate oxide integrity

HDP—high-density plasma
HEPA—high-efficiency particulate air (filter)
HF—high frequency
HMDS—Hexamethyldisilane, an adhesion promoter

IC—integrated circuit
ICP—inductively coupled plasma
IMD—intermetal dielectric
IMP—ionized metal deposition (same as IPVD)
INSOL—insoluble portion of polmer base in CA resist
IPVD—ionized PVD (same as IMP)

LDD—lightly doped drain
LF—low frequency
LLS—localized light scatterer
LOCOS—local oxidation of silicon
LPCVD—low-pressure chemical vapor deposition
LSS—implant range theory developed by Lindhard, Scharff, and Schiott

MBE—molecular beam epitaxy
MGS—metallurgical grade silicon
MOS—metal oxide semiconductor
MTF—modulation transfer function
MTTF—median time to failure

NMOS—N channel MOS transistor
NPN—bipolar transistor with N-type emitter and collector
NTD—neutron transmutation doping
NTRS—National Technology Roadmap for Semiconductors

OISF—oxidation-induced stacking fault
OPC—optical phase correction
OPD—optical path difference

PAC—photoactive compound
PAG—photo-acid generator
PEB—postexposure bake
PECVD—plasma-enhanced chemical vapor deposition
PMOS—P channel MOS transistor
PSG—phosphosilicate glass
PSM—phase shift mask
PVD—physical vapor deposition

QBD—charge to breakdown

RBS—Rutherford backscattering
RCA—a wafer cleaning process
RF—radio frequency, usually 13.56 Hhz
RIE—reactive ion etching
RTA—rapid thermal annealing
RTO—rapid thermal oxidation

SACVD—subatmospheric CVD
SC-1, SC-2—wafer cleaning solutions, part of RCA cleaning process
SCM—scanning capacitance microscope
SEM—scanning electron microscopy
SIA—Semiconductor Industry Association
SIMOX—process for SOI, named for "separation by implanted oxygen"
SIMS—secondary ion mass spectrometry
SMIF—standard mechanical interface (box)
SOG—spin-on glass
SOD—spin-on dielectric
SOI—silicon on insulator
SOL—soluble portion of polmer base in CA resist
SPEEDIE—Stanford Profile Emulator for Etching and Deposition in IC Engineering
SRH—Shockley, Read, Hall recombination
STM—Scanning tunneling microscope
SUPREM—Stanford University Process Engineering Models

TCA—trichloroethane
TCAD—technology computer-aided design
TED—transient-enhanced diffusion
TEM—transmission electron microscopy
TEOS—tetraethooxysilane, $Si(OC_2H_5)_4$
TXRF—Total X-ray fluorescence

ULSI—ultralarge-scale integration—usually > 10^6 components
UV—ultraviolet light, light with a wavelength of about 0.2 – 0.4μ

VLSI—Very large scale integration—usually > 10^5 components

XES—X-ray electron spectroscopy
XPS—X-ray photo-electron spectroscopy
XRF—X-ray fluorescence
XRD—X -ray diffraction

A.12 Tables in Text

A.13 Answers to Selected Problems

1.5. 4.6pA.

1.6. 2.15×10^5 Ωcm at room temperature.

1.12. 4.2×10^{-17} Farads.

3.1. $167°\text{Ccm}^{-1}$.

3.2. 0.109 gm.

3.3. f = 0.995.

3.4 3.82×10^{14} cm^{-3}.

4.1. 7.7%.

5.3. 0.15 μm.

5.4 $\lambda = 0.4$ μm

6.15. 0.5 μm.

6.16. $t_{<100>} = 1.12$ hours $t_{<111>} = 1.03$ hours

6.19. t = 225 hours.

7.2 16.66 μm.

7.3. (a) 1.75×10^{14} cm^{-2} (b) 0.44 μm (c) 75.75Ω/square

7.9. 0.72 μm.

7.17. 7.09.

8.2. $Q = 1 \times 10^{14}$ cm^{-2}.

8.3 $R^*_P + 4.3\Delta R^*_P$.

8.8 0.58 μm.

8.15. 94.4%.

9.6 1.4 μm min^{-1}.

9.9 0.94 μm min^{-1}

9.11 (a) 433 cm, 1.2×10^{-2} collisions; (b) 1.44 cm, 3.5 collisions; (c) 0.013 cm, 392 collisions; (d) 1.7×10^{-5} cm, 3.0×10^{5} collisions

10.2. 0.5 μm, 0.125 μm.

10.9. Chemical component = 0.55, Physical component = 0.45.

10.10. 2.5×10^{18} $\text{cm}^2\ \text{sec}^{-1}$

11.5. 1.3×10^{20} cm^{-3}

11.8 2.5 min.

Index

D

E

F

G

K

L

M